95

Tony Ivosic
87 B/EAST HILLS DR
SOMERS NY
10589
914 2776793

Bailey
and
Scott's

Diagnostic
Microbiology

Bailey and Scott's Diagnostic Microbiology

Sydney M. Finegold, M.D.,
SM(AAM), Diplomate, ABMM

Chief, Infectious Disease Section, Veterans
Administration Wadsworth Medical Center, Los
Angeles, California; Professor of Medicine and
of Microbiology and Immunology, School of
Medicine, University of California—Los Angeles

Ellen Jo Baron, Ph.D.,
RM(AAM)

Chief, Microbiology, North Shore University
Hospital, Manhasset, New York; Assistant
Professor of Pathology, Cornell University
Medical School, New York, New York

Seventh edition
With 232 illustrations and 207 color plates

The C. V. Mosby Company
St. Louis • Toronto • Princeton   1986

A TRADITION OF PUBLISHING EXCELLENCE

Editor: Dennis C. Carson
Assistant Editor: Elizabeth Raven
Project Editor: Mary Espenschied
Designer: Christine Leonard Raquepaw
Production: Susan Trail, Judy Bamert, Terry Silvey

Seventh Edition

The C.V. Mosby Company
11830 Westline Industrial Drive, St. Louis, Missouri 63146

Library of Congress Cataloging in Publication Data

Bailey, W. Robert (William Robert), 1917-
  Bailey and Scott's Diagnostic microbiology.

  Includes bibliographies and index.
  1. Diagnostic microbiology. I. Scott, Elvyn G.
II. Finegold, Sydney M., 1921-   . III. Baron,
Ellen Jo. IV. Title. V. Title: Diagnostic microbiology.
[DNLM: 1. Microbiological Technics. QW 25 B156d]
QR67.B33 1986 616′.01′028 85-32007
ISBN 0-8016-1582-8

C/VH/VH 9 8 7 6 5 4 3 2 1 02/C/272

To
Mary L. Finegold,
James C. Taylor, and
Alma and Lee Baron
with loving appreciation for
their constant guidance
and continued understanding

Contributors

W. Lawrence Drew, M.D., Ph.D.

Department of Microbiology and Infectious Diseases, Mount Zion Hospital and Medical Center, San Francisco, California; University of California—San Francisco

Martha A.C. Edelstein, B.A., MT(ASCP)

Infectious Disease Section, Veterans Administration Wadsworth Medical Center, Los Angeles, California

Lynne Shore Garcia, M.S., CLS(NCA), MT(ASCP)

Clinical Microbiology Laboratory, Medical Center, University of California—Los Angeles

Glenn D. Roberts, Ph.D.

Department of Laboratory Medicine, Section of Clinical Microbiology, Mayo Medical School, Mayo Clinic and Mayo Foundation, Rochester, Minnesota

Preface to Seventh Edition

With the change in authors (Ellen Jo Baron, Ph.D., replacing William J. Martin, Ph.D.), we have undertaken a total revision of *Diagnostic Microbiology*. We have invited several authorities to write individual chapters in addition to Lynne Shore Garcia, M.S., CLS(NCA), MT(ASCP), who has again provided a chapter on parasitology: W. Lawrence Drew, M.D., Ph.D. (virology), Martha A.C. Edelstein, B.A., MT(ASCP) (identification of anaerobes), and Glenn D. Roberts, Ph.D. (mycology).

The entire book has been rewritten from cover to cover. There is also a change in format, which we feel makes the book easier to use and more attractive (see How To Use This Book, pp. xiii-xiv). Color plates are scattered throughout the text, and a number of new photographs and illustrations have been added.

We have included, for the first time, information on virulence mechanisms and pathogenesis of infection. Chapters on epidemiology, DRGs, nosocomial infections, new and possible new agents of disease, and infection in the immunocompromised host have been added. There has been considerable expansion of the material on conventional and rapid biochemical methods, on nontraditional methods for detection and identification of pathogens, and on skin and soft tissue infections. Beyond this, all material has been expanded, updated, and reorganized.

Diagnostic Microbiology has a long tradition of excellent service to clinical microbiologists and others interested in medical microbiology. It began in 1940 as a manual entitled *Methods for Diagnostic Bacteriology* written by Isabelle G. Schaub and M. Kathleen Foley. At the time of the third edition of that work, in 1947, the name was changed to *Diagnostic Bacteriology.* In 1958, for the fifth edition, Elvyn G. Scott and W. Robert Bailey joined Schaub and Foley as co-authors. In 1962, Bailey and Scott became the sole authors and published the first edition of *Diagnostic Microbiology.* Subsequently, new editions have been published every four years. The fifth edition, in 1978, was written by Finegold, Martin, and Scott, and the sixth edition, in 1982, by Finegold and Martin. We are pleased to be a part of this heritage and are dedicated to doing our best to maintain the high standards of this work.

We gratefully acknowledge the assistance of many individuals, including readers who were kind enough to call our attention to errors in previous editions or to offer suggestions for improvement. We welcome especially your input on this new edition. Elvyn G. Scott has maintained a strong interest in this work and has kindly provided us with suggestions, advice, and encouragement; we are most appreciative. We would like to express our gratitude for the assistance of Diane Citron, Martha A.C. Edelstein, Paul Edelstein, Mary Finegold, Michael Finegold, Kimi Ishii, Meta Levi, Tomoko Sugano, Vera L. Sutter, James C. Taylor, Phyllis Vogel, and Hannah Wexler, who have helped in a variety of ways. We gratefully acknowledge, in addition, the advice of Renée Almon, Marjorie Berman, Victor Bokkenheuser, Marie Coyle, Richard D'Amato, Larry Drew, Richard Facklam, Susan Forlenza, Henry Isenberg, Michael Janda, Glenn Roberts, Mervin Silverberg, Carol Singer, Tsieh Sun, Katarina Szabo, and Mary Tyburski, who graciously consented to read certain chapters.

We incorporated suggestions from Mary Clancy, Carol Gagné, Janet Hindler, Clark Inderlied, Susan Kelley, and Kathy Whittaker. Most of the new photographs were taken by Mary Brown.

Sydney M. Finegold
Ellen Jo Baron

Preface to First Edition

Diagnostic Microbiology is the first edition of a new series and not a revision of the former publication *Diagnostic Bacteriology*, the latest edition of which we revised (1958). This new title derives in part from the fact that the new volume includes microorganisms other than bacteria. The reader will note, for example, that the former Society of American Bacteriologists has now become the American Society for Microbiology.

Since this book is designed to be used as a reference text in medical bacteriology laboratories and as a textbook for courses in diagnostic bacteriology at the college level, the material has been consolidated and placed in separate parts and chapters. The selected sequence will be commensurate with the needs of both the diagnostician and the student.

For purposes of orientation in taxonomy and ready reference, an outline of bacterial classification has been included. For the student beginning diagnostic work, some pertinent background information is presented on the cultivation of microorganisms, the microscopic examination of microorganisms, and the proper methods for collecting and handling specimens.

A number of chapters include recommended procedures for the cultivation of both the common and the rare pathogens isolated from clinical material and should serve to familiarize the microbiologist with the wide variety of pathogens that may be encountered. An additional chapter has been devoted to the methods employed in the microbiological examination of surgical tissue and autopsy material.

To effect further consolidation of the book's content, one part has been devoted to a series of chapters which cover the various groups of bacteria of medical importance—their taxonomic position, general characteristics, and procedures for their identification. The chapter on the enteric bacteria introduces the new classification of the family Enterobacteriaceae, outlines the group biochemical characteristics, and discusses the serological aspects. The chapter on the mycobacteria includes a discussion of the increasingly important unclassified (anonymous) acid-fast bacilli, giving the methods for their identification, certain cytochemical tests, and animal inoculation procedures.

The chapter on laboratory diagnosis of viral and rickettsial diseases includes a guide to the collection of specimens and offers recommendations for the appropriate time of collection. In the chapter on laboratory diagnosis of systemic mycotic infections, the biochemical approach in identifying the pathogenic fungi is brought to the reader's attention.

The remainder of the book includes prescribed tests for the susceptibility of bacteria to antibiotics, serological procedures on microorganisms and patients' sera, and a technical section on culture media, stains, reagents, and tests, each in alphabetical sequence.

We would like to express our gratitude to Mrs. Isabelle Schaub and to Sister Marie Judith for committing the continuation of the original publication, *Diagnostic Bacteriology*, to our care and responsibility. We also acknowledge the many kindnesses extended by a number of microbiologists and clinicians in permitting the use of published and unpublished materials.

W. Robert Bailey
Elvyn G. Scott

How To Use This Book

This edition of *Bailey and Scott's Diagnostic Microbiology* represents both a reorganization of the way in which subject material is presented and a major change in the appearance of the book. We have placed chapters of general importance to the practice of diagnostic clinical microbiology in Part I, including discussions of laboratory organization and safety, quality control, cost containment, and hospital epidemiology. Part II includes general methods used by microbiologists, including discussions of specimen procurement and transport, visual and serologic methods for detection of microorganisms, techniques and materials used for culture and identification of pathogenic microorganisms, new technological advancements (including the use of automation), and methods used for determining the effectiveness of antimicrobial therapy. Part III discusses the pathogenesis of infectious diseases in relation to specific sites within the body, highlighting the agents likely to be recovered from each organ system or type of specimen. Part IV details methods for identification of specific agents of infectious diseases. As in previous editions, formulas for media and stains are found in the final two chapters.

The format of this edition has been designed to aid students and technologists in using the material to best advantage. Utility of the book is enhanced by the features listed below.

1. All chapters are divided into numbered and lettered sections that follow a standard format. The title page for each chapter contains an outline listing the sections, enabling the reader to determine content of the chapter at a glance and to find the area of interest quickly.

2. Color plates are placed within or as close as possible to the chapter in which they are cited. The edge of the pages of color plates are colored black so that they can be easily located.

3. A second color has been added to highlight divisions of the book, to enhance the information presented in the illustrations, and to set off important material. All step-by-step test procedures, when at all possible, are presented on one page or on facing pages, so that they can be consulted during performance of the procedure.

4. The Glossary has been greatly expanded, and an Appendix has been added in which complete addresses of all suppliers are listed under product categories. Footnotes containing this information have thus been eliminated, and the names of commercial product suppliers are simply cited in the text in parentheses.

Contents

Color Plates

Part One

Organization and Function of the Clinical Microbiology Laboratory

1 Diagnostic Microbiology: Purpose and Philosophy

Clinical microbiologists are part of the health team and serve an important role in the diagnosis, management and prevention of infections in patients. Microbiologists should take pride in this role and should feel responsibility commensurate with it.

1.1. Purpose of Diagnostic Microbiology

The purpose of clinical microbiology is to work closely with clinicians and other health team members to provide diagnosis and optimum management of infectious disease in patients and to prevent the spread of infection to other individuals. In general, it is important to document the presence of infection, to determine its specific nature and to provide appropriate therapy early in the course of the illness. Early diagnosis and treatment are usually more urgent with infectious diseases than with any other type of disease process. In many infections, speedy treatment is crucial. Both mortality and morbidity may be reduced significantly if proper treatment is provided early. In others, hospitalization may be avoided or kept to a shorter time period if specific therapy is provided early. While the responsibility is large, the satisfaction that may be achieved in diagnosing and treating patients with infectious diseases can be great. It is very gratifying to see rapid improvement in a critically ill patient; all members of the health team share in this gratification.

1.2. Responsibility to the Clinician and Others

Microbiology laboratory service must be available at all times. This means that microbiologists must be on call if it is not reasonable to have the laboratory staffed at all times. Others may be able to set up certain types of specimens in the absence of the microbiologist, but the expertise of the microbiologist may be required to properly interpret a Gram stain or colonial morphology late at night. In assessing early findings, one should provide as much detail as possible and one should not hesitate to indicate the various possibilities as to the microbiologic diagnosis. The clinician sets up his or her own differential diagnosis based on the clinical picture, roentgenograms, blood studies, etc. The diagnostic possibilities, as seen by a competent microbiologist, are of paramount importance to the clinician in further narrowing down or substantiating a diagnosis. The microbiologist must be alert to unusual findings. As suggested earlier, speed is critical in serious illness caused by infectious agents. Good microbiologists can usually find one or more ways to expedite identification or probable identification of microorganisms in clinical specimens. If the health team is to function with maximum efficiency, the members of that team must communicate freely and frequently, particularly when dealing with seriously ill patients. The physician should lead in this respect, but if he or she does not, the others on the team should initiate communication when it may be helpful. Our primary concern always must be the patient.

The microbiologist can also be of service to the clinician by instructing him or her concerning the importance of proper specimen collection and transport and regarding specific techniques to be used. An interested physician can be taught how to judge the quality of a sputum specimen and how to interpret a Gram stain properly.

Microbiologists also have a responsibility to notify infection control personnel or epidemiologists and public health authorities. Urgent matters should be communicated by telephone.

The microbiologist also has an obligation to the patient aside from considerations of rapid, accurate diagnosis. Professionalism demands that microbiologists, as well as other members of the health team, not hesitate to deal with certain specimens or patients and that they respect the patient's rights with regard to sensitive information. At times the microbiologist may be pressured to release information on a patient to the patient, his or her family, or others; such pressure must be resisted. Demands of this nature should be referred to the physician.

1.3. Specimen Collection and Transport

Specimen collection and transportation are urgent considerations because the quality of a laboratory's work may be limited by the nature of a specimen and its condition on arrival in the laboratory. Chapter 6 will include a detailed discussion of correct collection and transportation methods.

Specimens should be obtained so as to preclude or minimize the possibility of introducing extraneous microorganisms that are not involved in the infectious process. The problem is greatest when the specimen may become contaminated with elements of the normal flora that may serve as pathogens in the entity being studied (e.g., *Klebsiella* as an oral cavity colonizer in a patient with pneumonia). Even normally sterile body fluids may be contaminated during specimen collection in such a way as to cause significant difficulty in interpretation. For example, consider a patient suspected of having bacterial endocarditis. Let us say that the patient does not actually have this disease, but that one or more blood cultures have become contaminated with coagulase-negative staphylococci during venipuncture. Since this organism can cause endocarditis (with some frequency in certain settings), this may lead to additional testing and prolongation of the hospital stay for the patient. Careful skin preparation before such procedures as blood cultures and spinal taps and techniques for bypassing areas of normal flora when this is important (e.g., percutaneous transtracheal aspiration in critically ill patients with pneumonia) will prevent many problems. Personnel must be instructed to label all specimens submitted to the laboratory with such data as the patient's name, hospital number, date and time, and exact nature and source of the specimen, as discussed in Chapter 3.

1.4. Noncultural Methods of Diagnosis

As noted above, the physician depends on data from many sources in arriving at tentative and definitive diagnoses. In addition to the usual medical history and physical examination, the competent clinician explores epidemiologic information (travel history; exposure to animals, ticks, or other vectors; illness in the family or neighborhood; previous illness in the patient that might have relapsed; etc.). He or she also obtains a number of laboratory tests (e.g., complete blood count, blood chemistry tests, liver function tests, spinal fluid examination) and special tests such as a chest roentgenogram, computerized tomography, radionuclide scans, ultrasound studies, etc. In the case of suspected infection, examination of direct preparations such as wet mounts, Gram stains, India ink preparations, and darkfield examinations may provide information quickly (see Chapter 7). The use of monoclonal antibodies or genetic probes may provide remarkable specificity in direct examination of clinical specimens (see Chapter 10). Certain skin tests may be useful diagnostically. Rapid examination for products of microorganisms (e.g., gas liquid chromatography for demonstration of volatile metabolic endproducts) may be helpful on occasion. Finally, the physician looks for an immunologic response to a given microorganism, usually in the patient's serum (see Chapter 12). This, of course, requires that an infection has been present sufficiently long that such a response could have taken place.

1.5. Rejection of Specimens

It is important that criteria be set up for specimen rejection; such criteria are indicated in appropriate places in this book. However, it is an important rule to always talk to the requesting physicians **before** rejecting specimens, since they are primarily responsible for the patients' welfare. They need support and advice. They may know or think they know that an unorthodox specimen may provide useful information. If this is not the case, the microbiologist must explain why it is not and must work with physicians to resolve the disagreement.

Frequently it is necessary and important to do the best possible job on a less than optimal specimen. It may be necessary to educate the clinician, and the best way to do this is to review individual specimens in a friendly and cooperative manner.

1.6. Extent of Identification Required

We lean heavily toward **definitive** identification. For example, identification to species within the *Bacteroides fragilis* group may be useful. *B. fragilis* and *B. thetaiotaomicron* are frequently found as pathogens, whereas recovery of *B. ovatus* may mean contamination of a specimen with normal bowel flora (or, in a blood culture, transient incidental bacteremia). Similarly, merely identifying an organism as "*Bacteroides ureolyticus* group" is inadequate. *B. gracilis* is more pathogenic and more resistant to antimicrobial agents than *B. ureolyticus*.

An outbreak of infantile diarrhea of serious proportion persisted for many months in a large general hospital in the southwestern United States because stool cultures did not reveal any pathogens. Until the *Escherichia coli* isolates were tested for enterotoxin production and found to be positive, all therapeutic and control measures attempted proved futile. Definitive identification of the unusual blood culture isolates from a number of outbreaks—and these were not really recognized initially as outbreaks—finally permitted determination that commercial intravenous fluid bottles were contaminated; this led to definitive control measures.[3] Many cases of bacteremia and many outbreaks across the country were attributable to this source.

Identification of a clostridial blood culture isolate as *Clostridium septicum* will alert the clinician to the possibility of malignancy in a patient because of the strong association between these two events.[1] Identification of an organism suspected initially of being *B. fragilis* in a patient with bacteremia of unknown source as actually being a *B. splanchnicus* could indicate that the source is probably in the gastrointestinal tract, whereas if it were *B. fragilis* it might also be in the genital tract or even another site.

Precise identification of organisms from a patient with two distinct episodes of infection at an interval of some months might permit establishing that the second infection represents a recurrence rather than a new infection, or it might permit excluding that possibility. Recurrent infection may suggest a foreign body or an abscess from prior surgery; in the absence of prior surgery, it suggests the possibility of malignancy or other underlying process. Definitive identification of an atypical mycobacterium may permit more accurate assessment as to whether the organism is truly involved in the disease, what the source might be, its drug susceptibility pattern, and the likelihood of its responding to the therapeutic regimen chosen.

In the case of certain organisms, especially the anaerobes, incomplete identification may lead to very serious errors in identification. Things that we learn in our first course of microbiology—that certain organisms produce spores, that some are gram positive and some are gram negative, and so on—do not necessar-

ily help with the anaerobes. It may be very difficult to demonstrate spores in sporulating anaerobes. Gram-positive anaerobes are very commonly decolorized and may appear gram negative, even early in the course of growth. Cocci may be mistaken for bacilli, or, more commonly, bacilli may be mistaken for cocci. It may even be difficult to define what an anaerobe actually is, considering that certain organisms, such as some clostridia (aerotolerant), are capable of relatively good growth under aerobic conditions. There are several outstanding examples in the literature of serious errors of this type in identification. For example, *B. melaninogenicus* has been incorrectly reported as being an anaerobic gram-positive streptococcus, and even such a great anaerobist as Prévot mistakenly classified as a *Fusobacterium (F. biacutum)* an organism subsequently shown to be gram positive and a *Clostridium*. Determination of the specific species of a group D *Streptococcus* (e.g., *S. bovis* as opposed to *S. faecalis*)[2] may permit the use of less toxic and less expensive therapeutic remedies. It may also have implications with regard to serious underlying disease. Organisms as diverse as *Listeria monocytogenes* and *Actinomyces viscosus* have been incorrectly identified as diphtheroids (even in reports in the literature) when shortcuts were taken.

Careful bacteriologic studies permit us to define the role of various organisms in different infectious processes, the prognosis associated with these, and so forth. Finally, definitive identification is important in educating clinicians as to the role of various organisms in infectious processes and, perhaps most important, prevents deterioration of the skills and interest of the microbiologist.

At the same time, certain shortcuts and use of limited identification procedures in certain cases are necessary in most clinical laboratories. Careful application of knowledge of the significance of various organisms in these situations and thoughtful use of limited approaches will keep expenses in line and keep the laboratory's workload manageable, while providing for optimum patient care.

1.7. Quantitation of Results

The concept of **quantitation** has not been adequately stressed in microbiology except in the case of urine cultures. Quantitation is useful in other situations as well. It may help to distinguish between an organism present as a "contaminant" and an organism actively involved in infection. It is often useful in determining the relative importance of different organisms recovered from mixed infections. Ordinarily, formal quantitation by dilution procedure or even by means of a quantitative loop is not necessary or desirable. Numbers of organisms present can be graded as "many" ("heavy growth"), "moderate numbers," or "few" ("light growth") on the basis of Gram stain appearance and the amount of growth on a plate. For example, does a given colony type extend to the secondary streak, tertiary streak, and so on? The Gram stain is important because differences in amount of growth or rate of growth of different organisms may be related to the fastidiousness of the organism.

1.8. Expediting Results

The need for **speed** in identification and susceptibility testing is another crucial area that has been neglected, as noted earlier. Few diseases are as dynamic and rapid acting as the infectious diseases. In certain serious infections, such as bacteremia, endocarditis, meningitis, and certain pneumonias, delay of a few hours (or even less in more critical cases) in providing proper therapy may lead to death. It is not always feasible or safe to try to "cover" all possible types of infecting organisms with antimicrobial therapy. Clearly, the clinician must use this type of empirical approach initially, but the microbiologist must be prepared to assist in choosing a rational approach through knowledge of the role of various organisms in different disease processes and through interpretation of direct smears. In such cases the microbiologist should offer something more than routine daily inspection and subculture so that any necessary or desirable modification of therapy can be made as soon as possible; of course, the clinician must communicate with the laboratory about problem cases. Cultures can be examined at 6-12 h intervals, and the processing can be speeded up considerably for selected cases (Chapter 4). Aside from lowering mortality and morbidity, rapid provision of data may shorten hospitalization and thus save money for the patient or the hospital. It may help avoid a surgical procedure.

A limited number of organisms are responsible for the majority of infections. Simple procedures (e.g., Gram stain, colony morphology, catalase, coagulase, bile solubility, oxidase, spot indole, and rapid susceptibility tests) often may provide accurate presumptive identification quickly. Automated rapid procedures can be very helpful.

Somewhat related to this point is the necessity for round-the-clock coverage, as indicated previously. Patients do develop pneumonia on Saturdays and Sundays, and they do go into septic shock after 5 PM and even between midnight and 7 AM. In one manner or another, **reliable** (and we emphasize reliable, because many times emergency laboratory technicians know little or no bacteriology) bacteriology must be available at all times. This includes setting up cultures, inspecting cultures set up earlier, and interpreting direct smears. A qualified microbiologist might be on call for problems encountered by the emergency laboratory crew. If available, infectious disease house officers may be able to set up certain special cultures, interpret Gram stains, and so forth.

In conclusion, we acknowledge that the ideal approach to microbiology can and should be modified according to circumstances. A large teaching hospital or clinic will need to do more, and should do more, than is done in smaller hospitals. In a very small community hospital, the services of a qualified consulting microbiologist should be sought. More must be done for the seriously ill patient, and it must be done as quickly as possible. Every patient has the right to optimal medical care, and therefore every hospital either must have all the necessary capabilities or must have access to them, and microbiologists must know when and how to refer specimens or cultures.

1.9. Interaction with the Clinician

Clinicians, like microbiologists, are human and vary considerably in intelligence, knowledge, character, conscientiousness, personality, and manners. Both clinicians and microbiologists should keep in mind that their primary purpose is to see that the patient is effectively treated. This will be best accomplished by wholehearted collaboration. Unfortunately, some clinicians—like some microbiologists— may be unreasonable at times. As with other interpersonal dealings in life, this may best be handled by a calm, patient, and pleasant attitude on the part of the one "under fire," demonstration of detailed knowledge of the microbiologic features of the case, and expression of a sincere interest in the problem and the patient's welfare. Demand by the physician for inappropriate cultures can often be countered by an explanation of why they would not be helpful (or perhaps might be misleading) and provision of key references from recent literature. In the final analysis, however, it must be remembered that the physician has the primary responsibility for the patient.

The microbiologist is in a position to provide invaluable service to the physician. This includes information on types of specimens that would be most helpful in a given situation, how to collect and transport them, what elements of the normal flora may be encountered, and whether they may be pathogenic under particular circumstances. Also important are interpretation of culture results, likely susceptibility patterns of isolates, and educational services not related to a specific patient.

In communicating with the physician, the microbiologist can avoid confusion and misunderstanding by not using jargon or abbreviations and by providing reports with clear-cut conclusions. Do not assume that the clinician is fully familiar with laboratory procedures or the latest taxonomic schemes. When feasible, provide interpretation on the written report, along with the specific results. However, **never provide only your interpretation** without the actual bacteriologic data (e.g., "Only normal flora isolated").

Monthly newletters may be used to supplement laboratory manuals in order to provide physicians with such material as details of your procedures, new nomenclature, and changes in usual susceptibility patterns of given organisms in your hospital's setting.

REFERENCES

1. Alpern, R.J., and Dowell, V.R. Jr. 1969. *Clostridium septicum* infections and malignancy. J.A.M.A. 209:385.
2. Facklam, R.R. 1980. Streptococci and aerococci. In Lennette, E.H., Balows, A., Hausler, W.J. Jr., and Truant, J.P., editors. Manual of clinical microbiology, ed. 3. American Society for Microbiology, Washington, D.C.
3. Maki, D.G., Rhame, F.S., Goldmann, D.A., and Mandell, G.L. 1973. The infection hazard posed by contaminated intravenous infusion fluid. In Sonnenwirth, A.C., editor. Bacteremia: laboratory and clinical aspects. Charles C Thomas, Publisher, Springfield, Ill.

BIBLIOGRAPHY

Neu, H.C. 1978. What should the clinician expect from the microbiology laboratory? Ann. Intern. Med. 89(Part 2):781.

2 Laboratory Safety

Microbiology laboratories are unique environments in relation to the safety of those who work within them. Clinical specimens received from patients pose a hazard to personnel because of infectious agents they may contain. Cultures of infectious agents, the products of many of the activities of clinical microbiologists, also pose a threat. Education of employees who routinely handle the potentially infectious agents and education (by means of biohazard notices as well as written and verbal instruction) for those people who have only limited exposure to the environment, such as custodial personnel, delivery personnel, and visitors, are the most important measures available for preventing laboratory acquired infection. Risks from a microbiology laboratory may extend to adjacent laboratories and to families of those who work in the microbiology laboratory. For example, Blaser and Feldman[1] noted that five of 31 individuals who contracted typhoid fever from proficiency testing specimens did not work in a microbiology laboratory. Two patients were family members of a microbiologist who had worked with *Salmonella typhi*, two were students whose afternoon class was in a laboratory where the organism had been cultured that morning, and one worked in an adjacent chemistry laboratory. In another incident, the wife and young son of one microbiologist became ill with typhoid due to

Salmonella of the same strain as was being tested in the microbiologist's laboratory. This microbiologist had worked with the organism during the day and then prepared dinner for the family that evening. Tragically, the microbiologist's wife died from her infection. The last several documented cases of smallpox in the world were acquired by employees working in a different area in the same building where a smallpox research laboratory was located. The principal investigator was so dismayed that his possibly deficient safety practices led to these smallpox cases that he committed suicide. It is the ultimate responsibility of the laboratory director or supervisor to insure that proper safety guidelines are adhered to.

2.1. General Safety Considerations

In addition to the threat of infection, microbiology laboratories also contain the safety risks associated with any laboratory or institutional environment, those of fire, electrical hazards, chemical hazards, environmental situations (slippery floors, faulty air-handling systems, etc.), radioactive materials, equipment malfunction, and dangers imposed by natural disasters. Each section of the microbiology laboratory should have a safety manual containing information about procedures to follow in case of fire, flood, earthquake, or other natural disaster, location of all safety equipment, and practices to follow in the event of a situation posing a safety hazard. These considerations are universal to all laboratories and are addressed in references on general laboratory safety. Guidelines for the storage of flammable materials and caustic chemicals have been delineated by the College of American Pathologists and should be strictly enforced. A good way to assure that all laboratory personnel are familiar with current safety practices is to hold periodic unannounced safety drills. By varying the hypothetical hazardous situation, the safety director allows all personnel the opportunity to become aware of their knowledge of proper ac-

tion in an emergency and to improve their performance before disaster strikes.

2.2. Biohazards and Practices Specific to Microbiology in General

The biohazards present in a clinical microbiology laboratory are a more specific concern of this text. Certain aspects of the organization, design, and functioning of such a laboratory should be accepted generally as good safety practices throughout all specialty areas of the laboratory.

2.2.a. Laboratory environment. The microbiology laboratory poses many hazards to unsuspecting and untrained people; therefore, access should be limited to those who have been informed of which actions they can perform safely. Visitors, especially small children, should be discouraged. Certain areas of high risk, such as the mycobacteriology and virology laboratories, should be closed to visitors. Custodial personnel should be trained to discriminate among the waste containers, dealing only with those that contain noninfectious material.

Care should be taken to prevent insects from infesting any laboratory areas. Mites, for example, have been known to crawl over the surface of media, carrying bacteria from colonies on one plate to other areas. Houseplants can serve as a source of such potential hazards, and should be carefully monitored for signs of infestation if they are not altogether excluded from the laboratory environment.

The air-handling system of a microbiology laboratory should convey air from low risk to higher risk areas. Ideally, the microbiology laboratory should be under negative pressure and air should not be recirculated after it passes through microbiology. The selected use of biological safety cabinets for those procedures that generate infectious aerosols is critical to laboratory safety. Many infectious diseases, such as plague, tularemia, brucellosis, histoplasmosis, viral encephalitis, tuberculosis, and Legionnaires' disease, are contracted by inhalation of the infectious particle, often present in a small droplet of liquid. If the droplet is between 2 and 5 μm in diameter, it may easily reach the alveolar spaces of the lung, where it may cause disease. Several common procedures used to process specimens for culture, notably mincing, grinding, vortexing, and preparing direct smears, are known to produce aerosol droplets. These procedures must be performed in a biological safety cabinet.

2.2.b. Biological safety cabinet. A biological safety cabinet is a device that encloses a workspace in such a way as to prevent workers from exposure to infectious disease agents. Air that has passed over the infectious material is sterilized, either by heat, ultraviolet light, or most commonly, by passage through a **high efficiency particulate air (HEPA)** filter that removes most particles larger than 0.3 μm in diameter. These cabinets are designated by class according to the degree of biological containment they afford. Class I cabinets allow room (unsterilized) air to pass into the cabinet and around the material within, sterilizing only the air to be exhausted (Figure 2.1). Class II cabinets sterilize air that flows over the infectious material, as well as air to be exhausted. The air flows in "sheets," which serve as barriers to particles from outside the cabinet, and which direct the flow of contaminated air into the filters (Figure 2.2). Such cabinets are called **laminar flow** biological safety cabinets. Type IIA cabinets have a fixed opening, and Type IIB cabinets have a variable sash opening through which the operator gains access to the work surface. Class III cabinets afford the most protection to the worker since they are completely enclosed, with negative pressure. Air coming into and going out of the cabinet is filter sterilized, and the infectious material within is handled with rubber gloves that are attached and sealed to the cabinet (Figure 2.3).

Most hospital clinical microbiology laboratory technologists use Class II cabinets for routine use. The use of biological safety cabinets for certain procedures will be discussed further

FIGURE 2.1
Class I biological safety cabinet.

FIGURE 2.2
Class II biological safety cabinet.

FIGURE 2.3
Class III biological safety cabinet.

FIGURE 2.4
An area of at least 3 feet from the front of a class II biological safety cabinet must be kept clear of people during operation.

below. The routine inspection and documentation of adequate function of these cabinets is a critical factor in an ongoing quality assurance program. Important to proper operation of laminar flow cabinets is maintenance of an open area for 3 feet from the cabinet during operation of the air-circulating system (Figure 2.4) to insure that infectious material is directed through the HEPA filter.

2.2.c. Protective clothing. Microbiologists should wear laboratory coats over their street clothes, and these coats should be removed before leaving the laboratory. If the laboratory protective clothing becomes contaminated with a pathogen, it should be autoclaved immediately and cleaned before reusing. Obviously, laboratory workers who plan to enter an area of the hospital in which patients are present, particularly patients at special risk of acquiring infection, such as intensive care units, the nursery, operating rooms, or areas in which immunosuppressive therapy is being administered, should take every precaution to cover their street clothes with clean or sterile protec-

tive clothing appropriate to the area being visited. Special protective clothing may be advisable for certain activities, such as working with radioactive substances or caustic chemicals.

2.2.d. Decontamination. All potentially infectious agents must be decontaminated before disposal. These include unused patient specimens as well as media that have been inoculated, whether pathogens have grown or not. Infectious material to be disposed of should be placed into containers that are labeled as to their biohazard risk. Certain instruments, such as scissors, forceps, and scalpel blade holders, should be placed into a closed metal container until they can be autoclaved. Sharp objects, needles and scalpel blades, should be inserted into a hard-sided puncture-proof container **without resheathing.** A suitable container is a hard plastic bottle with a small hole cut in the top to receive the items, or a small metal can with a similar hole. This container is clearly labeled as to contents, autoclaved, and discarded. Only needles that lock onto syringes or one-piece units should be used. Recapping needles with their protective sheaths after use has been shown to be a significant cause of accidental needle-puncture wounds in hospital and laboratory personnel.

Decontamination of potentially infectious material to be discarded from the microbiology laboratory is most often accomplished by steam sterilization in an **autoclave,** an instrument that uses moist heat at greater than atmospheric pressure to kill infectious agents. The pressure allows the steam to be heated above the boiling point, thus decreasing the time needed to sterilize by increasing the temperature. Material to be autoclaved should be loosely packed so that the steam can circulate freely around it. Material of potentially greater hazard, such as cultures and specimens from the mycobacteriology laboratory, is often autoclaved for 1 h instead of the usual 30-45 min autoclaving at 121° C and 15 pounds per square inch (psi) pressure. It is best to locate the autoclave within the laboratory; if infectious material must be transported for sterilization, however, it should be double-bagged and carried in leak-proof, autoclavable containers.

Autoclaves should be monitored regularly for adequate sterilization performance as part of regular quality control practice (discussed in Chapter 3). The proper loading and placement of material to be autoclaved does, however, help to determine whether material has been adequately sterilized. An important safety precaution for those operating an autoclave is to open the door slowly after completion of a cycle. Several workers have been severely burned by the rush of steam that escapes through the crack in the autoclave door as it is

first being opened. The use of a protective face mask for this procedure will prevent such burn incidents.

Workbenches and other horizontal surfaces should be decontaminated at least after every shift and immediately after every spill by washing with a liquid antiseptic agent, such as a phenolic compound, 70% ethanol, or a 0.5% solution of sodium hypochlorite (10% solution of household bleach in water). Diluted bleach is the most effective agent against viral contaminants, such as hepatitis B virus. For those laboratories in which viral contamination is a significant hazard, diluted bleach is recommended as the antiseptic of choice. It has recently been reported that 1.0 N NaOH is able to inactivate the infectious proteins called **prions** (discussed in Chapter 40) that may be the etiologic agents of Creutzfeldt-Jakob disease. Suppliers of commercially available disinfectants are listed in the Appendix. The longer the surface is allowed to remain wet with the agent, the more effective will be the antiseptic action. A minimum of 10 min is recommended. Germicides are not active unless they are in solution. Most disinfectants do not destroy bacterial spores, but these forms of pathogens do not usually pose a hazard to personnel. At least one commercially available disinfectant (Alcide) is moderately effective as a sporicidal agent. Alcide (Alcide Corporation) acts by releasing small quantities of microbicidal chlorine dioxide as it contacts the polysaccharides in bacterial cell walls. Additional contact allows additional release of active chlorite ion groups. This system thus delivers continuous antimicrobial action "on demand." It is good practice to wipe down the outside surfaces of other laboratory equipment, such as centrifuges, vortex mixers, telephones, and even fluorescent lamps above work surfaces, with disinfectant on a regular basis.

2.2.e. Personnel practices. Careful handling of infectious materials to prevent aerosol formation is an important aspect of microbiologic laboratory technique. If open flame burners are used, care must be taken to prevent spattering of material from inoculating needles and loops. The burner should be in a protective container to prevent accidental burns. Incinerator burners offer a less hazardous alternative to an open flame. Personnel should wear rubber gloves when handling material containing organisms that might cause disease if they penetrate through the skin. It is a good idea to wear gloves when handling large volumes of material, when performing procedures that require a significant amount of manipulation (such as grinding tissue or filtering feces), or when handling material from patients with particularly virulent or lethal infections. If the risk of aerosol infection is great, such as for tuberculosis, the addition of a molded surgical mask is recommended.

Mouth pipetting is strictly prohibited; mechanical devices (Figure 2.5) are used for drawing all liquids into pipettes. Eating, drinking, smoking, and applying cosmetics are strictly forbidden in work areas. Food and drink are stored in refrigerators and areas separate from the work area. All personnel should wash their hands with soap and water after handling infectious material and before leaving the laboratory area.

2.3. Classification of Biological Agents on the Basis of Hazard

The Centers for Disease Control publishes a booklet entitled *Classification of Etiologic Agents on the Basis of Hazard*,[2] which has served as a reference for assessing the relative risks of working with biological agents since 1969. Although many unusual agents will not be mentioned here, we will list a few of the more common agents likely to be encountered in clinical microbiology practice in the United States. An excellent source of more detailed information on handling of biohazardous material can be found in the 1984 booklet *Biosafety in Microbiological and Biomedical Laboratories*.[3]

2.3.a. Specific agents. Biosafety Level 1 agents include those that have no known patho-

FIGURE 2.5
Several devices used for drawing liquids into pipettes as alternatives to mouth pipetting.

genic potential for immunocompetent persons. These agents are useful in laboratory teaching exercises for beginning level students of microbiology. Level 1 agents include *Bacillus subtilis* and *Mycobacterium gordonae*. Precautions for working with Level 1 agents include standard good laboratory technique as described above in section 2.2.

Biosafety Level 2 agents are those most commonly being sought in clinical specimens. They include all of the common agents of infectious disease, as well as several more unusual pathogens. The most common causes of laboratory-acquired infection are: hepatitis B virus, *Coxiella burnetti*, *Brucella* species, *Francisella tularensis*, *Mycobacterium tuberculosis*, *Salmonella* and *Shigella* species, and arboviruses. Many other agents have been documented to cause laboratory-acquired infections. For handling clinical specimens suspected of harboring any of these pathogens, Biosafety Level 2 precautions are sufficient. This level of safety includes the principles outlined in section 2.2 above and the added measures of limited access to the laboratory during working procedures, training in the handling of pathogenic agents by laboratory personnel and direction by competent scientists, and the performance of aerosol-generating procedures in a biological safety cabinet.

Biosafety Level 3 procedures have been recommended for the handling of material suspected of harboring certain viruses, including vesicular stomatitis virus, certain arboviruses, and arenaviruses. These precautions, in addition to those undertaken for Level 2, include design and engineering features that increase the containment of potentially dangerous material and the requirement that personnel wear protective clothing and devices. Persons working with Biosafety Level 3 agents should have baseline sera frozen away for comparison to acute sera that may be drawn in the event of an unexplained illness.

Clinical laboratories will probably not encounter agents of Biosafety Level 4, which include only certain viruses of the arbovirus, arenavirus, or filovirus groups, none of which are commonly found in the United States. Biosafety Level 4 laboratories are maximum containment facilities; personnel and all materials are decontaminated before leaving the facility and all procedures are performed under maximum containment (pressure suits or cabinets).

2.4. Special Precautions for Specific Areas of Clinical Microbiology

2.4.a. Bacteriology and general accessioning. Guidelines for the laboratory should require that all respiratory tract specimens must be inoculated to media in a biological safety cabinet. All tissues, whether ground, minced, or touch-cultured, are handled in the cabinet. Any material from patients suspected of acquired immune deficiency syndrome (AIDS) or infectious hepatitis is handled within the safety cabinet. Inoculating material from Isolator tubes (described in Chapter 14) is also performed under laminar flow air handling conditions in the cabinet.

For handling potentially more infectious material, such as tissue from AIDS patients or

stool from patients with hepatitis, gloves should be worn. Specimen containers should be opened inside the biological safety cabinet. Always keep in mind that the outer surface of specimen containers may have been contaminated inadvertently with specimen. Work with hazardous specimens should be performed slowly and carefully to prevent accidental inoculation or production of aerosols.

Certain bacteria, when present on laboratory media after incubation, should be processed only within a biological safety cabinet. These include situations or colonies suspicious for *Yersinia pestis*, *Brucella* species, *Francisella tularensis*, *Rickettsia* and *Coxiella* species, *Bacillus anthracis*, and *Pseudomonas pseudomallei*. If production of aerosols is possible, *Neisseria gonorrhoeae*, *N. meningitidis*, and *Legionella* species should be manipulated in a cabinet.

2.4.b. Mycobacteriology. Processing of all specimens for mycobacteria should take place within a biological safety cabinet. Personnel may choose to wear face-molding masks as an added protective measure. All centrifugations should take place in sealed centrifuge safety cups. The placement of centrifuges under an exhaust system or within a biological safety cabinet will further decrease the hazards associated with centrifugation.

Laboratories that do not perform decontamination and concentration procedures may still be asked to perform a "stat" acid fast stain on the sputum of a patient suspected of active tuberculosis. Other laboratories may also wish to perform such stains rapidly. Liquefaction and concentration of sputum for direct acid fast staining (but not for subsequent culture) may be accomplished by adding an equal volume of 5% sodium hypochlorite solution (full-strength household bleach) to the specimen, capping the container tightly, agitating the suspension, and waiting 15 min before centrifugation. Mycobacteria are killed by this treatment.

2.4.c. Mycology. After inoculation, all plated media **must be sealed** to prevent accidental opening. Masking tape, certain cellophane tapes, and colored labeling tape have been found satisfactory (the tape must not lose its stickiness in a moist incubator). It is best to test a new batch of tape with uninoculated media before using it, as climatic conditions will alter the performance of tapes.

All moldlike fungi (those with aerial mycelia, as described in Chapter 43) must be manipulated under a biological safety cabinet. Many laboratories have been plagued by contaminating molds spread throughout all areas by spores from a single culture. When a mold appears on any medium within the laboratory, even if fungi are not being sought, the plate should be sealed immediately and only opened thereafter in the cabinet.

Any white, fuzzy fungus that appears on culture plates should be regarded with extreme suspicion as a possible dimorphic pathogen. Manipulations should be kept to a minimum and performed only by trained technologists with impeccable technique. Slide cultures should not be attempted for identification of fungi that grossly resemble the systemic pathogens *Blastomyces*, *Histoplasma*, and *Coccidioides*. Further discussion of handling such cultures can be found in Chapter 43.

2.4.d. Parasitology. The eggs of certain cestodes, if ingested during the infective stage, can cause disease. Microbiologists should exercise caution when handling suspected infected fecal material, and gloves should be worn if contact with infective material is possible. The use of a biological safety cabinet for handling most parasitic specimens is not necessary. However, for respiratory secretions that may harbor pathogens other than *Pneumocystis carinii* or flukes, manipulation under a safety cabinet is recommended. Cultures of the protozoan agents of primary meningoencephalitis (*Naegleria fowleri*, etc.) should be handled within a safety cabinet. Chapter 44 includes more discussion of handling of these agents.

2.4.e. Virology. All virology procedures performed in a routine clinical virology laboratory should be carried out within a biological safety cabinet. Specimens suspected of harboring hepatitis B or non-A, non-B virus should be handled with gloves. Technologists should hold a 4 × 4 inch square gauze pad soaked in 10% bleach solution so as to completely cover the rubber stopper of serum tubes or other containers as the stopper is pulled off to help to absorb droplets formed during removal of the tops of such containers. Special virology procedures, such as dissection of the heads of animals suspected of rabies infection, require stringent safety precautions. The precautions

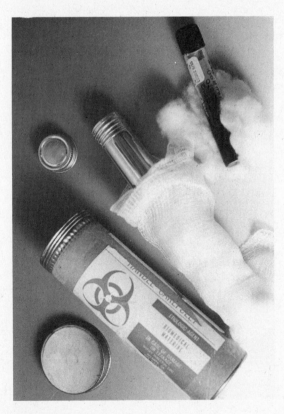

FIGURE 2.6
Proper containers for mailing etiologic agents.

necessary for laboratories performing routine virology will be further discussed in Chapter 41.

2.4.f. Serology. Sera can potentially transmit hepatitis, the most common cause of laboratory acquired infection. Gloves should be worn during manipulations that might allow skin contact with sera. The production of aerosols during the removal of tube tops or during other manipulations should be avoided; the disinfectant gauze pad described above is one effective method. If possible, procedures that generate aerosols, such as vortexing, pouring, shaking incubations, and washing steps for microtiter assays, should be performed in a biological safety cabinet. In reality, these precautions are rarely feasible, and the careful technique of laboratory workers is the best single safety measure available.

The availability of a proven effective and safe vaccine against hepatitis B should serve to significantly reduce the rate of laboratory acquired hepatitis. We recommend that all individuals who are required by their duties in the laboratory to have even moderate contact with sera receive the vaccine. **All sera and other body fluids should be handled as if they were infectious.**

2.5. Mailing Biologicals

Potentially infectious material must often be sent to distant laboratories for further studies. Etiologic agents, specimens, and biological materials may be shipped following the requirements of the Interstate Shipment of Etiologic Agents code. Cultures should be grown on solid media in a tube, preferably plastic, but most often glass. The cap must be sealed with waterproof tape. This primary container is packed in enough absorbent material to absorb the entire volume of the culture if it should leak or break; it is inserted into a second container, often a metal tube. The second container is capped, and is inserted into a shipping container, such as a cardboard mailing tube. Any labeling should be affixed to the outside of the secondary container. The mailing label is affixed to the shipping container along with an official Etiologic Agents label, available from CDC (Figures 2.6 and 2.7).

FIGURE 2.7
Label for etiologic agents and biomedical material.

REFERENCES

1. Blaser, M.J., and Feldman, R.A. 1980. Acquisition of typhoid fever from proficiency-testing specimens. N. Engl. J. Med. 303:1481.
2. Centers for Disease Control and National Institutes of Health. 1974. Classification of etiologic agents on the basis of hazard, ed. 4. U.S. Department of Health, Education, and Welfare, Public Health Service, Washington, D.C.
3. Centers for Disease Control and National Institutes of Health. 1984. Biosafety in microbiological and biomedical laboratories. H.H.S. Publication no. (CDC) 84-8395. U.S. Department of Health and Human Services, Public Health Service, Washington, D.C.

BIBLIOGRAPHY

College of American Pathologists. 1977. Safety inspection checklist. The College, Skokie, Ill.

Inderlied, C.B. 1985. The laboratory environment. In Wagner, K.P., and Kelley, S.G., editors. Clinical microbiology: listen, look, and learn series. Health and Education Resources, Inc., American Society for Microbiology, Washington, D.C.

Miller, B.M., editor. 1986. Laboratory safety: principles and practices. American Society for Microbiology, Washington, D.C.

Richardson, J.N., and Huffaker, R.H. 1980. Biological safety in the clinical laboratory. In Lennette, E.H., Balows, A., Hausler, W.J. Jr., and Truant, J.P., editors. Manual of clinical microbiology, ed. 3. American Society for Microbiology, Washington, D.C.

U.S. Department of Health and Human Services. 1982. Acquired immune deficiency syndrome (AIDS): precautions for clinical and laboratory staffs. M.M.W.R. 31:577.

3 Laboratory Organization and Quality Control

With the present and continuing reexamination of health care delivery by the medical, allied health, and governmental communities (see Chapter 4), it is incumbent on the microbiologist to ensure that the laboratory contributes to the highest quality of patient care by its expertise, its accuracy, its relevance, and the prompt reporting of its findings to the clinician. It is only by constant self-evaluation of the laboratory's performance through a quality control program that such a level of excellence can be developed and maintained. The ease with which technologists can perform to the best of their abilities and the extent to which they can work together as a team to accomplish the goal of high quality patient care are determined, in part, by the organization of both the physical environment and the workflow within the laboratory. This chapter discusses general considerations for specimen handling and reporting results that contribute to the overall **quality assurance** that technologists and physicians expect of the laboratory, as well as addressing some actual components of an active quality control program.

3.1. Specimen Accessioning

Laboratories should try to provide a central area to which all specimens are brought. This simplifies the delivery process and allows the laboratory to monitor and record all incoming specimens. The ability to determine whether a specimen has been received and at what point in the processing system a given specimen may be found is an important part of the overall organization of the laboratory. This may be called an "audit trail." It is at this point that specimens with requests for testing in more than one area of the laboratory can be divided, if necessary, or their proper routing can be arranged.

3.2. Specimen Identification

Proper identification of each specimen includes the patient's name and identification number. The specimen should be tightly capped and in the proper container. If the specimen is from a patient with an infectious disease of special concern, such as hepatitis or acquired immune deficiency syndrome (AIDS), the specimen should be bagged and labeled conspicuously with a warning, usually printed on yellow tape. Unfortunately, not all potentially harmful specimens are properly labeled; often a disease is unsuspected, as in many cases of tuberculosis, or the warning has been inadvertently forgotten. For this reason, all incoming specimens should be treated with a definite degree of suspicion and handled as though they may contain a hazardous agent. At the accessioning point, specific criteria for rejection of specimens should be enforced. Table 3.1 contains some suggested reasons for refusal to process a specimen. Other reasons for specimen rejection may be appropriate for individual laboratories. Under certain circumstances, such as receipt of an unlabeled specimen from a site that would be difficult or impossible to collect from again (cerebrospinal fluid, for example), there should be policies that would permit overriding the original rejection. One such policy might be the acceptance of an unlabeled specimen after the attending physician has personally come to the laboratory to identify and label the specimen and has signed a statement assuming responsibility for the proper identification.

3.3. Laboratory Requisition Form

The request slip accompanying the specimen must contain the patient's identification parameters, the patient's location, the date and time that the specimen was collected, the exact source and type of specimen, the requested studies, and other pertinent information (such as the antimicrobials the patient is receiving), as well as the physician responsible. It is very useful to include the time at which the specimen was received in the laboratory; many laboratories use a time-stamp machine for this purpose. A clean and legible request form is essential to optimal processing. The format of the request form can often influence the way in which physicians order tests. As mentioned in Chapter 4, listing a limited number of possible tests on the request form will contribute to limiting the test requests to those listed. The use of screening procedures and test panels dealing with a series of tests that might aid in identification of a particular infectious agent or type of infection may simplify the ordering process for physicians and clarify the request for the technologists. If the patient's diagnosis is included on the request, the laboratory can more easily determine which tests to perform to give the most useful information to the physician.

3.4. Reporting Results

Part of the organization of the microbiology laboratory must include a system for delivering results of test procedures to the physician (or patient-care unit). Certain information is important enough to warrant a telephone call. Suggested reports that ought to be relayed immediately include Gram stain results; positive direct visual preparations of any sort; positive antigen detection results from sterile body fluids; growth in blood cultures, cerebrospinal fluid, or from any sterile body fluid or tissue; positive acid fast smears; presence of organisms that would require the patient to be isolated, such as intestinal pathogens or *Staphylococcus aureus;* and growth of mycobacteria. It is

TABLE 3.1
Criteria for Rejection of Requests for Microbiologic Tests*

CATEGORY	CRITERION FOR REJECTION	ACTION
Identification	Discrepancy between patient identification on request form and on specimen container	Discuss with sender or return to sender for resolution. If discrepancy is unresolved, specimen is processed but no report issued.
	No identification on container	Do not process unless request form is wrapped around container. Write "Container not identified" on report form in such cases.
	Specimen source or type of culture ordered not on request form	Call physician or service for necessary information.
Specimen	Anaerobic culture request on	Cross anaerobic culture request off form.
	Sputum	Do not perform anaerobic cultures, except with microbiology staff approval. Explain reasoning to requesting physician.
	Midstream urine	
	Catheterized urine	
	Vaginal secretions	
	Prostatic secretions	
	Feces	
	Environmental material	
	Gastric washings	
	Bronchoscopic washings	
	Decubitus ulcer material	
	Throat material	
	Nose material	
	Skin material	
	Mouth material	
	Ileostomy material†	
	Colostomy material†	
	Fistula†	
	Specimen identified by anatomic site only (e.g., chest, leg, etc.)	Request additional information.
	Anaerobic culture request on swab material (unless swab has been submitted in anaerobic transport tube or bag)	Return request form to physician immediately, stamped "This specimen is unacceptable for culture of anaerobic bacteria because it was not transported under anaerobic conditions. Please submit syringe aspirate injected into anaerobic transport tube, or, if necessary, a swab in proper transport setup." Do not perform anaerobic culture unless physician insists it is not feasible to obtain another sample.
	Anaerobic culture request on unacceptable material (specified above) in anaerobic transport tube	Return request form to physician immediately, stamped "This specimen was submitted in an anaerobic transport tube for anaerobic culture. However, since this material is generally contaminated with normal flora anaerobes, no anaerobic culture was performed. Please contact laboratory to discuss obtaining a suitable specimen."

*Adapted from criteria in use at the Mayo Clinic.
†Refers to intraluminal material.

Continued.

TABLE 3.1
Criteria for Rejection of Requests for Microbiologic Tests—cont'd

CATEGORY	CRITERION FOR REJECTION	ACTION
Specimen—cont'd	Improperly collected sputum (i.e., saliva) for routine culture	Return request form to physician immediately, stamped "Improper specimen; please resubmit." Explain problem.
	Material received in fixative (e.g., formalin)	Notify physician and request new specimen. Stamp "Specimen unsatisfactory; please submit new specimen" on request form and return.
	Gram-stained smear of material from anus or rectum for gonococci	Cross Gram smear request off form.
	Dry swab	Notify physician and request new specimen. Stamp "Specimen unsatisfactory—dry swab; please submit new specimen" on request form and return.
	Blood culture with request for Gram-stained smears or cultures for mycobacteria (TB) or viruses	Cross request off form.
	Foley catheter tips	Discard sample. Explain problem.
	24 h urine or sputum collections for mycobacteria (TB) or fungi	Notify physician that 24 h collections are unacceptable and request three single-voided urine specimens or three consecutive, early morning, freshly expectorated sputa.
	Urine 　Held longer than 2 h at room temperature 　Improper container 　Leaking container	Return request form to physician immediately, stamped with "Improper specimen; please resubmit." Explain problem.
	Excess barium or oil in stool specimen for ova and parasites	Stamp "Exam for parasites unsatisfactory—oil (or barium) in excess" on report form and return.
	Less than one swab per request for bacterial, mycobacterial (TB), and fungal cultures	Call physician to request additional material. If additional material cannot be obtained, ask physician to state priorities for culture.
	Multiple urine, stool, sputum, and **routine throat specimens** on the same day from the same source (AFB requests excluded). Process all stool specimens received on children younger than 3 years	One specimen should be processed. Stamp duplicate request forms with "Multiple specimens received; one will be processed. Notify lab within 24 h if you wish the remaining specimens to be processed and explain circumstances."
	Specimen received grossly contaminated	Discard sample. Inform physician or nursing unit and request a repeat specimen.

equally important for the technologist to document what information was relayed by telephone, when this was done, and to whom. Other results are usually delivered in written form, either directly from the laboratory or via a computerized system of information process-

ing. Part of the quality control program of the laboratory should include periodic monitoring to insure that results are actually being delivered in a timely and accurate fashion. The work of the laboratory will only be worthwhile if it is useful in directing care for the patient. One aspect of the more careful scrutiny of hospital practices by government and other third-party payers (Chapter 4) has been a close examination of result reporting from laboratories to the patient care areas. Most administrative policies now require an interim or preliminary written report within 24 or at the most 48 h after specimen receipt. Those laboratories that enjoy hospital-wide on-line computer capability have a system in place that facilitates such reporting. Other laboratories must rely on multiple-copy report forms to accomplish this purpose.

Certain results are important to people other than physicians directly responsible for patients. Infection control practitioners monitor the incidence and spread of various infections throughout the hospital and must be given access to certain information, both on a daily basis and in cumulative fashion. Policies that govern which culture results must be telephoned directly to infection control practitioners should be clearly delineated. The laboratory also has an obligation to report certain infections, such as preventable venereal diseases, tuberculosis, agents of transmissible gastroenteritis, and diseases of grave concern such as botulism and plague, to the local public health authorities. All technologists should be informed as to which results require additional reporting, and standardized procedures should be established for this function. A laboratory may choose to selectively report certain other results, such as posting positive blood cultures from babies in the pediatric nurses' station. These laboratory results must be placed out of sight of all visitors.

3.5. Procedure Manual

Every laboratory must provide procedure manuals detailing all aspects of performance of procedures within that laboratory. Such manuals should be easily accessible at all times to the technologists who may wish to consult them. Manuals should discuss safety aspects of working within the laboratory, administrative and technical policies that must be followed by laboratory workers, as well as criteria for performance of all tests. The procedure manual should be the **working reference standard** for the entire staff. The manuals are reviewed regularly, at least annually, and the procedures are updated as they are modified or replaced. Documenting laboratory procedures, as is done by means of a manual, is as important as documenting the results of quality control procedures outlined below. The National Committee for Clinical Laboratory Standards has established guidelines for writing laboratory procedure manuals.[1] Those laboratories with computer-assisted word processing capability are at a great advantage in creating procedure manuals, as procedures can be easily updated, modified, and reprinted as necessary. In the laboratory of one of us (EJB), a copy of each procedure is given to a technologist being trained in the performance of that procedure. Deficiencies in the written procedure are immediately apparent at this time, and the written printout serves as a handy guideline for the technologist to use for making personal notes and comments to help in learning the new procedure.

3.6. Quality Control

A comprehensive quality control program will provide written records of the results of monitoring every procedure, instrument, and product used in the laboratory. Documentation of performance of quality control measures is as important as the performance itself. The written record for each laboratory procedure or function that is monitored should also contain a section that details any deviation from expected results, problems, or failures and the corrective actions taken in response to such problems. Incidents that occur in the laboratory that are not directly related to performance of tests, such as spills of infectious materials, personal injuries, abusive interactions between technologists and physicians, or any unusual occurrence, should also be documented. A special logbook for corrective actions is very helpful in documenting an ongoing quality control program's effectiveness.

Instrument checks should include preventive maintenance, temperature charts if applicable, and other records of performance. An example of a quality control log for an incubator is shown in Figure 3.1. All perishable products and all solutions must be labeled with the date of receipt or preparation, when they were first used, and the expiration date. All products, whether prepared in the laboratory or purchased from a commercial supplier, should be checked for proper performance. In the case of microbiological media, tests should include sterility and growth of microorganisms with both positive and negative outcomes.

Organisms for use in monitoring media performance can be stock cultures saved from actual patient isolates, but commercially obtained organisms are more standardized. Organisms

can be kept frozen indefinitely at $-70°$ C in skim milk (diluted 1:1 in distilled water and autoclaved at $121°$ C for 10 min) in small plastic freezer vials, or they may be maintained for quite some time on nutrient or blood agar slants under a layer of sterile mineral oil. Viability is prolonged when the media are prepared without added sodium chloride or carbohydrate. Alternatively, reference organisms can be purchased in lyophilized form, convenient for use in a quality control program, from several commercial suppliers (Bact-Chek, Roche Diagnostic Systems; BACTi Disks, Remel Laboratories; Bactrol Disks, Difco Laboratories; American Type Culture Collection [ATCC], and others listed in the Appendix).

Table 3.2 is an abbreviated list of the organisms to be tested and the results expected for some commonly used laboratory media. The bibliographic references cited at the end of this chapter contain more detailed lists of those media and reagents that should be evaluated and

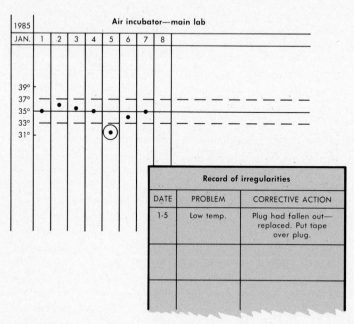

FIGURE 3.1
Example of incubator quality control performance record.

TABLE 3.2
Recommended Cultures for Monitoring Routine Culture Media, Stains, and Reagents*

MEDIUM OR TEST	CONTROL ORGANISM	EXPECTED RESULT
Acetate	E. coli	Growth, blue color
	S. flexneri	No growth
Arginine dihydrolase	E. cloacae	Positive
	P. vulgaris	Negative
Bile esculin agar	S. faecalis	Growth, blackening
	Viridans group streptococcus	No growth
Blood culture bottles		
Biphasic (vented)	H. influenzae	Growth on subculture
Anaerobic (unvented)	B. fragilis	Growth on subculture
Brain-heart infusion agar	C. albicans	Growth
with antibiotics	A. fumigatus	Inhibited
Brucella agar with laked	Peptococcus species	Growth (anaerobic)
blood, vitamin K_1, and		
hemin		
Catalase test	S. aureus	Positive
	Group A streptococcus	Negative
Chocolate agar	H. influenzae, S. pneumoniae,	Growth
	nutritionally variant strepto-	
	coccus	
Simmons citrate	K. pneumoniae	Positive
	E. coli	Negative
Coagulase test (rabbit	S. aureus	Clot
plasma)	S. epidermidis	No clot
CNA (colistin nalidixic acid)	S. faecalis	Growth
agar	P. aeruginosa	No growth
	S. aureus	Growth
CTA medium		
Glucose	N. gonorrhoeae	Acid (yellow)
Maltose	N. gonorrhoeae	No change
Sucrose	N. gonorrhoeae	No change
Lactose	N. lactamicus	Acid (yellow)
Differential carbohydrates	As indicated	
DNase agar	S. marcescens	Positive
	E. cloacae	Negative
Egg yolk agar (Nagler)	C. perfringens	Positive (anaerobic)
	B. fragilis	Negative (anaerobic)
EMB agar	E. coli	Growth, metallic sheen
	P. mirabilis	Growth, lactose negative (color-
		less colony)
FA test, group A streptococci	Group A streptococcus	Positive
	Group C streptococcus	Negative
Germ tube test	C. albicans	Positive
GN broth	S. typhimurium	Growth on subculture
	S. flexneri	Growth on subculture
Gram stain	S. aureus	Gram positive
	E. coli	Gram negative

*Media are checked on each new batch; sterility tests are performed on 5% of batches of 100 or fewer and 10 randomly selected plates or tubes from larger batches. They are incubated at 35° C or the temperature at which they will be used. Stains and reagents are tested when made or purchased. If they are not used frequently, test before each use. Test working solutions weekly and reagents daily for frequently used stains. *Continued.*

TABLE 3.2

Recommended Cultures for Monitoring Routine Culture Media, Stains, and Reagents—cont'd

MEDIUM OR TEST	CONTROL ORGANISM	EXPECTED RESULT
Hektoen agar	S. typhimurium	Growth, green colony with black center
	E. coli	Growth, orange colony (or no growth)
Hippurate hydrolysis	Group B streptococcus	Positive
	Group A streptococcus	Negative
Indole	E. coli	Positive
	K. pneumoniae	Negative
Kanamycin-vancomycin blood agar	B. fragilis	Growth (anaerobic)
	E. coli	Inhibited (anaerobic)
KCN	C. freundii	Growth
	S. typhimurium	No growth
Kit for identification of Enterobacteriaceae	Directions from manufacturer	
10% Lactose	A. calcoaceticus var. anitratus	Acid
	A. calcoaceticus var. lwoffi	Alkaline
L-J medium	M. tuberculosis (H37-RA strain)	Characteristic colonies
Lysine decarboxylase	S. typhimurium	Positive
	P. vulgaris	Negative
Motility medium	E. coli	Positive
	K. pneumoniae	Negative
Mueller-Hinton agar	S. aureus (ATCC 25923)	Acceptable zone sizes (see Chapter 13)
	E. coli (ATCC 25922)	
	P. aeruginosa (ATCC 27853)	
Nitrate reduction	P. aeruginosa	Positive, N_2
	A. calcoaceticus	Negative
	E. coli	Positive
O-F media		
Glucose	P. aeruginosa	Oxidizer (yellow)
Maltose	P. maltophilia	Oxidizer (yellow)
Ornithine decarboxylase	E. cloacae	Positive
	P. vulgaris	Negative
Optochin disk test	S. pneumoniae	≥14 mm zone (6 mm disk)
	S. mitis	<14 mm zone
Oxidase reaction	P. aeruginosa	Positive (blue)
	E. coli	No color change
Rice agar with Tween 80	C. albicans	Characteristic chlamydospores
	C. tropicalis	No chlamydospores
SAB agar with antibiotics	C. albicans	Growth
	A. fumigatus	Inhibited
Sheep blood agar	Group A streptococcus	Growth, beta hemolysis
	S. mitis	Growth, alpha hemolysis
Trypticase soy agar or broth	Group A streptococcus	Growth
TSI agar	P. mirabilis	K/AG, H_2S
	E. coli	A/AG
	P. aeruginosa	K/no reaction
Urea agar (Christensen)	P. vulgaris	Positive (red)
	E. coli	Negative
XLD agar	S. typhimurium	Growth, pink-red with black center
	E. coli	Yellow (or no growth)
Ziehl-Neelsen, fluorochrome stain	M. tuberculosis (H37-RA)	Positive acid-fast
	E. coli	Negative acid-fast

suggestions for organization of quality control programs. Selective media should be monitored for their ability to inhibit the expected organisms as well as for the growth of the sought-for organisms. Susceptibility testing procedures must be checked with organisms of known susceptibility, at least once for each lot of media used or often enough to insure correct results. The amount of quality control performed by a laboratory is dictated by the institution under which the laboratory is accredited, such as the Joint Commission on Hospital Accreditation, the College of American Pathologists, or the state in which the hospital functions. A laboratory must adjust its practices to satisfy the most stringent regulating agency. The documented recorded history of results within established limits can help to determine how often quality control procedures must be performed by any particular laboratory.

In addition to monitoring individual procedures, laboratories can monitor their overall performance by participating in a proficiency testing program. These programs are valuable for comparing one's results with those of many other laboratories, spotting errors in technique, and for learning to recognize unusual agents or rare results. A system of internal proficiency testing is easily accomplished by occasionally submitting the same sample, divided into two specimens, as a second specimen, unknown to the technologists. Lapses in consistency are often spotted in this way. The daily checking of reports by a supervisor or coworker can often catch errors before they have been released. Finally, occasional spot-checking of ongoing work by comparing cultures and work cards may point out potential sources of error.

The laboratory is often responsible for helping maintain quality control for other areas of the hospital. Monitoring the effectiveness of autoclaves in surgery, laundry, and other sections may be a function of the microbiology laboratory. Often the laboratory provides sterility checks for the pharmacy, blood bank, milk bank, dialysis service, and other areas. Unless there has been a documented epidemic, it is not recommended that routine sterility cultures of environmental surfaces be performed.

3.7. Statistics

Maintaining adequate records of specimens received, procedures performed, and results will be extremely helpful for determining staffing needs and organization of workload. Use of some method for assessing work accomplished, such as the College of American Pathologists workload unit recording system, will enable a laboratory to determine productivity, trends in test requests, and proper pricing structures. Other statistics that are helpful include cumulative susceptibility testing results. An updated compilation of these data, provided to physicians on a regular basis, preferably in a reduced format that allows physicians to carry the information in their white jacket pockets, will aid them in selecting the most efficacious antimicrobial agents, as well as alert them to new trends in susceptibility patterns among isolates from their institution. By comparing a particular organism's susceptibility pattern to the established norm, a technologist may find an error in identification or an unusual isolate that requires further study.

3.8. Information Processing

The number and diversity of the records and statistics that must be generated, evaluated, and stored by the microbiology laboratory have increased just as the technological advances have blossomed. Luckily, the development of information-processing systems suitable for use by the laboratory has also been occurring. It is hoped that microbiology laboratories can make use of some of the new technology to aid in the giant task of record-keeping. The use of computers for many tasks within the clinical microbiology laboratory is discussed in Chapter 4.

REFERENCE

1. Tentative guidelines for clinical laboratory procedure manuals. 1980. Villanova, Penn., National Committee for Clinical Laboratory Standards.

BIBLIOGRAPHY

Bartlett, R.C. 1974. Medical microbiology: quality, cost, and clinical relevance. John Wiley & Sons, New York.

Bartlett, R.C. 1985. Quality control in clinical microbiology. In Lennette, E.H., Balows, A., Hausler, W.J. Jr., and Shadomy, H.J., editors. Manual of clinical microbiology, ed. 4. American Society for Microbiology, Washington, D.C.

Blazevic, D.J., Hall, C.T., and Wilson, M.E. 1976. Cumitech 3, Practical quality control procedures for the clinical microbiology laboratory. In Balows, A., coordinating editor. American Society for Microbiology, Washington, D.C.

Miller, J.M. 1983. Quality control in the microbiology laboratory. Centers for Disease Control, U.S. Department of Health and Human Services, Public Health Service, Atlanta.

Miller, J.M., and Wentworth, B.B., editors. 1985. Methods for quality control in diagnostic microbiology. American Public Health Association, Washington, D.C.

4 Coping with DRGs: Cost
Containment Strategies
for Microbiology
Laboratories

4.1. Introduction

Diagnosis related groups (DRGs) were implemented in October, 1983, for many hospitals in the United States. The DRG system, officially enacted to stem the rising tide of Medicare health care costs, mandates that hospitals receive reimbursement for costs based primarily on the primary **diagnosis** given to a patient, rather than on the cost of medical care generated by that patient. A list of "diagnoses" is used to assess the amount of money paid to a hospital for each Medicare and Medicaid patient admitted. Variations in reimbursement are based on several factors, including the geographic location of the hospital, the prevailing costs of medical care, the type of patients seen at the hospital, and whether the hospital is a teaching hospital or a special care hospital. If a patient admitted for a coronary bypass operation develops a urinary tract infection and subsequent sepsis, the added laboratory, medication, and hospital day costs are not reimbursed. This system is also called **prospective payment.** It is immediately obvious that it is to a hospital's financial advantage to keep costs as low as possible. If the hospital can treat a patient for less money than the amount of prospective payment received, a hospital may even realize a profit. If one patient develops severe complications that substantially increase the total cost of that patient's stay, the hospital loses money.

Suddenly the laboratory, which previously had received reimbursement for all charged services and therefore served as a revenue-producing center for the hospital, became a potential drain on the hospital's resources, becoming a cost center. Many third-party payers (insurance companies) found it to their advantage to work out contracts with hospitals that resembled DRGs, such that hospitals without large numbers of Medicare patients still faced prospective payment reimbursement in some form. A few hospitals have closed, and many more have consolidated services to cut operating costs. Much care, including some surgery previously carried out in the hospital setting, has been shifted to outpatient units or the home and, when feasible, patients are discharged early to outpatient status or to home care. Even long-term intravenous antimicrobial therapy is being administered in the patient's home. Since physicians (pathologists, in particular, are involved) are now prohibited from billing Medicare or Medicaid patients for outside laboratory tests, there is a strong incentive provided for office-based laboratory testing. Accordingly, physicians' office laboratories have been expanded in many cases. Unfortunately, these laboratories are exempt from licensure requirements and from other regulations such as those requiring quality control (as long as such laboratories do not accept too many specimens from other physicians). The overall impact of DRGs on the health care delivery system in the United States has not been wholly realized; changes are continuing to occur.

The challenge that faces hospital-based microbiologists, as well as those working in referral laboratories that rely on reimbursement from health care providers, is to continue to deliver quality results under increasing budgetary constraints. Most laboratories have responded to this challenge, finding new (and sometimes better) ways to rapidly deliver quality work in a cost-efficient manner. Industry

has also responded by becoming more involved in developing rapid testing methods and pioneering ways to use new technology to the benefit of microbiology. The ultimate beneficiary of laboratory efforts is the patient; physicians and health care workers try to insure that he or she receives timely and appropriate treatment. The overall goal is quality patient care. Since the negative impact of slow or incorrect diagnosis of infectious disease is an increased hospital stay (at the attendant increased expenditure), changes made in microbiology to better serve the clinician and patient have a positive aspect that is multiplied in terms of cost benefits and quality health care. Strategies that can be employed to achieve these goals are the topic of this chapter. Numbers of rapid methods that have been discussed in other chapters throughout the book will be mentioned here in the context of application to particular situations. The precise performance of such tests, however, is not included here. Test methods are detailed in the appropriate later sections of this book. This chapter is intended as a sampler of ideas to serve as a basis upon which microbiologists can build, not an exhaustive catalogue of the available choices for altering test procedures to achieve maximum cost containment. Microbiologists, in choosing strategies that will work in their unique situations, are helping to shape the future of health care. Numbers of articles assessing the changing impact of DRGs on laboratory performance are published in the monthly *Medical Laboratory Observer* (Medical Economics Co., Oradell, NJ), which is playing an important role in reporting on the impact of DRGs to the paramedical community. Discussions of rapid methods for diagnosis of infectious diseases, presented at national and regional meetings of the American Society for Microbiology, American Society for Medical Technology, and the American Society of Clinical Pathologists, among others, as well as reports on the feasibility and validity of new methods published in numbers of journals cited throughout this text, are all sources of information and inspiration for microbiologists wishing to improve cost-effective performance.

4.2. General Approaches to Cost Savings

Knowledge about the true costs of microbiology laboratory procedures and information about the budget allocated to operations are essential in order for administrators of the laboratory to be able to monitor its costs and performance. It is important that laboratory administrators receive timely copies of the appropriate budget, broken down into divisions representing personnel costs, supplies, services, and overhead (if charged to the laboratory). With this information, planning for cost containment can be tailored to individual requirements and results of cost-cutting strategies can be monitored for their effectiveness. It is also essential to know the actual costs incurred in performance of each procedure. Bartlett et al.[1] and Garcia and Bruckner[4] have discussed procedures for gathering this information. An ongoing record of workload units (testing time, usually recorded in minutes) performed by technologists in each area of the microbiology laboratory is also important for assessing trends in workload, rearranging staffing patterns to fit the needs, and forecasting future developments, as well as for determining the technologist time expended on each procedure performed. The College of American Pathologists' workload recording units (CAP units) are widely used for this purpose.[2]

4.2.a. Education. The physician has the ultimate responsibility for patient care; all cost-generating procedures originate with a physician's orders. The first challenge that microbiologists face is that of educating physicians as to proper utilization of the services of the microbiology laboratory. Incoming physicians, those attending and those in training, should be presented with an orientation session detailing the functions and capabilities of the micro-

biology laboratory. Physicians should be aware of the hours during which microbiologists are available, the extent of diagnostic services provided, and the expected turnaround time for test results. Clinicians should be introduced to microbiologists with whom they may interact, so that communication can be open and often. A general orientation session presented to the house staff by the microbiologist should include suggestions for proper media, timing, and special requests for blood cultures, as well as other specimens that require advance notice or special handling. Microbiologists must also seek to learn from clinicians. Decisions as to elimination of tests, minimizing identification, hours that the laboratory should be open, etc., should be made jointly by knowledgeable physicians, such as infectious disease clinicians, and microbiologists so as to achieve cost containment without undue risk or discomfort to patients. Continuous dialogue between microbiologists and clinicians concerning proper utilization and interpretation of the laboratory's services should help to decrease excessive or inappropriate test requests. It is necessary to discuss proper laboratory utilization with the nursing staff as well. One strategy that pays off in terms of helping nurses and physicians to submit specimens properly for microbiologic analysis is the availability of a small, printed manual containing detailed instructions on proper submission of specimens, including containers, request forms, special handling requirements, timing and numbers of specimens to submit, and other information. Updated at least annually with procedural changes, such a book rapidly becomes an essential reference manual for nurses and clinicians, and the laboratory benefits both in decreased numbers of phone calls and in better quality of specimens. Some of the information to include in such a reference manual is found in Chapter 6.

A quarterly or semiannual publication originating in the microbiology laboratory that seems to impact positively on patient care and minimizing costs is the cumulative antimicrobial susceptibility statistics for the hospital. Information to include in this publication, which is best reduced to a pocket-sized folded card, could include maximum serum, urine, and cerebrospinal fluid levels achievable for appropriate antimicrobial agents, as well as some representative costs. By being aware of susceptibility patterns within the institution, clinicians can prescribe antimicrobial agents that are likely to be the most effective at the least cost. Although microbiology laboratories may have little input into the matter, the antimicrobial susceptibility results for third generation cephalosporins, broad spectrum penicillins, and more expensive aminoglycosides could be reported only for those bacteria that exhibit resistance to a predetermined group of first-choice antimicrobial agents, thus shaping the treatment patterns of physicians who consider in vitro susceptibility results in such decisions. Additionally, microbiologists should participate on those committees, usually consisting of representatives from the infectious disease service, medical and surgical services, and pharmacy, that choose which antimicrobial agents are routinely tested in the microbiology laboratory. By educating physicians as to appropriate use of antimicrobial agents, often in such subtle ways as reporting patterns, microbiologists are contributing to cost savings.

4.2.b. Limitations on testing. Laboratories can limit tests in several ways without harming patient care quality. As suggested by Ellner,[3] limits on the numbers of specimens in several categories (Table 4.1) that are accepted by the laboratory will contribute to more rational patient management. By offering test panels that automatically offer increasingly specialized tests based on the results of screening tests, laboratories can decrease the number of nonproductive tests run. For example, our laboratory (EJB) offers an Epstein-Barr viral (EBV) serology test panel. If the viral capsid antigen (VCA)-IgG level on a given sample is high, the

TABLE 4.1
Suggested Limits for Specimens Accepted for Microbiological Studies

SPECIMEN	LIMIT
Urine, stool, genital, sputum, wounds, upper respiratory area	One daily, maximum three weekly
Blood	Three daily, maximum six per patient admission
Stool for ova and parasites	Three per patient admission
Specimens for fungus culture and serology	Three per patient admission
Virus cultures	One of each type per patient admission
Sputum and gastric aspirate for mycobacteria	Three of each per patient admission
Urine or cerebrospinal fluid for mycobacteria	Infectious disease section approval required

Adapted from Ellner, P.D. 1985. A dozen ways to achieve more cost-effective microbiology. Med. Lab. Observer 17:40.

VCA-IgM test is automatically performed. Appropriate results in the preliminary tests then lead to performance of the EBV nuclear antigen (EBNA) serologic test. Other laboratories perform EBV specific serologies only after two negative heterophile test results and the presence of atypical lymphocytes in peripheral blood have been documented. A number of specimens are inappropriate for culture and may even yield misleading information. Foley catheter tip cultures; surface cultures of decubiti; anaerobic cultures from the vagina or cervix, perirectal abscesses, bowel contents, or oral sources; and cultures of periodontal material (except for specialized laboratories) do not contribute to good patient management and should be avoided. The laboratory should limit the testing of routine throat cultures to detection of beta hemolytic streptococci and respiratory viruses.

Cultures of material should be avoided if Gram stains or other direct visual examinations (Chapter 7) will yield sufficient diagnostic information. For example, a 10% potassium hydroxide (KOH) or calcofluor white wet preparation of scrapings from clinically compatible lesions on the tongue of a child suspected of having thrush or the vaginal wall of a woman suspected of candidal vaginitis, if positive, provides the diagnosis without culture. The presence of clue cells, lack of lactobacilli, increased pH, and disagreeable odor of vaginal discharge are indicative of bacterial vaginosis (nonspecific vaginitis), and cultures are unnecessary. The presence of multinucleated giant cells in a Tzanck preparation from a suspected herpetic vesicle precludes the necessity for culture.

Limitations that may be practiced within the laboratory should be undertaken only after careful study and discussions with clinicians to determine that no negative effect on patient care will result. The number of primary plates that are routinely inoculated with clinical material may be decreased. Stool cultures can be plated to two selective and differential media instead of three or four, in addition to blood and Campy and MacConkey agars (Chapter 17). It may be possible to eliminate inoculation of stool into enrichment broth for subsequent subculture if it can be shown that no significant additional isolates are recovered by this procedure. The number of media set up for cultivation of mycobacteria and fungi can be limited to support the growth of all etiologic agents in a more general sense. For example, instead of incubating separate sets of fungal media at 37° and 30° C, incubate one set of plates at 30° C, a temperature at which all fungi can grow. Biplates, such as anaerobic *Bacteroides* bile esculin and laked sheep blood with kanamycin and vancomycin, can be inoculated instead of two separate plates. Other cost-saving measures can be undertaken, depending on the individual situation present in each laboratory. Of course, the physicians must be kept well informed of laboratory policy so that special circumstances will be accommodated and patient care will not suffer.

4.2.c. Screening procedures. Tremendous cost savings can be achieved if specimens unlikely to yield diagnostic information are not processed beyond initial evaluation. The screening of expectorated sputum for the numbers of polymorphonuclear neutrophils and squamous epithelial cells per low power field is an effective way to improve the quality of sputum specimens received in the laboratory and to prevent unnecessary work. This approach should be extended to wound cultures received on swabs. Even when only one swab is received in the laboratory, both cultures and a Gram-stained smear may be prepared using the following method. The microbiologist vortexes the swab in 0.5 ml of the appropriate diluent (tryptic soy broth or brucella broth), places the swab into enrichment broth (thioglycolate), and inoculates several drops of material to the appropriate media and onto the surface of a slide with a sterile capillary pipette. The presence of polymorphonuclear neutrophils indicates an infectious process; the presence of squamous epithelial cells indicates surface skin contamination. The appearance of the Gram stain can further be used by technologists to determine the extent of definitive identification and susceptibility testing to be performed on the organisms recovered. The immediate information conveyed to physicians by the results of the Gram stain and the subsequent decrease in unnecessary studies performed on specimens of dubious value should far outweigh the inconvenience and time initially invested in the staining procedure.

A number of recent technical advances, including the use of bioluminescent analysis and colorimetric methods, have been directed toward screening urine (Chapter 18). Since the largest numbers of specimens received by many laboratories are urines, of which over half are culture negative or not diagnostically significant, a urine screening system can reduce unnecessary work. Physicians will benefit by receiving negative results one day sooner than by conventional culture, which should aid in preventing antibiotic overusage. A urine screen that has been evaluated for its applicability to the specific clinical milieu in which the laboratory functions should be considered.

New technologies are being applied to development of screening procedures for many other clinical specimens, although they have not received widespread acceptance yet. Tests should soon be available for rapid testing of stool filtrates for the presence of *Clostridium difficile* toxin, for example. Some tests on clinical specimens will have the greatest value as predictors of negative results, thus limiting the number of specimens that must be assessed by more cumbersome methods. Gas chromatography has long been studied as a means to quickly evaluate body fluids for the presence of bacterial metabolic products.

4.3. Rapid Detection of Etiologic Agents of Infection

4.3.a. Visual tests. As discussed throughout the book, there are numerous methods for rapidly detecting the presence of infectious agents or their products. The easiest to perform are direct wet preparations and simple stains. The Gram stain is probably the single most cost-effective test used in clinical microbiology. Some specific visual methods employ immunologic reagents coupled to marker substances. Examples include the rapid detection of *Chlamydia* elementary bodies by a monoclonal antibody conjugated with a fluorescein marker. Horseradish peroxidase, alkaline phosphatase, and other enzymatic markers have been used, particularly for detection of viral subunits, either nucleic acid sequences or surface proteins. Fluorescent reagents are available for specific staining of *Legionella* species, *Neisseria gonorrhoeae*, *Bordetella pertussis*, *Yersinia pestis*, *Francisella tularensis*, *Treponema pallidum*, *Bacteroides fragilis* and *B. melaninogenicus*, other bacteria, and a number of fungal and par-

asitic agents of infectious disease. For specimens that are suspected of harboring these agents, the use of rapid detection methods can save days and directly influence patient care.

4.3.b. Particle agglutination methods. Latex agglutination and staphylococcal coagglutination reagents coated with antibodies are available for rapid detection of many antigens. Group A beta hemolytic streptococci can be detected in throat swabbings within 15 min of collection of the specimen. Commercial kits are available for rapid detection of the antigens of the most common causes of meningitis, *Haemophilus influenzae* type b, *Neisseria meningitidis*, *Streptococcus pneumoniae*, and *S. agalactiae*. These tests may detect antigens in urine or serum as well. Cryptococcal antigen can be detected with more sensitivity using latex reagents than by India ink direct preparations. Latex tests for detection of rotavirus in stool filtrates have been compared favorably with electron microscopy and enzyme-linked immunosorbent assay (ELISA) methods. Latex reagents are also being evaluated for diagnosis of invasive staphylococcal disease (by quantitation of circulating teichoic acid antigens) and invasive *Candida* infections (by quantitation of circulating cell wall mannan).

4.3.c. Automation. The plethora of automated microbiology instruments allows rapid detection of the presence or absence of infectious agents and often yields identifications as well (Chapter 11). The use of such instruments can greatly increase microbiology laboratory productivity. Instruments developed to detect the presence of certain etiologic agents, particularly in urine, are the Vitek AMS, the Abbott MS-2, the new Hewlett-Packard instrument, and the General Diagnostics Autobac. Urines with numbers of microorganisms greater than 10^5/ml are identified within hours, all with greater than 95% sensitivity.

Radiometric and spectrophotometric detection of microbial metabolism, as used by the

Johnston Laboratories Bactec system, can significantly decrease the time to detection of mycobacteria in sterile body fluids and concentrated contaminated specimens and in some cases in blood. Other automated blood screening devices are being developed, utilizing colorimetric, electrical impedance, and other technological tools. The *Limulus* lysate test (Chapter 10), although somewhat labor intensive at this time, may be automated for detection of endotoxin. The Abbott Quantum makes use of ELISA technology to detect antigens of gonococci and chlamydia in genital swab specimens. An ELISA test is commonly used to detect the presence of rotavirus antigen in feces. Radioimmunoassay and ELISA methods can be used to rapidly diagnose hepatitis A and B.

4.3.d. Other strategies. Additional labor at the receiving end of a specimen may save time and effort later. Two such approaches are used for blood cultures, lysis-centrifugation (DuPont Isolator) and antimicrobial removal (Marion Antimicrobial Removal Device and Bactec resin bottles). Both systems entail additional initial processing of blood cultures (Bactec simply requires a separate culture collection bottle), but both systems decrease the time to detection of positive results. Rapid initiation of appropriate treatment based on blood culture results should save hospitals money and, more importantly, lead to more successful therapy of patients. Blood cultures not handled by an automated system or by direct plating may reveal positive results more rapidly if an early detection system is employed. These include internal subculture to agar that is enclosed within the system (Gibco biphasic bottle; Roche Septi-Check) and early external subculture or acridine orange stain. Almost 80% of all positive blood cultures will be detected within 24 h of collection if the vented or aerobic bottle is agitated during initial incubation and examined microscopically by acridine orange or subcultured within 6-12 h after receipt.

4.4. Speeding Up Identification Results

4.4.a. Noncommercial methods. Once microbial growth has occurred, several methods can be used to decrease the time required to ascertain identification and susceptibility results. Spot biochemical tests can reliably identify presumptively several bacteria. The most cost-effective measure available to microbiologists is to identify bacteria presumptively based on colony morphology and simple spot biochemical tests. Several organisms lend themselves to such methods. The indole and oxidase tests are two of the most useful and rapid tests available. Indole-positive, oxidase-negative, lactose-positive, nonmucoid, flat colonies on MacConkey agar can be reported as *Escherichia coli*. These organisms comprise a substantial percentage of the gram-negative bacilli isolated in most laboratories. Swarming *Proteus* species seen on blood agar may also be identified with spot indole. Indole-positive *Proteus* are *P. vulgaris*. Indole-negative strains are *P. mirabilis*. Colonies that morphologically resemble *Pseudomonas aeruginosa* may be identified presumptively based on beta hemolysis, blue-green pigment, characteristic odor, and positive oxidase spot test results. When assessing the results of cultures of genital specimens taken from sexually active adults, technologists may presumptively identify colonies of gram-negative diplococci growing on Thayer-Martin media that are oxidase positive as *Neisseria gonorrhoeae* or *N. meningitidis*. From cerebrospinal fluid and blood cultures, slightly beta hemolytic colonies of catalase-positive gram-positive short bacilli or coccobacilli can be presumptively identified as *Listeria monocytogenes* if they exhibit characteristic tumbling motility on wet preparation. A positive slide coagulase result on a colony of catalase-positive gram-positive cocci in clusters identifies the isolate as *Staphylococcus aureus*. Yeast cells from certain sources can be presumptively identified as *Candida albicans* if they form germ tubes within 3 h at 37° C in fetal bovine serum. The Quellung rapid serologic slide test can also be used to identify *Streptococcus pneumoniae* and *Haemophilus influenzae* type b.

Suspicious colonies on primary stool media can be subcultured to blood agar plates or to Kligler's iron or triple sugar iron agar slants immediately upon discovery. Rapid urease or phenylalanine tests can be set up at the same time to rule out certain nonpathogens. After 4-5 h incubation, enough of a film of growth will have occurred on the blood agar or the slant surface to allow the technologist to perform slide agglutination serologic typing tests.

Carbohydrate fermentation reactions of a number of non-Enterobacteriaceae can be determined within 4 h using a broth containing 20% carbohydrate, peptone, meat extract, and buffers, described in Chapter 9 (Procedure 9.9). Fastidious bacteria, including *Kingella* species, *Actinobacillus*, *Cardiobacterium*, DF-2, and *Neisseria*, can be rapidly identified biochemically using this medium.

Microbiologists should all have additional ideas about the implementation of rapid methods for identification that will fit into the workflow, capabilities, and needs of their individual situations. Many clinical situations exist in which rapid, presumptive information is more important than delayed, definitive information. It is important that the microbiologist ascertain from the consumers (the infectious disease specialists and other physicians that utilize laboratory results) which definitive results can be delayed or even deleted in exchange for early, presumptive information. An excellent plan for merging rapid methods into the workflow of a standard clinical microbiology laboratory was written by Pezzlo[8] as long ago as 1981. Other sources cited should be consulted for other ideas.

4.4.b. Commercial methods. More commercial systems for rapid identification of microorganisms exist than can be mentioned here. Many of them are discussed in Chapter 9. By using enzymatic substrates that yield a colored end product, the presence of enzymes can be used to identify bacteria even in the absence of growth. Rapid enzymatic or biochemical tests systems, made by Key Scientific, General Diagnostics, API, Innovative Diagnostics, Flow Laboratories, BBL Microbiology Systems, Remel Laboratories, Austin Biologicals, and many others, are available for preliminary screening and identification of most gram-negative bacilli, gram-negative cocci, anaerobic bacteria, and some gram-positive cocci. Immunologic reagents for identification of organisms by particle agglutination are also available. Such systems (as discussed in Chapter 25) for identification of beta hemolytic streptococci yield results within minutes or a few hours.

An important source of inoculum for direct application to commercial systems is blood culture broth. Broth from a positive blood culture medium may be inoculated directly to identification systems, such as rapid enzymatic test kits, or to coagulase plasma, depending on the Gram stain morphology. Even the particle agglutination identification systems have been shown to accurately identify organisms found in blood culture media when they are performed on properly prepared samples. One technique for preparing a sample suitable for biochemical inoculation is to remove 10 ml of the supernatant from a blood culture bottle shown to contain only one morphologic type of organism. The culture medium is centrifuged at 1,500 × g for 10 min to concentrate the bacteria, the supernatant is discarded, and the pellet is resuspended in distilled water (which serves to lyse blood cells). If desired, a second centrifugation can be performed to wash the bacteria free of blood cell components, but this has not usually been found to be necessary. This suspension is then inoculated to the rapid identification system of choice. Just as for suspicious colonies from stool cultures, blood culture broth may be plated to a blood agar plate and incubated for 3-4 h to allow a sufficient film of growth to develop. This film is removed with a cotton swab, emulsified in water or saline, and used to inoculate rapid systems.

The strategies and products mentioned here and in other sources that address cost containment should be evaluated for their utility in each laboratory, and their use should be considered where appropriate. It is possible that microbiology laboratories may have to respond to the DRG challenge by rearranging the workflow, expanding the hours of operation, and otherwise changing to conform to the times.

4.5. Speeding Up Susceptibility Results

The susceptibility of a microorganism to antimicrobial agents is even more important than the definitive identification in many cases. Several strategies have been developed to yield faster results in that area. Exhaustively reviewed by Isenberg and D'Amato,[5] rapid susceptibility testing methods range from reading disk diffusion agar plates after only 5 or 6 h incubation to direct inoculation of susceptibility testing media with specimen material. The most effective method for rapid susceptibility testing of isolated bacteria appeared to be that of Lorian,[7] in which isolated colonies were suspended in trypticase soy broth to a density equal to a McFarland 1.0 turbidity standard and the suspension was inoculated to Mueller-Hinton agar without preincubation. The standard zone sizes were used for interpretation of results, but Mueller-Hinton with 5% sheep blood was used for all gram-positive cocci. Qualitative results obtained after 5 h incubation agreed with conventional Bauer-Kirby disk diffusion determinations over 97% of the time for all organisms. Rapid methods have not been so standardized for quantitative susceptibility results. New technologies exploiting the ability of growing organisms to produce fluorescent marker metabolic end products or the technologic advances that allow laser imaging of tiny

amounts of bacterial mass are being actively pursued as possible candidates for rapid susceptibility testing use.

Direct susceptibility testing with urine has not yielded results that correlate well with conventional methods. Positive blood cultures, however, since they are almost universally monomicrobic, can be adapted for direct testing. Methods cited above for preparation of inocula for identification systems can also be used to prepare inocula for direct susceptibility testing. Greater than 95% agreement with interpretative results of conventional testing procedures can be achieved by dropping 2-3 drops of the well-agitated blood culture broth (Gram stained to ascertain the presence of only one morphologic type) directly to the surface of Mueller-Hinton agar. This inoculum is spread and further handled in the same manner as for standard disk diffusion. Results are thus available 1 day sooner than with conventional methods, which should always be performed to confirm rapid test findings. Another method for concentrating bacteria for inoculation into subsequent susceptibility testing systems is to inoculate 1 ml of the positive blood culture broth to an equal amount of Mueller-Hinton or tryptic soy broth and incubate the suspension for 1-2 h at 37° C. After this time, the turbidity of the suspension is adjusted to that of McFarland 0.5 and standard disk diffusion susceptibility testing procedures (as well as rapid identification procedures) are carried out. Even quantitative susceptibility testing can be speeded up, as reported by Kiehn et al.[6] A 1 ml suspension made of equal amounts of turbid blood culture broth and brain heart infusion broth, incubated for 3-6 h and diluted 1:500, can be used as the inoculum for a microbroth dilution susceptibility test with results that have greater than 98% agreement with conventional methods (within two dilutions). Of course, all of these strategies work only with rapidly growing organisms, and results must be confirmed with conventional methods on the following day.

The equivalent of direct susceptibility testing of at least two selected bacterial species can be accomplished extremely rapidly by using chromogenic substrates, as discussed in Chapter 13. The chromogenic cephalosporin **nitrocefin** can be used with pure culture material as well as with pelleted specimen material from cerebrospinal fluids, for example, for detection of beta lactamases. Such information should be generated for isolates of gonococci and *Haemophilus influenzae*. Detection of beta lactamases produced by staphylococci or *Bacteroides* may require increased reaction time, but the chromogenic substrate is still valuable for rapid detection of antimicrobial resistance. Other chromogenic substrates have been employed in other commercially produced rapid systems, usually impregnated on filter paper. Beta lactamases can be detected using other systems, such as acidometric or iodometric, but these methods are slightly more cumbersome than the single filter paper required for the chromogenic substrate tests. A rapid test for detection of the acetyltransferase enzyme that renders an organism resistant to chloramphenicol should be used to test isolates of *H. influenzae* from cerebrospinal fluid in areas where chloramphenicol resistance has been reported and where that agent is used in the initial treatment of meningitis. This test is also available as a filter paper–impregnated disk (Remel Laboratories). It is hoped that new detection systems for resistance to other agents will soon be available.

Automation has made a tremendous impact on susceptibility testing in microbiology. A number of systems are available, as detailed in Chapter 11, that yield qualitative and quantitative results within 4-6 h after the test is inoculated. Although certain types of resistance will not be detected with these systems as they are currently produced (such as inducible cephalosporinases and small numbers of methicillin-resistant staphylococci in a population of

bacteria), the information generated by such systems is extremely valuable. Special susceptibility tests that previously required hours of labor, such as synergism studies, can be performed easily with those automated systems that generate curves of bacterial growth as detected nephelometrically (Abbot MS-2, Autobac).

Use of the radiometric system (Bactec) for detection of metabolic activity has revolutionized susceptibility testing of mycobacteria. Results that used to require up to 3 weeks are now available in several days. The effect of combinations of antimycobacterial agents on growth of isolates can be assessed in this system as well.

4.6. Computerization

The final product of the labors of microbiologists is information and the thrust of this discussion has been toward strategies for decreasing the time until the information is available. The speed with which this information is generated will have no impact on patient care, however, if it is not quickly relayed to the physician with responsibility for patient care. It is in the rapid dissemination of information that the modern laboratory differs from those of the past. A computer system is essential for information storage, sorting, and retrieval.

Cost containment measures that can be aided by computerization include logging in of new specimens. A computer can flag a second specimen from the same patient on a single day to alert the laboratory to (probably) unnecessary test requests. Without an automated system, duplicate specimens are rarely recognized until the next day, after they have been inoculated, if they are discovered at all. A microbiology computer can be used to maintain inventory and avoid costly delays due to lack of products as well as loss of operating costs due to outdating or overstocking. The use of computers for direct test requesting and reporting will save technologist and clerical time. In addition, the information critical to patient care will reach the intended physician directly, without the possible misunderstandings that occur when messages are relayed by telephone or the costly delay while the proper party is being located. The computer can also be used to assess workload units of procedures, to effect direct billing and thus monitor laboratory usage, and to maintain quality control records. We (EJB) use a computer program to search our serology files for records of previous tests run on patient sera received for certain viral antibody tests. The system identifies sera that were previously tested and informs the technologist where the old serum is stored in the freezer so that it can be defrosted and tested with the current serum specimen. Of course, computers are valuable for preparing cumulative susceptibility data reports and for epidemiologic evaluation. Direct communication between microbiology instruments and laboratory computers can allow data to be transmitted easily after verification. Even if there is no computer access from the laboratory to the nursing stations, answers to telephone queries can be obtained much more quickly by finding the information on a laboratory computer than by leafing through a logbook for a patient's name or number.

Ultimately, it is computers that will help to effect the change in microbiology practices mandated by the need to control rising costs without adversely affecting patient care. The change from slow methods that require time for bacterial growth to more rapid methods for detection of pathogens and prediction of susceptibility patterns has begun late for microbiology in comparison to chemistry. Clinicians realize the value of rapid availability of results and will utilize the information for better patient care; they will demand more and better systems. Once hospital administrators also realize the cost benefit of rapid methods in mi-

crobiology, they will support more instrument acquisitions, which will spur the manufacturers to develop new and better systems. The revolution in microbiology, boosted by DRGs, has only begun.

REFERENCES

1. Bartlett, R.C., Kohan, T.S., and Rutz, C. 1979. Comparative costs of microbial identification employing conventional and prepackaged commercial systems. Am. J. Clin. Pathol. 71:194.
2. College of American Pathologists. 1985. Manual for laboratory workload recording method. The College, Skokie, Ill.
3. Ellner, P.D. 1985. A dozen ways to achieve more cost-effective microbiology. Med. Lab. Observer 17:40.
4. Garcia, L.S., and Bruckner, D.A. 1985. Microbiology's economics: dissecting procedures and costs. Med. Lab. Observer 17:51.
5. Isenberg, H.D., and D'Amato, R.F. 1984. Rapid methods for antimicrobic susceptibility testing. In Cunha, B.A., and Ristuccia, A.M., editors. Antimicrobial therapy. Raven Press, New York.
6. Kiehn, T.E., Capitolo, C., and Armstrong, D. 1982. Comparison of direct and standard microtiter broth dilution susceptibility testing of blood culture isolates. J. Clin. Microbiol. 16:96.
7. Lorian, V. 1977. A five hour disc antibiotic susceptibility test. In Lorian, V., editor. Significance of medical microbiology in the care of patients. Williams & Wilkins, Baltimore.
8. Pezzlo, M. 1981. Rapid methods in microbiology. III. Rapid methods for the identification of gram-negative organisms. Am. J. Med. Technol. 47:693.

BIBLIOGRAPHY

Bartlett, R.C. 1974. Medical microbiology: quality, cost and clinical relevance. John Wiley & Sons, New York.
Becker, B.L. 1985. Test menus and profiles: signs of change under DRG's. Med. Lab. Observer 17:26.
Doern, G.V., Scott, D.R., and Rashad, A.L. 1982. Clinical impact of rapid antimicrobial susceptibility testing of blood culture isolates. Antimicrob. Agents Chemother. 21:1023.
Everett, G.D., de Blois, S., Chang, P.F., and Holets, T. 1983. Effect of cost education, cost audits, and faculty chart review on the use of laboratory services. Arch. Intern. Med. 143:942.
Garcia, L.S. 1985. A cost containment checklist. Med. Lab. Observer 17:67.

Kaplan, R.L. 1981. Rapid methods in microbiology. II. Rapid identification of gram-positive organisms. Am. J. Med. Technol. 47:687.

Matsen, J.M. 1982. How rapid should rapid methods be? Clin. Microbiol. Newsletter 4:164.

Matsen, J.M., and Kelly, M.T. 1985. Practical clinical microbiology—laboratory perspectives for the era of prospective payment and DRG's. American Society for Clinical Pathology Commission on Continuing Education, Council on Microbiology, Chicago. (Workshop manual.)

Miller, J.M. 1984. The impact of DRG's on hospital laboratories. Clin. Microbiol. Newsletter 6:57.

Moore, H.B. 1981. Rapid methods in microbiology. IV. Presumptive and rapid methods in anaerobic bacteriology. Am. J. Med. Technol. 47:705.

Pezzlo, M.T. 1984. Detection of bacteriuria by automated methods. Lab. Med. 15:539.

Sanders, C.B., and Aldridge, K.E. 1983. The microbiology laboratory: garbage in, garbage out. Clin. Microbiol. Newsletter 5:123.

Tilton, R.C., editor. 1982. Rapid methods and automation in microbiology. American Society for Microbiology, Washington, D.C.

Winkel, P., and Statland, B.E. 1984. Assessing cost savings when unnecessary utilization of laboratory tests can be abolished. Am. J. Clin. Pathol. 82:418.

5 Hospital Epidemiology

5.1. Introduction

In addition to its important role in assisting in the diagnosis and guiding treatment of patients, the microbiology laboratory has the opportunity and responsibility to recognize infections of public health importance. The laboratory may identify infections that are capable of being spread from one individual to another, including tuberculosis, venereal disease and certain diarrheal diseases, among others. Data from clinical microbiology laboratories may suggest or document an epidemic outbreak in the community.

Of particular importance to the microbiology laboratories in hospitals is their role in identifying and investigating nosocomial infection. The balance of this chapter will be devoted to nosocomial infections.

5.2. Nosocomial Infections

Nosocomial infections are those that are acquired in the hospital setting (Chapter 23). These may, of course, first appear some time after a patient has been discharged from the hospital, depending on the incubation period of the infection in question. It may be difficult to distinguish between community-acquired and nosocomial infections inasmuch as incubation periods for many infections are variable or unknown. Identification by the laboratory of an unusual number of isolates of an uncommon

41

pathogen, of a number of strains of the same organism with an unusual antimicrobial susceptibility pattern or unique biochemical feature (e.g., lactose-positive *Proteus*), or clustering of isolates of a given type from an intensive care unit or other discrete area within the hospital, suggests the likelihood of an outbreak of nosocomial infection. The laboratory works closely with the infection control team to investigate the epidemiology of such outbreaks and to seek corrective measures. The laboratory assists in preventing infection of other patients and of hospital personnel by indicating which patients are likely to require isolation and by providing guidance in the use of disinfectants and sterilizing procedures.

5.2.a. Incidence. The National Nosocomial Infections Study (NNIS) carried out by the Centers for Disease Control indicates that 5%–6% of hospitalized patients develop nosocomial infection. It is estimated that the average nosocomial infection prolongs hospital stay by about 3.2 days and results in added direct charges of about $540 (based on 1977 figures). Thus, for the United States as a whole, nosocomial infections would cost over a billion dollars per year in direct costs alone. This does not take into account charges of physicians, loss of productivity, and costs of death. It appears that at least 1% of nosocomially infected patients die as a direct result of such infection and that nosocomial infection contributes to the deaths of an additional 2%–3% of infected patients.

Attack rates vary according to the type of hospital, with large referral hospitals having higher rates of nosocomial infection than small community hospitals. Large teaching hospitals have higher infection rates than small teaching hospitals. The difference in risk of infection is probably related to several factors—severity of the illness occasioning hospitalization, frequency of invasive diagnostic and therapeutic procedures, and variation in the effectiveness of infection control programs. Within hospitals,

surgical and medical services have the highest rates of infection, and pediatric and nursery units the lowest.

5.2.b. Epidemiology. Three principal factors determine the likelihood that a given patient will acquire a nosocomial infection: (1) susceptibility of the patient to the infection, (2) the virulence of the infecting organism, and (3) the nature of the patient's exposure to the infecting organism. In general, of course, hospitalized persons do have an increased susceptibility to infection, and it is not yet possible to immunize patients against nosocomial infections. Corticosteroids, cancer chemotherapeutic agents, and antimicrobial agents all contribute to the likelihood of nosocomial infection but are nonetheless important agents that are generally much more beneficial than harmful. It is also not possible to exert influence over the virulence of the infecting organisms. Patients with serious community-acquired infections are admitted to hospitals frequently. It is advisable in the case of an influenza epidemic to avoid hospitalizing patients without serious complications and who are not in real need of hospital care. Nonetheless, it is necessary to admit a number of patients and the disease may spread in this manner. Our best hope to minimize nosocomial infections is to eliminate sources of exposure and to interrupt means of spread of these organisms in the hospital environment.

The most important means of transmission of nosocomial infections is by contact, usually direct but sometimes indirect, as in the case of spread of infection by means of secretions. Infected patients are the primary source of organisms in nosocomial infections, although asymptomatic carriers may transmit such infection. **Handwashing** by personnel before and after contact with each patient is the most important way to prevent direct contact transmission of nosocomial infection. Appropriate isolation of infected patients is also important. The second most common means of spread of hospital-acquired infection is by contaminated vehicles or so-called common sources. Included here are contaminated food, water, medications or medical devices. Other types of materials in the hospital may serve as sources of nosocomial infection or as fomites. A recently described example was wet mattresses which served as environmental reservoirs of *Acinetobacter* which were involved in an outbreak of infections in a burn center. For the most part airborne spread of infection is not significant in the hospital setting, although it can be in situations such as influenza or pulmonary tuberculosis.

5.2.c. Types of nosocomial infection. Urinary tract infection, the most common type of hospital-acquired infection, accounts for some 40% of nosocomial infections. Surgical wound infections account for an additional 20%, lower respiratory tract infections (primarily pneumonia) account for 15%, and nosocomial bacteremia accounts for an additional 5%. Thus, these four categories together account for about 80% of nosocomial infections. Cutaneous infections account for an additional 5% of hospital-acquired infections. *Escherichia coli* is the most common pathogen isolated from urinary tract infections and is usually, but not always, of endogenous origin. Important factors in nosocomial urinary tract infection are manipulation of indwelling urinary catheters and other types of urologic manipulations carried out for diagnostic or therapeutic purposes. Surgical wound infections often involve indigenous flora, but *Staphylococcus aureus* and a number of different types of gram-negative aerobic or facultative bacilli are also important pathogens in this setting. Lower respiratory tract infection acquired in the hospital setting often is related to aspiration and thus involves normal oral flora; however, patients in the hospital setting commonly acquire nosocomial pathogens such as *S. aureus* and various gram-negative bacilli in their oral flora. If such patients should then aspirate, these organisms, in addition to anaerobes and streptococci from the indigenous

flora, may play a role in the subsequent aspiration pneumonia. Respiratory therapy procedures such as endotracheal suctioning or inhalation therapy may introduce nosocomial pathogens into the patient's respiratory tract. Contaminated vehicles such as medications or water used for inhalation therapy may also be responsible. Nosocomial bacteremia is most often related to the use of intravascular devices. These cannulae may be contaminated by direct contact spread via health care personnel or from the patient's own skin flora. Contaminated vehicles such as intravenous fluids or arterial pressure transducers are also important sources of nosocomial infections.

About two-thirds of nosocomial infections involve a single pathogen and about 20% involve multiple pathogens. Thus, pathogens are identified in 85% of nosocomial infections. Of these, about 85% are aerobic or facultative bacteria, and 7% fungi. The most frequently reported pathogens have been *Escherichia coli*, *Staphylococcus aureus*, enterococci and *Pseudomonas aeruginosa*. Additional pathogens, in order of frequency of isolation from nosocomial infections, are *Klebsiella* sp., coagulase-negative staphylococci, *Enterobacter* sp., *Proteus* sp., *Candida* sp., and *Serratia* sp. The frequency of isolation of different pathogens varies, of course, according to the service on which the patient is hospitalized and the site of infection. Various *Legionella* sp. have been implicated in outbreaks in hospitals, with the source of the organisms being the water system, air-conditioning system, or cooling tower in most cases. Major enteric pathogens such as *Salmonella* and *Shigella* may cause hospital outbreaks on occasion.

Many or most of the nosocomial pathogens, aside from those representing indigenous flora, are resistant to a number of antimicrobial agents. Methicillin-resistant *Staphylococcus aureus* infections, which initially were encountered primarily at large teaching hospitals, are increasing in frequency in small teaching hospitals and in nonteaching hospitals as well. Various gram-negative bacilli such as *Klebsiella pneumoniae, Serratia marcescens* and *Pseudomonas aeruginosa* are manifesting increased resistance to aminoglycosides, including amikacin. There has also been an increase in resistance of *Pseudomonas aeruginosa* to cefotaxime and moxalactam.

5.2.d. Control programs and role of microbiology laboratory. Hospital infection control programs are designed to detect and monitor hospital-acquired infections and to prevent them where possible. Hospitals have multidisciplinary infection control committees which should include a representative from the microbiology laboratory. Most hospitals have one or more infection control nurses who collect and analyze surveillance data, monitor patient care practices, and participate in epidemiologic investigations of problems. Some hospitals have physicians or sanitarians as hospital epidemiologists. Infection control personnel are responsible for systematic surveillance of patient disease in order to recognize problems of hospital-acquired infection and to detect epidemics as early as possible. The microbiology laboratory provides important data for this surveillance effort. Obviously, there must be good communication between laboratory personnel and the infection control team. It is desirable for infection control personnel to review the results of cultures in the laboratory on a daily basis. This provides a good opportunity for such people and laboratory microbiologists to exchange information and to learn to work together.

In the past, it was common for microbiology laboratories to culture the inanimate environment of the hospital as well as certain fomites routinely. It is now recognized that such activities done on a routine basis provide little or no useful information and are very time consuming and expensive. However, investigation of a specific problem of nosocomial infection may well be facilitated by cultures of the environment and personnel.

The prompt and accurate performance of routine microbiology procedures may be very helpful in infection control work. The importance of full identification of isolates is underlined by a recent report of an outbreak of bacteremia and meningitis due to *Streptococcus faecium* in a neonatal intensive care unit. Such outbreaks may not be recognized as outbreaks without full characterization of organisms. Beyond this, the microbiology laboratory must be able to adapt quickly to unexpected infection control problems. The laboratory may be asked to characterize organisms in detail, to perform additional susceptibility tests, and to screen a large number of specimens of various types for a particular pathogen. Infection control problems tend to occur suddenly and unexpectedly, and the microbiology laboratory must be prepared to react promptly and effectively in such situations. The laboratory director must assist the infection control team in planning strategies that are consistent with the resources of the laboratory. A laboratory should be prepared to ask for help from county or state health departments or other resources, when necessary. It is highly desirable for the laboratory to have contingency plans available for emergencies that might be anticipated. Obviously, laboratory budgets should be adequate to cover routine infection control testing as well as special tests and emergency procedures.

5.2.e. Reporting of results. As noted above, good infection control personnel review microbiology laboratory results on a daily basis, and this should include direct discussions between the two groups. Certain types of results should cause the microbiologist to initiate a phone call to the infection control team or infectious disease physicians, in addition to the attending physician. For example, all positive blood cultures, all positive spinal fluid cultures, all positive acid fast smears, isolations of enteric pathogens such as *Shigella*, and isolation of resistant organisms such as methicillin-resistant *Staphylococcus aureus* should be reported by phone. Isolation of a new or unusual pathogen should result in prompt relay of information to the infection control team.

Laboratory results should be kept in a readily accessible format such as a logbook if the laboratory is not computerized, and laboratory records, including microbiology work cards, should be kept on file for at least 2 years. Isolation of unusual organisms or organisms with unique susceptibility patterns are spotted readily. However, it may be much more difficult to recognize a cluster of cases of infection involving a common organism. Computers may be very useful for this purpose, as discussed in Chapters 4 and 11. Infection control personnel should be supplied with periodic computerized summaries of selective results. Tables indicating the frequency with which particular organisms have been isolated from various sites on specific wards or units and on specific services are very helpful. This type of data should be expressed in percentages. The antimicrobial susceptibility of various pathogens to the more commonly used antimicrobial agents should also be provided on a regular basis in tabular form. For this type of data to be useful, it is important to exclude repeat cultures of the same organism from the same patient.

5.2.f. Characterizing epidemic strains. A good system for typing microbial strains involved in outbreaks should be standardized, reproducible, sensitive, stable, readily available, inexpensive, applicable to a wide range of microorganisms and field tested in conjunction with epidemiologic investigation. No such ideal typing system is available, but it is important for us to appreciate the strengths and weaknesses of the systems that we use. Available typing methods include biological or biochemical typing (biotype), antimicrobial susceptibility patterns (antibiogram), serologic typing (serotype), bacteriocin typing (including both susceptibility to bacteriocin and production of bacteriocin), bacteriophage typing (phage type), plasmid analysis, restriction enzyme analysis of plasmid or chromosomal nucleic ac-

ids, transposon insertional mutagenesis, and nucleic acid homology. Biotyping and antibiograms are clearly suitable for all hospital clinical microbiology laboratories. Limited serologic typing may also be performed in clinical laboratories. For the most part, the other typing methods listed above are available only through reference or research laboratories.

Routine identification procedures, if organisms are identified to at least the species level, are very useful in permitting recognition of hospital-acquired infection outbreaks. As noted previously, full identification of streptococci permitted detection of a *Streptococcus faecium* outbreak in a neonatal intensive care unit. Failure to fully identify *Pseudomonas* species might lead to overlooking less commonly encountered species such as *Pseudomonas cepacia* or *P. maltophilia* as causes of an outbreak.

Commercially available biochemical test panels such as the API 20E, Micro-ID, and Enterotube II (Chapter 9) permit identification to species of the vast majority of fermentative gram-negative rods and, with the addition of a few other tests, also identify many nonfermenters. Such systems provide a computer data base into which biochemical profiles of large numbers of cultures have been entered (Chapter 9). These computerized systems employ "octal numbers" which have been used in epidemiologic investigations. Unfortunately, there is some problem with reproducibility of octal or biotype numbers. Some of the reasons for the lack of reproducibility are inexact descriptions of many of the taxonomic groups, variations in inoculum size, differences in temperatures and times of incubation and differences in media. Some of these factors apply more to interlaboratory discrepancies, but even within one laboratory there may be significant variation. Rigorous standardization of the test procedure, especially the inoculum, will provide better reproducibility with these systems. It must also be appreciated that certain of the reactions in these panels may be plasmid-mediated and therefore may be either acquired or lost by a strain during an outbreak of nosocomial infection. One should not assign too much significance to variations of just one or two tests in a biotype unless careful studies have been done to define the normal variation that can be expected in these cultures with the test being used. It is hoped that manufacturers of these commercial systems will ultimately provide us with standardized chemically defined media and reagents and carry out studies to examine the reproducibility of individual tests within and between laboratories.

Accurate reproducible susceptibility testing is important to the epidemiologist just as it is to the clinician. Recognition of outbreaks of infection due to gentamicin-resistant Enterobacteriaceae, methicillin-resistant *Staphylococcus aureus* and amikacin-resistant *Pseudomonas aeruginosa*, for example, is very important. In addition, antimicrobial susceptibility patterns may be useful as epidemiological markers in the same manner as biotyping. It is desirable to include, in the standard set of antimicrobial agents for testing, certain drugs such as nalidixic acid and streptomycin which are of proven epidemiological value. It must be remembered, however, that resistance to antimicrobial agents is often plasmid-mediated and therefore may be either lost or acquired by a strain during the course of an outbreak. The type of susceptibility test used and the method of reporting influence the degree to which antibiograms may be used successfully for epidemiologic purposes. Many laboratories use the Bauer-Kirby disk diffusion method (Chapter 13) for susceptibility testing. This method is standardized, reproducible, readily available and relatively inexpensive. However, it can be used only for rapidly growing bacteria. Reporting of results of such tests as resistant, susceptible or intermediate is much less useful to the infection control team than reporting of actual zone size measurements. With the Bauer-Kirby technique, however, degrees of resistance may not be appreciated. Absence of any

zone of inhibition might be seen for a strain with a minimum inhibitory concentration (MIC) of 16 µg/ml and with another for which the MIC was >1,024 µg/ml. Such striking differences in degree of resistance may well indicate entirely different strains for epidemiologic purposes, even though the species was identical. The mechanisms of resistance might well be different also. Broth dilution susceptibility testing is being used more widely now as a result of mechanization and commercialization. While differences in degrees of resistance, as in the example cited above, can readily be determined by this type of test, there are other problems. For example, an MIC of 8 µg/ml might actually be anywhere between 4 and 16 µg/ml. In this situation, an actual zone size measurement would provide less error.

When neither the antibiogram nor the biotype alone adequately characterizes a particular nosocomial strain, it may be useful to expand both typing systems by adding additional antimicrobial agents (or other substances with antimicrobial activity such as heavy metals) or additional biochemicals. One may also combine the results of biochemical and susceptibility testing to produce an "antibiotype."

Serologic typing is also potentially useful in hospital clinical microbiology laboratories and could be applicable to a broad range of microorganisms. However, its development as an epidemiologic tool is limited because of difficulties with mass production of antisera and with standardization of methods.

5.2.g. Special biotyping procedures. As indicated above, there are a number of other procedures aside from biotyping, antibiograms and serologic typing for characterization of epidemic strains. But, as noted, these procedures are primarily useful in reference laboratory or research settings. Bacteriophage typing, by definition, is limited to bacteria. It has been especially useful with *Staphylococcus aureus*, *Pseudomonas aeruginosa* and *Salmonella* species. Phage typing consists of spotting a series of bacteriophages on a "lawn" of the organism to be typed on an agar plate culture. Bacteriophages have a very specific host range, each one attacking only a particular type of a given organism such as *Staphylococcus aureus*. Thus there are a number of phages active against *S. aureus*, but each one lyses only particular types of *S. aureus*. From the pattern of lysis of the bacterium on the agar plate (see Figure 5.1), one can specify the phage type of a particular strain of *S. aureus*. If only phages numbered 52A and 80 among the whole set of phages used produce zones of lysis with a given strain of *S. aureus*, that strain is designated phage type 52A, 80. Bacteriocin typing is also limited to bacteria. **Bacteriocins** are a group of heterologous substances produced by bacteria that inhibit the growth of closely related species; they are usually proteins. There are two sys-

tems of bacteriocin typing: bacteriocin production, which involves determination of the inhibitory spectrum of bacteriocins produced by a strain to be typed, and bacteriocin susceptibility, in which the susceptibility of the strain to be typed to bacteriocins produced by a set of standard producer strains is determined.

Plasmids are extrachromosomal bits of genetic material that are able to self-replicate. Plasmids may be transferred from one bacterial cell to another by conjugation or transduction. Plasmid analysis has been used primarily to explain the occurrence of unusual or linked antibiotic resistance patterns. Plasmids themselves may be typed by means of restriction endonuclease digestion patterns. These restriction enzymes recognize specific nucleotide sequences in DNA and produce double-stranded cleavages. There are at least 36 of these enzymes for

FIGURE 5.1
Example of three *S. aureus* isolates with different phage typing patterns. The organisms are swabbed on agar plates to achieve confluent growth, and suspensions of several different bacteriophages are spotted on the agar surface in a standard pattern. The ability of particular phages to infect and lyse the staphylococci is detected by the presence of a lysed circle, or "plaque." The staphylococci are assigned phage types according to which phages can cause lysis. (Plates courtesy Henry Isenberg.)

which the specific recognition sequence and cleavage site has been defined. Mating experiments may be useful for assessing the stability of resistance (R) factors or plasmids in a bacterial population. It has been possible to show that plasmid or R factor epidemics occur in which a specific plasmid is transmitted from one genus of bacteria to another. Restriction enzyme analysis may also be used for characterizing strains of viruses. It has been used particularly for herpes simplex virus. Probably the ultimate test of genetic relatedness is the degree of chromosomal nucleic acid homology (Chapter 10), but at present the techniques are still so cumbersome that they have not been applied for epidemiologic purposes. Table 5.1 summarizes the various typing systems that have been found most useful for selected nosocomial pathogens.

5.2.h. Screening populations. When a hospital infection outbreak occurs, it may be necessary to determine the extent to which the infecting strain has spread among the patients. Thus, the laboratory may be required to screen a large number of patients in a short period of time. It is important to choose culture sites and culture media so as to avoid unnecessary effort. Sites known to be colonized by a particular pathogen should be selected for culture. In the case of a group B streptococcal outbreak, for example, good sources of cultures would be the umbilicus, throat and perhaps stool. In the case

of a staphylococcal outbreak in a nursery setting, cultures of the umbilicus and nose would be appropriate. For enteric gram-negative bacilli, throat and stool are the major reservoirs.

Selective media should be used to facilitate recovery of the organism being sought. In the case of an outbreak with an antibiotic resistant organism, the microbiologist may incorporate an appropriate concentration of the drug or drugs in question in appropriate plate media. With this approach, it is important to test each batch to be certain that it supports the growth of the epidemic strain that is being sought.

Occasionally, it is desirable to culture hospital personnel who may be involved in spreading an epidemic strain. It is important to culture only those individuals who are epidemiologically incriminated. Culturing large numbers of the medical staff indiscriminately is expensive, may yield misleading information, and causes anxiety and hostility.

Demonstration of bacteria on the hands of personnel may not only confirm the mechanism of cross infection but may serve as an important educational device to impress personnel with the importance of handwashing. A simple hand culturing procedure is to have personnel lightly touch their fingertips to the surface of an appropriate selective medium. Unfortunately, this technique is not very sensitive. Detection of hand colonization is much more likely if personnel vigorously wash their hands with 10 to

TABLE 5.1
Epidemiologic Typing Systems Most Useful for Nosocomial Pathogens

TYPING SYSTEM	MICROORGANISMS
Biotype	*Salmonella, Shigella,* other species of Enterobacteriaceae, *Pseudomonas,* fungi
Antibiogram	Enterobacteriaceae, *Pseudomonas* and other nonfermentative bacteria, *Staphylococcus*
Serotype	Viruses, Enterobacteriaceae, *Pseudomonas,* streptococci, *Legionella, Chlamydia*
Bacteriocin type	*Shigella, Pseudomonas, Serratia*
Bacteriophage type	*Staphylococcus, Pseudomonas, Salmonella, Mycobacterium*
Restriction enzyme analysis	Herpes simplex virus, adenovirus, (bacterial plasmids)

Modified from Aber, R.C., and Mackel, D.C. 1981. Epidemiologic typing of nosocomial microorganisms. Am. J. Med. 70:899.

20 ml of a nutrient broth. A good technique is to wash the hands in an ethylene oxide sterilized plastic bag or plastic glove containing the broth.

5.2.i. Storage of strains. It is important for microbiology laboratories to save unique isolates from patients so that they may be retrieved for further study if an epidemic is recognized later. Such organisms should be retained for at least a week in order to give the infection control team adequate time to review the situation to determine whether further analysis is indicated. Such storage, of course, is also valuable to clinicians who may wish to have additional identification procedures or susceptibility testing performed. Organisms that are documented as being involved in nosocomial infections and organisms with unique susceptibility patterns for the institution should be saved for extended periods of time.

5.3. Monitoring

Bacteriologic monitoring of personnel and of certain medical products or solutions is indicated on occasion.

5.3.a. Personnel monitoring. Some institutions require preemployment stool cultures on food handlers. This is of limited value. It is much more important to stress that food handlers submit cultures if they develop diarrhea. There should be no routine screening of personnel for nasal carriage of *Staphylococcus aureus*. A significant percentage of hospital personnel do carry this organism, but such individuals rarely shed enough organisms to pose a hazard and there is no simple way to predict which nasal carriers disseminate staphylococci. Culture of skin or other infections in members of the hospital staff is clearly an important function of the microbiology laboratory. The employee health service should be notified promptly of recovery of significant pathogens from such infections and of isolation of other organisms such as *Shigella* from stool cultures.

5.3.b. Monitoring of hospital supplies, water, etc. Because there have been a few outbreaks of nosocomial infection related to contaminated intravenous fluids and other commercial products, some hospitals have considered routine sampling of products before use. This is not practical and is not recommended. This type of contamination has typically involved only a small fraction of production lots, and the level of contamination is quite low. The quality control provided by the manufacturer is usually much more extensive than would be practical in the hospital microbiology laboratory. The better approach is for the infection control team to monitor patients for the development of nosocomial infections that might be related to the use of contaminated commercial products. In the event of an outbreak or an incident related to suspected contamination of commercial products, an appropriate microbiologic study is indicated. Most often, such infections are actually caused by in-use contamination of the system, rather than contamination during the manufacturing process. Suspect lots of fluid, catheter trays, etc. should be saved and the Food and Drug Administration notified if contamination is suspected.

Some hospitals prepare their own parenteral solutions, especially hyperalimentation fluids. Microbiologic testing is indicated as part of the quality control procedure. Since contamination of such fluids is generally rare and sporadic, it is not practical for most institutions to perform rigorous quality control to guarantee sterility of each lot that is produced. When culture is indicated, approximately 20 ml of fluid should be collected aseptically. A calibrated loop of 0.01 ml capacity may be used to inoculate the surface of a nutrient agar plate. The remaining fluid should be inoculated into a suitable nutrient broth. Hospitals that prepare infant formula should perform microbiologic studies to detect possible contamination. Several bottles of formula from each lot produced should be cultured by preparing a nutrient agar pour plate with 1 ml of milk. It has been suggested that no more than 25 colonies should be present after 48 h of incubation, and none of these should be potential pathogens such as *Staphylococcus aureus* or group A *Streptococcus*.

In the event of a *Legionella* outbreak, environmental sampling should be done. In particular, the potable water supply, the air-conditioning cooling towers, and other elements of the air-conditioning system should be cultured. Details of suitable procedures may be found in the laboratory manual by Edelstein.[2]

REFERENCES

1. Aber, R.C., and Mackel, D.C. 1981. Epidemiologic typing of nosocomial microorganisms. Am. J. Med. 70:899.
2. Edelstein, P.H. 1984. Legionnaires' disease laboratory manual. Document PB 84 156 827. National Technical Information Service, Springfield, VA.

BIBLIOGRAPHY

Archer, G.L., Dietrick, D.R., and Johnston, J.L. 1985. Molecular epidemiology of transmissible gentamicin resistance among coagulase-negative staphylococci in a cardiac surgery unit. J. Infect. Dis. 151:243.

Coudron, P.E., Mayhall, C.G., Facklam, R.R., Spadora, A.C., Lamb, V.A., Lybrand, M.R., and Dalton, H.P. 1984. *Streptococcus faecium* outbreak in a neonatal intensive care unit. J. Clin. Microbiol. 20:1044.

Dixon, R.E. 1980. Control of nosocomial and other infections acquired in medical-care institutions. In Lennette, E.H., Balows, A., Hausler, W.J. Jr., and Truant, J.P., editors. Manual of clinical microbiology, ed. 3. American Society for Microbiology, Washington, D.C.

Goldmann, D.A. 1980. Laboratory procedures for infection control. In Lennette, E.H., Balows, A., Hausler, W.J., Jr., and Truant, J.P., editors. Manual of clinical microbiology, ed. 3. American Society for Microbiology, Washington, D.C.

Jarvis, W.R., White, J.W., Munn, V.P., Mosser, J.L., Emori, T.G., Culver, D.H., Thornsberry, C., and Hughes, J.M. 1983. Nosocomial infection surveillance, 1983. M.M.W.R. 33:9SS.

Shands, K.N., Ho, J.L., Meyer, R.D., Gorman, G.W., Edelstein, P.H., Mallison, G.F., Finegold, S.M., and Fraser, D.W. 1985. Potable water as a source of Legionnaires' disease. J.A.M.A. 253:1412.

Smith, P.B. 1983. Biotyping—its value as an epidemiologic tool. Clin. Microbiol. Newsletter 5:165.

Part Two

Handling Clinical
Specimens for
Microbiological Studies

6

Selection, Collection, and Transport of Specimens for Microbiological Examination

6.1. Specimen Selection

The primary considerations here are that the specimen obtained be representative of the disease process and that sufficient material be collected to assure a complete and accurate examination. For example, a small amount of serous drainage from the surface of a diabetic foot ulcer with underlying osteomyelitis is not likely to yield organisms of the type found in the infected bone; indeed, it may yield no organisms at all. In the example cited, the ideal specimen would be a bone biopsy (to be studied histologically as well as bacteriologically). Although it may often not be feasible to obtain infected tissue, tissue is clearly the ideal specimen. Frankly purulent drainage is next in terms of desirability and is entirely satisfactory. In the case of a spreading lesion of the skin and subcutaneous tissue (such as progressive synergistic bacterial gangrene), material from the active margin of the lesion, rather than from the central portion of the lesion, is most likely to accurately reflect the true bacteriology of the process. Material obtained on a swab from a sinus tract opening often does not yield the true infecting organisms. A deep biopsy of the sinus tract would be much more reliable. Expectorated sputum, particularly if it is not a good purulent specimen with minimal salivary contamination, presents major problems—particularly since pneumonia is often a serious infection. Ways around this problem include obtaining blood cultures, examining pleural fluid when present, screening the sputum specimen under 100 × magnification to determine its quality (Chapters 4 and 7), and transtracheal aspiration. Material from normally sterile sites in the body always provides an excellent specimen if care is taken to avoid contamination with skin flora.

Since anaerobic bacteria may be involved in infections of any type anywhere in the body, one should always culture anaerobically specimens of any variety that are free of contamination with normal flora. Certain specimens are essentially always contaminated with normal flora and therefore should not ordinarily be cultured anaerobically: throat swabs, nasopharyngeal swabs, gingival swabs, expectorated sputum, sputum obtained by nasotracheal or orotracheal suction, specimens obtained via a bronchoscope, gastric contents, small bowel contents (the latter two types of specimens may yield valuable information on culture in the case of "blind loop" and similar syndromes), large bowel contents or feces (except for *Clostridium difficile*, *C. botulinum*), ileostomy and colostomy effluents, voided or catheterized urine, and vaginal or cervical swabs (except as discussed under specimen collection from patients with endometritis).

6.2. Collection Procedures

Generally, a report from the bacteriologic laboratory can indicate only what has been found by microscopic and cultural examination. An etiologic diagnosis is thus confirmed or denied. Failure to isolate the causative organism, however, is not necessarily the fault of inadequate technical methods; it is frequently the result of faulty collecting or transport technique. In a busy hospital the collection of specimens is too often relegated to persons who do not understand the requirements and consequences of such procedures. The microbiologist may also deserve criticism on occasion for neglecting to

provide adequate supplies or proper instructions, which may result in poorly collected samples. The following are **general considerations** regarding the collection of material for culture. Specific instructions for the handling of a variety of specimens are given in subsequent chapters.

Whenever possible, specimens should be obtained **before antimicrobial agents have been administered.** Often a purulent cerebrospinal fluid (CSF) reveals no bacterial pathogens on smear or culture when an antibiotic has been given within the previous 24 h. A patient with salmonellosis may have a negative stool culture if the specimen has been collected while he or she was receiving suppressive antibacterial therapy, only to reveal a positive culture several days after therapy has been terminated. If the culture has been taken after initiation of antibacterial therapy, the laboratory should be informed so that specific counteractive measures, such as adding penicillinase or merely diluting the specimen, may be carried out.

It is axiomatic that material should be collected where the suspected organism is **most likely to be found, with as little external contamination as possible.** The skin and all mucosal surfaces are populated with an indigenous flora and may often also acquire a transient flora or even become colonized for extended periods with potential pathogens from the hospital environment. The latter is particularly true of individuals who are quite ill, especially if they are receiving antimicrobial therapy (resistant organisms colonize as normal flora is suppressed). Accordingly, special procedures must be employed to help distinguish between organisms involved in an infectious process and those representing normal flora or "abnormal" colonizers that are not actually causing infection. Four major approaches are utilized to resolve this problem:

1. Cleanse the area with germicide using enough friction for mechanical cleansing as well. Start centrally and go out in

ever enlarging circles. Repeat this several times, using a new swab each time. Alcohol (70%) is satisfactory for skin, but a full 2 min of wet contact time is needed. Iodine (2%) and povidone-iodine work more quickly (1 min) and are effective against spore-forming organisms. Collection of normally sterile body fluids (such as joint, pleural, or cerebrospinal fluid) by percutaneous needle aspiration should always be preceded by thorough skin decontamination as described here.

2. Bypass areas of normal flora entirely (e.g., percutaneous transtracheal aspiration rather than coughed sputum).

3. Culture only for a specific pathogen (e.g., group A streptococci in the throat).

4. Quantitate culture results as a means of determining the likelihood of organisms being involved in infection (e.g., quantitative urine culture). Less formal quantitation may also be satisfactory and should **routinely** be used; this may involve grading on a scale of 4+ to 1+, or simply heavy growth, moderate growth, light growth, four colonies, and so forth (Chapter 8).

Another factor contributing to the successful isolation of the causative agent is the **stage of the disease** at which the specimen is collected for culture. Enteric pathogens are present in much greater numbers during the **acute,** or diarrheal, stage of intestinal infections and are more likely to be isolated at that time. Viruses responsible for causing meningoencephalitis are isolated from CSF with greater frequency when the fluid is obtained soon after the **onset** of the disease rather than when the symptoms of acute illness have subsided.

There are occasions when patients must participate actively in the collection of a specimen, such as a sputum sample. They should be given full instructions (Chapter 16), and cooperation should be encouraged by the ward attendant. Too often a container is placed on the patient's bedside table, with the only instructions being to "spit in this cup."

Another specimen for which proper collection procedures are essential for reliable culture results is the clean-catch, midstream urine specimen. These specimens, usually collected by the patient without the assistance of a trained medical care worker, often comprise a large portion of the specimens received by a clinical microbiology laboratory. Microbiologists may be asked to help prepare guidelines for proper specimen collection. The use of a printed card (bilingual, if necessary) with the procedure clearly described (see pp. 56-57 for example of such a card) can help to insure patient compliance. Separate cards should be given to males and females. Careful patient education should improve the quality of such urine specimens received by the laboratory.

Specimens should be of a **sufficient quantity** to permit complete examination and should be placed in sterile containers that avoid hazard to the patient, nurse, or ward messenger. A serious danger to the laboratory worker, as well as to all others involved, is the soiled outer surface of a sputum container, a leaking stool sample, or possible contact with blood-containing exudates. The hazard of spreading disease by inadequately trained nonprofessional workers is frequently overlooked. Its control requires continued education and constant vigilance by those in responsible and supervisory positions.

Provision must be made for the **prompt delivery** of specimens to the laboratory if the results of analysis are to be valid. It is difficult, for example, to isolate *Shigella* from a fecal specimen that has remained on the hospital ward too long, permitting overgrowth by commensal organisms and an increasing death rate of the shigellae. In some instances it may be necessary to take culture media and other equipment to the patient's bedside to ensure

PATIENT GUIDELINES FOR COLLECTION OF A URINE SPECIMEN

READ ENTIRE DIRECTIONS BEFORE STARTING PROCEDURE

Females

NOTE: Proper collection will help us to give useful results to your physician.

1. Prepare a sterile gauze pad (found on the shelf above the sink) for washing your vagina by wetting it in the sink and placing a small amount of soap on the surface so that it is sudsy. Prepare two more sterile gauze pads for rinsing by moistening them with warm water. Last, open the package of a fourth sterile gauze pad and leave it dry. Take the top off the plastic urine container and set it on the edge of the sink. Set the pads and the container in a row on the edge of the sink so that you can reach them while sitting on the toilet.

2. Pull your panties below your knees so that they will not interfere with your urine collection. With two fingers of one hand, hold the outer folds of your vagina apart. With the other hand, gently wash the vaginal area from the front to the back, using the soapy gauze pad. Discard the gauze in the wastebasket; do not throw it into the toilet.

3. Still holding the outer vaginal skin away from the opening through which you urinate, rinse the area from the front to the back, using first one moistened pad and then the second moistened pad. Last of all, dry the area from the front to the back with the dry gauze pad. Discard all gauze pads in the wastebasket.

4. Continue holding your outer vaginal folds apart and begin to urinate into the toilet. Lean slightly forward so that the urine flows directly down without running along the skin. After the first few teaspoons, place the sterile container under the stream of urine and collect the rest of your urine in the container. Even ¼ cup is an adequate sample for the test.

5. After you have finished, tighten the cap on the container securely and wash any spilled urine from the outside of the container. Make certain that your name is correctly written on the container.

6. Hand the filled and tightly capped container to the attendant in the outpatient laboratory area.

Males

1. Prepare a sterile gauze pad (found on the shelf above the sink) for washing your penis by wetting it in the sink and placing a small amount of soap on the surface so that it is sudsy. Prepare two more sterile gauze pads for rinsing by moistening them with warm water. Last, open the package of a fourth sterile gauze pad and leave it dry. Take the top off the plastic urine container and set it on the edge of the sink. Set the pads and the container in a row on the edge of the sink so that you can reach them while urinating.

2. Holding back your foreskin with one hand, if necessary, use the sudsy gauze pad to gently wash the end of your penis. Discard the gauze pad in the wastebasket; do not throw gauze pads into the toilet.

PATIENT GUIDELINES FOR COLLECTION OF A URINE SPECIMEN—cont'd

Males—cont'd

3. Continue holding back the foreskin and gently rinse the end of your penis, using first one moistened gauze pad and then the other, discarding them in the waste-basket when finished. Use the dry gauze pad to dry the end of your penis.
4. Continue holding back the foreskin and begin to urinate into the toilet. After the first few teaspoons, place the sterile container under the stream of urine and collect the rest of your urine in the container. Even ¼ cup is an adequate sample for the test.
5. After you have finished, tighten the cap on the container securely and wash any spilled urine from the outside of the container. Make certain that your name is correctly written on the container.
6. Hand the filled and tightly capped container to the attendant in the outpatient laboratory area.

prompt inoculation of the specimen. This is an unusual circumstance and requires prior arrangements with the laboratory.

Although most pathogenic microorganisms are not greatly affected by small changes in temperature, they are generally susceptible to drying out, particularly when on cotton applicator sticks. However, some bacteria, such as the meningococcus in CSF, are quite sensitive to low temperatures and require immediate culturing.

Specimens for gonococci can be inoculated directly onto selective media such as modified Thayer-Martin medium with carbon dioxide provided in a device (Transgrow) or by placing a generating tablet in a chamber (Figure 6.1) (Jembec; Chapters 8 and 19). Alternate methods include placing inoculated Thayer-Martin plates immediately into a candle jar (Figure 6.2).

Clinical material likely to contain abundant microbial flora may in most instances be held at 5° C in a refrigerator for several hours before culturing if it cannot be processed right away. This is particularly true with such specimens as

FIGURE 6.1
Modified Thayer-Martin medium in a square, plastic culture plate for transport and cultivation of *N. gonorrhoeae* (Neigon-Jembec, Flow Laboratories). A white tablet of bicarbonate is placed in a special well within the plate, the top is snapped shut, and the plate is sealed into a "Zip-Lock" plastic bag to maintain the increased CO_2 atmosphere during transport and incubation.

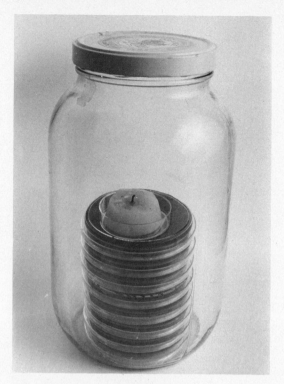

FIGURE 6.2
Thayer-Martin plates in a candle jar.

urine, feces, and material on swabs taken from a variety of sources, with the exception of wound cultures, which may contain oxygen-sensitive anaerobes. These should be inoculated promptly. Not only will refrigeration preserve the viability of most pathogens, it will minimize overgrowth of commensal organisms, increased numbers of which could make the isolation of a significant microbe more difficult. However, the sooner an organism leaving the sheltered environment of its host is transferred to an appropriate artificial culture medium, the better are the chances of its survival and subsequent multiplication.

Although not a function of specimen collection, it is an essential prerequisite that the **laboratory be given sufficient clinical information** to guide the microbiologist in selection of suit-

able media and appropriate techniques. Likewise, it is important for the clinician to appreciate the **limitations and potentials** of the bacteriology laboratory and to realize that a negative report does not necessarily invalidate the diagnosis. It is essential that close cooperation and frequent consultation among the clinician, nurse, and microbiologist be the rule rather than the exception.

Laboratory personnel should reject specimens not obtained in a proper manner and should be supported in this position by infectious disease clinicians or pathologists. In rejecting specimens, of course, the reasons should be explained to the requesting physician. Specimens should never be discarded before discussion with the requesting clinician. Some specimens, such as those taken at the time of surgery, are difficult or impossible to replace. Those specimens that cannot be replaced should be Gram stained and interpreted as carefully as possible. Guidelines for specimen rejection are discussed in Chapter 3.

6.2.a. Anaerobic collection procedures. Proper collection (that is, taking care to avoid inclusion of normal flora), cannot be overemphasized, because indigenous anaerobes are often present in such large numbers that even minimal contamination of a specimen with normal flora can give very misleading results and cause much wasted effort.

Coughed sputum is unsuitable, because it becomes contaminated with normal flora anaerobes on its passage through the mouth and pharynx. For the same reason, bronchoscopic specimens or those obtained by nasotracheal tube suctioning also should not be cultured anaerobically. The sampling tube always contacts normal flora on its downward path. The efficacy of a double lumen plugged catheter in preventing such contamination is questioned by some, but it may be possible to obtain reliable results by careful attention to detail in carrying out these procedures and by doing quantitative cultures. Adequate pleuropulmonary specimens for anaerobic culture can be obtained by transtracheal aspiration (TTA), thoracentesis or direct percutaneous needle puncture and aspiration of lung. Tracheostomy tube specimens may provide useful material when the tube is first placed; when it has been in place for a while there is inevitable contamination with oropharyngeal secretions, whether or not there is an inflated cuff.

Voided urine specimens are unsuitable for anaerobic culture because the distal portion of the urethra and the meatus are colonized with a normal flora containing anaerobes, which will contaminate urine passing through these areas. If a suprapubic bladder catheter or cystostomy or nephrostomy tube is in place, reliable urine specimens may be collected from these sites.

Endometritis presents a very difficult problem. Anaerobes are clearly very important in this infection. However, most cases of endometritis follow childbirth, and it has been demonstrated that in the postpartum period, **whether or not there is endometrial infection,** significant numbers of anaerobes and other organisms from the cervical and vaginal flora are found in the uterine cavity. There are not even quantitative differences between infected and uninfected patients. This situation may apply also in postabortal endometritis. Thus, one should obtain blood cultures and culture any better sources of material that may be available. Culture for the *Bacteroides fragilis* group may be useful. Since the presence of the *B. fragilis* group in this type of specimen indicates a poorer prognosis and since this organism is more resistant to antimicrobials than other anaerobes, it makes sense to determine whether it is present.

Infections of decubitus ulcers commonly involve anaerobic organisms, particularly when the decubitus is in the vicinity of the anus (sacral decubiti and decubiti of the hips and buttocks). Since these areas are subject to fecal contamination (this is how they become infected), the area must be thoroughly cleansed with an antiseptic agent before cultures are taken. Whenever possible, one should aspirate collections of pus from under skin flaps or from deep pockets, using a syringe and needle. The same considerations apply to other lesions in these areas (e.g., perirectal abscess).

Specimens that are normally sterile (such as spinal fluid and blood and joint fluid) may be collected in the usual fashion after thorough skin decontamination.

In general, material for anaerobic culture is best obtained using a needle and syringe. All air must be expelled from the syringe and needle (Plate 6.1). Use of swabs is a poor alternative because of excessive exposure of the specimen to the deleterious effects of oxygen and drying.

6.3. Specimen Transport

In the microbiologic examination of clinical specimens it is essential that the container bearing the specimen does not contribute its own microbial flora. Furthermore, the original flora should neither multiply nor decrease because of prolonged standing on the ward or prolonged refrigeration in the laboratory. In other words, **a sterile container should be used and the specimen should be plated as soon as possible.** Although these are not hard-and-fast rules, any deviation should be the responsibility of the microbiologist.

A variety of containers have been devised for collecting bacteriologic specimens. Many of these can be used repeatedly after proper sterilization and cleaning, whereas others must be incinerated after use. Apart from the sterile Pyrex Petri dish and its modern counterpart, the presterilized and disposable plastic dish, the most used (but not necessarily the most desirable) piece of collecting equipment is the cotton–, calcium alginate–, or Dacron (polyester)–tipped wooden applicator stick. These swabs are best prepared by autoclaving the wooden applicator sticks in Sörensen buffer, pH 7.2, for 5 min, drying them, and then tipping them with polyester batting,* calcium alginate (Colab Laboratories), or long-fibered medicinal cotton. One approach uses a sterile disposable culture unit (Culturette, Marion Scientific Corp.) (Figure 6.3). consisting of a plastic tube containing a sterile polyester-tipped swab and a small glass ampule of modified Stuart's holding medium. The unit is removed from its sterile envelope, and the swab is used to collect the specimen. It is then returned to the tube, the ampule is crushed, and the swab is forced into the released holding medium. This will provide sufficient moisture for storage up to 72 h at room temperature.

Some cotton used for applicators may contain fatty acids that may be detrimental to microbial growth. An excellent substitute is calcium alginate wool, derived from alginic acid, a natural plant product. This silky-fibered material dissolves in certain solutions that are compatible with bacterial preservation (such as dilute Ringer's solution with sodium hexametaphosphate) to form a soluble sodium algi-

nate. Calcium alginate–tipped wooden applicators or flexible aluminum nasopharyngeal swabs (Figure 6.4), as well as the citrate or hexametaphosphate diluents, are available commercially. Calcium alginate should not be used where herpes virus is anticipated, as it may inhibit replication of this virus.

A modification of the cotton applicator uses 28-gauge Nichrome or thin aluminum wire in place of the wooden stick. Because of its flexibility, the wire applicator is recommended for collecting specimens from the nasopharynx. To ensure that the small amount of cotton adheres to the wire during passage through the nasal tract, the end of the wire must be bent over and some collodion applied before the wrapping with cotton; otherwise, the outfit remains the same as that previously described. Commercially prepared sterile wire swabs also are available (Appendix).

A variety of transport media have been devised for prolonging the survival of microorganisms when a significant delay occurs between collection and culturing. Stuart and others[3] advocated a medium that has proved effective in preserving the viability of pathogenic agents in clinical material. The medium consists of buff-

---

*Dacron polyester filling, ½-pound bags, Sears, Roebuck and Co.

FIGURE 6.3
Sterile specimen collection unit consisting of a polyester swab with a plastic shaft inserted into a tight-fitting cap within a sterile tube (Culturette, Marion Scientific). After the specimen is collected, the glass ampule containing transport medium is broken to moisten and protect the specimen on the swab.

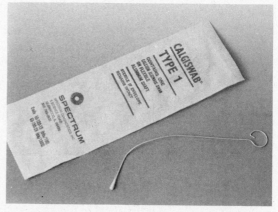

FIGURE 6.4
Calcium alginate nasopharyngeal swabs on a flexible wire that can be bent to conform to the shape of the nasal passage (Spectrum Diagnostics).

ered semisolid agar devoid of nutrients and containing sodium thioglycollate as a reducing agent and is used in conjunction with cotton swabs. Stuart's medium (available commercially) maintains a favorable pH and prevents both dehydration of secretions during transport and oxidation and enzymatic self-destruction of the pathogen present. However, the glycerophosphate present permits multiplication of certain organisms.

A report on a transport medium (available commercially) by Cary and Blair[1] (Figure 6.5) indicates that salmonellae and shigellae can be recovered from fecal specimens for as long as 49 days and *Vibrio cholerae* for 22 days; *Yersinia pestis* survives for at least 75 days. The medium itself remains good after storage at room temperature for longer than 1½ years.

Polyester-tipped swabs may be used for delayed recovery of group A streptococci from throat cultures. A report by Hosty and co-workers[2] indicates that the incorporation of a small amount of silica gel in the glass tube containing the polyester swab will further maintain

FIGURE 6.5
Small vial containing Cary-Blair medium for transport and maintenance of fecal specimens (Remel Laboratories).

the viability of group A streptococci in throat swabs for as long as 3 days before plating.

6.3.a. Anaerobic specimen transport. The collection of specimens for anaerobic culturing poses a special problem in that the conventional methods previously described will not lead to optimal recovery of these air-intolerant microorganisms. A crucial factor in the final success of anaerobic culturing is the transport of clinical specimens; the lethal effect of atmospheric oxygen must be nullified until the specimen has been processed anaerobically in the laboratory. We recommend using a double-stoppered collection tube or vial, gassed out with oxygen-free CO_2 or N_2 (Scott Laboratories, Gibco Diagnostics, and BBL) and containing an agar or broth indicator system (Plate 6.2).

One injects the specimen (pus, body fluid, or other liquid material) through the rubber stopper after first expelling all air from the syringe and needle. In the laboratory, the material is aspirated from the transport container by needle and syringe, inoculated to media, and incubated under anaerobic conditions. The syringe and needle, inserted into a rubber stopper, can be used for direct transport to the laboratory if the specimen can be processed within 30 min of collection. If only a swab specimen can be obtained, it may be collected on a swab that has been maintained in an anaerobic tube (Plate 6.3) and can then be transferred to a rubber-stoppered tube with a deep column of prereduced and anaerobically sterilized transport medium (several suppliers are listed in the Appendix). A convenient type of tube, stopper, and screw cap for laboratories wishing to make their own oxygen-free tubes is the Anaerobic Culture Tube, Hungate type, No. 2047-16125, available from Bellco Glass, Inc.

An Anaerobic Culturette (Marion Scientific Corp.) generates its own anaerobic atmosphere and contains a small amount of transport medium to prevent drying. The Bio-Bag (Marion Scientific Corp.) or GasPak Pouch (BBL Microbiology Systems) (Plate 6.4) offers remarkable flexibility. It is not only suitable for swabs (for short periods; no specific means are incorporated to maintain a moist environment, nor is there a holding medium), but it can also be used to transport specimens in plastic syringes and smaller specimens aspirated (through an attached syringe) into small-gauge sterile plastic tubing. It can also be used for tissue (placed first in a sterile tube or vial). Another versatile apparatus which has a self-contained reducing system, is the Vacutainer Anaerobic Transporter (BBL Microbiology Systems; Plate 6.5).

It is important to note that the materials recommended for anaerobic transport actually constitute ideal **universal transport setups**, since **all** types of microorganisms should survive well in them. It should be stressed that although the swab is the most widely used transport vehicle, it is preferable to submit a larger specimen whenever possible (e.g., a filled syringe or tube). When organisms may be scarce (as in some forms of tuberculosis), the larger the specimen the better. Throughout this text, specimen collection and handling methods are discussed in relation to the disease process or the etiologic agent. Procedures should be chosen based on the needs of the patients served by the laboratory.

6.4. Shipping Specimens

On occasion it is necessary to submit specimens to a **reference laboratory** in a distant city, thus requiring transportation by mail or express. If, for example, there is no viral diagnostic service available in the immediate area, it may be necessary to ship specimens at a low temperature to preserve their viability. This is especially true of virus-containing material, such as CSF, throat and rectal swabs, stools, and tissue, which should be refrigerated immediately and shipped in a Styrofoam box with commercial refrigerant packs (e.g., 3M Cryogel). Whole blood is **not** shipped. Rather, the serum is separated and sent in a sterile tube.

If a culture of an isolated organism is to be sent to a reference laboratory (state or public health laboratory), it is not necessary to send it in the frozen state.

In most instances microbiologic specimens can be satisfactorily shipped through the mails, provided that **special precautions** are taken against breakage and subsequent contamination of the mailing container. According to the Code of Federal Regulations,* a viable organism or its toxin or a diagnostic specimen of a volume less than 50 ml shall be placed in a securely closed, watertight specimen container, which is enclosed in a second durable watertight container. The entire space between the containers should contain sufficient absorbent material to absorb the entire contents in case of breakage or leakage. The containers are then enclosed in an outer shipping container of corrugated fiberboard, cardboard, wood, or such. The outer container shall be labeled with the Etiologic Agents/Biomedical Material red-and-white label (available commercially) (see Chapter 2 and Figure 2.6).

Double mailing containers must be used when the microbiologist considers the specimen to be of a hazardous nature or thinks it may constitute a definite danger to the person handling the container. This includes clinical specimens, cultures for identification, and so forth.

For the shipment of fecal specimens containing salmonellas or shigellas over long distances, the filter paper method may also be employed. In collecting the specimen by this technique, fresh fecal material must be spread fairly thinly over a strip of filter paper or clean blotting paper and allowed to dry at room temperature. Using forceps, the smeared strip is then folded inward from the ends in such a way that the fecal material is covered. The folded specimen may then be inserted in a plastic envelope (polyethylene is recommended) and placed in a container to conform with postal regulations. It is possible to ship a large num-

---

*Section 72.25 of Part 72, Title 42, amended.

ber of such specimens in one container through the mail. The pathogens are unaffected by this treatment, whereas the normal intestinal flora dies. On receipt at the laboratory the paper specimen may be cut into three pieces. One piece is placed in physiologic saline for suspension and direct plating, and the remaining pieces are placed in selenite and tetrathionate broths, respectively, for enrichment and subsequent plating.

When it is necessary to ship fecal specimens or when such specimens must be held for some time before culturing, it is recommended that they be placed in a preservative solution. Cary-Blair medium has proved satisfactory. It should be discarded if it becomes acid. Approximately 1 g of feces is emulsified in not more than 10 ml of preservative, and the preserved specimen is shipped in a heavy glass container (universal type) with a screw cap in the regular double mailing container just described.

6.5. Handling of Specimens in the Laboratory

In previous sections of this book the importance of a properly collected specimen was stressed and the responsibility of personnel in its collection was indicated. In the following section the subsequent handling of the specimen in the laboratory is considered. In addition, the responsibility of the laboratory worker is pointed out.

Since it is not always practical for many specimens to be inoculated as soon as they arrive in the laboratory, refrigeration at 4°-6° C offers a safe and dependable method of storing many clinical samples until they can be conveniently handled. However, some may require immediate plating (such as specimens that might contain gonococci or *Bordetella pertussis*), whereas others must be immediately frozen (e.g., stool that is to be held for subsequent attempts at *Clostridium difficile* toxin detection).

The length of time of refrigeration varies with the type of specimen: swabs from wounds (except for anaerobic cultures), the urogenital tract, throat, and rectum and samples of feces or sputum can be refrigerated for 2-3 h without appreciable loss of pathogens. Urine specimens for culture may be refrigerated at least 24 h without affecting the bacterial flora (except the tubercle bacillus, which may be adversely affected by the urine); on the other hand, CSF from a patient with suspected meningitis should be examined **at once.**

Specimens submitted for the isolation of virus should be refrigerated immediately; if they must be held for over 24 h, they should be frozen at −70° C, if possible. Specimens of clotted blood for virus serology may be refrigerated but never frozen, as discussed in Chapter 42.

Gastric washings and resected lung tissue submitted for culture of *Mycobacterium tuberculosis* should be processed soon after delivery, since tubercle bacilli may die rapidly in either type of specimen. Further discussion of handling material for mycobacterial culture is found in Chapter 41.

Pieces of hair or scrapings from the skin and nails submitted for the isolation of fungi may be kept at room temperature (protected from dust) for several days before inoculation. On the other hand, sputum, bronchial secretions, bone marrow, and purulent material from patients suspected of having systemic fungal infection should be inoculated to appropriate media as soon as possible, especially when the diagnosis of histoplasmosis is considered. Further guidelines for collection of specimens for fungal isolation are given in Chapter 43.

6.6. Inoculation of Primary Culture Media

Depending on the etiologic agents suspected, specimens are plated and inoculated to several growth media. Special media for unusual agents (e.g., Bordet-Gengou agar for *Bordetella pertussis*) are inoculated by request. Lab-

Text continued on p. 69.

TABLE 6.1
Selection of Primary Plating Media for Bacteriology Specimens*

SPECIMEN	DIRECT SMEAR	ROUTINE MEDIA	SUGGESTED ADDITIONAL MEDIA	SPECIAL SITUATIONS	COMMENTS
• Abscess/pus† (closed wound)	+	B, M, An, Thio.	As smear indicates; CNA		Wash any granules and "emulsify" in saline.
• Autopsy Blood, tissue			Follow procedure for "living" material		
Blood Peripheral blood		Choc, An	As smear indicates	Brucellosis, tularemia, cell wall-deficient bacteria, leptospirosis	Smear when evidence of growth
• Bone marrow		B, M, Choc			
Body fluids (except blood, CSF, urine)		Centrifuge fluids for 15 min at 2,500 rpm except when grossly purulent. Stain and culture sediment. Incubate supernatant for 24 h at 37° C. Filtration is also useful if the filter can be cultured directly.			
Bile	+	B, M, An, Thio	CNA, HE, XLD, GN		Do not use An if collected perorally.
Hematoma	+	Treat as abscess	CNA	PRAS if anaerobes suspected	
Joint	+	B, Choc, Thio	CNA	Brucellosis	
Pericardial, peritoneal	+	B, M, An, Choc, Thio	CNA		
Pleural empyema	+	B, M, An, Choc, Thio	CNA	Legionella pneumophila, Chlamydia in infants, Nocardia, Actinomyces	
Catheters Foley		Do not culture			
• Central venous pressure lines, umbilical or intravenous catheters		B	Thio		Roll segment back and forth across agar with sterile forceps 4 times; ≥ 15 colonies are associated with clinical significance. (See Chapter 14.)

Specimen		Collection/Processing	Media	Additional	Notes	Comments
• Central nervous system						
Brain tissue	+	Treat as abscess				
CSF, shunt, meningomyelocele, and ventricular fluid	+	If large enough volume, centrifuge for 15 min at 2,500 rpm, and smear, and culture sediment. Incubate supernatant for 48 h at 37° C.	B, Choc, Thio	As smear indicates: M, CNA, An	Leptospirosis	*Haemophilus influenzae* may not sediment at 2,500 rpm and may require 10,000 × g for 10 min. Alternatively, culture entire specimen.
Ear						
Internal	+		B, M, Choc, Thio	CNA	An if aspiration or biopsy material	
External	+		B, M, Choc	CNA		
Eye						
Conjunctiva	+		B, M, Choc, Thio	TM, CNA		
Other	+		B, M, Choc, An, Thio	CNA		
Genital tract—female						
• Amniotic fluid	+		B, M, TM, Choc, An, Thio	CNA		Should be collected without contamination by normal flora
Cervix	±		B, CNA, TM	Choc with 1% Iso-VitaleX, HBT	In pregnancy may include M	A small number of *Neisseria gonorrhoeae* are susceptible to vancomycin. Choc with 1% Iso Vitale X, especially when there is clinical evidence of gonorrhea and negative cultures (see Chapter 19).
• Cul de sac	+		B, M, Choc, TM, An, Thio	CNA, HBT		

Modified from Isenberg, H.D., Schoenknecht, F.D., von Graevenitz, A., and Rubin, S.J. 1979. Collection and processing of bacteriological specimens. Cumitech 9. American Society for Microbiology, Washington, D.C.

*B = blood agar, M = MacConkey agar, An = anaerobic blood agar, Choc = chocolate agar, Thio = thioglycolate broth, TM = Thayer-Martin agar, CNA = Columbia agar with colistin and nalidixic acid, HE = Hektoen enteric agar, XLD = xylose lysine deoxycholate agar, GN = gram-negative broth, HBT = human blood–Tween bilayer agar, Campy = *Campylobacter* agar.

†Bullets before entry indicate specimens that require immediate attention.

Continued.

TABLE 6.1
Selection of Primary Plating Media for Bacteriology Specimens—cont'd

SPECIMEN	DIRECT SMEAR	ROUTINE MEDIA	SUGGESTED ADDITIONAL MEDIA	SPECIAL SITUATIONS	COMMENTS
Genital tract—female—cont'd					
• Uterine material (endometrium, products of conception; fetus, placenta, lochia), tubes, ovaries	+	B, M, Choc, TM An, Thio	CNA, HBT		Anaerobic culture is done on material collected without contamination by vaginal flora.
Intrauterine device		Thio			
Urethra	±	TM	Choc with 1% IsoVitaleX	*Mycoplasma, Chlamydia* (nongonococcal urethritis)	Smears of urethral exudate that are positive for intracellular gram-negative diplococci from females are presumptively diagnostic and must be confirmed by culture.
Vagina (except cuff)	±	B, TM, CNA	HBT, Choc with 1% IsoVitaleX	B, M in pregnancy	Vaginal cuff infections are treated as Abscess/pus.
• Vulva (Bartholin abscess)	+	B, M, TM, An, Thio	CNA, Choc with 1% IsoVitaleX, HBT		
Genital tract—male					
Prostatic fluid	+	B, M, TM, Thio	CNA		
Testes and epididymis (aspirate)	+	B, CNA, TM, M			
Urethra	+	TM		*Chlamydia* (nongonococcal urethritis), *Mycoplasma*	
Intestinal tract					
Colostomy, ileostomy, feces, rectal swab	Presence of cells only (polymorphonuclear leukocytes)	B, M, HE, XLD, GN, Campy (42° C)		*Yersinia enterocolitica, Vibrio cholerae, V. parahaemolyticus, Neisseria gonorrhoeae* (rectal swab)	

Specimen		Media		Organisms	Comments
Gastric aspirate	+	B, M, Choc	CNA		May be submitted in young child in place of sputum.
Plastic prostheses	−	Thio			
Pus—closed wound		See Abscess/pus			
Respiratory tract					
Throat/pharynx	−	Streptococcal Selective Agar		Vincent's angina, N. gonorrhoeae, N. meningitidis, Corynebacterium diphtheriae	Routine culture for group A streptococci only. Incubate ANO_2 or use pour plate. If fluorescent antibody studies are done for group A streptococci, incubate swab for 2 h in Todd-Hewitt broth. May be submitted instead of sputum in cystic fibrosis.
Epiglottis	−	B, Choc	CNA		
Nasal sinus	+	B, M, Choc, An, Thio	CNA		
Nasopharynx	−	B, Choc	CNA		
Nose	+	B, CNA			
Oral cavity			Mannitol salt		
Pleural fluid		See Body fluids			Culture for yeast‡
Sputum	+	B, M, Choc	CNA	Mycoplasma, Nocardia	See Chapter 16.
Bronchial secretions	+	B, M, Choc	CNA		
Tracheal aspirate	+	B, M, Choc	CNA		
• Transtracheal aspirate	+	B, M, Choc, An, Thio	CNA	Mycoplasma	
Dental abscess	+	B, M, An, Thio	As smear indicates		
Skin					
• Deep wound (open)	+	B, M, An, Thio	CNA		
Superficial wound	+	B, M	CNA, Choc	Petechiae/pustules (Neisseria)	
Traumatized areas (burns, bites, decubitus ulcers)	+	B, M, Thio	As smear indicates; CNA, An	Foul-smelling or gas-containing lesions. Culture anaerobically	Quantitative culture of burn tissue may be useful (see Chapter 21).
Rash, nonpurulent lesions	+	B, M, Choc, Thio	CNA		Smear may be diagnostic, especially in meningococcemia.

‡See Chapters 16 and 43.

Continued.

TABLE 6.1
Selection of Primary Plating Media for Bacteriology Specimens—cont'd

SPECIMEN	DIRECT SMEAR	ROUTINE MEDIA	SUGGESTED ADDITIONAL MEDIA	SPECIAL SITUATIONS	COMMENTS
Tissue					
Surgical/biopsy	+	Grind with sterile Alundum (aluminum oxide) with a sterile mortar and pestle or sterile glass tissue grinder or homogenize (Chapter 21). Use enough broth to give a 10%-20% suspension.			
		B, M, An, Thio	CNA	Other media on the basis of history, body site, and smear (i.e., tularemia or brucellosis)	
Urine					
Clean-voided, catheterized, or ileal loop urine	±	B, M (See Chapter 18)	CNA	Leptospirosis	Gram stain on unspun urine may be useful in selected patients. It is not recommended as a routine procedure. (See Chapter 18.)
Suprapubic bladder tap; cystoscopy or ureterostomy urine	+	B, M, An, Thio (0.1 ml per plate)	CNA		

oratories in some geographic areas may choose to inoculate routinely media that other laboratories could not justify economically (e.g., selective agar for *Yersinia enterocolitica*). Table 6.1 suggests one approach to the inoculation of specimens for routine bacteriological studies. As discussed in Chapters 14 through 23, etiologic agents other than bacteria (fungi, viruses, parasites) must often be considered and sought in clinical specimens.

REFERENCES

1. Cary S.G., and Blair, E.B. 1964. New transport medium for shipment of clinical specimens. J. Bacteriol. 88:96.
2. Hosty, T.S., Johnson, M.B., Freear, M.A., Gaddy, R.E., and Hunter, F.R. 1964. Evaluation of the efficiency of four different types of swabs in the recovery of group A streptococci. Health Lab. Sci. 1:163.
3. Stuart, R.D., Tosach, S.R., and Patsula, T.M. 1954. The problem of transport of specimens for culture of gonococci. Can. J. Public Health 45:73.

BIBLIOGRAPHY

Amies, C.R. 1967. A modified formula for the preparation of Stuart's transport medium. Can. J. Public Health 58:296.

Bailey, W.R., and Bynoe, E.T. 1953. The "filter paper" method for collecting and transporting stools to the laboratory for enteric bacteriological examination. Can. J. Public Health, 44:468.

Forney, J.E., editor. 1968. Collection, handling, and shipment of microbiological specimens. Public Health Serv. Pub. No. 976, Nov. 1968. U.S. Government Printing Office, Washington, D.C.

Higgins, M. 1950. A comparison of the recovery rate of organisms from cotton-wool and calcium alginate wool swabs. Ministry Health Public Lab. Serv. Bull. 43.

Isenberg, H.D., Schoenknecht, F.D., von Graevenitz, A., and Rubin, S.J. 1979. Collection and processing of bacteriological specimens. Cumitech 9. American Society for Microbiology, Washington, D.C.

Pollock, M.R. 1948. Unsaturated fatty acids in cotton plugs. Nature 161:853.

Sachs, A. 1939. Difficulties associated with bacteriological diagnosis of bacillary dysentery. J. Roy. Army Med. Corps. 73:235.

Sutter, V.L., Citron, D.M., Edelstein, M.A.C., and Finegold, S.M. 1985. Wadsworth anaerobic bacteriology manual, ed. 4. Star Publishing Co., Belmont, Calif.

Washington, J.A. II. 1985. Bacteria, fungi and parasites. In Mandell, G.L., Douglas, R.G. Jr., and Bennett, J.E., editors. Principles and practice of infectious diseases, ed. 2. John Wiley & Sons, New York.

7 Optical Methods for Laboratory Diagnosis of Infectious Diseases

7.1. Introduction

Until the observations of van Leeuwenhoek during the late seventeenth century, the presence of infectious agents smaller than the human eye could see was only speculated upon. Since that time, however, the light microscope has become a most important tool for the diagnosis of infection. Even today, with the emphasis on rapid methods for diagnosis, many of which require complicated instruments or immunological reagents, simple visual inspection of clinical specimens obtained from patients is still the fastest and most specific way to immediately augment a physician's clinical diagnosis. Many infectious agents can be reliably identified with only a few simple stains and a basic microscope. The Gram stain is still the single most efficient and cost-effective test for rapid early diagnosis of bacterial infection. Methods discussed in this chapter include many common visual techniques that have been employed by microbiologists for decades as well as a few relatively recent innovations in microscopy. An excellent working microscopy manual is that by Robert F. Smith.[3]

7.2. Examination of Fresh Material

Most microscopic examinations of material are carried out with **brightfield microscopy,** in which the object to be viewed is illuminated with light from below the field of focus, usually provided by a coiled filament tungsten lamp. The glowing filaments are prevented from causing glare by focusing their light on the sub-stage condenser, rather than on the object (known as **Köhler illumination,** after the inventor of the method). Since most pathogens visible with the microscope are of a refractive index similar to that of aqueous suspending liquids, they are invisible unless they or the technique is modified. Closing the aperture of the condenser slightly may aid in detection of certain organisms, particularly protozoans and fungi, as the light will be hitting the edges of the object at a sharper angle, increasing contrast. For Köhler illumination, which assures the best brightfield viewing of unstained clinical material, the condenser should be properly focused. This is achieved by placing a slide on the stage and viewing it through the 10 × objective. After stopping down the radiant field diaphragm (the control in the base of the microscope where the light source is), the condenser is moved up or down until the leaves around the edge of the diaphragm are in sharp focus and the condenser is centered so that the circle of light is in the center of the field of view. At this point, the leaves of the radiant field diaphragm are opened until they just disappear from the field of view. The condenser aperture diaphragm must now be adjusted. For best viewing, the aperture should be closed slowly until the sharpest image is obtained. Since the human eye is most sensitive to green light, a green filter over the light source may enhance visualization.

For direct observation of unstained material, **phase contrast** microscopy may be helpful. In this lighting method, beams of light pass through the object and are partially deflected by different densities or thicknesses (refractive indices) of the object. These light beams are deflected again when they impinge on a special objective lens, increasing in light wave amplitude (and brightness) when aligning in phase, as when passing through material of uniform refractive index, and decreasing in amplitude (visualized as darkness) when out of phase, as when passing through areas of differing refractive index. Resolution for phase contrast microscopy is also heightened with the use of a green filter. In some laboratories, phase microscopic examination of bacterial colonies emulsified in water or saline or the supernatant of broth cultures (such as blood cultures), covered by a coverslip and examined under an oil immersion lens (1,000 ×) is performed routinely (Figure 7.1). With practice, microbiologists can learn to recognize morphologies, motility, and various other characteristics helpful in aiding early presumptive identification. The use of **immersion oil** to fill the space between the objective and the cover glass or object helps to keep light rays from dispersing and, since the oil is of the same refractive index as glass, prevents changes in wavelength due to changes in refractivity of the medium through which the light passes. Immersion oil is necessary to achieve enough resolution for the visualization of most bacteria; the 100 × objective is usually used for this purpose together with 10 × oculars (total magnification = 1,000 ×).

7.2.a. Direct examination of clinical specimens. Many clinical specimens may be examined under brightfield or phase contrast microscopy in their native state, preferably as soon as they are collected from the patient. Specimens that can be applied directly to the surface of a slide for this purpose include sputum, exudate from lesions, aspirated fluid, stool, vaginal discharge, and urine sediment. Material that is too thick to easily differentiate suspended material in can be diluted with equal parts of physiologic, sterile saline. It is best to prepare all slides made from fresh clinical material within a biohazard hood, since emulsifying material on the surface of a slide often creates aerosols. A coverslip is gently laid over the surface of the material and excess liquid is blotted from around the edges with a paper towel or tissue. This sort of preparation,

FIGURE 7.1
Blood culture broth positive for gram-negative bacilli; seen under phase contrast at 1,000 ×.

known as a **direct wet mount,** can be preserved for longer viewing time by ringing the edge of the coverslip with nail polish or histological mounting medium. Wet preparations are often used to detect motile trophozoites of fecal parasites such as *Giardia lamblia, Entamoeba histolytica,* and *Dientamoeba fragilis.* The eggs and cysts of other parasites, larvae, and adult worms are also often seen in wet mounts made from freshly passed stool. *Trichomonas vaginalis* can be seen moving in wet mounts prepared from vaginal discharge material or spun sediment from fresh urine specimens. Parasites can also be found in direct wet mounts made from material aspirated from the duodenum, lung, or abscess contents. Further discussion of detection of parasites from fresh clinical specimens is found in Chapter 44.

Stool may be examined directly by phase contrast microscopy for evidence of certain bacterial diseases as well as parasites. Experienced microbiologists can recognize the characteristic darting motility and short, curved morphology of *Campylobacter jejuni.* In areas of endemic cholera, the presence of *Vibrio cholerae* in stool can be established presumptively by microscopy.

Examination of blood, often diluted in saline, can establish the diagnosis of relapsing fever or leptospirosis, as discussed in Chapter 31. Microfilariae, including trypanosomes and hemoflagellates, may also be seen in direct preparations of blood.

7.2.b. Slightly modified direct preparations of clinical material. The use of **10% potassium hydroxide (KOH** preparation) will help to distinguish fungal elements in a direct wet preparation of clinical material. Proteinaceous components, such as host cells, are partially digested by the alkali, leaving intact the polysaccharide-containing fungal cell walls. The material to be examined, whether fluid or skin or nail scrapings, is added to a drop of 10% aqueous KOH on a glass slide (see also Chapter 46). The KOH may be preserved with 0.1% thimerosal (Sigma Chemical Co.) or its digestive capabilities may be enhanced by 40% dimethyl sulfoxide (DMSO), as suggested by

McGinnis.[2] A coverslip is laid over the preparation, and excess fluid is removed from the edges by gently pressing the slide, coverslip side down, on to several thicknesses of paper towels. If this procedure is followed, the slide may be examined several minutes later for the presence of fungal elements. Gentle heating may speed the activity of the KOH, but it is unnecessary and may be harmful to the specimen if overdone. A small amount of lactophenol cotton blue (available commercially) can be added to the 10% KOH for enhanced visibility of fungal elements, or lactophenol cotton blue may be used alone for wet mount preparations of fungi. One of the most exciting new stains for visualizing fungi and other microorganisms whose cell walls contain cellulose or chitin is calcofluor white, described below in section 7.4.c.

The presence of encapsulated yeast, suspicious for *Cryptococcus neoformans*, particularly in cerebrospinal fluid specimens, can be determined by adding equal parts of **India ink** (Pelikan brand) or **nigrosin** stain to the spun sediment of the spinal fluid. The polysaccharide capsules will exclude the particles of ink and the capsule will appear as a clear halo around the organisms. Direct visualization of fungi in clinical specimens will be further discussed in Chapter 43. Capsules of bacteria may also be demonstrated with India ink or nigrosin stains (Chapter 46), although these preparations are rarely used in laboratories today.

Lugol's iodine is often added to direct wet mounts of fecal material to aid the microscopist in differentiating parasitic cysts from host white blood cells. Many cysts will take up the iodine, appearing light brown in color. Other objects remain clear. The glycogen vacuole of cysts of *Iodamoeba bütschlii* is particularly visible after it absorbs the iodine. The use of iodine is delineated in Chapter 44.

Another simple stain, **Loeffler's methylene blue,** described in Chapter 46, may be added to wet mounts of feces (equal amounts of stain

and feces) for determination of the presence of leukocytes (Figure 7.2). The presence of many polymorphonuclear leukocytes is indicative of invasive disease such as bacterial dysentery or campylobacteriosis, as opposed to the noninflammatory nature of the diarrhea of most parasitic diseases or certain food poisonings.

By adding specific antiserum to a wet preparation of selected clinical material, certain organisms may be identified by a visible antigen-antibody reaction, the **quellung reaction.** Organisms with capsules, such as *Haemophilus influenzae* type b and *Streptococcus pneumoniae*, exhibit apparent capsular swelling in the presence of homologous antibody. Pathogens in cerebrospinal fluid and sputum can be identified rapidly by this method, although it is less commonly used today than it has been in the past, perhaps because of the recently developed antigen-detection reagents that utilize macroscopically visible endpoints (particle agglutination) instead of microscopically determined endpoints (discussed in Chapter 10).

7.2.c. Darkfield microscopy. Certain bacteria are so thin that they cannot be resolved in direct preparations, even with phase contrast microscopy. However, their characteristic motility is an important feature of presumptive identification. These bacteria, primarily spirochetes such as *Borrelia* and treponemes, are best visualized by **darkfield microscopy,** a method of allowing light to be reflected or refracted off the surface of the object, which appears brightly lit against a black background (Figure 7.3). Light from below the object is blocked in a central circle so that only light from the outer ring reaches the object at a sharp angle. The object reflects and scatters this light around the object's edges and the scattered light is viewed through the objective. Large, flat objects such as host cells and clear liquid will not refract much light, and will appear very dark. To control the path of light, a drop of immersion oil is placed on the top lens of the darkfield condenser, which is then

FIGURE 7.2
Loeffler's methylene blue stained preparation of feces from a patient with invasive bowel disease,
characterized by the presence of many leukocytes.

FIGURE 7.3
Darkfield microscopy.

slowly raised until the oil comes into contact
with the bottom of the slide containing the
specimen. The condenser height is adjusted
until the brightest light is visible reflecting off
the numerous small particles in the specimen.
The light coming into the condenser from below should be the brightest possible. It may be
helpful for the microbiologist to set the darkfield lighting with a sample slide of a scraping
made from the inside of one's cheek emulsified
in saline before the actual sample is obtained.
In that way, the delicate clinical material can
be examined without delay. This method is
used most often for the demonstration of motile
treponemes in exudate expressed from a primary chancre of syphilis. To best identify these
treponemes in darkfield preparations, oil is
used on the top of the coverslip to allow view-

ing with the oil immersion lens at 1,000 ×. Specimen collection and preparation are discussed in Chapter 19. Motile campylobacters in stool may also be seen under darkfield microscopy.

7.3. Examination of Fixed, Stained Material

Examination of stained material, either direct clinical specimens or samples of growth from cultures, is the most useful method for presumptive identification of bacteria and the presence of certain viruses and for definitive identification of most parasites and many fungi. Individual stains used for special purposes will be mentioned in this chapter and in Chapter 46, but specific procedures will usually be found in the sections of the book that detail techniques for handling specific specimens or identifying specific pathogens.

Stains are either (1) **simple,** consisting of the addition of one dye that serves to delineate morphology but renders all structures the same hue, or (2) **differential.** Differential stains consist of more than one dye added in several steps, and the stained structures are differentiated by color as well as by shape. Certain classical stains are commonly used in clinical microbiology and selected procedures for these stains will be discussed below. Formulas for all reagents not shown here are listed in Chapter 46, and procedures not listed here are found in the section of the book describing specific uses for certain staining methods.

7.3.a. Preparation of a "smear." Material to be stained is dropped (if liquid) or rolled (if present on a swab) onto the surface of a clean, dry glass slide. Once a swab has touched the surface of a nonsterile slide, it cannot be used for inoculating culture media. A sterile needle may be used to transfer a small amount of the bacterial growth from solid media to the surface of a slide. This material is emulsified in a drop of sterile water or saline on the slide. For very tiny colonies that might become lost in even a small drop of saline, a sterile wooden

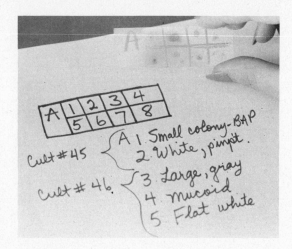

FIGURE 7.4
Preparation of a slide map for staining several colonies on one slide.

applicator stick can be used to touch the colony and obtain a bit of growth. This material is then rubbed directly onto the slide, where it can be easily seen. Bacterial morphology is well preserved with this technique. If more than one specimen is to be stained on the same slide, a wax pencil may be used to indicate divisions. It is helpful to draw a "map" of the slide so that different Gram stain results can be recorded in an organized fashion (Figure 7.4). In the case of certain critical specimens, such as cerebrospinal fluid, the use of alcohol-cleaned, sterilized slides is recommended. The material placed on the slide to be stained is allowed to dry or may be heated on a slide warmer to 60° C for at least 10 min to sterilize any pathogens that may be present. If the material is not heated, formalinized, or autoclaved, organisms may survive the staining procedure. Therefore, all stained slides should be treated as though they were potentially infectious, and should be discarded with other contaminated material after use. Flaming a slide by passing the slide through the blue flame of a Bunsen burner several times, until the slide is too hot to comfortably touch, will affix the material to the glass, but may not be bactericidal. Slides fixed in this way must be allowed to cool before they can be stained.

7.3.b. Gram stain. First devised by Hans Christian Gram during the late 19th century, the Gram stain can be used to effectively divide all bacterial species into two large groups: those that take up the basic dye, crystal violet (gram-positive), and those that allow the crystal violet dye to wash out easily with the decolorizer alcohol or acetone (gram-negative). The classic Gram stain procedure (Procedure 7.1) entails fixing the material to be stained, either by flaming as described above or by fixing in alcohol. Methanol fixation preserves the morphology of red blood cells as well as bacteria and is especially useful for examining bloody specimen material and blood culture supernatant fluid. Slides are overlayed with 95% methanol for 2 min, the methanol is allowed to run off, and the slides are air dried before staining.

After fixation, the first step in the Gram stain is the application of the crystal violet. After the crystal violet, a mordant, Gram's iodine, is applied to chemically bond the alkaline dye to the cell wall. The decolorization step distinguishes gram-positive from gram-negative cells. Probably because of increased lipid content of gram-negative cell walls, the alcohol or acetone allows increased permeability of the cell wall and the alkaline dye is washed out. The increased number of cross-linked teichoic acid residues found in gram-positive cell walls may also serve to enhance binding of the crystal violet. Gram-positive organisms that have lost cell wall integrity due to antibiotic treatment, old age, or action of autolytic enzymes will also allow the crystal violet to wash out with the decolorizer step. Animal cells, such as red and white blood cells, allow the stain to wash out with the decolorizer as well. At this stage, those organisms that stain gram-positive still retain the crystal violet and those that stain

gram-negative are clear. Addition of the counterstain, safranin (or carbol fuchsin, Chapter 46) will stain these clear organisms and cells pink or red. Although the counterstain may be taken up by the gram-positive organisms as well, their purple color will not be altered. Yeast cells also stain gram-positive, although fungal mycelia take up the Gram stain variably. Modifications of the classic Gram stain may be found in Chapter 46.

In addition to determining Gram reaction and morphology of isolated colonies of bacteria, the Gram stain should be used to examine clinical material directly. Sputum can be assessed for suitability for culture by determining the numbers of squamous epithelial cells and polymorphonuclear leukocytes present in the specimen (Chapter 16). If more than 10 epithelial cells are found in an average low power field (100 ×), a sputum sample can be assumed to be contaminated with normal oral flora and unsuitable for culture. The presence of few or no epithelial cells and more than 25 polymorphonuclear leukocytes represents a very good specimen. Obviously, patients with profound granulocytopenia will show few or no polymorphonuclear leukocytes; in sputum specimens from such patients the number of epithelial cells is used to judge the quality of the specimen. The numbers and morphologies of bacteria seen in direct smears of clinical material is very valuable for early clues as to cause of disease, as well as for comparison to the growth resulting after incubation. The presence of anaerobic organisms may be signaled, for example, by a culture showing many bacteria on Gram stain that yields light or no growth after aerobic incubation on standard media. Comparing Gram stain results to culture results is an excellent internal method for monitoring quality assurance. Several grading systems for reporting Gram stain results have been published, one of which is described in Table 7.1.

Unspun urine can also be Gram stained to determine the presence of significant bacteri-

PROCEDURE 7.1. CONVENTIONAL GRAM STAIN

1. Prepare reagents as follows:
   a. Crystal violet

Crystal violet, 90% dye content	10 g
Absolute methyl alcohol	500 ml

   b. Iodine

Iodine crystals	6 g
Potassium iodide	12 g
Distilled water	1,800 ml

   c. Decolorizer

Acetone	400 ml
Ethyl alcohol (95%)	1,200 ml

   d. Counterstain

Safranin, 99% dye content	10 g
Distilled water	1,000 ml

2. Fix material on slide as detailed in text. If slide is heat fixed, allow it to cool to the touch before staining.
3. Flood slide with crystal violet and allow to remain on the surface without drying for 10-30 seconds.
4. Rinse the slide with tap water, shaking off all excess.
5. Flood the slide with iodine and allow to remain on the surface without drying for twice as long as the crystal violet was in contact with the slide surface (20 seconds of iodine for 10 seconds of crystal violet, for example).
6. Rinse with tap water, shaking off all excess.
7. Flood the slide with decolorizer for 10 seconds and rinse immediately with tap water. Repeat this procedure until the blue dye no longer runs off the slide with the decolorizer. Thicker smears require more aggressive decolorizing. Rinse with tapwater and shake off excess.
8. Flood the slide with counterstain, allowing it to remain on the surface without drying for 30 seconds. Rinse with tap water and gently blot the slide dry with paper towels or bibulous paper or air dry. For very delicate smears, such as thin body fluids, air drying is the safest method.
9. Examine microscopically under an oil immersion lens at 1,000 × for white cells, bacteria, and other structures.

uria. A drop of well-mixed unspun urine is allowed to dry on the surface of a slide without being spread out. The presence of one or more bacteria in most oil immersion fields (1,000 ×) is indicative of over 100,000 organisms per milliliter of urine. Screening procedures for urine are discussed further in Chapter 18.

7.3.c. Acid fast stains. The cell walls of certain parasites and bacteria contain long chain (50-90 carbon atoms) fatty acids (mycolic acids),

TABLE 7.1
Grading System for Gram Stain Reporting of
Lower Respiratory Tract Secretions

Quantitative estimate derived from adding total scores	
10-25 neutrophils/10 × field	+1
>25 neutrophils/10 × field	+2
Mucus	+1
10-25 squamous cells/10 × field	−1
>25 squamous cells/10 × field	−2
Report; handling	
Oropharyngeal contamination, please repeat	≤0
Culture performed, general results only reported	1-2
Culture performed, complete workup	≥3

Modified from Bartlett, R.C. 1974. Medical microbiology: quality, cost, and clinical relevance. John Wiley & Sons, New York. p. 27.

lending them the property of resistance to destaining of basic dyes by acid alcohol. Thus, they are called "**acid fast.**" Mycobacteria such as *M. tuberculosis* and *M. marinum* (Plate 7.1) and coccidian parasites such as *Cryptosporidium* species (Plate 7.2) are characterized by their acid fast staining properties. The classic acid fast stain, Ziehl-Neelsen (Procedure 7.2), requires the addition of heat to allow the stain to enter the wax-containing cell wall. The cold Kinyoun acid fast stain modification is detailed in Chapter 41. Formulas are listed in Chapter 46. A modified acid fast stain has been developed for differentiating *Nocardia* species, filamentous, branching bacteria which contain fatty acid chains in their cell walls of approximately 50 carbon atoms, from similar non-acid fast actinomycetes. The *Nocardia* are decolorized by the standard acid alcohol step, but not by a milder decolorizer, 0.5%-1% sulfuric acid. These organisms are known as partially or weakly acid fast bacteria. A procedure for performing a partial acid fast stain is given in Chapter 33.

7.3.d. Methylene blue stain. A simple methylene blue stain of growth from Loeffler's agar slant cultures of possible diphtheria specimens may reveal characteristic metachromatic granules of *Corynebacterium diphtheriae*. This same stain will reveal the morphology of fusiform bacteria and of spirochetes in oral specimens.

7.3.e. Differential stains for parasites. Several differential stains are used to highlight the visibility and internal structures of cysts, trophozoites, or other forms of parasites, particularly those found in stool specimens. These stains, further described in Chapter 44, include Wheatley-Trichrome and iron hematoxylin. Toluidine O stain, used for rapid examination of respiratory tract material for the presence of *Pneumocystis carinii*, is described in Chapter 16. A rapid Gomori methenamine silver stain modification (also Chapter 16) has proved very valuable for the diagnosis of *P. carinii* in bronchial lavage and other specimens. Although such stains are usually performed by pathologists, microbiologists may be required to add these procedures to their protocols.

7.3.f. Differential stains for blood smears and tissue sections. Parasites that circulate in the bloodstream are often found within erythrocytes or free in the plasma. Several stains have been developed to help differentiate these parasites from human host cell components. The two stains most commonly used are Wright's and Giemsa (Chapter 46). Thin films of blood are fixed with methanol to preserve the red cell morphology so that the relationship of the parasites to the red cells can be clearly seen. The slides are then stained, revealing the nuclei and cytoplasmic features. To search a larger quantity of blood for the presence of parasites, a thick film may be prepared by placing a large drop of blood (the size of a nickel) in one area and defibrinating it by making ever-increasing circles from the center outward, using the edge of another glass slide. To visualize the parasites in such a thick smear, the red cells must be lysed with water. Preparation of stains of blood films is discussed in Chapter 44.

PROCEDURE 7.2. ZIEHL-NEELSEN ACID FAST STAIN

1. Prepare reagents as follows:
   a. Carbolfuchsin

Basic fuchsin	0.3 g
Ethanol (95%)	10 ml

   All ingredients are available from Sigma Chemical Co. or other chemical supply houses. Add together and mix. Add the fuchsin solution to 100 ml of 5% phenol solution in distilled water. This solution should then be placed on a stirring platform with a stir-bar in a 37° C incubator overnight; let the stain stand for several days, to allow all components to come into solution, before using the stain.

   b. Decolorizer

Ethanol (95%)	97 ml
Concentrated HCl	3 ml

   Add the hydrochloric acid to the ethanol slowly, working under a chemical fume hood.

   c. Counterstain

Methylene blue	0.3 g
Distilled water	100 ml

2. Use only new slides. Fix smears on heated surface (60° C for at least 10 min). Flood smears with carbolfuchsin and heat to almost boiling by performing the procedure on an electrically heated platform or by passing the flame of a Bunsen burner underneath the slides on a metal rack. Slides should steam.
3. Allow slides to sit for 5 min after heating; do not allow them to dry out.
4. Wash the slides in distilled water (tap water may contain acid fast bacilli). Shake off excess liquid.
5. Flood slides with decolorizer for approximately 1 min. Check to see that no more red color runs off the surface when the slide is tipped. Add a bit more decolorizer for very thick slides or those that continue to bleed red dye.
6. Wash thoroughly with water and remove the excess.
7. Flood slides with counterstain and allow to remain on surface of slides for 1 min.
8. Wash with distilled water and stand slides upright on paper towels to air dry. Do not blot dry.
9. Examine microscopically, screening at high power (400 ×) and confirming all suspicious organisms at 1,000 × with an oil-immersion lens.

The Giemsa stain is also used to visualize inclusions in virally or other infected cells, either directly from clinical material, such as the base of a suspected herpetic vesicle or a corneal scraping from a suspected case of *Chlamydia trachomatis* conjunctivitis, or for staining a monolayer of infected cell cultures, such as the McCoy cells of an in vitro *Chlamydia* culture (further developed in Chapter 38). The presence of other parasitic infections, such as toxoplasmosis in brain tissue, may be detected using the Giemsa stain. Neither the Wright's nor Giemsa stain will reliably stain fungal or bacterial elements, so they must be used in conjunction with other stains if the etiology of a suspected infection is totally unknown.

Other stains are used for special purposes, such as the iodine stain for the inclusions of chlamydia-infected monolayer cells, Seller's stain for the Negri bodies in rabies-infected tissues, and the Giménez stain for *Chlamydia* and *Legionella*. These stains are outlined in the chapters in which their use is described or in Chapter 46.

7.3.g. Fungal stains. Fungal elements can be seen in fixed material with several stains. The periodic acid–Schiff (PAS) is probably one of the best general stains since most fungal elements in clinical material (sputum, tissue, etc.) will take up the stain. Methenamine silver, in addition to staining certain parasites, will also stain fungal cell walls a dark blackish brown. This stain, however, usually takes increased

time to perform. The polysaccharide capsular material of certain fungi, notably *Cryptococcus neoformans*, stains bright pink with mucicarmine stain, which may prove useful for differentiating this fungus in tissue.

7.4. Fluorescence Microscopy

Certain dyes, called **fluors** or **fluorochromes**, have the property of becoming excited (raised to a higher energy level) after absorbing ultraviolet light (light of short wavelength). As the excited molecules return to their normal state, they release the excess energy in the form of visible light of longer wavelength than that which first excited them. This property of becoming self-luminous is called **fluorescence.** Modern microscopic methods have been developed to exploit the enhanced detection possible with this system. Figure 7.5 diagrams a modern fluorescence microscope, in which the light is emitted from above (epifluorescence). An excitation filter passes light of the desired wavelength to excite the fluorochrome, and a

FIGURE 7.5
Fluorescence microscope.

barrier filter in the objective prevents the exciting wavelengths from damaging the eyes of the observer. Fluorescing objects appear brightly lit against a dark background, with the color dependent on the dye being used. Many agents will absorb fluorescent dyes directly, as outlined below.

7.4.a. Acridine orange. The fluorochrome acridine orange binds to nucleic acid, either in the native or the denatured state. In some formulations of acridine orange, depending on the pH and concentration, the color of the fluorescence will vary. Acridine orange has been used as a viable dye, fluorescing green if the organism is alive and red if it is dead. Since the dye intercalates within nucleic acid, however, a viable organism will not remain alive for very long after staining. The use of acridine orange for highlighting bacteria in blood culture media (Procedure 7.3) has become widely accepted. Several studies have shown the staining of blood cultures with acridine orange to be as sensitive as blind subculture for initial detection of positive cultures.

7.4.b. Rhodamine-auramine. The mycolic acid in the cell walls of mycobacteria has an affinity for the fluorochromes auramine and rhodamine. These dyes will bind to mycobacteria, which appear bright yellow or orange against a greenish background. The counterstain, potassium permanganate, helps to prevent nonspecific fluorescence. All acid fast objects, including the sporozoan parasites, will stain with auramine or rhodamine as well. One widely used staining procedure, that of Truant,[4] is shown in Procedure 7.4.

An important aspect of the rhodamine-auramine stain is that slides may be restained with Ziehl-Neelsen or Kinyoun stain directly over the fluorochrome stain, as long as the oil has been removed. In this way, positive slides can be confirmed with the traditional stain, which will also aid in differentiating morphology.

7.4.c. Calcofluor white. The cell walls of fungi will bind the stain calcofluor white, greatly enhancing their visibility in tissue and other specimens. As described by Hageage and Harrington,[1] this stain is used in place of 10% KOH for initial examination of clinical material. It is also used to enhance visualization of morphologic elements of pure cultures of fungi. For many applications, it has supplanted the lactophenol cotton blue stain in some laboratories. Organisms fluoresce blue-white or apple green, depending on the light source (Plate

---

PROCEDURE 7.3. ACRIDINE ORANGE STAIN

1. Fix slide, either in methanol or with heat, as described above.
2. Flood slide with acridine orange stain (Chapter 46; also available from BBL Microbiology Products, Difco Laboratories, Remel Laboratories, and other suppliers). Allow stain to remain on surface of slide for 2 min without drying.
3. Rinse with tap water and allow the slide to air dry by leaning it upright to drain on paper towels.
4. Examine the slide microscopically under ultraviolet light with the same light source as that used for fluorescein. Bacteria will fluoresce bright orange against a green-fluorescing or dark background. The nuclei of blood cells may also fluoresce.

PROCEDURE 7.4. RHODAMINE-AURAMINE ACID FAST STAIN

1. Prepare reagents as follows:
   a. Rhodamine-auramine

Auramine O (C.I. 41000)	1.5 g
Rhodamine B (C.I. 45170)	0.75 g
Glycerol	75 ml
Melted phenol crystals	10 ml
Distilled water	50 ml

   Reagents are available from Sigma Chemical Co. and other chemical supply companies. Add the phenol and water together, then add the other ingredients. Place on a magnetic stirrer with a stir bar in the incubator. Allow to stir at 37° C overnight, or until all particulates are dissolved. Filter through glass wool and store in a brown glass bottle with a glass stopper. The stain is stable for at least 6 months in the refrigerator.

   b. Decolorizer

Hydrochloric acid (concentrated)	0.5 ml
Ethanol (70%)	100 ml

   c. Counterstain

Potassium permanganate	0.5 g
Distilled water	100 ml

   Mix together, filter through coarse filter paper or glass wool, and store in a brown glass bottle. The solution is stable at room temperature for 6 months.
2. Heat fix slides as described above.
3. Flood slides with rhodamine-auramine. Allow the stain to remain on the slide for 15 min. Do not allow the surface to dry.
4. Rinse the slides with distilled water and shake off excess liquid.
5. Flood slides with decolorizer for 2-3 min. Slide will still appear pink.
6. Rinse thoroughly with distilled water, shake off excess.
7. Flood slides with counterstain for 3-4 min. Do not allow slides to dry.
8. Rinse thoroughly with distilled water and allow to air dry as described above for other acid fast stains.
9. Examine microscopically under the same ultraviolet light source as used for fluorescein. Acid fast bacilli will be visible as bright yellow-orange organisms against a green background. Slides can be screened on high power (400 ×) and verified under oil immersion.

Modified From Truant, Brett, and Thomas. 1962. Henry Ford Hosp. Med. Bull. 10:287.

PROCEDURE 7.5. EXAMINING CLINICAL MATERIAL FOR THE PRESENCE OF FUNGAL ELEMENTS

1. Prepare calcofluor white stain as follows:

   Calcofluor white M2R (Polysciences or Sigma Chemical Co.)   0.1 g

   Evans blue (Sigma)   0.05 g

   Distilled water   100 ml

   Mix thoroughly and store in a brown bottle at room temperature. The solution is stable for 1 year.

2. Add one drop of the calcofluor white solution and one drop of 10% KOH (described above) to the specimen to be examined on a clean glass slide. Place a coverslip over the material and turn the slide face down on several thicknesses of paper toweling, pushing gently to flatten the coverslip down and express excess fluid out from the edges of the coverslip and into the paper towels.

3. Examine the slide under ultraviolet light, using a K530 excitation filter and a BG 12 barrier filter, as for fluorescein. Other filter combinations that produce light of blue-white wavelength such as a G-365 excitation filter and an LP 420 barrier filter can be used.

4. Fungal elements will appear apple green (or blue-white, depending on the filter combination used), with a much dimmer reddish tinted fluorescing background.

7.3). The modification of the stain that we suggest is outlined in Procedure 7.5. The fluorescent stain and the KOH are added separately, since they tend to precipitate if combined and stored as a single solution.

7.5. Antibody-Conjugated Stains

The most specific detectors are antibodies that bind tightly to antigens against which they are directed (Chapter 12). Antibodies can be produced against entire classes of agents that share common antigens or against specific determinants, such as the carbohydrate that is common to the cell walls of *Streptococcus pyogenes*. If antibodies are conjugated to a dye that allows their reactive sites to interact with the homologous antigens, they serve as visible flags for the presence of that antigen. Several of the dyes that are commonly bound to antibodies are described below.

7.5.a. Fluorescein-conjugated stains. Antibodies bound to the fluorochrome **fluorescein isothiocyanate (FITC)** are used to visualize many bacteria in direct specimens. Fluorescein fluoresces an intense apple green when excited. Examples include *Bordetella pertussis* in nasopharyngeal smears from children suspected of having whooping cough, and *Legionella* species in respiratory specimens or tissue of patients with Legionnaires' disease. Monoclonal antibodies (described in Chapter 10) have been successfully conjugated to fluorescein for detection of chlamydiae; herpes, respiratory syncytial, and rabies viruses; treponemes and other pathogens in directly stained clinical material. Other fluorescein-conjugated antibodies are used to identify pure cultures of organisms, such as certain *Actinomyces* species, *Streptococcus pyogenes* (Plate 7.4), *Neisseria gonorrhoeae* and others. As more monoclonal antibodies are developed, more conjugated stains will be produced for the rapid, direct detection of pathogens in clinical material.

7.5.b. Enzyme-conjugated stains. For those laboratories that do not have access to a fluorescent microscope, enzymes that catalyze the production of a colored precipitin product are an excellent alternative conjugate for specific antibody detector reagents. Horseradish peroxidase is a small enzyme that produces an orange-brown precipitate as its easily visible endpoint. Conjugated to antibodies, it is known as **immunoperoxidase stain,** and it is used to detect cytomegalovirus and other virus proteins or nucleic acids in cells. Although primarily used to detect viral antigens, other antigens could easily be detected with this system. Other enzymes have been conjugated to antibodies. Alkaline phosphatase produces a blue precipitate as its endproduct, and it, too, has been used as a detector for viral antigens, as well as inclusions of chlamydiae.

7.5.c. Biotin-avidin-enzyme-conjugated stains. Single-stranded nucleic acid probes (described in Chapter 10), antimicrobial antibodies, or antibiotin antibodies can be bound to the small molecule, biotin. This molecule has a strong affinity for the protein avidin, which has four binding sites. Thus, biotin bound to avidin or antibody can be complexed to fluorescent dyes or to color-producing enzymes to form specific detector systems. Products are available for the detection of nucleic acids of cytomegalovirus, herpes I and II viruses, hepatitis B virus, adenovirus 2, Epstein-Barr virus, and *Chlamydia.*

7.6. Electron Microscopy

The electron microscope uses electrons instead of light to visualize small objects; thus the resolution is increased relative to the shortness of the wavelength of the electron beams. Instead of lenses, the electrons are focused by electromagnetic fields and form an image on a fluorescent screen, like a television screen. Many new morphologic features of bacteria, bacterial components, fungi, and parasites have been discovered using electron microscopy. For routine microbiological diagnosis, however, the greatest use of electron microscopy has been for detection of viral causes of gastroenteritis. All enteric viruses can be identified in either direct electron microscopic preparations of fecal material or by immune electron microscopy, in which fecal samples are mixed with specific antiviral antibody before staining. Since an electron microscope is a major capital investment, few laboratories have the capability to use these techniques on a routine basis.

REFERENCES

1. Hageage, G.J. Jr., and Harrington, B.J. 1984. Use of calcofluor white in clinical mycology. Lab. Med. 15:109.
2. McGinnis, M.R. 1980. Laboratory handbook of medical mycology. Academic Press, New York.
3. Smith, R.F. 1982. Microscopy and photomicrography: a practical guide. Appleton-Century-Crofts, New York.
4. Truant, J.P., Brett, W.A., and Thomas, W. Jr. 1962. Fluorescence microscopy of tubercle bacillus stained with auramine and rhodamine. Henry Ford Hosp. Med. Bull. 10:287.

BIBLIOGRAPHY

Douglas, S.D. 1980. Microscopy. In Lennette, E.H., Balows, A., Hausler, W.J. Jr., and Truant, J.P., editors. Manual for clinical microbiology, ed. 3. American Society for Microbiology, Washington, D.C.
Goodman, N.L. 1985. Direct microscopy in diagnosing fungal disease. Diagn. Med. 8:14.
McCarthy, L.R., and Senne, J.E. 1980. Evaluation of acridine orange stain for detection of microorganisms in blood cultures. J. Clin. Microbiol. 11:281.
Yong, D.C.T., and Peter, J.B. 1984. Using DEM to detect pediatric viral gastroenteritis. Diagn. Med. 7:45.

8 Cultivation and Isolation of Viable Pathogens

Although future trends in clinical microbiology are clearly pointing in the direction of developing rapid, non-growth-dependent methods for detecting the presence of infectious agents, the isolation and identification of viable pathogens is still the "gold standard" for diagnosis of infectious diseases today. A pure culture of a clone of identical cells has been necessary for performing biochemical differentiation tests and susceptibility studies, since single cells are impossible to work with easily, and mixed cultures yield no useful or even misleading information. In the late nineteenth century, the invention in Robert Koch's laboratory by Frau Hesse of solid agar aided the development of the newly burgeoning science of clinical microbiology. Before solid media plates were available, microbiologists had to rely on the method developed by Lister, employing the principle of limiting dilutions from cultures in broth media for obtaining pure isolates with which to work. General concepts applicable to the in vitro cultivation of pathogens are outlined below.

Methods used to create optimal conditions for the cultivation of pathogens have been developed over years of experimentation. At this time, commercially produced environmental systems, artificial media, cell culture lines, and all other items necessary for the practice of clinical microbiology are readily available to microbiologists in the industrialized world. Laboratorians in less well-developed parts of the world may still need to bleed their own sheep (or themselves) and perform other basic tasks necessary to practice diagnostic microbiology, but most microbiologists now purchase the majority of the materials needed for cultivation, identification, and susceptibility testing of pathogenic microorganisms.

8.1. Artificial Media

8.1.a. General concepts of artificial media.
Over the years varied strategies have been developed for the cultivation of pathogens. Ingredients necessary for the growth of pathogens can be supplied by a living system, as in the human or animal host or in cell culture, or by mixing together the required nutrients in an artificial system. During the nineteenth century, media were prepared in glass containers, from which the phrase *in vitro* (which means "in glass") originated. To encourage the growth of particular organisms from a milieu containing only a few of the desired organisms among large numbers of normal flora, various kinds of laboratory-prepared nutrient-containing solutions were concocted, and called **enrichment media.** An example of such a medium is selenite broth, which encourages the growth of small numbers of stool pathogens and suppresses the growth of the much larger numbers of normal stool organisms. A second class of artificial media is called **supportive.** These media contain nutrients that allow most nonfastidious organisms to grow at their natural rates, without affording any particular organism a growth advantage (except for the organism's own metabolism) on the medium. Examples of supportive media are nutrient agar and brain heart infusion agar. Media containing one or more agents inhibitory to all organisms except the organism being sought were developed, first using dyes that exhibited antibacterial characteristics, later using antibiotics, and still later

incorporating components that take into consideration certain metabolic activities of the organisms sought. Such media are known as **selective media,** since they select for certain organisms to the disadvantage of others. An example of a selective medium is phenylethyl alcohol agar, which inhibits the growth of aerobic and facultatively anaerobic gram-negative rods and allows gram-positive cocci to grow. The third type of medium, **differential,** employs some factor or factors that allows colonies of organisms that possess certain metabolic characteristics to be morphologically distinguished from those organisms that have different characteristics. The most supportive differential medium is sheep blood agar, which allows many organisms to grow and additionally allows different organisms to be distinguished on the basis of their hemolytic reactions against the sheep red blood cells, production of pigment, etc. (discussed in more depth in Section 8.3.a). Table 8.1 lists a number of media that are commonly used in clinical microbiology, along with

the ingredients that allow for differential or selective ability.

8.1.b. Preparation of dehydrated artificial media that require autoclaving. Dehydrated media powders should be kept in their original bottles with the caps tightly closed. The date received and the date first opened for use should be recorded on the bottle itself. Media makers should always **read the label** before preparing any media. Media should be prepared in clean glassware that has been rinsed in distilled or deionized water. To avoid boiling over during heating, a vessel holding a liquid solution to be autoclaved should never be filled more than two-thirds full. The proper amount of powder is weighed onto paper and poured into the container in which it is to be prepared. Distilled water is added next with vigorous swirling to achieve an even suspension. If other liquid ingredients are to be added, they should be incorporated at this point. If the solution is clear, as most broths usually are, it requires no further manipulation before autoclaving; how-

TABLE 8.1
Primary Plating Media

MEDIUM	COMPONENTS/COMMENTS	PRIMARY PURPOSE
Bacteroides bile esculin agar (BBE)	Trypticase soy agar base with ferric ammonium citrate, enriched with hemin (5 mg/ml). Bile salts and gentamicin act as inhibitors.	Selective and differential for *Bacteroides fragilis* group
Bile esculin agar (BEA)	Nutrient agar base with ferric citrate. Hydrolysis of esculin by group D streptococci imparts a brown color to medium; sodium desoxycholate inhibits many bacteria.	Differential isolation and presumptive identification of group D streptococci
Bismuth sulfite agar (BS)	Peptone agar with dextrose and ferrous sulfate. Gram-positive organisms and other Enterobacteriaceae inhibited by bismuth sulfite and brilliant green.	Selective for isolation of *Salmonella* from stool
Blood agar	Trypticase soy agar base or beef heart infusion base with 5% sheep blood.	Cultivation of fastidious microorganisms, determination of hemolytic reactions
Bordet-Gengou agar	Potato-glycerol based medium enriched with 15%-20% defibrinated blood. Contaminants inhibited by methicillin (final concentration of 2.5 µg/ml).	Isolation of *Bordetella pertussis*

Continued.

TABLE 8.1
Primary Plating Media—cont'd

MEDIUM	COMPONENTS/COMMENTS	PRIMARY PURPOSE
Buffered charcoal yeast extract agar (BCYE)	Yeast extract, agar, charcoal and salts supplemented with L-cysteine HC1, ferric pyrophosphate, ACES buffer, and alpha-ketoglutarate.	Selective for *Legionella* sp.
Campy-blood agar	Contains vancomycin (10 mg/liter), trimethoprim (5 mg/liter), polymixin B (2,500 U/liter), amphotericin B (2 mg/liter), and cephalothin (15 mg/liter) in a *Brucella* agar base with sheep blood	Selective for *Campylobacter* sp.
CDC anaerobic blood agar	Trypticase soy agar with 5% sheep blood enriched with hemin, L-cystine, and vitamin K_1.	Isolation of anaerobic organisms
Cefsulodin-irgasan-novobiocin (CIN) agar	Peptone base with yeast extract, mannitol, and bile salts. Supplemented with cefsulodin, irgasan and novobiocin; neutral red and crystal violet indicators.	Selective for *Yersinia* sp.
Chocolate agar	Peptone base, enriched with solution of 2% hemoglobin or IsoVitaleX (BBL).	Cultivation of *Haemophilus* and *Neisseria* sp.
Columbia colistin-nalidixic acid (CNA) agar	Columbia agar base with 10 mg colistin/liter, 15 mg nalidixic acid/liter, and 5% sheep blood.	Selective isolation of gram-positive cocci
Cooked meat (CM; also called chopped meat)	Solid meat particles initiate growth of bacteria, reducing substances lower oxidation-reduction potential (Eh).	Cultivation of anaerobic organisms
Cycloserine-cefoxitin fructose agar (CCFA)	Egg yolk base with fructose, cycloserine (500 mg/liter), and cefoxitin (16 mg/liter) added to inhibit stool flora. Neutral red indicator.	Selective for *Clostridium difficile*
Cystine-lactose-electrolyte-deficient (CLED) agar	Peptone base agar with lactose and L-cystine; bromthymol blue indicator inhibits swarming of *Proteus* sp.	Isolation and enumeration of bacteria in urine
Cystine-tellurite blood agar	Infusion agar base with 5% sheep blood. Reduction of potassium tellurite by *Corynebacterium diphtheriae* produces black colonies.	Isolation of *C. diphtheriae*
Dermatophyte test medium (DTM) agar	Nutrient base with glucose and phenol red indicator. Contaminants inhibited by cycloheximide, gentamicin, and tetracycline.	Isolation and identification of dermatophytes
Eosin methylene blue (EMB) agar (Levine)	Peptone base with lactose and sucrose. Eosin and methylene blue as indicators.	Isolation and differentiation of lactose-fermenting and non-lactose-fermenting enteric bacilli
Gram-negative broth (GN)	Peptone base broth with glucose and mannitol. Sodium citrate and sodium desoxycholate act as inhibitory agents.	Selective (enrichment) liquid medium for enteric pathogens
Hektoen enteric (HE) agar	Peptone base agar with bile salts, lactose, sucrose, salicin, and ferric ammonium citrate. Indicators include bromthymol blue and acid fuchsin.	Differential, selective medium for the isolation and differentiation of *Salmonella* and *Shigella* from other gram-negative enteric bacilli
Kanamycin-vancomycin laked blood agar (KVLB)	*Brucella* agar base with kanamycin (75 μg/ml), vancomycin (7.5 μg/ml), vitamin K_1 (10 μg/ml) and 5% laked blood.	Selective isolation of *Bacteroides* sp.

TABLE 8.1
Primary Plating Media—cont'd

MEDIUM	COMPONENTS/COMMENTS	PRIMARY PURPOSE
Lombard-Dowell agar	Casein digest agar enriched with hemin (10 mg/liter), vitamin K_1 (10 mg/liter), L-cystine (0.4 g/liter), and yeast extract.	Isolation of anaerobic organisms
Lowenstein-Jensen (L-J) agar	Egg-based medium; contaminants inhibited by malachite green.	Isolation of mycobacteria
MacConkey agar	Peptone base with lactose. Gram-positive organisms inhibited by crystal violet and bile salts. Neutral red acts as indicator.	Isolation and differentiation of lactose fermenting and non-lactose-fermenting enteric bacilli
Mannitol salt agar	Peptone base, mannitol, and phenol red indicator. Salt concentration of 7.5% inhibits most bacteria.	Selective isolation of coagulase-positive staphylococci
Middlebrook 7H10 agar	Complex base with albumin, salts, enzymatic digest of casein enrichment, and malachite green inhibitor.	Isolation of and antimicrobial susceptibility testing of mycobacteria
Mycosel or mycobiotic agar	Peptone base with glucose; contaminants inhibited by chloramphenicol and cycloheximide.	Isolation of dermatophytes
New York City (NYC) agar	Peptone agar base with cornstarch, supplemented with yeast dialysate, 3% hemoglobin, and horse plasma. Antibiotic supplement includes vancomycin (2 μg/ml), colistin (5.5 μg/ml), amphotericin B (1.2 μg/ml), and trimethoprim (3 μg/ml).	Selective for *Neisseria gonorrhoeae*
Petragnani agar	Coagulated-egg medium with malachite green to inhibit commensals.	Isolation of mycobacteria
Phenylethyl alcohol (PEA) agar	Nutrient agar base. Phenylethanol inhibits growth of gram-negative organisms.	Selective isolation of gram-positive cocci
Sabouraud dextrose agar	Peptone base agar. Final pH of medium (5.6) favors growth of fungi over bacteria.	Isolation of dermatophytes
Salmonella-Shigella (SS) agar	Peptone base with lactose, ferric citrate, and sodium citrate. Neutral red acts as indicator; inhibition of coliforms by brilliant green, bile salts.	Selective for *Salmonella* and *Shigella* sp.
Schaedler agar	Peptone and soy protein base agar with yeast extract, dextrose, and buffers. Addition of hemin, L-cystine, and 5% blood enriches for anaerobes.	Nonselective medium for the recovery of anaerobes and aerobes
Selenite broth	Peptone base broth. Sodium selenite toxic for most Enterobacteriaceae.	Enrichment for isolation of *Salmonella*
Streptococcal selective agar (SSA)	Contains crystal violet, colistin, and trimethoprim-sulfamethoxazole in 5% sheep blood agar base.	Selective for *Streptococcus pyogenes*
Tetrathionate broth	Peptone base broth. Bile salts and sodium thiosulfate inhibit gram-positive organisms and Enterobacteriaceae.	Selective for *Salmonella* and *Shigella*
Thayer-Martin agar	Blood agar base enriched with hemoglobin and supplement B; contaminating organisms inhibited by colistin, nystatin, vancomycin, and trimethoprim.	Selective for *Neisseria gonorrhoeae* and *N. meningitidis*

Continued.

TABLE 8.1
Primary Plating Media—cont'd

MEDIUM	COMPONENTS/COMMENTS	PRIMARY PURPOSE
Thioglycolate broth	Pancreatic digest of casein, soy broth, and glucose enrich growth of most microorganisms. Thioglycolate and agar reduce Eh.	Supports growth of anaerobes, aerobes, microaerophilic, and fastidious microorganisms
Thiosulfate citrate-bile salts (TCBS) agar	Peptone base agar with yeast extract, bile salts, citrate, sucrose, ferric citrate, and sodium thiosulfate. Bromthymol blue acts as indicator.	Selective for *Vibrio cholera*
Transgrow agar	Thayer-Martin agar packaged in 1.2 dram bottle for increased surface area and easier transport of specimens.	Selective for *Neisseria gonorrhoeae*
Vaginalis (V) agar	Columbia agar base supplemented with 5% human blood.	Selective and differential for *Gardnerella vaginalis*
Xylose lysine desoxycholate (XLD) agar	Yeast extract agar with lysine, xylose, lactose, sucrose, and ferric ammonium citrate. Sodium desoxycholate inhibits gram-positive organisms; phenol red acts as indicator.	The isolation and differentiation of *Salmonella* and *Shigella* from other gram-negative enteric bacilli

FIGURE 8.1
Gauze-covered nonabsorbable cotton plug and aluminum foil cover for flasks used in media preparation.

ever, most agar solutions require heating almost to the boiling point, with constant agitation, to achieve an even solution. The use of a stirrer-hot plate and a magnetic stir-bar will greatly increase the efficiency of this stage of media making. The hot solution must be watched extremely carefully as soon as tiny bubbles begin to appear, as these media tend to boil over very easily. Some media are ready to be dispensed at this point.

If the medium is to be sterilized by autoclaving, it is capped with either a plastic screw cap or a plug. A good plug can be made from a large wad of nonabsorbable cotton wrapped in a one-layer thick square of gauze. For autoclaving flasks of agar which are to be poured into plates by hand, we have found a large square of aluminum foil molded to the shape of the flask to be an excellent cover which can be removed and replaced many times and allows the neck of the flask to remain sterile until the foil is lifted off (Figure 8.1). The solutions are placed in the autoclave and sterilized; the timing of the sterilization should start from the moment the temperature reaches 121° C. Very large quantities of media may require a longer sterilization time than is recommended on the package label. Once the sterilization cycle is completed, the autoclave chamber is slowly returned to atmospheric pressure, to prevent the liquid from boiling over. Autoclaved media should not be kept in the autoclave once the pressure has equalized, since prolonged heat may alter some of the ingredients.

Autoclaving can be a dangerous activity; all of the safety precautions outlined in Chapter 2 and the quality control practices outlined in Chapter 3 should be carefully adhered to by operators. Autoclave performance should be monitored for microbial killing regularly and during every use (with autoclave tape, for example) for achievement of proper temperature. Media removed from the autoclave should be placed into a 55° C water bath to cool before any supplements are added or before plates are poured. Liquid media or media which are not to be dispensed may be allowed to cool on the benchtop. Agar will tend to settle to the bottom of a flask during autoclaving, so all flasks should be swirled in a large circle on the bench top (to avoid making bubbles) before pouring. If a few bubbles appear on the surface of a freshly poured plate, they can be removed by quickly passing the flame from a Bunsen burner over the surface. We have found that leaving the covers of Petri dishes slightly ajar allows contaminants to reach the agar surfaces. Our recommendation is to leave tops closed and incubate plates overnight after they have set, to remove surface moisture and detect contamination.

8.1.c. Methods of sterilization other than autoclaving. Media that contain serum or certain proteins are often sterilized by **inspissation**. In this intermittent sterilization method, the media are placed in a chamber through which steam continuously flows for approxi-

mately 30 min each day for several successive days. Loeffler agar and Lowenstein-Jensen agar are prepared using this method. The previous edition of this book contains a complete procedure for using an autoclave for inspissation sterilization. Delicate media may also be sterilized by allowing the flasks or tubes to remain in a chamber through which steam actively flows. Such a chamber, the Arnold steam sterilizer, is also often used to remelt media that have been prepared in advance and allowed to harden. This method is particularly useful for pouring fresh agar plates made from previously prepared agar deep tubes, to which a sterile, nonautoclavable additive such as blood is added immediately before pouring. Plates that are uncommonly used but that require fresh enrichments (egg yolk agar, Bordet-Gengou, etc.) can be prepared as needed from agar deep tubes, which have a much longer shelf life than poured plates.

Carbohydrate solutions and other liquids

FIGURE 8.2
Use of a membrane filter system to sterilize nonautoclavable solutions.

that may be denatured by heat can be **filter sterilized.** By injecting the liquid through a syringe containing a membrane filter with pores no larger than 0.2 or 0.45 μm in diameter, most bacteria are trapped (Figure 8.2). Disposable closed membrane filtration systems are available commercially (Appendix).

Most hospitals use **gas sterilization** for instruments and equipment. This method uses ethylene oxide to destroy bacteria and spores. Microbiologists may make use of the gas sterilizer to process reusable plasticware and instruments. Gas sterilization takes much longer than the other methods described, usually requiring an overnight cycle and aeration time for the ethylene oxide to diffuse away.

8.2. Conditions Necessary for Growth of Pathogens

In order for bacteria or fungi to multiply on or in artificial media, they must have available the required nutrients, a permissive temperature, enough moisture in the medium and in the atmosphere, the proper gaseous atmosphere, proper salt concentration, an appropriate pH, and there must be no growth-inhibiting factors (such as other bacteria or fungi or artificial compounds that antagonize growth).

8.2.a. Establishing atmospheric conditions required for growth of pathogens. Pathogenic organisms are either **aerobic,** utilizing oxygen as a terminal electron acceptor and showing good growth in an atmosphere of room air, **anaerobic,** relatively intolerant to the presence of oxygen, or **microaerophilic,** growing best in atmospheres of reduced oxygen tension. Aerobic organisms can be incubated in room air without much difficulty. Most clinically significant "aerobic" organisms are actually **facultatively anaerobic;** they grow under either aerobic or anaerobic conditions. True aerobic organisms include *Pseudomonas* species, members of the Neisseriaceae family, *Brucella* species, *Bordetella* species, and *Francisella* species, as well as mycobacteria, filamentous fungi, and others.

To achieve an atmosphere of incubation other than room air, several strategies have been developed. Organisms that grow best with greater CO_2 concentrations than are found in room air, called **capnophilic,** may be incubated in an atmosphere of 5%-10% CO_2 in a special incubator with sealed doors. Gas of the proper mixture is fed into the incubator automatically from nearby cylinders. The CO_2 concentration should be checked on a routine basis. By placing inoculated cultures into a sealable container and evacuating the room air down to a negative pressure of 25 pounds of mercury, replacing it with a commercially produced artificial mixture of gases placed under pressure in a gas cylinder, microbiologists can produce any desired atmosphere. Three evacuation-replacement cycles are usually necessary to remove all residual normal atmosphere. Sealable plastic bags into which the components of a CO_2 and H_2 generating system and an indicator of the proper atmosphere can be placed are also available commercially for the production of specialized atmospheres of incubation (Bio-Bag, Marion Scientific Co., and GasPak Pouch, BBL Microbiology Systems). The Bio-Bag has been designed for creating either anaerobic or capnophilic atmospheres; the GasPak Pouch is available for anaerobic incubation only. These bags are especially convenient for incubating primary plates from important cultures or in other circumstances where few plates are used. These bags accommodate only a few culture plates each, but all plates can be examined through the plastic without opening the bag. Some organisms that appear to be microaerophilic or capnophilic are actually **humidophilic;** they require increased moisture in the atmosphere.

Pathogenic campylobacters require a high carbon dioxide content (5%-10%) and no more than 6% oxygen. This atmosphere can be achieved safely by using a premixed gas for evacuation-replacement or by creating the atmosphere in a sealed jar or plastic bag with a commercially available self-contained generator system. These generator systems, which are similar to those available for creating an anaerobic atmosphere in a closed container, consist of an envelope that contains the components of a small hydrogen (and sometimes a CO_2) generating system. Chemical components required to catalyze the reaction between hydrogen and oxygen, forming water, removing oxygen, and thus creating the anaerobic atmosphere in such a system (alumina-coated palladium pellets), may be incorporated into the generator or supplied separately. For production of an atmosphere conducive for growth of campylobacters, the external catalyst is unnecessary. Other methods for creating the atmosphere required by campylobacters are discussed in Chapter 30.

The proper atmosphere for microaerophilic organisms requires an oxygen tension lower than that of room air. A CO_2 concentration of approximately 3% can be achieved in a **candle jar.** A small white wax candle is lit in a jar with a sealable lid, such as a commercial mayonnaise jar (Figure 6.3 in Chapter 6). The candle uses up just enough oxygen before it goes out (from lack of oxygen) to lower the O_2 tension. The products of combustion are CO_2 and water, both growth factors for the organisms. The candle jar is often used to cultivate *Neisseria gonorrhoeae*. A self-contained culture medium and increased carbon dioxide producing system has been developed for culturing gonococci. A tablet of sodium bicarbonate (such as Alka-Seltzer) dissolves in the moisture created by sealing the medium in a zip-lock plastic bag and produces enough CO_2 to allow growth of the pathogen (this is further discussed and illustrated in Chapter 6). Microaerophilic conditions can also be created by adding a small concentration of agar to a liquid medium. By preventing oxygen at the surface from being dispersed throughout the liquid by inhibiting circulating convection currents, the agar serves to create a mini-microaerophilic environment about 1-2 cm below

the surface of the medium. *Leptospira* species are cultivated in this way.

8.2.b. Methods for establishing anaerobic atmospheric conditions for incubation of primary culture plates. The most commonly used system for creating specialized anaerobic and capnophilic atmospheres is the anaerobic jar. Available anaerobic jars include the GasPak (BBL Microbiology Systems), and those made by Scott Laboratories and Oxoid U.S.A. Both systems utilize a clear, heavy plastic jar with an airtight lid that is clamped down to prevent leakage (Figure 8.3).

Anaerobic jars are used primarily with plated media. The introduction of a gas mixture

FIGURE 8.3
GasPak anaerobic jar (BBL Microbiology Systems) containing inoculated plates, gas-generating envelope, catalysts, and indicator strip.

containing H_2 into a jar is followed by catalytic conversion of the oxygen in the jar with hydrogen to water, thus establishing anaerobiosis. A catalyst composed of palladium-coated alumina pellets held in a wire mesh is preferred, since there is no explosion hazard with this "cold" catalyst and it is more convenient to use. However, the pellets can be inactivated by excess moisture and H_2S. Therefore, they should be reactivated **after each use** by heating the basket or sachet of pellets to 160° C in a drying oven for 1½-2 h. It is convenient to have a few extra baskets or sachets of catalysts for this purpose. Reactivated catalysts should be stored in a dry area until used. We do not recommend the use of jars without catalysts.

Anaerobic jars can be set up by two different methods. The easiest method utilizes a commercially available H_2 and CO_2 generator envelope, which is activated by simply adding 10 ml of water. The open envelope is placed in the jar with the inoculated plates, water is added, and the jar is sealed. Production of heat within a few minutes (detected by touching the top of the jar) and subsequent development of moisture on the walls of the jar are indications that the catalyst and generator envelope are functioning properly. Reduced conditions are achieved in 1-2 h, although the methylene blue or resazurin indicators take longer to decolorize. Alternatively, the "evacuation-replacement" system may be used. Air is removed from the sealed jar by drawing a vacuum of 25 inches of mercury. This process is repeated two times, filling the jar with an oxygen-free gas such as N_2 between evacuations. The final fill of the jar is made with a gas mixture containing 80%-90% N_2, 5%-10% H_2, and 5%-10% CO_2. Carbon dioxide is included since many anaerobes require it for maximal growth. The atmosphere in the jars should be monitored by including an indicator to check anaerobiosis. Anaerobiosis is achieved more quickly by the evacuation-replacement method. However, both methods give comparable yields of anaer-

obes from clinical specimens if the specimen is properly transported and set up in jars immediately after plates are streaked.

Stringent anaerobic conditions required by some organisms are attainable in an enclosed system, called a **glovebox** or an **anaerobic chamber.** Made of molded or flexible clear plastic, these chambers allow materials to enter through an airlock. The operator uses gloves or sleeves that form airtight seals around his or her arms to handle items inside the chamber (Figure 8.4). Media stored in the chamber are kept oxygen-free and thus able to support the growth of even the most oxygen-sensitive anaerobic organisms. For practical purposes, most pathogenic anaerobes can tolerate a minimal amount of room air. Methods that make use of fresh media and that allow inoculated cultures to be brought under anaerobic conditions quickly (oxygen-reduction potential less than -10 mV), such as the anaerobic jars or plastic pouches discussed above, should be adequate for isolation of most clinically significant anaerobes.

Anaerobic incubation may also be carried out in tubes. Tubed media produced under anaerobic conditions are called **prereduced anaerobically sterilized (PRAS)** media.

8.2.c. Prereduced anaerobically sterilized (PRAS) and roll-tube techniques. PRAS tubes are made by combining the constituents of the media, boiling the liquid to remove dissolved air, and then gassing-out with an oxygen-free gas. During the remainder of the media-making process (sterilization, inoculation, and subculture), air is prevented from gaining entrance into the containers by a gassing procedure or by keeping the container stoppered or sealed. To lower the Eh of the media, a reducing agent is added before sterilization. Details of PRAS media preparation and inoculation are given in the VPI *Anaerobe Laboratory Manual* by Holdeman, Cato, and Moore.[1] PRAS media are available from commercial sources.

PRAS tubes can be inoculated by either the

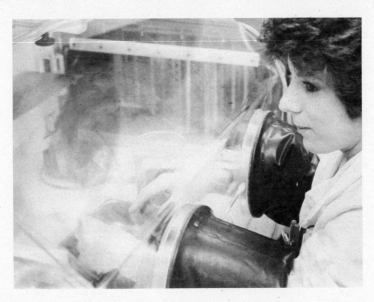

FIGURE 8.4
Anaerobic chamber (Anaerobe Systems). The rubber sleeves form airtight seals around the operator's arms, allowing the operator to work without gloves.

closed or open methods. In the closed method, also known as the Hungate method, a syringe and needle are used to inoculate through the rubber seal. Biochemical testing for speciation may be done by this technique; the PRAS II system (Scott Laboratories) is excellent for this purpose.

PRAS tubes can also be inoculated by the open method which consists of removing the rubber stopper and inserting a cannula that has oxygen-free gas flowing from the tip. While the tube is open, inoculation can be accomplished by loop or Pasteur pipette. Special equipment can be purchased for the inoculating procedure (Bellco Glass and Kontes), or a simple inoculating device can be made using a bent needle attached to tubing and connected to a ring stand. The PRAS tube is held by an adjustable laboratory clamp containing an aluminum test tube cap within which the tube is placed. Some batches of tungsten wire may oxidize PRAS media. It is therefore advisable to use platinum wires and loops for PRAS techniques.

Organisms can be grown in or on a thin layer of agar that covers the inside walls of tubes, achieved by the roll-tube technique (the tubes are rolled and cooled until the melted agar forms the thin layer referred to), although colonies are difficult to subculture and differentiate. It is our feeling that roll-tube methods are not as practical for clinical work as the other methods discussed here. Cultivation of anaerobes will be further discussed in Chapters 20 and 34.

8.2.d. Temperatures of incubation. Human pathogens generally multiply best at temperatures similar to those in the host. Isolation of most pathogens, therefore, can be carried out using incubators of only two temperatures: 35° C, close to the normal human body temperature, and 30° C, the temperature of the surface of the body. With the few exceptions noted below, all bacteria and viruses of pathogenic importance may be isolated from cultures incubated at 35° C. Material from lesions suspected of being infected with *Mycobacterium mar-*

inum, blood and urine being tested for lepto-spires, and all cultures from which fungi are being sought should be incubated at 30° C. Recovery of certain organisms can be enhanced by incubation at unusual temperatures; *Campylobacter jejuni* grows at 42° C, although most other fecal pathogens cannot. Incubation at this temperature, therefore, acts as an enrichment procedure. Cold enrichment for *Listeria* and *Yersinia enterocolitica* utilizes the same principle.

The temperature of incubators should be monitored by checking each area of the incubator where cultures will be placed, since temperature variations do occur within incubators. The humidity can be controlled automatically by feeding water from an external source into the system as needed, or manually by placing a large pan filled with water on the bottom shelf of the incubator. A little detergent in the water will discourage contaminants.

8.2.e. pH of artificial media. Although commercially produced dehydrated powders are so consistent that even the ultimate pH is usually correct, the hydrogen ion concentration should be checked using a pH meter. Especially after altering the pH of a medium with additives or for special uses, the pH should be reestablished. It is important to remember that pH electrodes are calibrated according to temperature; thus the pH reading of a hot solution will be different than that taken at room temperature. If the calibration temperature for the electrode cannot be adjusted, then the pH must be measured at approximately 28° C, or room temperature. Solid media pose an additional problem, since the pH is best adjusted while the media are still in liquid form and thus hotter than 50° C. A surface electrode may be used to measure the pH of agar, but these electrodes are very expensive and the agar must be set, which makes it difficult to alter the pH if needed. A workable strategy is to allow a small quantity of the molten agar to solidify in a tiny beaker or plastic cup. The pH of

this material can be easily determined with a regular pH electrode thrust into the agar after it has been vigorously broken up with a tongue depressor. The moisture in the medium will be enough to allow proper operation of the pH meter.

8.3. Characteristics of Certain Commonly Used Artificial Media

Only a few of the hundreds of available media will be mentioned here, as a sample of the types of media available. The choices of which media should be used to culture clinical specimens will be discussed in the chapters in Part III that detail laboratory handling of specimens and in chapters in Part IV that deal with individual isolates. Complete descriptions of the composition and use of these and other media are found in the *Difco Manual* (Difco Laboratories), *Scott Manual* (Scott Laboratories), *Oxoid Manual* (Oxoid U.S.A.), and the *GIBCO Technical Manual* (GIBCO Laboratories).

8.3.a. Blood agar. Most specimens received in a clinical microbiology laboratory are plated onto blood agar, since it supports all but the most fastidious clinically significant isolates and since most microbiologists have become adept at making decisions about the identification of bacteria from their colonial morphologies on blood agar. These media consist of a base containing a protein source, such as tryptones, soybean protein digest (containing a slight amount of natural carbohydrate), sodium chloride, agar, and 5% defibrinated blood. In the United States, the blood source is usually sheep, whereas horse blood is often used in Europe. The ability of certain bacteria to produce extracellular enzymes that act on the red cells to lyse them completely (beta hemolysis), to produce a greenish discoloration around the colony (alpha hemolysis), or to have no effect (sometimes called gamma hemolysis) is determined on blood agar (Plate 8.1). Production of hemolysins by bacteria is dependent on many environmental factors, such as pH and atmosphere of incubation. Microbiologists often use colony morphology and hemolysin production as initial screening tests to assist in the decisions of what further steps may be necessary for identification of an isolate. To accurately read the hemolytic reaction on a blood agar plate, the technologist must hold the plate up to the light and observe the plate with the light coming from behind. If the loop used to streak the culture on the blood agar has been stabbed into the medium to cause certain organisms to grow below the surface, production of oxygen-sensitive beta hemolysin by those isolates that produce it may be enhanced. Alternatively, plates may be incubated anaerobically to demonstrate oxygen-sensitive hemolysis. Hemolytic patterns on blood agar are discussed further in Chapter 25.

In special circumstances, blood other than sheep blood may be desirable. For example, the pigment of the pigmented *Bacteroides* species appears most regularly and rapidly when rabbit blood is used; this rabbit blood is **laked** (frozen and thawed to partially damage the erythrocyte cell walls). For work with anaerobes, we recommend *Brucella* agar base supplemented with hemin (5 μg/ml) and vitamin K_1 (10 μg/ml). This medium is suitable for non-anaerobes as well. In addition, there are two selective media that should be considered along with phenylethyl alcohol agar: (1) *Bacteroides* bile esculin agar (BBE) and (2) kanamycin-vancomycin laked rabbit blood agar (KVLB).

8.3.b. *Bacteroides* bile esculin agar (BBE). BBE agar is useful for the rapid isolation and presumptive identification of the *B. fragilis* group. It contains 100 μg/ml of gentamicin, which inhibits most aerobic organisms; 20% bile, which inhibits most anaerobes except for the *B. fragilis* group and a few other species; and esculin, which aids in detecting the *B. fragilis* group which are usually esculin positive. Other non–*B. fragilis* group organisms that may rarely grow on this medium are *Fusobac-*

terium mortiferum, Klebsiella pneumoniae, Enterococcus, and yeast. However, unlike the *B. fragilis* group, their colony size is less than 1 mm in diameter.

8.3.c. Kanamycin-vancomycin laked rabbit blood agar (KVLB). KVLB agar is useful for the rapid isolation of *Bacteroides* sp. The medium contains 75 μg/ml kanamycin, which inhibits most aerobic, facultative, and anaerobic gram-negative rods except for *Bacteroides*, and 7.5 μg/ml vancomycin, which inhibits most gram-positive organisms. The laked blood allows earlier pigmentation of the pigmented *Bacteroides* sp. However, many strains of *B. asaccharolyticus* and *B. gingivalis* will not grow on this medium because of their susceptibility to vancomycin. Yeast and other kanamycin-resistant organisms sometimes grow on this medium; therefore, one should Gram stain and check the aerotolerance of all isolates.

8.3.d. Chocolate agar. This medium uses the same base as blood agar. Originally, red blood cells were added to the molten base and the temperature was raised enough to partially lyse the cells (around 85° C), causing the medium to turn a chocolate-brown color. Now, hemoglobin and the other nutrients present in the lysed red cells, hemin (also known as "X" factor) and the coenzyme nicotine adenine dinucleotide (called "V" factor), are added as supplements to a nutritionally rich agar base. *Neisseria gonorrhoeae* and *Haemophilus* species, among other fastidious organisms, will grow only in the presence of the nutrients supplied by chocolate agar. Chocolate agar has been modified to be selective for pathogenic Neisseriaceae by the addition of antibiotics, including colistin (to inhibit other gram-negative bacteria), vancomycin (to inhibit gram-positive bacteria), and nystatin or anisomycin (to inhibit yeast). The most widely used formula is that of Thayer and Martin. Thayer-Martin agar incorporates nystatin to inhibit yeasts. Modified Thayer-Martin (MTM) includes trimethoprim to inhibit *Proteus*. The most common modification is Martin-Lewis agar, which substitutes anisomycin (characterized by a longer shelf life and greater activity against yeast) for nystatin. Other modifications are available. Chapters 19, 26, and 45 also mention these media.

8.3.e. MacConkey agar. The most commonly used primary selective and differential agar, MacConkey agar contains crystal violet dye to inhibit the growth of gram-positive cocci and the pH indicator neutral red to impart differential characteristics. Gram-negative bacilli grow readily; lactose fermenters produce acid products of metabolism that cause the pH of the medium close to the colony to fall. The neutral red then turns red at the acid pH (Plate 8.2). Nonlactose fermenters remain colorless and translucent.

8.3.f. Columbia CNA agar with blood. Columbia agar base is a nutritionally rich formula containing three peptone sources. The added 5% defibrinated blood provides more nutrients and the capability of displaying hemolytic reactions. The antibacterial agents colistin (10 µg/ml) and nalidixic acid (15 µg/ml) completely suppress the growth of Enterobacteriaceae and *Pseudomonas* species while allowing staphylococci, streptococci, and enterococci to grow. Certain gram-negative organisms such as *Gardnerella vaginalis* and some *Bacteroides* species can grow very well on Columbia CNA with blood.

8.3.g. Brain heart infusion media. Another nutritionally rich formula, brain heart infusion (BHI) can be used to grow a variety of microorganisms, either in a liquid form as a broth or hardened with agar, with or without added blood. Key ingredients include infusion from several animal tissue sources, added peptone, phosphate buffer, and a small concentration of dextrose. The carbohydrate provides a readily accessible source of energy for the organisms. Brain heart infusion broths are often used as blood culture media and as basal media for many metabolic tests, particularly for identifi-

cation of streptococci. The usual base for blood agar plates is heart infusion agar, but BHI, trypticase soy agar, or *Brucella* agar are preferred by many workers.

Brain heart infusion agar with 5%-10% sheep blood and the antimicrobial agents chloramphenicol (16 µg/ml) and gentamicin (5 µg/ml) will inhibit the growth of bacteria while allowing the growth of even the most fastidious dimorphic fungi. This agar should be used as a primary plating medium for the growth of fungi, since it has been shown to yield better recovery than the previously recommended Sabouraud dextrose (described below).

8.3.h. Sabouraud dextrose agar. Developed for the cultivation of pathogenic fungi, particularly the agents of superficial mycoses, this medium contains peptones, dextrose, and agar. It is recommended only for primary isolation of dermatophytes at this time, with the addition of the antimicrobial agents cycloheximide (0.5 µg.ml) and chloramphenicol (16 µg/ml). Subcultures of fungi originally isolated on BHI may exhibit more standard morphology on Sabouraud dextrose; thus it is still useful for identification of molds once they have been isolated. The final pH, around 5.6, is much lower than that of most media and tends to inhibit the growth of bacteria.

8.3.i. Hektoen enteric agar. This medium is included as an example of a selective, differential agar that is not autoclaved. The concentrations of bile salts and the dyes bromthymol blue and acid fuchsin are high enough to inhibit the growth of most normal fecal flora, while inhibiting the growth of *Salmonella* and *Shigella* species only slightly. Because so few organisms can grow on the medium, it is unnecessary to sterilize it prior to dispensing plates. Lactose fermenting organisms, by lowering the pH of the medium in the area of colonies, turn the colonies yellow. The addition of ferric ammonium citrate, a source of iron common to many media formulas, allows the production of H_2S from sodium thiosulfate to be visualized by formation of a black precipitate around colonies.

8.3.j. Lowenstein-Jensen agar. This medium was developed as a selective enrichment agar for mycobacteria. The dye malachite green inhibits the growth of contaminants that are able to survive the initial specimen processing. Lowenstein-based media are the only commonly used formulas that require the addition of homogenized eggs, which necessitates sterilization by inspissation. The utilization of egg protein by some mycobacteria results in production of niacin, an important differentiating characteristic. Many modifications of the basic media are used, including those of Gruft (added antibiotics and ribonucleic acid growth factor) and Wallenstein (added glycerol). Use of these media is mentioned in Chapter 41.

8.3.k. Middlebrook agars and broths. These media, made of more defined components than egg base media, are also used for cultivation of mycobacteria. The malachite green and low pH serve to inhibit contaminants and the clear nature of the agar allows technologists to observe colony morphology easily. Middlebrook formulas are also used for antimicrobial susceptibility testing of mycobacteria, since the antimicrobial agents would be damaged by the repeated heating used to prepare inspissated egg base media. The enrichment supplements of oleic acid, albumin, dextrose, and catalase must be added to support the growth of most mycobacteria.

8.3.l. Phenylethyl alcohol agar. By adding the chemical phenylethyl alcohol to a peptone and beef extract base, an agar is created that inhibits the growth of gram-negative bacteria. The addition of 5% sheep blood provides nutrients for streptococci and staphylococci. This medium is also used to cultivate anaerobic gram-negative organisms, which are not inhibited by the alcohol. After preparation, phenylethyl alcohol plates smell like roses.

8.3.m. PPLO agar. An enrichment medium for mycoplasma (formerly called **pleuropneumonia-like organisms, PPLO**), this formula contains slightly less agar than most bacteriological media and is prepared at a slightly higher pH. Beef heart infusion, peptones, and the added nutrients of serum or ascitic fluid allow the mycoplasma to grow as small colonies with dense centers. Agents to inhibit contaminants, such as penicillin and crystal violet, can be added.

8.3.n. Streptococcal selective agar. Recently improved, streptococcal selective agar (SSA) is available commercially. A modification of sheep blood agar, this medium contains crystal violet, trimethoprim-sulfamethoxazole, and colistin in concentrations adequate to inhibit most streptococci except for *Streptococcus pyogenes* and *S. agalactiae*. Beta hemolysis is readily observed. The medium is effective for primary plating of throat swabs for detection of group A streptococci (also discussed in Chapter 25).

8.3.o. Xylose-lysine-desoxycholate agar. Like Hektoen agar, xylose-lysine-desoxycholate (XLD) agar is selective for *Shigella* and *Salmonella* and is not autoclaved. The salts inhibit many Enterobacteriaceae and gram-positive organisms. The phenol red indicator accounts for the differentiation of nonlactose-fermenters (*Shigella* and *Salmonella*) as colorless (pale pink) colonies. Ferric ammonium citrate allows the visualization of H_2S producing organisms as colonies with black centers. Organisms that ferment the carbohydrates in the medium (xylose, lactose, and sucrose) produce yellow colonies.

8.3.p. Thioglycolate broth. The most commonly used enrichment broth in clinical microbiology, thioglycolate, uses 0.075% agar to prevent convection currents from carrying atmospheric oxygen throughout the broth. Thioglycolic acid also acts as a reducing agent, further lowering the oxidation-reduction potential of the medium. With the addition of many nutrient factors, casein, yeast and beef extracts, vitamins, and others, this medium enhances the growth of most pathogenic bacteria. Other nutrient supplements, an oxidation-reduction indicator (resazurin), dextrose, vitamin K_1, and hemin, have been added for various modified formulas. Experienced technologists can visualize the difference between the diffuse, even growth of gram-negative, facultative bacilli and the discrete, puffball-type growth of gram-positive cocci. Strict aerobes, such as pseudomonads and yeast, tend to grow in a thin layer on the surface of the broth (Figure 8.5). For cultivation of anaerobes, the BBL Microbiology Systems product BBL 135C supplemented with hemin (5 µg/ml), vitamin K_1 (0.1 µg/ml), and sodium bicarbonate (1 mg/ml) is best.

8.3.q. GN broth. Used as a selective broth for the cultivation of salmonellas and shigellas from stool specimens and rectal swabs, GN (which stands for gram negative) broth contains several active ingredients. Sodium citrate and sodium desoxycholate (a bile salt) destroy gram-positive organisms and inhibit the early multiplication of coliforms. The addition of more mannitol than dextrose serves to encourage the growth of mannitol-fermenting pathogens and discourage the growth of *Proteus* species. The medium is buffered to remain at neutral pH, even after production of acid metabolites by bacterial growth. To obtain the optimal benefit of the selective nature of GN broth, it should be subcultured 6-8 h after initial inoculation and incubation. After this time, the coliforms begin to overgrow the pathogens.

8.3.r. Chopped meat broth. With or without added glucose, this medium is used to enrich and preserve the growth of anaerobic organisms. The pieces of meat provide protein substrates for proteolytic enzymes, serve as reducing substances to maintain the low oxidation-reduction potential, and somehow prevent rapidly growing bacteria from overgrowing slower forms. A mineral oil or vaspar overlay on a chopped meat culture of an anaerobic bacterium will allow many anaerobes to remain viable for many months. Chopped meat need not be incubated anaerobically to support the growth of anaerobes.

8.3.s. *Trichomonas* medium. Developed for isolation of human protozoa, this medium contains antibiotics such as chloramphenicol, to inhibit growth of contaminating bacteria. The pH, around 6.0, favors the growth of trichomonads. Nutrients are provided by peptones, maltose, and cysteine.

• • •

There are many other media available that can be used to cultivate pathogens. We have mentioned examples of supportive, enrichment, selective, and differential media. Our basic recommendations for handling specimens are covered in Part III. However, for an individual laboratory, the ultimate choice of which primary and secondary media to use for inoculating clinical specimens will depend on the patient population served by the laboratory, the extent of services offered by the laboratory, and the cost-benefit ratio of each additional

FIGURE 8.5
Growth of gram-negative bacilli (left tube), gram-positive cocci (center tube), and yeast (right tube) in thioglycolate broth.

medium. The laboratory director often needs to make hard decisions about limiting the numbers of media used to obtain the most generally beneficial results. Some of these issues are addressed in Chapter 4.

8.4. Using Streak Plates to Isolate and Enumerate Growth of Pathogens

Inocula are usually spread over the surface of agar plates in a standard pattern, so that the quantity of bacterial growth can be deter-

mined, either semiquantitatively or relatively. A useful streaking pattern is illustrated in Figure 8.6. The relative numbers of organisms in the original specimen can be estimated based on the extent of growth of colonies past the original area of inoculation. For some viscous specimens, such as sputum, and for some highly selective media, such as stool agars, better isolation of all colony types can be achieved if the technologist returns the loop to the original inoculum area on the plate several times

FIGURE 8.6
Streaking pattern for primary inoculation of plates to achieve isolated colonies. Growth in the initial half of the plate only is semiquantitated as $1+$ or $2+$ (sparse); growth into the third quadrant is reported as $3+$ (moderate); and growth into the fourth quadrant is reported as $4+$ (heavy). If numbers of colonies can be counted, this number should be reported.

FIGURE 8.7
Inoculation of plates streaked with a calibrated loop.

during the initial streaking pattern. We have found that flaming the loop between streaking areas is not necessary for most specimens. It may be beneficial, however, to flame the inoculating loop between streaking areas when the original inoculum is material from an already growing bacterial colony.

Streaking plates with a measured amount of inoculum, such as that found in a standard calibrated loop (used to quantify colony-forming-units [CFU] in fluid specimens like urine), should be done to facilitate ease of counting colonies. For this reason, the inoculum may be spread out more evenly over the entire plate (Figure 8.7).

8.5. Cell Cultures for Cultivation of Pathogens

Although fungi and most bacteria grow readily on artificial media, certain pathogens require factors provided only by living cells. Often, these organisms are obligate intracellular parasites, but occasionally they are not, although scientists have been unable to isolate the critical growth factors needed to support growth on wholly artificial media. An example of a pathogen of the latter type is *Legionella*

pneumophila, which was isolated in chicken embryo culture before the necessary growth factors were discovered and incorporated into artificial media by scientists at the Centers for Disease Control in Atlanta. All viruses and chlamydiae are obligate intracellular parasites, growing outside of the host only in tissue cultures or cell cultures. These media are made up of layers of living cells, growing on the surface of a solid matrix, such as the inside of a glass tube or the bottom of a plastic flask (Figure 8.8). Pathogenic viruses are cultivated in clinical microbiology laboratories on cell cultures of two types, **primary cell lines** and **continuous cell lines.** Primary cell lines are produced by cutting up fresh tissue, often kidney, into tiny pieces. When treated with the proteolytic agent trypsin, the tissue pieces break up into individual cells, which are seeded into a flask or tube containing growth-supportive media (formulas are given in Chapter 45). The cells attach to the inside bottom of the container and multiply until they reach a single layer, a **monolayer,** of confluent growth. Normal cells are inhibited from growing on top of each other. Fibroblast cells, such as human foreskin primary cell line, are spindle shaped

FIGURE 8.8
Tissue culture flask used for maintaining cell lines.

FIGURE 8.9
Monolayer of uninoculated human fibroblasts, visualized at 400 ×.

FIGURE 8.10
Monolayer of African green monkey kidney cells, visualized at 400 ×.

(Figure 8.9). Cells from other tissue sources, such as kidney cells, may be shaped more irregularly, like polygons (Figure 8.10). Primary cell lines usually carry the same number of chromosomes as the natural cells from which they were derived, the **diploid** number of normal somatic cells, and they will multiply for only approximately 50 generations before they begin to die off. If cells are obtained from a malignant tissue source, such as a human epithelial cell cancer, they will multiply indefinitely in cell culture and they often contain aberrations in the number of chromosomes they possess (**aneuploid**). Such cell cultures are called continuous cell lines.

In addition to their use for cultivation of viruses, tissue cultures may be used for other purposes in clinical microbiology. Several cell lines, including Hep-2, HeLa, and Vero, have been used for detection of the cytotoxin of *Clostridium difficile* (Chapter 17). Chlamydiae are cultivated on a special cell line, McCoy cells, the monolayer of which is treated with cycloheximide to prevent multiplication before the specimen is inoculated. Isolation of chlamydiae is discussed in Chapter 38. Maintenance and inoculation of the tissue culture lines used for routine clinical virology are reviewed in Chapter 42.

8.6. Use of Experimental Laboratory Animals for Isolation and Identification of Human Pathogens

Clinical microbiologists used to rely heavily on inoculation of experimental animals for the isolation and identification of infectious agents. Today, such activities are usually confined to research facilities or public health laboratories. For this reason, animal inoculation techniques will not be mentioned extensively in the rest of this book, unless their application is particularly important for clinical diagnosis. An abbreviated summary of the animals and agents that have been commonly used for diagnosis is shown in Table 8.2.

TABLE 8.2
Animals Used for Diagnosis

ANIMAL	ROUTE OF INOCULATION	AGENT SOUGHT
Guinea pig	Subcutaneous	*Francisella tularensis*
	Eye	*Shigella*
		Escherichia coli (invasiveness)
	Intradermal	*Corynebacterium diphtheriae* (virulence)
	Intraperitoneal	Many viruses
		Clostridia
		F. tularensis
		Leptospira
		Mycobacterium tuberculosis
		Nocardia
		Spirillum minus
		Yersinia pestis
Mouse	Intracerebral	*Cryptococcus neoformans*
	Subcutaneous	*Bacillus anthracis*
	Intraperitoneal	*Borrelia*
		Clostridia
		C. neoformans
		Histoplasma capsulatum
		Nocardia
		S. minus
		Toxoplasma gondii
		Coccidioides immitis
		Blastomyces dermatitidis
Suckling mouse	Intraperitoneal	Coxsackie A virus
		Enterotoxigenic *E. coli*
Hamster	Intradermal	*Leishmania tropica, L. braziliensis*
	Intraperitoneal	*L. donovani*
		Clostridia
		Leptospira
Rabbit	Eye	*Listeria*
		Shigella, E. coli (invasiveness)
	Intradermal	*C. diphtheriae* virulence
Rat	Intraperitoneal	*Borrelia*
		Toxoplasma
		Y. pestis
Embryonated hen's eggs	Yolk sac	Viruses
		Rickettsia
		Chlamydia

REFERENCE

1. Holdeman, L.V., Cato, E.P., and Moore, W.E.C. 1977. Anaerobe laboratory manual, ed. 4. Anaerobe Laboratory, Virginia Polytechnic Institute and State University, Blacksburg, Va.

BIBLIOGRAPHY

Anonymous. 1984. Difco manual. ed. 10. Difco Laboratories, Detroit.

Anonymous. 1982. The Oxoid manual, ed. 5. Oxoid Ltd., Basingstoke, U.K.

Anonymous. 1983. Products for microbiology: technical manual. GIBCO Laboratories, Madison, Wisc.

Emmons, C.W., Binford, C.H., Utz, J.P., and Kwon-Chung, K.J. 1977. Medical mycology, ed. 3. Lea & Febiger, Philadelphia.

Estevez, E.G. 1984. Bacteriologic plate media: review of mechanisms of action. Lab. Med. 15:258.

Isenberg, H.D., Washington, J.A. II., Balows, A., and Sonnenwirth, A.C. 1985. Collection, handling, and processing of specimens. In Lennette, E.H., Balows, A., Hausler, W.J. Jr., and Shadomy, H.J., editors. Manual of clinical microbiology, ed. 4. American Society for Microbiology, Washington, D.C.

Joklik, W.K. 1980. The nature, isolation, and measurement of animal viruses. In Joklik, W.K., Wilda, H.P., and Amos, D.B., editors. Zinsser microbiology, ed. 17. Appleton-Century-Crofts, New York.

MacFaddin, J.F. 1985. Media for isolation-cultivation-identification-maintenance of medical bacteria, vol. 1. Williams & Wilkins, Baltimore.

Phillips, E., and Nash, P. 1985. Culture media. In Lennette, E.H., Balows, A., Hausler, W.J. Jr., and Shadomy, H.J., editors. Manual of clinical microbiology, ed. 4. American Society for Microbiology, Washington, D.C.

Smith, T.F. 1981. Viruses. In Washington, J.A. II, editor. Laboratory procedures in clinical microbiology. Springer-Verlag, New York.

Sutter, V.L., Citron, D.M., Edelstein, M.A.C., and Finegold, S.M. 1985. Wadsworth anaerobic bacteriology manual, ed. 4. Star Publishing Co., Belmont, Calif.

Washington, J.A. II. 1981. Initial processing for cultures of specimens. In Washington, J.A. II, editor. Laboratory procedures in clinical microbiology. Springer-Verlag, New York.

9 Conventional and Rapid Microbiological Methods for Identification of Bacteria and Fungi

Cultivation and identification of specific pathogens from material collected from patients suspected of having infection is still the most reliable diagnostic tool, even though it is not the fastest. In some cases (such as with *Rickettsia* species) recovery of the infecting organisms is difficult or (such as with *Treponema pallidum*) impossible. In those cases, reliance must be placed on serologic or other methods for diagnosis. However, until molecular biological techniques have advanced to the point that the microorganisms contributing to infectious diseases can be pinpointed by totally individual genetic markers, definitive diagnosis of most infections continues to require isolation of an etiologic agent. Chapter 8 discussed various growth media and strategies for encouraging the growth of cultivatable microorganisms. This chapter will discuss basic morphologic clues and enzymatic and biochemical tests that are used to identify such pathogens once they have been isolated. In addition, we will mention some of the rapid methods and basic concepts of the commercial systems that are currently available for performing biochemical and enzymatic tests. Certain of the biochemical tests used to identify bacteria are also used for identification of some fungi. Biochemical or enzymatic methods that are applicable only to fungal isolates will also be mentioned.

Identification of viruses does not depend primarily on biochemical or enzymatic means, but relies more heavily on the specific damage inflicted on the growth pattern of tissue culture cells by invasion and proliferation of viruses. Fungi and eukaryotic parasites are identified primarily by visualizing characteristic morphologic features of the parasites themselves. Techniques for identification of these agents will be discussed in Chapters 42 to 44. In addition, there are many new methods based on antigenic detection and molecular manipulations that are not covered in this chapter, several of which are discussed in Chapter 10.

9.1. Basic Approaches to Identification of Pathogens

General strategies for determining the category of pathogen isolated and for deciding which further tests are needed for identification will be discussed in this section.

9.1.a. Preliminary identification of colonies growing on solid media. Since most clinical specimens are inoculated onto and into several media, including some selective or differential agars (Chapter 8), the first clue to identification of an isolated colony is the nature of the medium on which the organism is growing. For example, with rare exceptions such as enterococci (described in Chapter 25), only gram-negative bacteria grow well on MacConkey agar or other selective/differential agars for gram-negative bacteria. Plates that contain substances inhibitory to gram-negative bacteria, such as Columbia agar with colistin and nalidixic acid, support growth of gram-positive organisms. Most bacteria and fungi will proliferate on nutrient or supplemented media, such as 5% sheep blood agar, chocolate agar, and brain heart infusion agar.

Moldlike fungi, of course, produce fuzzy or fluffy growth due to their aerial hyphae. If a fuzzy colony is noted on agar plates (Figure 9.1), the plate should be placed into a biological safety cabinet before the plate is opened for further examination. All bacterial colonies

FIGURE 9.1
A moldlike fungus is growing among the bacterial colonies on this primary blood agar plate inoculated with sputum. The plate must be examined in a biohazard hood to avoid dissemination of the fungus.

should be subcultured to other media, and the fungus can then be studied by methods outlined in Chapter 43. Before removing the plate from the cabinet, it should be sealed on two sides with tape to prevent dissemination of spores. Such precautions decrease the chances of laboratory acquisition of systemic fungal infection and prevent contamination of other media during subsequent plate handling or incubation.

It is unwise to place total confidence on colonial morphology for preliminary identification of isolates on primary media, since a microorganism may produce a colony that is not different from colonies of many other species. Yeast colonies often resemble those of staphylococci, for example. Unless colony morphology is distinctive (such as that of typical *Pseudomonas aeruginosa*, Chapter 28) or growth appears on selective media, the cellular morphology of the microorganism must be determined. Even colonies on selective media usually require some additional verification (for example, *Listeria monocytogenes* colonies are indistinguishable from those of *Streptococcus agalactiae;* Chapter 33). Examination of a wet preparation

of bacterial colonies under oil immersion (1,000 ×) magnification, with or without phase microscopy, can rapidly provide many clues as to possible identity. For example, a wet preparation prepared from a translucent, alpha hemolytic colony on blood agar may yield cocci in chains, a strong indication that the bacteria are probably streptococci; or long, thin, uniform, chaining rods, suspicious for lactobacilli. Motility can often be detected by this initial examination; the presence of yeast cells, mimicking bacterial colonies, can also be discovered. The preparation of direct wet mounts is discussed in Chapter 7.

9.1.b. Gram stain morphology for initial identification of bacteria: classical and nontraditional methods. The microbiologist should perform a Gram stain of material from isolated colonies (described in Chapter 7) to gain the most valuable cellular morphologic information. Most bacteria can be divided into four distinct groups: gram-positive cocci, gram-negative cocci, gram-positive bacilli, and gram-negative bacilli. Some species are morphologically indistinct and are described by combining the above terms, such as "gram-negative coccobacilli" or "gram-variable bacilli." Other morphological shapes encountered include curved rods and spirals. Identification procedures are based on the cellular morphology of bacteria. Once this basic information is known, definitive identification can proceed (Figure 9.2).

Gram stain results are not always indicative of the cell wall structure of the organism. For example, certain gram-positive bacteria (and fungi) lose some of their cell wall integrity with age or under adverse conditions (such as exposure to antimicrobial agents) and appear to stain gram-negative. Many *Bacillus* species appear gram-negative on stains, resulting in incorrect additional tests for speciation (and much confusion), and some clostridia (which also possess gram-positive-type cell walls)

FIGURE 9.2
Flow chart illustrating basic identification parameters for bacteria.

never stain gram-positive. To try to capture the proper stain reaction of an organism suspected of being gram-positive, it may be useful to stain a very young broth subculture. If this fails, there are at least two nonstain systems available to aid in determination of true Gram stain reaction. The reagent L-alanine-4-nitroanilide (**LANA**) has been shown by Carlone et al.[2] to differentiate Gram reactivity of aerobic and facultatively anaerobic organisms. This reagent is commercially available impregnated in cotton swabs (Remel Laboratories), which turn yellow when touched to the colony of a gram-negative

bacterium. The KOH test has also been used successfully for problem organisms. Halebian et al.[3] have discussed its usefulness. A loop of growth from a colony of the organism is emulsified on the surface of a glass slide in a suspension of 3% potassium hydroxide (**KOH**). The suspension is stirred continuously for 60 seconds, after which the loop is gently pulled from the suspension. Gram-negative cell walls are broken down, releasing viscid chromosomal material, which causes the suspension to become thick and stringy (Figure 9.3). Although useful, neither of these tests is foolproof, as re-

FIGURE 9.3
The KOH test. Addition of 3% KOH to a gram-negative bacillus causes release of viscous nuclear material.

FIGURE 9.4
Susceptibility to vancomycin (impregnated in a filter paper disk) can differentiate gram-positive bacilli (upper half of plate) from gram-negative bacilli (no zone of inhibition, lower half of plate).

viewed by von Graevenitz and Bucher.[6] Many gram-positive bacteria (with a few exceptions, such as certain lactobacilli) are susceptible to vancomycin, an antimicrobial agent that acts on the gram-positive cell wall. Inhibition of growth by vancomycin at concentrations as low as 3 μg/ml can often presumptively identify a gram-negative-staining organism as gram-positive, saving a technologist from performing inappropriate tests that yield confusing results. Certain gram-negative organisms, notably *Moraxella* and *Acinetobacter* species, may be vancomycin susceptible. The vancomycin screening test can be easily performed by heavily inoculating the organism onto a portion of the surface of a sheep blood agar plate and placing a 5 μg vancomycin disk (available from Anaerobe Systems, Scott Laboratories, and other disk manufacturers, commonly used for assisting in Gram reaction determination with anaerobic bacteria) on the inoculated agar surface. Any zone of inhibition after overnight incubation is usually indicative of a gram-pos-

itive bacterium (Figure 9.4). Conversely, with a few exceptions, most truly gram-negative organisms are resistant to vancomycin and susceptible to colistin or polymyxin at 10 μg/ml.

9.2. Extremely Rapid Biochemical or Enzymatic Tests That Can Be Performed on Single Colonies Growing on Primary Media

All of the tests described here can be performed directly with inocula from colonies seen on primary isolation plates. They all take less than an hour, and most of them take only a minute or two. Such tests can help the technologist place an isolate of known morphology into a further subdivision, thus directing the additional procedures needed for identification (Figure 9.2) and providing valuable tentative or preliminary identification in cases of serious infection. In addition to those tests mentioned here, there are others in use in laboratories around the world; still others are constantly being developed.

6.1

6.2

6.3

6.4

PLATE 6.1. Eliminating air bubbles from syringe and needle to protect anaerobes in specimen from exposure to oxygen.

PLATE 6.2. Injecting specimen into gassed-out tube.

PLATE 6.3. Swab in anaerobic atmosphere. Companion tube on right (shown with specimen on swab in place) contains prereduced nonnutritive semisolid transport medium.

PLATE 6.4. The Bio-Bag (Marion Scientific) containing one inoculated agar plate that has been incubated in the self-contained anaerobic atmosphere.

6.5

PLATE 6.5. The Vacutainer Anaerobic Transporter (Becton-Dickinson Laboratories). The inner tube contains the specimen, which is brought into contact with the anaerobic atmosphere in the outer tube by depressing the plunger.

7.1

7.2

PLATE 7.1.   Acid fast stain of *Mycobacterium marinum* from skin lesion.
PLATE 7.2.   Acid fast stain of *Cryptosporidium* in unconcentrated stool.

7.3

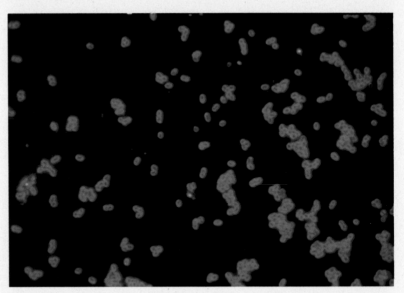

7.4

PLATE 7.3. Fungal elements stained with calcofluor white.
PLATE 7.4. Fluorescent antibody–stained *Streptococcus pyogenes* from pure culture.

8.1

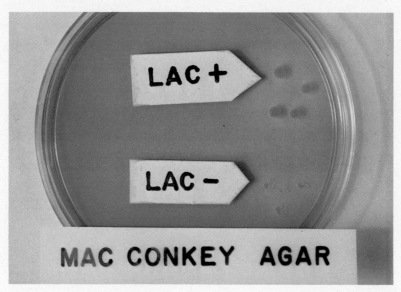

8.2

PLATE 8.1.   Sheep blood agar plate exhibiting all three types of hemolysis.
PLATE 8.2.   Appearance of lactose-fermenting and non-lactose-fermenting colonies on MacConkey agar.

9.1

9.2

9.3

9.4

PLATE 9.1. Kovac's oxidase test. A purple color results when a small portion from a colony of an oxidase positive organism is rubbed onto filter paper saturated with the oxidase reagent. (From Baron. 1985. Clinical microbiology, vol. 3: Listen, look, and learn. Health and Education Resources, Bethesda, Md.)

PLATE 9.2. Spot indole test. A blue-green color results when a small portion from a colony of an indole positive organism is rubbed onto filter paper saturated with the indole reagent. (From Baron. 1985. Clinical microbiology, vol. 3: Listen, look, and learn. Health and Education Resources, Bethesda, Md.)

PLATE 9.3. Moeller's decarboxylase broth media. (From Baron. 1985. Clinical microbiology, vol. 3: Listen, look, and learn. Health and Education Resources, Bethesda, Md.)

PLATE 9.4. Examples of inoculated triple sugar iron agar slants. (From Baron. 1985. Clinical microbiology, vol. 3: Listen, look, and learn. Health and Education Resources, Bethesda, Md.)

9.5

9.6

9.7

9.8

PLATE 9.5. Multitest media (R/B System, Flow Laboratories) that allows aerobic reactions on the slant and anaerobic reactions in the pinched-off base of the tube. (From Baron. 1985. Clinical microbiology, vol. 3: Listen, look, and learn. Health and Education Resources, Bethesda, Md.)

PLATE 9.6. Example of a microdilution tray identification/susceptibility system format (American MicroScan). (From Baron. 1985. Clinical microbiology, vol. 3: Listen, look, and learn. Health and Education Resources, Bethesda, Md.)

PLATE 9.7. The Minitec system (BBL Microbiology Systems), which employs filter-paper disks impregnated with substrates.

PLATE 9.8. The API (Analytab Products, Inc.) miniaturized identification system. (From Baron. 1985. Clinical microbiology, vol. 3: Listen, look, and learn. Health and Education Resources, Bethesda, Md.)

ENTEROTUBE

9.9

9.10

MICRO-ID

9.11

N. meningitidis

9.12

PLATE 9.9. The Enterotube II (Roche Diagnostics) miniaturized identification system. (From Baron. 1985. Clinical microbiology, vol. 3: Listen, look, and learn. Health and Education Resources, Bethesda, Md.)

PLATE 9.10. The Uni-NF-Tek plate, an example of the Flow (Flow Laboratories) miniaturized identification system.

PLATE 9.11. The Micro-ID (General Diagnostics) miniaturized identification system. (From Baron. 1985. Clinical microbiology, vol. 3: Listen, look, and learn. Health and Education Resources, Bethesda, Md.)

PLATE 9.12. The RapID N/H (Innovative Diagnostics) miniaturized identification system.

FIGURE 9.5
Catalase test. Bubbles of gas are released when a catalase positive organism is emulsified in a drop of hydrogen peroxide on a slide.

PROCEDURE 9.1. CATALASE TEST

1. With a loop or sterile wooden stick, transfer a small amount of pure growth from the agar onto the surface of a clean, dry glass slide.
2. Immediately place a drop of 3% hydrogen peroxide (H_2O_2) onto a portion of a colony on the slide.
3. Observe for the evolution of bubbles of gas, indicating a positive test (Figure 9.5).

9.2.a. Catalase test. The catalase test is useful for the identification of many bacteria and will be mentioned several times in the chapters in Part IV. For example, streptococci do not possess the enzyme catalase, which catalyzes the liberation of water and oxygen from hydrogen peroxide, a metabolic endproduct toxic to bacteria. All members of the staphylococci, however, are catalase positive. Catalase reactions can also differentiate *Listeria monocytogenes* (catalase positive) from beta hemolytic streptococci. Most *Neisseria* species are catalase positive. The test can be performed with a very small amount of growth removed from an agar surface (Procedure 9.1).

It has been recommended that the test be performed only on isolates grown on non-blood-containing media. Although red blood cells contain some catalase, a technologist can distinguish the very weak reaction of contaminating red blood cells by performing a control slide catalase test with a small loopful of the blood-containing agar on the same slide with the organism. If the catalase reaction from the colony is much stronger than that from the agar alone, the test can be considered positive.

9.2.b. Slide coagulase test (clumping factor test). Gram-positive cocci that are catalase positive belong to the family Micrococcaceae, which includes the staphylococci (Chapter 24). The slide coagulase test (Procedure 9.2) is used to quickly screen for isolates of *Staphylococcus aureus*, which are almost always coagulase positive. Although other species of staphylococci

PROCEDURE 9.2. SLIDE COAGULASE (CLUMPING FACTOR) TEST

1. Place a drop of coagulase plasma (rabbit plasma with EDTA or citrate, available commercially from BBL Microbiology Systems, Difco Laboratories, GIBCO Laboratories, and others) on a clean, dry glass slide.
2. Place a drop of distilled water or saline next to the drop of plasma as a control.
3. With a loop, straight wire, or wooden stick, emulsify an amount of the isolated colony being tested in each drop, inoculating the water or saline first. Try to create a smooth suspension.
4. Observe for clumping in the coagulase plasma drop and a smooth, homogeneous suspension in the control. Clumping in both drops indicates that the organism autoagglutinates and is unsuitable for the slide coagulase test.

PROCEDURE 9.3. SPOT OXIDASE TEST

1. Prepare a solution of 1% tetramethyl-p-phenylenediamine dihydrochloride (available from Kodak Chemicals, Sigma Chemical Co., and other suppliers) in sterile distilled water each day. To eliminate some work, 50 mg reagent powder can be weighed into each of a large number of plastic, snap-top tubes at one sitting. Each day of use, 5 ml of water is added to one tube (to a predrawn line, for example), which is discarded after that day's use.
2. Place a filter paper circle into a sterile plastic disposable Petri dish and moisten the filter paper with several drops of the fresh reagent.
3. Remove a small portion of the colony to be tested (preferably not more than 24 h old) with a platinum wire or wooden stick and rub the growth on the moistened filter paper.
4. Observe for a color change to blue or purple (Plate 9.1) within 10 seconds (timing is critical).

PROCEDURE 9.4. SPOT INDOLE TEST

1. Prepare indole reagent (1% paradimethylaminocinnamaldehyde, available from Sigma Chemical Co. and other chemical supply houses, dissolved in 10% [vol/vol] concentrated hydrochloric acid). Store in a dark bottle in the refrigerator.
2. Each day, saturate a qualitative filter paper (Whatman No. 1 is fine) in the bottom of a Petri dish with the reagent.
3. Using a wooden stick or loop, rub a portion of the colony on the filter paper. Rapid development of a blue color indicates a positive test. Most indole positive organisms will turn blue within 30 seconds.

may be coagulase positive (*S. intermedius* and *S. hyicus* ss. *hyicus*), they are not clinically important agents of human disease.

Clumping factor is a cell-associated substance that binds plasma fibrinogen, causing agglutination of the organisms by binding them together with aggregated fibrinogen. Not all *S. aureus* strains produce this substance. The reaction must be read within 10 seconds, and the inclusion of an autoagglutination control will decrease the number of false positive results. Rabbit coagulase plasma with EDTA or citrate is preferable to human plasma, which may contain substances inhibitory to the reaction.

9.2.c. Oxidase test. Performed to presumptively identify *Neisseria* species and to initially characterize gram-negative bacilli, the oxidase test indicates the presence of the enzyme cytochrome oxidase. This iron-containing porphyrin enzyme participates in the electron transport mechanism and in the nitrate metabolic pathways of some bacteria. Although the test can be performed by flooding the agar surface of an inoculated plate with the reagent after incubation (Chapter 26), it is most easily interpreted when carried out by the Kovac's method (Procedure 9.3).

If an iron-containing wire is used to transfer growth, a false positive reaction may result; therefore, platinum wire or wooden sticks are recommended. Certain organisms may show slight positive reactions after the initial 10 seconds have passed; such results are not considered definitive. Passing a culture several times on artificial media and testing a very fresh subculture may sometimes induce an organism that displays a questionable or negative reaction to display its true oxidase positivity. Several manufacturers, including Marion Scientific, Difco Laboratories, General Diagnostics, Austin Biological Laboratories, and others, produce oxidase test systems consisting of reagent-impregnated filter-paper strips or disposable glass ampules containing small amounts of reagent. Such systems yield results comparable to the conventional test and save preparation time.

9.2.d. Spot indole test. Organisms that produce the enzyme tryptophanase are able to degrade the amino acid tryptophan into pyruvic acid, ammonia, and the product indole. Indole is detected by its combination with the indicator aldehyde to form a colored endproduct (Procedure 9.4 and Plate 9.2). This test can be used to differentiate swarming *Proteus* species from one another and to presumptively identify *Escherichia coli*. It has also been found useful for examining anaerobic organisms.

9.2.e. Bile solubility test. *Streptococcus pneumoniae* possesses a very active autocatalytic enzyme which lyses the organism's own cell wall during cell division. Under the influence of a bile salt (sodium deoxycholate), the organisms rapidly autolyze. Procedure 9.5 outlines the performance of this test. Other alpha hemolytic streptococci do not possess such an active enzyme and will not dissolve in bile. The bile solubility test may not always work, since old colonies may have lost their active enzyme. Therefore, non-bile-soluble streptococci that resemble pneumococci should be further identified by another method (see Chapter 25).

9.2.f. Spot urease test. *Proteus* species, *Klebsiella* species, some *Citrobacter* species, some *Haemophilus* species, the yeast *Cryptococcus neoformans*, and several other bacteria and fungi produce the enzyme urease, which hydrolyzes urea into ammonia, water, and carbon dioxide. The alkaline endproducts cause the indicator phenol red to change from yellow to pink. This test can be used to screen lactose negative colonies on differential media plated with material from stool specimens, helping to differentiate *Salmonella* and *Shigella* species, which are urease negative, from the urease positive nonpathogens. (Note that *Yersinia enterocolitica*, a stool pathogen, is also urease positive.) This recently described test is outlined in Procedure 9.6.

9.2.g. Rapid thermonuclease test. Another way to distinguish between *Staphylococcus aureus* and coagulase negative staphylococci (particularly useful for supernatants of blood culture broths growing gram-positive cocci in clusters, for which rapid presumptive identification is essential) is the demonstration of the production of a thermostable deoxyribonuclease by *S. aureus* (Procedure 9.7). Only plates from the manufacturer mentioned have been found to perform satisfactorily in this particular procedure.

9.2.h. Miscellaneous rapidly determined information. Colonial morphology, fluorescence under ultraviolet light *(Bacteroides mel-*

FIGURE 9.6
Bile solubility test. Within 15 min after placing a drop of bile reagent on a colony of *Streptococcus pneumoniae*, the colony dissolves.

PROCEDURE 9.5. BILE SOLUBILITY TEST

1. Make a solution of bile salt (10% sodium deoxycholate, available from Difco Laboratories, Sigma Chemical Co., and other sources, in distilled water) and store it at room temperature. The reagent is good for 6 months.
2. Select a well-isolated suspicious colony from a blood agar or chocolate agar plate and place 1 drop of the reagent directly upon the colony.
3. Keeping the plate very level, to prevent the reagent from running and washing a nonpneumococcal colony away, producing a false-positive result, allow the reagent to dry. Placing the plate in an aerobic incubator will speed up this process.
4. When the reagent has dried (in approximately 15 min), examine the area for the absence or flattening of the original colony (Figure 9.6), indicators of bile solubility. Ascertain that an alpha hemolytic streptococcal colony has not merely been washed to another portion of the plate by making certain that the bile drop has remained where it was placed (the blood under the drop becomes slightly hemolyzed).

PROCEDURE 9.6. SPOT UREASE TEST

1. Make a solution of the urea reagent (10% urea agar base, available from BBL Microbiology Systems and Difco Laboratories, in distilled water) and store it in the refrigerator.
2. Place a filter paper circle (the filter paper must be catalog No. F2315-50, American Scientific Products) in the bottom of a Petri dish and moisten with several drops of the reagent.
3. Rub a portion of the colony to be tested onto the moist filter paper using a wooden stick or loop. Observe for a color change from yellow to pink or red, which may take as long as 2 min. The pink endproduct indicates that urease activity was present.

Modified from Qadri, S.M.H. et al. 1984. J. Clin. Microbiol. 20:1198.

PROCEDURE 9.7. RAPID THERMONUCLEASE TEST

1. Boil approximately 2 ml of blood culture broth (can be mixed or unmixed) in a water bath or microwave oven for 15 min. The red cells will clot in the bottom of the tube. Allow the tube to cool to room temperature.
2. Punch a well in DNAse test agar (Thermal agar, available from Edge Diagnostics) with the large end of a Pasteur pipette or a plastic drinking straw, remove the agar plug, and fill the well with the heated and cooled supernatant above the red cell clot (approximately 2 drops). A positive control, a negative blood culture seeded with *S. aureus* and passed to a new negative blood culture weekly, should be included each time the test is performed.
3. Incubate the plate at 37° C in an upright position and inspect the plate after 1 h and again after 2 h for the presence of a pink zone around the well of a positive fluid. The pink halo, evidence of the breakdown of DNA, is indicative of *S. aureus*, which produces a thermostable nuclease. A small, clear zone around a well is not indicative of a positive test, as some coagulase negative staphylococci can degrade the dye without denaturing the DNA.
4. The plate may be refrigerated and reused several times.

Modified from Madison, B.M., and Baselski, V.S. 1983. J. Clin. Microbiol. 18:722; and Ratner, H.B., and Stratton, C.W. 1985. J. Clin. Microbiol. 21:995.

aninogenicus), pigment production (*Pseudomonas, Chromobacterium,* etc.), spreading (*Capnocytophaga, Proteus,* etc.), pitting of agar (*Eikenella corrodens*), hemolytic reaction on blood agar, odor, and many other characteristics mentioned throughout the text are very helpful in narrowing down identification possibilities.

9.3. Conventional Metabolic Biochemical Tests

A relatively small proportion of the total genetic makeup of bacteria is involved in production of the enzymes that metabolize various substrates. These enzymes have traditionally been used as markers for separating species groups. If an organism possessed a given enzyme and was able to utilize a substrate, an endproduct would be formed that changed the pH of the medium, causing a visual color change in a pH indicator substance. In some cases, the organism's ability to grow in a medium could be detected by increased turbidity or the presence of colonies on the surface. This approach has been modified in many ways in recent years, but it is still used for identification of unusual pathogens, difficult-to-speciate pathogens, and as the standard against which all other metabolic test methods are compared. There are many conventional tests other than those described in this chapter; some of them will be mentioned in later sections of the book. Detailed explanations of the principles of metabolic reactions can be found in other references, such as *Manual of Clinical Microbiology,* ed. 4, edited by Lennette et al. (American Society for Microbiology, Washington, D.C.), *Zinsser Microbiology,* edited by Joklik et al. (Appleton-Century-Crofts, Norwalk, Conn.), *Microbiology, Including Immunology and Molecular Genetics,* ed. 4, edited by Davis et al. (Harper & Row, New York), and other sources.

9.3.a. Oxidation and fermentation tests. The metabolic pathways used by a microorganism during utilization of a substrate for production of cell building material and for energy (usually with the concomitant production of acid byproducts) can be either **oxidative** or **fermentative.** Oxidation occurs when the organism uses oxygen as a terminal electron acceptor. This reaction can be observed on the surface of agar slants or in the surface layer of liquid media loosely capped to allow diffusion of air. Fermentation occurs in the absence of oxygen. During fermentation, the organism often produces large amounts of organic acids. Fermentation can be demonstrated by overlaying substrate-containing media with mineral oil or a petroleum jelly (Vaseline) and paraffin combination (vaspar) to exclude oxygen. A special medium containing low concentrations of peptone (oxidative-fermentative [O-F] medium, described in Chapter 28) has been developed for testing this aspect of the metabolism of bacteria. In either case, the final endproducts are detected by noting a change in the color of the pH indicator incorporated into the media. It is clear that the pH at which the indicator changes color will substantially affect the outcome of the test. For that reason, the indicator given for a particular medium formula must not be modified. Many substrate utilization tests rely on either bromcresol purple, which changes from purple to yellow at pH 6.3, Andrade's acid fuchsin indicator, which changes from pale yellow to pink at pH 5.5, or phenol red, which changes from red to yellow at pH 7.9. Formulas for the preparation of media containing certain of these indicators are found in Chapter 45.

9.3.b. Hydrolysis tests. An enzyme that breaks down a substrate by adding the components of water to key bonds within the substrate molecule is called a **hydrolyzing** enzyme. The products are measured by some visual reaction. Substrates for such enzymes that are commonly used in differentiating species include sodium hippurate, which can be broken down by *Listeria, Streptococcus uberis,* and group B streptococci (*S. agalactiae,* Chapter 25); deoxyribonucleic acid (DNA), which can be hydrolyzed by certain Enterobacteriaceae, certain species of staphylococci (see 9.2.g), and other microorganisms; urea (mentioned above in part 9.2.f); and esculin, which is hydrolyzed by *Listeria monocytogenes*, group D streptococci, some viridans streptococci, and some anaerobes, among others. Hydrolysis of starch, casein, and lecithin is also used for differentiation of species. Certain mycobacteria can be identified by their ability to hydrolyze the detergent, polysorbate-80 (Tween-80). These media can all be purchased, either fully prepared or in dry powder form. Uses of hydrolysis tests for identifications are described throughout the book.

9.3.c. Amino acid degradation. Enzymes formed by some organisms either **deaminate, dihydrolyze,** or **decarboxylate** amino acids, breaking them down into smaller components. The amino acid substrates tested often include lysine, arginine, ornithine, tryptophan (described above in 9.2.d), and phenylalanine. Certain mycobacteria can be differentiated by their ability to deaminate pyrazinamide. Some of these amino acid–degrading enzymes are active in the absence of oxygen; therefore, such tests are often carried out in the deep butts of agar tubes or in liquid media overlaying with vaspar to prevent the products of more active oxidative enzymes from obscuring the results. One such commonly used system is that of Moeller (Plate 9.3). Amino acids (lysine, arginine, and ornithine) are incorporated into broth media containing 0.05% glucose, to allow the organisms to begin growth, and bromocresol purple indicator. Along with each amino acid being tested, a control tube of the glucose-containing broth base without amino acid is inoculated to serve as a standard against which to compare the color of the indicator. In the case of most of the amino acid degradation reactions, the endproducts (such as ammonia) are alkaline and the color indicator changes to its original color: bromcresol purple turns to purple and phenol red changes to red. Phenylala-

nine deamination, on the other hand, occurs in air and is measured by the production of a green reactant after the addition of 10% ferric chloride. The media for performing all of the tests mentioned here are commercially available (Appendix).

9.3.d. Single substrate utilization. Many organisms can be recognized by their ability to grow in the presence of only a single compound that supplies enough of the organism's nutrient needs. Substrates that can fulfill this function and are helpful in differentiating microorganisms include citrate, malonate, and acetate. Growth on a substrate-containing agar slant, with or without a pH indicator, is used as the endpoint of this test. Another variant of this test, used to determine whether a yeast is able to grow with only a single carbohydrate or nitrate, is called an **assimilation** test. Filter paper disks impregnated with the substrate are placed on the surface of a Petri dish of agar without nutrients that has been streaked with a suspension of the yeast being tested so as to obtain confluent growth. The yeast grows around the disks that contain substrates that it can utilize, or assimilate.

9.3.e. Nitrate reactions. Nitrate serves as the source of nitrogen for many bacteria and fungi, but it must be broken down. The first step in nitrate utilization is reduction to nitrite by removal of one oxygen molecule. The Enterobacteriaceae and many other gram-negative bacilli, mycobacteria, and fungi reduce nitrate to nitrite. Certain microorganisms are able to further reduce nitrite to nitrogen by replacing the remaining oxygens with hydrogens. Some *Pseudomonas* species and other nonfermentative gram-negative bacilli possess this capability, as do other species. The classical nitrate reduction test is described in Procedure 9.8. The ability of yeasts to utilize nitrate can be determined by the same method used for assimilation tests.

9.3.f. Triple sugar iron agar and Kligler's iron agar reactions. Reactions of bacteria in

118 Handling Clinical Specimens for Microbiological Studies

PART TWO

PROCEDURE 9.8. CONVENTIONAL NITRATE REDUCTION TEST

1. Grow the organism in 5 ml of nitrate broth (commercially available) for 24-48 h. A small inverted tube, called a **Durham tube,** may be placed into the broth to trap bubbles of nitrogen gas that may be formed by nitrite-reducing organisms.
2. Prepare the reagents that combine with the nitrite to form colored endproducts:
Reagent A
Sulfanilic acid
Acetic acid (5 M) 4 g / 500 ml

Reagent B
N,N-dimethyl-1-naphthylamine 3 ml
Acetic acid (5 M) 500 ml
3. Add 3 drops of reagent A and then 3 drops of reagent B to the suspension of organisms in broth.
4. Wait 5 min for the production of a red color, indicating the presence of the nitrate reduction product, nitrite.
5. An organism may reduce nitrite all the way to nitrogen gas, thus yielding a negative (colorless) reaction in the first part of the nitrate test. The gas may not have collected in the Durham tube, necessitating the final step in the nitrate test. The presence of unreduced nitrate can be detected by adding a pinch of zinc powder (commercially available) to the broth if the red color did not develop within 5 min after the initial reagents were added. Zinc can itself reduce nitrate; if the organism has not attacked the nitrate, it will be reduced by the zinc to form nitrite, which can then react with reagents A and B to yield a red color. This red color after the addition of zinc indicates a negative test result.

Kligler's iron agar (**KIA**) or triple sugar iron agar (**TSIA**) can be used to direct the initial identification of gram-negative bacilli, particularly members of the Enterobacteriaceae (Chapter 27). KIA and TSIA can detect three primary characteristics of a bacterium: the ability to produce gas from the fermentation of sugars, the production of large amounts of hydrogen sulfide gas (as visualized by the formation of a black iron-containing precipitate), and the ability to ferment lactose in KIA or lactose and sucrose in TSIA. A small amount of growth from a pure colony is picked onto a straight wire and inoculated to these media by streaking the surface of the slant and stabbing the butt of the tube all the way to the bottom. Only the tops of colonies growing on selective agar should be touched, since inhibited flora may still be present and viable. For the same reason, the needle or loop should not be cooled in the agar of any selective medium. Gas formation is usually visualized as bubbles and cracks in the medium, caused by the pressure of the gas formed in the agar. Therefore, the inoculating wire must be stabbed down the center of the agar butt of the tube; careless inoculation may allow the wire to form a channel in the agar along the inside glass wall of the tube through which the newly formed gas may escape, preventing its detection. The presence of oxygen in the atmosphere is necessary for the proper reaction to occur on the slant; therefore caps must be very loose if screw-capped tubes are used.

Both TSIA and KIA contain a limiting amount of glucose and a tenfold greater lactose concentration. Enterobacteriaceae and other glucose fermenters first begin to metabolize glucose, as glucose utilizing enzymes are present constitutively and the bacteria can gain the most energy from using the simplest sugar. All other sugars must be converted to glucose before they enter the Embden-Meyerhof pathway. Glucose utilization occurs both aerobically on the slant where oxygen is available as a terminal electron acceptor, and in the butt where conditions are anaerobic. Once a glucose fermenting bacterium has reduced all of the available glucose to pyruvate, it will further metabolize pyruvate via the aerobic Krebs cycle (on the slant) to produce acid endproducts. The acid in the medium causes the pH indicator, phenol red, to assume a yellow color. Thus, after 6 h of incubation, both the slant and butt of a TSIA or a KIA that has been inoculated with a glucose fermenter will appear yellow. If the organism cannot ferment glucose, the **butt** will remain red (indicating no change in pH) or become alkaline (may be indicated by a red color slightly deeper than that of the original medium), demonstrating that the organism is not a member of the Enterobacteriaceae.

After depletion of the limited glucose, an organism that is able to do so will begin to utilize lactose or sucrose. Since there is 10 times as much lactose (and sucrose in TSIA) as glucose in the agar, the organism will have enough substrate to continue making acid end products. The slant and butt of the TSIA or KIA will remain yellow after 18-24 h incubation. This reaction is called acid over acid (A/A) and the organism is identified as a lactose fermenter. The production of gas will cause the medium to break up or to be pushed up the tube, so that a gas-producing lactose fermenter will give an A/A plus gas reaction.

If the organism being tested cannot use the lactose in the medium, it must produce energy in a less efficient way by using the proteins and amino acids in the medium as nutrient sources. Protein metabolism occurs primarily on the surface of the slant where oxygen is plentiful. The byproducts of peptone breakdown (such as ammonia) are alkaline and cause the phenol red indicator to revert back to its original red color. After 18-24 h incubation of a nonlactose fermenter, the TSIA or KIA will thus show a red slant; the butt remains yellow due to the early anaerobic glucose metabolism. This reaction is called alkaline over acid (Alk/A or K/A).

Glucose nonfermenters may also produce alkaline products from peptone utilization on the slant. Such reactions will be alkaline over alkaline (Alk/Alk or K/K) or alkaline over no change (Alk/NC). Plate 9.4 shows several different possible reactions in TSIA.

Either lactose fermenters or nonlactose fermenters can produce hydrogen sulfide, and the black precipitate may mask the true color of the butt. In this case, the ability to ferment or oxidize glucose can be tested by inoculating the organism into **oxidative-fermentative** media (Chapter 28). These media are prepared with a low peptone concentration so that the pH change that occurs after metabolism of glucose will not be affected by the alkaline products formed from peptone utilization.

The initial reaction of an inoculum from a pure culture of a bacterial strain in TSIA or KIA gives a microbiologist a great deal of information about what the genus might be, and further tests are often chosen based on this reaction. Although these media are used primarily for gram-negative bacilli, the ability of one species of gram-positive bacilli, *Erysipelothrix rhusiopathiae*, to produce hydrogen sulfide is often detected in TSIA. *Bacillus* species that are inoculated to TSIA or KIA because they are initially thought to be gram-negative bacilli will usually yield an acid slant over a slightly orange (or no change in color) butt. Subtle patterns and colors of reactions, such as a cherry-red slant and very little gas (suggestive of *Serratia* species) or a very dark red slant (suggestive of *Proteus, Providencia,* or *Morganella* species), can be recognized by experienced technologists and serve to guide the choice of further tests.

9.4. Modifications of Conventional Biochemical Tests

A number of modifications of conventional biochemicals have been used in recent years to facilitate inoculation of media, to decrease the incubation time, to automate the procedure, or to systematize the determination of species based on reaction patterns. Some of these systems will be described briefly in this chapter.

9.4.a. Modified conventional biochemical test systems that utilize small volumes. A number of conventional methods can be made to yield more rapid results by heavily inoculating a very small volume of substrate. Used successfully for rapid identification of *Neisseria* species, the method of Kellogg described in Cumitech 4[5] uses this principle. A modification of the Kellogg broths (Procedure 9.9) has been used for rapid determination of carbohydrate reactions of fastidious gram-negative bacilli. The reagents can be used to test most bacteria, including *Neisseria* species.

Many tests, including hippurate hydrolysis, nitrate reduction, urease production, decarboxylations, and deaminations, have been modified for rapid results. For these tests, small volumes of media are inoculated with heavy suspensions of the organism to be tested. Media manufacturers (Appendix) produce many such reagents. In several cases commercial suppliers (including Remel Laboratories, Austin Biological Laboratories, and others) produce reagent-impregnated paper disks or filter paper strips to be eluted in a small volume of water or saline to form the test substrate. Key Scientific Products was one of the first commercial suppliers of single substrates for elution. In the Key system, compressed tablets

that could be stored at room temperature are added to small volumes of water as needed to produce the substrates for specific reactions. All of these systems obviate the need for the technologist to prepare these media in the usual way. The test organism can then be suspended directly in the substrate. Such small volume, singly performed tests are extremely useful for differentiating two similar species that differ in only one characteristic or for ruling out an organism that is characterized by a single parameter. One example is the use of a rapid urease test that can help eliminate certain nonpathogens from further biochemical testing as possible stool pathogens, many of which (except for *Y. enterocolitica*) are urease negative. The nitrate test for mycobacteria has been adapted to this format, as has the niacin test (Chapter 41). Other tests have also been adapted for rapid determination with filter paper reagents.

9.4.b. Multitest systems. The simplest multitest system consists of a conventional-type format that can be inoculated once to yield more than one result. By combining reactants, for example, one substrate can be used to determine indole and nitrate results; indole and motility results; motility, indole, and ornithine; or other combinations. These systems are commercially available (powder or prepared media). The R/B system (Flow Laboratories) incorporates several media within one uniquely designed tube (Plate 9.5).

In a widely used type of identification system, conventional biochemicals have been put up in smaller volumes and packaged so that they can be inoculated easily with one manipulation instead of several. When used in conjunction with a computer-generated data base (described below), the biochemical patterns generated can be used to predict species identification with much more precision than obtainable using conventional methods with fewer parameters. Two manufacturers (American MicroScan and MicroMedia Systems) pro-

PROCEDURE 9.9. RAPID CARBOHYDRATE FERMENTATION REACTION TEST

1. Prepare buffered indicator solution as follows:

KH_2PO_4	0.01 g
K_2HPO_4	0.04 g
KCl	0.80 g
Phenol red	0.004 g (or 0.4 ml of a 1% aqueous solution)
Distilled water	100 ml

   Adjust the pH to 7.0; sterilize by passing the solution through a 0.2 μm diameter pore size membrane filter, and store in a tightly capped brown bottle in the refrigerator (4° C).

2. Prepare 20% stock carbohydrate solutions as follows:

Peptone	10 g
Meat extract	3 g
NaCl	5 g
Distilled water	1,000 ml

   Add 20 g of the appropriate carbohydrate (glucose, sucrose, etc. available from Difco Laboratories) to 100 ml of the peptone broth solution, adjust to pH 7.0, and filter sterilize as above One portion of the peptone broth should be retained without carbohydrate to serve as a control. These solutions may be stored frozen in small aliquots.

3. Place 0.1 ml of the indicator buffer solution in a plastic or glass disposable culture tube (10 × 75 mm diameter) for each carbohydrate to be tested and for one control. Make an extremely heavy suspension of a pure culture of the organism to be tested in each of the indicator buffer tubes (should be milky).

4. Add 1 drop (approximately 0.04 ml) of the appropriate carbohydrate stock solution to each suspension. Add 1 drop of peptone broth without carbohydrate to one suspension to serve as a negative control.

5. Cap the tubes and incubate them in a water bath or heating block at 35° C for up to 4 h, observing periodically for a change in indicator from red to yellow. Many reactions will be positive within 30 min; questionable reactions may require up to 24 h for full development. The control tube should remain red.

Modified from Brown. 1974. Appl. Microbiol. 27:1027, and Hollis et al. 1980. J. Clin. Microbiol. 12:620.

duce conventional biochemicals in microdilution trays (Plate 9.6) that are shipped to the user in a frozen state and maintained frozen until they are thawed, inoculated, and used. These systems require overnight incubation, as do conventional biochemicals. The addition of reagents for the demonstration of endproducts of reactions is necessary. The Sceptor system (BBL Microbiology Systems) is also based on a microdilution array, but the substrates are dried in the trays, which are rehydrated with a suspension of the organism during inoculation.

The Minitek system (also BBL Microbiology Systems) incorporates a microbroth format and allows the user to determine which reactions are to be tested by arbitrarily adding substrate-impregnated filter paper disks to wells in a plastic tray (Plate 9.7). Many different groups of bacteria, including Enterobacteriaceae, anaerobes, and *Neisseria* species, can be tested in the versatile Minitek system. If heavy inocula are used to inoculate the Minitek wells, results may be available within 4 h.

The API 20E for identification of gram-negative bacilli, API 20S for identification of streptococci, API 20C for yeast identification, and API 20A for identification of anaerobes (Analytab Products) incorporate dried reagents in plastic cupules into which a suspension of the test organism is placed (Plate 9.8). With a heavy inoculum, results may be read after 4-6 h incubation in some cases. The API Rapid E for Enterobacteriaceae, Rapid NFT for nonfermentative gram-negative bacilli, and Rapid Strep for streptococcal identification systems (also Analytab Products) use the same format, although a number of chromogenic substrates (described below) are incorporated as differential reactants to allow more rapid results (4 h). The API systems have been adopted by large numbers of laboratories since their introduction in the late 1970s. Because of an extensive computer-generated data base incorporating the results of 21 test results (including the oxidase reaction that is performed separately), use of the API system for identification of Enterobacteriaceae has facilitated the recognition of several of the new species of Enterobacteriaceae and has allowed laboratories to designate species to a more precise level (based on biotype) than was previously possible in a cost-effective manner.

Innovative formats for conventional biochemicals are found in several other systems. The Enterotube II (for lactose fermenters) and Oxi-Ferm (for nonfermenters), produced by Roche Diagnostics, are contained within a large tube. A colony is picked onto the end of a long inoculating needle that is drawn through a series of substrate-containing agar compartments in the plastic tube (Plate 9.9). The Enteric-Tek for Enterobacteriaceae, Uni-Yeast-Tek for yeast, Anaerobe-Tek for identification of anaerobes, and Uni-N/F-Tek for nonfermentative gram-negative bacilli (Flow Laboratories) employ substrate-containing media in pie-shaped wedges in a circular plastic tray (Plate 9.10). Substrates incorporated into agar plates allow many bacteria to be tested at one time in a cost-effective manner (Cathra Repliscan II System, MCT Diagnostics).

In recent years several of the multitest systems have been adapted to yield results more rapidly, often without requiring overnight incubation. The Micro-ID system (General Diagnostics) was one of the first to exploit the principle that bacterial enzymes can act in the absence of actual viable growth or multiplication. The detection of **preformed enzymes** relies on the inoculation of substrate-containing solutions with an extremely heavy suspension of the organism, resembling the turbidity of skim milk (around 1×10^9 bacteria per milliliter). Enough of the enzyme will be present in this volume of organisms to cause the substrate reaction to occur, even if the organisms are no longer alive. The Micro-ID system uses a number of substrates that detect preformed enzymes in addition to conventional tests for identification of Enterobacteriaceae. The test organism suspension is inoculated to plastic wells, the tray is incubated, and the entire tray is tipped to allow reactants in a separate chamber to mix with the suspension (Plate 9.11). Results are available after 4 h incubation. Tests of this sort (several have been mentioned above) yield results after several hours of incubation instead of the overnight incubation required by many conventional methods.

Newer biochemical test systems may also utilize chromogenic substrates. Chromogenic substrates are acted upon by enzymes to form colored products; a separate visual indicator system is unnecessary. Because most of the enzymes being detected by their activity on chromogenic substrates are preformed, results are available within 4 h for most systems using these substrates. Identification systems that utilize a large number of chromogenic substrates include the RapID ANA anaerobic identification panel and the RapID N/H panel for identification of *Neisseria* and *Haemophilus* species, produced by Innovative Diagnostics (Plate 9.12). Rapid Strep and Staph-Ident systems by Analytab Products and several other *Neisseria* and *Haemophilus* identification systems also utilize chromogenic substrates.

Systems that include susceptibility testing as well as identification parameters on the same tray (including those produced by American MicroScan and MicroMedia Systems) must be incubated overnight to allow enough growth of the organism for accurate test results. Changes in the technology of microbiology are being contemplated, however, that will shorten incubation time by relying on parameters other than growth for measurement of an organism's reaction to an antimicrobial substrate, as further discussed in Chapter 13.

9.4.c. Automated microbial identification systems. Although they are discussed in more detail in Chapter 11, the most widely used automated identification systems are mentioned briefly here. Systems that utilize a microdilution tray format have been automated to allow hands-off or partially manual reading of results. The MicroScan (American MicroScan) and Sceptor systems (BBL Microbiology Systems) both employ readers that interface with the data base for computer-assisted identification. The Sceptor system includes an automated filling device for rehydrating the wells with a suspension of the test organism. API-compatible systems (UniScept Plus and Aladin, Analytab Products) also incorporate an automated reader that interfaces with their extensive data base.

The Autobac IDX (General Diagnostics)

was one of the first automated susceptibility systems. It has been modified to provide bacterial identification. Organisms are inoculated into plastic cuvettes containing various inhibitory substances. After 3-6 h incubation, the identification of a test organism is determined by its growth pattern in the presence of the different antibacterial agents, as measured by light-scatter photometry. The AutoMicrobic System (Vitek Systems) determines the growth of the test strain within tiny substrate-containing wells on a plastic card by measuring turbidity. Once the card has been inoculated, the instrument performs all readings without operator assistance; results are available within 4-6 h incubation. Cards are available for identification of gram-negative fermenters and nonfermenters, yeast, staphylococci, and streptococci, some of which require longer incubation periods for final results. The Avantage system (Abbott Laboratories) utilizes a plastic cartridge with a number of wells containing lyophilized substrates that is manually inoculated in one step. The instrument monitors turbidity over time, yielding results based on kinetic patterns of growth and metabolism. Separate reagent cartridges are available for identification of yeasts, nonfermenting gram-negative bacilli, and Enterobacteriaceae.

9.5. Computer-Assisted Data Base Systems

The principles upon which computer-assisted data base systems for identification of species are based are simple. The first step in developing a data base is to accumulate a large number of organisms of known species. Each strain is subjected to an identical battery of biochemical and enzymatic tests. The reactions are recorded as positive ($+$) or negative ($-$) and the cumulative results of each test are expressed as a percentage of each genus or species that possesses that characteristic. For example, suppose that 100 different known *Escherichia* strains and 100 known *Shigella* strains are tested in four biochemicals, yielding the results

TABLE 9.1

Generation and Utilization of Genus-Identification Data Base Probability: Percent Positive
Reactions for 100 Known Strains

ORGANISM	BIOCHEMICAL PARAMETER			
	LACTOSE	SUCROSE	INDOLE	ORNITHINE
Escherichia	91	49	99	63
Shigella	1	1	38	20

TABLE 9.2

Generation and Utilization of Genus-Identification Data Base Probability: Probability that
Unknown Strain X Is a Member of the Known Genus Based on Results of Each Individual
Parameter Tested

ORGANISM	BIOCHEMICAL PARAMETER			
	LACTOSE	SUCROSE	INDOLE	ORNITHINE
X	%+	%+	%−	%+
Escherichia	.91	.49	.01	.63
Shigella	.01	.01	.62	.20

Probability that X is *Escherichia* = .91 × .49 × .01 × .63 = .002809
Probability that X is *Shigella* = .01 × .01 × .62 × .20 = .000012

illustrated in Table 9.1. Now an unknown organism, X, is tested in the same four biochemicals, yielding results as follows: lactose +, sucrose +, indole −, and ornithine +. The results of testing the known strains are now converted to the percentage probability that the unknown strain X is a member of one of the known genera based on each separate test result (Table 9.2). If *Escherichia* sp. are 91% lactose positive, then the probability that X is an *Escherichia* based on lactose alone is 0.91. If *Shigella* sp. are 38% indole positive, then the probability that X is a *Shigella* based on indole alone is 0.62 (1.00 [all *Shigella*] − 0.38 [percent of positive *Shigella*] = 0.62 [percent of *Shigella* that are indole negative]). The probabilities are then multiplied to achieve a calculated likelihood that X is one or the other of the two genera. Ultimately, X is more likely to be an *Escherichia*, with a probability of 357:1 (1 divided by 0.0028). This is still a very

unlikely probability, but we have tested only four parameters, and the indole, a very important one, was atypical. As more parameters are added to the formula, the importance of just one test decreases and the overall pattern prevails. It is obvious that with typical organisms being tested for 20 or more reactions, a computer must be used to generate the probabilities. The more organisms in the data base, the more precise will be the genus or species designations derived. All commercial suppliers of multicomponent biochemical test systems provide their customers with a computer, a computer-derived code book, or access to a telephone inquiry center for matching profile numbers to species. By adding large numbers of organisms to the data base, unusual patterns can be recognized. In some cases, new species or unusual species involved in an unsuspected epidemic have been discovered in this way.

REFERENCES

1. Brown, W.J. 1974. Modification of the rapid fermentation test for *Neisseria gonorrhoeae*. Appl. Microbiol. 27:1027.
2. Carlone, G.M., Valadez, M.J., and Pickett, M.J. 1983. Methods for distinguishing gram-positive from gram-negative bacteria. J. Clin. Microbiol. 16:1157.
3. Halebian, S., Harris, B., Finegold, S.M., and Rolfe, R.D. 1981. Rapid method that aids in distinguishing gram-positive from gram-negative anaerobic bacteria. J. Clin. Microbiol. 13:444.
4. Hollis, D.G., Sottnek, F.O., Brown, W.J., and Weaver, R.E. 1980. Use of the rapid fermentation test in determining carbohydrate reactions of fastidious bacteria in clinical laboratories. J. Clin. Microbiol. 12:620.
5. Kellogg, D.S. Jr., Holmes, K.K., and Hill, G.A. 1976. Cumitech 4. Laboratory diagnosis of gonorrhea. Coordinating editors, Marcus, S., and Sherris, J.C. American Society for Microbiology, Washington, D.C.
6. von Graevenitz, A., and Bucher, C. 1983. Accuracy of the KOH and vancomycin tests in determining the Gram reaction of non-enterobacterial rods. J. Clin. Microbiol. 18:983.

BIBLIOGRAPHY

Blazevic, D.N., and Ederer, G.M. 1975. Biochemical tests in diagnostic microbiology. John Wiley & Sons, New York.

D'Amato, R.F., McLaughlin, J.C., and Ferraro, M.J. 1985. Rapid manual and mechanized/automated methods for the detection and identification of bacteria and yeasts. In Lennette, E.J., Balows, A., Hausler, W.J. Jr., and Shadomy, H.J., editors. Manual of clinical microbiology, ed. 4. American Society for Microbiology, Washington, D.C. (Extensive reference list included.)

LeBeau, L.J. 1983. Roots of automation in microbiology; an introduction. Am. J. Med. Tech. 49:299. (Entire issue devoted to automation in microbiology.)

Paik, G. 1980. Reagents, stains, and miscellaneous test procedures. In Lennette, E.H., et al., editors. Manual of clinical microbiology, ed. 3. American Society for Microbiology, Washington, D.C.

Washington, J.A. II, editor. 1985. Laboratory procedures in clinical microbiology, ed. 2. Springer-Verlag, New York.

10 Nontraditional Methods for Identification and Detection of Pathogens or Their Products

The microbiologist has traditionally sought to isolate pathogenic organisms in pure culture in an artificial environment outside the human host. In this way, the morphology, biochemical activity, and antimicrobial susceptibility pattern of each organism could be examined and evaluated. In the case of viral diseases, identification of the pathogen required recognition of a particular cytopathic effect in a predefined cell culture medium, a criterion that demanded a high degree of sophistication in the laboratory and often a fairly long incubation period. Only by definitive identification could the cause of an infection or disease be ascertained. A second and less satisfying method for diagnosis of disease has been the demonstration (by showing a significant rise in titer) of a specific humoral antibody response to the organism in question. For efficient serological diagnosis, therefore, the clinician must be able to narrow down the possible causes of disease so that the appropriate antigens can be chosen to test against the patient's serum specimens, since testing sera against all possible antigens would be prohibitive. It often takes 2 weeks or longer for antibodies to appear. As more patients survive with compromised immune systems such that their antibody production is severely curtailed or absent, the use of rising serologic titers for diagnosis has become less universally applicable. In addition, it has been shown that many patients will exhibit a nonspecific rise in antibodies in response to certain antigenic stimuli, confounding the interpretation of serological tests.

Modern science has developed many new techniques, unthought of in the days of Pasteur, to aid laboratorians in this time of need. The needs are for more rapid specific diagnostic tests, obviating the classic waiting period for growth of microorganisms, and for tests that detect antigens of pathogens without waiting for an antibody response. This chapter briefly describes several of these new methods in a general sense.

10.1. *Limulus* Amebocyte Lysate Assay

Within the hemolymph (bloodlike circulating fluid) of the horseshoe crab, *Limulus polyphemus*, are numerous circulating cells called **amebocytes.** It was found by Levin and Bang in 1964 that the lysate of these amebocytes would gel in the presence of minute amounts of **lipopolysaccharide** (**endotoxin**) from the cell walls of gram-negative bacteria. The role that endotoxin plays in the pathogenesis of infections caused by gram-negative bacilli is discussed in Chapter 14. The test for gelation of this material, known as the *Limulus* amebocyte lysate (LAL) assay, has been used by industry to detect gram-negative bacterial contamination in a wide range of products, including injectables and other parenterally administered products, and has been modified for use with body fluids from patients to detect circulating endotoxin, a tangible sign of gram-negative bacterial infection. The gelation of the lysate is specific for endotoxin and sensitive to <0.1 ng of endotoxin per milliliter. Kits for performing the test, including special endotoxin-free tubes and diluent, are commercially available (Appendix). The lysate is provided lyophilized. After addition of diluent, a measured amount of the fluid to be tested is added and the lysate solution is incubated for ½-4 h at 37° C in a water bath. The presence of any gel indicates that endotoxin was present in the sample and the strength of the gel is related to the concentration of endotoxin.

Fluids that have been tested by the LAL include cerebrospinal fluid, plasma and serum, joint fluid, urine, and cervical and urethral discharge from patients with gonorrhea. The LAL test, however, has not been widely adopted in clinical microbiology laboratories. Problems of nonspecific positive reactions, particularly with plasma, serum, and other sterile body fluids, have precluded its routine use in most situations. Performance of the LAL assay requires meticulous attention to technique, as any contaminating endotoxin (such as is found in almost all tap water and often in washed glassware) will yield a false-positive result. Whether the LAL test can be adapted for rapid and accurate clinical testing has not been determined.

10.2. Particle Agglutination

10.2.a. Latex agglutination. Antibody molecules can be bound in a random alignment to the surface of latex beads (Figure 10.1). Since the number of antibody molecules bound to each latex particle is large, the potential number of antigen binding sites exposed is also large. If antigen is present in a solution being tested, the antigen will bind to the combining sites of the antibody exposed on the surfaces of the latex beads, forming cross-linked aggregates of latex beads and antigen. The large size of the latex bead enhances the ease with which the agglutination reaction is recognized. The pH, osmolarity, and ionic concentration of the solution will influence the amount of binding that occurs, so that conditions under which latex agglutination procedures are carried out must be carefully standardized. Additionally, many constituents of body fluids have been found to cause false positive agglutination in the latex agglutination systems available. To counteract this problem, it is recommended that all specimens be pretreated with ethylene

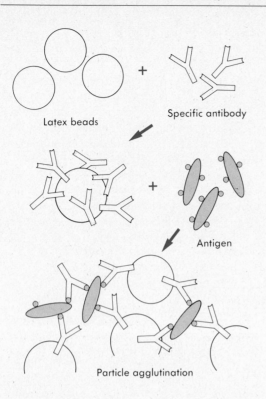

Latex beads

Specific antibody

Antigen

Particle agglutination

FIGURE 10.1
Alignment of antibody molecules bound to the surface of a latex particle and latex agglutination reaction.

diamine tetraacetic acid (EDTA) to extract the antigen before testing, as suggested for cerebrospinal fluid and outlined in Chapter 15. A similar pretreatment protocol is included as a standard step in the procedure in some of the commercial systems. Commercial systems should be used intact, following the manufacturer's recommendations, to insure accurate results. Either a solid, particulate antigen, such as whole bacteria, or soluble antigen, such as capsular polysaccharide, can cause particle agglutination. Microorganisms or their antigenic determinants for which commercial latex agglutination reagents are available include *Haemophilus influenzae* type b, *Neisseria meningitidis*, *N. gonorrhoeae*, *Streptococcus pneumoniae*, *S. pyogenes*, *S. agalactiae*, other beta hemolytic streptococci, *Staphylococcus aureus*, and *Cryptococcus neoformans*. The individual products are discussed in those chapters that deal with the organisms being sought, particu-

larly Chapters 15 and 25. A latex test for the detection of *Clostridium difficile* enterotoxin in stool supernatant is available from Marion Scientific.

Several companies have marketed systems for the detection of antigen of group A beta hemolytic streptococci directly in material on a throat swab. The swabs are treated with an extraction fluid to dissolve the antigen in a liquid suspension. The liquid is then added to the antibody-coated latex reagent; agglutination indicates that the antigen was present in the throat of the patient in some concentration. The specificity of these tests for streptococcal pharyngitis has been reported to be quite high (Chapter 16), although the results vary according to the reference procedure used for comparison. Latex agglutination products are also available for the detection of antibodies to streptococcal structural and extracellularly released antigens, as discussed in Chapters 12 and 25.

FIGURE 10.2
Coagglutination.

10.2.b. Coagglutination. Similar to latex agglutination, coagglutination utilizes antibody bound to a particle to enhance visibility of the agglutination reaction between antigen and antibody. In this case, the particles are killed and treated *S. aureus* organisms (Cowan I strain), which contain a large amount of an antibody-binding protein, **protein A,** in their cell walls. In contrast to latex particles, these staphylococci bind only the base of the heavy chain portion of the antibody, leaving both antigen binding ends free to form complexes with specific antigen (Figure 10.2). Several commercial suppliers have prepared coagglutination reagents for identification of streptococci, including Lancefield groups A, B, C, D, F, and G, *S. pneumoniae, N. meningitidis, N. gonorrhoeae,* and *Haemophilus influenzae* types b, a, and c-f, as detailed in Chapters 15 and 25. The coagglutination reaction is highly specific, but may not be as sensitive for detecting small quanti-

ties of antigen in cerebrospinal fluid as latex agglutination.

10.2.c. Liposome-enhanced latex agglutination. One commercial supplier (Cooper Biomedical Co.) has made use of the ability of phospholipid molecules to form small closed vesicles under certain controlled conditions. These vesicles, consisting of a single lipid bilayer, are called **liposomes.** Reactive chemical groups and other molecules can be bound to the surface of the liposomes, which can then act as agglutinating particles in a reaction. By combining liposomes containing reactive molecules on their surfaces and latex particles that harbor antibody binding sites on their surfaces, reagents are created that transform a rather weak antigen-antibody particle agglutination reaction into a stronger, more easily visualized reaction. The liposomes can change shape to present the greatest surface area (and binding sites) to the latex particles. This test is diagrammed in Chapter 12 (Figure 12.6) and can be seen in detail there.

10.3. Countercurrent Immunoelectrophoresis (CIE)

With some exceptions (such as *S. pneumoniae* serotypes 7 and 14), most bacterial antigens are negatively charged in a slightly alkaline environment, while antibodies are neutral. This principle is exploited by CIE assays, in which solutions of antibody and body fluid to be tested are placed in small wells cut into a slab of agarose (a gelatinlike matrix through which molecules can diffuse readily) on a glass surface (Figure 10.3). Since several wells can be cut in one agarose slab, small portions of a single body fluid specimen may be tested against several different antibodies. A paper or fiber wick is used to connect the two opposite sides of the agarose to troughs of buffer, carefully formulated for each antibody-antigen system. When an electric current is applied through the buffer, the negatively charged antigen molecules (if they are present) migrate toward the positive electrode and thus toward the wells on the other side of the slab. The neutrally charged antibodies are carried toward the negative electrode by the flow of the slightly alkaline buffer. At some point between the wells a zone of equivalence occurs, and the antigen-an-

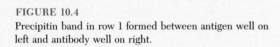

FIGURE 10.3
Apparatus for performing counterimmunoelectrophoresis.

FIGURE 10.4
Precipitin band in row 1 formed between antigen well on left and antibody well on right.

tibody complexes form a visible precipitin band (Figure 10.4). The entire procedure usually takes about 1 h.

Any antigens for which antisera are available can be tested by CIE. The sensitivity appears to be about the same as that of coagglutination, detecting approximately 0.01-0.05 mg antigen per milliliter, which translates to about 10^3 organisms per milliliter of fluid. Bands are often difficult to see, and the agarose gel may require overnight washing in distilled water to remove nonspecific precipitin reactions. Testing positive and negative controls is especially critical, since sera may contain nonspecifically reacting agents that form nonstable complexes in the gel. CIE is more expensive (because of the initial capital outlay and the large quantities of antigen and antibody that must be used) than either latex particle agglutination or coagglutination.

10.4. Enzyme-Linked Immunosorbent Assay (ELISA)

The principles of ELISA systems were first explored during the 1960s by investigators searching for a substitute for radioimmunoassay procedures, which required radioisotope-labeled substrates and an elaborate instrument for counting radioactive emissions (discussed in Chapter 11). The basic ELISA detection system consists of antibodies bonded to enzymes that remain able to catalyze a reaction that yields a visually discernible endproduct while attached to the antibody. Furthermore, the antibody binding sites remain free to react with their specific antigen. The use of enzymes as labels has several advantages. The enzyme itself is not changed during activity; it can catalyze the reaction of a large number of substrate molecules, greatly expanding the reaction and thus enhancing the possibility of detection. Enzyme conjugated substrates are quite stable, unlike radioactive substrates, and can be stored for relatively long time periods. Additionally, the formation of a colored endproduct allows direct observation of the reaction or measurement with a simple instrument.

Most ELISA systems developed for detection of infectious agents consist of antibody directed against the agent in question firmly fixed to a solid matrix, either the inside of the wells of a microdilution tray or the outside of a spherical plastic or metal bead, or some other solid matrix. Such systems are called **solid phase immunosorbent assays (SPIA)**. If antigen is present in the fluid to be tested, stable antigen-antibody complexes form when the fluid is added to the matrix. Washing steps to remove nonspecifically adsorbed molecules are very important in ELISA tests. A second antibody against the antigen being sought is then added to the system. This antibody has been complexed to an enzyme, such as alkaline phosphatase or horseradish peroxidase, that catalyzes a reaction that yields a colored endpoint. If the antigen is present on the solid matrix, it will now bind the second antibody, forming a sandwich with antigen in the middle. After washing has removed unbound labeled antibody, the addition of the substrates for the enzyme completes the reaction, and the visually detectable endpoint will appear wherever the enzyme is present (Figure 10.5). Because of the expanding nature of the reaction, even minute amounts of antigen (<1 ng antigen/ml) can be detected. The system just described requires a specific enzyme-labeled antibody for each antigen tested. It is simpler to use an indirect assay that uses a second unlabeled antibody to bind to the antigen-antibody complex on the matrix. A third antibody, labeled with enzyme and directed against the nonvariable F_c portion of the unlabeled second antibody, can then be used as the detection marker for a number of different antigen-antibody complexes.

Although this simplified explanation may serve as a guideline, there are many other aspects of ELISA testing to consider. Excellent discussions of methodology and possible future developments are presented by Yolken.[2,3] The

FIGURE 10.5
Principle of solid-phase enzyme immunosorbent assay.

use of monoclonal antibodies (described below) has helped increase the sensitivity of currently available ELISA assays, but many infectious agents including viruses, bacteria, fungi, and *Mycoplasma*, are still not efficiently detected by ELISA. Systems commercially available and gaining acceptance for routine diagnostic testing include those for detection of rotavirus, hepatitis B antigens, *N. gonorrhoeae* antigens in swabs from genital sites, *Chlamydia trachomatis* in swabs from eyes and genital sites, Epstein-Barr virus antigens, respiratory syncytial virus, and adenoviruses. Because ELISA assays still require several hours, they are not the systems of choice when extremely rapid results are required, as for specific diagnosis of meningitis. Development of more sensitive assay systems will enhance the speed and utility of ELISA testing and greatly expand the number of agents that can be reliably detected with this technology. Although some ELISA tests are developed for visual reading of results, most systems rely on automated spectrophotometric reading of endpoints. The instruments used for such readings are discussed in Chapter 11.

10.5. Monoclonal Antibodies: Preparation and Utilization

One of the largest drawbacks to any of the systems that utilize antibodies as reagents has been the requirement for large quantities of rather pure, high avidity, high affinity antibody molecules. Previous technologies thus required immunization of either many small animals or several large animals with the antigen being sought, repeated bleedings, and subsequent purification of the antigen elicited. Different animals reacted with different antibody responses to the same antigen, resulting in a lack of uniform reagents and the necessity to continually retest the antibody for reactivity in a given system. Additionally, some antigens, such as *N. meningitidis* group B, were poor immunogens, and good antibodies were impossible to obtain in any quantity.

The ability to create an immortal cell line, producing large quantities of a completely characterized and highly specific antibody, known as a **monoclonal antibody,** has revolutionized the science of immunologic testing. Monoclonal antibodies are produced by the daughter cells (clones) of a single hybrid cell, the product of fusion of an antibody-producing lymphocyte and an immortal malignant antibody-producing lymphocyte cell. One technique for the production of such a clone of cells, called **hybridoma cells,** is illustrated in Figure 10.6. A mouse is immunized with the antigen for which an antibody is to be created. The animal responds by producing many antibodies to the antigenic determinants injected. The mouse's spleen, which contains antibody-producing plasma cells, is removed and emulsified so that single antibody-producing cells can be separated and placed into individual wells of a microdilution tray. These cells cannot remain viable in cell culture for very long. They must be fused together with cells that are able to survive and multiply in tissue culture, the immortal cells of a **myeloma** (malignant tumor of antibody-producing plasma cells). The special myeloma tumor cells used for hybridoma production possess a very important defect, however. They are deficient in the enzyme hypoxanthine phosphoribosyltransferase. This defect leads to their inability to survive in a medium containing hypoxanthine, aminopterin, and thymidine (HAT medium). Antibody-producing spleen cells, however, possess the enzyme. Thus, fused hybridoma cells survive in the selective medium and can be recognized by their ability to grow indefinitely in the medium. Unfused antibody-producing lymphoid cells will die after several multiplications in vitro because they are not immortal, and unfused myeloma cells will die in the presence of the toxic enzyme substrates. The only surviving cells will be true "hybrids." The growth medium supernatant from the microdilution tray wells in which the hybridoma cells are

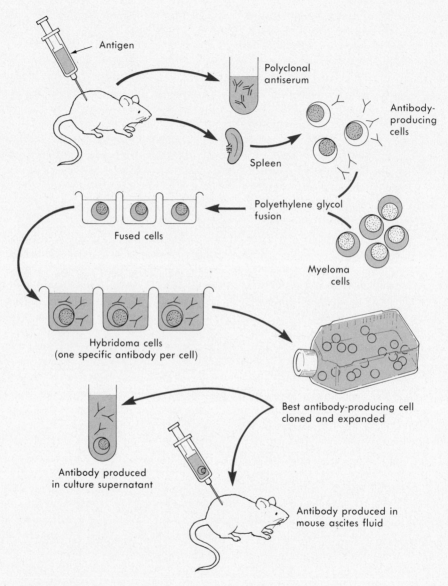

FIGURE 10.6
Production of a monoclonal antibody.

growing is then tested for the presence of the desired antibody. Many such cell lines are usually examined before a suitable antibody is found, since it must be specific enough to bind only the type of antigen to be tested, but not so specific that it binds only the antigen from the particular strain with which the mouse was first immunized. When a good candidate antibody-producing cell is found, the hybridoma cells are either cultured in large numbers in cell cultures in vitro, or they are reinjected into the peritoneal cavities of many mice, where the cells multiply and produce large quantities of antibody in the ascitic fluid that is formed. Ascitic fluid can be removed from mice many times over the animal's lifetime. Since all of the cells are derived from a single cell producing one antibody molecule type, the antibody is called **monoclonal.**

Monoclonal antibodies have been successfully used in commercial systems for the detection of certain infectious agents. For example, a monoclonal antibody to a protein of *C. trachomatis* has been conjugated to a fluorochrome dye, allowing the visual detection, under fluorescence microscopy, of the elementary bodies and inclusions present in clinical material from patients infected with chlamydiae (see Chapter 38). Monoclonal antibodies to the *N. meningitidis* group B capsular polysaccharide have been bound to latex particles to create a reagent that can detect the presence of this organism in cerebrospinal fluid, urine, and other body fluids. Many other commercial products utilizing monoclonal antibodies are being developed.

10.6. Genetic Probes: Preparation and Utilization

Even more specific than antibody reagents are nucleic acid probes, discrete sequences of single-stranded DNA or RNA that form strong covalently bonded hybrids with the specific complementary strand of nucleic acid. Methods are available that allow isolation of nucleic acid sequences from cultures of clones of a known bacterial species that constitute a single gene or locus, specific for the whole species or a gene that is common to all pathogenic organisms within the species. An example of a method for preparation of a DNA probe for a segment of the chromosome of a virus is illustrated in Figure 10.7. The chromosomal nucleic acid from a prototype virus is released by lysing the virions. Bacterial endonuclease restriction enzymes are used to cut the DNA into small segments, which are inserted into a circular strand of plasmid DNA. The plasmid has been chosen for its ability to multiply to large numbers once it has entered the cytoplasm of its bacterial host cell. The expanded plasmids are released from the bacteria and isolated based on their molecular weight and charge. The particular fragments of DNA that match that found in the virus are then isolated by using the same restriction endonucleases, purified, and labeled with either a **radioisotope** (often ^{32}P) or **biotin,** a small molecule that can be covalently bound to the DNA without destroying its ability to hybridize with complementary DNA. The biotinylation method of labeling nucleic acid probes was developed as recently as 1981 by Langer et al.[1] Bacterial or eukaryotic organism nucleic acid can be isolated and cloned as well.

The material to be tested (either a culture of unknown microorganism or clinical material that may contain the organisms being sought) is affixed to a solid matrix, usually some sort of filter. After the material suspected of containing the gene or nucleic acid sequence being sought has been applied, the filter is treated to render the double-stranded DNA single-stranded. The probe, a small piece of labeled single-stranded DNA, is then allowed to react with the material on the filter. If complementary sequences are present, the probe DNA will form strong bonds and remain on the filter, even when the filter is washed extensively to remove unbound DNA and nonspecifically

Virus

Free viral DNA

Restriction
endonuclease
treatment

Insert desired
fragment into
plasmid vector

Plasmid multiplies
in bacterial host

Plasmids isolated

DNA probe fragment
purified

Avidin

Biotin

or

DNA probes labeled

Fragments dissociated
into single-stranded

FIGURE 10.7
Production of a radioactive or biotin-avidin labeled single-stranded nucleic acid probe for a specific
segment of DNA from a specific virus. The isolated viral DNA is inserted into a plasmid vector, which
is expanded by multiplication within a bacterial host.

bound DNA (Figure 10.8). The labeled DNA probe is now treated to allow visualization (Figure 10.9). If the label is radioactive, the filter is covered with a piece of film; the film develops a dark spot wherever the bound probe is present on the filter underneath. In the case of biotin-labeled probes, a second protein, avidin, which binds tightly to biotin, is added to the matrix. Avidin can be attached to a number of different marker materials, including enzymes such as horseradish peroxidase, alkaline phosphatase, fluorescent dyes, radioisotope-labeled molecules, or electron-dense markers like ferritin. Thus the exact location of the bound DNA probe can be determined by the visualization of the avidin-bound marker. Plate 10.1 illustrates the use of a biotin-avidin-horseradish peroxidase probe used to detect the antigen of herpes simplex virus in infected cells on a filter.

Advantages of the nucleic acid probe systems include the ability of the DNA probe to detect sequences among a mixture of many other genes and molecules, the stability of DNA (allowing the material to remain on the filter for a long period before the test must be performed) and the ability of the probe to detect DNA from nonviable material. For example, a drop of fecal material may be placed on a filter, allowed to dry, and the filter then can be carried or mailed to a distant laboratory for testing at some future date. Conversely, because growth is not necessary, the material can be tested immediately. The biotin-avidin system obviates the need for radioactive materials, but it is not as sensitive. Many workers are actively seeking ways to improve this technology. Gen-Probe has developed a new approach utilizing ribosomal RNA detection that has significantly increased sensitivity and speed, can give quantitative results, and does not require a solid matrix for testing. A currently available

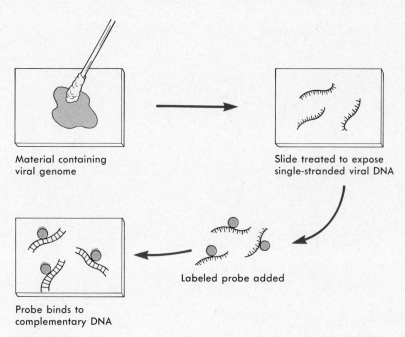

Material containing
viral genome

Slide treated to expose
single-stranded viral DNA

Labeled probe added

Probe binds to
complementary DNA

FIGURE 10.8
Detecting genetic material using a labeled nucleic acid probe.

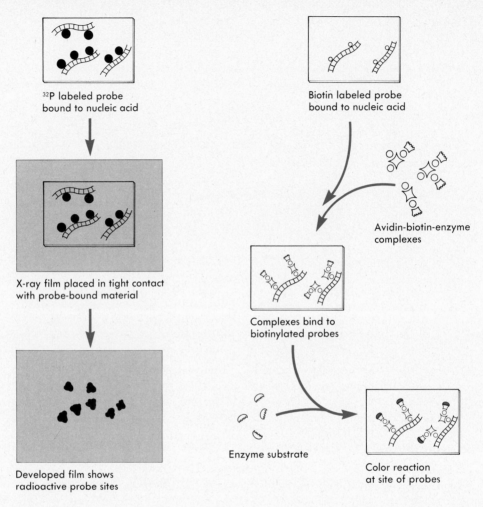

FIGURE 10.9
Detection of labeled nucleic acid probe using radiography or colorimetric enzymatic detection system.

commercial system (Enzo Patho-Gene, Enzo Biochem) can detect DNA sequences of herpes simplex viruses I and II, cytomegalovirus, hepatitis B virus, Epstein-Barr virus, adenovirus, and *Chlamydia* species, making use of biotin-avidin-horseradish peroxidase labeling techniques.

10.7. DNA-DNA Hybridization (Figure 10.10)

Another development that utilizes much of the same technology as that described above for genetic probes is DNA or nucleic acid hybrid-

ization. Used primarily to determine the relatedness of two different bacterial clones, this method exploits the ability of single-stranded DNA to bind to complementary sequences. Clones from a single colony of a known bacterium are grown in a medium containing radiolabeled substrates that are incorporated into the bacterial DNA during growth. These known bacteria are then lysed to release their DNA, which is treated with endonucleases to cleave it into small fragments. These fragments are then heated or chemically treated to cause

FIGURE 10.10

DNA-DNA hybridization to determine the amount of relatedness between the genomes of two bacterial clones.

them to dissociate and become single-stranded. The bacteria to be compared to the known strain are cloned, cultured in unlabeled media, and attached to a filter matrix and treated so that their double-stranded DNA also dissociates into single strands. The known labeled fragments of single-stranded DNA are allowed to react with the DNA of the unknown strain on the filter, and unbound DNA is washed off. The labeled DNA pieces will bind (or hybridize) only to DNA that is an exact match, so the amount of labeled DNA left on the filter after washing will define how closely related the genetic material of the two strains are. If both clones are derived from the same original colony, there should be 100% relatedness. Workers have defined a species as those bacteria with very similar morphologic and biochemical characteristics that exhibit ≥ 70% genetic relatedness by DNA-DNA hybridization.

10.8. Future Uses of New Technology

DNA hybridization technology has been used extensively to determine the relatedness of bacterial clones. It is in this manner that many species of bacteria have been characterized and given new designations. For the first time, the relatedness of two biochemically similar bacterial groups can be determined at the genetic level. As a consequence, several historically characterized species have been broken down into many different new species, such as some groups within the genus *Enterobacter*, and other species have been combined (for example, all *Salmonella* species have been shown to be so closely related genetically that they belong to a single species). By using these new tools, scientists will probably redefine many of the bacterial taxa that are familiar to microbiologists and physicians. It is likely that confusion over nomenclature will continue for many years to come.

By using the technological methods described above, either singly or in combination, microbiologists will be able to diagnose many infections without the time-consuming requirement of culturing the pathogen in the laboratory. The development of nucleic acid probes for gene-size sequences of DNA and the ability to create infinite amounts of antibody of great specificity offer to students of infectious diseases the promise of exquisitely sensitive and specific reagents. It is currently possible to detect the presence of the gene that codes for resistance to a particular antibiotic in nonviable bacteria that have been affixed to a filter. Even the ability of certain colonies of bacteria to produce a particular toxin can be detected with DNA probe methods. Additional commercial systems for applications such as those mentioned here will be available in the near future.

Immunologic reagents of very good sensitivity can be developed by binding monoclonal antibodies to particles for agglutination. These techniques are also rapid, since there is no requirement for attachment of the antigen to a matrix. In the case of ELISA assays, the use of monoclonal antibody reagents allows testing of specific small antigens, such that two closely related pathogens may be differentiated. The future of microbiology is certain to include a large number of non-growth-dependent rapid testing methods for the presence of pathogens in clinical specimens. Many of these methods will make use of the technological breakthroughs described above, often combined with instruments to further automate the processes, as discussed in Chapter 11. Microbiologists, who have traditionally taken great pride in the fact that their judgment and interpretation are still necessary for laboratory diagnosis of infectious diseases, will have to learn to trust results obtained by nontraditional approaches, sacrificing the satisfaction of seeing colonies and cytopathic effect for the worthwhile goal of better patient care through more rapid diagnosis. However, there will always be a place for traditional microbiology.

REFERENCES

1. Langer, P.R., Waldrop, A.A., and Ward, D.C. 1981. Enzymatic synthesis of biotin-labeled polynucleotides: novel nucleic acid affinity probes. Proc. Natl. Acad. Sci. 78:6633.
2. Yolken, R.H. 1982. Enzyme immunoassays for the detection of infectious antigens in body fluids: current limitations and future prospects. Rev. Infect. Dis. 4:35.
3. Yolken, R.H. 1985. Solid-phase enzyme immunoassays for the detection of microbial antigens in body fluids. In Lennette, E.H., Balows, A., Hausler, W.J. Jr., and Shadomy, H.J., editors. Manual of clinical microbiology, ed. 4. American Society for Microbiology, Washington, D.C.

BIBLIOGRAPHY

Berry, A.J., and Peter, J.B. 1984. DNA probes for infectious disease. Diagn. Med. 7:62.
Conway de Macario, E., and Macario, A.J.L. 1983. Monoclonal antibodies for bacterial identification and taxonomy. Am. Soc. Microbiol. News 49:1.
Kaplan, S.L. 1983. Antigen detection in cerebrospinal fluid—pros and cons. Am. J. Med. 75(suppl. 1B):109.
McCarthy, L.R. 1983. The impact of new technology on clinical microbiology. Clin. Microbiol. Newsletter 5:68.
Olsiewski, P.J., Thalenfeld, B.E., and Engelhardt, D.L. 1984. Applications of nonradioactive DNA probe technology. Am. Clin. Prod. Rev. October, 1984.
Tenover, F.C. 1985. DNA probes for infectious diseases. Clin. Microbiol. Newsletter 7:105.
Tompkins, L.S. 1985. DNA methods in clinical microbiology. In Lennette, E.H., Balows, A., Hausler, W.J. Jr., and Shadomy, H.J., editors. Manual of clinical microbiology, ed. 4. American Society for Microbiology, Washington, D.C.

11 Principles of Automated Methods for Diagnostic Microbiology

Since Isenberg et al. pioneered the development of an automated system for antimicrobial susceptibility testing in the 1960s,[3] the acceptance and utilization of instrumentation for clinical microbiology have become realities. More than one third of all hospital microbiology laboratories now use a radiometric method (Bactec, Johnston Laboratories) for detecting positive blood cultures. Many other instruments for the identification and susceptibility testing of microorganisms, the detection of antigens and microbial products in human clinical material, and the measurement of antimicrobial agents in body fluids are being used in laboratories throughout the United States and Europe. Some of the more commonly used instruments with applications directly related to diagnostic microbiology are mentioned in this chapter. Since the field is expanding so rapidly, there will be many more automated systems available by the time this book is published. In addition to outlining the principles employed by some of the new microbiology instruments, we will mention some of the promising new directions that are being explored for diagnosis of infectious diseases.

11.1. Basic Principles Employed by Common Automated Systems for Detection and Identification of Viable Pathogens

11.1.a. Turbidity as an indicator of growth. Pasteur initially made use of the fact that microbes would multiply in liquid medium until their presence could be detected visually as an increase in turbidity. Turbidity is actually the ability of particles in suspension to refract and deflect light rays passing through the suspension, such that the light is reflected back into the eyes of the observer. Some of the instruments that measure turbidity determine the **optical density (OD)**, a measurement of turbidity, by comparing the amount of light that passes through the suspension (the percent transmittance) to the amount of light passing through a control suspension without particles. A photoelectric sensor, or photometer, converts the light that impinges on its surface to an electrical impulse, which can be quantified. A second type of turbidity measurement is obtained by **nephelometry**, or **light scatter.** In this case, the photometers are placed at angles to the suspension, and the scattered light, generated by a laser or incandescent bulb, is measured. The amount of light scattered is dependent on the number and size of the particles in

suspension. Turbidity measurements are used to determine whether an organism is present in a clinical specimen (such as in the detection of clinically significant urinary tract infections by the MS-2 and Avantage instruments of Abbott Laboratories, the AutoMicrobic System of Vitek Systems, and the Autobac IDX of General Diagnostics) or to determine whether a particular strain of bacterium or yeast can grow in the presence of specific growth inhibitors, including antimicrobial agents. In the case of the Autobac IDX, the substrates are introduced into medium in cuvettes by elution from filter paper disks; the other systems use lyophilized substrates. Most automated susceptibility testing systems make use of turbidometric or nephelometric measurements of growth. Table 11.1 lists the automated systems most commonly used for detection of microbial growth.

For measurement of turbidity of a suspension to be accurate, the particles must either remain in suspension or must be agitated before measurement if the photometers are aimed horizontally. Automated systems that utilize turbidity measurements usually must include an automated agitation device. The Autobac IDX, Avantage, and MS-2 systems, all of which use cuvettes containing growth medium,

TABLE 11.1
Automated Microbiology Systems that Measure Growth or Metabolism

PRINCIPLE	APPLICATION(S)	INSTRUMENT(S)
Nephelometry or colorimetry (cuvettes)	1. Growth detection 2. Identification 3. Susceptibilities	Autobac IDX-C (General Diagnostics) AutoMicrobic System (Vitek Systems) MS-2 (Abbott Laboratories) Uniscept (Analytab Products)
Nephelometry or colorimetry (microdilution format)	1. Identification 2. Susceptibilities	Micro-Coder I (Micro-Media Systems) MicroScan (MicroScan) Pasco (Difco Laboratories) Precept (Austin Biological Laboratories) Sceptor (BBL Microbiology Systems) Sensititre (Gibco Laboratories)
Video image analysis (cuvettes)	1. Identification 2. Susceptibilities	Aladin (Analytab Products)

utilize an incubator-shaker module. Another way to circumvent the problem is to measure the turbidity in the medium from the bottom. Those susceptibility testing systems that employ microdilution plates have adopted this method (Table 11.1). For example, the MicroScan system uses fiberoptics to deliver an equal amount of light to the bottom of each microdilution well; the light transmitted is determined by photometric measurements from above (Figure 11.1). Other systems may use a single light source and move all wells of the microdilution plate through its path.

Certain systems quantitate the number of microorganisms in the specimen by turbidity measurements. The AutoMicrobic System (Vitek Systems) for example, pulls body fluid such as urine into the growth wells on a plastic card (Plate 11.1) by suction (another instrument is necessary to fill the cards). The wells are arranged in such a way that the body fluid is serially diluted as it fills successive wells. After a relatively short incubation period, the turbidity in the wells is measured and compared to wells containing no growth substances. The ability of an organism to grow in only certain wells is then used to determine the number of colony-forming units (CFU) present in the initial specimen. Susceptibilities can be determined by inoculating a suspension of the isolated organism into a second card of antimicrobial agent-containing wells and measuring turbidity after incubation. A classic 1975 paper by Thornsberry et al.[6] describes parameters to examine in evaluating an automated susceptibility testing system.

11.1.b. Colorimetric determinations for microbial identification. Several systems use a modification of conventional biochemical testing (Chapter 9) that relies on the color changes of pH indicators in media to indicate the presence of metabolic endproducts. The change in wavelength of light transmitted through the growth cuvette or well is measured by a photoelectric cell. Detection of microbial metabolism by measuring colored endproducts or indicators is called **colorimetry.** AutoMicrobic System cards with growth substance–containing wells are inoculated with clinical specimens (primarily urine) or bacterial or yeast suspensions made from pure cultures for identification. The overnight-incubation UniScept Plus API system utilizes color changes that indicate substrate utilization in plastic cuvettes, a small-volume modification of conventional biochemical testing. Makers of identification and susceptibility microdilution systems (such as MicroScan) have chosen to place turbidity and colorimetry determination tests on the same tray. Other manufacturers, including those of Micro-Coder I (Micro-Media Systems), Sceptor (BBL Microbiology Systems), Pasco (Difco

FIGURE 11.1
Diagram of delivery of light to microdilution wells by fiberoptics, as utilized by MicroCoder identification and susceptibility testing system (MicroScan).

Laboratories), Precept (Austin Biological Laboratories), and Sensititre (Gibco Laboratories) provide separate trays for identification and susceptibility testing. Table 11.1 contains a partial list of systems that use automated measurement of turbidity or color change for microbial growth detection, identification, or susceptibility testing.

In addition to the instrumentation required for automatic reading of results, several of these systems require a rehydrating apparatus. API 3600, Sensititre, and Sceptor systems (Table 11.1) are distributed dry, which increases shelf life and allows room-temperature storage. Dry panels, however, must be rehydrated, a task that is easily automated but that requires another instrument.

11.1.c. Detection of microbial growth by measuring radioactive metabolites. The Bactec system (Johnston Laboratories) measures the production of radioactive carbon dioxide gas by organisms that metabolize ^{14}C-labeled substrates (glucose, amino acids, and alcohols). Blood (or sterile body fluid) for routine culture is inoculated into bottles that contain the labeled substrates. The media are agitated, preferably on a rotary shaker (also supplied by the manufacturer) during a preliminary incubation period. At predetermined time intervals thereafter, the bottles are placed into the monitoring module (Figure 11.2), where they are automatically moved past a detector. The detector inserts two needles through a rubber septum seal at the top of each bottle (Figure 11.3) and draws out the gas which has accumulated above the liquid medium, replacing this headspace gas with fresh gas of the same mixture (aerobic or anaerobic). If metabolism of the labeled substrates has occurred, ^{14}CO$_2$ will be detected as it passes through an ionization chamber. Any level of radiation (above a preset baseline that accounts for the metabolism of cellular elements in the blood) is considered to be suspicious for microbial growth. The computerized data-handling section of the instrument will light a red indicator light on a front panel as it detects bottles with radioactivity above a certain level and will automatically print out the

FIGURE 11.2
A technologist places blood culture bottles containing radioactive substrates on the Bactec instrument (Johnston Laboratories).

FIGURE 11.3
The detector module of the Bactec instrument, in which gas above the medium is removed and measured for radioactivity and fresh gas is substituted.

values of relative radiation detected in the headspace of each bottle. The microbiologist then retrieves the suspicious bottles and continues processing (as described in Chapter 14).

Modifications of the basic principle have increased the capabilities of the Bactec system. Currently, more than 100 laboratories use the instrument to identify pathogenic *Neisseria* species. Labeled substrates that are utilized by only one species of *Neisseria* are incorporated into special media. After 3 h incubation, the organism can be identified by its ability to utilize the appropriate substrate, producing measurable $^{14}CO_2$. In addition, the instrument has been used successfully to detect the presence of *Mycobacterium tuberculosis* and other mycobacteria in clinical specimens. Sterile body fluids are inoculated directly, and urine and sputum specimens are inoculated after decontamination and concentration into Bactec bottles containing ^{14}C-labeled growth factors utilized only by mycobacteria. Detection of products of metabolism of these substrates by mycobacteria may be possible within 10 days of inoculation. Because of certain technical considerations, it is still recommended that standard cultures on solid media be inoculated along with Bactec cultures. If growth is detected radiometrically, a subculture from the initial medium into a second medium that contains *p*-nitro-alpha-acetyl-beta-hydroxy-propiophenone (NAP) can differentiate *M. tuberculosis* and *M. bovis*, which are susceptible to the agent, from other mycobacteria, which exhibit radiometric evidence of growth within 3 days. Mycobacterial susceptibility testing has also been performed acceptably using the radiometric Bactec system; this provides results more rapidly than conventional methods. The use of the Bactec instrument for mycobacteriology is discussed further in Chapter 41.

The original Bactec included very little computerized data management and required that laboratories use radioactive substances, which are difficult to discard in many localities

and to which technologists object. In the newest modifications of the system, a computerized data handling and retrieval system has been incorporated that greatly simplifies the daily maintenance and handling of cultures. A second and more major change involves the substitution of infrared detection for radiometric detection of gaseous metabolic endproducts, obviating the handling problems associated with radioisotopes. These modifications should add to the practicality of this instrument. The overall detection of positive cultures by the infrared device is statistically equivalent to that of the radiometric method.

11.1.d. Bioluminescence assays for viable organisms. The glowing cold light produced in firefly tails is the endproduct of a chemical reaction, the conversion of the substrate luciferin to oxyluciferin and light, catalyzed by the enzyme luciferase, and driven by the dephosphorylation of adenosine triphosphate (ATP). The light generated by this reaction can be measured directly with a **luminometer,** similar to a photometer. The amount of light (measured in photons) produced by the reaction taking place in an excess of luciferin is directly proportional to the amount of ATP present in the solution. Unlike a photometric system, however, there is no need for an exogenous light source. ATP is present within all living cells, and by selectively releasing the ATP from bacterial cells only, the number of colony forming units in a clinical specimen can be estimated. At least three systems have employed this principle for screening urine specimens for bacteria: the Lumac Bacteriuria Screening System (3M Medical Products), the Monolight (Analytical Luminescence Laboratory), and the Turner Luminescent System (Turner Designs). The Lumac system is unavailable for clinical microbiology laboratories at this writing, although modifications are being explored. These systems require several steps, including the lysis of somatic cells to release nonbacterial ATP and the subsequent lysis of bacteria and measurement of the resulting bacterial ATP. The Lumac and Turner systems measure bacterial ATP after a short incubation period, whereas the Monolight assays the bacterial ATP directly. In any case, those urines without evidence of bacteria in counts above a certain number can be immediately reported out as negative at the threshold level predetermined by the system. These systems have shown excellent correlation to culture methods when 10^5 CFU/ml is chosen as the threshold number above which a urine is considered to be positive (and thus must be plated). It should be noted that in certain types of urinary tract infection a threshold of 10^2 CFU/ml is appropriate; the luminescent systems currently available would not be satisfactory for screening urines in this category.

11.1.e. Colorimetric particle detection for urine screening. One of the newest technologies developed to rapidly determine whether a urine specimen contains significant numbers of bacteria is the Bac-T-Screen Bacteriuria Detection Device (Figure 11.4; Marion Scientific). With this system, a measured amount of urine is drawn through a paper filter by vacuum suction. Particles such as bacteria and white blood cells adhere to the filter while crystals and nonsignificant particles are washed through. A stain is then passed through the filter imparting color, the depth of which is dependent on the number of stainable particles (Figure 11.5). The filter paper is then manually inserted into another section of the instrument, where a photometer compares the color to a preset standard. The filter may also be examined visually. Urines that stain at a level below the control can be considered negative and need not be plated. At a threshold of 10^5 CFU/ml, this system compares very well with conventional plating. Some laboratories have reported problems with clogging and a small percentage of false negatives.

Individual considerations such as patient

FIGURE 11.4
The Bac-T-Screen bacteriuria detection device (Marion Scientific).

population, budget constraints, need for rapid results, and many other factors (including the 10^2 CFU/ml threshold mentioned above) will determine whether a laboratory can benefit from any particular automated system for detection of significant urinary tract infections. Other aspects of urinary tract infections, including the appropriate use of screening systems, are discussed in Chapter 18. Considerations that laboratories must face concerning cost containment are discussed in Chapter 4.

11.1.f. Electrical impedance as an indicator of microbial growth. Although systems employing electrical impedance have not been used widely in clinical laboratories, there is a great theoretical advantage to being able to detect the presence of multiplying yeast or bacteria by measuring the changes in the flow of

FIGURE 11.5
A Bac-T-Screen filter through which urine to be tested and stained has been passed. The stain only binds to particles; thus the depth of the red color is indicative of the number of particles (bacteria or leukocytes) in the specimen.

an electric current passing through the medium in which a specimen is being incubated (**impedance changes**). With continuous monitoring, the first sign of impedance change indicating microbial growth could be instantly recorded, unlike most of the other currently available systems that require periodic monitoring with manual or mechanical manipulation. Positive blood cultures, monitored by impedance, could be detected and reported in the middle of the night, without the presence of a technologist. Currently, trials are in progress with impedance devices produced in England by Malthus Instruments and Orbec, Ltd. for monitoring blood and urine specimens for bacteria.

11.1.g. Replica plating system for bacterial identifications and susceptibilities. The replica plating system (Cathra Repliscan II, MCT Diagnostics) makes use of the Steers-Foltz repli-

cator (described in Chapter 13), a device that can deposit a reproducible small inoculum from a suspension of bacteria in a discrete position on the surface of an agar plate. Inocula from approximately 35 separate bacterial suspensions can be deposited on each of any number of agar plates, containing media for assessing substrate utilization as well as agar dilution susceptibilities (described in Chapter 13). By recording, storing, and interpreting the results with computer-assisted data systems, technologists can perform rapid and cost-effective identifications and susceptibilities; this will be useful primarily for laboratories that must process large numbers of isolates daily.

11.2. Automated Microbiology Support Systems

A number of instruments have been developed to aid microbiologists by automating certain tasks; often such automation increases reproducibility and consistency. For example, an automated agar sterilizer, Petri dish filler, liquid media dispenser, and colony counter are marketed by New Brunswick Scientific Co. Once the medium has been prepared, an automated plate inoculator (Spiral System Instruments) may be used to distribute the inoculum in a spiral pattern, producing isolated colonies near the outer edge. This manufacturer also markets a colony counter that uses computerized data processing.

Several companies produce devices that fill microdilution trays or make serial twofold dilutions in microdilution trays. Systems such as the Dynatech MIC-2000 (Figure 11.6) and the Twelve-way Inoculating Made Easy (T.I.M.E.; Dynatech Laboratories), HandiSpense and automated 96-well microdilution plate filling device (Bellco Glass), and the Pro/Pette (Cetus Corp.) can be used to fill microdilution plates for bacterial susceptibility testing and identification systems or for the new immunoassay methods (described below).

FIGURE 11.6
The Dynatech microdiluter (Dynatech Laboratories) used to make serial two-fold dilutions in microdilution trays.

11.3. Antigen and Microbial Product Detection

In addition to identifying, quantifying, and determining susceptibilities of microorganisms, microbiologists are increasingly diagnosing disease by identifying microbial constituents (antigens) or products of microbial metabolism in specimens obtained from the infected host. Antimicrobial agents with sufficient toxicity to require therapeutic monitoring also require detection and quantitation. Widely used methods that require instrumentation will be described here.

11.3.a. Gas-liquid chromatography. In **gas-liquid chromatography (GLC)** a liquid sample is passed through a matrix that differentially separates its constituents. The volatile components of the sample are carried along with a flow of specially prepared heated gas through a long, narrow **column** packed with resin or some other material that differentially slows down the rate of travel of the components based on their sizes, molecular weights, or charges. As the various components reach the end of the column, their presence is detected by a change in the temperature or ionization potential, and

their relative amounts are plotted on a recording chart as peaks. GLC applications for diagnostic microbiology are increasing. GLC was first used by microbiologists to identify anaerobic bacteria by separating and identifying the metabolic endproducts of carbohydrate fermentation or amino acid degradation. Different species of anaerobic bacteria yield different endproducts or different relative amounts of these endproducts, primarily volatile fatty acids and nonvolatile organic acids. The GLC patterns obtained from culture supernatants are often definitive (further discussed in the anaerobe laboratory manuals by Holdeman et al.[2] and by Sutter et al.[5]). New uses for GLC include the rapid detection of infection involving anaerobic organisms (with information on the specific organisms involved) and the identification of mycobacteria isolated from clinical specimens, such as described by Tisdall and coworkers.[7] Bacterial vaginosis, a nonpurulent infection of the vaginal tract characterized by decreased numbers of lactobacilli and increased numbers of anaerobes, often in concert with *Gardnerella vaginalis* (Chapters 19 and 39), can be diagnosed by detecting an increased ratio of succinic to lactic acid in GLC profiles prepared from vaginal discharge material, as described by Spiegel et al.[4] How much is gained by GLC analysis over diagnosis by clinical and conventional microbiologic means remains to be better defined. Any gas liquid chromatograph instrument can be used for microbiological assays, since the level of sensitivity required is not great. Computers may be used to start and stop the GLC analysis, to control the baseline, and to identify and quantify the peaks representing the various endproducts.

11.3.b. High-performance liquid chromatography. The column packing material in **high-performance liquid chromatography (HPLC)** consists of special resins that bear a number of ion-exchange groups on their surfaces, such that constituents in the sample undergoing HPLC are preferentially retained in the column based on their affinity for the charged ionic groups. Components with the weakest attraction for the resin will flow through the column fastest and **elute** (appear at the other end) first. This process is known as **ion-exchange chromatography,** the same principle as that used to separate IgG from IgM by elution from a column (Chapter 12). HPLC, by using newly developed column packing material, high pressure to force the sample through the column, and liquid buffer carriers at room temperature instead of hot gas, has decreased analysis time and improved resolution compared with GLC. Uses of HPLC for microbiology are just being developed. It is currently being used by some medical centers to determine the levels of antimicrobial agents, including chloramphenicol, flucytosine, vancomycin, aminoglycosides, and others, in body fluids, as well as for other therapeutic drug monitoring. Products of microbial metabolism may also be detected using HPLC.

11.4. Immunologic Detection Methods for Antigen or Antibody

All of the automated immunologic detection methods in use rely on the same principle, the ability of an antigen and its homologous antibody to bind to each other selectively and with high affinity (discussed in Chapter 12). If either component is labeled in such a way that it can be recognized and quantified, the amount of the other component can be accurately determined. The methods are suitable for detection and quantitation of either antibodies to infectious agents or antigens of various sorts, not limited to microbial antigens. With the advent of monoclonal technology (discussed in Chapters 10 and 12), the possibilities for sensitivity and broad applicability of immunologic methods are practically infinite.

11.4.a.   Counterimmunoelectrophoresis.

The simplest method for determining the presence of cross-reacting antigen or antibody is to visually observe the product of the reaction between an antigen and its bound antibody. Originally performed in liquid with whole bacterial cells (agglutination, Chapter 12), the procedure was modified by Ouchterlony for performance in a semisolid gel matrix. Antigen and antibody were placed in wells cut into the agarose or agar surface of the matrix and they slowly diffused toward each other. If they cross-reacted, they bound one another to form a precipitin reaction, visible as a white line in the gel somewhere between the two wells (Plate 11.2). Counterimmunoelectrophoresis merely adds an electric current to help move the antigen and antibody toward each other more quickly. Since there is really no automation involved in this technique, it is discussed in more depth in Chapter 10.

Counterimmunoelectrophoresis is specific, but it requires enough material to produce a visible reaction. In numerous situations, only minute amounts of the substance being sought are present in the patient. In other cases, the subject of the assay is a molecule too small to yield a visible precipitin reaction. Therefore, more sensitive immunoassays were developed.

11.4.b.   Nephelometry.
Antigen-antibody complexes in solution may be too small to see easily with the naked eye, but they do alter the turbidity of the suspension as measured photometrically. **Nephelometry** (described above in 11.1.a) measures the increased light scatter of a solution as the complexes form; the kinetics of this change can be determined quite quickly when the photometric results are analyzed by computer. Although more widely used in chemistry laboratories than in microbiology laboratories, nephelometry has been used to measure immune complexes and the presence of antibodies to several substances.

11.4.c. Radioimmunoassay.
The main difference among various sophisticated immunoassay systems in use today is the choice of label. The first such methods employed radioisotopes, either tritium (^3H), iodine (^{125}I), cobalt (^{57}Co), or carbon (^{14}C), to label antigen

molecules of the same substance being measured in the assay. **Radioimmunoassay (RIA)**, as the method is called, relies on the competitive binding to antibody of labeled antigen, provided by the assay, and unlabeled antigen, present in the unknown patient sample. When all three components are present in the system, an equilibrium exists, dependent on the amount of unlabeled antigen. The more unlabeled (patient) antigen that is added, the less the labeled antigen will be bound to the antibody. When the antigen-antibody complexes are precipitated out of solution and the amount of radioactive label in the precipitate is determined, the unlabeled antigen present in the sample being assayed can be quantified. In practice, a standard curve is first created by adding known amounts of unlabeled antigen to the system. The amount of radiolabel present in the precipitate of the test solution is compared to values obtained from the standard curve to provide quantitative results.

Although RIA is an immunoassay procedure, it is used more widely for detection of circulating proteins, hormones, and drugs than for diagnosis of infectious diseases, and thus its primary application seems to be in chemistry laboratories. RIA is being used in a limited way in infectious disease diagnosis to detect antigens of and antibodies to the hepatitis viruses, enteroviruses, and *Legionella*, as well as to determine the presence of immune complexes and to measure the amount of antimicrobial agents in patients' body fluids. RIA techniques are highly specific and sensitive, but they require very expensive instruments and highly skilled technologists. The radioisotopes have a relatively short half-life. Additionally, the institution must be licensed and willing to deal with the use and disposal of radioactive substances. At least two alternatives to radioactive labels are being promulgated, as described below.

11.4.d. Enzyme-linked immunosorbent assay. By using enzymes instead of isotopes as labels for antigen or antibody, many of the disadvantages of RIA can be overcome. Instead of a radioactive substance, the antigen (or antibody) is bound to an enzyme that can react with a substrate to yield a colored endproduct. Horseradish peroxidase (which yields a yellow-brown precipitate) and alkaline phosphatase (which yields a blue precipitate) are often chosen. The use of biotin-avidin complexes (described in Chapter 10) for binding enzyme can greatly increase the affinity of the reactants and the speed and intensity of the result. The reagents have a long half-life, and the sensitivity of the assays is similar to that of RIA.

Enzyme-linked immunosorbent assay (ELISA) systems are gaining wide usage in microbiology laboratories. The basic principles of ELISA assays that can be performed without automation are described in Chapter 10. For most clinical applications, however, the changes being detected are so subtle that computer analysis of results is required. Standard commercially produced immunoassay kits that rely on competitive binding, removal of free substrate from the bound complexes before measurement, and comparison of results to a standard curve, as in RIA, are available for the detection of antibodies to viruses, bacteria, and parasites. However, they are primarily used for monitoring levels of drugs, including antimicrobials.

The most commonly used systems use a direct determination of the amount of bound, labeled substance after unbound constituents have been removed by a washing step. Sensitive photometers that can determine slight differences in color are coupled with computers to automatically compare results to standards. Most of the systems are prepared in microdilution plates, but other configurations are used. In many commercial systems, antigen-antibody complexes are bound to a solid phase, either the inside of the microdilution well, a plastic paddle, or a plastic bead. This simplifies washing and allows easier manipulation. Table 11.2 lists products available currently that employ

TABLE 11.2
Automated Microbiology Systems That Use ELISA Technology

MATRIX	SUBJECT	MANUFACTURER(S)
Plastic bead	Gonococci, *Chlamydia*, hepatitis ag*; rubella, hepatitis ab†	Quantum System (Abbott Laboratories)
Metal bead	*E. histolytica*, rubella, *Treponema*, *Toxoplasma*, cytomegalovirus, herpes, Epstein-Barr virus, varicella-zoster virus ab; rotavirus ag	Bio-Enzabead (Litton Bionetics)
Microdilution well	Rubella, *Toxoplasma*, cytomegalovirus, herpes virus ab; respiratory syncytial virus, varicella-zoster virus, herpes virus ag	Microwell Test System (Ortho Diagnostic Systems)
	Epstein-Barr virus, human T cell leukemia virus (HTLV III) ab	EIA Plate Kit (DuPont Co.)
	Mumps, *Mycoplasma*, *Chlamydia*, herpes, measles, rubella, cytomegalovirus, varicella-zoster, *Toxoplasma* ab	EIA System (Whittaker M.A. Bioproducts)
Plastic disk	*Toxoplasma*, rubella, cytomegalovirus, *E. histolytica*, *Treponema*, herpes ab; hepatitis, *Chlamydia*, herpes ag	Cordia Systems (Cordis Laboratories)

ag, antigen.
†*ab*, antibody.

ELISA technology for detection of microbial antigens or antibodies. In addition to the ELISA readers provided by most manufacturers of the reagents, several companies including Dynatech Laboratories and Bio-Tek Instruments produce computerized, programmable reader instruments for determining and printing results from any microdilution format assay system.

A modification of ELISA assays is widely used for monitoring levels of drugs, including antimicrobials. The enzyme-multiplied immunoassay, marketed by Syva Company as EMIT, uses an enzyme bound to a molecule identical to the agent being sought as the third constituent in a competitive assay. The agent, if present in the patient's sample, will bind to antibody, allowing the free enzyme-agent complex to react with its substrate to produce a color change. If the patient's specimen contains only small amounts or none of the agent being tested for, the enzyme-agent complex is free to bind to the antibody. When bound to antibody, the enzyme changes conformation, reducing enzyme activity. This commercial system, used to monitor aminoglycoside levels and to detect varous proteins, is very specific and correlates well with RIA methods.

11.4.e. Fluorescent immunoassays. Fluorescent molecules are also used as substitutes for radioisotope or enzyme labels in several automated systems. In contrast to ELISA systems, **fluorescent immunoassays (FIA)** require only minimal incubation times, no buffered substrate, and fewer washing steps. Current uses in microbiology encompass only the measurement of levels of antimicrobial agents present in body fluids, although other applications are in the development stages. Commercially available systems include the Optimate (Ames Division of Miles Laboratories), which uses a fluorogenic substrate (umbelliferone) bound to molecules of the agent being assayed to compete with free molecules of the agent for antibody-binding sites. The more competing free agent (from patient serum), the more fluorescence can be produced by an exogenous enzyme acting on the unbound substrate-agent complex. In another system, the International Diagnostic Technology FIAX system, fluorescent-labeled and patient-unlabeled substance compete for antibody (or antigen, if antibody is being assayed) bound to a plastic paddle. This relatively simple system accurately detects antibodies to *Toxoplasma*, rubella virus, cytomegalovirus, and herpes virus, as well as to other proteins. The TD$_X$ System from Abbott Laboratories uses a fluorescence polarization format for a competitive therapeutic drug-monitoring assay. A molecule identical to that being assayed is bound to fluorescein, a fluorescent dye. Under polarized light, the amount of fluorescence emitted is dependent on the amount of rotation of the fluorescein-drug complex; the more rotation, the less fluorescence. The conjugated drug and the free drug in the patient sample compete for antibody-binding sites. As the fluorescein complex is bound, it will fluoresce with greater polarization, since its rotation is slowed by the antibody. This sensitive and specific assay is available for monitoring levels of aminoglycosides and vancomycin, as well as many other compounds.

Besides those mentioned, many more fluorescent immunoassay systems are available or in the development stage. Microbiologists can keep abreast of such prospects by occasionally chatting with their cohorts in clinical chemistry. Exciting future applications of FIA as a more rapid and equally sensitive substitute for ELISA for diagnosis of infectious diseases are on the horizon.

11.5. Possible Future Directions in Clinical Microbiology

Every month suggestions for new ways to utilize technology for diagnosis of infectious disease or identification of pathogens are published. Identification of mycobacteria, traditionally a time-consuming and difficult process, has been the target of several investiga-

tors. Wieten and others[8] have suggested the use of pyrolysis mass spectrometry, the analysis of the degradation products of a substance being heated in a vacuum, for species identification of mycobacteria. In limited trials, samples of nonviable isolates yielded results that corresponded well to biochemical methods. Brennan and co-workers[1] have tried to identify non-*M. tuberculosis* mycobacteria using thin-layer chromatography. For this method, extracts of the organisms are spotted on the surface of a thin semisolid gel matrix and subjected to an electrical field that moves the components on the basis of molecular weight and charge. Species are identified by the final pattern formed by the constituents. By using such techniques, new species of existing organisms may also be discovered.

Several groups of investigators are exploring the use of fluorescent probes as indicators of metabolic processes. In these applications, the fluorescent label is bound to substrate. Slight changes in substrate conformation or quantity can be measured very sensitively with these labels, which can detect metabolic activity at much lower levels than present pH indicators. Future applications would include identification and susceptibility results available within hours at levels of sensitivity that approach the current conventional methods. DNA and other nucleic acid probes are discussed in Chapter 10.

Applications of technologies being used by other scientific disciplines, such as flow cytometry, laser imaging, and crossed immunoelectrophoresis, may revolutionize the practice of clinical microbiology in the years ahead. It is beyond the scope of this book to try to discuss them all.

11.6. Computerization in Microbiology

Very few of the automated systems described above or in other areas of the book would be possible without computerization. Microprocessor-controlled mechanical functions, such as moving a culture bottle into position for removing headspace gas or shining a beam of light through a solution in a plastic well to determine the turbidity of the solution, are integral to the new microbiology systems. Even more obvious is the computer-controlled recording and integration of data, which are stored and printed, often as directly reportable results. Aside from their important place as the central processing units of almost all automated instruments, however, computers can perform an even more fundamental role in facilitating smooth functioning of the laboratory.

As evidenced by its valued presence in many institutions, a microbiology computer or a laboratory computer with microbiology functions (Figure 11.7) can perform multiple tasks. Only some of them will be listed here and other uses are discussed in Chapters 3 and 4; individual laboratories will constantly find new uses for their computers. Word-processing programs can be used in microbiology for a number of administrative functions. Besides the ob-

FIGURE 11.7
In the laboratory of one of us (E.J.B.) a computer is used for word processing (laboratory manuals) and for recording all serology test requests and results.

vious ones of facilitating correspondence and writing manuscripts, a word processor is invaluable for preparing and updating procedure manuals. As changes are implemented, they can be written into the program, distributed to all technologists, and then reformatted for automatic inclusion in the manual. Quality control recording sheets and records can be generated with such a program, changing parameters as necessary. Ongoing records of quality control discrepancies can be placed into the program and then printed out as a single report when needed.

Programs are available for inventory control that can greatly reduce time and anxiety associated with ordering and maintaining supplies, a continuing headache in most laboratories. Supply orders can be documented and initiated on the computer, which could then be programmed to flag certain dates for checking on backorders or initiating inquiries. As supplies are received, they are logged into the system.

Computers can be used to calculate workload units such as those utilized by the College of American Pathologists (discussed in Chapter 4). Raw data can be entered daily as numbers of specimens processed or numbers of tests performed and the calculations can be analyzed and stored for later retrieval. Cost accounting of procedures can be facilitated by computer-assisted data processing. Computers with graphics capabilities can visually display such data, to help spot trends and highlight areas in which workload is changing.

Computers can also directly decrease the manual labor involved in logging in new specimens by printing labels for culture media, printing up work cards, and notifying the laboratory if a request for processing a particular specimen is repeated within a specified number of days. A computer in the accessioning area can even perform automatic billing of tests.

The maintenance of records of results, both identifications and susceptibilities, is critical for epidemiologic surveillance and for monitoring patient progress. Myriad computer systems have capabilities for data storage and retrieval. Reports can be generated, cataloguing susceptibility results of isolates sorted by source, species, doctor, ward, and any other parameter. Unusual susceptibility patterns or those that do not match the supposed identification of the isolate can be flagged. Results of cultures can be studied in many ways, allowing microbiologists access to information that could be gathered previously only by great effort.

In addition to the management functions, the computer can aid in reporting results. Results immediately accessible to the patient units will have much greater impact on patient care, as well as cut down on communication lags and errors. It is estimated that systems in operation at several large institutions have saved at least 1 h per physician per day. Physicians could even request tests by computer, gaining valuable time and cutting transcription errors. Laboratory computers that interface with hospital computers can deliver patient demographic data directly to the laboratory and provide direct billing capability. Epidemiologic data entered in the laboratory could be retrieved by nurse epidemiologists in another location for more efficient operation. In the ultimate computerized laboratory, results generated by instruments automatically would be updated to the patient's charts, even during the middle of the night.

REFERENCES

1. Brennan, P.J., Heifets, M., and Ullom, B.P. 1982. Thin-layer chromatography of lipid antigens as a means of identifying nontuberculous mycobacteria. J. Clin. Microbiol. 15:447.
2. Holdeman, L.V., Cato, E.P., and Moore, W.E.C., editors. 1977. Anaerobe laboratory manual, ed. 4. Virginia Polytechnic Institute and State University, Blacksburg, Va.
3. Isenberg, H.D., Reichler, A., and Wiseman, D. 1971. Prototype of a fully automated device for determination of bacterial antibiotic susceptibility in the clinical laboratory. Appl. Microbiol. 22:980.
4. Spiegel, C.A., Amsel, R., Eschenbach, D., et al.: 1980. Anaerobic bacteria in nonspecific vaginitis. N. Engl. J. Med. 303:601.
5. Sutter, V.L., Citron, D.M., Edelstein, M.A.C., and Finegold, S.M. 1985. Wadsworth anaerobic bacteriology manual. Star Publishing Co., Belmont, Calif.
6. Thornsberry, C., Gavan, T.L., Sherris, J.C., Balows, A., Matsen, J.M., Sabath, L.D., Schoenknecht, F., Thrupp, L.D., and Washington, J.A. II. 1975. Laboratory evaluation of a rapid, automated susceptibility testing system: report of a collaborative study. Antimicrob. Agents Chemother. 7:466.
7. Tisdall, P.A., DeYoung, D., Roberts, G.D., and Anhalt, J.P. 1982. Identification of clinical isolates of mycobacteria with gas-liquid chromatography: a 10-month follow-up study. J. Clin. Microbiol. 16:400.
8. Wieten, G., Haverkamp, J., Henk, L.C., et al. 1981. Pyrolysis mass spectrometry: a new method to differentiate between the mycobacteria of the 'tuberculosis complex' and other mycobacteria. J. Gen. Microbiol. 122:109.

BIBLIOGRAPHY

Ackerman, B.H., Berg, H.G., Strate, R.G., et al. 1983. Comparison of radioimmunoassay and fluorescent polarization immunoassay for quantitative determination of vancomycin concentrations in serum. J. Clin. Microbiol. 18:994.
Barry, A.L., Jones, R.N., and Gavan, T.L. 1978. Evaluation of the Micro-Media System for quantitative antimicrobial drug susceptibility testing: a collaborative study. Antimicrob. Agents Chemother. 13:61.
Bruckner, D.A., Hindler, J.A., Martin, W.J., and Palmer, R. 1982. Comparison of radioimmunoassay with a new immunofluorescent method (FIAX) for measuring tobramycin in serum. Antimicrob. Agents Chemother. 21:107.
Buchanan, A.G., Witwicki, E, and Albritton, W.L. 1983. Serum aminoglycoside monitoring by enzyme immunoassay, biological, and fluorescence immunoassay procedures. Am. J. Med. Tech. 49:437.
Delaney, C.J., Opheim, K.E., Smith, A.L., and Plorde, J.J. 1982. Performance characteristics of bioassay, radioenzymatic assay, homogeneous enzyme immunoassay, and high performance liquid chromatography for determination of serum gentamicin. J. Clin. Microbiol. 21:19.
Filburn, B.H., Shull, V.H., Tempera, Y.M., et al. 1983. Evaluation of an automated fluorescence polarization immunoassay for vancomycin. Antimicrob. Agents Chemother. 24:216.
Fitzgibbon, R.J. 1984. Clinical laboratory reference. Medical Economics Books, Oradell, N.J.

Gavan, T.L., Jones, R.N., and Barry, A.L. 1980. Evaluation of the Sensititre system for quantitative antimicrobial susceptibility testing: a collaborative study. Antimicrob. Agents Chemother. 17:464.

Gerson, B. 1984. Fluorescence immunoassay. J. Clin. Immunoassay 7:73.

Gorbach, S.L., Mayhew, J.W., Bartlett, J.G., et al. 1976. Rapid diagnosis of anaerobic infection by direct gas-liquid chromatography of clinical specimens. J. Clin. Invest. 57:478.

Hale, D.C., Wright,, D.N., McKie, J.E., et al. 1981. Rapid screening for bacteriuria by light scatter photometry (Autobac); a collaborative study. J. Clin. Microbiol. 13:147.

Isenberg, H.D. 1984. Automated methods of bacterial susceptibility testing. Ann. N.Y. Acad. Sci. 428:236.

Isenberg, H.D., and D'Amato, R.F. 1984. Rapid methods for antimicrobic susceptibility testing. In Cunha, B.A., and Ristuccia, A.M., editors. Antimicrobial therapy. Raven Press, New York.

Isenberg, H.D., and D'Amato, R.F. 1985. New methods for the detection of bacteria and fungi. Lab. Med. 2:1.

Isenberg, H.D., and MacLowry, J.D. 1976. Automated methods and data handling in bacteriology. Ann. Rev. Microbiol. 30:483.

Isenberg, H.D., Gavan, T.L., Sonnenwirth, A., et al. 1979. Clinical laboratory evaluation of automated detection/identification system in analysis of clinical urine specimens. J. Clin. Microbiol. 10:226.

Kuhn, P.J. 1984. Comparing the new automated microbiology systems. Med. Lab. Observer 16:118.

Looney, C.E. 1984. High-sensitivity light scattering immunoassays. J. Clin. Immunoassay 7:90.

Malloy, P.J., Miceika, B.G., and Ducate, M.J. 1983. Automated methods in microbiology: II. Identification and susceptibility testing. Am. J. Med. Tech. 49:313.

Miceika, B.G., Malloy, P.J., and Ducate, M.J. 1983. Automated methods in microbiology: I. Bacterial detection systems. Am. J. Med. Tech. 49:305.

Morgan, M.A., Horstmeier, C.D., DeYoung, D.R., and Roberts, G.D. 1983. Comparison of a radiometric method (Bactec) and conventional culture media for recovery of mycobacteria from smear-negative specimens. J. Clin. Microbiol. 18:384.

Narayan, S. 1983. Chromatography: III. Ion-exchange chromatography. J. Clin. Lab. Automation 3:225.

Ryan, K.J. 1981. What to look for in a clinical microbiology laboratory computer system. Clin. Microbiol. Newsletter 3:165.

Shekarchi, I.C., Sever, J.L., Nerurkar, L., and Fuccillo, D. 1984. Comparison of enzyme-linked immunosorbent assay with enzyme-linked fluorescence assay with automated readers for detection of rubella virus antibody and herpes simplex virus. J. Clin. Microbiol. 21:92.

Smith, P.B., Gavan, T.L., Isenberg, H.D., Sonnenwirth, A., Taylor, W.I., Washington, J.A. II, and Balows, A. 1978. Multi-laboratory evaluation of an automated microbial detection/identification system. J. Clin. Microbiol. 8:657.

Spiegel, C.A., Malangoni, M.A., and Condon, R.E. 1984. Gas-liquid chromatography for rapid diagnosis of intra-abdominal infection. Arch. Surg. 119:28.

Tracy, R.P., and Young, D.S. 1983. Two-dimensional gel electrophoresis: methods and potential applications in the clinical laboratory. J. Clin. Lab. Automation 3:235.

Ulrich, P.G., and Wannlund, J.C. Bioluminescence in the microbiology laboratory. Am. Clin. Prod. Rev., November 1984, p. 50.

Witebsky, F.G., Silva, C.A., Selepak, S.T., et al. 1983. Evaluation of four gentamicin and tobramycin assay procedures for clinical laboratories. J. Clin. Microbiol. 18:890.

12 Diagnostic Immunologic Principles and Methods

Infectious diseases can be definitively diagnosed in only three ways: (1) by documenting the presence in the patient of an agent known to cause the disease, either by visualizing the agent directly in clinical material obtained from the patient or by cultivating the agent in the laboratory (within an animal host or in vitro); (2) by detecting a specific product of the infectious agent in clinical material obtained from the patient, a product that could not have been produced without the agent's presence; and (3) by detecting an immunologic response specific to the infecting agent in the patient's serum. Detection of the agent by visualization or cultivation is the focus of much of this text, covered extensively in Parts II and III. Detection of products of the agent is addressed in Chapter 10 and again as this diagnostic method relates to individual pathogens. Methods for documenting the presence of an immune response will be described in this chapter.

12.1. General Features of the Immune Response

12.1.a. Categories of immune responses. The human specific immune responses are simplistically divided into two categories. **Cell-mediated immune responses,** which are carried out by special lymphocytes of the T (thymus-derived) class, include production of activator chemicals that induce other cells to attack and kill pathogens readily as well as the direct attacking and killing of pathogens (or host cells damaged or infected by pathogens) by the T lymphocytes themselves. Although diagnosis of certain diseases may be aided by measuring the cell mediated immune response to the pathogen, such tests are carried out by skin tests or at specialized immunology laboratories, rather than by clinical microbiologists, and are beyond the scope of this book. **Antibody-mediated immune responses** are those produced by specific proteins generated by lymphocytes of the B (bone marrow–derived) class. Because these proteins have immunologic function and because they fold into a globular structure in the active state, they are called **immunoglobulins.** Immunoglobulins, also called **antibodies,** since they are produced against a particular foreign structure or "body," attach to offending agents or their products and thus aid the host in removing the agents. These agents need not be pathogenic microorganisms, as the immune system is also effective against some tumor cells, transplanted (nonself) tissue, pollen, and other foreign substances. Books by Roitt et al. and Bellanti (see bibliography) are among several excellent sources of information about the human immune response. This chapter will deal only with the detection of antibodies produced against infectious agents, although many of the techniques employed may be used for the detection of other types of antibodies.

Antibodies are either secreted into the blood or lymphatic fluid (and sometimes other body fluids) by the B lymphocytes, or they remain attached to the surface of the lymphocyte or other effector cells. Because the mediators of this category of immune response chiefly circulate in the blood, this type of immunity is also called **humoral immunity.** For purposes of determining whether an antibody has been produced against a particular agent by a patient, the patient's **serum** (or occasionally the plasma) is tested for the presence of the antibody. The study of the diagnosis of disease by

measuring antibody levels in serum is thus called **serology.**

12.1.b. Characteristics of antibodies. Antibodies are produced against a specific small chemically and physically defined substance recognized as foreign by the host, called an antigen or an antigenic determinant. By a genetically determined mechanism, normal humans are able to produce antibodies specifically directed against almost all the antigens with which they might come into contact throughout their lifetimes. Antigens may be part of the physical structure of the pathogen or they may be a chemical produced and released by the pathogen. One pathogen may contain or produce many different antigens that the host will recognize as foreign, so that infection with one agent may cause a number of different antibodies to appear. *Streptococcus pyogenes* is an example of a pathogen that induces production of several different antibodies (Figure 12.1). In addition, some antigenic determinants of a pathogen may not be available for recognition by the host until the pathogen has undergone a physical change. For example, until a pathogenic bacterium has been digested by a human polymorphonuclear neutrophil, certain antigens deep within the cell wall are not "visible" to the host immune system. Once the bacterium is broken down, these new antigens are revealed and antibodies can be produced against them. For this reason, a patient may produce different antibodies at different times during the course of a single disease.

Antibodies function by attaching to the surface of pathogens and making the pathogens more amenable to ingestion by phagocytic cells (**opsonizing antibodies**) or by attaching to the surface of pathogens and contributing to their destruction by the lytic action of **complement** (**complement-fixing antibodies**). Although humans produce several different classes of antibodies, differentiated by their structures, diagnostic serologic methods have been primarily developed to measure only two antibody

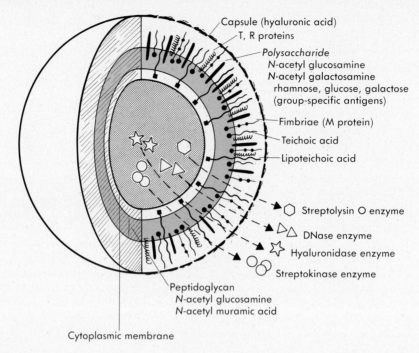

FIGURE 12.1
Streptococcus pyogenes contains many antigenic structural components and produces several antigenic enzymes, each of which may elicit a specific antibody response from the infected host.

FIGURE 12.2
Structure of immunoglobulin M.

FIGURE 12.3
Structure of immunoglobulin G.

classes, immunoglobulin M (IgM) and immunoglobulin G (IgG). The basic structure of an antibody molecule is comprised of two mirror-images, each made up of two identical protein chains. At the terminal ends are the antigen-binding sites, which specifically attach to the antigen against which the antibody was produced. Depending on the specificity of the antibody, antigens of some similarity, but not identical, to the inducing antigen may also be bound. The complement-binding site is found in the center of the molecule in a structure that is similar for all antibodies of the same class. In most cases, the first antibody produced in response to a foreign agent is IgM. Thus, presence of IgM is usually indicative of recent infection and active infection. IgG antibody may persist long after infection has run its course. The IgM antibody type (Figure 12.2) consists of five identical proteins with the basic antibody structures linked together at the bases, leaving 10 antigen-binding sites available. The second antibody class, IgG, consists of one basic antibody molecule with two binding sites (Figure 12.3). The differences in the size and conformation between these two classes of im-

munoglobulins result in differences in activities and functions.

12.1.c. Features of the humoral immune response useful in diagnostic testing. Normal humans produce both IgM and IgG in response to most pathogens. The larger number of binding sites on IgM molecules can help to more quickly clear the offending pathogen, even though each individual antigen-binding site may not be the most efficient for attaching the antigen. Over time, the cells that were producing IgM switch to producing IgG, often more specific for the antigen (also called more **avid**). The IgG has only two binding sites, but it can bind complement. When IgG has bound to an antigen, the base of the molecule may be left projecting out in the environment. Structures on the base attract and bind phagocytic cell membranes, increasing the chances of engulfment and destruction of the pathogen by the host cells. In most cases, IgM is produced by a patient only after the first interaction with a given pathogen and is no longer detectable within a relatively short period afterward. For serologic diagnostic purposes, one important difference between IgG and IgM is that IgM cannot cross the placenta of pregnant women. Therefore, any IgM detected in the serum of a newborn baby must have been produced by the baby itself. IgM, because of its shape, cannot bind complement. Other differences between IgG and IgM are exploited to separate them so that the presence of one class of antibody in a patient's serum will not interfere with testing for the presence of the other class. A second encounter with the same pathogen will usually induce only an IgG response. Because the B lymphocytes retain memory of this pathogen, however, they can respond more quickly and with larger numbers of antibodies than at the initial interaction. This response is called the **anamnestic response.** The relative humoral responses over time are illustrated in Figure 12.4.

FIGURE 12.4
Relative humoral response to antigen stimulation over time.

12.1.d. Interpretation of serologic tests. A central dogma of serology is the concept of **rise in titer.** The **titer** of antibody is the reciprocal of the highest dilution of the patient's serum in which the antibody is still detectable. Patients with large amounts of antibody have high titers, since antibody will still be detectable at very high dilutions of serum. Serum for antibody levels should be drawn during the acute phase of the disease (when it is first discovered) and again during convalescence (usually at least 2 weeks later). These specimens are called **acute and convalescent sera.** For some infections, such as Legionnaires' disease, hepatitis, and others, titers may not rise until months after the acute infection. Accurate results useful for diagnosis of many infections are only achieved when acute and convalescent sera are tested concurrently in the same system, since variables inherent in the procedures and laboratory error can easily result in differences of one doubling (or twofold) dilution in the results obtained from even the same sample tested at the same time.

Patients with intact humoral immunity will develop increasing amounts of antibody to a disease-causing pathogen over several weeks. If it is the patient's first encounter with the pathogen and the specimen has been obtained early enough, no antibody will be present at the onset of disease. In the case of a second encounter the patient's serum will usually contain measurable antibody during the initial phase of disease and the level of antibody will quickly increase, due to the anamnestic response. For most pathogens, an increase in the patient's titer of two doubling dilutions (for example, from a positive result at 1:8 to a positive result at 1:32) over several weeks is considered to be diagnostic of current infection. This is called a **fourfold rise in titer.**

With most diseases, there exists a spectrum of responses from infected humans, such that a person may develop antibody from subclinical infection or after colonization by an agent without actually having disease. In these cases, the presence of antibody in a single serum specimen or a similar titer of antibody in paired sera may merely indicate past contact with the agent and cannot be used to accurately diagnose a recent disease. On the other hand, patients may respond to an antigenic stimulus by producing antibody that can cross-react with other antigens. These antibodies are nonspecific and thus they may cause misinterpretation of serologic tests. For the vast majority of serologic procedures for diagnosis of recent infection, therefore, testing both acute and convalescent sera is the method of choice. Except for detecting the presence of IgM, the testing of a single serum can only be recommended in certain cases, such as for diagnosis of recent infection with *Mycoplasma pneumoniae* and viral influenza B, where high titers may indicate recent infection. Cumitech 15, by Chernesky, Ray, and Smith,[1] contains an excellent discussion on the collection and interpretation of paired sera for immunologic testing.

If the infecting or disease-causing agent is extremely rare and people without disease would have no chance of developing an immune response, such as the rabies virus or the toxin of botulism, the presence of specific antibody in a single serum specimen can be diagnostic. There are, in addition, a number of circumstances when serum is tested only to determine whether a patient is "**immune,**" i.e., has antibody to a particular agent either in response to a past infection or to immunization. These tests can be performed with a single serum sample. Correlation of the results of such tests with the actual immune status of individual patients must be performed to determine the level of detectable antibody present that corresponds to actual immunity to infection or reinfection in the host. For example, very sensitive tests can detect the presence of very tiny amounts of antibody to the rubella virus. Certain people, however, may still be susceptible to infection with the rubella virus with such small amounts of circulating antibody, and a higher level of antibody may be required to assure protection from disease. Depending on the etiologic agent, even low levels of antibody may protect a patient from pathologic effects of disease, although they may not prevent reinfection. As more sensitive testing methods are developed, and these types of problems become more common, microbiologists will need to work closely with clinicians to develop guidelines for interpreting the results of serologic tests as they relate to the status of individual patients.

12.2. Principles of Serologic Test Methods

Antibodies can be detected in many different ways. In some cases, antibodies to an agent may be detected in more than one way, but the different antibody detection tests may not be measuring the same antibody. For this reason, the presence of antibodies to a particular pathogen as detected by one method may not correlate with the presence of antibodies to the same agent detected by another test method. This concept will become clearer after antibody detection methods have been discussed.

Slide agglutination tests are the easiest to perform and in some cases are the most sensitive tests currently available. Either artificial carriers, such as latex particles or treated red blood cells, or biological carriers, such as whole bacterial cells, can present an antigen that will bind with antibody produced in response to that antigen when it was introduced to the host. Reagents for many of the following tests are commercially available; selected suppliers are listed in the Appendix.

12.2.a. Direct whole pathogen agglutination for antibody detection. The most basic tests for antibody are those that measure the antibody produced by a host to determinants on the surface of a bacterial agent in response to infection with that agent. Specific antibodies bind to surface antigens of the bacteria in a thick suspension and cause the bacteria to clump together in visible aggregates (Figure 12.5). Such antibodies are called **agglutinating antibodies**, and the reaction is called **bacterial agglutination**. Electrostatic and other forces influence the formation of aggregates in solutions, so that certain conditions are usually necessary for good results. Since most bacterial surfaces exhibit a negative charge, they tend to repel each other. Performance of agglutination tests in sterile physiologic saline (0.85% sodium chloride in distilled water), which has free positive ions present in the solution, will enhance the ability of antibody to cause aggregation of bacteria. Bacterial agglutination tests can be performed on the surface of glass slides or in tubes. Tube agglutination tests are often more sensitive, since a longer incubation period, allowing more antigen and antibody to interact, can occur. The small volume of liquid used for slide tests requires a rather rapid reading of the result, before the liquid has evaporated.

Examples of bacterial agglutination serologic tests are the tests for antibodies to *Francisella tularensis* and *Brucella* species, usually part of a panel of so-called **febrile agglutinin** tests. Bacterial agglutination tests are often used to diagnose diseases in which the bacterial agent is difficult to cultivate in vitro. Diseases commonly diagnosed by this technique include Legionnaires' disease, listeriosis, tetanus, yersiniosis, leptospirosis, brucellosis, and tularemia. The reagents necessary to perform many of these tests are commercially available, singly or as complete systems (Appendix). Agglutination tests for certain diseases such as typhoid fever have become less useful with the ability of most laboratories to culture and identify the causative agent. Furthermore, the typhoid febrile agglutinin test (called the Widal test) is often positive in patients with infections caused by other bacteria, due to cross-reacting antibodies or to previous immunization against typhoid. We recommend that appropriate specimens from patients suspected of having

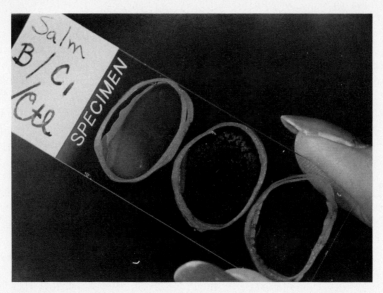

FIGURE 12.5
An example of a slide agglutination test. An organism that biochemically resembles a *Salmonella*
species is emulsified in several drops of saline on a slide. Drops of antiserum prepared against specific
Salmonella serotypes are added to the suspension; the organism agglutinates in the presence of
homologous antiserum (center circle).

typhoid fever be cultured for the presence of
salmonellae (stool, urine, or blood as appropriate; discussed in Chapters 14, 17, and 18) and
that reliance not be placed on febrile agglutinins for diagnosis of this disease.

Whole cells of parasites, including *Plasmodium, Leishmania,* or *Toxoplasma gondii,* have
also been used for direct detection of antibody
by agglutination. In addition to using the actual
infecting bacteria or parasites as the agglutinating particles for the detection of antibodies,
certain bacteria may be agglutinated by antibodies produced against another infecting
agent. Many patients infected with one of the
Rickettsia produce antibodies that can agglutinate bacteria of the genus *Proteus.* Tests for
these cross-reacting antibodies are called the
Weil-Felix tests. Although these antibodies are
also produced in response to bacterial infection, their presence has been used traditionally
as presumptive serologic evidence of rickettsial

disease. As newer, more specific serologic
methods of diagnosing rickettsial disease become more widely available, the use of the
Proteus agglutinating tests should be discontinued.

12.2.b. Latex particle agglutination tests.
Recently, several serologic procedures have
been developed for the detection of antibody
via the agglutination of an artificial carrier with
antigen bound to its surface. As noted in Chapter 10, similar systems employing artificial carriers coated with antibodies are commonly
used for detection of microbial antigens. As discussed in Chapters 15, 16, and elsewhere, antigens of streptococci, *Cryptococcus neoformans,* agents of bacterial meningitis, and other
etiologic agents can be detected using latex and
staphylococcal particle agglutination systems.
The size of the carrier enhances the visibility of
the agglutination reaction, and the artificial nature of the system allows the antigen bound to

the surface to be extremely specific. Complete systems for the use of latex or other particle agglutination tests are commercially available for the accurate and sensitive detection of antibody to cytomegalovirus and rubella virus, and other systems are in the evaluation stage. Staphylococci containing protein A have occasionally been used as antibody-capture reagents, or to remove IgG from serum that also contains IgM. Although latex particle agglutination tests have been developed for detecting antibodies to gonoccoci, they have not been found to be as reliable as other tests for gonorrhea. Latex tests for antibodies to *Coccidioides*, *Sporothrix*, *Echinococcus*, and *Trichinella* are available, although they are not widely used because of the uncommon occurrence of the corresponding infection or its limited geographic distribution. Results of latex agglutination tests are dependent on several factors, including the amount and avidity of antigen conjugated to the carrier, the time of incubation together with patient's serum (or other source of antibody), and the microenvironment of the interaction (including pH, tonicity, protein concentration, etc.). Commercial tests have been developed as systems, complete with their own diluents, controls, and containers. For accurate results, they should be used as units, without modifications. If tests have been developed for use with cerebrospinal fluid, for example, they should not be used with serum unless the product insert or the technical representative has certified such usage.

A modification of latex agglutination procedures involves the use of a liposome particle (described in Chapter 10) coated with antihuman immunoglobulin added to the suspension of latex particles coated with the specific antigen. If antibodies are present in a serum specimen they will bind to the latex particle. The liposomes will then bind to the antibodies, increasing the size of the agglutinated particles and thereby enhancing the sensitivity of the test (Figure 12.6). These reagents are commercially available (Cooper Biomedical Co.) for the detection of antibodies to streptolysin O and deoxyribonuclease produced in response to infection with *S. pyogenes* and for the detection of the heterophile antibodies produced by some patients with infectious mononucleosis.

12.2.c. Hemagglutination tests for antibody detection. Treated animal red blood cells have also been used as carriers of antigen for agglutination tests, called **indirect hemagglutination** or **passive hemagglutination** tests, since it is not the antigens of the blood cells themselves but the passively attached antigens that are being bound by antibody. The most widely used of these tests are the microhemagglutination test for antibody to *Treponema pallidum* (MHA-TP, so-called because it is performed in a microtiter plate), the hemagglutination treponemal test for syphilis (HATTS), the passive hemagglutination tests for antibody to extracellular antigens of streptococci, and the rubella indirect hemagglutination tests, all of which are available commercially. Certain reference laboratories, such as the Centers for Disease Control, also perform indirect hemagglutination tests for antibodies to some clostridia, *Pseudomonas pseudomallei*, *Bacillus anthracis*, *Corynebacterium diphtheriae*, *Leptospira*, and the agents of several viral and parasitic diseases.

12.2.d. Flocculation tests for antibody detection. In contrast to the aggregates formed when particulate antigens bind to specific antibody, the interaction of soluble antigen with antibody results in the formation of a **precipitate,** a concentration of fine particles, usually visible only because the precipitated product is forced to remain in a defined space within a matrix. Although the **precipitin test** is not used for serological determinations directly, two variations are widely used. In **flocculation tests,** the precipitin endproduct forms macroscopically or microscopically visible clumps. The Venereal Disease Research Laboratory

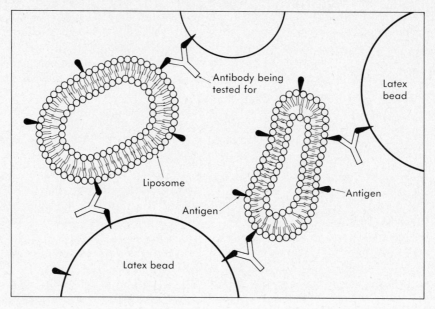

FIGURE 12.6
Diagram of liposome-latex agglutination reaction.

test, known as the **VDRL,** is the most widely used flocculation test. Patients infected with pathogenic treponemes, most commonly *T. pallidum,* the agent of syphilis, form an antibodylike protein called **reagin,** that binds to the test antigen, **cardiolipin-lecithin-coated cholesterol** particles, causing the particles to flocculate. Since reagin is not a specific antibody directed against *T. pallidum* antigens, the test is not highly specific, but it is a good screening test, detecting over 99% of cases of secondary syphilis. Very early in the infection, the VDRL test is still negative. Conditions and infections other than syphilis can cause a patient's serum to yield a positive result for the VDRL test, called a **biologic false positive** test (discussed in Chapter 19). The VDRL is the single most useful test available for testing cerebrospinal fluid in cases of suspected neurosyphilis, although it may be falsely positive in this disease. The performance of the VDRL

test requires scrupulously clean glassware and exacting attention to detail, including numerous daily quality control checks. In addition, the reagents must be prepared fresh each time the test is performed, patients' sera must be inactivated by heating for 30 min at 56° C before testing, and the reaction must be read microscopically. For these reasons, it is being supplanted in many laboratories by a qualitatively comparable test, the **rapid plasma reagin,** or **RPR** test. The RPR test is commercially available as a complete system containing positive and negative controls, the reaction card, and the prepared antigen suspension. The antigen, cardiolipin-lecithin-coated cholesterol with choline chloride, also contains charcoal particles to allow for macroscopically visible flocculation. Sera are tested without heating, and the reaction takes place on the surface of a specially treated paper card, which is then discarded (Figure 12.7). The RPR test

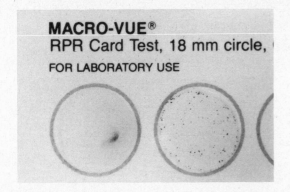

MACRO-VUE®
RPR Card Test, 18 mm circle,
FOR LABORATORY USE

FIGURE 12.7
Rapid plasma reagin test for syphilis. (Courtesy Hynson, Westcott, & Dunning.)

is not recommended for testing cerebrospinal fluid. All procedures are standardized and clearly described in product inserts, and these procedures should be strictly adhered to. The failure of the RPR test to detect minimally reactive sera in one statewide proficiency testing survey was shown to be due to deficiencies in technique used, rather than deficiencies in the reagents or the test system itself. An excellent set of guidelines for acceptable test performance was published by Neimeister and co-authors.[2] Overall, the RPR appears to be a more specific screening test for syphilis than the VDRL and it is certainly easier to perform. Flocculation tests are also performed to detect antibodies to *Trichinella;* reagents are commercially available.

12.2.e. Countercurrent immunoelectrophoresis for antibody detection. The second variation of the classic precipitin test has been widely used to detect small amounts of antibody. This test takes advantage of the net electric charge of the antigens and antibodies being tested in a particular test buffer. Because the antigen and antibody being sought migrate toward one another in a semisolid matrix under the influence of an electrical current, the method is called **countercurrent immunoelec-**trophoresis, or simply **counterimmunoelectrophoresis (CIE).** The principles of this test were outlined in Chapter 10; the same methodology is used to identify specific antigen or antibody. When antigen and antibody meet in optimal proportions, a line of precipitation will appear. Since all variables, such as buffer pH, type of gel or agarose matrix, amount of current, amounts and concentrations of antigen and antibody, size of antigen and antibody inocula, and placement of these inocula, must be carefully controlled for maximum reactivity, CIE tests are difficult to develop and perform. Other methods for detection of antibody to infectious agents are more commonly used in most diagnostic laboratories. A very sensitive, but not very specific, commercially available test employs CIE for detection of antibody to *Entamoeba histolytica* in patients suspected of having invasive, extraintestinal amebic disease, primarily liver abscess.

12.2.f. Hemagglutination inhibition tests for viral antibodies. Many human viruses have the ability to bind to surface structures on red blood cells from different species. For example, rubella virus particles can bind to human type O, goose, or chicken erythrocytes and cause agglutination of the red blood cells. Influenza and parainfluenza viruses agglutinate guinea pig, chicken, or human O erythrocytes; many arboviruses agglutinate goose red blood cells; adenoviruses agglutinate rat or Rhesus monkey cells; mumps virus agglutinates chicken or goose cells; measles virus binds red blood cells of monkeys; and herpes and cytomegaloviruses agglutinate sheep red blood cells. Serologic tests for the presence of antibodies to these viruses exploit the agglutinating properties of the virus particles. Patients' sera that have been treated with kaolin or heparin-magnesium chloride (to remove nonspecific inhibitors of red cell agglutination and nonspecific agglutinins of the red cells) are added to a system that contains the virus suspected of causing disease. If antibodies to the virus are present, they will form complexes and block the binding sites on the viral surfaces. When the proper red cells are added to the solution, all of the virus particles will be bound by antibody, preventing the virus from agglutinating the red cells. Thus the patient's serum is positive for **hemagglutination inhibiting antibodies.** As for most serologic procedures, a fourfold increase in such titers is considered diagnostic. The hemagglutination inhibition tests for most agents are performed only at reference laboratories. Procedures for performing such tests are delineated in the *Manual of Clinical Immunology* (American Society for Microbiology). Rubella antibodies, however, are often detected with this method in routine diagnostic laboratories. Several commercial rubella antibody detection systems are available.

12.2.g. Neutralization tests. To test for certain antibodies, the ability of a patient's serum to block the effect of the antigenic agent can be evaluated. In the case of viruses, antibody that destroys the infectivity of the virus is called **neutralizing antibody**. The serum to be tested is mixed with a suspension of infectious virus particles of the same type as those with which the patient is suspected of being infected. A control suspension of viruses is mixed with normal serum. The virus suspensions are then inoculated into a cell culture system that supports growth of the virus. The control cells will display evidence of virus infection. If the patient's serum contains antibody to the virus, that antibody will bind the virus particles and prevent them from invading the cells in culture. The antibody has **neutralized** the infectivity of the virus. These tests are technically demanding, time consuming, and are performed only in those laboratories that routinely perform virus cultures.

Antibodies to bacterial toxins and other extracellular products that display measurable activities can be tested in the same way. The ability of a patient's serum to neutralize the erythrocyte lysing capability of streptolysin O, an extracellular enzyme produced by S. *pyogenes* during infection, has been used for many years as a test for previous streptococcal infection. After pharyngitis with streptolysin O–producing strains, most patients show a high titer of the antibody **antistreptolysin O (ASO)**. Streptococci also produce the enzyme **deoxyribonuclease B (DNase B)** during infections of the throat, skin, or other tissue. A neutralization test that prevents activity of this enzyme, the anti-DNase B test, has also been used extensively as an indicator of recent or previous streptococcal disease. The use of particle agglutination (latex or indirect hemagglutination) tests for the presence of antibody to many of the streptococcal enzymes has replaced the use of these neutralization tests in many laboratories.

12.2.h. Complement fixation for antibody detection. One of the classic methods for demonstrating the presence of antibody in a patient's serum has been the **complement fixation test (CF)**. This test consists of two separate systems, the first (the indicator system) consisting of a combination of sheep red blood cells, complement-fixing antibody (IgG) raised against the sheep red blood cells in another animal, and an exogenous source of complement (usually guinea pig serum). When these three components are mixed together in optimum concentrations, the anti–sheep erythrocyte antibody will bind to the surface of the red cells and the complement will then bind to the antigen-antibody complex, ultimately causing lysis of the red cells. For this reason, the anti–sheep red cell antibody is also called **hemolysin.** The second system consists of the antigen suspected of causing the patient's disease and the patient's serum. These components are added to a suspension of the sheep erythrocytes, hemolysin, and a critical amount of complement. For the CF test, these two systems are tested in sequence (Figure 12.8). The patient's serum is first added to the putative antigen; then the limiting amount of complement is added to the solution. If the patient's serum contains antibody to the antigen, these antigen-antibody complexes will bind all of the complement added. In the next step, the sheep red blood cells and the hemolysin (indicator system) are added. Only if the complement has not been bound by a complex formed with antibody from the patient's serum will the complement be available to bind to the sheep cell-hemolysin complexes and cause lysis. A positive result, meaning the patient does possess

complement-fixing antibodies, is revealed by failure of the red cells to lyse in the final test system. Lysis of the indicator cells indicates lack of antibody, and a negative CF test.

This test has been used over the years for the detection of many types of antibodies, particularly antiviral, although it requires many manipulations, at least 48 h for both stages of the test to be completed, and often yields nonspecific results. Many new systems both for improved recovery of pathogens or their products and for more sensitive and less demanding pro-

FIGURE 12.8
Complement fixation test.

cedures for detection of antibodies, described in this chapter as well as in Chapters 8, 10, and 11, have gradually been introduced to replace the CF test. At this time, CF tests are performed chiefly for diagnosis of unusual infections; these tests are done primarily in reference laboratories. This test is still probably the most common method for diagnosis of infection due to the common respiratory viruses, influenza A and B, parainfluenza, adenovirus, and respiratory syncytial virus, as well as for diagnosis of mycoplasma infection and Q fever. It is recommended that laboratories without experience in performing these tests not adopt complement fixation tests for routine diagnostic testing when other, less demanding, procedures are available.

12.2.i. Enzyme-linked immunosorbent assays. The number of antibody detection tests developed utilizing **enzyme-linked immunosorbent assay (ELISA)** technology is expanding rapidly. ELISA methods for antibodies to infectious agents are sensitive and specific. As described more thoroughly in Chapter 10, the presence of specific antibody is detected by its ability to bind a second antibody conjugated to a colored or fluorescent marker. Various enzyme-substrate systems and the use of avidin-biotin to bind marker substances were also discussed in Chapter 10. The antigen to which the antibodies bind, if they are present in patients' sera, is either attached to the inside of wells of a microtiter plate or onto the surface of beads or plastic paddles. Although the sensitivity of certain particle-agglutinating tests is greater than ELISA tests for antibody at the current time, ELISA methodology is being rapidly improved. Once many of the disadvantages of this method have been overcome (some are mentioned below), it is probable that these systems will be the most commonly used antibody detection systems; this may happen in the near future. Currently, ELISA test procedures require several incubation periods and washes that must be performed manually. However,

the potential for more complete automation of these procedures is great. Advantages are that tests can be performed easily on many serum samples at the same time, and the colored or fluorescent endproducts are easily detected by instruments, removing the element of subjectivity inherent in so many serological procedures that rely on a technologist's interpretation of a reaction. Disadvantages include the need for some special equipment; the fairly long reaction times (hours instead of minutes); the relative endpoint of the test (that relies on measuring the amount of a visible endproduct that is not dependent on the original antigen-antibody reaction itself, but on a second enzymatic reaction), as compared with a directly quantitative result; and the requirement for batch processing to insure that performance of the test is cost-effective. Possibly as a result of the measurement of the endpoint of a secondary reaction, ELISA methods do not generate a true titer result, another major disadvantage of the system. A general discussion of the principles of automated ELISA readers currently available is found in Chapter 11. Commercial microdilution systems are available for the detection of antibody specific for hepatitis virus antigens, herpes simplex virus I and II, respiratory syncytial virus, cytomegalovirus, human T-cell lymphotropic virus III (HTLV III, the etiologic agent of AIDS), rubella virus (both IgG and IgM), *E. histolytica,* and *Toxoplasma gondii.* Reliability of the results of these tests is variable. ELISA systems with the solid phase represented by a bead of metal or glass are available for detection of antibody to rubella virus, cytomegalovirus, herpes simplex virus, *T. gondii, T. pallidum, E. histolytica,* and HTLV III.

12.3. Indirect Fluorescent Antibody Tests and Other Immunomicroscopic Methods

Perhaps the serologic method most widely applied for the detection of diverse antibodies is that of **indirect fluorescent antibody** determination **(IFA)**. For tests of this type, the antigen against which the patient makes antibody (such as whole *Toxoplasma* organisms or viruses in infected tissue culture cells) is affixed to the surface of a microscope slide. The patient's serum to be tested is diluted and placed on the slide, covering the area in which antigen was placed. If antibody is present in the serum, it will bind to its specific antigen. Unbound antibody is then removed by washing the slide. In the second stage of the procedure, antihuman globulin (which may be directed specifically against IgG or IgM) conjugated to a dye that will fluoresce when exposed to ultraviolet light (discussed in Chapter 7) is placed on the slide. This conjugated marker for human antibody will bind to the antibody already bound to the antigen on the slide, and will serve as a marker for the antibody when viewed under a fluorescent microscope (Figure 12.9). Commercially available systems include the slides with the antigens, positive and negative control sera, diluent for the patients' sera, and the properly diluted conjugate. As with other commercial products, IFA systems should be used as units, without modifying the manufacturers' instructions. After they have been stained, the slides are covered with a drop of buffered glycerol and a glass coverslip is applied. The fluorescence does not fade appreciably for several days if the slides are kept refrigerated in the dark, but it is best to examine them immediately after staining. Such slides cannot be used as permanent mounts, since the fluorescence does fade with time. Currently, commercially available IFA tests include those for antibodies to *Legionella* species; *T. gondii;* varicella-zoster virus; cytomegalovirus; Epstein-Barr virus capsid antigen, early antigen, and nuclear antigen; herpes simplex I and II; rubella virus; *Mycoplasma pneumoniae; T. pallidum* (the fluorescent treponemal antibody absorption test,

FIGURE 12.9
Indirect fluorescent antibody test for *Toxoplasma gondii* antibodies. *Toxoplasma* organisms affixed to the slide bind specific antibodies in the patient's serum. Antihuman antibody conjugated with fluorescein binds in turn to the bound patient's antibodies, causing the organisms to fluoresce.

FTA-ABS); and several rickettsiae. Most of these tests, if performed properly, give extremely specific and sensitive results, although tests for herpes simplex II virus antibodies may yield cross-reactive results when herpes simplex I virus antibodies are present. They can be performed rapidly and are cost-effective with only a few samples, in contrast to ELISA.

Antibodies may be conjugated to other markers in addition to fluorescent dyes. This technology has been called **colorimetric immunologic probe detection.** Recently, the use of enzyme-substrate marker systems has expanded. Horseradish peroxidase, alkaline phosphatase, and avidin-biotin conjugated enzyme labels have all been used as visual tags for the presence of antibody. These reagents have the advantages of allowing the preparation of permanent mounts, since the reactions do not fade with storage, and of requiring only a standard light microscope for visualizing results.

12.4. Radioimmunoassay

This automated method of detecting antibodies is usually not performed in a serology laboratory, but in a chemistry laboratory. **Radioimmunoassay (RIA)** is primarily used to measure antigens (notably certain hormones or proteins) in serum samples. The techniques can be used to determine the quantity of antibody as well. For diagnosis of infectious diseases, RIA tests are primarily used to detect antibody to hepatitis B viral proteins. As described in Chapter 11, radioactively labeled antibody competes with the patient's unlabeled antibody for binding sites on a known amount of antigen. A reduction in radioactivity of the antigen-patient antibody complex compared to the radioactive counts measured in a control test with no antibody is used to quantitate the amount of patient antibody bound to the antigen. It is hoped that development of new marker substances, such as enzyme and substrate systems, chemiluminescence, and fluorescence (see 12.5 below), will eventually produce tests as sensitive as RIA without the dangers of radioactive reagents.

12.5. Fluorescence Immunoassays

Because of the inconveniences associated with radioactive substances and scintillation counters, **fluorescence immunoassays (FIA)** were developed. Using fluorescent dyes or molecules as markers instead of radioactive labels, these tests are based on the same principle as RIA. The primary difference is that in RIA systems the competitive antibody is radioactively labeled and in FIA the antigen is fluorescence labeled. Binding of patient antibody to a fluorescent-labeled antigen can reduce or **quench** the fluorescence, or binding can cause fluorescence by allowing conformational change in a fluorescent molecule. These principles and others can be employed for diagnostic tests. Chapter 11 describes the principles involved in the fluorescence immunoassay reader for microbiological determinations. Systems are commercially available to measure antibody to rubella, cytomegalovirus, toxoplasma, and herpes simplex I and II.

12.6. Separating IgM from IgG for Serologic Testing

Since IgM is usually produced only during a patient's first exposure to an infectious agent, the detection of specific IgM can help the clinician a great deal in establishing a diagnosis, especially for diseases that may have less well-characterized clinical presentations, such as toxoplasmosis, or those for which rapid therapeutic decisions may be required. Pregnant women who are exposed to rubella and develop a mild febrile illness can be tested for the presence of antirubella IgM. If positive, damage to the fetus is possible and the option of elective termination of pregnancy should be offered. Given the technical difficulty and limited availability of rubella IgM tests, many physicians prefer to demonstrate seroconversion by hemagglutination inhibition, indirect fluorescent antibody, or complement fixation tests as evidence for current rubella infection. An additional reason to measure IgM alone is for the diagnosis of neonatal infections. Since IgG can readily cross the placenta, newborn babies will carry titers of IgG nearly identical to those of their mothers. Accurate serologic diagnosis of infection in neonates requires either demonstration of a rise in titer (which takes time to occur) or the detection of specific IgM directed against the putative agent. This IgM would have to be of fetal origin, since the molecule does not cross the placental barrier. Agents that are difficult to culture or those that adult females would be expected to have encountered during their lifetimes, such as cytomegalovirus, herpesviruses, *Toxoplasma*, rubella virus, or *T. pallidum*, are those for which specific identification of fetal IgM is most often used. The names of some of the tests for these agents have been grouped together with the acronym TORCH (*Toxoplasma*, rubella, cytomegalovirus, and herpes). These tests should be ordered separately, depending on the clinical illness of a newborn suspected of having one of these diseases. However, infected babies often appear clinically the same as those without any of these infections.

Several methods have been developed to measure only the specific IgM in sera that may also contain specific IgG. In addition to using a labeled antibody specific for only IgM as the marker in the assays described above, the immunoglobulins can be separated from each other by physical means. Centrifugation through a sucrose gradient, performed at very high speeds, has been used in the past to separate IgM, which has a greater molecular weight, from IgG. This method is time consuming and requires a very expensive ultracentrifuge. Most laboratories use a commercially available system that uses the principle of ion exchange (Figure 12.10). Serum is placed on a column of QAE-Sephadex A-50 (an ion exchange resin that binds proteins on the basis of

attracting molecules of opposite electrical charge). Both immunoglobulins will initially bind to the resin. A solution of buffer at pH 7.0 is run through the column and IgG, because of its relatively lesser negative charge, is washed through (eluted) with the buffer. A second buffer of pH 4.2 is then run through the column to elute the more negatively charged IgM. The commercially available IgM isolation system (Isolab, Inc.) recovers more than 80% of the IgM present in the original serum, with very little contaminating IgG. Since the serum must be washed through the column with buffer, the IgM solution in the **eluate** (fluid collected from the column) is more dilute than in the original serum (usually 1:10, depending on the volume of serum originally placed on the column) and the pH will be acidic. The pH should be adjusted back to neutral before the

FIGURE 12.10
Separation of IgM from human serum by passing the serum through an ion exchange column.

eluate is tested serologically. Newer systems that require less manipulation are available. It is even possible, using a specially designed filtration system concentrator, to reconstitute the concentration of IgM in the eluate to that of the original serum. An added bonus of the IgM separation column is that **rheumatoid factor**, IgM antibodies produced by some patients against their own IgG, will often bind to the IgG molecules being washed through the column and be removed along with the IgG. These rheumatoid factors can cause nonspecific and interfering results with many serologic tests, and their presence should be taken into account. There are many cases in which serologic tests can yield false positive and false negative results. Other considerations, including patient history and clinical situation, must be employed in diagnosis of neonatal infection. Culturing the agent from patient material from infants suspected of having herpes or cytomegalovirus infection is still the most reliable diagnostic method.

REFERENCES

1. Chernesky, M.A., Ray, C.G., and Smith, T.F. 1982. In Drew, W.L., editor. Laboratory diagnosis of viral infections. Cumitech 15. American Society for Microbiology, Washington, D.C.
2. Neimeister, R.P., Teschemacher, R., Yankevitch, I.J., and Cocklin, J. 1975. Proficiency testing, trouble shooting and quality control for the RPR test. Am. J. Med. Technol. 41:13.

BIBLIOGRAPHY

Bellanti, J.A. 1985. Immunology III: basic processes, ed. 3. W.B. Saunders Co., Philadelphia.

Carter, J.B., Biesecker, J.L., and Rippey, J.H. 1983. Immunoserology review or "the modern serology lab." American Society of Clinical Pathologists, Commission on Continuing Education, Council on Immunopathology, Chicago, p. 53.

Johnson, R.B., and Libby, R. 1980. Separation of immunoglobulin M (IgM) essentially free of IgG from serum for use in systems requiring assay of IgM-type antibodies without interference from rheumatoid factor. J. Clin. Microbiol. 12:451.

Nichols, W.S. and Nakamura, R.M. 1980. Agglutination and agglutination inhibition assays. In Rose, N.R., and Friedman, H., editors. Manual of clinical immunology, ed. 2. American Society for Microbiology, Washington, D.C.

Noonan, K.D. 1984. Latex agglutination testing: the importance of the microenvironment. Clin. Microbiol. Newsletter 6:20.

Palmer, D.F. 1980. Complement fixation test. In Rose, N.R., and Friedman, H., editors. Manual of clinical immunology, ed. 2. American Society for Microbiology, Washington, D.C.

Roitt, I.M., Brostoff, J., and Male, D.K. 1985. Immunology. Gower Medical Publishing, Ltd., London. (Distributed by C.V. Mosby Co., St. Louis.)

Stevens, R.W. 1980. Particle agglutination tests in the rapid serodiagnosis of bacterial infections. Clin. Immunol. Newsletter 1:1.

13 Methods for Testing Antimicrobial Effectiveness

Isolating an infectious agent from a patient with disease is often not sufficient for determining proper therapy. Many bacteria and some fungi manifest resistance to antimicrobial agents and some viruses have already developed resistance to the newest antiviral agents. Patterns of resistance are constantly changing. No matter how rapidly new therapeutic agents are introduced, the microbes seem to be able to overcome them. Even the pneumococcus, which for decades was invariably susceptible to penicillin G at levels of less than 0.04 U/ml, has developed resistance to this drug in some strains.

Since the susceptibility of bacteria, fungi, and viruses to antimicrobial agents cannot be predicted, testing individual pathogens against appropriate antimicrobial agents is often necessary. The appropriate agent (with the most activity against the pathogen, the least toxicity to the host, appropriate pharmacologic characteristics, and most economical) can then be chosen, allowing a more certain therapeutic outcome. Table 13.1 lists some commonly used antimicrobial agents and the types of etiologic agents against which they are usually effective. The ultimate therapeutic outcome depends on many more variables, of course. The underlying disease and condition of the host, the use of indicated drainage and debridement procedures, the pharmacologic properties of the antimicrobial agent, additional therapeutic agents

TABLE 13.1
Selected General Categories of Antimicrobial Agents Used to Treat Systemic Bacterial Infection

GRAM-NEGATIVE ORGANISMS OTHER THAN *PSEUDOMONAS AERUGINOSA*	*PSEUDOMONAS AERUGINOSA*	GRAM-POSITIVE BACILLI AND STAPHYLOCOCCI	ENTEROCOCCI	ANAEROBES	NONENTEROCOCCAL STREPTOCOCCI
Aminoglycosides	Aminoglycosides	Cephalosporins	Ampicillin	Broad-spectrum penicillins	Penicillins
Broad-spectrum penicillins	Broad-spectrum penicillins	Erythromycin	Penicillin and amino-glycoside combination	Cefoxitin	
Cephalosporins	Cefoperazone	Penicillins	Vancomycin	Chloramphenicol	
Cotrimoxazole	Ceftazidime	Vancomycin		Clindamycin	
Imipenem	Imipenem			Imipenem	
Tetracyclines	Monobactams			Metronidazole	

being given, and other factors will exert a strong influence on the ultimate outcome. Microbiologists can only recommend therapeutic agents based on their in vitro activities. The clinician must make the final choice based on his or her knowledge of all the pertinent facts. At times, an antimicrobial agent that shows poor in vitro activity against an organism is used in a patient with good results; the opposite effect may also occur. One important concept that must be stressed is that in vitro susceptibility tests cannot be performed on mixed cultures; only pure cultures will yield valid results. With these caveats in mind, we have catalogued the antimicrobial susceptibility testing methods currently in widespread use among microbiologists in the United States.

The term **antibiotic** has been defined as a chemical produced by a microorganism that inhibits the growth of other microorganisms. Antibiotics modified by chemical manipulations are still considered to be antibiotics. An **antimicrobial agent** is active against microorganisms and may be produced either naturally by microorganisms or synthetically by scientists in laboratories. The term **chemotherapeutic agent** has been used to refer to synthetic and other antimicrobial agents and also to refer to agents that act against human cells, such as immune modulators and anticancer drugs. The subterms **antiviral agent** and **antifungal agent** are more specific terms that fall into the general category of antimicrobial agents, as we refer to them here.

13.1. Nonautomated In Vitro Susceptibility Testing

During the days soon after the discovery of sulfonamides and penicillin, pathogenic organisms were rarely tested for their susceptibility to drugs. Patients were treated empirically and the organisms were often susceptible. It was not until resistance began to emerge, soon after the agents were introduced, that microbiologists began to test an infecting organism against antimicrobial agents. The classic method used for in vitro testing was that of broth dilution, which yields a quantitative result for the amount of antimicrobial agent that is needed to inhibit growth of a specific microorganism.

For many types of susceptibility testing, a standard inoculum of bacteria must be used. The number of bacteria in a liquid medium can be determined by counting individual cells in a microscopic counting chamber, called a Petroff-Hausser chamber, by measuring the optical density of a broth culture of the bacteria and comparing it to the number of colonies found on subculture to solid agar, by growing the organisms to stationary phase (when their numbers level out at approximately 1×10^9 bacteria per milliliter), or by visually comparing the turbidity of the liquid medium to a standard that represents a known number of bacteria in suspension. Turbidity standards (Figure 13.1) can be prepared by mixing chemicals that precipitate to form a solution of reproducible turbidity. Such solutions, using barium sulfate, were developed by **McFarland** to approximate numbers of bacteria in solutions of equal tur-

FIGURE 13.1
McFarland standards numbers 0.5, 1, and 3.

TABLE 13.2
McFarland Nephelometer Standards

	TUBE NUMBER									
	1	**2**	**3**	**4**	**5**	**6**	**7**	**8**	**9**	**10**
Barium chloride (ml)	0.1	0.2	0.3	0.4	0.5	0.6	0.7	0.8	0.9	1
Sulfuric acid (ml)	9.9	9.8	9.7	9.6	9.5	9.4	9.3	9.2	9.1	9
Approx. cell density ($\times 10^8$/ml)	3	6	9	12	15	18	21	24	27	30

PROCEDURE 13.1. PREPARATION OF McFARLAND NEPHELOMETER STANDARDS

1. Set up 10 test tubes or ampules of equal size and of good quality. Use new tubes that have been thoroughly cleaned and rinsed.
2. Prepare 1% chemically pure sulfuric acid.
3. Prepare 1% aqueous solution of chemically pure barium chloride.
4. Add the designated amounts of the two solutions to the tubes as shown in Table 13.2 to make a total of 10 ml per tube.
5. Seal the tubes or ampules. The suspended barium sulfate precipitate corresponds approximately to homogenous *Escherichia coli* cell densities per milliliter throughout the range of standards, as shown in Table 13.2.

---

bidity, as determined by colony counts (Table 13.2). They are prepared as detailed in Procedure 13.1.

13.1.a. Bacterial broth dilution methods. A complete protocol for performing these tests is found in the **National Committee for Clinical Laboratory Standards (NCCLS)** publication, *M7-T, Tentative Standard—Methods for Dilution Antimicrobial Susceptibility Tests for Bacteria That Grow Aerobically.*[14] We will describe the basics of the procedures, but the reader is referred to the NCCLS publications and other references cited at the end of this chapter for more complete details. For broth dilution methods, decreasing concentrations of the antimicrobial agent(s) to be tested, usually prepared in twofold dilutions, are placed in tubes of a broth medium that will support the growth of the test microorganism. The most commonly used broth for these tests is Mueller-Hinton (available commercially) supplemented with the cations magnesium and calcium (formulas in Chapter 45). For broth dilution susceptibility testing of staphylococci against methicillin, oxacillin, nafcillin, or cephalosporins, 2% sodium chloride must be added to the cation-supplemented Mueller-Hinton broth.

The antimicrobial agents are prepared in concentrated solution in diluent and then diluted to the appropriate concentrations in broth. The diluents used for the commonly tested antimicrobial agents are shown in Table 13.3. Preparation of the antimicrobial agents must take into consideration that the laboratory standard powder obtained from the manufacturer (some of these are listed in Table 13.4),

TABLE 13.3
Solvents and Diluents for Preparation of Stock Solutions of Antimicrobials

ANTIMICROBIAL	SOLVENT*	DILUENT*
Amoxicillin	Phosphate buffer, pH 6.0, 0.1 M	Phosphate buffer, pH 6.0, 0.1 M
Ampicillin	Phosphate buffer, pH 8.0, 0.1 M	Phosphate buffer, pH 6.0, 0.1 M
Cephalothin†	Phosphate buffer, pH 6.0, 0.1 M	Water
Chloramphenicol and erythromycin	Ethanol	Water
Moxalactam (diammonium salt)‡	0.04 N HCl (let sit for 1.5-2 h)‡	Phosphate buffer, pH 6.0, 0.1 M
Nalidixic acid	½ volume of water, then add NaOH 1 M, dropwise to dissolve	Water
Nitrofurantoin§	Phosphate buffer, pH 8.0, 0.1 M	Phosphate buffer, pH 8.0, 0.1 M
Rifampin	Methanol	Water (with stirring)
Sulfonamides	½ volume hot water and minimal amount of 2.5 M NaOH to dissolve	Water
Trimethoprim	0.05 N lactic or hydrochloric acid, 10% of final volume	Water (may require heat)

From National Committee for Clinical Laboratory Standards. 1983. Methods for dilution antimicrobial susceptibility tests for bacteria that grow aerobically; tentative standard. M7-T 3-31. Permission to reproduce this table has been granted by the Committee. NCCLS is not responsible for errors or inaccuracies. The most current edition of the standard is available from NCCLS, 771 E. Lancaster Ave., Villanova, PA 19085.

*These solvents and diluents are for making *stock solutions* of antimicrobials requiring other than aqueous (water) reagents. They can be further diluted as necessary in water or broth. The products known to be suitable for water solvents and dilution are amikacin, azlocillin, bacitracin, carbenicillin, cefamandole, cefotaxime, cefoperazone, clindamycin, cloxacillin, colistin, dicloxacillin, gentamicin, kanamycin, lincomycin, methicillin, mezlocillin, nafcillin, netilmicin, oxacillin, penicillin, piperacillin, polymyxins, spectinomycin, streptomycin, tetracyclines, ticarcillin, tobramycin, trimethoprim (if lactate) and vancomycin.

†Solubilize all other cephalosporins and cephamycins (unless manufacturer indicates otherwise) in phosphate buffer, pH 6.0, 0.1 M and further dilute in sterile distilled water.

‡The diammonium salt of moxalactam is very stable, but is almost pure R isomer. Moxalactam clinical is a 1:1 mixture of R and S isomers. Therefore, dissolve the salt in 0.04 N HCl and allow it to react for 1½-2 h to convert it to equal parts of both isomers.

§Alternatively, dissolve nitrofurantoin in dimethyl sulfoxide (DMSO).

usually at no cost, often does not consist of 100% active compound. The **specific activity** is the amount, in μg/mg, of active antimicrobial agent in the powder. For example, if the microbiologist receives 100 mg of rifampin powder that possesses a specific activity of 950 μg/mg, or 95%, there is actually only 950 μg of active drug in every 1000 μg of powder. The microbiologist must add a little extra powder to the solution to obtain the activity desired. To make a solution containing 1,280 μg/ml rifampin, assuming an activity of 950 μg/mg, a simple calculation is performed.

$$\frac{950}{1000} = \frac{1280}{x}, \qquad x = 1347$$

For every 1,280 μg of active rifampin desired, 1,347 μg of powder of 95% activity must be added to the diluent. This makes sense since the extra powder includes the inactive components. The weight of rifampin powder to be added per ml diluent is then multiplied times the number of ml of diluent desired, to determine how much total powder to weigh. Since the antimicrobial agent is diluted in broth and serial twofold dilutions are then prepared, the initial amount of solution is usually not more

TABLE 13.4
Manufacturers of Commonly Used Antimicrobial Agents (Sources of Laboratory Reference Standard Powders)

ANTIMICROBIAL AGENT	MANUFACTURER
Amikacin	Bristol Laboratories, Syracuse, N.Y.
Amoxicillin	Bristol Laboratories, Syracuse, N.Y.
	Beecham Laboratories, Bristol, Tenn.
Amphotericin	Squibb & Sons, Inc., Princeton, N.J.
Ampicillin	Bristol Laboratories, Syracuse, N.Y.
	Beecham Laboratories, Bristol, Tenn.
Azlocillin	Miles Pharmaceutical, West Haven, Conn.
Aztreonam	Squibb & Sons, Inc., Princeton, N.J.
Bacitracin	The Upjohn Company, Kalamazoo, Mich.
Carbenicillin	Pfizer, Inc., Quality Control Section, Terre Haute, Ind.
Cefaclor	Lilly Research Laboratories, division of Eli Lilly & Co., Indianapolis, Ind.
Cefamandole	Eli Lilly & Co., Indianapolis, Ind.
Cefazolin	Eli Lilly & Co., Indianapolis, Ind.
	Smith, Kline & French Laboratories, Philadelphia, Pa.
Cefoperazone	Pfizer, Inc., Quality Control Section, Terre Haute, Ind.
Cefoxitin	Merck Institute for Therapeutic Research, Rahway, N.J.
Cefotaxime	Hoechst-Roussel, North Somerville, N.J.
Cefsulodin	Abbott Laboratories, North Chicago, Ill.
Ceftazidime	Glaxo, Research Triangle Park, N.C.
Ceftizoxime	Smith, Kline & French Laboratories, Philadelphia, Pa.
Cephalexin	Lilly Research Laboratories, division of Eli Lilly & Co., Indianapolis, Ind.
Cephalothin	Lilly Research Laboratories, division of Eli Lilly & Co., Indianapolis, Ind.
Cephradine	Smith, Kline & French Laboratories, Philadelphia, Pa.
Chloramphenicol	Parke Davis and Co., Detroit, Mich.
	Lederle Laboratories, Pearl River, N.Y.
Cinoxacin	Lilly Research Laboratories, division of Eli Lilly & Co., Indianapolis, Ind.
Clindamycin	The Upjohn Company, Kalamazoo, Mich.
Cloxacillin	Bristol Laboratories, Syracuse, N.Y.
Colistin	Parke Davis and Co., Detroit, Mich.
	Warner Lambert Co., Ann Arbor, Mich.
Dicloxacillin	Bristol Laboratories, Syracuse, N.Y.
Doxycycline	Pfizer, Inc., Quality Control Section, Terre Haute, Ind.
Erythromycin	Eli Lilly & Co., Indianapolis, Ind.

TABLE 13.4

Manufacturers of Commonly Used Antimicrobial Agents (Sources of Laboratory Reference Standard Powders)—cont'd

ANTIMICROBIAL AGENT	MANUFACTURER
Flucytosine (5-fluorocyto-sine)	Hoffman-La Roche, Inc., Nutley, N.J.
Gentamicin	Schering Corporation, Bloomfield, N.J.
Imipenem	Merck Institute for Therapeutic Research, Rahway, N.J.
Kanamycin	Bristol Laboratories, Syracuse, N.Y.
Ketoconazole	Janssen Pharmaceutica, Inc., New Brunswick, N.J.
Lincomycin	The Upjohn Company, Kalamazoo, Mich.
Methicillin	Bristol Laboratories, Syracuse, N.Y.
Metronidazole	G.D. Searle & Co., Skokie Ill.
Mezlocillin	Miles Pharmaceuticals, West Haven, Conn.
Minocycline	Lederle Laboratories, Pearl River, N.Y.
Moxalactam	Lilly Research Laboratories, division of Eli Lilly & Co., Indianapolis, Ind.
Nafcillin	Wyeth Laboratories Inc., Philadelphia, Pa.
Nalidixic acid	Sterling-Winthrop Research Institute, Rensselaer, N.Y.
Neomycin	The Upjohn Company, Kalamazoo, Mich.
Netilmicin	Schering Corporation, Bloomfield, N.J.
Nitrofurantoin	Norwich Pharmacal Company, Norwich, N.Y.
Norfloxacin	Merck Institute for Therapeutic Research, Rahway, N.J.
Nystatin	E.R. Squibb & Sons, Inc., Princeton, N.J.
Oxacillin	Bristol Laboratories, Syracuse, N.Y.
Penicillin	Wyeth Laboratories Inc., Philadelphia, Pa.
	Bristol Laboratories, Syracuse, N.Y.
Piperacillin	Lederle Laboratories, Pearl River, N.Y.
Polymyxin B	Pfizer, Inc., Quality Control Section, Terre Haute, Ind.
	Sigma Chemical Co., St. Louis, Mo.
Rifampin	Ciba Pharmaceutical Co., Summit, N.J.
Sisomicin	Schering Corporation, Bloomfield, N.J.
Spectinomycin	The Upjohn Company, Kalamazoo, Mich.
Streptomycin	Pfizer, Inc., Quality Control Section, Terre Haute, Ind.
Sulfadiazine	ICI Americas Inc., Wilmington, Del.
Sulfamethoxazole	Burroughs Wellcome Co., Research Triangle Park, N.C.
	Hoffman-La Roche, Inc., Nutley, N.J.

Continued.

TABLE 13.4
Manufacturers of Commonly Used Antimicrobial Agents (Sources of Laboratory
Reference Standard Powders)—cont'd

ANTIMICROBIAL AGENT	MANUFACTURER
Sulfisoxazole	Hoffman-La Roche, Inc., Nutley, N.J.
Tetracycline	Bristol Laboratories, Syracuse, N.Y.
	Lederle Laboratories, Pearl River, N.Y.
Ticarcillin	Beecham Laboratories, Bristol, Tenn.
Tobramycin	Lilly Research Laboratories, division of Eli Lilly & Co., Indianapolis, Ind.
Trimethoprim	Burroughs Wellcome Co., Research Triangle Park, N.C.
	Hoffman-La Roche, Inc., Nutley, N.J.
Vancomycin	The Upjohn Company, Kalamazoo, Mich.
	Lilly Research Laboratories, division of Eli Lilly & Co., Indianapolis, Ind.

than 2 ml. NCCLS M7-T also describes preparation of antimicrobial agent solutions.[14]

A standard inoculum of the microorganism (often 1×10^6 organisms per milliliter, a 1:500 dilution of a suspension of turbidity equal to a McFarland standard 1.0, Table 13.2) is added to an equal volume (often 1 ml) of each concentration of antimicrobial agent and to a tube of the growth medium without antimicrobial agent, which serves as a growth control (Figure 13.2). Notice that adding a bacterial suspension will dilute both the suspension and the concentration of antimicrobial agent in the tube; this must be taken into account during preparation of the inoculum and of the dilutions of antimicrobial agents. An uninoculated tube of medium is incubated to serve as a negative growth control. After sufficient incubation (usually overnight), the tubes are examined for turbidity, indicating growth of the microorganism. The organism will grow in the control tube, and in any other tube that does not contain enough antimicrobial agent to inhibit growth. The lowest concentration of the agent that inhibits growth of the organism, as detected by lack of visual turbidity (matching the negative growth control) is designated the **minimum in-**hibitory concentration (MIC). If the concentration of antimicrobial agent represented by the MIC can be readily achieved in the **patient's serum** by normal routes of delivery, the organism is said to be **susceptible** to that agent. Most clinicians try to achieve a concentration of antimicrobial agent at the site of infection that is four times the in vitro MIC of the microorganism being tested although this is not always feasible or necessary. The level of agent attained in the urine, cerebrospinal fluid, other body fluid, or in an abscess may be very much different, however, and such differences must be considered when therapy is being chosen. If the MIC is above the achievable level or within a range toxic to the host, the microorganism is said to be **resistant** to the antimicrobial agent. Thus, susceptibility and resistance are functions of the site of the infection, the microorganism, and the antimicrobial agent being tested. The **breakpoint** of an antimicrobial agent is the concentration that can be achieved in the serum with optimal therapy (Table 13.5). One can find several different versions of breakpoints. We use the FDA version in package inserts for each drug when available. Organisms with MIC's below the breakpoint are

TABLE 13.5
"Breakpoints"* for Activity of Antimicrobial Agents

DRUG	BREAKPOINT†
Penicillin G	32
Ampicillin	16
Carbenicillin, ticarcillin	128
Piperacillin, mezlocillin, azlocillin	128
Cephalexin	8
Cephalothin	16
Cefazolin	32
Cefaclor	8
Cefamandole	32
Cefoxitin	32
Cefotaxime	32
Oxacillin, nafcillin	12
Cefoperazone	32
Moxalactam	32
Chloramphenicol	24
Clindamycin	4
Erythromycin	4
Metronidazole	16
Tetracycline	8
Doxycycline	4
Amikacin	24
Gentamicin	8
Tobramycin	8
Kanamycin	24
Vancomycin	16

*The term "breakpoint" as used here means a concentration of an antimicrobial agent in blood that can be achieved with maximal therapy.
†Levels expressed as µg of drug/ml, except for penicillin G, which is expressed as units of drug/ml.

considered "susceptible." Certain antimicrobial agents are less active at an acid pH, such as might be found within an abscess. These factors also contribute to the efficacy of treatment. The results of in vitro tests are subject to many variables, such as inoculum size, the rate of growth of the bacterium, the incubation period, the nature of the medium used, and the stability of the antimicrobial agent. By using standard methods, as detailed in NCCLS M7-T, microbiologists can deliver consistent results that can serve to aid clinicians in their choices

of therapeutic regimens. Figure 13.2 illustrates a procedure commonly used to determine the MIC of an antibiotic against a test organism.

The MIC measures the ability of the antimicrobial agent to inhibit multiplication of the organism. Thus, organisms in the inoculum may be merely inhibited by the antimicrobial agent and will be able to recommence growing if the antimicrobial influence is removed. In that case, the antimicrobial agent is said to be **bacteriostatic,** or inhibitory. For certain serious infections, such as endocarditis and meningitis, and perhaps osteomyelitis, and in patients who lack a well-functioning immune system, it may be important to determine the ability of an agent to actually kill the infecting organism.

To measure the ability of the antimicrobial agent to kill the microorganism, the **bactericidal activity** test is performed using the same broth dilution susceptibility testing system. When the initial microorganism suspension is being inoculated into the tubes of broth, a measured portion is removed from the growth control tube immediately after it was inoculated and this aliquot is plated to solid agar for determination of actual **colony forming units (CFU)** in the inoculum. The technologist determines this number by counting the number of colonies present after overnight incubation of the agar plate and multiplying times the dilution factor. For example, a 0.001 ml calibrated loop can be used to streak a plate for CFU from dilutions made from the growth control tube. If there were 5×10^5 organisms per milliliter in the test tubes, there should be around 250 colonies on a subculture plate made from a 1:2 dilution of the growth control tube (0.001 ml of a suspension of 2.5×10^5 organisms contains 2.5×10^2 organisms). The 1:2 dilution is necessary in order to be able to count the colonies on the plate. It is possible to accurately count colonies numbering from 30-300 on a subculture plate, but counting a greater number of colonies is time-consuming and often inaccur-

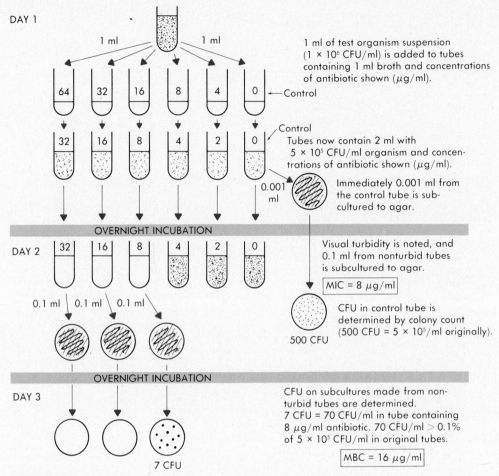

DAY 1

1 ml   1 ml

64   32   16   8   4   0   ←——Control

1 ml of test organism suspension
(1 × 10⁶ CFU/ml) is added to tubes
containing 1 ml broth and concentrations
of antibiotic shown (μg/ml).

32   16   8   4   2   0

Control
Tubes now contain 2 ml with
5 × 10⁵ CFU/ml organism and concentrations of antibiotic shown (μg/ml).

0.001 ml

Immediately 0.001 ml from
the control tube is sub-
cultured to agar.

OVERNIGHT INCUBATION

DAY 2   32   16   8   4   2   0

Visual turbidity is noted, and
0.1 ml from nonturbid tubes
is subcultured to agar.

MIC = 8 μg/ml

0.1 ml   0.1 ml   0.1 ml

CFU in control tube is
determined by colony count
(500 CFU = 5 × 10⁵/ml originally).

500 CFU

OVERNIGHT INCUBATION

DAY 3

CFU on subcultures made from nonturbid tubes are determined.
7 CFU = 70 CFU/ml in tube containing
8 μg/ml antibiotic. 70 CFU/ml > 0.1%
of 5 × 10⁵ CFU/ml in original tubes.

MBC = 16 μg/ml

7 CFU

FIGURE 13.2
Determining MIC and MBC for one organism and one antibiotic.

ate. After the MIC has been determined, a
known quantity (often 0.1 ml) of inoculum from
each of the tubes of broth that showed no visible turbidity after overnight incubation is subcultured to solid agar plates. The small amount
of the antimicrobial agent that is carried over
with this inoculum is easily removed by diffusion into the agar. The number of colonies that
grow on this subculture after overnight incubation is then counted and compared to the
number of CFU/ml in the original inoculum.

Within those tubes that showed no turbidity,
microorganisms were either still viable or they
were killed by the antimicrobial agent. Since
even bactericidal drugs do not always totally
sterilize a bacterial population, the lowest concentration of antimicrobial agent that allowed
less than 0.1% of the original inoculum to survive is said to be the **minimum bactericidal
concentration (MBC)**, also called the **minimum
lethal concentration (MLC)** (illustrated in Figure 13.2). For our example, the MBC would be

TABLE 13.6
Activity of Antimicrobial Agents Against
Bacteria

AGENTS THAT ARE USUALLY BACTERICIDAL	AGENTS THAT ARE USUALLY BACTERIOSTATIC
Aminoglycosides	Chloramphenicol (also
Cephalosporins	bacteriocidal in some
Metronidazole	cases)
Penicillins	Nalidixic acid
Polymyxins	Sulfonamides
Rifampin	Tetracyclines
Vancomycin	

Note: Erythromycin and clindamycin can act as
bactericidal or bacteriostatic agents.

the tube from which less than 50 CFU grew. The technologist must be careful that the original inoculum is great enough to measure a 99.9% lethal effect by the techniques being used in the test. For example, if the original inoculum contained only 10^4 CFU/ml, it would require the subculture of a 1 ml aliquot to yield the number of colonies (greater than 10 CFU) required to demonstrate less than 0.1% survival. One milliliter can be subcultured by pour plate, but it is a cumbersome task.

Certain antimicrobial agents are bactericidal in activity; they cause irreversible damage to bacteria. Other agents are known to be bacteriostatic, inhibiting growth by preventing multiplication, but not causing death. In some cases, drugs that are primarily bacteriostatic may be bactericidal against a given type of organism. The general category of certain antimicrobial agents is shown in Table 13.6. When an agent that has known bactericidal properties exhibits an in vitro MBC that is very much greater than its MIC (requires a great deal more antimicrobial agent to kill the bacteria than to merely inhibit growth; differences of 32 times are sometimes cited) against a bacterial strain, the strain is said to be **tolerant.** Laboratory techniques play a large part in determining whether a bacterial strain is designated as tolerant, as has been pointed out by Taylor and others.[25] The clinical importance of tolerance, if any, has never been established.

Ellner and Neu have proposed reporting susceptibility results in a way that combines the MIC and the achievable peak antimicrobial agent level in a single value, the **inhibitory quotient (IQ).** The IQ is the ratio of the average peak achievable level in the clinical specimen from which the bacterium was isolated (urine, blood, bile, cerebrospinal fluid) to the actual MIC. For example, clindamycin achieves an average peak level of about 5 µg/ml in serum. If the MIC of clindamycin for a *Staphylococcus aureus* strain isolated from blood is 0.5 µg/ml, then the IQ is 5 divided by 0.5, or 10. These authors believe that an IQ 4 to 8 times the MIC can generally provide adequate treatment. No matter how a laboratory reports the results of quantitative susceptibility tests, the most important factor is the acceptance of the results by clinicians and the influence of those results on the treatment of patients.

The MICs and MBCs of a given antimicrobial agent can be determined for any bacterium that is able to grow in liquid media. The optimal temperature for such tests is 35° C, since methicillin-resistant *Staphylococcus aureus* only exhibits that resistance at 35° C or below. Many bacteria require a medium different from cation-supplemented Mueller-Hinton broth or special supplements added to the standard broth to achieve good growth. For example, streptococci are often tested in Todd-Hewitt broth. Certain fastidious bacteria require the addition of horse serum, rabbit serum, or special commercially produced nutrient supplements, such as Fildes' extract (Difco) or Iso-VitaleX (BBL Microbiology Systems).

The methods outlined above can be used to test many types of bacteria, aerobic and anaerobic, but they are time consuming and very labor intensive. For each combination of bacterium and antimicrobial agent, a complete set of tubes must be prepared. It would be prohibitive to test more than a few antimicrobial agents against each isolate. Clinicians, however, have to choose from among numerous possible agents; a more practical method had to be adopted. The development of agar dilution and disk diffusion methods, described below, was one solution to the problem. A more recent innovation has been the adaptation of macrobroth dilution methods to a microbroth format, saving in reagents and technologist time.

The adaptation of the macrobroth dilution test to a microdilution format, which utilizes plastic microdilution trays (Figure 13.3), has made routine reporting of MIC results possible for many laboratories. Although a few large centers still prepare their own microdilution plates to save money and allow flexibility in the antimicrobial agents being tested, most laboratories buy commercially prepared plates. MIC

microdilution trays purchased as commercial systems have the advantage of being prepared in great quantities under very strict quality control standards to assure consistent performance. Their disadvantages include high cost and a predetermined format. Even anaerobic susceptibility testing trays are commercially available; they must be reduced in an anaerobic atmosphere (Chapter 8) before being inoculated and then incubated anaerobically for 48 h. The microbroth systems designed for aerobic organisms are read after overnight (18-24 h) incubation. All plates are viewed manually on a light box or read from the bottom with a mirror reader (Figure 13.4). Automated readers are described in Chapter 11.

Some systems are prepared complete by the manufacturer, shipped frozen to the consumer, and stored in the freezer until thawed and used. Such systems are easy to inoculate, often including a disposable plastic inoculating apparatus that requires only one manipulation to inoculate all 96 wells on the microdilution plate. However, they may suffer from degra-

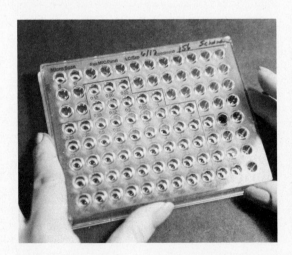

FIGURE 13.3
Plastic microdilution tray used for microbroth dilution antibiotic susceptibility testing. Antimicrobial agents are arranged in linear arrays of serial twofold dilutions.

FIGURE 13.4
Reading microbroth dilution results using a magnifying mirror reader.

dation of the antimicrobial agents if major temperature variations are encountered during shipping and storage. A second type of commercial microbroth system consists of dried or lyophilized antimicrobials. The organism suspension or another diluent may be used to rehydrate the wells. If any number of such plates must be inoculated, some mechanical or instrumental device is necessary. Because of the small volume of medium in the wells, the incubating plates must be protected from dehydration by sealing them with a plastic tape, incubating them in a small humidified chamber (Figure 13.5), or stacking them.

Although microdilution plates are prepared using the same growth medium and the same antimicrobial agent concentrations as macrobroth methods, there is one important differ-

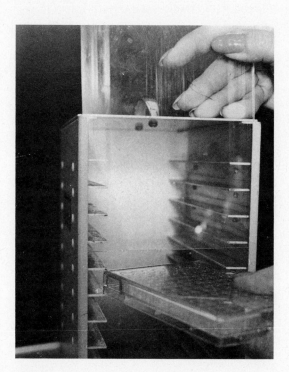

FIGURE 13.5
Incubating microdilution trays in a humidified chamber.

ence. The true inoculum of bacteria, still 5×10^5/ml, is considerably decreased per microdilution well because of the small volume being tested. These wells usually hold only 0.1 ml, effectively reducing the final inoculum to 5×10^4 CFU per well. This number may not include a sufficient number of colony forming units to allow expression of resistance shared by only a small proportion of the total organisms present in the primary isolate. This small, resistant population of organisms may contribute to cases of treatment failure with antimicrobial agents that appeared to be effective by in vitro microdilution MICs. The small inoculum also makes MBC testing difficult, as the numbers of CFU may not be great enough to determine 99.9% killing. We recommend that microbroth dilution methods be used for determining MICs only and that MBC results be reported from macrobroth tube susceptibility tests only.

As for all laboratory tests, susceptibility test results must be monitored and evaluated using standard quality control strains of bacteria. By testing strains with known MICs, technologists can uncover breaks in technique or problems with media or reagents. NCCLS recommends routine testing of *Escherichia coli* American Type Culture Collection (ATCC) 25922, *Pseudomonas aeruginosa* ATCC 27853, *Staphylococcus aureus* ATCC 29213, and *Streptococcus faecalis* ATCC 29212, since their MICs all fall within a measurable range. NCCLS M7-T discusses performance of quality control procedures.

Organisms for which standardized procedures have not been agreed upon can be tested for in vitro susceptibility to selected agents. However, in the absence of standards, results should be interpreted with caution. The filamentous bacteria, particularly *Nocardia* species, may be tested using agar dilution methods; other methods have also been used. Since the methods are so specialized, susceptibility testing of clinically important isolates should be performed only by reference laboratories that have experience in such procedures.

13.1.b. Bacterial disk diffusion methods.

As more antimicrobial agents became available for treating a wide variety of bacteria, the limitations of the macrobroth dilution method became apparent. Before microdilution technology was available, methods were developed for testing an isolate against more than one antimicrobial agent, such as inoculating the surface of an agar plate with the organism to be tested, placing small glass or metal cylinders into the agar to create tiny wells above the agar surface, and placing suspensions of antimicrobial agents into the cylinders. The antimicrobial agent would diffuse into the medium in a circle around the cylinder, inhibiting the growth of the organism wherever the concentration of drug was high enough. Large zones indicated more effective antimicrobial activity. No zone indicated complete resistance. In this crude way, several agents could be tested against one isolate at the same time. This method was modified in 1947 by Bondi and others[5] by incorporating the antimicrobial agent into filter paper disks. The use of disks allowed a large number of identical tests to be prepared in advance and stored for future use. It was not until the landmark study by Bauer, Kirby, Sherris, and Turck[3] in 1966 that the use of filter paper disks for susceptibility testing was standardized and correlated with MICs using a large number of bacterial strains. The disk diffusion susceptibility test, as the method of Bauer, Kirby, Sherris, and Turck was designated, yields qualitative results that correlate well with the quantitative results obtained by MIC tests.

These authors chose concentrations of antimicrobial agents to incorporate into the filter paper disks that showed the best results (clearest, within acceptable size, and most consistent zones of inhibition). They then tested many strains of rapidly growing bacteria, such as Enterobacteriaceae and staphylococci, by both broth dilution and by spreading the bacteria on the surface of Mueller-Hinton agar plates, pressing the disks onto the inoculated plate surfaces, incubating the plates overnight at 35° C, and measuring the zone of inhibition of growth around each disk (Figure 13.6). For each combination of antimicrobial agent and bacterial species tested, a regression analysis was performed, plotting the zone size in millimeters against the MIC (Figure 13.7). Breakpoint zone diameters were chosen that corresponded to the MICs that fell into the susceptible and resistant ranges, based on **achievable serum levels.** For a small group of organisms, the zone size did not correlate well with the MIC. For this reason, zone sizes that fell within an arbitrarily selected middle range were designated "**intermediate.**" For bacteria whose zones fell in this range, the MIC could not be predicted or the organism was **moderately susceptible** to the agent being tested. The latest modifications of the agar disk diffusion testing procedure have been published in NCCLS M2-A3, the current state of the art in such matters; a "moderately susceptible" category has been established for certain penicillins and cephalosporins.[15]

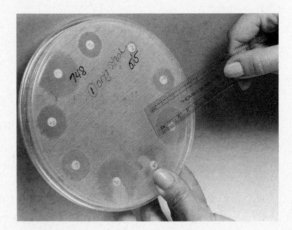

FIGURE 13.6
Measuring zones of inhibition on a disk diffusion susceptibility test plate.

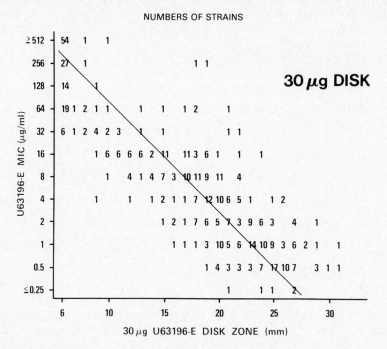

FIGURE 13.7
Example of a regression analysis plot for a series of organisms of the same species tested for MICs by broth dilution compared with disk diffusion zone diameters. (From Jones, R.N., Thornsberry, C., and Barry, A.L. In vitro antimicrobial susceptibility testing using 30 μg and 75 μg U63196-E (Cefpimizole AC-1370) disks. Diagn. Microbiol. Infect. Dis. 3:87, 1985.

The agar disk diffusion test is still used by many laboratories in the United States and around the world, for it is the easiest to perform and standardization is not difficult. The results can also be directly correlated to MIC values. Each time a new antimicrobial agent is developed and released for clinical use, a large number of organisms must be tested in the manner described here to establish interpretive zone sizes for the agent. Unless zone sizes have been specifically established for a species of bacterium, microbiologists may not test an isolate of that species by the agar disk diffusion method because the results will not correlate with known MIC values. It must also be remembered that the designations "susceptible" and "resistant" relate to achievable serum levels; antimicrobial agents that are excreted

through the kidneys achieve much higher concentrations in urine than are obtainable in serum, such that an isolate from a urinary tract infection that is "resistant" by agar disk diffusion may be "susceptible" to the same antimicrobial agent in the urine. For the same reason, the zone sizes that have been established for antimicrobial agents that are used primarily or exclusively for treatment of urinary tract infections, such as nalidixic acid, cinoxacin, nitrofurantoin, trimethoprim, and sulfisoxazole, correspond to levels of antimicrobial agent achievable in urine only.

Interpretation of the results of the disk diffusion test depends on proper performance of the test. The variables that influence the outcome include the depth, pH, cation content, supplements, and source of the Mueller-Hinton agar; the age and turbidity of the bacterial inoculum; the way in which the inoculum is spread on the plate, including the type of cotton swab used for spreading; the temperature, atmosphere, and time of incubation; the method of reading results; the antimicrobial content of the disks, their age and storage conditions; and more. For these reasons, performance of the test must strictly adhere to the NCCLS guidelines.

Laboratories can monitor their performance by periodically testing the recommended quality control strains *Staphylococcus aureus* ATCC 25923, *Escherichia coli* ATCC 25922, and *Pseudomonas aeruginosa* ATCC 27853. For monitoring disks that contain combination antibiotics (such as Augmentin, the beta lactam amoxicillin plus the beta lactamase inhibitor, clavulanic acid), *E. coli* ATCC 35218 is used. Sulfonamide drugs are tested with *Streptococcus faecalis* ATCC 29212 to determine that the

Mueller-Hinton agar does not itself contain sulfonamide-inhibiting substances. The NCCLS publication M2-A3 describes all aspects of performance of this test.[15] An excellent troubleshooting guideline for tracing sources of error in the disk diffusion test was written by Miller and colleagues.[13]

Modifications of the standard disk diffusion test have been adopted for testing several commonly isolated bacteria: *Haemophilus* species, *Neisseria gonorrhoeae*, and *Streptococcus pneumoniae*. Table 13.7 summarizes some of these considerations. Methicillin-resistant *Staphylococcus aureus* poses special problems for susceptibility testing. Mueller-Hinton agar should contain 4% NaCl to obtain the most reliable results. Plates should be incubated at 35° C or slightly lower for at least 24 h, and zones of inhibition around methicillin and oxacillin disks should be examined carefully under **reflected** light for a slight haze of growth; such a

TABLE 13.7
NCCLS Recommendations for Disk Diffusion Testing of Fastidious Aerobic Bacteria*

| ORGANISM† | MEDIUM, SUPPLEMENT | DISK (CONTENT) | ZONE (mm) BREAKPOINT FOR | |
			SUSCEPTIBLE	RESISTANT
H. influenzae	MHA, 1% hemoglobin or 5% lysed horse blood plus 1% IsoVitaleX (BBL) or 1% Supplement VX (Difco)	Ampicillin (10 μg) Penicillin (10 U)	≥20 ≥20 (standard breakpoints appear to apply for chloramphenicol, tetracycline, and trimethoprim-sulfamethoxazole)	≤19 ≤19
S. pneumoniae	MHA, 5% sheep blood	Oxacillin (1 μg) (to screen for penicillin resistance)	≥20	≤12
N. gonorrhoeae	GC Agar Base (Difco), 1% IsoVitaleX or Supplement VX	Penicillin (10 U)	≥20	≤19

From Hindler, J. 1983. Strategies for antimicrobial susceptibility testing of fastidious aerobic bacteria. Am. J. Med. Tech. **49**:761.
*As modified from NCCLS protocol M2-A3.
†Inoculum preparation: suspend overnight growth from plate into MHB to obtain turbidity equivalent to a McFarland 0.5 standard. Incubation: overnight at 35° C in CO_2 for *N. gonorrhoeae*. CO_2 is usually not necessary for *H. influenzae* and *S. pneumoniae*.

haze indicates a resistant subpopulation and the organism should be reported as "resistant." Strains of *S. aureus* (and perhaps coagulase negative staphylococci) resistant to methicillin or oxacillin are likely to be resistant to all penicillinase-resistant penicillins (cloxacillin, nafcillin) and to all classes of cephalosporins, and should be reported as such. Enterobacteriaceae, *Aeromonas, Acinetobacter, Pseudomonas,* staphylococci, enterococci, nonenterococcal streptococci, and *Listeria monocytogenes* can be tested against selected antimicrobial agents by the standard disk diffusion method.[15] If the organism is unable to grow satisfactorily after overnight incubation on Mueller-Hinton agar, 5% defibrinated sheep blood may be added to the agar without appreciably affecting the overall results.

An unusual test that can be performed by the disk diffusion method is the determination of penicillin resistance of *S. pneumoniae* by the organism's inhibition by a 1 μg oxacillin disk. Zones less than 20 mm diameter indicate that the pneumococcus is resistant or relatively resistant to penicillin.

Certain results obtained in vitro are known to be unreliable. For example, cephalosporins are therapeutically ineffective against methicillin-resistant staphylococci that appear to be susceptible to cephalosporins in vitro. All oxacillin or methicillin resistant staphylococci should be reported as resistant to cephalosporins or the unwary physician may be misled. Although *Salmonella typhi* is inhibited by aminoglycosides in vitro, these agents are ineffective for treating typhoid fever. Aminoglycosides may inhibit enterococci in vitro, but they are not ever recommended alone for the treatment of enterococcal infections. Disk diffusion susceptibility testing, while the most standardized and commonly used method in the United States, is still a demanding test, fraught with pitfalls that, if not circumvented, can render the results less than totally reliable. Barry and

Thornsberry discuss performance of the disk diffusion test in the current American Society for Microbiology Manual of Clinical Microbiology.[2]

13.1.c. Agar dilution methods. In addition to broth dilution MICs, another method for testing the MICs of a large number of isolates against many concentrations of several antimicrobial agents is that of **agar dilution.** For this method, concentrations of antimicrobial agents are incorporated into agar plates, one plate for each concentration to be tested. The organisms to be tested are diluted to a slightly greater turbidity than that of a McFarland 0.5 standard, and an aliquot of each suspension is placed into one well of a replicating inoculator device (called a **Steers-Foltz replicator,** Plate 13.1). This device has metal prongs that are calibrated to pick up a small amount of the bacterial suspension (usually 0.001 ml) and deliver it to the agar surface. At least 25 different strains can be placed in the wells of the inoculator for delivery to each plate in a single manual movement. In this manner, approximately 1×10^5 CFU are delivered in a discrete drop to the surface of agar plates containing different concentrations of antimicrobial agents. After overnight incubation, the organisms will grow on those plates that do not contain enough antimicrobial agent to inhibit them. The lowest concentration of agent that allows less than 3 CFU or only a slight haze to grow is the MIC. MBC results cannot be determined using this technique. NCCLS publication M7-T[14] describes performance of this test in detail.

Although agar dilution susceptibility testing is not commonly used by clinical laboratories for testing aerobic organisms, it is a good research laboratory technique for testing anaerobic bacteria and also is used as a reference method against which other methods are compared for testing anaerobic bacteria. As described in NCCLS publication M11-A,[16] the reference test is performed much like the aerobic test with several important modifications. Agar plates must be prepared fresh the same day as they are inoculated, using Wilkins-Chalgren agar (available commercially). The bacteria are brought to turbidity in *Brucella* broth or Schaedler broth before being placed in the inoculator wells. Plates are inoculated quickly and immediately placed into an anaerobic atmosphere for incubation (as described in Chapter 8) and MIC results are read after 48 h of incubation. It must be noted that this NCCLS procedure is a reference procedure and should **not** be used for testing susceptibility of clinical isolates for purposes of guiding therapy—not all anaerobes are able to grow on Wilkins-Chalgren agar and some that do grow do not grow well. Accordingly, the inoculum is relatively small and the organisms may be susceptible to lower levels of drug than when tested with other media. This procedure may be used with *Brucella* base blood agar with reliable results.

13.1.d. Agar dilution susceptibility testing of mycobacteria. Although the frequency with which most bacterial populations produce a mutation that leads to resistance to an antimicrobial agent is usually 1 in 10^6, it is 10 times greater for mycobacteria. Thus, primary treatment of mycobacterial disease should include combinations of two or more agents and susceptibility testing methods should allow recognition of 1% resistance in the population. The antimicrobial agents tested against these organisms are listed in Table 13.8. Secondary agents are tested when an isolate is found to be resistant to the first choice agents, those considered to be primary. The recommended method, the proportion method, is a modified agar dilution susceptibility test. Performance of this test is detailed in the book by Vestal[27] and in Roberts's chapter in Washington's *Laboratory Procedures in Clinical Microbiology.*[20]

Since isolation of mycobacteria can take as long as several weeks and since primary resistance to the first choice antimycobacterial agents is becoming more common, we recommend that susceptibility testing be performed directly on specimens that are discovered to harbor acid fast bacilli, as seen on examination of the concentrate (detailed in Chapter 41). More commonly, however, the presence of mycobacteria will be discovered by isolation of the organisms on culture. The procedures for testing such isolates against primary drugs (**indirect susceptibility testing**) are included here, as well as modifications for **direct** testing of positive specimens.

For testing mycobacteria, Middlebrook 7H11 agar (Chapter 45) containing antimicrobial agents is prepared in quantity, and 5 ml is poured into each section of divided Petri dishes (Felsen quadrant plates) as outlined in Table 13.9. A number of whole Petri plates are

TABLE 13.8

Antimicrobial Agents Used for Testing Mycobacterial Susceptibilities

Primary drugs	Secondary drugs
Isoniazid	Capreomycin
Ethambutol	Cycloserine
Streptomycin	Ethionamide
Rifampin	Kanamycin
Pyrazinamide	p-Aminosalicylic acid

TABLE 13.9

Concentrations of Antimicrobial Agents Used in Middlebrook 7H11 Agar Quadrants for Susceptibility Testing of Mycobacteria

PLATE	QUADRANT	ANTIMICROBIAL AGENT
1	I	None (control)
	II	Isoniazid (0.2 μg/ml)
	III	Isoniazid (1 μg/ml)
	IV	Ethambutol (10 μg/ml)
2	I	None (control)
	II	Streptomycin (2 μg/ml)
	III	Streptomycin (10 μg/ml)
	IV	Rifampin (1 μg/ml)
3	I	p-Aminosalicylic acid (2 μg/ml)
	II	p-Aminosalicylic acid (10 μg/ml)

poured containing drug-free Middlebrook 7H11, to serve as growth controls for determining CFU. These plates can be stored refrigerated, tightly wrapped in plastic, for up to a maximum of 4 weeks before they are inoculated. As in preparing any solution of antimicrobial agent, the specific activity must be taken into account, as described in 13.1.a. Another method for incorporating antimycobacterial agents into agar is to pour the molten agar into the quadrants over antimicrobial agent–impregnated filter paper disks, as described by Wayne and Krasnow,[29] outlined in Table 13.10 (Plate 13.2). These plates must be incubated overnight to allow diffusion of the antimicrobial agent throughout the agar in the quadrant. They may then be refrigerated, but it is best to inoculate them within a few days after preparation. This technique of preparing antimicrobial agent solutions using filter paper–impregnated disks as the source of the drug is called **disk elution.** It is also used for testing anaerobes; see 13.1.e below.

Preparation of the inoculum for indirect mycobacterial susceptibility testing against the primary drugs is outlined in Procedure 13.2.

Mycobacteria tend to grow in serpentine fashion, called **cords,** consisting of many individual organisms bound together. It is necessary to attempt to break up these cords as much as possible to accurately determine the number of resistant bacteria in a population. The use of Tween-containing media and glass beads for vortexing bacterial suspensions helps to break up the cords. As for all procedures involving mycobacteria, these manipulations must be carried out within a biological safety cabinet, described in Chapter 2. Only reference laboratories should be used to test secondary drugs.

If acid fast bacilli are seen on the concentrated direct smear, material from the concentrate can be diluted in Middlebrook 7H9 as shown in Table 13.11 and then inoculated onto quadrants for susceptibility testing as outlined in Procedure 13.2.

In reporting results of the drug susceptibility tests, the report should include:

1. Type of test—direct or indirect
2. Number of colonies on control quadrant
3. Number of colonies on drug quadrant
4. Concentration of drug in each quadrant

From these data, a rough approximation of

TABLE 13.10

Disk Contents for Preparation of Disk-Elution Mycobacterial Susceptibility Test Plates Using Middlebrook 7H11 Agar

PLATE	QUADRANT	DISK	FINAL CONCENTRATION (μg/ml)
1	I	None (control)	0
	II	Isoniazid (1 μl)	0.2
	III	Isoniazid (5 μl)	1
	IV	Rifampin (5 μl)	1
2	I	None (control)	0
	II	Ethambutol (25 μl)	5
	III	Streptomycin (10 μl)	2
	IV	Streptomycin (50 μl)	10
3	I	None (control)	0
	II	p-Aminosalicylic acid (10 μl)	2
	III	p-Aminosalicylic acid (50 μl)	10

PROCEDURE 13.2. INDIRECT MYCOBACTERIAL SUSCEPTIBILITY TESTING

1. Suspend a wooden stickful or a loopful of growth in 5 ml of Middlebrook 7H9 broth (commercially available) containing 5 glass beads, 1-2 mm in diameter. Vortex for 15 seconds. Allow the solution to settle for 10-15 min after vortexing to discourage aerosol dissemination. Either adjust turbidity directly, if culture is fresh, or allow culture to incubate for 7 days.

2. Vortex several times for 15 seconds each to break up cords. Adjust turbidity to that of a McFarland 0.5 standard.

3. Dilute this suspension 1:100 (0.05 ml into 5 ml) and then 1:100 again, to make a final dilution of 1:10,000 in Middlebrook 7H9 broth.

4. Inoculate 0.1 ml of each of the two dilutions (the 10^{-2} and 10^{-4}) onto each quadrant of the drug-containing plates and to two whole plates with drug-free media. Tilt the plates gently to spread the 0.1 ml drop around; do not allow it to pool up around the edges. By spreading the 0.1 ml onto the surface of a whole plate for the growth controls, the actual number of colonies can usually be counted. Leave the plates upright in the safety cabinet with tops slightly ajar for about 10 min to allow the inoculum to dry.

5. Tape the plates closed on two sides with clear cellophane tape to prevent accidental opening, and then place the plates, stacked two high, four plates each into polyethylene plastic bags, sealed with tape.

6. Incubate the plates in 5%-10% CO_2 at 37° C for a maximum of 3 weeks, or until colonies can be counted. Record growth as 4+ (>500 CFU), 3+ (200-500 CFU), 2+ (100-200 CFU), 1+ (50-100 CFU), and the actual number if <50 CFU.

7. Using the number of CFU on the growth control plates from the 10^{-4} dilution, estimate whether or not >1% of the inoculum grew on any drug-containing quadrant.

Modified from Vestal, A.L. 1975. Procedures for the isolation and identification of mycobacteria. DHEW publication no. (CDC) 77-8230. Centers for Disease Control, Atlanta.

TABLE 13.11
Dilution of Concentrate for Inocula

NO. OF ACID FAST BACILLI PER OIL IMMERSION FIELD	CONTROL QUADRANT 1	CONTROL QUADRANT 2	DRUG QUADRANTS
Less than 1	Undiluted	10^{-2}	Undiluted
1-10	10^{-1}	10^{-3}	10^{-1}
More than 10	10^{-2}	10^{-4}	10^{-2}

the percentage of organisms resistant to the drug may be calculated as follows:

$$\frac{\text{No. of colonies on drug quadrant}}{\text{No. of colonies on control quadrant}} \times 100 =$$

% resistance at that drug concentration

Refer to previously cited manual[27] and reference 29 for examples and photographs of these drug susceptibility tests.

Radiometric growth detection (described in Chapter 11) has recently been modified for detection and susceptibility testing of *Mycobacterium tuberculosis* and other mycobacteria. Such testing yields results in several days, as compared with several weeks required for agar dilution methods. Antimicrobial agents are incorporated into bottles containing radioactive substrates (Johnston Laboratories) and growth of the mycobacteria, indicating resistance, is detected by measuring the amount of radioactive gas produced by the bacteria. Further discussion of radiometric detection of growth of mycobacteria is found in Chapter 41. Although the technology has not been adopted by large numbers of laboratories, preliminary reports are promising.

13.1.e. Broth-disk elution methods. Using drug-impregnated filter paper disks as the source of antimicrobial agent for broth or agar dilution testing, disk elution is used not only for testing mycobacteria but is commonly used for testing anaerobic bacteria. Anaerobes can also be tested by using macrobroth or microbroth dilution or agar dilution procedures. There are also special standarized disk diffusion tests for anaerobes, but these are too cumbersome for routine use. Additional details are in the *Wadsworth Anaerobic Bacteriology Manual*.[24] For most laboratories, the broth-disk elution method or a microbroth procedure using commercially available frozen drug-containing trays would be most practical for susceptibility testing of anaerobes. As first described by Wilkins and Thiel,[30] the disk elution method used brain-heart infusion broth that required inoculation under anaerobic conditions and an-

aerobic incubation. This method proved too cumbersome for most laboratories and was modified by Kurzynski and others to allow inoculation and incubation to be performed in air. Helstad and others have since refined the method,[9] which is outlined in Procedure 13.3.

At least two automated susceptibility testing systems, Autobac (General Diagnostics) and MS-2 (Abbott Laboratories) use the disk elution technique for susceptibility testing of aerobes. These instruments are described in Chapter 11. Automated susceptibility testing instruments are mentioned briefly below.

13.1.f. In vitro fungal susceptibility testing methods. Because fungi are large cells with more variation in size than bacteria, preparation of a standard suspension of known CFU is difficult. Primarily for this reason, fungal susceptibility testing is difficult to perform and is thus much less standardized than are bacterial methods. Although possible for yeast, establishing a standardized inoculum for filamentous fungi is beyond the capability of most laboratories. Basically, fungi are tested by the macrobroth dilution method against amphotericin B and 5-fluorocytosine, the two most commonly used antifungal agents. Methods for testing the newer imidazoles, ketoconazole, miconazole, and clotrimazole, are not well described. Special media are necessary for fungal susceptibility testing; such testing is best left to a reference laboratory.

Disk diffusion tests for testing 5-fluorocytosine have been described by Utz and Shadomy,[26] but they are not widely accepted. A good discussion of current methods can be found in the chapter by Shadomy, Espinel-Ingroff, and Cartwright.[23]

13.1.g. In vitro viral susceptibility testing methods. Although not routinely performed, even by laboratories that perform routine viral cultures, viral susceptibility testing is a procedure that has been described and will undoubtedly become more widely used in the future. As shown by Howell and Miller,[11] routine testing of herpes simplex isolates against acyclovir

PROCEDURE 13.3. ANAEROBIC SUSCEPTIBILITY TESTING BY BROTH-DISK ELUTION

1. Prepare enriched (supplemented) thioglycolate broth without indicator (Chapter 45) in 16 × 100 mm glass screw-cap test tubes, 5 ml broth per tube. Just before use, the media should be boiled for 5 min to drive off oxygen and cooled to room temperature.
2. Add the appropriate number of drug-impregnated disks, as shown in Table 13.12. Although a 2 h diffusion period was originally recommended, this has not been found to be essential for good results.
3. Prepare the inoculum directly from colonies on agar. Suspend enough growth in 5 ml of freshly boiled thioglycolate to approximate the turbidity of a 0.5 McFarland standard. If there are insufficient isolated colonies for direct inoculation, colonies may be incubated overnight in supplemented thioglycolate broth to achieve enough turbidity. Add 2 drops of inoculum to each tube of broth with disks and to one tube of drug-free broth as a growth control.
4. Tighten caps, gently invert tubes two or three times to mix, and incubate 18-24 h at 37° C. (Occasionally, 48 h incubation is required.) Interpret the anaerobic isolate to be resistant to all antimicrobial agents in which growth (measured by visual turbidity) is equal to or greater than 50% of that found in the control tube. For most isolates, there will be no visible growth in tubes containing an antimicrobial agent to which the isolate is susceptible. If the interpretation of the test is unclear for any single antimicrobial agent, report the organism as resistant to that agent or repeat the test.

can be accomplished without much difficulty. With increasing use of antiviral agents, such as amantadine for influenza A and the antiherpetic agents (acyclovir, arabinoside-A, ribavirin, etc.), the testing of viral isolates for resistance will undoubtedly become necessary to assist clinicians in choices of therapy. Briefly, supernatant from a tissue culture known to be producing infectious virus is inoculated into several wells of freshly passed tissue culture cells, some control wells without drug and some wells containing dilutions of the antiviral agent being tested. After sufficient incubation to produce cytopathic effect in the control wells, the wells containing antiviral agent are examined. The concentration of antiviral agent that reduces the number of tissue culture infec-

tive doses can be identified. Arbitrary numbers of infected cells can be chosen to approximate different levels of antiviral activity. For herpes cultures, results may be available as quickly as within 24 h.

13.2. Serum Bactericidal Levels

In addition to determining in vitro susceptibility test results for isolates from patients receiving antimicrobial therapy, a laboratory can measure the activity of the patient's own serum against his or her specific pathogen. The lowest dilution of patient's serum that kills a standard inoculum of the organism is called the **serum bactericidal level (SBL)**. Originally described by Schlichter and MacLean,[21] the test was used to measure the antibacterial level of

TABLE 13.12

Preparation of Broth-Disk Elution Tubes for Anaerobic Susceptibility Testing

ANTIMICROBIAL AGENT	DISK CONTENT (μg)	NO. DISKS/5 ml	FINAL CONCENTRATION (μg/ml)
Ampicillin	10	2	4
Carbenicillin	100	6	120
Cefoperazone	75	4	60
Cefoxitin, cefamandole, cefotaxime	30	3	18
Chloramphenicol	30	3	18
Clindamycin (for oral	10	2	4
therapy)	2	4	1.6
	2	8	3.2
Mezlocillin	75	4	60
Moxalactam	30	3	18
Metronidazole	80	1	16
Penicillin	10 U	1	2 U
Ticarcillin	75	4	60

From Sutter, V.L., Citron, D.M., Edelstein, M.A.C., and Finegold, S.M. 1986. Wadsworth anaerobic bacteriology manual, ed. 4. Star Publishing Co., Belmont, Calif.

serum from rabbits being treated with penicillin for experimental endocarditis. Still known as the **Schlichter test** in some laboratories, it has been modified to serve as a broad guideline to aid clinicians in deciding whether a patient is being given effective therapy for a serious infection. This test has been particularly recommended for assessing treatment of endocarditis, although Coleman, Horwitz, and Andriole[7] were unable to establish an association between serum bactericidal concentrations and therapeutic outcome. The paper by these authors contains references to many earlier studies. Wolfson and Swartz[32] also discuss many aspects of the serum bactericidal test.

Despite the controversy associated with this test, some still feel that it can serve to provide general guidelines for the clinician treating such conditions as osteomyelitis or bacterial endocarditis or in therapy of patients with cancer or other immunosuppressive disorders. Various elements of performance of the test may vary among laboratories; they include the inoculum (stage of growth, number of CFU), the diluent

(broth, diluted human serum), method of subculture, timing of serum collection, and others. Blood for testing should be collected approximately 15 min before the next dose of antimicrobial agent is administered (**trough** or **valley** level) and approximately 30 min after the antimicrobial agent has been administered to the patient (**peak** level). Because of the problems in standardizing pooled human sera, we suggest that those wishing to use the test use broth diluent. A concise discussion of the variables involved in the serum inhibitory and bactericidal tests can be found in the references by Washington[28] and Witebsky.[31] Another method is described by Schoenknecht, Sabath, and Thornsberry.[22]

Often the results of tests of this type are not clearcut. Each laboratory must decide how skipped tubes and inconsistent results should be handled. Possible strategies include performing tests in duplicate or repeating the entire procedure. Most studies have suggested that an SBL of greater than or equal to 1:8 corresponds to adequate therapy. The most conservative values suggested for determining therapeutic efficacy are that the patient's serum yield a peak titer of greater than or equal to 1:64 and a trough of greater than or equal to 1:32. Because methods for obtaining such values differ among laboratories, a consensus has not been reached. The NCCLS has formed a subcommittee to establish standardized procedures for serum inhibitory and bactericidal testing procedures.

13.3. In Vitro Synergism and Antagonism

When combinations of two or more antimicrobial agents provide more antimicrobial activity against a pathogen than the total additive effect of the agents given separately, the agents are said to be **synergistic.** Combinations of antimicrobial agents are advisable for treating serious infections, for infections in hosts with compromised immune systems, for treating infections due to organisms known to develop resistance to one agent, and for certain mixed infections. In contrast, when one agent diminishes the activity of a concurrently administered second antimicrobial agent, their activity is said to be

antagonistic. Antagonism may occur, for instance, if a growth-inhibiting agent, such as chloramphenicol, is administered with an agent such as penicillin, which requires actively growing bacteria for bactericidal activity. The antagonism in the example cited is primarily of the nature of **slower** bactericidal activity; such slowing of bactericidal activity may be significant in meningitis, for example. Synergism and antagonism of two antimicrobial agents against a particular bacterium can be measured by performing an in vitro test using a checkerboard format, as illustrated in Figure 13.8.

If only two agents are being assessed for synergism, **time kill curves** may provide the most clinically relevant answer. In such tests, as in simple MIC determinations for combinations of agents, the antimicrobial agents are added to broth in fractions of the MIC, which was established in a previous test. For example, drug A is tested at one fourth of its MIC and drug B is added to drug A at one half, one fourth, and one eighth of its MIC (when tested separately). The definition of synergy is that the sum of the fractions for an effective combi-

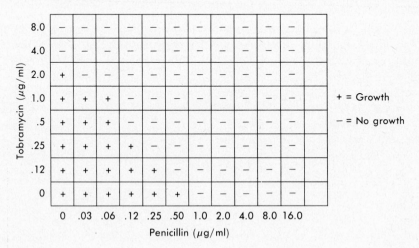

FIGURE 13.8
Checkerboard microdilution format used for testing synergism of two antimicrobial agents against a bacterium.

nation is less than unity. The reverse combinations of antimicrobial agents are also tested, as are the antimicrobial agents alone. The inoculum is added as for MIC tests, and samples of the suspensions are removed at intervals during incubation for subculture to determine CFU. If there is a decrease of CFU corresponding to $\frac{1}{100}$ of the CFU found on subculture from a tube containing the most effective drug tested singly, synergism is assumed.

Serious infections caused by enterococci, the most penicillin-resistant streptococci, are often treated with combinations of a penicillin and an aminoglycoside. Although time kill curves of the organism against combinations of the two antimicrobial agents being used would give the most specific information about synergism, a screening procedure has been suggested. By determining whether the isolate is resistant to a very high concentration of aminoglycoside, a prediction can be made as to the organism's probable response to such combination therapy. For example, the isolate is tested in a broth dilution system against 2,000 µg/ml streptomycin. If the enterococcus is resistant to this amount, it can be assumed that there will be no synergism.

Synergism with three or more agents can be performed, but the methods are too cumbersome for routine use. Berenbaum[4] and Schoenknecht and others [22] discuss the theory of such tests. Methods for synergism testing are described in the book edited by Lorian (listed in the Bibliography) as well as in many other publications. Recent discussions of methods are found in the papers by Marymount and Marymount[12] and Norden.[17]

13.4. Rapid Tests for Antimicrobial Susceptibility

Certain bacteria are resistant to some penicillin and cephalosporin antibotics due to their production of the enzyme **beta lactamase.** This enzyme binds to antibiotics that possess a beta lactam ring (Figure 13.9) and, in most cases,

ultimately opens the ring, inactivating the antibiotic. Although it is not the only resistance mechanism against beta lactam antibiotics, it is a very important one. The presence of beta lactamase, either in body fluid, culture supernatant, or directly within bacterial cells, can be demonstrated with a very rapid test, the **beta lactamase test.** The substrate can be a penicillin or a cephalosporin, since both classes of antibiotic may be affected by these enzymes. Several methods have been used to detect beta lactamases, as described in the *Manual of Clinical Microbiology.*[22] For example, products of penicillin breakdown can reduce iodine bound to starch, causing loss of the color of the starch-iodine compound. Hydrolysis of penicillin into acid products by the enzyme has been measured by a color change in a pH indicator (phenol red) from red to yellow. The most sensitive method, however, is detection of the enzyme by its ability to hydrolyze the beta-lactam ring of a **chromogenic cephalosporin** (a cephalosporin that is a visibly colored compound, yellow in its complete state and red if the beta lactam ring is broken). This compound, called nitrocefin (Glaxo), has a very high affinity for most bacterial beta lactamases. The compound is commercially available impregnated onto filter paper disks or strips (Cefinase, BBL Microbiology Systems). A small amount of growth of the organism to be tested is rubbed on the filter paper. Development of a red color within a

Basic cephalosporin

FIGURE 13.9
The beta lactam ring.

maximum of 30 min indicates presence of beta lactamase. The test is useful for testing isolates of gonococci, *Staphylococcus aureus*, most *Bacteroides* species (*Bacteroides gracilis* is often resistant to a number of beta lactam drugs but is nitrocefin negative), and *Haemophilus* species. (*H. influenzae* may, of course, be ampicillin-resistant by a mechanism other than beta lactamase production and would thus be beta lactamase negative as well.) The nitrocefin test is the only beta lactamase test that can detect beta lactamases of all of the aforementioned species. Presumptive tests may be performed on cerebrospinal fluid sediment and blood culture supernatant as long as appropriate negative controls are also tested concurrently.

A second rapid test can be used to detect chloramphenicol resistance among *Haemophilus*. If the organisms possess chloramphenicol acetyltransferase, the enzyme will modify a substrate (acetyl-S-coenzyme A), the breakdown product of which can induce a chromogenic indicator substance to turn yellow. The reagents for this test are commercially available as filter paper disks (C.A.T., Remel Laboratories). Results are obtained within 30 min. *Haemophilus* isolates from cerebrospinal fluid and blood should be tested upon initial isolation, since the incidence of chloramphenicol resistance appears to be increasing, although it is still very low.

Several other strategies can be used to determine susceptibility results more rapidly than is possible with conventional methods. Agar disk diffusion results on plates prepared in the standard manner may be read quite accurately after only 5-6 h incubation in many cases. The use of a heavy inoculum, described by Lorian (discussed in more detail in Chapter 4) allowed accurate readings within 5 h of inoculating pure cultures to plates. Some workers have used tetrazolium dye, a compound that is reduced to purple by metabolizing bacteria, to delineate zones of inhibition on agar disk diffusion plates after 6½ h incubation. By increasing the initial inoculum, broth dilution tests may be modified to yield faster results. The most radical method for obtaining rapid results, however, is the inoculation of susceptibility testing media with material from the clinical specimen itself. Although results using inocula from body fluids and urines have not correlated well with conventional methods, they do yield general information. Tests performed on positive blood culture broth, however, have given satisfactory results. As detailed in Chapter 4, susceptibility tests may be set up directly or within a few hours of detection of a positive blood culture.

By far the most accepted methods for obtaining rapid susceptibility results are the automated systems. The Automicrobic System (Vitek Systems), the Autobac IDX (General Diagnostics), and the MS-2 and Avantage (Abbott Laboratories) have utilized small cuvettes or growth wells in which the test organism is incubated. Growth is determined photometrically by a measurement of turbidity. Each of these systems yields accurate results in 3-6 h. Several other manufacturers have automated parts of the methods used for testing MICs in microdilution trays. Although most of the systems require overnight incubation, including Micro-Media Systems, American MicroScan, Sceptor (BBL Microbiology Systems), Uniscept (API), and Pasco (Difco Laboratories), at least one system provides results in 5 h (Sensititre, GIBCO Laboratories). General principles of such systems are discussed in Chapter 11. New methods being developed include the use of fluorogenic compounds to measure growth, laser imaging of growth in wells, and fluorescence markers as probes for actively growing cells. The ability to deliver susceptibility determinations to the physician within the first few hours of discovery of the infectious process is the ultimate goal of such studies.

13.5. Measurement of Antimicrobial Agent Levels in Body Fluids

The measurement of the amount of antimicrobial agent in the serum or body fluid of a patient is performed for two reasons. First, it is the best method for determining whether an effective level of antimicrobial agent is being achieved. Although serum is usually tested, levels of agents in cerebrospinal fluid or other body fluids may not correlate with serum levels. For some drugs, impaired renal function and other conditions may lead to excessive serum levels with conventional dosage. Second, several agents, notably the aminoglycosides, are therapeutically effective at concentrations very close to those that may be toxic to the host. The administration of these agents should be carefully monitored by determining serum levels. The dosage can be adjusted to prevent toxicity while maintaining adequate therapeutic levels.

Methods for measuring the concentrations of these agents in body fluids are constantly being improved and refined. Originally, all assays were performed as **bioassays,** using an indicator strain of bacterium sensitive to the drug being evaluated. Known concentrations of the drug were impregnated into filter paper disks or placed in wells on the surface of an agar plate that had been seeded with an inoculum of an organism known to be sensitive to that drug. The patient's serum or other body fluid was also placed on similar disks or in similar wells in duplicate. By comparing the sizes of zones of inhibition of the bacterial strain around the known amounts of drug to the zones formed around the patient specimen, a good estimate of the amount of the antimicrobial agent present in the specimen could be determined. This method worked well with single agents but became difficult to perform when a patient was receiving multiple agents. At first, organisms that were resistant to every antimicrobial agent except the one being tested were

sought. Eventually, however, technological advances allowed the development of automated methods.

Most antimicrobial agent levels are performed by gas liquid chromatography, high pressure liquid chromatography, fluorescence polarization immunoassay, radioimmunoassay or some other type of competitive binding immunoassay, or some other form of immunoassay. Discussion of the princples of some of the instruments involved is found in Chapter 11.

The results of tests for levels of antimicrobial agents, also called **therapeutic drug monitoring (TDM),** are used to modify treatment being administered to patients with infectious diseases. The same automated test systems, however, are also used to monitor therapy with many other agents, including antiepileptic, antiarrhythmic, antineoplastic, and antidepressant compounds. For this reason, such testing is usually performed in the chemistry section of the laboratory, rather than microbiology. The immunoassays being developed for TDM are much more specific and easier to perform than were the bioassays, and they have the advantage of yielding results within hours, rather than requiring overnight incubation. Publications by Anhalt,[1] Buchanan et al.,[6] Edberg et al.,[8] Pezzlo,[18] and Pippenger[19] discuss various aspects of TDM testing.

REFERENCES

1. Anhalt, J.P. 1981. Liquid chromatographic assay of antibiotics. Clin. Microbiol. Newsletter 3:159.
2. Barry, A.L., and Thornsberry, C. 1985. Susceptibility testing: diffusion test procedures. In Lennette, E.H., Balows, A., Hausler, W.J., Jr., and Shadomy, H.J., editors. Manual of clinical microbiology, ed. 4. American Society for Microbiology, Washington, D.C.
3. Bauer, A.W., Kirby, W.M.M., Sherris, J.C., and Turck, M. 1966. Antibiotic susceptibility testing by a standardized single disk method. Am. J. Clin. Pathol. 45:493.
4. Berenbaum, M.C. 1978. A method for testing for synergy with any number of agents. J. Infect. Dis. 137:122.

5. Bondi, A., Spaulding, E.H., Smith, E.D., and Dietz, C.C. 1947. A routine method for the rapid determination of susceptibility to penicillin and other antibiotics. Am. J. Med. Sci. 214:221.

6. Buchanan, A.G., Witwicki, E., and Albritton, W.L. 1983. Serum aminoglycoside monitoring by enzyme immunoassay, biological, and fluorescence immunoassay procedures. Am. J. Med. Tech. 49:437.

7. Coleman, D.L., Horwitz, R.I., and Andriole, V.T. 1982. Association between serum inhibitory and bactericidal concentrations and therapeutic outcome in bacterial endocarditis. Am. J. Med. 73:260.

8. Edberg, S.C., Barry, A.L., and Young, L.S. 1984. Cumitech 20. Therapeutic drug monitoring: antimicrobial agents. American Society for Microbiology, Washington, D.C.

9. Helstad, A.G., Hutchinson, M.A., Amos, W.P., and Kurzynski, T.A. 1984. Evaluation of two broth disk methods for antibiotic susceptibility testing of anaerobes. Antimicrob. Agents Chemother. 26:601.

10. Hindler, J. 1983. Strategies for antimicrobial susceptibility testing of fastidious aerobic bacteria. Am. J. Med. Tech. 49:761. (Entire issue devoted to susceptibility testing.)

11. Howell, C.L., and Miller, M.J. 1984. Rapid method for determining the susceptibility of herpes simplex virus to acyclovir. Diagn. Microbiol. Infect. Dis. 2:77.

12. Marymount, J.H., and Marymount, J. 1981. Laboratory evaluation of antibiotic combinations; a review of methods and problems. Lab. Med. 12:47.

13. Miller, J.M., Thornsberry, C., and Baker, C.N. 1984. Disk diffusion susceptibility test troubleshooting guide. Lab. Med. 15:183.

14. National Committee for Clinical Laboratory Standards. 1983. Methods for dilution antimicrobial susceptibility tests for bacteria that grow aerobically. M7-T 3:31. Order no. M7-T, available from NCCLS, 771 East Lancaster Avenue, Villanova, PA 19085. (Enclose check for $15.00 with your order, plus $5.00 for overseas postage.)

15. National Committee for Clinical Laboratory Standards. 1984. Performance standards for antimicrobial disk susceptibility tests, ed. 3, M2-A3 4:369. Order no. M2-A3, available from NCCLS, 771 East Lancaster Avenue, Villanova, PA 19085. (Enclose check for $15.00 with your order, plus $5.00 for overseas postage.)

16. National Committee for Clinical Laboratory Standards. 1985. Reference agar dilution procedure for antimicrobial susceptibility testing of anaerobic bacteria; approved standard. Order no. M11-A, available from NCCLS, 771 East Lancaster Avenue, Villanova, PA 19085. (Enclose check for $15.00 with your order, plus $5.00 for overseas postage.)

17. Norden, C.W. 1982. Problems in determination of antibiotic synergism in vitro. Rev. Infect. Dis. 4:276.

18. Pezzlo, M. 1983. Assay of antimicrobial agents. Am. J. Med. Tech. 49:779.

19. Pippenger, C.E. 1983. The future role of the clinical laboratory in therapeutic drug monitoring. Am. J. Med. Tech. 49:565.

20. Roberts, G.D. 1981. Mycobacteria and nocardia. In Washington, J.A. Jr., editor. Laboratory procedures in clinical microbiology. Springer-Verlag, New York.

21. Schlichter, J.G., and MacLean, H. 1947. A method for determining the effective therapeutic level in the treatment of subacute bacterial endocarditis with penicillin: a preliminary report. Am. Heart J. 34:209.

22. Schoenknecht, F.D., Sabath, L.D., and Thornsberry, C. 1985. Susceptibility tests: special tests. In Lennette, E.H., Balows, A., Hausler, W.J. II, and Shadomy, H.J., editors. Manual of clinical microbiology, ed. 4. American Society for Microbiology, Washington, D.C.

23. Shadomy, S., Espinel-Ingroff, A., and Cartwright, R.Y. 1985. Laboratory studies with antifungal agents: susceptibility tests and bioassays. In Lennette, E.H., Balows, A., Hausler, W.J. Jr., and Shadomy, H.J., editors. Manual of clinical microbiology, ed. 4. American Society for Microbiology, Washington, D.C.

24. Sutter, V.L., Citron, D.M., Edelstein, M.A.C., and Finegold, S.M. 1985. Wadsworth anaerobic bacteriology manual, ed. 4. Star Publishing Co., Belmont, Calif.

25. Taylor, P.C., Schoenknecht, F.D., Sherris, J.C., and Linner, E.C. 1983. Determination of minimum bactericidal concentrations of oxacillin for Staphylococcus aureus: influence and significance of technical factors. Antimicrob. Agents Chemother. 23:142.

26. Utz, C., and Shadomy, S. 1977. Antifungal activity of 5-fluorocytosine as measured by disc diffusion susceptibility testing. J. Infect. Dis. 135:970.

27. Vestal, A.L. 1975. Procedures for the isolation and identification of mycobacteria. DHEW publication no. (CDC) 77-8230. Centers for Disease Control, Atlanta.

28. Washington, J.A. II. 1981. Bactericidal tests. In Washington, J.A. II, editor. Laboratory procedures in clinical microbiology. Springer-Verlag, New York.

29. Wayne, L.G., and Krasnow, I. 1966. Preparation of tuberculosis susceptibility testing medium by means of impregnated discs. Am. J. Clin. Pathol. 45:769.

30. Wilkins, T.D., and Thiel, T. 1973. Modified broth-disk method for testing the susceptibility of anaerobic bacteria. Antimicrob. Agents Chemother. 10:926.

31. Witebsky, F.G. 1984. Serum inhibitory and bactericidal titrations. ASCP Check Sample MB 84-7 (MB-138). American Society of Clinical Pathologists, Traverse City, Mich.

32. Wolfson, J.S., and Swartz, M.N. 1985. Serum bactericidal activity as a monitor of antibiotic therapy. N.
Engl. J. Med. 312:968.

BIBLIOGRAPHY

Isenberg, H.D., and D'Amato, R.F. 1984. Rapid methods
for antimicrobic susceptibility testing. In Cunha, B.A.,
and Ristuccia, A.M., editors. Antimicrobial therapy.
Raven Press, New York.

Lorian, V., editor. 1984. Antibiotics in laboratory medicine. Williams & Wilkins, Baltimore.

Willett, H.P. 1980. The action of chemotherapeutic agents.
In Joklik, W.K., Willett, H.P., and Amos, D.B., editors.
Zinsser microbiology, Appleton-Century-Crofts, New
York.

Part Three

Etiologic Agents
Recovered from
Clinical Material

14 Microorganisms Encountered in the Blood

Microorganisms present in the circulating blood, whether continuously or transiently, are a threat to every organ in the body. Invasion of the bloodstream by microorganisms per se, aside from the problems of disseminating infection and involving and affecting the function of implanted foreign bodies (e.g., heart valves and artificial joints), may have serious immediate consequences, including shock, disseminated intravascular coagulation (DIC), and death. Thus, bacteremia constitutes one of the most serious situations in infectious disease. The expeditious detection and identification of blood-borne pathogens is one of the most important functions of the microbiology laboratory. Positive blood cultures may help provide a clinical diagnosis as well as a specific etiologic diagnosis. Pathogens of all four major groups—bacteria, fungi, viruses, and parasites—may be found in circulating blood during the course of disease. Bacteria, on the other hand, may also be recovered from peripheral blood in the absence of disease. After any loss of the integrity of the capillary endothelial cells, a few bacteria may enter the bloodstream and live for a short time until the primary defense systems of a healthy host (phagocytic cells or antibody and complement) destroy them. Eukaryotic parasites may also be found transiently in the bloodstream as they migrate to the environment of choice. Their presence, however, can-

not be considered to be consistent with a state of good health. Table 14.1 shows the most common microorganisms isolated from blood during a 2-year period at one major medical center. The kinds of microorganisms isolated from blood cultures vary depending on the patient population served by an institution.

14.1 Parasitic Infections

14.1.a. Pathogenic mechanisms. Parasites that infect cellular components may cause disease by disrupting the normal function of the infected cells. Invasion of the phagocytic cells of the reticuloendothelial system, as occurs in visceral leishmaniasis, renders those cells less able to fulfill their role as nonspecific immune responders. Proliferation of infected mononuclear phagocytes in the liver, spleen, and bone marrow, leads to enlargement of the liver and spleen and contributes to the anemia and leukopenia seen in patients with this infection. Primary growth of *Trypanosoma cruzi* in the human host occurs in various host cells that are initially penetrated. When the parasites mature to the trypomastigote stage and burst out of the host cells, a generalized parasitemia results. Although able to multiply in any organ, the organisms prefer to invade muscle (including heart muscle) and nerve tissue; the cycle then repeats itself. Damage to the host is probably due to both its own inflammatory response attempting to localize or destroy infected tissue, and to rupture of infected host cells during the release of trypomastigotes. The most important consequences of the disease are congestive heart failure and cardiac arrhythmias relating to cardiac muscle and its conducting tissue involvement, and dilation of the esophagus and colon, probably related to neuronal involvement.

Tachyzoites of the parasite *Toxoplasma gondii* may be found in circulating blood. They invade cells within lymph nodes and other organs, including lung, liver, heart, brain, and eye. The resulting cellular destruction ac-

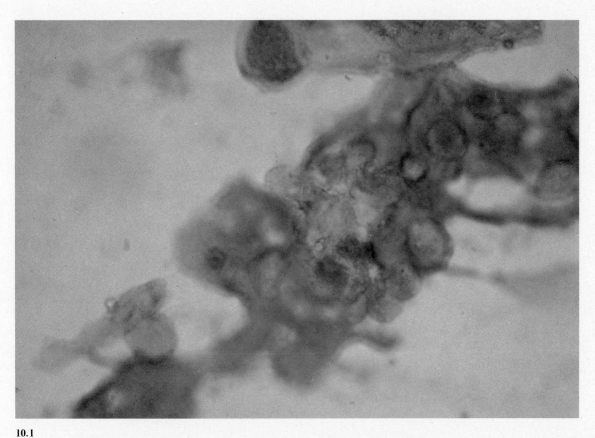

10.1

PLATE 10.1. Direct detection of herpes simplex virus on a vaginal smear. A herpes simplex specific biotinylated DNA probe (Enzo Biochem) complexes to homologous viral DNA sequences in the nuclei of infected cells. Avidin complexed to horseradish peroxidase serves as the visual marker, causing the nuclei of infected cells to appear red. (Courtesy Enzo Biochem, Inc.)

11.1

11.2

PLATE 11.1. Plastic card containing dried substrate in tiny wells. The tray is filled with a suspension of urine or an organism by vacuum suction, incubated and interpreted automatically (AutoMicrobic System, Vitek Systems).

PLATE 11.2. Ouchterlony gel diffusion reaction; antiserum in center well and antigens in outside wells. The continuous precipitin line indicates immunologic identity.

13.1

PLATE 13.1. Steers replicator apparatus used for performing agar dilution susceptibility tests.

13.2

PLATE 13.2. *Mycobacterium tuberculosis* susceptibility test (organism is INH resistant).

TABLE 14.1

Microorganisms Isolated from Blood Cultures Monitored from 1975-1977 at the University of Colorado and the Denver Veterans Administration Hospitals

ORGANISM	NUMBER OF TRUE SEPTICEMIAS	NUMBER OF CONTAMINANTS	ORGANISM	NUMBER OF TRUE SEPTICEMIAS	NUMBER OF CONTAMINANTS
Escherichia coli	113	2	*Peptococcus* species	7	1
Staphylococcus aureus	68	23	*Eubacterium* species	7	1
Streptococcus pneumoniae	43	0	*Candida parapsilosis*	7	0
Klebsiella pneumoniae	40	0	*Listeria monocytogenes*	7	0
Pseudomonas aeruginosa	36	0	*Clostridium* species	6	3
Bacteroides fragilis	30	0	*Cryptococcus neoformans*	6	0
Enterococci	26	4	Other gram-negative rod nonfermenters	6	0
Streptococcus pyogenes	18	1	Other *Candida* species	5	0
Other Enterobacteriaceae	17	0	*Bacteroides* species	5	0
Candida albicans	15	0	*Fusobacterium necrophorum*	5	0
Other streptococci	14	3	*Acinetobacter calcoaceticus*	5	0
Torulopsis glabrata	14	1	*Haemophilus influenzae*	5	0
Proteus mirabilis	14	0	*Candida tropicalis*	3	4
Viridans streptococci	13	12	*Propionibacterium acnes*	1	73
Serratia marcescens	13	1	*Mucor* species	1	0
Enterobacter aerogenes	11	2	Other	8	8
Streptococcus agalactiae	11	0			
Staphylococcus epidermidis	10	153			
Peptostreptococcus species	9	0			
Clostridium perfringens	8	8			
Neisseria gonorrhoeae	8	0			
Corynebacterium species	7	26			

Modified from Weinstein, M.P., Reller, L.B., Murphy, J.R., and Lichtenstein, K.A. 1983. The clinical significance of positive blood cultures: a comprehensive analysis of 500 episodes of bacteremia and fungemia in adults. I. Laboratory and epidemiologic observations. Rev. Infect. Dis. **5**:35.

counts for the manifestations of toxoplasmosis.

Malarial parasites invade host erythrocytes and hepatic parenchymal cells. The significant anemia and subsequent tissue hypoxia that may result from destruction of red cells by the parasite is a major cause of morbidity. The host's immunologic response is to remove the parasites and damaged red blood cells; the immune response may also have deleterious effects.

Although microfilariae are seen in peripheral blood during infection with *Dipetalonema, Mansonella, Loa loa, Wuchereria,* or *Brugia,* it is the adult worm that elicits the inflammatory response, primarily in lymphatics, that causes the distinctive lesions of filariasis related to lymphatic obstruction.

14.1.b. Detection. Parasites in the bloodstream are usually detected by direct visualization. Those parasites for which diagnosis is routinely dependent on observation of the organism in peripheral blood smears by a technologist include *Plasmodium, Trypanosoma,* and *Babesia.* Patients with malaria or filariasis may display a periodicity in their episodes of fever that allows the physician to time the collection of blood for visual examination for parasites for optimal results. Further discussion of life cycles of blood-borne parasites and techniques for examination of blood for their presence can be found in Chapter 44. Serological tests for diagnosis of infection due to blood-borne parasites are also useful, as will be detailed in Chapter 44.

14.2. Virus Infections

14.2.a. Pathogenic mechanisms. Although many viruses do circulate in the peripheral blood at some stage of disease, the primary pathology relates to infection in the target organ or cells. Those viruses that preferentially infect blood cells are Epstein-Barr virus and cytomegalovirus, which invade lymphocytes, and the newly recognized lymphadenopathy-associated virus (LAV) or human T cell leukemia virus III (HTLV III), which involves only certain T lymphocytes. The pathogenesis of viral diseases of the blood is the same as that of viral diseases of any organ; by diverting the cellular machinery to create new viral components, the virus may prevent the host cell from performing its normal function, thus depriving the host of the necessary product or function of that cell. The cell may be destroyed or damaged by viral replication, and immunologic responses of the host may also contribute to the pathology of the resulting disease.

14.2.b. Detection. Although many viral diseases have a viremic stage, recovery of virus particles or detection of circulating viruses has been used routinely in the diagnosis of only a few diseases. Detection of viral antigen by immunologic methods has gained widespread use for diagnosis of hepatitis B. By using an enzyme-linked immunoassay (ELISA) procedure (Chapter 12), the surface antigen (HbsAg) and early antigen (HbeAg) can be quantitatively measured in serum. Separation of the buffy coat cells from blood using a Ficoll-Hypaque gradient allows this virus-rich component to be inoculated into tissue culture for isolation of cytomegalovirus. Most recently, the discovery of a viral etiology for acquired immune deficiency syndrome (AIDS) has led to the development of ELISA and other methods for the detection of HTLV III antibody. Methods for the detection of viruses in the bloodstream will be discussed in Chapter 42.

14.3. Fungal Infections

14.3.a. Pathogenic mechanisms. Fungemia is usually a serious condition, occurring primarily in immunosuppressed patients and those with serious or terminal illness. The fungi do not invade blood cells, but their presence in the blood usually indicates a focus of infection elsewhere in the body. The large size and sterol-containing cell walls of fungi make them particularly insensitive to the primary host defenses, antibody and phagocytic cells. Fungi in the bloodstream can be carried to all organs of the host, where they may grow, invade normal tissue, and elaborate toxic products. Fungi gain entrance to the circulatory system via loss of integrity of the gastrointestinal or other mucosa, through damaged skin, secondary to involvement of the lung or other organ, or by means of intravascular catheters. Several outbreaks of systemic *Rhizopus* infection were traced to the use of bandage material contaminated with spores of the fungus. Systemic fungal diseases that begin as pneumonia disseminate from the lungs, which serve as the portal of entry. Arthroconidia of *Coccidioides immitis* and microconidia of *Histoplasma capsulatum* and *Blastomyces dermatitidis* are ingested by alveolar macrophages in the lung. These macrophages carry the fungi to nearby lymph nodes, usually the hilar nodes. The fungi multiply within the macrophages and ultimately are released into the circulating blood, from which they go on to seed other organs or are destroyed by the body's defenses. Further discussion of the mycoses is found in Chapter 43.

14.3.b. Culture. Even though all disseminated fungal disease is preceded by fungemia, recovery of the microorganisms from blood cultures has not been common. One reason for this may be that cultures are not often taken at the fungemia stage because presence of the disease has not yet been recognized. More importantly, methods for culture of fungi from blood have not been ideal.

Many fungi can be recovered in standard blood culture media if the bottle has been vented to allow sufficient oxygen in the atmosphere for fungal growth. Fungi may grow slowly and poorly in the media that best support bacterial growth, however, and the ideal temperature for certain fungal forms (30° C) is lower than that recommended for optimal bacterial isolation. Although yeasts have been isolated from routine blood culture media, only rarely have filamentous fungi been recovered with the routine systems. Until recently, the best medium for the recovery of fungi from

FIGURE 14.1
Biphasic blood culture bottle, containing an agar slant that can be immersed in broth if the bottle is tipped.
(Courtesy GIBCO Laboratories.)

blood has been a biphasic system. The biphasic bottle contains an agar slant partially immersed in broth (Figure 14.1). Higher isolation rates and decreased time to recovery are achieved with brain heart infusion agar and broth incubated at 30° C than with other media. The bottle requires adequate ventilation, since pathogenic fungi grow best in the usual atmospheric oxygen tension. Even with such a system, optimal recovery rates for fungi have not been achieved. Several medical centers have now reported increased numbers of fungal isolations with the use of commercially available lysis-centrifugation system, the DuPont Isolator (section 14.5.c.).

Blood specimens for detection of fungemia are collected in the same manner as for bacterial culture. Using conventional media, vented and incubated at 30° C, many yeasts will be isolated within a week. Faster detection may occur with the radiometric detection system (discussed below). However, for recovery of blood-borne fungi, the lysis-centrifugation system has been most efficacious.

14.3.c. Antigen detection. Because many patients with systemic or invasive fungal infections are immunosuppressed and do not produce appreciable antibodies, detection of circulating fungal antigens or other cell wall components may be a more fruitful diagnostic method than searching for the presence of antibodies. This procedure might also give positive results early in the illness, before there has been time for an antibody response. This concept is being explored for diagnosis of several of the common fungal diseases, and tests employing it have been marketed for aiding diagnosis of at least two mycotic diseases. The presence of mannan antigen, one of the polysaccharides found in *Candida albicans* cell walls, has been noted in the serum of some severely ill patients with invasive disease. A commercially available latex agglutination test (Cand-Tec, Ramco Laboratories) can be used to detect circulating mannan in serum, thus suggesting systemic infection with *C. albicans.* A sensitive latex particle agglutination test is also available for detection of the polysaccharide capsular antigen of *Cryptococcus neoformans* in serum or cerebrospinal fluid (Calas, Meridian Diagnostics, and Crypto-Test, M.A. Bioproducts). Quantitation of this antigen can be followed sequentially to determine the effectiveness of antifungal therapy.

14.4. Bacterial Infection

14.4.a. Pathogenic mechanisms. Bacteria in the bloodstream, bacteremia, may indicate the presence of a focus of disease, such as pneumonia or liver abscess, or may merely represent transient release of bacteria into the bloodstream, such as occurs after vigorous toothbrushing by a normal person. Septicemia or sepsis indicates a situation in which bacteria or their products (toxins) are causing harm to the host. Unfortunately, clinicians often use the terms interchangeably. Signs and symptoms of septicemia may include fever or hypothermia, chills, hyperventilation and subsequent respiratory alkalosis, skin lesions, change in mental status, diarrhea, etc. More serious manifestations include hypotension or shock, disseminated intravascular coagulation (DIC), and major organ system failure.

Shock is the gravest complication of septicemia. In septic shock, the presence of bacterial products and the host's responding defensive components act to shut down major host physiological systems. Manifestations include drop in blood pressure, rise in heart rate, impairment of function of vital organs (brain, kidney, liver, and lungs), acid-base problems, and bleeding problems. Gram-negative bacteria and certain other microorganisms contain a substance in their cell walls, endotoxin, that has a strong effect on several physiological functions. This substance, a lipopolysaccharide (LPS) composing part of the cell wall structure (Figure 14.2), may be released during the normal growth cycles of bacteria or after the destruction of bacteria by host defenses. Endotoxin (or the lipoidal disaccharide core of the LPS, Lipid A) has been shown to mediate a number of systemic reactions, including a drop in circulating granulocytes, a febrile response, and the activation of complement and certain blood-clotting factors.

Although most gram-positive bacteria do not contain endotoxin, some produce exotoxins, and in any case, the effects of their presence in the bloodstream may be equally devastating to the patient. The disastrous complication of disseminated intravascular coagulation, in which numerous small blood vessels become clogged with clotted blood, can occur with septicemia involving any circulating pathogen, including parasites, viruses, and fungi, although it is most often a consequence of gram-negative bacterial sepsis.

14.4.b. Organisms commonly isolated from blood. The commonest portals of entry for sep-

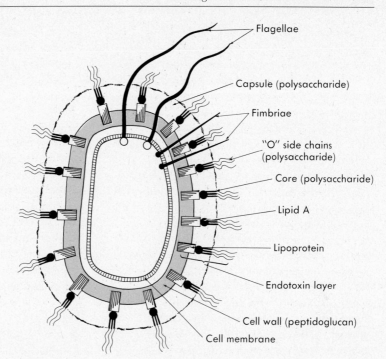

FIGURE 14.2
Gram-negative cell wall structure.

Flagellae

Capsule (polysaccharide)

Fimbriae

"O" side chains (polysaccharide)

Core (polysaccharide)

Lipid A

Lipoprotein

Endotoxin layer

Cell wall (peptidoglucan)

Cell membrane

ticemia are the genitourinary tract (25%), respiratory tract (20%), abscesses (10%), surgical wound infections (5%), biliary tract (5%), miscellaneous sites (10%), and uncertain sites (25%). The organisms most commonly isolated from blood are gram-negative rods, including the Enterobacteriaceae and *Pseudomonas* species, organisms most likely to be inhabitants of the hospital environment and thus to colonize the skin and gastrointestinal tracts of hospitalized patients (Table 14.1). Factors contributing to initiation of such infections are immunosuppressive agents, widespread use of broad-spectrum antibiotics that suppress the normal flora and allow the emergence of resistant strains of bacteria, invasive procedures that allow bacteria access to the interior of the host, more extensive surgical procedures, and prolonged survival of debilitated and seriously ill patients.

With the ever-increasing use of intravenous catheters, intraarterial lines, and vascular prostheses, organisms found as normal inhabitants

of the human skin are able to gain access to the bloodstream and to find a surface on which to multiply. Heart valves may represent such a surface. Endocarditis occurs when colonies of bacteria (vegetations) are present on a heart valve. Constant shedding of bacteria into the bloodstream is one of the usual consequences of endocarditis. In such a setting, *Staphylococcus epidermidis* and other coagulase negative staphylococci have been increasingly detected. The isolation of coagulase negative staphylococci with the same biochemical and antibiotic susceptibility patterns from more than one blood culture from a patient should alert the clinician to the possibility of a clinically significant isolate. *S. epidermidis* is also the most common etiologic agent of prosthetic valve endocarditis, with *Staphylococcus aureus* the second most common. *S. aureus* is an important cause of septicemia without endocarditis, in association with other foci such as abscesses, wound infections, and pneumonia.

Immunocompromised hospitalized patients

tend to become colonized with bacteria that are relatively antibiotic resistant, such as *Serratia marcescens*, *Enterobacter* species, and *Pseudomonas aeruginosa*. Another such bacterium, much less commonly encountered, is *Corynebacterium* group JK. This organism should be suspected if a diphtheroid-like bacterium isolated from blood displays an unusually broad antibiotic resistance pattern, often being sensitive only to vancomycin. *Corynebacterium* JK is extremely virulent and must not be dismissed as a contaminant.

The primary causes of infectious endocarditis are the viridans streptococci, comprising a large number of species, described in Chapter 25. These organisms are normal inhabitants of the oral cavity or gastrointestinal tract, often gaining entrance to the bloodstream because of gingivitis or dental manipulation. Heart valves, especially those that have been previously damaged, present convenient surfaces for attachment of these bacteria. The resulting vegetations ultimately seed bacteria into the blood at a slow but constant rate. Identification of these streptococci may be useful, as certain species (such as *Streptococcus intermedius*), may be associated with increased frequency of metastatic abscess formation. *Streptococcus sanguis I* and *II* and *Streptococcus mutans* are most frequently isolated from streptococcal endocarditis. Other agents of infectious endocarditis are as follows:

Streptococcus sanguis I and II
Streptococcus mutans
Streptococcus intermedius
Nutritionally deficient streptococci
Enterococci
Streptococcus bovis
Other streptococci
Staphylococcus aureus
Staphylococci (coagulase negative)
Salmonella species
Serratia marcescens
Other Enterobacteriaceae

Pseudomonas species
Haemophilus species
Unusual gram-negative bacilli (*Actinobacillus*, *Cardiobacterium*, etc.)
Bacteroides fragilis
Other *Bacteroides* species
Fusobacterium species
Other anaerobes
Candida parapsilosis
Candida tropicalis
Other yeast species
Coxiella burnetii
Chlamydia species
Other (including polymicrobial infectious endocarditis)

The group D streptococci are normal gastrointestinal flora but may be found in the oral cavity as well. Their involvement in bacteremia is usually related to infection of the genitourinary tract or to intraabdominal infection involving bowel flora. The presence of *Streptococcus bovis*, a nonenterococcal group D streptococcus, is significantly associated with large bowel carcinoma; clinicians should be notified of this association when this organism is isolated from blood. Identification of this group D streptococcus as *S. bovis* is also important in that infection with this organism (including endocarditis) will respond to penicillin G, whereas enterococcal endocarditis requires the addition of an aminoglycoside.

Septicemia occurs in 25%-30% of patients with pneumococcal pneumonia, and is usually the most reliable way to establish the diagnosis. The prognosis is poorer in patients with pneumococcal pneumonia complicated by sepsis. Because the organisms produce an autolytic enzyme, early subculture of blood culture broths (before 18 h) is necessary. *Streptococcus pneumoniae* grows extremely well in biphasic media, as described below.

Haemophilus influenzae infections may be accompanied by septicemia. The organism requires an enriched medium, such as chocolate agar, and 10% CO_2 for growth. *Haemophilus parainfluenzae* can also be recovered from blood, particularly as an etiologic agent of endocarditis. This organism grows as large clumps of filamentous rods, which may appear branched in the original stains from broth. Other *Haemophilus* species, including *Haemophilus aphrophilus* and *Haemophilus paraphrophilus*, may also cause bacteremia and endocarditis. Arterial embolization is relatively common in endocarditis involving *Haemophilus* species. All of the *Haemophilus* species grow sparsely in blood culture broth and often do not exhibit visually discernible turbidity. For this reason, blind stains or subcultures are essential. Unless such subcultures are made to a medium such as chocolate agar and incubated under 5%-9% CO_2, the organism can be overlooked.

Listeria monocytogenes is a cause of septicemia in immunosuppressed patients, alcoholics, and pregnant women. The bacterium may resemble a diphtheroid or coccus on Gram stain, but grows on 5% sheep blood agar as a translucent, moderately beta hemolytic colony, resembling group B streptococci. *Listeria* must be distinguished from diphtheroids and from groups B and D streptococci. It displays a characteristic tumbling motility at room temperature but not at 35° C.

Anaerobic organisms also cause septicemia. *Bacteroides fragilis* is the most common anaerobe isolated from blood. *Clostridium perfringens*, however, can cause rapidly fatal disease and must be presumptively identified by Gram stain appearance and gas and hemolysis in the bottle so that clinicians can be alerted to the possibility of the presence of this virulent bacterium in the bloodstream. In one large recently reported study, however, *Clostridium perfringens* was judged to be a significant isolate (representing true infection) only 50% of the time. The isolation of *C. septicum* may be indicative of malignancy, particularly in the cecum or elsewhere in the gastrointestinal tract of the patient. Chapters 34 to 37 discuss the anaerobic organisms in detail.

An organism associated with fulminant septicemia, often in splenectomized or compromised patients, although rarely isolated, is DF-2. DF-2 is normal oral flora of dogs; 12 of 20 reported cases of DF-2 infection were associated with dog contact or dog bites. A fastidious fermentative gram-negative bacillus, DF-2 will grow in conventional blood culture media. Subcultures may require as long as 4 days before colonies are visible. The organism is described in Chapter 29.

Almost every recognized bacterial species has been implicated as a cause of bacteremia; it is beyond the scope of this text to mention them all here. Certain organisms that require special techniques for isolation are mentioned below. Other bacteria that may grow in routine culture media include *Rothia dentocariosa*, *Campylobacter* species (especially *Campylobacter fetus*), *Alcaligenes* species, *Cardiobacterium hominis*, *Chromobacterium* species, *Eikenella corrodens*, *Flavobacterium* species, and *Mycoplasma*. If these less common organisms are suspected by the clinician, the laboratory can be alerted to hold the blood culture media for an extended period of time past the first week.

Although *Yersinia pestis*, the agent of plague, and *Francisella tularensis*, the agent of tularemia, may grow in routine blood culture media, diagnosis by blood culture is not recommended for two reasons: (1) These organisms are fastidious in their growth requirements and often require prolonged incubation time for detection. The serious nature of the diseases, however, precludes such a slow method of diagnosis. Serologic methods are more reliable and rapid. If an organism resembling *Y. pestis* or *F. tularensis* is isolated from blood, the physician should be notified and the organism should be forwarded to the nearest public health facility that can handle such an isolate. (2) These pathogens are classified as class three etiologic agents (extremely hazardous) and require special containment facilities for their manipulation. Chapter 2 discusses some aspects of laboratory safety in relationship to handling such hazardous agents.

14.4.c. Timing and quantity of blood for conventional culture. Conditions in which bacteria are only transiently present in the bloodstream include manipulation of infected tissues, instrumentation of contaminated mucosal surfaces, and surgery involving nonsterile sites. These backgrounds may also lead to significant septicemia. Incidental, transient bacteremia may occur spontaneously or with such minor events as chewing food. Bacteria can be found intermittently in the blood of patients with undrained abscesses. During early stages of typhoid fever, brucellosis, and leptospirosis, bacteria are continuously present in the bloodstream. The causative agents of meningitis, pneumonia, pyogenic arthritis, and osteomyelitis are often recovered from blood during the early course of these diseases. In the case of transient seeding of the blood from a sequestered focus of infection, such as an abscess, bacteria are present in the blood prior to the febrile episode. If a regular periodicity of fevers can be established, then the most advantageous time to draw blood cultures will be just before the anticipated rise in temperature.

In bacterial endocarditis and other endovascular infections, organisms are released into the bloodstream at a fairly constant rate so that timing of cultures is not important. Many studies have shown that the likelihood of recovering a pathogen is increased as the volume of blood cultured increases, provided that there is adequate dilution of such blood to negate the effect of normal antibacterial substances and antimicrobial agents that may be present. When a patient's condition requires institution of therapy as rapidly as possible, the luxury of

time for the collection of multiple blood culture samples is lacking. A compromise that has been generally accepted is to collect 30 ml of blood at one time, 10 ml from each of **three separate venipunctures from three different sites, using three separate needles and syringes,** before the patient is given antimicrobial therapy. For initial evaluation of fever of unknown origin, four separate blood cultures, two drawn on each of 2 days, will detect most causative agents. The large study reported by Weinstein et al.[4] revealed that 99.3% of 500 episodes of septicemia were identified by the first two blood cultures, comprising 30 ml total volume of blood cultured. In another study, in 98% of patients with infective endocarditis who had not received antimicrobial agents, two blood cultures established the diagnosis. If therapy can be delayed, three separate blood collections of 10 ml each, and a second set of three cultures taken on the second day (if necessary), will detect most etiologic agents of endocarditis, even for patients who have received prior antibiotic therapy. This presumes use of setups adequate for growth of the organism involved.

It is not safe to take large samples of blood from children, particularly young infants. Fortunately, infants with septicemia usually yield large numbers of bacteria per milliliter of blood. For infants and children, only 1-5 ml of blood need be drawn for bacterial culture.

14.4.d. How to draw blood for conventional culture. Since the media into which blood specimens are placed have been developed as enrichment broths to encourage the multiplication of even one bacterium, it follows that these media will enhance the growth of any stray contaminating bacterium, such as a normal inhabitant of human skin. Because of the rising incidence of true infections caused by bacteria that normally are nonvirulent indigenous microflora of a healthy human host, interpretation of the significance of growth of such bacteria in blood cultures has become in-

---

PROCEDURE 14.1. DRAWING BLOOD FOR CULTURE

1. Choose the vein to be drawn by touching the skin before it has been disinfected.
2. Cleanse the skin over the venipuncture site in a circle approximately 5 cm in diameter with 70% alcohol, rubbing vigorously.
3. Starting in the center of the circle, apply 2% iodine (or povidone iodine) in ever-widening circles until the entire circle has been saturated with iodine. Allow the iodine to remain on the skin for at least 1 min. The timing is critical; a watch or timer should be used.
4. If the site must be touched by the phlebotomist after preparation, the phlebotomist must disinfect the fingers used for palpation in identical fashion.
5. Insert the needle into the vein and withdraw blood.
6. After the needle has been removed, the site should be cleansed with 70% alcohol again, as many patients are sensitive to iodine.

---

creasingly difficult. To help clinicians determine whether an *S. epidermidis*, other coagulase negative staphylococcus, *Corynebacterium* species, or *Propionibacterium acnes* is a true pathogen or an inadvertently introduced skin contaminant, blood cultures are drawn from separate sites, even when more than one blood culture is to be drawn at one time, such as prior to instituting emergency therapy. Only recovery of identical "nonvirulent" bacteria from multiple cultures is considered to be indicative of infection. Quantitation of bacteremia may be helpful.

Another strategy is to reduce the risk of introducing contaminants into blood culture media by careful skin preparation. Procedure 14.1 details the steps necessary for drawing blood for culture. Laboratories that recover "contaminants," as determined by clinical evaluation of the patients' conditions, at rates greater than 3% should suspect improper phlebotomy techniques and should institute measures to reeducate the phlebotomists in proper skin preparation methods. It is undesirable to draw blood through a vascular shunt or catheter, since

these prosthetic devices may harbor colonizing bacteria that are not present in the circulating blood of the patient, and blood obtained through the foreign material would yield false positive results. It is also recommended to draw blood below an existing intravenous line, if possible, since blood above the line will be diluted with the fluid being infused.

If the blood for culture is not being inoculated directly into broth media, it must be transported with an anticoagulant. Heparin, ethylenediaminetetraacetate (EDTA), and citrate have been found to be inhibitory to a number of organisms; thus, sodium polyanethol sulfonate (SPS, Liquoid) in concentrations of 0.025%-0.03% is the best anticoagulant for blood.

14.4.e. How to culture intravenous catheter tips. When colonization of an indwelling catheter is suspected of being the focus for septicemia, the catheter tip may be cultured to determine its status. As first reported by Maki and co-workers,[2] the number of colony-forming units (CFU) of bacteria on the catheter directly relates to whether it is the source of the infec-

FIGURE 14.3
Method for culturing intravenous catheter tip.

tion. The skin around the catheter is carefully disinfected with an iodine preparation, and the catheter is removed. A short section (approximately 2 inches), including the area directly beneath the skin, is aseptically cut off and sent to the microbiology laboratory in a sterile container without liquid. This section of catheter is rolled across the surface of an agar plate with sterile forceps (as shown in Figure 14.3). After overnight incubation, the colonies are counted. Fifteen or more CFU correlates well with the catheter tip being the source of infection.

14.4.f. Conventional blood culture media, additives, and dilution factors. The diversity of bacteria that are recovered from blood requires an equally diverse armamentarium of media to enhance the growth of these bacteria. Basic blood culture media contain a nutrient broth and an anticoagulant. The numbers of different broth formulations available are staggering, including those that can be prepared by the laboratory in-house and those that are commer-

cially prepared. Most blood culture bottles available commercially contain tryptic soy broth, brain heart infusion, supplemented peptone, or thioglycolate broth. More specialized broth bases include Columbia or *Brucella* broth. Growth of cell wall–deficient bacteria may be enhanced by the addition of osmotic stabilizers such as sucrose, mannitol, or sorbose, to create a hyperosmotic (hypertonic) medium. Media without such osmotic additives are known as isotonic. The hypertonic bottles are difficult to inspect visually for evidence of bacterial growth, as red cells in the media become partially lysed and no longer sediment to the bottom, giving a muddy appearance to the broth. Such media are more useful when blood culture systems do not rely on visual evidence of growth as the only indication for further examination, such as the radiometric growth detection system described below.

The anticoagulant in blood culture media must not harm the bacteria and must prevent clotting of the blood, which would entrap bacteria and prevent their detection. The most commonly used preparation in blood culture media today is 0.025%-0.03% SPS. In addition to its anticoagulant properties, SPS is also anticomplementary, antiphagocytic, and interferes with the activity of certain antimicrobial agents, the aminoglycosides. SPS may, however, inhibit the growth of a few microorganisms such as some strains of *Neisseria* species, *Gardnerella vaginalis*, *Streptobacillus moniliformis*, and all strains of *Peptostreptococcus anaerobius*. The addition of 1.2% gelatin has been shown to counteract this inhibitory action of SPS.

Penicillinase may be added to blood culture media to specifically inactivate certain penicillins and other beta lactam antibiotics in the blood of patients. After addition of penicillinase, an equivalent amount of the penicillinase should be cultured on the surface of a chocolate agar plate to rule out the possibility that a contaminant has been introduced to the blood culture via the additive. The use of penicillinase has been largely superseded in recent years by the availability of a resin-containing medium that inactivates most antibiotics nonselectively by adsorbing them to the surface of the resin particles. Several studies have detailed faster and increased recovery of pathogens from patients receiving antibiotics when blood was cultured with the aid of resin-containing systems. When the Antimicrobial Removal Device (ARD, Marion Laboratories), a resin-containing bottle into which blood from patients receiving antibiotics is drawn, is used with conventional manual blood culture systems, it is necessary to perform the additional manipulations of rotating the blood with the resin and then centrifuging the blood to remove the resin particles before inoculating the culture media. This device has been shown to remove at least 25 antimicrobial agents from blood; its use may be associated with inhibition of some strains of bacteria.

In addition to volume of blood cultured and type of media chosen, the dilution factor for the blood in the medium must be considered. To conserve space and materials, it is desirable to combine the largest feasible amount of blood from the patient (usually 10 ml) with the smallest amount of medium that will still encourage the growth of bacteria and dilute out or inactivate the antibacterial components of the system. For this purpose, a 1:10 ratio (1:5 at a minimum) of blood to medium has been found to be most advantageous.

14.4.g. Incubation conditions for conventional blood cultures. The atmosphere in commercially prepared blood culture bottles is usually of a very low oxidation-reduction potential, allowing most facultative and some anaerobic organisms to multiply. To encourage the growth of strict aerobes, such as yeast and *P. aeruginosa*, transient venting of the bottles with a sterile, cotton-plugged needle is necessary. For optimal recovery of pathogens, therefore, the use of two different bottles of blood culture media, one vented and one unvented, is recommended.

14.4.h. Detecting growth in conventional blood cultures. Most clinical laboratories report a positive blood culture rate of greater than 8%. Five percent or more of positive blood cultures will yield anaerobic bacteria. Restricted patient populations may influence the rate of positive cultures reported from smaller hospitals and clinics.

After 6-18 h of incubation, most bacteria are present in numbers large enough to detect by blind subculture or acridine orange viable stain (discussed in Chapter 7). Constant agitation of the bottles during initial incubation will enhance the growth of the facultative bacteria, which are the most common isolates. Agitation does not allow the red cells to settle in the media, however, so that gross visual detection of growth is not possible soon after the initial incubation with agitation.

Blind subcultures after the first 6-12 h of incubation are performed by aseptically removing a few drops of the well-mixed medium and spreading this inoculum onto a chocolate blood agar plate, which is incubated in 5%-10% CO_2 at 35° C for 48 h. Bottles are then reincubated without agitation for 7 days unless the patient's condition requires special consideration, as discussed below. Growth of anaerobic bacteria can be detected by visual inspection with such success that blind anaerobic subcultures are not recommended. After 48 h incubation, a second blind subculture or acridine orange stain should be performed.

Bottles should be examined visually at least daily. Growth is usually indicated by hemolysis of the red cells, gas bubbles in the medium, turbidity, or appearance of small colonies in the broth or on the surface of the sedimented red cell layer (Plate 14.1) (occasionally along the walls of the bottle). When macroscopic evidence of growth is apparent, a Gram stain of a drop of medium will be more rewarding. Methanol fixation of the smear preserves bacterial and cellular morphology, which may be especially valuable for detecting gram-negative bacteria among red cell debris. Examination of the positive broth under phase microscopy will reveal details of morphology and motility that may aid the clinician in making an early decision regarding treatment. As soon as a morphologic description can be tentatively assigned to a pathogen detected in blood, the physician should be given all of the available information. Determining the clinical significance of an isolate is the physician's responsibility. If no organisms are seen on microscopic examination of a bottle that appears positive, subcultures should be performed anyway.

14.4.i. Procedures for handling positive blood cultures. Subcultures from blood cultures suspected of being positive, whether proven by microscopic visualization or not, should be made to a variety of media so as to be able to support the growth of most bacteria, including anaerobes. Initial subculture may include chocolate blood agar, 5% sheep blood agar, MacConkey agar (if gram-negative bacteria are seen), anaerobic supplemented blood agar, and a selective medium for *Bacteroides* species, such as *Bacteroides*-bile-esculin agar (Chapter 34). The incidence of polymicrobic bacteremia/fungemia ranges from 3%-20% of all positive blood cultures. For this reason, samples must be streaked for isolated colonies. Restreaking positive bottles a second time at the end of the incubation period to detect further organisms past the original subculture is of questionable value and is not recommended.

A number of rapid tests for identification and presumptive antimicrobial susceptibilities can be performed from the broth blood culture, if a unimicrobic infection is suspected (based on microscopic evaluation). A suspension of the organism that approximates the turbidity of a 0.5 McFarland standard, achieved directly from the broth, or by centrifuging the broth and resuspending the pelleted bacteria, can be used to inoculate Mueller-Hinton agar plates for the Bauer-Kirby susceptibility test or for performing dilution antimicrobial susceptibilities. These suspensions may also be used to set up preliminary biochemical tests such as coagulase, thermostable nuclease, esculin hydrolysis, bile solubility, or antigen detection by fluorescent-antibody stain or agglutination procedures for gram-positive bacteria and oxidase and rapid biochemicals such as API Rapid E, Minitek, or Micro-ID (see Chapters 9 and 10) for gram-negative bacteria. Presumptive results must be verified with conventional procedures using pure cultures. Chapter 4 also includes some discussion of rapid methods of handling positive blood cultures.

All isolates from blood cultures should be stored for an indefinite period, preferably by freezing at −70° C in 10% skim milk. Storing an agar slant of the isolate under sterile mineral oil at room temperature is a good alternative to freezing. It is often necessary to compare separate isolates from the same patient or isolates of the same species from different patients, sometimes even months after the bacteria were isolated.

14.4.j. Culturing suspected contaminated banked blood, plasma, or other infused fluids. When an infusion is suspected of being the source of bacteremia or fungemia, it must be cultured in a manner similar to that used for blood. Since contamination is usually random and rare, the routine monitoring of intravenous fluids and banked blood is not rational. However, in cases of suspected contamination, the fluid, plasma, or other blood product is aseptically aspirated into a syringe and 5-10 ml is aseptically introduced into each of two blood culture bottles. One bottle is incubated at room temperature to enhance the growth of psychrophilic (cold-loving) gram-negative bacilli, which have been implicated as the cause of fatal transfusion reactions, and the other bottle is incubated at 35°-37° C. The normal visual and cultural methods used to detect positive cultures are then followed.

A number of infections have been documented to be transmitted by blood transfusions or needle contact, including malaria, trypanosomiasis, toxoplasmosis, cytomegalovirus disease, AIDS, hepatitis, and bacterial endocarditis. Gram-negative bacteria are most often implicated in contaminated intravenous fluids, although the possibility exists for any organism to multiply in a suitable environment and subsequently be injected into a compromised host.

14.4.k. Special problems and unusual microorganisms. Special handling may be required for recovery of *Brucella* species from blood; septicemia occurs only during the first 3 weeks of illness. Best recovery is obtained with *Brucella* or trypticase soy broth, and the use of biphasic media may enhance growth of the bacteria. The bottles should be continuously vented and incubated in 10% CO_2 at 37° C for at least 4 weeks. Blind subcultures should be performed at 4 days and weekly thereafter onto *Brucella* blood agar plates and incubated as above. *Brucella* species may grow slowly, so cultures must be incubated for longer than average time periods. Cultures should be handled in a biological safety cabinet.

Visualization is diagnostic for 70% of cases of febrile disease caused by *Borrelia* species. The organisms may be seen in direct wet preparations of a drop of anticoagulated blood diluted in saline as long, thin, unevenly coiled spirochetes that seem to push the red blood cells around as they move. Thick and thin smears of blood, prepared as for malaria testing (described in Chapter 44) and stained with Wright's or Giemsa stain, are also quite sensitive for the detection of *Borrelia*.

Leptospirosis can be diagnosed by isolating the causative spirochete from blood during the first 4-7 days of illness. Media with up to 14% (vol/vol) rabbit serum, such as Fletcher's, Tween 80–albumin, or Ellinghausen, McCullough, Johnson, Harris (EMJH) semisolid media are recommended (described in Chapters 31 and 45). After adding 1-3 drops of fresh or SPS-anticoagulated blood to each of several tubes with 5 ml of culture medium, the cultures are incubated for 5-6 weeks at 28°-30° C in air in the dark. Leptospires will grow 1-3 cm below the surface, usually within 2 weeks. The organisms remain viable in blood with SPS for 11 days, allowing for transport of cultures from distant locations. Direct darkfield examination of peripheral blood is not recommended, since many artifacts are present that may resemble spirochetes.

One of the agents of rat-bite fever, *Streptobacillus moniliformis*, may be recovered in blood cultures. Concentrations of SPS greater than 0.025% will inhibit the growth of this organism, however, so the addition of 1.2% gelatin to commercial media is recommended.

These organisms will grow in conventional media after several days of incubation, visible as "puffball" colonies on the surface of the red cell layer. Cell wall–defective forms may require the use of hypertonic media for recovery.

Mycobacterium avium-intracellulare has been isolated increasingly often from the blood of patients suffering from AIDS. By the time the infection is discovered, the bacteria are usually circulating in great numbers. Although holding conventional media for several weeks will allow these slow-growing bacteria to be detected, the use of special media, such as Middlebrook 7H9 broth with 0.05% SPS or brain heart infusion broth with 0.5% Tween-80, with or without a Middlebrook 7H11 agar slant, has given faster results. The newer methods of detection, radiometric and lysis-centrifugation (described below), have been shown to greatly shorten the time required for mycobacterial cultures to become positive.

Certain streptococci are unable to multiply without the addition of 0.001% pyridoxal hydrochloride (also called thiol or vitamin B_6). These streptococci are known as "nutritionally variant" or "satelliting" streptococci. Although human blood introduced into the blood culture medium will provide enough of the pyridoxal to allow the organisms to multiply in the bottle, standard sheep blood agar plates may not support their growth. Subculturing the broth to a 5% sheep blood agar plate and overlaying a streak of *S. aureus* to produce the supplement will generally demonstrate colonies of the streptococci growing as tiny "satellites" next to the streak, as shown in Chapter 25 (Plate 25.1). Some commercially supplied media may be supplemented with enough pyridoxal (0.001%) to support growth of nutritionally variant streptococci.

14.5. New and Nonconventional Methods for Detecting Bacteremia

14.5.a. Antimicrobial removal device. By drawing blood into a vial containing anticoagu-

lant, a cationic resin, and a polymeric adsorbent resin, antimicrobial agents present in the blood can be removed before the blood is introduced into culture media. The vial is commercially available (ARD, Marion Laboratories). Blood must be rotated in the vial with the resins for 15 min, centrifuged to remove the resins, and then inoculated into the media of choice. This device can remove up to 100 μg of most antibiotics. Although there are studies that imply no significant advantage with this system, most workers have found increased and faster isolation of pathogens from the blood of patients being treated with antimicrobial agents. Negative aspects include inhibition of the growth of some strains of gram-negative bacilli.

14.5.b. Radiometry. More than one third of all hospital microbiology laboratories use this automated system, marketed commercially as Bactec (Johnston Laboratories). The blood culture media are produced to contain radiolabeled metabolites (^{14}C-labeled glucose, amino acids, and alcohols). When bacteria or fungi grow in the medium, they metabolize the ^{14}C substrates and release $^{14}CO_2$ into the atmosphere above the medium, where it is trapped in the head space of the bottle. The Bactec instrument inserts a sterilized needle into the bottle and samples a portion of the atmosphere periodically. The presence of $^{14}CO_2$ indicates that metabolism is occurring and that therefore there are viable microorganisms in the bottle. The blood cultures are always agitated during early incubation to facilitate the growth of aerobic and facultative organisms. Additionally, the radiometric reading must be monitored, since a minimal amount of metabolism by the human blood cells in the culture medium is common. A resin-containing broth medium is also available for the Bactec; it removes antimicrobial agents by adsorption. No further manipulations are required to use this medium after the blood specimen is introduced into the broth.

The intervals at which the radiometric detection is carried out, the levels of radioactivity considered to be suspicious, the timing and number of blind subcultures to perform, the gas mixture to reintroduce into the head space after sampling, and other considerations must be determined for each laboratory to best serve the needs of the physicians and patients. This system is explained in more detail in Chapter 11.

Problems encountered with the Bactec system include false positives due to inappropriate threshold values, false positives due to carryover of organisms from positive bottles to adjacent culture bottles by inadequately sterilized sampling needles, false negatives because of failure of certain microorganisms to metabolize detectable levels of labeled substrates, and disposal of the radioactive media at the end of the incubation period. Regulations governing the disposal of the media vary among states.

Advantages of the Bactec system are more rapid detection time for many pathogens, availability of an antimicrobial-removal additive for the medium, the ability to monitor growth without visual inspection or subculture, the automated handling of large numbers of blood culture bottles, allowing the use of hypertonic media, and the potential to tie the system into a management information processing data base for monitoring results and generating statistical reports for both historical and epidemiological studies.

The manufacturers of Bactec have introduced a modification of the system that relies on the infrared detection of CO_2 elaborated by bacterial and fungal metabolism rather than on the detection of radioisotopes. This new system should alleviate many of the problems associated with the handling of radioactive materials necessary with current methods. In several trials, the new detection system has yielded results identical to those with the radiometric instrument. The ability to detect growth of certain organisms by nonradiometric means is still being improved.

14.5.c. Lysis-centrifugation.

In order to rapidly remove pathogens from the blood and its antibacterial properties and antimicrobial agents, Sullivan, Sutter, and Finegold[3] introduced a system that employed lysis of blood cells and filtration of the hemolyzed suspension to trap the bacteria on the filter. Although the technology was cumbersome, the results were rewarding. This filtration system was the forerunner of the lysis-centrifugation system developed by Dorn et al.[1], commercially available as the Isolator (E. I. DuPont de Nemours & Co.). The Isolator consists of a double-stoppered tube containing saponin to lyse blood cells, polypropylene glycol to decrease foaming, SPS as an anticoagulant, EDTA to chelate calcium ions and thus inhibit the complement cascade and coagulation, and a small amount of an inert fluorochemical (Fluorinert, 3M Co., St. Paul, Minn.) to cushion and concentrate the microorganisms during a 30 min centrifugation at $3,000 \times g$ (Figure 14.4). The bottom stopper is slanted at the angle of centrifugation, allowing the sediment to be cushioned by Fluorinert at all times. After centrifugation of the solution is completed, the supernatant is discarded, the sediment containing the pathogens is vigorously vortexed, and the entire sediment is plated to solid agar.

Benefits of this system include the more rapid and greater recovery of certain microorganisms, the presence of actual colonies for direct identification and susceptibility testing after initial incubation, the ability to quantify the colony forming units present in the blood, rapid detection of polymicrobial bacteremia, increased recovery of filamentous fungi and yeasts, dispensing with the need for a separate antibiotic-removal step, the ability to choose special media for initial culture setup based on clinical impression (such as direct plating onto media supportive of *Legionella* species or *Mycobacterium* species), and possible greater recovery of intracellular pathogens due to lysis of host cells.

Shortcomings of the system seem to be a relatively high rate of plate contamination, multiple manipulations with the attendant risk of needle-puncture injury, and failure of the system to detect certain bacteria, such as *S. pneumoniae*, *L. monocytogenes*, and anaerobic bacteria, as well as conventional systems. With the introduction of a semiautomated system for removal of the supernatant and aspiration of the sediment (Isostat, DuPont Co.) some of

the negative aspects associated with manipulating the tube are eliminated. The combination of an Isolator tube and an anaerobic broth blood culture bottle would be a very good system.

14.5.d. Self-contained subculture. A recent modification of the biphasic blood culture medium is the Septi-Chek system (Roche Diagnostics), consisting of a conventional blood culture broth bottle with an attached chamber

FIGURE 14.4
DuPont Isolator lysis-centrifugation tube.

FIGURE 14.5
Self-contained subculture system for blood cultures.

containing a three-sided slide coated with choc-olate, MacConkey, and malt agars (Figure 14.5). To subculture, the entire broth contents are allowed to contact the agar surfaces by in-verting the bottle, a simple procedure that does not require opening the bottle or using needles. The large volume of broth that is sub-cultured and the ease of subculture allow faster detection time for many organisms than is pos-sible with conventional systems. The Septi-Chek system appears to enhance the recovery of S. pneumoniae but does not efficiently re-cover anaerobic isolates.

14.5.e. Detection of microorganisms through changes in electrical impedance. The passage of electric current through a liquid me-dium can be measured. Electrodes placed in the broth can continuously monitor electrical impedance, even overnight when no technolo-gists are present. The Bactometer is currently the only commercially available instrument in the United States for this purpose. Initial impedance changes occur at a microbial colony count of approximately 5×10^5, the same level of growth at which turbidity is first discernible. This system and others that detect microbial growth through changes in electrical conductiv-ity or microcalorimetry (heat given off during bacterial metabolism) have not enjoyed wide use in clinical laboratories yet.

14.5.f. Other nonculture methods for de-tecting bacteremia. In addition to testing for circu-lating antigens using latex agglutination pro-cedures, available for some yeasts, group B streptococci, H. influenzae type b, S. pneu-moniae, staphylococcal teichoic acids, and Neis-seria meningitidis, counterimmunoelectropho-resis (CIE) has been used with varying success for determining the presence of antigens in serum. Cross-reacting substances may block re-actions in some cases, or cause nonspecific ag-glutination. These techniques are discussed in Chapter 10.

The lysate from amebocytes of Limulus po-lyphemus, the horseshoe crab, will gel in the presence of as little as 0.1 ng of endotoxin. This highly sensitive test, the Limulus amebocyte lysate assay, can be used to detect circulating lipopolysaccharides (LPS) in patients with gram-negative bacteremia. Sites of gram-nega-tive bacterial infection other than blood may also cause a positive test result with serum. Al-though often used as an emergency test to di-agnose gram-negative bacterial meningitis, the amebocyte lysate assay is not commonly used to diagnose bacteremia, in part because of its nonspecific nature in blood testing.

Detecting the presence of metabolic end products of microbial activity in serum using gas liquid chromatography (GLC) has been ex-plored. Some success in detecting products of anaerobic metabolism has been reported. A promising use of GLC may be its ability to de-tect metabolic products of mycobacteria, organ-isms whose diagnosis by conventional methods is extremely time consuming. The use of GLC in clinical microbiology is discussed in Chapter 11.

REFERENCES

1. Dorn, G.L., Haynes, J.R., and Burson, G.G. 1976. Blood culture technique based on centrifugation: devel-opmental phase. J. Clin. Microbiol. 3:251; clinical eval-uation 3:258.
2. Maki, D.G., Weise, C.E., and Sarafin, H.W. 1977. A semiquantitative culture method for identifying intra-venous catheter-related infection. N. Engl. J. Med. 296:1305.
3. Sullivan, N.M., Sutter, V.L., and Finegold, S.M. 1975. Practical aerobic membrane filtration blood culture technique: development and procedure. J. Clin. Micro-biol. 1:30.
4. Weinstein, M.P., Reller L.B., Murphy, J.R., and Lich-tenstein, K.A. 1983. The clinical significance of positive blood cultures: a comprehensive analysis of 500 epi-sodes of bacteremia and fungemia in adults. I. Labora-tory and epidemiologic observations. Rev. Infect. Dis. 5:35.

BIBLIOGRAPHY

Balows, A., and Sonnenwirth, A.C. 1983. Bacteremia: laboratory and clinical aspects. Charles C Thomas, Publisher, Springfield, Ill.

Balows, A., and Tilton, R.C., editors. 1983. Proceedings of a symposium. Body fluids and infectious diseases: clinical and microbiologic advances. Am. J. Med. 75:1.

Berlin, O.G.W., Zakowski, P., Bruckner, D.A., and Johnson, B. L. Jr. 1984. New biphasic culture system for isolation of mycobacteria from blood of patients with acquired immune deficiency syndrome. J. Clin. Microbiol. 20:572.

Blazevic, D.J., McCarthy, L.R., and Morello, J.A. 1982. Minimum guidelines for blood cultures. Clin. Microbiol. Newsl. 4:85.

Farrar, W.E. 1985. Leptospira species (leptospirosis). In Mandell, G.L., Douglas, R.G. Jr., and Bennett, J.E., editors. Principles and practice of infectious diseases, ed 2. John Wiley & Sons, New York.

Henry, N.K.,Grewell, C.M., Van Grevenhof, P.E., et al. 1984. Comparison of lysis-centrifugation with a biphasic blood culture medium for the recovery of aerobic and facultatively anaerobic bacteria. J. Clin. Microbiol. 20:413.

Moody, J.A., Fasching, C.E., Shanholtzer, C.J., et al. 1984. Evaluation of new blood culture processing system. J. Clin. Microbiol. 20:351.

Reller, L.B., Murray, P.R., and MacLowry, J.D. 1982. Cumitech 1A. Blood cultures II. Washington, J.A. II, coordinating editor. American Society for Microbiology, Washington, D.C.

Scheld, W.M., and Sande, M.E. 1985. Endocarditis and intravascular infections. In Mandell, G.L., Douglas, R.G. Jr., and Bennett, J.E., editors. Principles and practice of infectious diseases, ed 2. John Wiley & Sons, New York.

Tilton, R.C. 1982. The laboratory approach to the detection of bacteremia. Ann. Rev. Microbiol. 36:467.

Washington, J.A. II. 1978. The detection of septicemia. CRC Press, West Palm Beach, Fla.

15 Microorganisms Encountered in the Cerebrospinal Fluid

15.1. Introduction

15.1.a. Anatomy and physiology of the cerebrospinal fluid. Fully surrounding the brain and spinal cord, the cerebrospinal fluid (CSF) has several functions. It cushions the bulk of the brain and provides buoyancy, reducing the effective weight of the brain by a factor of 30. The CSF, through its circulation around the entire brain, ventricles, and spinal cord, carries essential metabolites into the neural tissue and cleanses the organs of wastes. Every 3-4 h, the entire volume of CSF is exchanged. The CSF is produced by the choroid plexus, specialized secretory cells located centrally within the brain in the third and fourth ventricles (fluid-filled cavities within the brain). The fluid travels around the ouside areas of the brain within the subarachnoid space, driven primarily by the pressure produced initially at the choroid plexus. The subarachnoid space is the intervening space between the **pia mater,** the tissue layer immediately covering the brain, and the **arachnoid,** a membrane loosely covering the brain and part of the spinal cord. Attachment between these two membranes is mediated by a thin network of fibers. The membranes surrounding the brain, the pia mater and the arachnoid, are collectively called the **leptomeninges.** All of the membranes surrounding the brain, including the **dura,** which covers the leptomeninges, are called the **meninges.** The portion of the arachnoid that covers the top of the brain contains special structures, **arachnoid villi,** that absorb the spinal fluid and allow it to pass into the blood.

Infection within the subarachnoid space or throughout the leptomeninges is called **meningitis.** With bacterial meningitis, cerebrospinal fluid usually contains large numbers of inflammatory cells (greater than $1,000/mm^3$), primarily polymorphonuclear neutrophils, shows a decreased glucose level relative to the serum glucose level (the normal ratio of CSF to serum glucose is approximately 0.6), and an increased protein concentration (normal protein is 15-50 mg/100 ml in adults and as high as 170 mg/100 ml, with an average of 90 mg/100 ml, in newborns). Most infectious agents reach the leptomeninges via hematogenous spread, entering the subarachnoid space through the choroid plexus or through other blood vessels of the brain. Meningitis can be either acute, usually caused by an encapsulated bacterial species, or chronic, caused by *Mycobacterium tuberculosis*, other bacteria, or fungi. Table 15.1 lists

TABLE 15.1
Etiologic Agents of Acute Meningitis

ACUTE BACTERIAL MENINGITIS	ACUTE NONBACTERIAL MENINGITIS
Streptococcus pneumoniae	*Cryptococcus neoformans*
Haemophilus influenzae	*Naegleria* or *Acanthamoeba*
Neisseria meningitidis	*Candida*
Streptococcus agalactiae (group B streptococci)	Viruses (usually enteroviruses)
Gram-negative bacilli, including *Flavobacterium meningosepticum*	*Angiostrongylus cantonensis*
Listeria monocytogenes	*Toxoplasma gondii*
Staphylococci	
Leptospira	
Treponema pallidum	
Mycobacterium tuberculosis	

some of the more common causes of acute meningitis. Inflammation of brain parenchyma, called **encephalitis,** is usually a result of viral infection. Concomitant inflammation of the meninges often occurs with this condition, which is then called **meningoencephalitis,** although the cellular infiltrate is more likely to be lymphocytic. Early in the course of viral encephalitis or when much tissue damage occurs as a part of encephalitis, however, the nature of the inflammatory cells found in the cerebrospinal fluid is no different from that associated with bacterial meningitis; typically, cell counts are much lower. In the past, patients who showed symptoms of meningitis and yielded cerebrospinal fluid samples that failed to grow a bacterial agent in culture were said to be suffering from **aseptic meningitis.** The other possibility to consider in the case of a patient who had received antibiotics previously, of course, is that of partially treated bacterial meningitis. With the advent of improved technology and availability of viral cultures, many instances of "aseptic meningitis" can now be assigned a viral etiology. Aseptic meningitis may also be due to tumor, cysts, chemicals, sarcoidosis, or other noninfectious causes.

15.1.b. Pathogenesis and epidemiology of meningeal infections. Most cases of meningitis caused by bacteria or encephalitis caused by viruses share the same pathogenesis. The etiologic agent impinges on the mucous membranes of the nasopharynx and oropharynx, attaches with the aid of an adherence mechanism (discussed in Chapter 16), and multiplies at the initial site. The organism somehow invades or is carried across tissue into the bloodstream, where it disseminates throughout the system during a bacteremic or viremic phase. Humoral immunity presumably intervenes at this stage in patients who are protected; the antibodies bind to the bacterial capsules and promote phagocytosis by opsonization. The microorganism enters the CSF through loss of capillary integrity or through some other mechanism, and multiples within the CSF, initially free of harmful antibodies or phagocytic cells. Organisms that can adhere to mucosal epithelium and evade destruction by possessing an antiphagocytic capsule are the best pathogens. In patients with impaired host defenses, other etiologic agents can gain a foothold and cause disease. Patients with prosthetic devices, particularly central nervous system shunts, are at increased risk of developing meningitis due to less "virulent" species, such as organisms that comprise the normal skin flora, aerobic and anaerobic diphtheroids and *Staphylococcus epidermidis*. Staphylococci may possess specialized virulence factors that allow them to colonize artificial surfaces. The "slime" or noncapsular polysaccharide produced by some staphylococci seems to help these bacteria adhere to smooth plastic and glass surfaces.

Viruses may enter the central nervous system through the bloodstream, but they may also travel along the nerves that lead to the brain (e.g., herpes simplex) or via the olfactory tract (e.g., adenovirus). Infections adjacent to the brain such as sinusitis and subdural abscess may also lead to meningitis. Patients with meningitis or encephalitis present with fever, stiff neck, headache, nausea and vomiting, sensory deprivations, and change in mental status.

Which etiologic agents are involved as the cause of any occurrence of bacterial meningitis is dependent on several factors, but age of the patient is most prominent. Ninety-five percent of all cases in the United States occur in children less than 5 years. In children in the United States between the ages of 1 month and 6 years, *Haemophilus influenzae* type b is the most common agent, although *Neisseria meningitidis* is more common among British children of the same age. From age 6, patients are more likely to develop meningococcal or pneumococcal meningitis. Ninety-five percent of all cases are due to *H. influenzae* type b, *N. meningitidis*, and *Streptococcus pneumoniae*.

The age group with the highest prevalence

of meningitis is that of the newborn, with a concomitant increased mortality rate (as high as 20%). Organisms causing disease in the newborn are different from those that affect other age groups; many of them are acquired by the newborn during passage through the mother's vaginal vault. Neonates are likely to be infected with, in order of incidence, group B streptococci, *Escherichia coli*, other gram-negative bacilli, *Listeria monocytogenes*, and other organisms. The prevalence of these organisms is probably due to the immature immune system of neonates, the organisms present in the colonized female vaginal tract, as well as to the increased permeability of the blood-brain barrier of newborns. *Flavobacterium meningosepticum* has been associated with nursery outbreaks of meningitis. The organism is presumably acquired nosocomially, since it is a normal inhabitant of water in the environment.

Lack of demonstrable humoral antibody against *H. influenzae* type b in children has been associated with increased incidence of meningitis. Most children develop measurable antibody by age 5. The importance of antibody is also a factor in adults, since military recruits without antibody to *N. meningitidis* are more likely to develop disease. *N. meningitidis* has been associated with epidemic meningitis among young adults in crowded conditions (e.g., military recruits and college dormitory mates). Meningococcal meningitis is endemic in certain areas of central Africa and Nepal. Visitors planning to visit these areas are urged to receive meningococcal vaccine. The *Morbidity and Mortality Weekly Report*, published by the Centers for Disease Control, furnishes physicians with an annual guide to recommendations for precautions to be taken by travelers.

Factors that predispose adults to meningitis are often the same factors that increase the likelihood that the adult will develop pneumonia or other respiratory tract colonization or infection, since the respiratory tract is the primary portal of entry for many etiologic agents of meningitis. Alcoholism, splenectomy, diabetes mellitus, prosthetic devices, and immunosuppression contribute to increased risk. Important causes of meningitis in the adult, in addition to the meningococcus in young adults, include pneumococci, *L. monocytogenes*, and less commonly *Staphylococcus aureus* and various gram-negative bacilli. The latter organisms lead to meningitis via hematogenous seeding from various sources, including urinary tract infections.

The sequelae of acute bacterial meningitis in children are frequent and serious. Seizures occur in 20%-30% of patients seen at large urban hospitals, and other neurologic changes are common. Acute sequelae include cerebral edema, hydrocephalus, cerebral herniation, and focal neurologic changes. Permanent sensorineural deafness occurred in 10% of children who recovered from bacterial meningitis studied at one institution. It has also been reported that more subtle physiological and psychological sequelae follow an episode of acute bacterial meningitis. It can be appreciated that even though the mortality from such infections has dropped from 90%-100% in the preantibiotic era to 3%-30% today, the morbidity associated with meningitis today is still significant.

Chronic meningitis often occurs in patients who are immunocompromised in some way, although this is not always the case. Etiologic agents of chronic meningitis are as follows:

Mycobacterium tuberculosis
Cryptococcus neoformans
Coccidioides immitis
Histoplasma capsulatum
Blastomyces dermatitidis
Candida species
Miscellaneous other fungi
Nocardia
Actinomyces
Treponema pallidum
Brucella
Salmonella
Rare parasites—*Toxoplasma gondii*, cysticercus, *Paragonimus westermani*

Patients experience an insidious onset of disease, with fever, headache, stiff neck, nausea and vomiting, lethargy, confusion, and mental deterioration. Symptoms may persist for a month or longer before treatment is sought. The CSF usually manifests an abnormal number of cells (usually lymphocytic), elevated protein, and some decrease in glucose content. The pathogenesis of chronic meningitis is similar to that of acute disease.

Although not directly an infection of the CSF, brain abscesses may occasionally cause changes in the CSF and clinical symptoms that mimic meningitis. Brain abscesses may also rupture into the subarachnoid space producing a severe meningitis with high mortality. If anaerobic organisms or viridans streptococci are recovered from CSF cultures, the diagnosis of brain abscess must be entertained. Immunosuppressed patients may show a rapidly progressive fungal infection of the nasal sinuses or palatal region that travels directly to the brain.

Viral encephalitis, which cannot always be distinguished from meningitis clinically, is common in the warmer months. The primary agents are enteroviruses (coxsackievirus A and B, echoviruses), mumps virus, herpes simplex virus, and arboviruses (togavirus, bunyavirus, equine encephalitis, other encephalitis viruses). Other viruses, such as measles, cytomegalovirus, lymphocytic choriomeningitis, Epstein-Barr, hepatitis, varicella-zoster, rabies, and myxo- and paramyxoviruses, are less commonly encountered. The preceding viral illness or exposure history are important considerations in establishing an etiology by clinical means.

Parasites can cause meningoencephalitis, brain abscess, or other central nervous system infection via two routes. The free-living amebae, *Naegleria fowleri* and *Acanthamoeba* species, invade the brain directly through the nasal mucosa. These organisms are acquired by swimming or diving in natural freshwater ponds and lakes, especially those with stagnation. Other parasites reach the brain via hematogenous spread. Immunosuppressed patients are likely to acquire toxoplasmosis, the agent of which grows intracellularly and destroys brain parenchyma. Toxoplasmosis is a common central nervous system affliction in patients with acquired immune deficiency syndrome (AIDS; discussed further in Chapter 23). *Entamoeba histolytica* and *Strongyloides stercoralis* have been visualized in brain tissue, and the larval form of *Taenia solium* (the pork tapeworm), called a **cysticercus,** can travel to the brain via the bloodstream and grow in that site, causing symptoms of chronic meningitis and displacing normal tissue. Amebic brain infection and cysticercosis cause changes in the CSF that mimic meningitis.

15.2. Collection, Transport, and Initial Handling of Specimens

CSF is usually collected by aseptically inserting a needle into the subarachnoid space at the level of the lumbar spine. Three or four tubes of CSF should be collected and immediately labeled with the patient's name. Tube number 3 or 4 is used for cell count and differential. If a small capillary blood vessel is inadvertently traversed during the spinal tap (lumbar puncture), blood cells picked up from this source will usually be absent from the last tube collected; comparison of counts between tubes 1 and 4 is usually of interest. The other tubes can be used for both microbiological and chemical studies. In this way, a larger proportion of the total fluid can be concentrated, facilitating detection of infectious agents present in low numbers, and the supernatant can still be used for other required studies. Microbiologists should periodically monitor the sterile tubes used in lumbar puncture kits prepared at their institutions by processing filter-sterilized negative CSF as a quality control check. CSF collecting tubes have been known to harbor nonviable bacteria, which can cause false-positive Gram stain results.

The volume of CSF is critical for detection of certain microorganisms, such as *Mycobacte-*

rium tuberculosis and *Cryptococcus neoformans.* At least 10 ml of CSF is recommended for analysis of CSF suspected of containing these pathogens by centrifugation and subsequent culture. When an inadequate volume of CSF is received, the physician should be consulted as to the order of priority of laboratory studies.

Cerebrospinal fluid should be hand-delivered **immediately** to the laboratory. Specimens should never be refrigerated. If they are not being processed immediately, they should be incubated or left at room temperature. One exception to this rule involves CSF for viral studies. These specimens may be refrigerated for up to 24 h after collection or frozen at $-70°$ C if a longer delay is anticipated until they are inoculated. Cerebrospinal fluid for viral studies should never be frozen at temperatures that are warmer than $-70°$ C. Certain agents, such as *S. pneumoniae,* may not be detectable after an hour or longer unless antigen detection methods are used. Prompt examination by microbiologists can often determine the etiologic agent within as short a time as 30 min, helping the clinician to direct or correct therapy. Cerebrospinal fluid is one of the few specimens handled by the laboratory for which information relayed to the clinician can directly affect therapeutic outcome. Such specimens should be processed immediately upon receipt in the laboratory and all results should be telephoned to the physician as soon as they are available.

Initial processing of CSF for bacterial, fungal, or parasitic studies includes centrifugation of all specimens greater than 1 ml volume for at least 15 min at 1500 x g. Specimens in which cryptococci or mycobacteria are suspected must be handled differently. Discussions of techniques for culturing CSF for fungi are found in Chapter 43, and methods for isolating mycobacteria are detailed in Chapter 41. The supernatant is decanted into a sterile tube, leaving approximately 0.5 ml fluid in which to vortex the sediment before it is inoculated to media or examined visually. This mixing of the sediment is critical. Laboratories that use a sterile capillary pipette to remove portions of the sediment from underneath the supernatant will miss a significant number of positive specimens. The sediment must be thoroughly mixed **after** the supernatant has been removed. Either vortexing or forcefully aspirating the sediment up and down into a sterile pipette several times will adequately disperse the organisms that remained adherent to the bottom of the tube after centrifugation. The supernatant can be used to test for the presence of antigens or for chemistry evaluations (protein, glucose, lactate, etc.). Even if there is no immediate use for the supernatant, it should be kept as a safeguard. Later, supernatants from culture-negative CSF can be pooled, filter sterilized, and used as a diluent for other tests or for quality control.

15.3. Visual Detection of Etiologic Agents of Meningitis

15.3.a. Direct wet preparation. Amebae are best observed by examining thoroughly mixed sediment as a wet preparation under phase contrast microscopy (Chapter 7). If a phase contrast microscope is not available, observing under light microscopy with the condenser closed slightly is an alternative technique. Amebae are recognized by typical slow, methodical movement in one direction by advancing pseudopodia. The organisms may require a little time under the warm light of the microscope before they begin to move. They must be distinguished from motile macrophages which occasionally occur in CSF. Following up a suspicious wet preparation, a trichrome stain (Chapter 44) can help differentiate amebas from somatic cells (Plate 15.1) The pathogenic amebas can be cultured on a lawn of *Klebsiella pneumoniae*, as outlined below.

15.3.b. India ink preparation. *Cryptococcus neoformans*, because of the large polysaccharide capsule that serves as a virulence mechanism in the pathogenesis of meningitis, can often be visualized by the India ink stain. A drop of CSF sediment is mixed with one third volume of India ink (Pelikan Drawing Ink, Block, Gunther, and Wagner; available at art supply stores). The India ink can be protected against contamination by adding 0.05 ml thimerosal (Merthiolate, Sigma Chemical Co.) to the bottle when it is first opened. After mixing the CSF and ink to make a smooth suspension, a coverslip is applied to the drop and the preparation is examined under high-power magnification (400 ×) for characteristic encapsulated yeast cells, which can be confirmed by examination under oil immersion (1000 ×) (Figure 15.1). The inexperienced microscopist must be careful not to confuse white blood cells with yeast. The presence of encapsulated buds, smaller than the mother cell, is diagnostic. All requests for India ink preparations should automatically include performance of a cryptococcal latex agglutination test, as outlined below. This test is more sensitive than India ink, es-

FIGURE 15.1
Encapsulated budding cells of *Cryptococcus neoformans* seen in an India ink preparation made from infected cerebrospinal fluid (1,000 ×).

pecially considering that patients with crypto-coccal meningitis may yield only one yeast cell per 20 ml CSF.

15.3.c. Stained smear of sediment. The classic stain, the Gram stain, must be performed on all CSF sediments. After thoroughly mixing the sediment, a heaped drop is placed on the surface of a sterile or alcohol-wiped slide. Applying a second heaped drop in the same area after the first drop has dried will increase the concentration of material that can be thoroughly examined. The sediment should never be spread out on the slide surface, as this merely increases the difficulty of finding small numbers of microorganisms. False positive smears have resulted from inadvertent use of contaminated slides. The use of a steel autoclavable slide holder is recommended (Figure 15.2). The drop of sediment is allowed to air dry, is heat or methanol fixed, and stained by either Gram or acridine orange stain (Chapter 7). The acridine orange fluorochrome stain may allow faster examination of the slide under high power magnification (400 ×), and thus a more

FIGURE 15.2
Stainless steel autoclavable glass microscope slide holder, suitable for autoclaving cleaned slides.

thorough examination. The brightly fluorescing bacteria will be easily visible. All suspicious smears can be restained by the Gram stain (directly over the acridine orange stain) to confirm morphology of any organisms seen. Based on demographic and clinical patient data and Gram stain morphology, the etiology of the majority of cases of bacterial meningitis can be presumptively determined within the first 30 min after receiving the specimen. Acid fast smears are handled differently, as discussed in Chapter 41.

15.3.d. Quellung reaction. Serologic identification of either *H. influenzae* type b, *S. pneumoniae*, or *N. meningitidis* in CSF can be made using the quellung reaction (Chapter 12) after the organism has been presumptively identified by Gram stain morphology. A drop of undiluted antiserum is mixed with a drop of the unstained sediment and a drop of saturated aqueous methylene blue dye on a slide, and a coverslip is applied to the wet preparation. The light is adjusted by closing the condenser and the organisms are observed for an apparent capsular swelling, a visual artifact of the reaction between capsular polysaccharide antigen and antibody. Sera are available from Difco Laboratories and the Centers for Disease Control. This test is rarely performed today, having been supplanted by the direct antigen detection systems discussed below.

15.4. Syphilis Serology

Diagnosis of neurosyphilis is based on several parameters, including the number and types of white and red cells present in the patient's CSF, patient history and epidemiological factors, levels of protein and glucose, and the VDRL test. The VDRL test (Chapter 12) is the only useful test for detecting antibodies directed against *Treponema pallidum* in CSF. A positive CSF VDRL is still not diagnostic in itself, as patients with successfully treated neurosyphilis may retain a positive CSF VDRL even years later.

15.5. Detection of Antigen in CSF

The availability of reagents and complete systems for the rapid detection of antigen in CSF is an exciting use of the new technology (principles of these methods were discussed in Chapter 10). Countercurrent immunoelectrophoresis (CIE), although the first widely accepted method for rapid antigen detection from CSF, has been largely replaced by the more sensitive and simpler techniques of latex agglutination and coagglutination, although CIE may be used in some laboratories for detection of antigen to *Listeria monocytogenes*, for which no latex tests are available. There are four commercial systems available at the time of writing of this chapter for testing CSF samples for the presence of antigen (Table 15.2). All systems utilize the principle of an antibody-coated particle that will bind to specific antigen, resulting in macroscopically visible agglutination. The soluble capsular polysaccharide produced by the most common etiologic agents of meningitis and the group B streptococcal polysaccharide are well suited to serve as bridging antigens. The particle used for each system is listed in Table 15.2, as are the antigens for which reagents are available. The systems differ in that certain antibodies are polyclonal and others are monoclonal (Chapter 10), and not all systems detect all antigens.

Reagents for the detection of the polysaccharide capsular antigen of *Cryptococcus neoformans* are available from M.A. Bioproducts and Meridian Diagnostics. Interference with the reaction may occur if patients possess rheumatoid factor. For CSF specimens that yield positive results for cryptococcal antigen, a second latex agglutination test for rheumatoid factor should be performed. A positive rheumatoid factor test renders the cryptococcal latex test uninterpretable, and the results should be reported as such, unless the rheumatoid factor antibodies can be diluted out. The commercial test systems incorporate rheumatoid factor testing in their protocol. Specimens that contain large amounts of capsular antigen may yield a false-negative reaction due to a prozone phenomenon. Especially if the India ink preparation is positive, CSF should be diluted out for testing with latex antigen detection reagents.

In general, the commercial systems have been developed for use with CSF, urine, or serum, although results with serum have not been as critical diagnostically as those with CSF. Soluble antigen from several infective agents tends to concentrate in the urine during some illnesses, so that urine may be an effective diagnostic body fluid in those cases. Urine, however, does seem to produce a higher incidence of nonspecific reactions than either

TABLE 15.2
Direct Antigen Detection Systems for Etiologic Agents of Meningitis

TEST	MANUFACTURER	PARTICLE	DETECTION OF			
			H. INFLUENZAE b	*S. PNEUMONIAE*	*N. MENINGITIDIS*	*S. AGALACTIAE*
Bactigen	Wampole Laboratories	Latex	+	+	A,B,C,Y	—
Directogen	Hynson, Westcott & Dunning	Latex	+	+	A,B,C	+
Phadebact	Pharmacia Diagnostics	Staphylococci	+	+	+	+
Wellcogen	Wellcome Diagnostics	Latex	+	+	A,C,Y,W135	+

serum or CSF. The manufacturers' directions must be followed for performance of antigen detection test systems for different specimen types. Although some of the systems require pretreatment of samples, usually heating for 5 min, not all manufacturers recommend such a step. The reagents, however, may yield false positive or cross-reactions unless specimen pretreatment is performed. Interference by rheumatoid factor and other substances, more often present in body fluids other than CSF, has also been reported. The method of Smith and coworkers [2] has been shown to effectively reduce a substantial portion of nonspecific and false-positive reactions, at least for tests performed with latex particle reagents. This pretreatment, called rapid extraction of antigen procedure (REAP; Procedure 15.1), is recommended for those laboratories that use commercial body fluid antigen detection kits. Certain commercial systems have such an extraction procedure included in their protocols.

Once the fluid sample has been treated, it is mixed with a drop of the particle reagent and observed for a very short time for agglutination in one specific antibody-coated reagent and no reaction with the other reagents. Advantages of this system over conventional culture are that specimens containing only nonviable organisms due to previous therapy and those with small numbers of organisms that are near the sensitivity of Gram stain can be rapidly identified as having antigen present. The greatest advantage is that a specific etiologic agent can be identified within minutes of receiving the specimen. Confirmation of identification of organisms seen on Gram stain can be accomplished, as well as the detection of an etiologic agent in smear-negative specimens. The systems are not substitutes for properly performed smears and cultures, but they provide an important additional diagnostic test to aid clinicians in initial management of serious meningitis.

15.6. Culture for Etiologic Agents of CSF Infection

After vortexing the sediment and preparing smears, several drops of the sediment should be inoculated to each medium. Routine bacteriologic media should include a chocolate agar plate, 5% sheep blood agar plate, and an enrichment broth, usually thioglycolate without

---

PROCEDURE 15.1. RAPID EXTRACTION OF ANTIGEN PROCEDURE (REAP)

1. Pipette 0.05 ml fluid to be tested (CSF, serum, or urine) into a 1.5 ml plastic conical microcentrifuge tube.
2. Add 0.15 ml of 0.1 M ethylenediaminetetraacetic acid (EDTA, Sigma Chemical Co.) to the microcentrifuge tube, close the cap tightly, and vortex the tube.
3. Heat in a dry bath (available from instrument supply companies) for 3 min at 100° C.
4. Centrifuge the tubes for 5 min at $13,000 \times g$ in a tabletop microcentrifuge. Be certain that the instrument used achieves the required centrifugal force.
5. Remove the supernatant with a capillary pipette and use one drop of this solution as the test sample in the antigen detection test, following the manufacturer's instructions for performance of the test.

Modified from Smith et al. 1984. J. Clin. Microbiol. 20:981-984.

indicator. The plates should be incubated at 37° C in 5%-10% CO_2 for at least 72 h. If a CO_2 incubator is not available, a candle jar (Chapter 8) can be used. The broth should be incubated in air at 37° C for at least 5 days. The broth cap must be loose to allow free exchange of air. If organisms morphologically resembling anaerobic bacteria are seen on the Gram stain, an anaerobic blood agar plate may be inoculated additionally. If the Gram stain revealed large, regular gram-negative rods, a Mac-Conkey plate should be added to the initial media. The authors of Cumitech 14[1] recommend that penicillinase (Difco Laboratories or BBL Microbiology Systems) be added to culture media if patients have received prior antibiotic therapy. One drop of penicillinase is mixed with the drop of inoculum on each plate, and another drop of penicillinase is added to the broth tube in which the specimen is to be incubated as well as to a second thioglycolate tube that serves as a sterility control for the penicillinase. These media will support the growth of almost all bacterial pathogens and several fungi.

Cultures specifically for detection of fungi or mycobacteria are handled in a biological safety cabinet. The symptoms of chronic meningitis that prompt a physician to request fungal cultures are the same as those for tuberculous meningitis, which should always be sought by the laboratory if chronic or fungal meningitis is suspected. Two drops of the well-mixed sediment should be inoculated to a non–blood containing medium (brain heart infusion with gentamicin and chloramphenicol, as discussed in Chapter 8) plate or slant and a brain heart infusion or inhibitory mold agar slant or plate. Addition of a third medium such as Mycosel or Mycobiotic (selective agar, Chapter 8) is recommended. The material can be deposited on the agar surface without spreading for isolation. Fungal media should be incubated in air at 30°

C for 4 weeks. If possible, it is best to inoculate two sets of media and incubate one set at 30° C and one set at 35° C. As discussed in Chapter 41, centrifugation may not effectively sediment mycobacteria; other methods are suggested.

The free-living amebas can be co-cultivated on artificial media if they are supplied with a living nutrient, such as *Klebsiella pneumoniae*. This procedure should be tried if amebic meningoencephalitis is suspected (Procedure 15.2).

Cerebrospinal fluid may be inoculated directly to tissue culture for detecton of viral agents. Diagnosis of viral encephalitides is often accomplished by isolation of the virus from a throat culture, feces culture, or blood, so these specimens should be submitted in addition to CSF for identification of an etiologic agent. Methods for cultivation of viruses from such specimens are discussed in detail in Chapter 42. Briefly, 0.25 ml of CSF per tube is inoculated into tubes of primary monkey kidney, Hep-2 continuous cell line, and human fetal diploid foreskin fibroblast cell cultures. These culture systems are incubated at 35° C in air for varying amounts of time, depending on the cell culture system. Further details of viral isolation procedures are found in Chapter 42.

15.7. Other Diagnostic Techniques

Certain agents of encephalitis or meningitis can only be detected by examining brain tissue. Brain biopsy specimens are submitted for histopathologic evaluation. Direct smears can be stained with fluorescent or horseradish peroxidase conjugated antibodies for rapid detection of herpes viruses, varicella-zoster, and rabies. Stained smears can be used to visualize *Toxoplasma gondii* and other parasites, as well as the characteristic inclusions of cytomegalovirus and herpes. These diagnostic procedures are usually performed by pathologists rather than microbiologists. Peroxidase- and fluorescein-

**PROCEDURE 15.2. MONAXENIC CULTIVATION OF *NAEGLERIA FOWLERI*
AND *ACANTHAMOEBA* SPECIES**

1. Prepare a nonnutritive agar as follows:

Bacto agar (Difco Laboratories)	2 g
Distilled water	100 ml

   Dissolve the agar in the water and autoclave for 10 min at 121° C. Allow to cool to 56° C, mix thoroughly, and pour five 100 mm diameter Petri plates, 20 ml agar per plate. Allow the plates to harden.

2. Make Page's ameba saline solution as follows*:

NaCl	0.120 g
$MgSO_4 \cdot 7H_2O$	0.004 g
$CaCl_2 \cdot 2H_2O$	0.004 g
Na_2HPO_4	0.142 g
KH_2PO_4	0.136 g

   Dissolve each salt (available from any chemical supply company) in 10 ml of distilled water in 16 × 125 mm screw cap test tubes. These tubes may be kept refrigerated for months. In a 100 ml Erlenmeyer flask or bottle, add 1 ml of each of the five salt solutions. Add 95 ml distilled water.

3. Make a thick suspension (approximately equal to a McFarland 3.0 turbidity) of a fresh subculture (overnight) of *Klebsiella pneumoniae* in 1 ml Page's saline.

4. Place a single drop of the centrifuged CSF sediment in the center of each of two nonnutrient agar plates.

5. Place 3 drops of the *Klebsiella* suspension directly on top of the drop of CSF sediment on each plate.

6. Seal the edges of each plate with cellophane tape to prevent drying, and incubate in air at 37° C for 14 days.

7. Examine the surface of the agar with the low power objective of a microscope (100 ×) daily for motile amebas. Amebas may become visible within 48 h.

8. If viable amebas are found, they may be fixed and permanently stained by emulsifying a loopful scraped from the surface of the plate in a tiny amount of Page's saline in a small test tube.

9. Add 3 parts polyvinyl-alcohol (PVA; Chapter 44), and prepare a thin smear as for staining PVA-fixed fecal specimens.

10. Stain the smear with trichrome stain (Chapter 44) and observe for trophozoites.

Modified from the procedure of Dr. J.J. Napolitano, Adelphi University, Long Island, N.Y.
*Modified from Page, F.C. 1976. An illustrated key to freshwater and soil amoeba. Freshwater Biological Association Scientific Publication 34, Ferry Moose Ambeside, Cumbria, England.

conjugated antibodies have been used for the successful detection of *Toxoplasma*-infected cells in sections made from brain tissue.

Other new approaches are being explored for diagnosis of meningitis. Although it is not widely used, the *Limulus* amebocyte lysate test for lipopolysaccharide (Chapter 10) has proven to be very sensitive for diagnosis of meningitis caused by gram-negative bacteria, including *E. coli*, *H. influenzae*, and *N. meningitidis*. Since *Listeria* also contains endotoxin, though a gram-positive organism, the *Limulus* test might also yield positive results with this etiologic agent. Enzyme-linked immunosorbent assay (ELISA) procedures (Chapter 10) have also been adapted for diagnosis of meningitis. Systems are being manufactured for detection of *H. influenzae*, *S. pneumoniae*, and *N. meningitidis* antigens. An ELISA system has been shown to reliably detect antigens of *M. tuberculosis* in CSF. Because of the slow growth of this organism and the lack of any rapid procedures for its detection, such tests are highly desirable. No commercial systems are currently available. Gas-liquid chromatography and electron-capture chromatography have been evaluated for rapid detection of etiologic agents of disease in CSF. Although reports are promising, these methods are not yet available for routine testing.

REFERENCES

1. Ray, C.G., Wasilauskas, B.L., and Zabransky, R.J. 1982. Laboratory diagnosis of central nervous system infections. In McCarthy, L.R., editor. Cumitech 14. American Society for Microbiology, Washington, D.C.
2. Smith, L.P., Hunter, K.W. Jr., Hemming, V.G., and Fischer, G.W. 1984. Improved detection of bacterial antigens by latex agglutination after rapid extraction from body fluids. J. Clin. Microbiol. 20:981.

BIBLIOGRAPHY

Conly, J.M., and Ronald, A.R. 1983. Cerebrospinal fluid as a diagnostic body fluid. Am. J. Med. 75:102.
Greenlea, J.E. 1985. Anatomic considerations in central nervous system infections. In Mandell, G.L., Douglas, R.G. Jr., and Bennett, J.E., editors. Principles and practice of infectious diseases, ed 2. John Wiley & Sons, New York.
Kuhn, P.J. 1983. Meningitis and encephalitis: are we doing all we can? Diagn. Med. 6:36.
McGee, Z., and Kaiser, A.B. 1985. Acute meningitis. In Mandell, G.L., Douglas, R.G. Jr., and Bennett, J.E., editors. Principles and practice of infectious diseases, ed 2. John Wiley & Sons, New York.
Swartz, M.N. 1984. Bacterial meningitis: more involved than just the meninges. N. Engl. J. Med. 311:912.

16 Microorganisms Encountered in the Respiratory Tract

16.1. Introduction

16.1.a. General considerations, anatomy, and normal state of the respiratory tract. The respiratory tract begins with the nasal or oral passages and extends past the nasopharynx and oropharynx to the trachea and then into the lungs. The trachea divides into bronchi, which subdivide into bronchioles, the smallest branches of which terminate in the alveoli. Several mechanisms serve to nonspecifically protect the respiratory tract from infection, including the hairs, convoluted passages, and mucus lining of the nasal turbinates; secretory IgA and nonspecific antibacterial substances (lysozyme) in respiratory secretions; the cilia and mucus lining the trachea; and reflexes such as cough, sneeze, and swallow. These mechanisms serve to prevent foreign objects or organisms from entering the bronchi and gaining access to the lungs, which should be sterile in the healthy host. Once particles that have escaped the airflow turbulence and the mucociliary sweeping activity enter the alveoli, alveolar macrophages ingest them and carry them to the lymphatics. In addition, normal flora of the nasopharynx and oropharynx help to prevent colonization of the respiratory tract by pathogenic microorganisms.

16.1.b. Flora of the respiratory tract. Those bacteria that can be isolated as part of the normal flora of healthy hosts are listed in

TABLE 16.1
Organisms Commonly Present in the Nasopharynx and Oropharynx of Healthy Humans

RARELY PATHOGENS	POSSIBLE PATHOGENS
Nonhemolytic streptococci	*Acinetobacter*
Staphylococci	Viridans streptococci
Micrococci	Beta hemolytic streptococci
Corynebacterium species	*Streptococcus pneumoniae*
Coagulase negative staphylococci	*Staphylococcus aureus*
Neisseria species, other than *N. gonorrhoeae* and *N. meningitidis*	*Corynebacterium diphtheriae*
	Neisseria meningitidis
Lactobacillus species	*Cryptococcus neoformans*
Veillonella species	*Mycoplasma* species
Spirochetes	*Haemophilus influenzae*
	Haemophilus parainfluenzae
	Branhamella catarrhalis
	Candida albicans
	Herpes simplex virus
	Enterobacteriaceae
	Mycobacterium species
	Pseudomonas species
	Filamentous fungi
	Klebsiella ozaenae
	Eikenella corrodens
	Bacteroides species
	Fusobacterium species
	Peptostreptococcus species
	Actinomyces species

Table 16.1. In addition, Table 16.1 lists many species that may cause disease under certain circumstances but are often isolated from the respiratory tracts of healthy persons. Under certain circumstances, for unknown reasons—perhaps due to previous damage by a viral infection, loss of some host immunity, or because of physical damage to the respiratory epithelium (from smoking, for example)—these colonizing organisms go on to cause disease. Organisms isolated from normally sterile sites in the respiratory tract by methods that avoid contamination with normal flora (discussed in Chapters 6 and 34) should be definitively identified and reported to the clinician.

Certain microorganisms are considered to be etiologic agents of disease if they are present in any numbers in the respiratory tract because they possess virulence factors that are expressed in every host. These are listed in the box on p. 239. Many selective media have been designed to isolate these organisms, even in the presence of normal flora. This chapter will discuss such methods, as well as strategies to follow for handling of specimens received from the respiratory tract.

16.1.c. Pathogenic mechanisms employed by agents of respiratory tract infections. Microorganisms cause disease primarily by only a few pathogenic mechanisms. As these mechanisms relate to respiratory tract infections, they will be discussed briefly. For any organism to cause disease, it must first be able to gain a foothold within the respiratory tract in order to grow to sufficient numbers to produce symptoms. Therefore most etiologic agents of respiratory tract disease must first adhere to the mucosa of the respiratory tract. The presence of normal flora and the overall state of the host affect the ability of microorganisms to adhere. Surviving or growing on host tissue without causing overt harmful effects is called **colonization.** Except for those microorganisms that are breathed directly into the lungs, all etiologic agents of disease must first colonize the respiratory tract to some degree before they can cause harm.

Bacteria that possess specific adherence factors include *Streptococcus pyogenes*, whose cell wall contains lipoteichoic acids and certain proteins (M protein and others), visible as a thin layer of fuzz surrounding the bacteria. Other bacteria that possess lipoteichoic acid adherence complexes are *Staphylococcus aureus* and certain viridans streptococci. Many gram-negative bacteria, particularly Enterobacteriaceae, *Legionella* species, *Pseudomonas* species, *Bordetella pertussis*, and *Haemophilus* species (and *Actinomyces* species, which are gram positive), adhere by means of protein-

DEFINITE RESPIRATORY TRACT PATHOGENS

Corynebacterium diphtheriae (toxin-producing)
Neisseria gonorrhoeae
Mycobacterium tuberculosis
Mycoplasma pneumoniae
Chlamydia trachomatis
Bordetella pertussis
Legionella species
Pneumocystis carinii
Nocardia species
Histoplasma capsulatum
Coccidioides immitis
Cryptococcus neoformans (may also be recovered from patients without disease)
Blastomyces dermatitidis
Viruses

VERY RARE

Francisella tularensis
Bacillus anthracis
Yersinia pestis
Pseudomonas pseudomallei
Coxiella burnetti
Chlamydia psittaci
Brucella species
Salmonella species
Pasteurella multocida
Parasites
Klebsiella rhinoscleromatis

aceous fingerlike surface structures called **fimbriae** (Figure 16.1). Fimbriae are often also called **pili,** although this is technically the term for a similar structure that participates in sexual interaction rather than strict adherence. Viruses possess either a hemagglutinin (influenza viruses) or other protein that mediates their attachment to host epithelium.

The production of extracellular toxin was one of the first pathogenic mechanisms discovered among bacteria. It has been appreciated more recently that certain fungi may also produce toxins that may play a role in human disease, but there have been no proven toxins among those fungi that cause respiratory disease. *Corynebacterium diphtheriae* is a classic example of a bacterium that produces disease due to the action of extracellular toxin. Once the organism colonizes the upper respiratory epithelium, it elaborates a toxin that is disseminated systemically, adhering preferentially to central nervous system cells and muscle cells of the heart. Systemic disease characterized by myocarditis and local disease leading to respiratory distress (see below) can follow, as can peripheral neuritis. Growth of *C. diphtheriae* causes necrosis of the epithelial mucosa, characterized by a **diphtheritic (pseudo) membrane,** which may extend from the anterior nasal mucosa to the bronchi or be limited to any area between, most often to the tonsillar and peritonsillar areas. The membrane may cause sore throat and interfere with respiration and swallowing. Although nontoxic strains of *C. diphtheriae* can cause disease, it is much milder than the version mediated by toxin. The toxin gene is carried into the bacteria by phage, as mentioned in Chapter 33.

Some strains of *Pseudomonas aeruginosa* produce a toxin very similar to diphtheria toxin. Whether this toxin actually contributes to the pathogenesis of respiratory tract infection with *P. aeruginosa* has not been verified. *Bordetella pertussis,* the agent of whooping cough, also produces toxins. The role of these toxins in production of disease is not clear.

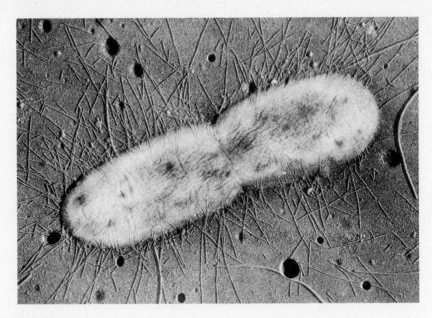

FIGURE 16.1

Fimbriae of *Escherichia coli*, extending as thin projections from the cell periphery. (Courtesy A. Ryter, Institut Pasteur. From Boyd, R.F. 1984. General microbiology. The C.V. Mosby Co., St. Louis.)

They may act to inhibit the activity of phagocytic cells or to damage cells of the respiratory tract. *S. aureus* and beta hemolytic streptococci produce extracellular enzymes that act to damage host cells or tissues. Extracellular products of staphylococci aid in production of tissue necrosis and destruction of phagocytic cells, contributing to the commonly seen phenomenon of abscess formation associated with infection caused by this organism. Although *S. aureus* can be recovered from throat specimens, it has not been proven to cause pharyngitis. Enzymes of streptococci, including hyaluronidase, allow rapid dissemination of the bacteria. Many other etiologic agents of respiratory tract infection also produce extracellular enzymes and toxins.

In addition to adherence and toxin production, pathogens cause disease by merely growing in host tissue, interfering with normal tissue function and attracting host immune effectors, such as neutrophils and macrophages. Once these cells begin to try to destroy the invading pathogens and repair the damaged host tissue, an expanding reaction ensues with more nonspecific immunological factors being attracted to the area, increasing the amount of host tissue damage. Respiratory viral infections usually progress in this manner, as do many types of pneumonias, such as those caused by *Streptococcus pneumoniae*, *S. pyogenes*, *Staphylococcus aureus*, *Haemophilus influenzae*, *Neisseria meningitidis*, *Branhamella catarrhalis*, *Mycoplasma pneumoniae*, and most gram-negative bacilli. Aspiration of minor amounts of oropharyngeal material, as occurs often during sleep, plays an important role in the pathogenesis of many types of pneumonia.

The ability to evade host defense mechanisms is another virulence mechanism that certain respiratory tract pathogens possess. *S. pneumoniae*, *N. meningitidis*, *H. influenzae*, *K. pneumoniae*, mucoid *P. aeruginosa*, *Crypto-*

coccus neoformans, and others possess polysaccharide capsules that serve both to prevent engulfment by phagocytic host cells and to protect somatic antigens from being exposed to host immunoglobulins. The capsular material is produced in such abundance by certain bacteria, such as pneumococci, that soluble polysaccharide antigen particles can bind host antibodies, blocking them from serving as opsonins. Proof that the capsular polysaccharide is the principal virulence mechanism of *H. influenzae*, *S. pneumoniae* and *N. meningitidis* was established when vaccines consisting of capsular antigens alone were shown to protect individuals from disease.

Some respiratory pathogens evade the host immune system by multiplying within host cells. *Chlamydia trachomatis*, *Chlamydia psittaci*, and all viruses replicate within host cells. They have evolved methods for being taken in by the "nonprofessional" phagocytic cells of the host to achieve their required environment, which is protected from host humoral immune factors and other phagocytic cells until the host cell becomes sufficiently damaged that it is recognized as foreign and attacked. A second category of agents of respiratory tract disease is actively taken up by phagocytic host cells, usually macrophages, within which they are able to multiply. *Legionella*, *Listeria*, some *Salmonella* species, *Pneumocystis carinii*, and *Histoplasma capsulatum* are some of the more common intracellular parasites and *Mycobacterium tuberculosis* is the classic representative of an intracellular pathogen. In primary tuberculosis, the organism is carried to an alveolus in a **droplet nucleus,** a tiny aerosol particle containing as few as one tubercle bacillus (the minimum infective dose). There it is phagocytized by alveolar macrophages, which carry it to the nearest lymph node, usually in the mediastinal or hilar chains. In the node the organisms slowly multiply within macrophages, destroying them and being taken up by other phagocytic cells in turn. Within the protected environment of the macrophages, which are somehow prevented by the bacteria from accomplishing lysosomal fusion, tubercle bacilli multiply to a critical mass, which spills out of the destroyed macrophages through the lymphatics into the bloodstream, producing bacteremia and carrying tubercle bacilli to many parts of the body. In most cases, the host immune system reacts sufficiently at this point to kill most of the bacilli; a small reservoir of live bacteria may be left, usually in the apical portion of the lung. These bacilli are walled off, and a subsequent insult to the host, either immunologic or physical, may cause breakdown of the focus of latent tubercle bacilli, allowing active multiplication and disease. In certain patients with primary immune defects of some type, the initial bacteremia seeds bacteria throughout a host which is unable to control them, leading to disseminated or **miliary** tuberculosis. Growth of the bacteria within host macrophages and histiocytes in the lung causes an influx of more effector cells, including lymphocytes, neutrophils, and histiocytes, eventually resulting in granuloma formation, then tissue destruction and cavity formation. The lesion is characteristically a semisolid, amorphous tissue mass resembling semisoft cheese, from which it receives the name **caseation necrosis.** The infected tissue can extend into bronchioles and bronchi, from which bacteria are disseminated via respiratory secretions, coughing, etc., to the next victim and also to other portions of the patient's own lungs.

16.2. Upper Respiratory Tract Infections

Microorganisms that cause disease in the upper respiratory tract, the nasopharynx and pharynx, must come into contact with the mucosal epithelium, adhere, and multiply. They are carried in by aerosols in the case of *N. meningitidis*, *Bordetella pertussis*, *C. diphtheriae*, and many viruses. They may be passed in secretions, either by intimate contact or through crowded conditions or poor hygiene. *Myco-*

plasma species and *S. pyogenes* are often passed in this way. Although a large number of species of bacteria and fungi may be isolated from specimens taken from the upper respiratory tract, very few organisms have been shown to cause true disease in that area.

16.2.a. Etiologic agents of nasopharyngeal and oropharyngeal infections. The most commonly sought bacterial pathogen is *S. pyogenes*, or group A beta hemolytic streptococcus, the agent that leads to poststreptococcal sequelae such as acute rheumatic fever and glomerulonephritis. The organism not uncommonly causes **suppurative (pyogenic)** infections of the sinuses and middle ear and cellulitis as secondary pyogenic sequelae after an episode of pharyngitis. Accordingly, streptococcal pharyngitis is usually treated to prevent both the suppurative and nonsuppurative sequelae, as well as to decrease morbidity. Rare cases of pharyngitis caused by groups B, C, and G and by nonhemolytic members of these groups of streptococci (including group A) have been reported. Although bacteria other than group A streptococci may cause pharyngitis, this occurs only rarely, and laboratories should not look for other agents except in special circumstances and after discussion with the clinician involved.

Although much less common than streptococcal pharyngitis, *C. diphtheriae* can still be isolated from patients with sore throat, as well as more serious systemic disease. Other *Corynebacterium* species (*C. ulcerans*, *C. hemolyticum*, and *C. pyogenes*) can cause pharyngitis with or without membrane formation or associated rash, but such infections are rare. *Neisseria meningitidis* can be recovered from the nasopharynx of carriers, although it does not cause significant disease at this site. *Neisseria gonorrhoeae*, however, can cause an exudative pharyngitis which is especially prevalent among men who engage in homosexual practices. In disseminated gonococcal disease, the organism may be isolated from throat cultures as well. Gonococcal pharyngitis is not always sympto-

matic. Although *H. influenzae*, *Staphylococcus aureus*, and *Streptococcus pneumoniae* are frequently isolated from nasopharyngeal and throat cultures, they have not been shown to cause pharyngitis, except for *S. aureus* in the immunosuppressed patient. Carriage of any of these organisms, as well as *N. meningitidis*, may have clinical importance for some patients or their contacts. Especially in patients with cystic fibrosis, throat cultures may yield etiologic agents of pneumonia that cannot be isolated from sputum because of overgrowth by other bacteria. As in all other situations, communication between microbiologists and physicians clarifies the relevance of such findings. Cultures of specimens obtained from the anterior nares often yield *S. aureus*. The carriage rate for this organism is especially high among health care workers.

Mycoplasma pneumoniae may, rarely, cause pharyngitis and can be isolated from nasopharyngeal swabs. Such a swab may also be the specimen of choice for isolation of *Chlamydia trachomatis* from suspected cases of pneumonia, especially in very young babies. A number of viruses cause exudative pharyngitis or rhinitis, including rhinoviruses, adenoviruses, respiratory syncytial virus, influenza and parainfluenza viruses, coronaviruses, coxsackieviruses, cytomegalovirus, and Epstein-Barr virus. Additionally, *H. influenzae* (and occasionally other organisms) causes a serious epiglottitis that can rapidly lead to airway obstruction if not treated. The combined efforts of certain anaerobic oral flora causes an exudative pharyngitis known as **Vincent's angina** that may be characterized by a membrane-type lesion similar to that of diphtheria (the foul odor noted in patients with Vincent's angina helps to differentiate the two syndromes). Peritonsillar abscesses are common features of this syndrome. Evidence suggests that *Fusobacterium necrophorum* is a key pathogen in this setting, but other anaerobes may also be involved.

Immunosuppressed patients, including very

young babies, may develop oral candidosis, called **thrush.** Oral thrush can extend to produce esophagitis, a common finding in AIDS and other immunosuppressed patients. Oral mucositis or pharyngitis in the granulocytopenic patient may be caused by Enterobacteriaceae, *S. aureus,* or *Candida* species. It is manifested by erythema, sore throat, and possibly exudate or ulceration. Herpes simplex virus can cause painful lesions in the mouth and the oropharynx, another condition that is also prevalent among immunosuppressed patients.

A very rare form of chronic, granulomatous infection of the nasal passages, including the sinuses and occasionally the pharynx and larynx, is rhinoscleroma. Associated with *Klebsiella rhinoscleromatis,* the disease is characterized by nasal obstruction appearing over a long period of time, caused by tumorlike growth with local spread. Another species, *K. ozaenae,* can also be recovered from upper respiratory tract infections. This organism may contribute to the condition called **ozaena,** characterized by a chronic, mucopurulent nasal discharge (often foul-smelling, due to secondary low-grade anaerobic infection).

16.2.b. Collection and transport of specimens. Although the general concepts of collection and transport of specimens were covered in Chapter 6, a few specific comments are appropriate here. Either cotton-, Dacron-, or calcium–alginate tipped swabs are suitable for collection of most upper respiratory tract microorganisms. Calcium alginate may be toxic, however, to some *Chlamydia* species. If the swab remains moist, no further precautions need to be taken for specimens that are inoculated within 4 hours of collection. After that period, some kind of transport medium to maintain viability and prevent overgrowth by contaminants should be used. Swabs for detection of group A streptococci only are the exception. This organism is highly resistant to desiccation and will remain viable on a dry swab for as long as 48 hours. Throat swabs of this type can be easily placed in glassine paper envelopes for mailing or transport to a distant laboratory. Throat swabs are adequate for recovery of adenoviruses and herpes viruses, *C. diphtheriae, Mycoplasma, Chlamydia,* yeast, and *Haemophilus* species. Nasopharyngeal swabs are better suited for recovery of respiratory syncytial virus, parainfluenza virus, *Bordetella pertussis, Neisseria* species, and the viruses causing rhinitis. Although modified Stuart's transport medium, as is often used in commercially produced swab systems, will preserve most viruses for a short time, nasopharyngeal swabs should ideally be transported in veal infusion broth or other protein-containing fluid if they are not being cultured within a few hours. They should be refrigerated, **not frozen.** Recovery of *C. diphtheriae* is enhanced by culturing both throat and nasopharynx. Transport media should be used as discussed in Chapter 6. Aspirated nasopharyngeal secretions collected in a soft rubber bulb are the best specimens for *B. pertussis.* Specimens for *B. pertussis* should ideally be inoculated directly to fresh culture media at the patient's bedside. If this is impossible, transport for less than 2 h in 1% casamino acid media (described below in Procedure 16.1) is acceptable.

16.2.c. Direct visual examination of upper respiratory tract specimens. A Gram stain of material obtained from upper respiratory secretions or lesions can do very little to help with diagnosis. Yeastlike cells can be identified, helpful in identifying thrush, and the characteristic pattern of fusiforms and spirochetes of Vincent's angina may be visualized. Plain Gram's crystal violet (allowed to remain on the slide for 1 min before rinsing with tap water) can be used to identify the agents of Vincent's angina as well as the Gram stain. For other causes of pharyngitis, Gram stains are unreliable. Direct smears of exudate from membranelike lesions to differentiate diphtheria from other causes of such membranes are not reliable and are not recommended. Fungal ele-

PROCEDURE 16.1. DIRECT FLUORESCENT ANTIBODY STAIN
FOR *BORDETELLA PERTUSSIS*

1. Prepare casamino acid transport and holding medium. Add 1 g casamino acids (commercially available) to 100 ml distilled water in acid-washed glassware. Adjust pH to 7.2 and dispense in 0.5 ml amounts in acid-washed screw capped 12 × 75 mm tubes. Tighten caps and autoclave 20 min. This medium can be stored for 1 year at refrigerator temperature.
2. Immediately after collection, insert nasopharyngeal swab or material obtained by aspiration into cool casamino acid medium. Incubate the specimen for 1 h at 35° C.
3. With a sterile capillary pipette, place a heaped drop of the well-mixed medium onto each of two circles of a clean glass slide suitable for fluorescent staining. Allow the smears to air dry and reapply material for a total of three applications. Heat fix the slide. Remove a known positive and a known negative control slide (prepared from stock cultures) from the freezer at the same time, following an identical procedure for each slide.
4. Place a drop of fluorescein-conjugated anti-*Bordetella pertussis* antibody to completely cover one of the smears and place a drop of fluorescein-conjugated normal rabbit serum over the second control smear. Incubate at room temperature in a humidified chamber in the dark (placing the slide on a broken wooden applicator stick in a Petri dish with a moist gauze pad [Figure 16.2] works well) for 30 min.
5. Rinse the slides two times in phosphate buffered saline, pH 7.5 (commercially available), allowing them to remain in the second buffer rinse for 10 min, and then rinse in distilled water.
6. Mount with glycerol buffered mounting fluid, pH 8.5 (commercially available), and examine under ultraviolet light for bright fluorescing coccobacilli with bright rims and darker centers. The patient control smear should show no fluorescence, and the known positive smear should yield brightly fluorescing short bacilli and coccobacilli.

Modified from Anhalt. 1981. In Washington, J.A. Jr., editor: Laboratory procedures in clinical microbiology. Springer-Verlag, New York; and Parker and Linneman. 1980. In Lennette, E.H., et al., editors: Manual of clinical microbiology, ed. 3. American Society for Microbiology, Washington, D.C.

ments, including yeast cells and pseudohyphae, may be visualized with a 10% KOH preparation or with calcofluor white fluorescent stain, as described in Chapter 7. Direct examination of material obtained from the nasopharynx of suspected cases of whooping cough using a fluorescent antibody stain has been shown to yield some early positive results. The stain should be performed as outlined in Procedure 16.1.

Direct fluorescent antibody smears similar to those described for pertussis have been used

FIGURE 16.2
Use of a gauze pad, a broken wooden applicator stick, and a Petri dish to make a moist chamber suitable for incubating slides during a fluorescent antibody staining procedure.

to identify group A beta hemolytic streptococci in throat specimens. This technology has largely been supplanted by direct detection of antigen, for which a large number of commercial products are available. Direct antigen detection systems will be discussed below. Fluorescent antibody stain reagents are also commercially available for detection of herpes simplex antigen, influenza virus (rarely used), adenovirus, parainfluenza virus, and respiratory syncytial virus (M.A. Bioproducts). Our hospital virology laboratory (under the direction of Dr. Paul Swenson, E.J.B.) has had very good results in detecting respiratory syncytial infections directly from smears using commercially available reagents (Burroughs-Wellcome).

16.2.d. Culturing upper respiratory tract specimens. Classically, throat swabs have been plated onto 5% sheep blood agar (trypticase soy base). Other animal blood cells will serve to provide the necessary nutrients required by the usual pathogens being sought (primarily *S. pyogenes*), but sheep blood does not support

growth of the beta hemolytic bacteria, *Haemophilus haemolyticus* and *H. parahaemolyticus*. Thus these organisms will not be mistaken for possible beta hemolytic streptococci if sheep blood agar is used. The use of a sheep blood agar plate for isolation of *S. pyogenes* has the drawback of requiring overnight growth for colony formation and further manipulations of beta hemolytic growth for definitive identification. If sufficient numbers of pure colonies are not available for antigenic typing, a subculture requiring additional growing time is necessary. New selective agars (such as Strep Selective Agar, BBL Microbiology Systems, mentioned in Chapter 8) have been developed that suppress the growth of almost all normal flora and beta hemolytic streptococci except for groups A and B. By placing a 0.04 unit differential bacitracin filter paper disk (Taxo A, BBL or Bacto Bacitracin, Difco Laboratories) directly on the area of initial inoculation, presumptive identification of *S. pyogenes* can be made after overnight incubation (Plate 16.1; all group A and a very small percentage of group B streptococci are susceptible). If preferred, direct antigen detection tests (coagglutination or latex agglutination, Chapters 12 and 25) can also be carried out from the more isolated beta hemolytic colonies that appear after overnight incubation on selective agar. Further discussion of procedures for identification of beta hemolytic streptococci is found in Chapter 25.

Cultures for *C. diphtheriae* should be plated onto sheep blood agar or streptococcal selective agar as well as to special media for recovery of the agent of diphtheria, since streptococcal pharyngitis is in the differential diagnosis of diphtheria and since dual infections do occur. These special media include a Loeffler's agar slant and a cystine-tellurite agar plate (Chapter 45). Identification of the organism is discussed in Chapter 33. Recovery of this organism is enhanced by culturing specimens from both throat and nasopharynx of infected patients.

Freshly prepared Bordet-Gengou agar (Chapter 45) is the medium of choice for isolation of *B. pertussis*. A modified medium designed for isolation of *Legionella* species, buffered charcoal yeast extract agar with 3 μg/ml lincomycin and 80 μg/ml anisomycin has also been shown to yield good recovery of *B. pertussis*, as reported by workers at the Centers for Disease Control.[4] Jones and Kendrick[5] have also reported excellent recovery on a blood-free medium containing charcoal, heart infusion base, 2% agar, and 0.3 U/ml penicillin. Stauffer and others showed best recovery of *B. pertussis* when this medium was supplemented with 40 μg/ml cephalexin.[10] Since the charcoal medium developed for *Legionella* is more readily available, it would appear to be a useful substitute. Specimens should be plated directly onto media, if possible, as the organisms are extremely delicate. Technologists should utilize both fluorescent antibody smears and cultures to achieve maximum detection. The yield of positive isolations from clinical cases of pertussis seems to vary from 20%-98%, depending on the stage of disease, previous treatment of the patient, and laboratory techniques.

Specimens received in the laboratory for isolation of *N. meningitidis* (for detection of carriers) or for *N. gonorrhoeae* should be plated to a selective medium, either modified Thayer-Martin or Martin-Lewis agar (Chapter 8). After 48 h incubation in 5%-10% CO_2, typical colonies of *Neisseria* species will be visible. Further identification procedures for these bacteria are discussed in Chapter 26.

Clinical specimens from cases of epiglottitis (swabs obtained by a physician) should be plated to sheep blood agar, chocolate agar (for recovery of *Haemophilus* species), and a streptococcal selective medium if desired. Since *S. aureus* and *S. pneumoniae* may, rarely, cause this disease, their presence must be sought.

16.2.e. Nonculture methods for detecting agents of pharyngitis. One of the major improvements in clinical microbiology in recent years has been the development of rapid methods for antigen detection that obviate the need for culture. Identification of group A streptococcal antigen in throat specimens has benefitted greatly from these developments. At least 10 commercial products are available, employing latex agglutination or enzyme immunoassay technologies, that allow detection of group A streptococcal antigen within as short a time as 10 min. Although the specific procedures vary with the products, several generalizations can be made. Throat swabs are incubated in some type of acid reagent or enzyme to extract the group A specific carbohydrate antigen. It seems that Dacron swabs are most efficient at releasing antigen, although other types of swabs may yield acceptable results. Wooden handles seem to interfere with extraction. It is best to follow the recommendations of the manufacturer of the extraction kit to achieve optimal results. For kits such as Streptex (Burroughs-Wellcome Co.), Directogen (Hynson, Westcott & Dunning), and D.A.I. (Direct Antigen Identification, Difco Laboratories), swabs are incubated in extraction fluid for 45-60 min at 37° C. The extraction fluid is then added to latex particles coated with antibody (usually polyclonal) which agglutinate in the presence of the antigen to form a visible positive reaction. Kits such as PathoD$_X$ (Diagnostic Products), Detect-A-Strep (Antibodies Incorporated), another form of Directogen (Hynson, Westcott & Dunning), and Culturette Brand Ten-Minute Group A Strep ID (Marion Scientific) require shorter incubation periods. The Ventrescreen Strep A assay (Ventrex Laboratories) is the only currently available enzyme immunoassay. Antigen is enzymatically extracted from swabs with a 5 min incubation at room temperature. The antigen is then bound to a plastic bead, which acts as the solid phase for the immunoassay. The antibody-binding step requires a 30 min room temperature incubation. Alkaline phosphatase enzyme is used as the visual indicator (Chapter 12). In most laboratory comparisons between a rapid method and conventional culture methods for detecting the presence of group A streptococci in throat swabs, the commercial kits have shown excellent sensitivity and exquisite specificity. There have been doubts expressed, however, about their overall ability to detect all clinically important streptococcal infections. Such systems are discussed further in Chapter 25. In those situations in which rapid results are important (such as physicians' offices), information about the presence of other organisms is not required, and the number of positive results allows the test to be cost effective. A commercial screening test for group A streptococci in throats may be the method of choice.

Rapid nonmicroscopic detection methods for the other agents of upper respiratory tract infections are not so well developed as those for *S. pyogenes*. It is possible that the Chlamydiazyme test (Abbott Laboratories), used primarily for detection of antigen in genital tract specimens, may be modified for use with nasopharyngeal swabs to detect *Chlamydia pneumonia*. Several manufacturers are actively engaged in developing such assays for detection of agents of respiratory tract infections and the next several years should be exciting, highlighted by the introduction of many new products that allow direct detection of antigens in numerous types of clinical material. Nucleic acid probes, discussed in Chapter 10, are also being developed for commercial application.

16.3. Acute Lower Respiratory Tract Infections

The etiologic agents of community-acquired pneumonia vary with the age and state of health of the patient. Pneumonias among patients with various types of immunosuppressive factors are discussed in Chapter 23. Among previously healthy patients 2 months to 5 years old, viruses, including respiratory syncytial, parainfluenza and influenza, and adenoviruses, are the most common etiologic agents of lower respiratory tract disease. In addition to pneumonia, which indicates involvement of the lung parenchyma, viruses cause bronchiolitis and bronchitis. The latter infections may manifest as croup. Presumably, growth of viruses in host cells disrupts the function of the latter and encourages the influx of nonspecific immune effector cells which exacerbate the damage. Damage to host epithelial tissue by virus infection is known to predispose patients to secondary bacterial infection, as reviewed by Mills.[6] Children suffer less commonly from bacterial pneumonia, usually caused by *H. influenzae*, pneumococci, or *S. aureus*. Neonates may acquire lower respiratory tract infections with *Chlamydia trachomatis* or *Pneumocystis carinii* (which may indicate an immature immune system or other immune defect).

The most common etiologic agent of lower respiratory tract infection among adults younger than 30 years old is *Mycoplasma pneumoniae*. This organism is transmitted via close contact. Contact with secretions seems to be more important than inhalation of aerosols for dissemination. Once they contact respiratory mucosa, *Mycoplasma* are able to adhere to and colonize respiratory mucosal cells. Both a protein adherence factor and gliding motility may be determinants of virulence. Once oriented in their preferred site between the cilia of respiratory mucosal cells, *Mycoplasma* multiply and somehow destroy ciliary function. Cytotoxins produced by *Mycoplasma* may account for the cell damage they inflict.

Lower respiratory tract infections in older patients are due most commonly to bacterial infection, with *S. pneumoniae* most prevalent (causing 80% of all community acquired bacterial pneumonia). Aspiration pneumonia occurs in the community setting and involves primarily oral anaerobes and viridans streptococci but may also involve *Staphylococcus aureus* or gram-negative rods such as *K. pneumoniae*, other Enterobacteriaceae, and *Pseudomonas* species, particularly in patients with recent hospital or nursing home experience. *H. influenzae*, *Legionella* species, *Acinetobacter*, *B. catarrhalis*, meningococci, and other agents may also be implicated. In the hospital setting, pneumonia involves many of these same agents. Aspiration pneumonia is probably the major type of hospital-acquired pneumonia, followed by pneumococcal disease. *Legionella* has been implicated in a number of hospital outbreaks.

For many of the agents of purulent pneumonia, colonization of the upper respiratory tract is followed by migration of the organisms through the mucociliary layer of the bronchi toward the lungs. Aspiration of oropharyngeal contents, often not overt, plays an important role in the pathogenesis of many different types of pneumonia. Aided by gravity and often by loss of some host nonspecific protective mechanism, the organisms reach lung tissue, where they multiply and attract host responder cells. The buildup of cell debris and fluid contributes to the loss of lung function and thus to the pathology. Agents with polysaccharide capsules, such as pneumococci, *Klebsiella* species, *Haemophilus* species, certain S. *aureus*, and cryptococci, seem more able to avoid phagocytosis and thus more likely to cause pneumonia in patients without adequate humoral immunity in the form of specific antibody.

Adults may suffer from viral pneumonia caused by influenza, adenovirus, varicella, rubeola, or respiratory syncytial virus, particularly during epidemics. After viral pneumonia, particularly influenza, secondary bacterial disease caused by beta hemolytic streptococci, pneumococci, S. *aureus*, *B. catarrhalis*, *H. influenzae*, and *N. meningitidis* is more likely. Unusual causes of acute lower respiratory tract infection include *Actinomyces* and *Nocardia* species; the agents of plague, tularemia, melioidosis *(Pseudomonas pseudomallei)*, *Brucella*, *Salmonella*, *Coxiella burnetti* (Q fever), *Bacillus anthracis*, and *Pasteurella multocida*. *Paragonimus westermani*, *Entamoeba histoly-*

tica, *Ascaris lumbricoides*, and *Strongyloides* species (the latter may cause fatal disease in immunosuppressed patients) may rarely be recovered from sputum. A high index of suspicion by the clinician is usually a prerequisite to a diagnosis of parasitic pneumonia in the United States. Psittacosis should be ruled out as a cause of acute lower respiratory tract infection in patients who have had recent contact with birds. *Histoplasma capsulatum*, *Blastomyces dermatitidis*, *Paracoccidioides brasiliensis*, *Coccidioides immitis*, and *Cryptococcus neoformans*, and occasionally *Aspergillus fumigatus* may cause acute pneumonia. In the immunosuppressed patient, these fungi, as well as other *Aspergillus* species, *Candida*, zygomycetes, and other fungi, may cause pulmonary infection.

As noted above, pneumonia secondary to aspiration of gastric or oral secretions is rather common. It happens most often during a loss of consciousness as might occur with anesthesia or a seizure or after alcohol or drug abuse, but other patients, particularly among geriatric groups, may also develop aspiration pneumonia. Neurologic disease or esophageal pathology and periodontal disease or gingivitis are other important background factors. The oral black-pigmenting *Bacteroides* species, *Bacteroides oris*, *B. buccae*, *B. disiens*, *B. gracilis*, fusobacteria, and anaerobic and microaerophilic streptococci are the most common agents, but, as noted, S. *aureus* and various Enterobacteriaceae and *Pseudomonas* may also be acquired in this way. The anaerobic agents possess many factors that may enhance their ability to produce disease, such as extracellular enzymes and capsules. It is their presence, however, in an abnormal site within the host and lowered oxidation-reduction potential secondary to tissue damage that probably contributes most to their pathogenicity.

Non-aspiration pneumonia in hospitalized patients is associated most commonly with *P. aeruginosa*, S. *aureus*, *Klebsiella* species, and other Enterobacteriaceae. Some of these pneumonias are secondary to sepsis, and some are related to contaminated inhalation therapy equipment. Other aspects of pneumonia among hospitalized patients, as well as other groups at increased risk of developing respiratory tract disease, are discussed in Chapter 23.

16.4. Chronic Lower Respiratory Infections

Mycobacterium tuberculosis is the most likely etiologic agent of chronic lower respiratory tract infection, but fungal infection and anaerobic pleuropulmonary infection may also run a subacute or chronic course. Mycobacteria other than *M. tuberculosis* (MOTT) may also cause such disease, particularly *M. avium-intracellulare* and *M. kansasii.* Mentioned above as possible causes of acute, community-acquired lower respiratory tract infections, fungi and parasites are more commonly isolated from patients with chronic disease. *Actinomyces* and *Nocardia* may also be associated with gradual onset of symptoms. Agents of chronic disease in compromised hosts are discussed in Chapter 23. The pathogenesis of many of the infections caused by agents of chronic lower respiratory tract disease is characterized by the requirement for some breakdown of cell-mediated immunity in the host or the ability of these agents to avoid being destroyed by host cell-mediated immune mechanisms. This may be by an effect on macrophages, by the ability to mask foreign antigens, sheer size, or by some other factor, allowing them to grow within host tissues without eliciting an overwhelming local reaction.

16.5. Laboratory Diagnosis of Lower Respiratory Tract Infections

16.5.a. Collection and transport of specimens. Lower respiratory tract secretions will be contaminated with upper respiratory tract secretions, especially saliva, unless they are collected using some invasive technique. For this reason, sputa are among the least clinically relevant specimens received for culture in microbiology laboratories, as well as being among the most numerous and time consuming. When hospital laboratories began to reject some sputum samples based on visual examination of predominant cell types (as discussed below), the numbers of acceptable specimens received by the laboratory dramatically increased. It is possible, therefore, for microbiologists and clinicians to influence the quality of specimens received for culture. Good sputum samples are dependent on thorough patient education and the presence of a health care worker to oversee all phases of the collection process. Patients should be instructed to provide a deep cough specimen. The material should be expelled into a sterile container, with an attempt to minimize contamination with saliva. Specimens should be transported to the laboratory immediately, as even a moderate amount of time at room temperature can result in loss of some etiologic agents of respiratory tract infection.

Patients who are unable to produce sputum may be assisted by respiratory therapy technicians, who can use postural drainage and thoracic percussion to stimulate production of acceptable sputum. Alternatively, an **aerosol-induced specimen** may be collected. Particularly useful for obtaining material suitable for isolation of the agents of mycobacterial or fungal disease, aerosol-induced specimens are collected by allowing the patient to breathe aerosolized droplets of a solution of 15% sodium chloride and 10% glycerine for approximately 10 min, or until a strong cough reflex is initiated. The lower respiratory secretions obtained in this way appear watery, resembling saliva. They are, however, usually adequate for culture and should be accepted in the laboratory without prescreening.

Another specimen for isolation of acid fast bacilli that may be collected from patients who are unable to produce sputum, particularly young children, is the **gastric aspirate.** Before the patient has arisen in the morning, a nasogastric tube is inserted into the stomach and contents are withdrawn (on the assumption that acid fast bacilli from the respiratory tract were swallowed during the night and will be present in the stomach). The relative resistance of mycobacteria to acidity allows them to remain viable for a short period. Gastric aspirate specimens must be delivered to the laboratory immediately so that the acidity can be neutralized. Due to the presence of mycobacteria in tap water, acid fast smears from gastric aspirates are often falsely positive, and ordinarily should not be examined.

Patients with tracheostomies are unable to produce sputum in the normal fashion, but nurses can easily collect lower respiratory tract secretions in a Lukens trap (Figure 16.3). These specimens (called **tracheostomy aspirates** or **tracheal aspirates**) should be treated as sputum (without microscopic screening, discussed below) by the laboratory. Patients with tracheostomies rapidly become colonized with gram-negative bacilli and other nosocomial

FIGURE 16.3
Tracheal secretions received in the laboratory in a Lukens trap.

pathogens. Such colonization per se does not have clinical relevance, but these organisms may be aspirated and cause pneumonia. Thus there is real confusion for microbiologists and clinicians trying to ascertain the etiologic agent of disease in these patients.

When pleural empyema is present, thoracentesis may be used to obtain infected fluid for direct examination and culture. This constitutes an excellent specimen that accurately reflects the bacteriology of an associated pneumonia. Laboratory examination of such material is discussed in Chapter 21. Blood cultures, of course, should always be obtained from patients with pneumonia. Physicians sometimes attempt to obtain more representative specimens via a bronchoscope than are possible with noninvasive techniques. Bronchial secretions are often obtained by instilling a small amount of sterile physiologic saline into the bronchial tree and withdrawing the fluid when purulent secretions are not visualized. Such **bronchial washing** specimens will still be contaminated with upper respiratory tract flora, such as viridans streptococci and *Neisseria* species. Recovery of potential pathogenic organisms from bronchial washings should be attempted, however, since such specimens may be more diagnostically relevant than sputa. A deeper sampling of desquamated host cells and secretions is also obtained via bronchoscopy and is called **bronchial lavage**. Lavages are especially suitable for detecting *Pneumocystis* cysts and fungal elements.

The specimen obtained by only moderately invasive means that is best suited for microbiologic studies is that obtained via a **protected catheter bronchial brush**. A small brush that holds 0.01 to 0.001 ml of secretions is placed within a double cannula. The end of the outermost tube or cannula is closed with a removable plug made of polyethylene glycol. Once the cannula has been inserted to the proper area, the inner cannula is pushed out, dislodging the protective plug as it is extruded. Then the brush is extended beyond the inner cannula. The specimen is collected and the brush is withdrawn into the inner cannula, which is withdrawn into the outer cannula to prevent contamination as it is removed. The contents of the bronchial brush may be suspended in 1.0 ml of broth solution with vigorous vortexing and then inoculated onto culture media by technologists using a 0.01 ml calibrated inoculating loop. Specimens obtained via doublelumen protected catheters have been stated by some workers to be suitable for anaerobic as well as aerobic cultures. Colony counts of greater than 1000 organisms per milliliter in the broth diluent (or 10^6/ml in the original specimen) have been considered to correlate with infection, as reported by Pollock and associates.[8] However, other studies question the validity of this procedure, even when cultures are done quantitatively. Furthermore the tiny sample and its aeration are problems with the technique.

Several invasive procedures are used to collect specimens when definitive results are necessary or when anaerobic bacteria are being sought. Percutaneous **transtracheal aspirates (TTA)**, as mentioned in Chapter 6, are obtained by inserting a small plastic catheter into the trachea via a needle previously inserted through the skin and cricothyroid membrane. This invasive procedure, although somewhat uncomfortable for the patient and not suitable for all patients (it cannot be used in uncooperative patients, in patients with bleeding tendency, or with poor oxygenation) guarantees a specimen uncontaminated by upper respiratory tract flora and undiluted by added fluids, provided that care is taken to keep the catheter from being coughed back up into the pharynx. Anaerobic agents of actinomycosis and aspiration pneumonia can best be isolated from transtracheal aspirate specimens. For patients with pneumonia, a **thin needle aspiration** of material from the involved area of the lung may be performed, often without fluoroscopy. If no

material is withdrawn into the syringe after the first try, approximately 3 ml of sterile saline can be injected and withdrawn into the syringe. Patients with emphysema, uremia, thrombocytopenia, or pulmonary hyptertension may be at increased risk of complication (primarily pneumothorax or bleeding) from this procedure. The specimens obtained are very small in volume, and protection from aeration is usually impossible. Transbronchial biopsies are used more for histologic diagnosis than for culture. Direct examination of such specimens for agents such as *Pneumocystis* is often positive.

The most invasive procedure for obtaining respiratory tract specimens is the **open lung biopsy.** Performed by surgeons, this method is used to procure actual lung tissue. Biopsy specimens are extremely helpful for diagnosis of severe viral infections, such as herpes pneumonia, for rapid diagnosis of *Pneumocystis* pneumonia, and for other hard-to-diagnose pneumonias. Some groups feel that *Pneumocystis* infection may be diagnosed as readily by the much less invasive bronchial lavage procedure as from lung biopsy specimens, particularly from patients with AIDS.

16.5.b. Direct visual examination of lower respiratory tract specimens. Lower respiratory tract specimens can be examined by direct wet preparation for some parasites and by special procedures (see below) for *Pneumocystis*. Fungal elements can be visualized under phase microscopy with 10% KOH or calcofluor white (Chapter 7). If pneumococci or *Haemophilus influenzae* type b are suspected, a portion of purulent material may be mixed with an equal amount of antiserum for performance of the Quellung test, described in Chapter 7. For most other evaluations, the specimen must be fixed and stained. Bacteria and yeasts can be recognized on Gram stain. One of the most important uses of the Gram stain, however, is to evaluate the quality of expectorated sputum received for routine bacteriologic culture. As mentioned in Chapter 7 (Table 7.1) and in Cumitech 7 by Bartlett et al.,[2] a portion of the specimen consisting of purulent material is chosen for the stain. An acceptable specimen will yield less than 10 squamous epithelial cells per low power field (100 ×). The number of white cells may not be relevant, since many patients are severely neutropenic. On the other hand, the presence of greater than or equal to 25 polymorphonuclear leukocytes per 100 × field, together with few squamous epithelial cells, assures one of an excellent specimen (Plate 16.2). The presence of ciliated columnar bronchial epithelial cells or goblet cells in specimens obtained by bronchoscopy may also be indicative of a deep specimen. Only expectorated sputa are suitable for rejection based on microscopic screening. However, it is important to realize that in *Legionella* pneumonia, sputum may be scant and watery with few or no host cells. Such specimens may still often be positive by direct fluorescent antibody stain and culture, and should not be subjected to screening procedures.

In addition to the Gram stain, respiratory specimens may be stained for acid fast bacilli with either the classic Ziehl-Neelsen or the Kinyoun carbol fuchsin stain (Chapters 7, 41, and 46). Auramine or auramine-rhodamine are also used for detection of acid fast organisms. Because they are fluorescent, these stains are more sensitive than the carbol fuchsin formulas and are preferable for rapid screening. Slides may be restained with the classic stains directly over the fluorochrome stains as long as all of the immersion oil has been removed carefully with xylene. When results are needed urgently, material may be stained unconcentrated, as described in Chapter 7. All of the acid fast stains will also reveal *Cryptosporidium* species if they are present in the respiratory tract, as may occur in immunosuppressed patients.

Immunosuppressed patients are often at risk of infection with *Pneumocystis carinii*. Al-

though the modified Gomori methenamine silver stain procedure (Procedure 16.2) yields the best results, it takes approximately 1 h of technologist time to perform and may not be suitable as an emergency procedure, especially on nights or weekends. A fairly rapid stain, toluidine blue O, has been used in many laboratories with great success. This stain is outlined in Procedures 16.3 and 44.19.

Direct fluorescent antibody stain (available from several suppliers mentioned in Chapter 39) has been used for detection of *Legionella* species in lower respiratory tract specimens. Sputum, pleural fluid, aspirated material, and tissue are all suitable specimens. Polyclonal antibody reagents and a monoclonal antibody directed against all serotypes of *Legionella pneumophila* are used, since there are so many different serotypes of legionellae. A nucleic acid probe capable of detecting certain species of *Legionella* is under study now and should be available commercially soon.

Direct fluorescent antibody reagents (commercially available) are also used to detect antigens of a number of viruses, including herpes simplex, cytomegalovirus, adenovirus, and respiratory syncytial virus. Procedures similar to those described above for fluorescent antibody staining for *B. pertussis* will yield good results. Commercial suppliers of reagents provide procedure information for each of the tests available. Fluorescent antibody reagents have recently been reintroduced for detection of *Bacteroides fragilis* and *Bacteroides melaninogenicus* and certain cross-reacting *Bacteroides*. Transtracheal aspirate material and pleural fluid would be suitable for such a stain. As stated above, the use of both ELISA and immunofluorescent reagents for diagnosis of chlamydial pneumonia is being explored in research laboratories and should be available soon.

16.5.c. Culture of lower respiratory tract specimens. Most of the commonly sought etiologic agents of lower respiratory tract infection

PROCEDURE 16.2. GOMORI METHENAMINE SILVER STAIN (GMS)
(80° C METHENAMINE SILVER NITRATE STAIN)

1. Prepare reagents as follows:
   a. Chromic acid (10% solution)

Chromic acid (Fisher Scientific)	100 g
Distilled deionized water	1,000 ml

   Weigh out 100 g chromic acid and dissolve in 1 liter distilled water. Solution usable for up to 1 year.

   b. Methenamine (3% solution)

Hexamethylenetetramine (Fisher Scientific)	12 g
Distilled deionized water	400 ml

   Weigh out 12 g hexamethylenetetramine and dissolve in 400 ml distilled water. Solution usable for up to 6 months.

   c. Silver nitrate (5% solution)

Silver nitrate (Fisher Scientific)	5 g
Distilled deionized water	100 ml

   Weigh out 5 g silver nitrate and dissolve in 100 ml distilled water. Solution is usable for up to 6 months.

   d. Stock methenamine-silver nitrate

Methenamine (3% solution)	400 ml
Silver nitrate (5% solution)	20 ml

   A white precipitate forms when reagents are added together, but immediately clears with mixing. Store at 4° C. The solution is usable for up to 1 month.

   e. Borax (5% solution)

Borax (sodium borate) (Fisher Scientific)	5 g
Distilled deionized water	100 ml

   Dissolve sodium borate in distilled water. Solution usable for up to 1 year.

   f. Sodium bisulfite (1% solution)

Sodium bisulfite (Fisher Scientific)	5 g
Distilled deionized water	500 ml

   Weigh out sodium bisulfite and add to distilled water. Solution usable for up to 1 year.

   g. Gold chloride (0.2% solution)

Gold chloride (chloroauric acid; Sigma Chemical Co.)	0.5 g
Distilled deionized water	250 ml

   Weigh out gold chloride and add to distilled water. Solution usable for up to 1 year.

Modified by Lynne Garcia and the UCLA parasitology laboratory from Pintozzi, R. 1978. J. Clin. Pathol. 31:803.

Continued.

PROCEDURE 16.2. GOMORI METHENAMINE SILVER STAIN (GMS)
(80° C METHENAMINE SILVER NITRATE STAIN)—cont'd

    h. Sodium thiosulfate (2% solution)

        Sodium thiosulfate (Fisher Scientific)   10 g

        Distilled deionized water   500 ml

      Solution usable for up to 1 year.

    i. Stock light green solution

        Light green SF-Yellowish (Harleco)   0.2 g

        Distilled deionized water   100 ml

        Glacial acetic acid   0.2 ml

      Solution usable for up to 1 year.

    j. Working light green solution

        Stock light green solution   10 ml

        Distilled deionized water   40 ml

      Solution usable for up to 1 month.

    k. Fill two Coplin jars each with absolute ethanol and 95% ethanol. These jars may be sealed with screw caps and the reagents can be reused until they become cloudy.

    l. Fill two Coplin jars with xylene. These jars may be sealed and the xylene can be reused.

2. Immediately before each staining procedure, prepare working methenamine-silver nitrate as follows:

    Stock methenamine-silver nitrate   37.5 ml

    Distilled deionized water   37.5 ml

    Borax (5% solution)   3 ml

This solution must be prepared fresh in a Coplin jar for each set of slides stained. It is not reusable, even for a second staining procedure performed immediately afterward.

3. Staining procedure

    a. Turn on water bath allowing 45-60 min to reach 80° C.

    b. Prepare smears and air dry. Heat fix all smears at 70° C for 10 min on a heating block.

    c. Fix smears in absolute methanol for a minimum of 3 min.

    d. Place two Coplin jars, one containing 5% chromic acid (approximately 50 ml) and the other containing working methenamine solution into 80° C water bath for 5 min.

    e. Place smears into heated 5% chromic acid. Incubate in water bath at 80° C for 2 min.

    f. Remove slides from chromic acid and place in Coplin jar with distilled water. Rinse slides in three changes of distilled water.

    g. Place slides in 1% sodium bisulfite for 30 seconds.

    h. Rinse in three changes of distilled water.

PROCEDURE 16.2. GOMORI METHENAMINE SILVER STAIN (GMS)
(80° C METHENAMINE SILVER NITRATE STAIN)—cont'd

i. Place slides in heated methenamine working solution. Incubate in water bath at 80° C for 4½ min.

j. Place slides in Coplin jar with distilled water. Rinse in three changes of distilled water.

k. Wipe the back of slides with a paper towel to remove excess methenamine.

l. Tone in 0.2% gold chloride for 30 seconds; background lightens in this step.

m. Rinse in three changes distilled water.

n. Place slides in 2% sodium thiosulfate for 30 seconds to remove unreduced silver.

o. Rinse in three changes of distilled water.

p. Counterstain in light green working solution for 30 seconds.

q. Rinse in three changes of distilled water.

r. Dehydrate and clear for 30 second intervals in two changes each of 95% ethanol, 100% ethanol, and xylene, respectively.

s. Place coverslips on slides with Permount while the slides are still wet with xylene. Slides are ready to be read.

4. Interpretation: Background will be green and *Pneumocystis* cysts will appear gray to black. They are spherical, may be punched in and cup shaped, and may show black parentheses-like structures in the center (Plate 16.3). The cysts tend to occur in groups, often surrounded by foamy looking green exudative background material.

---

will be isolated on the commonly used media: 5% sheep blood agar, MacConkey agar, and chocolate agar. Because of contaminating oral flora, sputum specimens, specimens obtained by bronchial washing and lavage, and tracheal aspirates are not inoculated to enrichment broth or incubated anaerobically. Only specimens obtained by percutaneous aspiration (including transtracheal aspiration) and perhaps by protected bronchial brush are suitable for anaerobic culture. Transtracheal and percutaneous lung aspiration material may be inoculated to enriched thioglycolate as well as to solid media. For suspected cases of Legionnaires' disease, buffered charcoal yeast extract agar (BCYE; Chapters 39 and 45) and selective

BCYE are inoculated. Pertussis media, as mentioned above, may also be inoculated.

Contaminated specimens received for isolation of mycobacteria must be decontaminated and concentrated before they are inoculated to media (discussed in Chapter 41). The radiometric detection system (Bactec, Johnston Laboratories) has been used with good success for more rapid detection of growth of mycobacteria, especially *M. avium-intracellulare*, than can be achieved with conventional cultures. Specimens are inoculated to special media for mycoplasma isolation (Chapter 38). For isolation of the dimorphic fungi, material should be inoculated to brain heart infusion agar as well as to infusion or Sabouraud's heart infusion

PROCEDURE 16.3. TOLUIDINE BLUE O STAIN FOR DETECTION OF *PNEUMOCYSTIS* IN RESPIRATORY SECRETIONS

1. Prepare stain solutions A and B.
   Solution A: Sulfation reagent
   a. Add 15 ml 1 N NaOH to 35 ml ether (USP) in a separating funnel and shake vigorously for 1 min. Release the stopcock occasionally to relieve pressure. Drain the NaOH phase out the bottom of the funnel. Repeat this procedure once again to remove impurities and preservatives from the ether.
   b. Add 10 ml distilled water to the 35 ml ether (USP) in the separating funnel and shake vigorously for 1 min. Release the stopcock occasionally to relieve pressure. Repeat this procedure once again. The ether should be fully saturated with water at this point. Allow the two solutions to separate and discard the water layer (the lower phase) by allowing it to run out the bottom of the funnel. Allow a few milliliters of the ether phase to run out also, to ensure that no water is left.
   c. Transfer the remaining 25 ml of water-saturated ether to a 100 ml Erlenmeyer flask immersed in an icewater bath. Allow to cool for 5 min. Place the ice bath under a chemical fume hood. Slowly add 25 ml concentrated sulfuric acid while continuously shaking the flask. Mix contents well and pour the reagent into a Coplin jar. The solution may be stored at room temperature for as long as 6 weeks, providing the jar is sealed with stopcock grease to prevent evaporation.
   Solution B: Toluidine blue O
   a. In a Coplin jar under a fume hood, place:

Toluidine blue O (Fisher Scientific Co.)	0.06 g
Distilled water	15 ml

   Swirl vigorously to dissolve the dye in the water. Add, in order:

Hydrochloric acid (concentrated)	0.5 ml
Absolute ethanol	35 ml

   Screw the cap of the Coplin jar tightly closed. The stain solution can be kept at room temperature and reused for 6 months.

Modified by Beverly Tenenbaum, North Shore University, Manhasset, N.Y. from procedures published in Cumitech 7,[2] Settnes and Larsen,[9] and by Chalvardjian and Grawe.[3]

PROCEDURE 16.3. TOLUIDINE BLUE O STAIN FOR DETECTION
OF *PNEUMOCYSTIS* IN RESPIRATORY SECRETIONS—cont'd

2. Make smears of the material to be stained. Choose mucoid-appearing flecks from bronchial washing material. Bronchial lavage specimens should be centrifuged for 10 min at 1500 × g. The sediment is then used to prepare smears. If open lung or transbronchial biopsy tissue is available, touch the cut surface of tissue to the slide, squeezing the tissue down to express infectious agents. Allow the smears to air dry. Stain a known positive control slide with each patient specimen run.
3. Fix slides for 1 min in absolute ethanol. Allow to dry.
4. Place slides in solution A for 5 min, dipping them twice when they are initially immersed.
5. Place them into a Coplin jar filled with tap water for 5 min to rinse off solution A. Dip the slides twice during this rinse.
6. Place slides into solution B for 3 min.
7. Dehydrate slides by dipping them for 30 seconds into each of 2 jars of isopropyl alcohol (99%).
7. Clear slides by dipping them into a jar of xylene.
8. Mount coverslips with Permount or similar mounting medium. Slides can be examined immediately.
9. Observe for cysts of *Pneumocystis*, which appear reddish blue or purple against a blue background. The organisms are often seen in clumps, particularly in areas of frothy looking material (Plate 16.4). Cysts are occasionally punched in, appearing crescent shaped.
10. If the background also appears purple, making it difficult to differentiate cysts, a second smear can be prepared with the addition of a drop of sterile defibrinated sheep blood mixed gently with the material on the slide before it dries. The blood cells seem to alter the staining characteristics of the background, rendering it more greenish and allowing the cysts to stand out.

agar (SABHI) with sheep blood and Mycobiotic or Mycosel (or some inhibitory mold agar), as discussed in Chapters 8 and 43.

Patients with cystic fibrosis may yield such numerous colonies of mucoid *Pseudomonas aeruginosa* that other growth is obscured. For such specimens, selective agar, mentioned in Chapter 23, should be inoculated. The isolation of *Haemophilus* species in specimens containing large numbers of normal flora can be facilitated by placing a 10 U bacitracin disk in the primary inoculum on the chocolate agar plate (George Tortora, personal communication). This may be particularly valuable with sputum specimens received from patients with cystic fibrosis.

Viruses and chlamydiae require tissue culture techniques, detailed in Chapters 38 and 42. Specimens for viral culture should be placed in a protein-containing transport medium such as Minimum Essential Medium in Eagle's Buffered Salt Solution (commercially available, Appendix) with amphotericin B or veal infusion broth and refrigerated (never frozen) until they can be cultured. Chlamydia cultures are transported as stated above.

16.5.d. Nonculture methods for diagnosing lower respiratory tract infections. In addition to direct fluorescent antibody staining of lower respiratory tract secretions, several other non-culture techniques have been utilized. Traditional serology, of course, is valuable for retrospective diagnosis of respiratory tract infections (Chapter 12). A recently introduced enzyme immunoassay for the detection of *B. pertussis* antibodies (Labsystems) may be helpful in timely diagnosis of pertussis. Gas-liquid chromatography has been used to analyze fluids for the presence of metabolites of pneumococci, mycobacteria, and other pathogens (see Chapter 11). Although the idea is promising, there are no practical schemes in general use for diagnosing lower respiratory tract infection in this way. Elevated pleural fluid lactic acid levels are indicative of bacterial empyema (Chapter 21), but there is a little overlap with malignant pleural effusion. Testing clinical material directly for antigens of common pathogens, an approach that has succeeded for detection of group A streptococci in throat swabs, shows promise for diagnosis of pneumonia. The problems of nonspecific reactivity and masking of reactions by mucus and other factors have not been fully resolved. Electron microscopy has been used for detection of virus particles, although these procedures are limited to a few very specialized laboratories. DNA hybridization, a promising technique for detection of viral and other microbial gene sequences in clinical material, discussed in Chapter 10, has been used by a number of workers. These **in situ hybridization** procedures utilizing biotinylated or other DNA probes have successfully visualized herpes simplex, varicella-zoster, adenovirus, and cytomegalovirus infected cells in sections from lungs and in cell layers. Within a relatively short time, such probes for all types of microbes will be widely available for use with clinical material by microbiologists.

REFERENCES

1. Anhalt, J.P. 1981. Fluorescent antibody procedures and counterimmunoelectrophoresis. In Washington, J.A. Jr., editor. Laboratory procedures in clinical microbiology. Springer-Verlag, New York.
2. Bartlett, J.G., Brewer, N.S., and Ryan, K.J. 1978. Cumitech 7. Laboratory diagnosis of lower respiratory tract infections. In Washington, J.A. II, coordinating editor. American Society for Microbiology, Washington, D.C.
3. Chalvardjian, A.M., and Grawe, L.A. 1963. A new procedure for the identification of *Pneumocystis carinii* cysts in tissue sections and smears. J. Clin. Pathol. 16:383.
4. Hayes, P.S., Feeley, J.C., Johnson, S.E., et al. 1985. Use of charcoal yeast extract agar for the isolation of *Bordetella pertussis*. Abstracts, Annual Meeting of the American Society for Microbiology. C 188.

5. Jones, G.L., and Kendrick, P.L. 1969. Study of a blood-free medium for transport and growth of *Bordetella pertussis*. Health Lab. Sci. 6:40.

6. Mills, E.L. 1984. Viral infections predisposing to bacterial infections. Ann. Rev. Med. 35:469.

7. Parker, C.D., and Linnemann, C.C. Jr. 1980. *Bordetella*. In Lennette, E.H., et al. Manual of clinical microbiology, ed 3. American Society for Microbiology, Washington, D.C.

8. Pollock, H.M., Hawkins, E.L., Bonner, J.R., et al. 1983. Diagnosis of bacterial pulmonary infections with quantitative protected catheter cultures obtained during bronchoscopy. J. Clin. Microbiol. 17:255.

9. Settnes, O.P., and Larsen, P.E. 1979. Inhibition of toluidine blue O stain for *Pneumocystis carinii* by additives in the diethyl ether. Am. J. Clin. Pathol. 72:492.

10. Stauffer, L.R., Brown, D.R., and Sandstrom, R.E. 1983. Cephalexin-supplemented Jones-Kendrick charcoal agar for selective isolation of *Bordetella pertussis*: comparison with previously described media. J. Clin. Microbiol. 17:60.

BIBLIOGRAPHY

Browning, R.J. 1983. Diagnosing pulmonary diseases: a clinician's perspective. Diagn. Med. 6:39 and 6:62.

Gilligan, P.H., and Schidlow, D.V. 1984. The role of *Pseudomonas cepacia* in pulmonary disease of cystic fibrosis patients. Clin. Microbiol. Newsletter 6:42.

Harrison, H.R. 1982. The current status of the diagnosis of chlamydial respiratory infections. Clin. Lab. Med. 2:371.

Hildreth, S.W., Hall, C.B., and Menegus, M.A. 1983. Respiratory syncytial virus. Clin. Microbiol. Newsletter 5:93.

McDougall, J.K., Beckman, A.M., Galloway, D.A., et al. 1985. Defined viral probes for the detection of HSV, CMV, and HPV. In Kingsbury, D.T., and Falkow, S., editors. Rapid detection and identification of infectious agents. Academic Press, New York.

Parker, R.H. 1983. *Hemophilus influenzae* respiratory infection in adults. I. Recognition and incidence. Postgrad. Med. 73:179.

Parker, R.H., 1983. *Hemophilus influenzae* respiratory infection in adults. II. Treatment guidelines. Postgrad. Med. 73:187.

Welch, D.F. 1984. Clinical microbiology of cystic fibrosis. Clin. Microbiol. Newsletter 6:39.

von Graevenitz, A. 1983. Which bacterial species should be isolated from throat cultures? [Editorial] Eur. J. Clin. Microbiol. 2:1.

17 Microorganisms Encountered in the Gastrointestinal Tract

17.1. Anatomy and General Features of the Gastrointestinal Tract

The gastrointestinal tract (Figure 17.1) is actually in continuation with the external environment. Ingested material that enters the gastrointestinal tract passes through the esophagus into the stomach, through the duodenum, the jejunum, the ileum, and finally through the cecum and colon to the anus. During passage, fluids and other components are both added to this material (as secretory products of individual cells and as enzymatic secretions of glands and organs) and removed from this material by absorption through the gut epithelium. The duodenum, jejunum, and ileum are collectively called the **small intestine,** and the cecum and colon comprise the **large intestine.** The nature of the epithelial cells lining the gastrointestinal tract varies with the segment; the small intestine is lined with small projections, called **villi,** that greatly increase the surface area. The function of villi is to absorb fluids and nutrients from the intestinal contents. Other cells of the small intestine secrete fluids and metabolites into the lumen. Many of the cells in the lining of the large intestine are mucus secreting, and there are no villous projections into the lumen. The remaining excess fluid within the gastrointestinal tract is reabsorbed by the cells lining the large intestine before waste is finally discharged through the anus. The lining of the

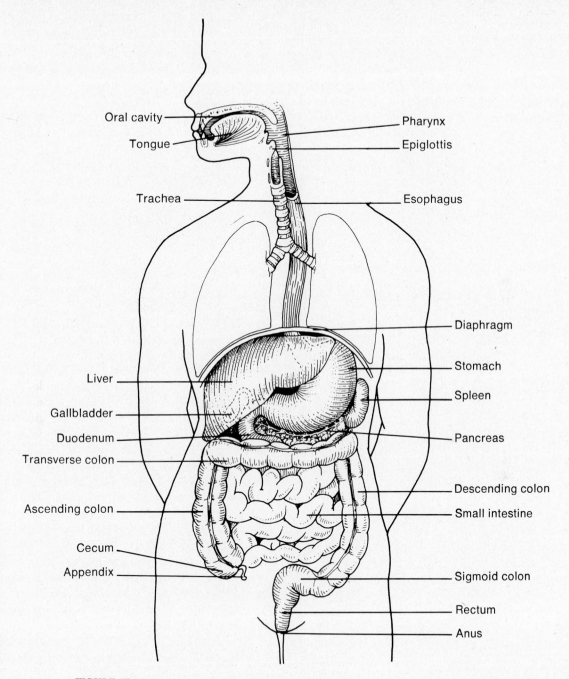

FIGURE 17.1
General anatomy of the gastrointestinal tract. (From Broadwell, D.C., and Jackson, B.S. 1982.
Principles of ostomy care. The C.V. Mosby Co., St. Louis.)

gastrointestinal tract, including the cells and their closely adjacent secretions, is called the **mucosa.** Because of the differing nature of the mucosal surfaces of various segments of the bowel, different infectious disease processes tend to occur in each segment. The appendix, a long, narrow tube of bowel tissue, extends from the cecum near the ileum. The appendix may become inflamed and even gangrenous when there is stasis within its lumen or when there is an adjacent inflammatory process. Appendicitis is the most common initial event leading to intraabdominal abscesses in children. Infections of the appendix are discussed in Chapter 20.

The gastrointestinal tract contains a vast and diverse normal flora. Although the acidity of the stomach prevents any significant colonization in a normal host, many species can survive passage through the stomach to become resident within the lower intestinal tract. Normally, the upper small intestine also contains only a sparse flora (10 to 10^3 bacteria per milliliter, primarily streptococci, lactobacilli, and yeasts), but by the time the distal ileum is reached, counts are about 10^6 to 10^7 per milliliter, and Enterobacteriaceae and *Bacteroides* are present. In the case of certain types of pathology (e.g., bleeding or obstructing peptic ulcer) there may be much higher bacterial counts and a more diverse flora in the stomach and duodenum. This has implications in the case of a patient who suffers a perforated peptic ulcer. Babies usually are colonized by normal human epithelial flora (staphylococci, *Corynebacterium* species, etc.) and other gram-positive organisms (bifidobacteria, clostridia, lactobacilli, streptococci) within a few hours of birth. As more bacteria are swallowed, the content of the intestinal flora changes. The normal flora of the adult large bowel, predominantly anaerobic species, including *Bacteroides, Clostridium, Peptostreptococcus, Bifidobacterium, Eubacterium,* and others, is established relatively early in life. The anaerobes outnumber the

aerobes, primarily *Escherichia coli*, other Enterobacteriaceae, enterococci, and other streptococci, by 1000:1. The number of bacteria per gram material within the lumen of the bowel increases steadily as material approaches the sigmoid colon (the last segment). Eighty percent of the dry weight of feces from a healthy human consists of bacteria, which can be present in numbers as high as 10^{11} to 10^{12} per gram. After antimicrobial therapy, the large bowel may become colonized with nosocomial pathogens such as *Staphylococcus aureus, Pseudomonas aeruginosa,* and other resistant gram-negative bacilli. This influences the flora of any subsequent intraabdominal infection.

17.2. Pathophysiology of Gastrointestinal Infections

17.2.a. Role of the normal flora in host defense. The normal flora is an important factor in the response of the host to introduction of a potentially harmful microorganism. It has been shown that whenever a reduction in normal flora occurs, due to antibiotic treatment or to some host factor, resistance to gastrointestinal infection is significantly reduced. The most common example of the protective effect of normal flora is the development of the syndrome **pseudomembranous colitis (PMC).** Caused by the toxins of the anaerobic organism *Clostridium difficile* and occasionally other clostridia and *Staphylococcus aureus*, this inflammatory disease of the large bowel (Plate 17.1) seldom occurs except after antimicrobial or antimetabolite treatment has altered the normal flora. Almost every antimicrobial agent and several chemotherapeutic agents have been associated with the development of cases of PMC. *C. difficile*, either present in small numbers in the normal host or resident in the hospital environment, from which it colonizes hospitalized patients, is suppressed by normal flora. When normal flora are reduced, *C. difficile* is able to multiply and produce its toxins (discussed below). Thus, this syndrome is also known as "antibiotic-associated colitis." Other microorganisms that may gain a foothold when released from selective pressure of normal flora include *Candida* species, staphylococci, *Pseudomonas* species, and various Enterobacteriaceae as noted above.

17.2.b. Nonspecific host defense mechanisms. Several other factors contribute to host resistance to disease. The acidity of the stomach effectively restricts the number and types of organisms that enter the lower gastrointestinal tract. Normal peristalsis helps to move organisms along, allowing them little chance to adhere to the mucosa. The mucus layer coating the epithelium entraps microorganisms and helps to propel them along. The normal flora, of course, prevents colonization by potential pathogens. Secretory IgA and phagocytic cells within the gut help to destroy etiologic agents of disease, as do eosinophils (particularly active against parasites). For a microorganism to cause gastrointestinal infection, it must possess one or more factors that allow it to overcome these host defenses, or it must enter the host at a time when one or more of the innate defense systems is inactive. For example, certain stool pathogens are able to survive gastric acidity only if the acidity has been reduced by bicarbonate or other buffer or by cimetidine and similar medications. Pathogens taken in with milk have a better chance of survival, since milk neutralizes stomach acidity. Organisms such as *Mycobacterium tuberculosis* and *Shigella* are able to withstand exposure to gastric acids, and thus require much smaller infectious inocula than acid-sensitive organisms such as *Salmonella*.

17.2.c. Pathogenic mechanisms of agents of gastrointestinal infections. Etiologic agents of gastrointestinal infection are known to cause disease in only four ways: (1) by producing a toxin that affects fluid secretion, cell function, or neurologic function; (2) by growing within or close to intestinal mucosal cells and destroying them, thus disrupting function; (3) by invading the mucosal epithelium, causing cellular destruction and occasionally invading the bloodstream and going on to systemic desease; and (4) by adhering to intestinal mucosa, thus preventing the normal functions of absorption and secretion. Since the normal adult gastrointestinal tract receives up to 8 liters of fluid daily in the form of ingested liquid and the secretions of the various glands that contribute to digestion (salivary glands, pancreas, gallbladder, and stomach), of which all but a small amount must be reabsorbed, it is obvious that any disruption of the normal flow or resorption of fluid will have a profound effect on the host.

"Food poisoning" may occur as a result of the ingestion of toxins produced by microorganisms. The microorganisms usually produce their toxins in consumables before they are ingested; thus the patient ingests **preformed** toxin. Although strictly speaking these syndromes are not gastrointestinal infections but intoxications, they are acquired by ingestion of microorganisms or their products and will be considered in this chapter. It is possible, particularly in staphylococcal food poisoning and botulism, that the causative organisms are not present in the bowel of the patient at all.

17.2.d. Gastrointestinal or systemic diseases associated with toxin-producing microorganisms. One of the most potent **neurotoxins** known is produced by the anaerobic organism, *Clostridium botulinum*. This toxin acts to prevent the release of the neurotransmitter acetylcholine at the cholinergic nerve junctions, causing flaccid paralysis. The toxin acts primarily on the peripheral nerves but also on the autonomic nervous system. Patients exhibit descending symmetrical paralysis and ultimately die from respiratory paralysis unless they are given mechanical ventilation. In most cases, patients who develop botulism have ingested the preformed toxin in food (home-canned tomato products and canned cream-base foods are often implicated) and the disease is considered to be an intoxication, although *C. botulinum* has been recovered from the stools of a number of adult patients. A relatively recently recognized syndrome, **infant botulism,** is a true gastrointestinal infection. It is probable that the flora of the normal adult bowel usually prevents colonization by *C. botulinum,* whereas the organism is able to multiply and produce toxin in the infant bowel. Infant botulism is not uncommon; babies acquire the organism by ingestion, although the source of the bacterium is not always clear. There has been an association with honey and corn syrup; it is recommended that babies under 9 months of age not be fed honey. The effect of the toxin is the same, whether it is ingested in food or produced within the bowel.

Other bacterial agents of food poisoning that produce neurotoxins include *Staphylococcus aureus* and *Bacillus cereus.* Toxins produced by these organisms cause vomiting, independent of other actions on the gut mucosa. Staphylococcal food poisoning is one of the most commonly reported categories of food-borne disease. The organisms grow in warm food, primarily meat or dairy products, and produce the toxin. Onset of disease is usually within 2-6 h of ingestion. *B. cereus* produces two toxins, one of which is preformed, called the **emetic toxin,** because it produces vomiting. The second type, probably several enterotoxins (discussed below), causes diarrhea. Often acquired from rice, *B. cereus* has also been associated with cooked meat, poultry, vegetables, and desserts. Perhaps the most common cause of food poisoning is type A *Clostridium perfringens,* which produces toxin in the host after ingestion. It causes a relatively mild, self-limited (usually 24 h) gastroenteritis, often in outbreaks in hospitals. Meats and gravies are common offending foods. Investigations of outbreaks of food poisoning due to preformed toxin ingestion are carried out by public health laboratories and should not be attempted by clinical laboratories.

The second category of toxins, **cytotoxins,** act to disrupt the structure of individual intestinal epithelial cells. When these cells are destroyed, they slough from the surface of the mucosa, leaving it raw and unprotected. The secretory or absorptive functions of the cells are no longer performed. The damaged tissue evokes a strong inflammatory response from the host, further inflicting tissue damage. Patients often shed numerous polymorphonuclear neutrophils and blood into the stool, experience pain, cramps, and an urgent need to defecate even though there is little material in the bowel (tenesmus). The term **dysentery** refers to this destructive disease of the mucosa, almost exclusively occurring in the colon. Cytotoxin has not yet been shown to be the sole virulence factor for any etiologic agent of gastrointestinal disease; most agents produce a cytotoxin in conjunction with another factor. *E. coli* strains seem to possess virulence mechanisms of many types; some strains produce a cytotoxin that destroys epithelial cells and blood cells. *C. difficile* produces such a cytotoxin, the presence of which is a most useful marker for diagnosis of pseudomembranous colitis (PMC). (The *C. difficile* cytotoxin assay is described below.) *Shigella dysenteriae, Staphylococcus aureus, C. perfringens,* and *Vibrio parahaemolyticus* produce cytotoxins that probably contribute to the pathogenesis of diarrhea, although they may not be essential for initiation of disease. Other vibrios, *Aeromonas hydrophila,* a relatively newly described agent of gastrointestinal disease, and *Campylobacter jejuni,* the most common cause of gastrointestinal disease in many areas of the United States, have been shown to produce cytotoxins. The role that these toxins actually play in the pathogenesis of the disease syndromes is not yet delineated. With the exception of the cytotoxin of *C. difficile,* routine tests for cytotoxins are not available.

Enterotoxins cause an alteration in the metabolic activity of intestinal epithelial cells, resulting in an outpouring of electrolytes and fluids into the lumen. They act primarily in the jejunum and upper ileum, where the majority of the fluid transport takes place. The stool of patients with enterotoxic diarrheal disease involving the small bowel is profuse and watery, and polymorphonuclear neutrophils and blood are not prominent features. The classic example of an enterotoxin is that of *Vibrio cholerae*, called **choleragen** (Figure 17.2). This toxin consists of two subunits, A and B. The A subunit is composed of one molecule of A_1, the toxic moiety, and one molecule of A_2, which binds an A_1 subunit to five B subunits. The B subunits bind the toxin to a receptor (a ganglioside, an acidic glycolipid) on the intestinal cell

membrane. Once the toxin binds, it acts on adenylate cyclase enzyme, which catalyzes the transformation of adenosine triphosphate (ATP) to cyclic adenosine monophosphate (cAMP). Increased levels of cAMP stimulate the cell to actively secrete ions into the intestinal lumen; to maintain osmotic stabilization, the cells then secrete fluid into the lumen. The fluid is drawn from the entire fluid store of the body. Patients therefore can become dehydrated very rapidly, as mentioned in Chapter 30. Oral fluid replacement with a glucose-containing electrolyte solution will adequately treat most patients with cholera, since fluid reabsorption can be coupled to glucose transport into the cells. *V. cholerae* must be able to multiply to sufficient

1. Cholera toxin binds to cell membrane via B subunits.

2. B subunits change conformation to allow A subunits to enter membrane.

3. A subunits dissociate and A_1 activates adenylate cyclase.

FIGURE 17.2
Diagrammatic representation of the structure and action of cholera toxin.

numbers to produce toxin in the infected host. To this end, the bacteria possess motility and adherence factors, as discussed below. *V. cholerae* inhabit sea and stagnant water and are spread in contaminated water. They have been isolated from coastal waters of several states, and there have been a few cases of cholera reported that were acquired in the United States.

Other organisms also produce a choleragen-like enterotoxin. A group of vibrios similar to *V. cholerae* but serologically different, known as the **noncholera vibrios,** produce disease clinically identical to cholera, effected by a very similar toxin. The heat labile toxin (LT) elaborated by certain strains of *E. coli*, called **enterotoxigenic *E. coli* (ETEC)**, is very similar to choleragen, sharing cross-reactive antigenic determinants. The enterotoxins of some *Salmonella* species (including *S. arizonae*), *Vibrio parahaemolyticus*, the *Campylobacter jejuni* group, *Clostridium perfringens*, *C. difficile*, *Bacillus cereus*, *Aeromonas*, *Shigella dysenteriae*, and many other Enterobacteriaceae also cause positive reactions in at least one of the tests for enterotoxin. The exact contribution of these enterotoxins to the pathogenicity of each of these stool pathogens remains to be elucidated.

Certain strains of *E. coli*, in addition to producing a heat-labile toxin similar to choleragen (LT), also produce a heat stable toxin (ST) with other properties. Although ST also promotes fluid secretion into the intestinal lumen, its effect is mediated by activation of guanylate cyclase, resulting in increased levels of cyclic guanylate monophosphate (GMP), which yields the same net effect as increased cAMP. Tests for ST include ELISA, immunodiffusion, and the classic suckling mouse assay, in which culture filtrate is placed into the stomach of a suckling mouse and the intestinal contents are later measured for fluid volume increase.

Several tests are available for the detection of enterotoxin, although these are not performed in routine diagnostic microbiology laboratories. The classic test is the "ligated rabbit ileal loop test." For this test, a rabbit is anesthetized, and a long section of the ileum is pulled out through an incision in the abdominal wall. Several sections of ileum are tied off (ligated) with heavy suture material, each about 4 inches long, so that they resemble a string of sausages. An equal portion of the culture filtrate to be tested, a known positive filtrate for enterotoxin, and a negative control of the culture medium only are injected into the lumens of separate ligated loops with a needle and syringe. The ileum is placed back into the rabbit and the incision is stitched or stapled together. Within a period of hours, the rabbit is sacrificed and the intestinal loops are examined. Those loops that received toxin are found to be distended with fluid that has been secreted into the loop, whereas the loops without enterotoxin will show no distension, resembling the control loops. Several different fluids may be tested for enterotoxin in the same rabbit.

Other tests for enterotoxin include the Chinese hamster ovary (CHO) cell assay and the Y-1 adrenal cell assay, tissue culture assays in which a tissue culture consisting of CHO cells or Y-1 adrenal cells, known to be sensitive to the action of enterotoxin, are exposed to test fluids and examined for evidence of damage (rounding up). Since choleragen is toxigenic, specific antibodies have been produced against it. Thus, antibody can be used to specifically identify the antigen. The most common tests are of the immunodiffusion type. No easily performed test is generally available, although ELISA procedures and molecular probes have been developed.

17.2.e. Gastrointestinal infections associated with destruction of cell function without toxins. Organisms that multiply within certain cells of the mucosa, disrupting normal function of those cells, can cause diarrheal disease. Viruses probably act in this manner, multiplying within cells of the small bowel. Diarrhea of viral etiology is not associated with the presence of blood and white cells. Hepatitis A, B, non-A non-B, rotavirus, Norwalk-like agents, and occasionally adenovirus have been associated with diarrheal symptoms in infected patients, whereas the role of other viruses, such as coxsackievirus and echoviruses, in the etiology of diarrhea has not been established. Viral diarrhea may be the second most common infectious disease among people in the United States (after upper respiratory tract infections). Nursery and day-care center outbreaks of rotavirus diarrhea have been reported. Although young children are at most risk, close adult contacts may also become infected. Rotaviruses and Norwalk-like agents are both visualized by electron microscopy within the absorptive cells at the ends of the intestinal villi, where they mutliply and destroy cellular function. The villi become shortened and inflammatory cells infiltrate the mucosa, further contributing to the pathologic condition. Hepatitis viruses have not been found in intestinal cells, but it is possible that some multiplication occurs there, since diarrhea is a common early symptom of hepatitis. Other viruses, particularly enteroviruses, can be recovered from feces, although the disease-producing activity occurs in other sites. Chapter 42 discusses recovery of viruses from stool for diagnosis of viral disease. The etiology of diarrhea associated with an overgrowth of *Candida* species in the bowel, especially in patients taking broad spectrum antibiotics, has not been established. It is **not** due to *Candida* and probably is similar to other types of antibiotic-associated diarrhea without PMC. Filamentous fungi may, on occasion, be associated with altered gastrointestinal function, particularly in immunosuppressed patients.

17.2.f. Gastrointestinal infections associated with invasive microorganisms. Certain parasites, particularly *Entamoeba histolytica*

and *Balantidium coli,* invade the intestinal epithelium of the colon as a primary site of infection. The ensuing amebic dysentery is characterized by blood and **numerous white blood cells,** and the patient experiences cramping and tenesmus. Other parasites that are acquired by ingestion, such as *Schistosoma* species and *Trichinella*, may cause transient bloody diarrhea and pain during migration through the intestinal mucosa to their preferred sites within the host.

Bacteria that invade the epithelial cells also produce symptoms of dysentery. The most common etiologic agent is *Shigella*, although strains of *E. coli* called **enteroinvasive** may be associated with an identical syndrome. The bacteria penetrate the superficial layers of the mucosa, rarely passing into deeper host tissues. Invasiveness, then, is a virulence factor for these organisms. The classic test for invasiveness is the **Sereny test,** in which a suspension of the organism is placed within the conjunctival sac of a guinea pig or rabbit. Within a short time, an invasive organism will penetrate the epithelial cells, causing a purulent and exudative conjunctivitis. A modified ELISA for detecting enteroinvasive *E. coli* and virulent *Shigella* has recently been described by Pál et al.[2]

Other bacteria not only invade superficial epithelia but may invade the blood vessels to disseminate systemically. Certain *Salmonella* species, such as *S. typhi, S. enteritidis*, and *S. choleraesuis,* are more likely to do this. *S. typhi* and *S. choleraesuis* are etiologic agents of **enteric fever,** systemic diseases characterized by fever, headache, vomiting, and sometimes constipation (rather than diarrhea). The organisms can be recovered from the blood, stool, and, occasionally, the duodenal fluid of patients with this syndrome. Invasiveness is also thought to contribute to the pathogenesis of disease associated with species of vibrios, campylobacters, *Yersinia enterocolitica, Plesiomonas shigelloides*, and *Edwardsiella tarda*.

Unusual agents and those that have not been cultured, such as the mycobacteria that may be associated with Crohn's disease (Chapter 41), the bacteria associated with Whipple's disease (Chapter 40), and the spirochetal organisms possibly linked to gastroenteritis (Chapter 40), are also candidates as invasive etiologic agents of gastrointestinal disease. Occasionally, stool cultures from patients with diarrheal disease yield heavy growths of organisms such as *Pseudomonas* species or *Klebsiella pneumoniae*, not usually found in such numbers as normal flora. There is no definitive evidence that these organisms actually contribute to the pathogenesis of the diarrhea.

17.2.g. Gastrointestinal infections associated with adherent microorganisms. *Giardia lamblia* has become increasingly more common as an etiologic agent of gastrointestinal disease in the United States. Excreted into freshwater by natural animal hosts such as the beaver, the organism can be acquired by drinking stream water or even city water in some localities, particularly in the Rocky Mountain states, as well as throughout the world. The organism, a flagellated protozoan, adheres to the intestinal mucosa of the small bowel, possibly by means of a ventral sucker, destroying the ability of the mucosal cells to participate in normal secretion and absorption. There is no evidence of invasion or toxin production.

Yet another virulence mechanism for *E. coli* may be adherence. Certain strains have been implicated as etiologic agents of malabsorption diarrhea; the strains have no other detectable pathogenic mechanisms, but are able to multiply in close proximity to the intestinal epithelial cells. Such a disease has been documented by electron microscopic studies in both rabbits and humans. *Cryptosporidium* and *Isospora* species, etiologic agents of diarrhea in animals and poultry and more recently recognized as causing human disease, probably also act by adhering to intestinal mucosa and disrupting

function. Cryptosporidia are not uncommonly seen in the diarrhea of patients with acquired immune deficiency syndrome (AIDS), as well as in the feces of people with animal exposure; both cryptosporidia and *Isospora* may cause severe, protracted diarrhea in AIDS patients.

17.2.h. Other infectious causes of gastrointestinal disease. Agents of sexually transmitted disease may cause gastrointestinal symptoms when they are introduced into the colon via sexual intercourse. *Mycobacterium avium-intracellulare* (Chapter 41) may be transmitted in this way, going on to cause devastating systemic disease in patients with AIDS. Homosexual practices predispose people to such infections as gonococcal and herpetic proctitis, syphilis, and others. Chapter 23 contains further discussion of patients at risk for these and other causes of gastrointestinal disease. The pathogenesis of infections due to *Dientamoeba fragilis* and *Blastocystis hominis* (a possible coccidian etiologic agent of human diarrheal disease) is not well documented, although these organisms are associated with gastrointestinal symptoms.

17.3. Collection and Transport of Stool Specimens

Specimens that can be delivered to the laboratory within 1 h may be collected in a clean waxed cardboard or plastic container. Stool for direct wet mount examinations, *C. difficile* toxin assays, concentration for detection of ova and parasites, immunoelectron microscopy for detection of viruses, and ELISA or latex agglutination test for rotavirus must be sent to the laboratory without any added preservatives or liquids. Volume of stool at least equal to the size of a walnut is necessary for most procedures. If a delay longer than 2 h is anticipated for stools for bacterial culture, the specimen should be placed in transport media. For bacterial culture, Cary-Blair transport media has been shown to best preserve the viability of intestinal pathogens, including *Campylobacter* and *Vibrio* species. Some workers recommend reducing the agar content of Cary-Blair medium from 0.5% to 0.16% for maintenance of *Campylobacter*. Buffered glycerol transport medium does not maintain these bacteria. Several manufactureres produce a small vial of Cary-Blair with a self-contained plastic scoop suitable for collecting samples. *Shigella* species are delicate; best recovery is obtained by inoculating media directly at the bedside. If direct plating is not convenient, a transport medium of equal parts of glycerol and 0.033 M phosphate buffer (pH 7.0) will support viability of *Shigella* better than will Cary-Blair. For this purpose, maintenance of the glycerol transport medium at refrigerator or freezer temperatures will yield better results. For detection of ova and parasites, polyvinyl alcohol (PVA) fixative is recommended (Chapter 44). One part fecal material should be added to three parts PVA. PVA vials are available commercially. Stools for virus culture must be refrigerated if they are not inoculated to media within 2 h. A rectal swab, transported in modified Stuart's transport medium, is adequate for recovery of most viruses from feces. Stools received for detection of *C. difficile* cytotoxin should be frozen, preferably at $-70°$ C, but at least at $-20°$ C, until they are tested. Stool may be defrosted, centrifuged, and filtered (as described in Procedure 17.1 below), and the filtrate can be refrozen without affecting the results (although there is some loss of titer).

If an etiologic agent is not isolated with the first culture or visual examination, two additional specimens should be submitted to the laboratory over the next few days. Since organisms may be shed intermittently, collection of specimens at different times over several days should enhance recovery. Certain infectious agents, such as *Giardia*, may be very difficult to detect, requiring the processing of multiple specimens over many weeks or duodenal aspirates (in the case of *Giardia*) until the organism is found.

If stool is unavailable, a rectal swab may be substituted as a specimen for bacterial or viral culture but it is not as good, particularly for diagnosis in adults. For suspected *Campylobacter*, the swab must be placed in transport medium immediately to avoid drying. Swabs are not acceptable for detection of parasites or viral antigens. The swab should be placed in the transport media mentioned above.

Other specimens that may be obtained for diagnosis of gastrointestinal tract infection include duodenal aspirates (usually for detection of *Giardia* or *Strongyloides*), which should be immediately examined by direct microscopy for presence of motile trophozoites, cultured for bacteria, and placed into PVA fixative. The laboratory should be informed in advance that such a specimen is going to be collected, so that the specimen can be processed and examined effectively. The "string test" has proven useful for diagnosis of duodenal parasites such as *Giardia* and for isolation of *Salmonella typhi* from carriers and patients with acute typhoid fever. A weighted gelatin capsule containing a tightly wound length of string is swallowed by the patient, leaving the end of the string protruding from the patient's mouth. After a predetermined time period, during which the capsule reaches the duodenum and dissolves, the string is pulled back out, covered with duodenal contents. This string must be delivered immediately to the laboratory. In the laboratory, the technologist strips the mucus and secretions that are attached to the string with sterile gloved fingers, depositing some material on slides for direct examination, some material into fixative for preparation of permanent stained mounts, and inoculating some material to appropriate media for isolation of bacteria.

Biopsy material and material from mucosal lesions may be obtained from patients during proctoscopy or sigmoidoscopy. Such material is often fixed for histologic and pathologic examinations. Microbiologists should handle such material as if it were feces, staining or culturing as requested.

17.4. Direct Detection of Agents of Gastroenteritis in Feces

A direct wet mount (Chapter 7) of fecal material, particularly with liquid or unformed stool, is the fastest method for detection of motile trophozoites of *Dientamoeba fragilis*, *Entamoeba*, *Giardia*, and other intestinal parasites (that may not contribute to disease, but may alert the microbiologist to the possibility of finding other parasites), such as *Entamoeba coli*, *Endolimax nana*, *Chilomastix mesnili*, and *Trichomonas hominis*. Occasionally, the larvae or adult worms of other parasites may be visualized. Experienced observers can also see the refractile forms of cryptosporidia and many types of cysts on the direct wet mount. Examination of a direct wet mount of fecal material taken from an area with blood or mucus, with the addition of an equal portion of Loeffler's methylene blue (Chapter 46), is helpful for detection of fecal leukocytes, which may aid in differentiating among the various types of diarrheal syndromes discussed above. If they are plentiful, the ova of intestinal parasites will be seen. Under phase and darkfield microscopy, the darting motility and curved forms of *Campylobacter* may be observed in a warm sample. Water, which will immobilize *Campylobacter*, should not be used. Trained observers working in endemic areas can recognize the characteristic appearance and motility of *V. cholerae*.

Immune electron microscopy is a very rapid method for detecting rotavirus and Norwalk-like agents. Details of the procedures are discussed in Chapter 42. For most laboratories, electron microscopy is unavailable, and rotavirus is detected using a solid phase ELISA procedure or a latex agglutination test. Several manufacturers produce systems for detection of the antigen of rotavirus, including a microwell

plate system (M.A. Bioproducts, Inc.), a plastic bead system (Rotazyme, Abbott Laboratories), and a latex agglutination system (Rotalex, Orion Research). For the immunoassay systems, the feces are diluted to suspend the viral antigens, the solid material is removed by filtration or centrifugation, and the filtrate is added to the immunoassay solid phase on which antibody to rotavirus has been adsorbed. After an attachment step, excess material is washed off and an enzyme-conjugated antibody is added. If viral antigens were present, the conjugate will adhere to the solid phase as well. With the addition of the proper substrate, the enzyme will effect a visible color change (further discussed in Chapter 12). Instructions for each of the commercial systems vary, but the results have been uniformly good, with detection of rotavirus by ELISA comparable to electron microscopy in sensitivity. The latex agglutination test exhibits similar sensitivity with a much less complex system. This high sensitivity is probably a result of the huge numbers of virus particles that are shed in the feces of patients with infection.

Feces may be Gram stained for detection of certain etiologic agents. Although gram-negative bacilli cannot be differentiated, sheets of polymorphonuclear neutrophils and many clumps of typical gram-positive cocci are indicative of staphylococcal infection (Plate 17.2). Many thin, comma-shaped gram-negative bacilli may indicate *Campylobacter* infection (if vibrios have been ruled out), and large numbers of gram-positive bacilli, large and thin with parallel walls, may be suggestive of overgrowth by *Clostridium difficile* (Plate 17.3). Acid fast stain should be used to detect *Cryptosporidium* species and mycobacteria. *Isospora* are also acid fast. Examination of fixed fecal material for parasites by trichrome or other stains is thoroughly covered in Chapter 44. It is recommended that a permanent stained preparation be made from all unformed stool specimens received in the laboratory for detection of parasites.

14.1

PLATE 14.1. Many colonies of *Staphylococcus aureus* on layer of settled red blood cells in blood culture bottle.

15.1

PLATE 15.1. Trichrome stained preparation of *Naegleria fowleri* isolated from cerebrospinal fluid and grown on a lawn of Enterobacteriaceae.

16.1

A

16.2   B

PLATE 16.1.   Primary streptococcal selective agar (BBL Microbiology Systems) culture plate from a
throat specimen that contained many group A beta hemolytic streptococci. Growth of the bacteria is
inhibited in zone surrounding the 0.04-unit bacitracin disk.

PLATE 16.2.   Gram stain of sputum specimens (400 ×). **A,** This specimen contains numerous
polymorphonuclear leukocytes and no visible squamous epithelial cells, indicating that the specimen is
acceptable for routine bacteriologic culture. **B,** This specimen contains numerous squamous epithelial
cells and rare polymorphonuclear leukocytes, indicating an inadequate specimen for routine
bacteriologic culture.

16.3

16.4

PLATE 16.3. Cysts of *Pneumocystis carinii* in bronchial lavage, stained with modified Gomori methenamine silver stain (1,000 ×).

PLATE 16.4. Toluidine blue O stained cysts of *Pneumocystis carinii* in smear made from centrifuged sediment from bronchial lavage specimen (1,000 ×).

17.1

17.2

PLATE 17.1. Autopsy specimen of colon showing multiple yellow, elevated plaques indicative of the inflammatory exudate of pseudomembranous colitis.
PLATE 17.2. Gram stain of stool with staphylococcal enterocolitis.

17.3

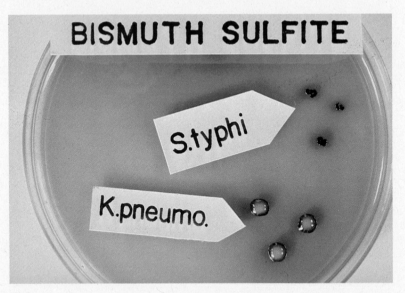

17.4

PLATE 17.3. Gram stain of stool with *Clostridium difficile* pseudomembranous colitis.
PLATE 17.4. The appearance of colonies of *Salmonella typhi* on bismuth sulfite agar.

18.1

PLATE 18.1. Filter paper used to detect pyuria and bacteriuria by staining trapped particles (Bac-T-Screen, Marion Laboratories). Amount of color yielded by specimen (center circle) is compared to control color samples around the edge of the specimen circle.

17.5. Culture of Fecal Material for Isolation of Etiologic Agents of Gastrointestinal Disease

As outlined in Chapter 6, fecal specimens for culture should be inoculated to several media for maximum yield, including solid agar and broth. The choice of media is arbitrary and based on the particular requirements of the clinician and the laboratory. Recommendations are given below.

17.5.a. Cultures for bacterial etiologic agents. Stools received for routine culture in most clinical laboratories in the United States should be examined for the presence of *Campylobacter*, *Salmonella*, and *Shigella* species under all circumstances. If the incidence of *Yersinia enterocolitica* gastroenteritis is high enough in the area served by the laboratory, this agent should also be routinely sought. Special procedures for detection of vibrios, *C. difficile*, and mycobacteria should be carried out on request. It is the decision of the microbiologist, with input from clinicians, as to whether or not detection of *Aeromonas* species should be part of a routine stool culture. Two strategies for such detection are mentioned below.

Specimens received for detection of the most commonly isolated Enterobacteriaceae, *Salmonella* and *Shigella* species, should be plated to a supportive medium, a slightly selective and differential medium, and a moderately selective medium. A highly selective medium may be included under certain circumstances, but does not seem to be cost effective for most microbiology laboratories. Blood agar (tryptic soy agar with 5% sheep blood) is an excellent general supportive medium (Chapter 8). Blood agar medium will allow growth of yeast species, staphylococci, and enterococci, in addition to gram-negative bacilli. If there is a predominance of a gram-positive organism, it will be detected on the blood agar. Another benefit of blood agar is that it will allow oxidase testing of colonies. We recommend that several colonies (that do not resemble *Pseudomonas*) from the third or fourth quadrant be routinely screened for production of cytochrome oxidase (Chapter 9). If large numbers of *Aeromonas*, *Vibrio*, or *Plesiomonas* species are present, they will be detected by their positive oxidase reaction.

If a more selective agar for detection of gram-positive organisms is desired, Columbia base agar with colistin and nalidixic acid (CNA) would be a good choice (Chapter 8). For routine cultures, however, detection of small numbers of gram-positive organisms does not seem warranted. The moderately selective agar should support growth of most Enterobacteriaceae, vibrios, and other possible pathogens, MacConkey agar seems to work very well. Some laboratories use eosin–methylene blue (EMB), which is slightly more inhibitory. All lactose negative colonies are tested further (Chapter 27), ensuring adequate detection of most vibrios and most pathogenic Enterobacteriaceae. Lactose-positive vibrios (*V. vulnificus*), some *Aeromonas*, and *Plesiomonas* species will not be distinctive on MacConkey agar.

The specimen should also be inoculated to a moderately selective agar such as Hektoen enteric (HE) or xylose-lysine desoxycholate (XLD) media. These media inhibit growth of most Enterobacteriaceae, allowing *Salmonella* and *Shigella* species to be detected. Colony morphologies of lactose negative, lactose positive, and H_2S-producing organisms are outlined in Chapter 8. The highly selective media brilliant green (BG) or bismuth sulfite (BS) may be used for detection of *Salmonella* species; they should be heavily inoculated, since they are quite inhibitory. *S. typhi* will often display silver metallic colonies with black halos surrounding them on BS (Plate 17.4), whereas salmonellas show pink colonies on BG. Other potential pathogens do not survive on these agars. All these media are incubated at 35°-37° C in air and examined at 24 and 48 h for suspicious colonies.

Cultures for isolation of *Campylobacter jejuni* and *C. coli* should be inoculated to Campy-blood agar (further discussed in Chapter 30). *Brucella* broth base has yielded less satisfactory recovery of *Campylobacter* species. Commercially produced agar plates for isolation of campylobacters are available from several manufacturers. These plates are incubated in a microaerophilic atmosphere at 42° C and examined at 24 and 48 h for suspicious colonies (Chapter 30).

Vibrios that are etiologic agents of gastroenteritis may be detected by screening all oxidase positive colonies growing on blood agar. Many vibrios are beta hemolytic. For specific detection of *V. cholerae* and other vibrios, thiosulfate-citrate-bile salts-sucrose agar (TCBS, Chapter 45) is recommended. The agar is heavily inoculated with feces, as are the moderately selective media, and incubated in air at 35°-37° C for up to 48 h. Either large, flat yellow or olive green colonies should be further tested. Chapter 30 contains identification procedures for vibrios likely to be isolated from feces.

A special medium has been developed for recovery of *Yersinia enterocolitica*. Often called CIN agar, this medium is made from a peptone agar base with mannitol, neutral red, crystal violet, and the antimicrobial agents cefsulodin, 3, 3′, 4′, 5-tetrachlorosalicylanilide (irgasan), and novobiocin (Chapter 45). CIN agar is available commercially as powder or plates. The specimen is streaked on the agar and the plate is incubated at room temperature for 48 h. Colonies of *Y. enterocolitica* appear bright pink with a red center. Very few other organisms will grow on CIN agar, although some *Aeromonas* species have been found to grow very well on some formulations of this medium. If *Aeromonas* is suspected as the etiologic agent of diarrheal disease, we recommend inoculation of CIN agar at 37° C in addition to other media. A blood agar medium containing ampicillin has been used for selective recovery of *Aeromonas* with good success.

Enrichment broths are often used for enhanced recovery of *Salmonella*, *Shigella*, and *Campylobacter*, although *Shigella* does not often survive enrichment. Gram-negative broth (Hajna GN, Chapter 45) or selenite F broth (Chapter 45) yield good recovery. An enrichment broth that increases the yield of positive cultures for *Campylobacter* species is Campy-thioglycolate (Chapter 30). Enrichment broths for Enterobacteriaceae should be incubated in air at 35° C for 12-18 h and then several drops should be subcultured to at least two selective medium plates. Enrichment broth for *Campylobacter* is refrigerated overnight or for a minimum of 8 h before a few drops are plated to campylobacter agar and incubated as above. *Yersinia enterocolitica* also can be "cold enriched." A swab of fecal material is inoculated to a tube of 5 ml of phosphate-buffered saline (pH 7.2) and the tube is refrigerated for up to 21 days. A few drops are subcultured to CIN agar every 4 days and incubated as above. Such a cold enrichment procedure is most useful for epidemiologic studies, since results may not be known soon enough to benefit an individual patient. Alkaline peptone water (Chapter 45) has been shown to adequately enrich for vibrios. After 8 h incubation, several drops from the broth should be inoculated to TCBS and incubated as above (also discussed in Chapter 30).

Clostridium difficile may be recovered by plating stool to cycloserine cefoxitin egg fructose agar (CCFA, Chapter 45). Two or three drops (or 0.1 g) of stool are inoculated to CCFA agar and streaked for isolation. Plates are incubated anaerobically (Chapters 8 and 34) for 48 h and examined for characteristic large (4 mm diameter) yellow colonies with an opalescent sheen. *C. difficile* is one of the most oxygen-sensitive of the clinically important clostridia. For this reason, it may fail to grow from material inoculated to plates in the air and incubated in an anaerobic jar or plastic bag. Best recovery is obtained on plates inoculated with fecal material in an anaerobic chamber (Chapter 35). *C. difficile* colonies will fluoresce yellow-green under ultraviolet light and they exhibit a very strong horse manure-like odor. *C. difficile* can be presumptively identified on the

PROCEDURE 17.1. *CLOSTRIDIUM DIFFICILE* CYTOTOXIN ASSAY

1. Prepare growth medium as follows:

Eagle's minimum essential medium with Hanks' balanced salt solution (without glutamine)	500 ml bottle
Fetal bovine serum	50 ml
L-glutamine	5 ml

   All of these products are available from Flow Laboratories. Fetal bovine serum, obtained in 100 ml bottles, must be heat inactivated at 56° C for 30 min before using for the first time. The L-glutamine is purchased in 100 ml amounts and stored at −20° C in 5 ml aliquots. One aliquot can be defrosted and added to growth medium each time it is prepared.

   To the above solution, add 5 ml of penicillin-streptomycin-amphotericin B (100 ×; M.A. Bioproducts). Mix thoroughly and dispense the solution aseptically into bottles containing 100 ml each. Freeze these bottles at −20° C. Thaw in a 37° C water bath before use.

2. Prepare maintenance medium as follows:

Modified Eagle's minimum essential medium with Earl's salts and Hepes buffer (without sodium bicarbonate and glutamine	500 ml bottle
Fetal bovine serum	10 ml
L-glutamine	5 ml
Penicillin-streptomycin-amphotericin B	5 ml

   Add the above components aseptically, mix thoroughly, and store the solution frozen at −20° C in 100 ml amounts.

3. Prepare trypsin solution as follows:

2.5% trypsin in modified Hanks' balanced salt solution without magnesium and calcium (10 ×) (Flow Laboratories)	20 ml
Hanks' balanced salt solution	180 ml

   Add the two solutions aseptically, mix thoroughly, and store at −20° C in 3 ml aliquots. Defrost aliquots in a 37° C water bath before use.

4. Prepare stool specimens for assay by mixing formed stools with an equal volume of Hanks' balanced salt solution or phosphate buffered saline (0.01 M, pH 6.9). Liquid stools may be handled without dilution. A maximum of 5 ml of stool material is centrifuged at 2500 × g for 20 min. The supernatant (approximately 2 ml fluid) is passed through a sterile, disposable 0.45 μm membrane filter. The filtrate should be crystal clear and may be slightly yellow. The filtrate may be frozen at −20° C until tested, although freezing at −70° C is preferable.

Continued.

PROCEDURE 17.1. *CLOSTRIDIUM DIFFICILE* CYTOTOXIN ASSAY—cont'd

5. For each stool filtrate to be tested, two sterile 12 × 75 mm plastic snap-top tubes are labeled. One tube is "T" for toxin and the second tube is "A" for antitoxin. Add 0.15 ml growth medium to tube "A" and 0.10 ml growth medium to tube "T." Add 0.05 ml stool filtrate to tube "A" for each set, mix thoroughly and transfer 0.1 ml to the corresponding "T" tube. Tube "A" thus contains a 1:4 dilution of the filtrate and tube "T" contains a 1:5 dilution. Add 0.1 ml *C. difficile* antitoxin diluted 1:25 in phosphate buffered saline (Department of Anaerobic Microbiology, Attn.: Tracy Wilkins, VPI & SU, Blacksburg, VA 24061) to tube "A".

6. Prepare the following control mixtures in small plastic tubes:
   0.1 ml toxin (also obtained from VPI) and 0.1 ml antitoxin (neutralization control)
   0.1 ml toxin and 0.1 ml growth medium (toxin control)
   0.1 ml antitoxin and 0.1 ml growth medium (antitoxin control)
   0.2 ml growth medium (cell culture control)

7. Working in a laminar flow biosafety cabinet, aseptically pipette all of the fluid medium from above the cell monolayer of a 75 ml flask of Hep-2 cells (available from Flow Laboratories). Add 10 ml Hanks' balanced salt solution without calcium and magnesium. Swirl the flask gently, aseptically aspirate off the entire fluid medium, and discard it.

8. Add 3 ml trypsin solution and rotate this solution over the entire monolayer. Remove 2 ml and incubate the flask with the remaining 1 ml trypsin for 5-10 min at 37° C until the monolayer can be seen to have come off (floating cells).

9. Resuspend the cells by agitating the flask and add 8 ml growth medium to dilute out the effects of the trypsin. These suspended cells are used in the toxin assay.

10. Add 0.1 ml of the cell suspension to each of enough wells of a 96-well flat-bottomed well microdilution plate (Falcon Plastics) to accommodate all of the controls and filtrates to be tested.

11. Add 0.1 ml from each "A" tube, each "T" tube, and each control tube to separate wells containing cell suspensions. We have not found it necessay to preincubate the cell suspensions before adding the filtrates.

12. Cover the plate with a sterile seal and incubate overnight at 37° C in an air incubator that does not have too much humidity.

13. Read the plates on an inverted microscope, observing for cytopathic effect, evidenced by rounding up of the cells. Positive cytotoxicity is indicated by 100% rounding of cells. Figures 17.3 and 17.4 show the appearance of the monolayer before and after the effects of the cytotoxin.

FIGURE 17.3
Appearance of healthy Hep-2 cell monolayer.

FIGURE 17.4
Appearance of Hep-2 cell monolayer damaged by the effects of the cytotoxin of *Clostridium difficile*.

PROCEDURE 17.1. *CLOSTRIDIUM DIFFICILE* CYTOTOXIN ASSAY—cont'd

14. Interpretation of the results is as follows:

    Controls should all yield confluent monolayers without rounding, except for the toxin control, which should show 100% cytotoxicity.

    Negative filtrates will yield confluent monolayers without rounding of cells in both "A" and "T" wells of the assay.

    Positive filtrates will show rounding of cells and cytotoxicity in the "T" wells, but no rounding in the "A" wells, indicative of specific inhibition of cytoxocity by antitoxin.

    Filtrates which show cytotoxicity in both "A" and "T" wells are **cytotoxic** themselves (they contain a nonspecific factor toxic to the Hep-2 cells). This toxic reaction must be diluted out to determine the true presence of *C. difficile* toxin.

    Results are reported as the dilution at which the stool is positive for cytotoxin. For the assay described here, positive results are detected at 1:10.

15. Nonspecific toxicity can be removed in two ways. The first is to freeze and thaw the filtrate once again, which may remove these factors. The second is to dilute the filtrate (perform a titration assay). Dilute toxic stool filtrates in growth medium, making a series of dilutions including 1:2, 1:4, 1:8, 1:16, 1:32, and 1:64. Test these diluted specimens in the standard cytotoxin assay described above. Toxic stools can be titrated and retested the next time the assay is performed. Results of toxic filtrates are reported out by stating the dilution at which the nonspecific toxicity is removed, revealing toxicity that is inhibited by antiserum, such as "filtrate toxic at 1:10, *C. difficile* toxin present at 1:20" or by stating the highest dilution at which a toxic reaction is evident, such as "nonspecific toxicity present at 1:40, no *C. difficile* toxin detected at higher dilutions."

basis of colony and Gram stain morphology. Definitive identification is outlined in Chapter 35. Although detection of *C. difficile* in stool of patients with diarrhea may be suggestive of PMC, detection of the toxin in stool filtrates (Procedure 17.1) and especially visualization of pseudomembranes or plaques on the bowel mucosa of the patient (Plate 17.1) by colonoscopy or proctoscopy are more diagnostic of the syndrome. In addition, other clostridia have occasionally been implicated as etiologic agents of PMC

Mycobacterium avium-intracellulare complex organisms may be isolated from the stool of patients with AIDS, and intestinal tuberculosis may still be suspected in some unusual cases. Methods for culturing acid fast bacilli from feces are discussed in Chapter 41. It is not recommended that clinical microbiology laboratories process stool for *M. tuberculosis*, since the procedure is so cumbersome. Reference laboratories are better equipped for such requests.

17.5.b. Cultures for viral etiologic agents. In addition to the viral agents of gastroenteritis, rotavirus, and Norwalk-like agent, whose detection is by latex agglutination, enzyme immunoassay, or electron microscopy, as discussed above, many viral agents of disease are routinely sought in feces. Fresh feces or rectal swabs are inoculated to antibiotic-containing media (Chapter 45) for 30 min before inoculating to tissue culture (Chapter 42). Choice of tissue culture is determined by the etiologic agents sought, but feces are usually inoculated to primary monkey kidney, human fetal diploid fibroblast, and a human epithelial continuous cell line (Chapter 42).

17.6. Detection of *Clostridium difficile* Cytotoxin

Detection of the cytotoxin of *C. difficile* is the most specific laboratory diagnostic test presently available for antibiotic-associated PMC, although there are patients without PMC or even diarrhea who nevertheless yield toxin-producing *C. difficile* organisms from fecal cultures and whose stool contains cytotoxin. With a less cytotoxin-sensitive cell line, however, such as HeLa cells or Hep-2 cells, the detection of toxin is generally a good indicator of the disease. Even laboratories that do not routinely utilize tissue culture methods can adapt this procedure to their schedules. The serology laboratory of one of us (EJB), which had never even seen a tissue culture assay before, routinely performs the *C. difficile* cytotoxin assay (Procedure 17.1) twice weekly with excellent results.

Although it is possible to maintain a cell line in the laboratory, cell lines are also available commercially. Recently, a prepared microdilution tray containing tissue culture cells has been made available for the *C. difficile*

toxin assay (Bartels Immunodiagnostics). With the availability of this system, the cytotoxicity assay is within the ability of most clinical microbiology laboratories. The number of requests for the assay and economic considerations are among the factors to consider in deciding whether to offer such a test in house or to send specimens to a reference laboratory. A procedure for passage and maintenance of Hep-2 cells, a recommended cell line for the cytotoxic assay, is detailed in Chapter 42. We maintain the cell line in one tissue culture flask (75 ml), incubated in a small air incubator at 37° C. The modified maintenance procedure used in our laboratory (EJB) is detailed in Procedure 17.2. All manipulations must be carried out in a biological safety cabinet to minimize contamination of the tissue culture. Cells are passed to a new flask each time the tissue culture assay is performed and once on Fridays to allow viability over the weekend, for a maximum of three times weekly. A latex agglutination method for detection of *C. difficile* enterotoxin (Marion Scientific) is promising. An ELISA test is also available but has not been widely evaluated.

The cytotoxic assay detailed in Procedure 17.1 has been developed over months of trial and error, and it differs from other published methods in several ways. Individual laboratories will have to work out their own solutions to problems that arise, such as how many cells to place into each well of the microdilution plate, and whether the cells must be added first and allowed to settle before the toxin is added. The choice of which cell line to use for the assay is important. Chinese hamster ovary cells have been shown by Murray and Weber[1] to be more susceptible to the toxin than were Hep-2 cells. For our laboratory (EJB), Hep-2 cells yield acceptable sensitivity. Once an initial cell line is purchased, it may be maintained by serial passage for many generations, as outlined in Procedure 17.2.

PROCEDURE 17.2. MAINTENANCE OF HEP-2 CELL CULTURE LINE

1. Cells are maintained by "feeding" on Monday, Wednesday, and Friday afternoons.
2. Working in the laminar flow biological safety cabinet, the technologist aseptically pipettes the fluid medium from above the monolayer and discards this fluid.
3. The technologist then adds 20 ml of maintenance medium.
4. The flask is tightly capped, and the culture is incubated in air at 37° C.
5. Each Thursday after the cells have been trypsinized and prepared for the cytotoxin assay as described above, 2 ml of the cell suspension is pipetted into each of two new 75 ml plastic tissue culture flasks (Falcon Plastics).
6. To each flask, add 18 ml growth medium. Incubate the flasks, tightly capped, at 37° C in air for 24 h.
7. Aseptically pipette the fluid from above the monolayer and discard the fluid. Replace the growth medium with 20 ml maintenance medium. Incubate the tightly closed flasks in air at 37° C until they are "fed" again or used to perform the cytotoxin assay. We have successfully maintained the same cell line for at least 1 year in this manner. Further hints for cell culture techniques and freezing cell cultures are found in Chapter 42.

REFERENCES

1. Murray, P.R., and Weber, C.J. 1983. Detection of *Clostridium difficile* cytotoxin in Hep-2 and CHO cell lines. Diagn. Microbiol. Infect. Dis. 1:331.
2. Pál, T., Páscsa, A.S., Emödy, L., Vörös, S., and Sélley, E. 1985. Modified enzyme-linked immunosorbent assay for detecting enteroinvasive *Escherichia coli* and virulent *Shigella* strains. J. Clin. Microbiol. 21:415.

BIBLIOGRAPHY

Du Pont, H.L., and Pickering, L.K. 1980. Infections of the gastrointestinal tract. In Greenough, W.B., and Merigan, T.C., editors. Current topics in infectious disease. Plenum Publishing Co., New York.

Guerrant, R.L. 1985. Principles and definition of syndromes of gastrointestinal infections and food poisoning. In Mandell, G.L., Douglas, R.G. Jr., and Bennett, J.E., editors. Principles and practice of infectious diseases, ed 2. John Wiley & Sons, New York.

Guerrant, R.L. 1985. Inflammatory enteritides. In Mandell, G.L., Douglas, R.G. Jr., and Bennett, J.E., editors. Principles and practice of infectious diseases, ed 2. John Wiley & Sons, New York.

Guerrant, R.L., and Hughes, J.M. 1985. Nausea, vomiting, and noninflammatory diarrhea. In Mandell, G.L., Douglas, R.G. Jr., and Bennett, J.E., editors. Principles and practice of infectious diseases, ed 2. John Wiley & Sons, New York.

Middlebrook, J.L., and Dorland, R.B. 1984. Bacterial toxins: cellular mechanisms of action. Microbiol. Rev. 48:199.

Rolston, K.V.I., and Hopfer, R.L. 1984. Diarrhea due to *Plesiomonas shigelloides* in cancer patients. J. Clin. Microbiol. 20:597.

Sack, R.B., Tilton, R.C., and Weissfeld, A.S. 1980. Laboratory diagnosis of bacterial diarrhea. In Rubin, S.J., editor. Cumitech 12. American Society for Microbiology, Washington, D.C.

18

Microorganisms Encountered in the Urinary Tract

18.1. Introduction

18.1.a. General considerations, anatomy, and normal flora. The urinary tract consists of the kidneys, the ureters, the bladder, and the urethra (Figure 18.1). Although the urethra hosts a resident microflora that colonizes its transitional epithelium, consisting of coagulase-negative staphylococci, viridans and nonhemolytic streptococci, lactobacilli, diphtheroids (*Corynebacterium* species), nonpathogenic *Neisseria* species, transient gram-negative aerobic bacilli (including Enterobacteriaceae), anaerobic cocci, *Propionibacterium* species, anaerobic gram-negative cocci and bacilli, commensal *Mycobacterium* species, commensal *Mycoplasma* species, and occasional yeasts, all areas of the urinary tract above the urethra in a healthy human are sterile. Because noninvasive methods for collecting urine must rely on a specimen that has passed through a contaminated milieu, interpretation of the results of cultures of such specimens requires that some discriminatory criteria be used. The use of quantitative cultures for diagnosis of urinary tract infections, first popularized by Kass[2,3] has been modified to include separate quantitative criteria to be applied to different types of patients. Quantitative cultures of urine are still critical for diagnosis of UTI; however, the classical criterion of greater than 10^5 colony forming units of bacteria per milliliter of urine as highly indicative of infection must be modified

279

FIGURE 18.1
Overview of the anatomy of the urinary tract. (From Potter, P.H., and Perry, A.G. 1985. Fundamentals of nursing. The C.V. Mosby Co., St. Louis.)

for different patient categories. This chapter will deal with various aspects of urinary tract infection and its laboratory diagnosis.

18.1.b. Epidemiology and pathogenesis of urinary tract infections (UTI). UTI are primarily of two types: cystitis, which is infection of the bladder, and pyelonephritis, which is infection of the renal parenchyma. Pyelitis and ureteritis do occur but are not commonly diagnosed as such. Urethritis, which is very common, is generally discussed as a sexually transmitted disease (Chapter 19), although the acute urethral syndrome (see below) is not usually placed in the sexually transmitted category, strictly speaking. Urinary tract infections are more common in women than in men, due at least partially to the short female urethra and its proximity to the anus. Additionally, sexual

activity serves to increase the chances of bacterial contamination of the female urethra, pregnancy causes anatomical and hormonal changes that favor development of urinary tract infections, and changes in the genitourinary tract mucosa related to menopause may play a role. Colonization of the introitus by coliforms is a major background factor for recurrent bladder infection in females. It is estimated that approximately 20% of all women have a urinary tract infection at least once, with the incidence increasing with age. Among **asymptomatic** females of childbearing age or older, a culture yielding greater than 10^5 organisms per milliliter of a single bacterial species is very likely to correspond to UTI. If a repeat specimen also yields the same result with the same organism, presence of infection is 95% certain. The incidence of urinary tract infection among males is extremely low until after age 60; prostatic hypertrophy then contributes to development of UTI. Bacterial prostatitis contributes to the problem of recurrent cystitis in males. Any anatomic barrier to free flow of urine through the urinary tract contributes to development of UTI; involved are prostatic hypertrophy, neurogenic disorders, tumors, and stones. Previous infection with certain urea-splitting organisms, notably *Proteus* and related species, is often associated with the formation of urinary stones, which further predispose the patient to infection. The introduction of a foreign body into the urinary tract, especially one that remains in place for a time (such as a Foley catheter) carries a substantial risk of leading to infection. As many as 20% of all hospitalized patients who receive short-term catheterization develop a UTI. Consequently, UTI is the most common nosocomial infection in the United States and the infected urinary tract is the most common source of bacteremia.

Most infections involving the kidneys are acquired by the **ascending route (bacteria migrate from the bladder to reach the tissues of the kidneys).** However, yeast (usually *Candida albicans*), *Mycobacterium tuberculosis*, *Salmonella* species, *Leptospira* species, or *Staphylococcus aureus* in the urine often indicate pyelonephritis acquired via **hematogenous spread,** or the **descending route.**

Among the bacteria most commonly isolated from patients (overwhelmingly women) suffering from community acquired acute cystitis are *Escherichia coli, Klebsiella* species, other Enterobacteriaceae, and *Staphylococcus saprophyticus.* Hospitalized patients are most likely to be infected by *E. coli, Klebsiella* species, *Proteus mirabilis,* other Enterobacteriaceae, *Pseudomonas aeruginosa,* and enterococci. Other less commonly isolated agents are other gram-negative bacilli such as *Acinetobacter* and *Alcaligenes* species, other *Pseudomonas* species, *Citrobacter* species, *Gardnerella vag-*

inalis, beta hemolytic streptococci, and *Neisseria gonorrhoeae. Trichomonas vaginalis* may occasionally be observed in urinary sediment and *Schistosoma haematobium* can lodge in the urinary tract and release eggs into the urine.

In most hospitalized patients, UTI is preceded by urinary catheterization or other manipulation of the urinary tract. Although the pathogenesis of catheter-associated UTI is not fully understood, certain possibilities have been discussed. It is certain that soon after hospitalization, patients become colonized with bacteria endemic to the institution, often gram-negative aerobic and facultative bacilli carrying resistance markers. These bacteria colonize patients' skin, gastrointestinal tract, and mucous membranes, including the anterior urethra. With insertion of a catheter, the bacteria may be pushed along the urethra into the bladder or, in the case of an indwelling catheter, may migrate along the track between the catheter and the urethral mucosa, gaining access to the bladder. There has been some suggestion that nosocomial UTIs caused by certain bacteria, notably *Serratia marcescens*, are more likely to result in secondary bacteremia.

Certain women are more likely to suffer from chronic or recurrent UTIs. Several studies by Leffler and Svanborg-Eden[4] and Svanborg-Eden and Jodal[6] have shown stronger binding of *E. coli* isolated from infected urine to the genitourinary tract epithelial cells of infection-prone women than to noninfected controls. The organisms themselves may have adherence mechanisms that allow them to adhere well. Mechanisms by which other common etiologic agents of UTI produce disease are not yet well understood. It is probable that their presence induces an inflammatory response, which in turn causes tissue destruction and the characteristic pain, burning, and urinary frequency of acute cystitis. Damage to renal parenchyma that occurs in pyelonephritis results in flank pain, fever and other systemic symptoms, or sometimes no symptoms until much damage has occurred.

Another urinary tract infection that has only recently been fairly well understood is the **acute urethral syndrome,** studied by Stamm.[5] Women, primarily young, sexually active women, experience dysuria, frequency, and urgency but yield fewer than 10^5 organisms per milliliter urine on culture. As many as one third of all women who seek medical attention for complaints of symptoms of acute cystitis fall into this group. Although *Chlamydia trachomatis* and *N. gonorrhoeae* urethritis, anaerobic infection, genital herpes, and vaginitis account for some cases of acute urethral syndrome, most of these women are infected with organisms identical to those that cause cystitis, but in numbers less than 10^5/ml urine. One must use a cutoff of 10^2/ml, rather than 10^5/ml, in this group, but must insist on concomitant pyuria. The leukocyte esterase test (discussed below) is not sensitive enough for determining pyuria in these cases. Approximately 90% of these women have pyuria, an important discriminatory feature of infection. Recognition of this large class of patients with UTI that do not fit into classic categories has led to a reexamination of the criteria used to discriminate between urine specimens from patients with infection and those specimens from which culture results indicate only contamination.

Patients with true UTI whose urine may yield fewer numbers of bacteria than the classic 10^5/ml include infants and children, catheterized patients, patients who have received antibacterial agents previously, patients who consume large amounts of liquid and thus dilute bladder urine, symptomatic patients (usually with pyuria), patients with urinary obstruction that may prevent organisms from being excreted, and patients with pyelonephritis acquired from hematogenous spread (particularly yeast, *S. aureus*, and *M. tuberculosis* infections). For this reason, good communication between clinicians and microbiologists is essen-

tial for proper interpretation of urine culture results. If laboratorians also quantitate polymorphonuclear neutrophils in urine, as they should, the diagnostic value of a urine specimen is increased significantly.

18.2. Collection and Transport of Urine Specimens

Prevention of contamination by normal vaginal, perineal, and anterior urethral flora is the most important consideration for collection of a clinically relevant urine specimen. The least invasive procedure, that of the **clean-catch, midstream urine specimen collection,** must be performed carefully for optimal results, especially in females. Good patient education is essential. A method for collection of such a specimen is detailed in Chapter 6. Collection of reliable urine specimens from male patients is not difficult, as outlined in Chapter 6. If the clinician wishes to determine whether UTI in a male is localized to the bladder or the prostate using a noninvasive procedure, the "three-glass" collection procedure may be used. The first specimen collected is the initial 5-10 ml voided; this represents the "urethral" specimen. The next ounce or so of voided urine is discarded, and then an additional 10 ml is collected (the **"midstream"** specimen). After the bladder has been emptied, the patient is given a prostatic massage and the third specimen is the next 10 ml of urine and prostate secretions that accumulate. A higher count of organisms in the third specimen of urine than in the first indicates prostatic infection. Some physicians prefer to culture expressed prostatic secretions separately and then obtain another 10 ml urine specimen following this.

Slightly more invasive, urinary catheterization may allow collection of bladder urine with less urethral contamination. There is the risk, however, that urethral organisms will be introduced into the bladder with the catheter. **Suprapubic bladder aspiration,** withdrawal of bladder urine directly into a syringe through a percutaneously inserted needle, insures a contamination-free specimen. This procedure can be performed with very little risk in infants, small children, and adults with full bladders.

Urine, being an excellent supportive medium for growth of most bacteria, must be immediately refrigerated or preserved. Bacterial counts in refrigerated (4° C) urine remain constant for as long as 24 h. A urine transport tube, B-D Urine Culture Kit (Becton Dickinson Vacutainer Kits) containing boric acid, glycerol, and sodium formate, has been shown to preserve bacteria without refrigeration for as long as 24 h when greater than 100,000 organisms per milliliter were present in the initial urine specimen, as reviewed by Weinstein.[8] The system may inhibit the growth of certain organisms, and it must be used with 3-5 ml of urine. Another preservative system (Sage Products) may be less toxic to bacteria, although counts failed to remain completely stable for periods longer than 4 h. A new lyophilized system may prove to be more beneficial, but for populations of patients from whom colony counts of less than 100,000 organisms per milliliter might be clinically significant, the current preservative is not recommended. None of the kits has any advantage whatever over refrigeration except, perhaps, convenience.

18.3. Rapid Screening Tests for UTI

As many as 60%-80% of all urine specimens received for culture by the average hospital laboratory may contain only contaminants or no etiologic agents of infection. Procedures developed to quickly identify those urine specimens that will be "negative" on culture, to thus circumvent excessive use of media, technologist time, and the overnight incubation period, are discussed in this section. The Gram stain is the easiest and least expensive, and probably the most sensitive and reliable, screening method for identifying urine specimens that contain $>10^5$ colony-forming units (CFU) per milliliter. As outlined by Washington et al.,[7] a drop of

well-mixed urine is allowed to air dry. The smear is stained and examined under oil immersion (1,000 ×). Presence of at least one organism per field (examining 20 fields) correlates with significant bacteriuria ($>10^5$ CFU/ml). The presence of pus cells could also be detected in this way. Most microbiologists, for reasons that are not clear, are unwilling to adopt this procedure as part of the routine laboratory examination of urine specimens.

Several chemical tests, impregnated onto paper strips, can be used to assess parameters that may indicate UTI. The **Griess test** for presence of nitrate reducing enzymes, produced by the most common urinary tract pathogens, has been incorporated onto a paper strip that also tests for leukocyte esterase, an enzyme produced by polymorphonuclear neutrophils. These strips are available commercially (LN Strip and Chemstrip 9, Bio-Dynamics). Triphenyltetrazolium chloride is reduced by a number of commonly encountered urinary tract pathogens and can be impregnated into a strip test, but this test has not achieved wide usage. The sensitivity of these screening tests is not great enough to recommend their use (as a stand-alone test) in most circumstances.

Two automated methodologies have been used for screening urine specimens. The detection of bacterial adenosine triphosphate (ATP) by measuring light emitted by the reaction of luciferin-luciferase has been exploited by several companies (Chapter 11). After somatic cell ATP is removed by selectively disrupting somatic cells enzymatically, the bacterial cells are lysed and the released ATP is allowed to drive the light-producing reaction. Photons are measured, correlating with the numbers of bacteria present in the sample. The Turner System (Turner Designs) requires measurements to be made before and after a short incubation period, which allows bacteria to multiply. The Microscreen System (Analytical Luminescence Laboratory) measures the amount of ATP in the bacteria in the sample directly. These systems are somewhat expensive and do take time, and therefore are not suitable for every laboratory. Improvements in the ease of their use and decreasing test time will serve to make the luminescent tests more attractive to laboratories for screening urine specimens prior to culture in the future.

The Bac-T-Screen Bacteriuria Detection Device (Marion Laboratories) uses a different approach (Figure 18.2). Urine is forced through a filter paper, which retains both neutrophils and microorganisms. A dye is then added to the filter paper to visualize the particulate matter that has adhered. The intensity of color relates to the number of particles (Plate 18.1). This procedure, which takes less than 2 min, has been shown by Davis and co-workers[1] to detect 95% of all positive urine specimens, even if 100 organisms per milliliter are considered to be significant. The detection of pus cells as well as bacteria and yeast probably accounts for the increased sensitivity of this system at low numbers of CFU. Organisms likely to be associated with false negative results include enterococci and *Pseudomonas aeruginosa;* the reason for this is not known.

Screening of urine can also be accomplished simply by enumerating polymorphonuclear neutrophils (PMNs) in uncentrifuged specimens, which correlates fairly well with the number of PMNs excreted per hour, the best indicator of the state of the host. Patients with more than 400,000 PMNs excreted into the urine per hour are likely to be infected, and

FIGURE 18.2
The Bac-T-Screen bacteriuria detection instrument (Marion Laboratories).

the presence of more than 10 PMNs/mm^3 correlates very well with this excretion rate and with infection. This test can be performed using a hemocytometer, but it is not easily incorporated into the workflow of most microbiology laboratories. The standard urinalysis (usually done in hematology or chemistry sections) includes an examination of the **centrifuged** sediment of urine for enumeration of PMNs, results of which do not correlate well with either PMN excretion rate or the presence of infection.

Given the importance of the 10^2/ml count and the PMN count, the screening systems mentioned above, other than Gram stain, PMN count, and perhaps the Bac-T-Screen device, should not be used. In general, there is a cost advantage to screening only in laboratories receiving a large number of inappropriate specimens; accordingly, education of physicians is one important approach. Good medical practice and cost-effective microbiology dictate that only urine from patients with symptoms of UTI plus a selected group expected to have asymptomatic bacteriuria (e.g., patients in the first trimester of pregnancy) should be cultured. Other situations in which patients with no symptoms of UTI might be cultured include bacteremia of unknown source, patients with urinary tract obstruction, follow-up after removal of an indwelling urinary catheter, and follow-up of previous therapy. It must also be remembered that screening may delay culture results, especially if one of the rapid, automated instruments for urine culturing is used.

18.4. Methods for Culturing Urine and Interpretive Criteria

18.4.a. Routine culture. Once it has been determined that a urine specimen should be cultured for isolation of the common agents of UTI, a measured amount of urine is inoculated to each of the appropriate media. The urine should be mixed thoroughly before plating. The plates can be inoculated using disposable

sterile plastic tips with a displacement pipetting device, calibrated to deliver a constant amount, but this method is somewhat cumbersome. Most commonly, microbiologists use a **calibrated loop** designed to deliver a known volume, either 0.01 or 0.001 ml of urine. These loops, made of platinum or other material, can be obtained from a number of laboratory supply companies (Appendix). They must be inserted into the urine in a cup **vertically** or they will pick up more than the desired volume of urine. A widely used method is described in Procedure 18.1. The choice of which media to inoculate is dependent upon the patient population served and the preference of the microbiologist. The use of a 5% sheep blood agar plate and a MacConkey agar plate will allow detection of most gram-negative bacilli and staphylococci. Enterococci and other streptococci, however, may be obscured by heavy growth of Enterobacteriaceae. The addition of a selective plate for gram-positive organisms, such as Columbia colistin-nalidixic acid agar (CNA) or phenylethyl alcohol agar (Chapter 8) may add discriminatory capability but also adds cost to the procedure. We (EJB) routinely inoculate urine specimens to a MacConkey and a CNA plate. Any urine specimens received from female patients (who may be infected with *Staphylococcus saprophyticus*, which is somewhat inhibited on CNA) or that were collected by any technique other than clean-catch, midstream urine collection are additionally inoculated to sheep blood agar. For our hospital, this system works well.

18.4.b. Interpreting culture results. For routine urine cultures, growth of more than three species is usually considered as indicative of contamination. For such cultures, the organisms are minimally identified (such as lactose-positive gram-negative rods and coagulase-negative staphylococci) and enumerated. Susceptibility tests are not performed. Plates from such cultures are held, however, as there are situations in which growth of more than three or-

PROCEDURE 18.1. INOCULATING URINE WITH A CALIBRATED LOOP

1. Flame the inoculating loop (usually calibrated to deliver 0.001 ml). Place it upright without touching any surface to cool.
2. Mix the urine thoroughly and remove the top of the container. If the urine is in a small diameter tube, the surface tension will alter the amount of specimen picked up by the loop. A quantitative pipette should be considered if the urine cannot be transferred to a larger container.
3. Insert the loop vertically into the urine (Figure 18.3) to allow urine to adhere to the loop.
4. Spread the loopful of urine over the surface of the agar plate as shown in Figure 18.4
5. Without reflaming, insert the loop vertically into the urine again for transfer of a loopful to a second plate. Repeat for each plate.
6. Incubate plates for at least 18 h at 35°-37° C in air. Colonies are counted on each plate. The number of CFU is multiplied by 1000 (if a 0.001 ml loop was used) or by 100 (if a 0.01 ml loop was used) to determine the number of microorganisms per milliliter in the original specimen.
7. Reincubate plates with no growth or tiny colonies for an additional 24 h, because antimicrobial treatment or other factors may inhibit initial growth, before discarding plates.
8. It is desirable to store the loop (handle down) in a test tube taped to the wall, rather than flat on the bench, in order to prevent bending which would destroy the calibration.

ganisms may be significant (e.g., patients with Foley catheters) and the physician always has the option of calling the laboratory to request more definitive studies. Growth of less than 10,000 CFU/ml of one or two organisms may indicate infection. The organisms are identified, but susceptibility studies are not performed unless the clinician notifies the laboratory to do so. One or two strains growing in numbers greater than 10,000/ml are identified and tested for antimicrobial susceptibilities. A pure culture of *Staphylococcus aureus* is considered to be significant regardless of the number of CFU, and susceptibility tests are performed. The presence of yeast in any number is reported to physicians, and pure cultures of a yeast are identified as to species.

18.4.c. Unusual etiologic agents of UTI. Culture methods for isolation of mycobacteria, *Haemophilus influenzae, Leptospira, Gardnerella vaginalis, Trichomonas vaginalis,* and other more rarely encountered agents of UTI are discussed in the appropriate other areas of this book. *Salmonella* are recovered during the early stages of typhoid fever; their presence should be immediately reported to the physician. If anaerobes are suspected, percutaneous bladder tap should be done by the physician unless urine can be obtained from the upper urinary tract (e.g., from a nephrostomy tube). Most important for detecting such agents is communication to the laboratory by the clinician that such an agent is suspected. However, the laboratory can exert some initiative here as

Loop is touched to the center of the plate, from which the inoculum is spread in a line across the diameter of the plate.

Without flaming or re-entering urine, loop is drawn across the entire plate, crossing the first inoculum streak numerous times to produce isolated colonies.

FIGURE 18.3
Method for inserting a calibrated loop into urine to ensure that the proper amount of specimen will adhere to the loop.

FIGURE 18.4
Method for streaking with calibrated urine loop to produce isolated colonies and countable CFUs of organisms.

well. In cases of "sterile pyuria," Gram stain may reveal unusual organisms with distinctive morphology (*H. influenzae* and anaerobes, for example). Presence of any organisms on smear that do not grow in culture is an important clue to the cause of the infection. The laboratory can then take the action necessary to optimize chances for recovery, whether it includes inoculating a special medium or examining a spun sediment under phase contrast microscopy.

18.4.d. Antibody-coated bacteria test. Developed in 1974, the **antibody-coated bacteria test** is used in an attempt to determine whether a patient is suffering from bladder infection (cystitis) or renal tissue infection (pyelonephritis), using a noninvasive technique. Previous methods required collection of urine directly from the renal pelvis, bilateral ureteral catheterization after bladder washout, or direct tissue biopsy. Since simple bladder infection can usually be effectively treated by administration of a single large dose of an appropriate

antimicrobial agent, it is important to be able to differentiate such an infection from one that requires more prolonged therapy. Incidentally, many clinicians use response to single dose treatment as a means of distinguishing between upper and lower tract infection. The antibody-coated bacteria test consists of washing the centrifuged sediment of urine containing large numbers of bacteria and then staining the washed bacteria with fluorescein-conjugated antihuman globulin. The bacterial cells are again washed to remove nonspecifically bound conjugate and the bacteria are examined under ultraviolet light. If at least one-fourth of the bacteria are fluorescent, indicating the presence of human immunoglobulin on their surface, the test is considered positive and the patient is considered to have a more deep-seated infection than cystitis. Although not difficult to perform, lack of standardization among laboratories and lack of uniformly available reagents have caused confusion in interpretation of results among different laboratories. Furthermore, there may be both false positive and false negative results. The test has not been widely accepted, primarily because patients can be given a short course of therapy empirically. Those who show bacteriologic and symptomatic cure are then assumed to have had uncomplicated bladder infection. This test seems to be useful in certain settings, but, in its present state, is not warranted for general testing.

18.5. Automated Nonscreening Methods for Laboratory Diagnosis of UTI

Several instruments have been developed for the "hands-off" detection of bacteriuria. The principles employed by these systems are described in Chapter 11. The Autobac (General Diagnostics) uses a series of nephelometric determinations over time to identify numbers of bacteria in urine. The urine specimen is introduced to the instrument in a cuvette, which allows the urine to be diluted out into growth media. Cuvettes containing different substrates can be inoculated with diluted specimen. During incubation with shaking, growth in the cuvette is periodically monitored by measuring the amount of light scatter that occurs in the growth wells compared to a control well. An internal computer processes the information and generates results. Within 6 h, most negative urine specimens can be identified. Those urine specimens that contain significant counts of bacteria (CFU $>10^5$) are usually identified within 3 h. Preliminary identification of the organisms is achieved by determining in which substrates growth occurred. Note that urine containing less than 10^5 CFU/ml will not be considered positive with such a system.

The AutoMicrobic System (Vitek Systems) is the most labor-free screening system. Once the urine is introduced into the tiny wells of a plastic substrate card by vacuum suction and the card is placed into the instrument, it is incubated and examined periodically by measuring the amount of light that passes through the individual wells. The wells contain substrates that can be utilized by only certain etiologic agents of UTI. After 6-8 h, microorganisms will grow in the appropriate substrate wells and be detected by increased turbidity. The internal computer issues a colony count and a preliminary identification of the agent or agents identified. In this system as well, low counts of bacteria or yeast will be considered negative urine cultures.

The MS-2 (Abbott Laboratories Diagnostics Division) uses a cuvette system similar to that of the Autobac. Growth in various wells is identified by the amount of light that can be transmitted through the cuvettes. Measurements are taken periodically, and increased turbidity is assessed in comparison with control cuvettes. Urine specimens can be screened within 3 h, as is true in most cases for the other automated systems. It is possible that with this system the sensitivity for the lower limit of detection may be adjusted for fewer CFU than for some of the other instruments, though such parameters have not been studied.

Since most clinical laboratories receive more urine specimens than specimens from any other category, it is important that laboratories develop an efficient, cost-effective way of handling them. It seems that some form of preliminary screening system to rule out negative cultures, combined with a standard method for quantifying and identifying significant etiologic agents of UTI, will be of most benefit to the patients being served. Strategies employed by laboratories in hospitals that must cut costs without sacrificing patient-relevant quality are discussed in Chapter 4.

REFERENCES

1. Davis, J.R., Stager, C.E., and Araj, G.F. 1984. Laboratory evaluation of a bacteriuria detection device for urine screening. Am. J. Clin. Pathol. 31:48.
2. Kass, E.H. 1956. Asymptomatic infections of the urinary tract. Trans. Assoc. Am. Physicians 69:56.
3. Kass, E.H. 1960. The role of asymptomatic bacteriuria in the pathogenesis of pyelonephritis. In Quinn, E.L., and Kass, E.H., editors: Biology of pyelonephritis. Little, Brown & Co., Boston.
4. Leffler, H., and Svanborg-Eden, C. 1981. Glycolipid receptors for uropathogenic *Escherichia coli* on human erythrocytes and uroepithelial cells. Infect. Immun. 34:920.
5. Stamm, W.E. 1980. Causes of the acute urethral syndrome in women. N. Engl. J. Med. 303:409.
6. Svanborg-Eden, C., and Jodal, U. 1979. Attachment of *Escherichia coli* to urinary sediment epithelial cells from UYIT-prone and healthy children. Infect. Immun. 26:837.
7. Washington, J.A. II, White, C.M., Laganiere, M., and Smith, L.H. 1981. Detection of significant bacteriuria by microscopic examination of urine. Lab. Med. 12:294.
8. Weinstein, M.P. 1983. Evaluation of liquid and lyophilized preservatives for urine culture. J. Clin. Microbiol. 18:912.

BIBLIOGRAPHY

Bartlett, R.C. 1984. Urine screening—to screen or not to screen. Clin. Microbiol. Newsletter 6:29.

Edberg, S.C. 1981. Methods of quantitative microbiological analyses that support the diagnosis, treatment, and prognosis of human infection. CRC Crit. Rev. Microbiol. 8:339.

Fihn, S., and Stamm, W.E. 1983. Management of women with acute dysuria. In Rund, D.A., and Wolcott, B.W., editors: Emergency medicine annual, vol. 2. Appleton-Century-Crofts, East Norwalk, Conn.

Gabre-Kidan, T., Lipsky, B.A., and Plorde, J.J. 1984. *Haemophilus influenzae* as a cause of urinary tract infections in men. Arch. Intern. Med. 144:1623.

Platt, R. 1983. Quantitative definition of bacteriuria. Am. J. Med. 75:44.

Stamm, W.E., and Turck, M. 1983. Urinary tract infection. Year Book Medical Publishers Inc., Chicago.

Stamm, W.E. 1983. Measurement of pyuria and its relation to bacteriuria. Am. J. Med. 75:53.

Stamm, W.E. 1983. Interpretation of urine cultures. Clin. Microbiol. Newsletter 5:15.

Thomas, V.L. 1983. The antibody-coated bacteria test: Uses and findings. Lab Management, 21:39.

Wright, D.N., and Matsen, J.M. 1984. Diagnosing urinary tract infection. Diagn. Med. 7:44.

19 Genital and Sexually Transmitted Pathogens

19.1. Normal and Pathogenic Flora of the Genital Tract

The lining of the normal human genital tract is a mucosal layer made up of transitional, columnar, and squamous epithelial cells. A variety of species of commensal bacteria colonize these surfaces, causing no harm to the host except under abnormal circumstances, and helping to prevent the adherence of pathogenic organisms. Normal urethral flora include coagulase negative staphylococci and corynebacteria, as well as a number of anaerobes. The vulva and penis, especially the area underneath the prepuce (foreskin) of the uncircumcised male, may harbor *Mycobacterium smegmatis* along with other gram-positive bacteria. The flora of the female genital tract (Figure 19.1) varies with the pH and estrogen concentration of the mucosa, which is dependent on the age of the host. Prepubescent and postmenopausal women harbor primarily staphylococci and corynebacteria, the same flora present on surface epithelium, while women of reproductive age may harbor large numbers of facultative bacteria such as Enterobacteriaceae, streptococci, and staphylococci, as well as anaerobes such as lactobacilli, anaerobic non-spore-forming bacilli and cocci, and clostridia. The numbers of anaerobic flora remain constant throughout the monthly cycle. Many women carry group B beta hemolytic streptococci (*Streptococcus aga-*

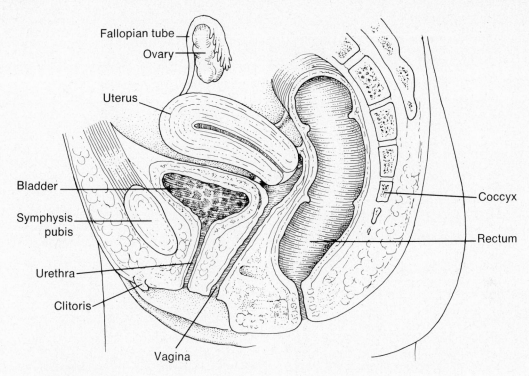

FIGURE 19.1
Diagrammatic representation of the female genital tract. (From Broadwell, D.C., and Jackson, B.S. 1982. Principles of ostomy care. The C.V. Mosby Co., St. Louis.)

lactiae), which may be transmitted to the neonate as it passes through the birth canal, causing devastating systemic disease. Treatment of the mother to prevent carriage of the organism is not feasible, and whether or not a colonized infant will become ill cannot be predicted. Although yeast (acquired from the gastrointestinal tract) may be transiently recovered from the female vaginal tract, they are not normal flora of the genital tract. Lactobacilli are the predominant organisms in secretions from normal, healthy vaginas (Figure 19.2).

Infections of the genital tract in normal females above or below child-bearing age are often a result of irritation or a foreign body and are caused by the same organisms that cause skin wound infections. Genital tract infections caused by sexually transmitted agents in chil-

dren (preadolescents) are most often the result of sexual abuse. The laboratory should treat specimens from such patients with extreme care, carefully identifying and documenting all isolates, since medicolegal implications exist.

Chlamydia trachomatis, Gardnerella vaginalis, Neisseria gonorrhoeae and *meningitidis, Ureaplasma urealyticum, Mycoplasma hominis,* and other organisms may be acquired as people engage in sexual activity. The organisms may exist in the genital tract in the absence of any noticeable pathology. Although the role of *M. hominis* in the pathogenesis of genital infection is unclear, it has been associated with infections in females, such as pelvic inflammatory disease, pyelonephritis, and postpartum fever. *U. urealyticum* is related to nongonococcal urethritis in males and perhaps to low birth weight

FIGURE 19.2
Predominance of lactobacilli in Gram stain from healthy vagina.

of the babies of infected females. Organisms recovered from the genital tract that are usually considered to be pathogens include the following:

Bacteria
    Chlamydia trachomatis
    Gardnerella vaginalis
    Haemophilus ducreyi
    Mycoplasma hominis
    Neisseria gonorrhoeae
    Neisseria meningitidis
    Ureaplasma urealyticum
Fungi
    Candida species
    Other yeast
Viruses
    Cytomegalovirus
    Herpes simplex virus
Protozoans
    Trichomonas vaginalis

In addition, a number of other agents cause genital tract disease but are not routinely isolated from clinical specimens; included are the viruses of molluscum contagiosum and genital warts (condylomata acuminata), *Calymmato-bacterium granulomatis* (Chapter 39), *Trepo-*

nema pallidum (Chapter 31), and ectoparasites such as scabies and lice (Chapter 44). Infections with more than one agent are not uncommon. Such dual or concurrent infections should always be considered.

Homosexual practices and increasingly common heterosexual practices of anal-genital intercourse have allowed a number of gastrointestinal and systemic pathogens to also be considered etiologic agents of sexually transmitted diseases (STD). The intestinal protozoa *Giardia lamblia*, *Entamoeba histolytica*, and *Crypto-sporidium* sp. (Chapter 44) are significant causes of STD, especially among homosexual populations. In the same group of patients, fecal pathogens such as *Salmonella*, *Shigella* (both discussed in Chapter 27), and *Campylo-bacter* (Chapter 30) are often transmitted sexually. Oral-genital practices probably allow *N. meningitidis* (Chapter 26) to colonize and infect the genital tract. Viruses shed in secretions or present in blood (cytomegalovirus, hepatitis B and non-A non-B, and the human T cell lymphotropic virus [HTLV III] of acquired immune deficiency syndrome [AIDS]) are increasingly being spread by sexual practices. The spectrum of diseases (not normally considered to be sexually transmitted) that accompanies AIDS is discussed in Chapter 23.

Certain pathogens are usually sought in specimens from lesions on surface epithelium of or near the genital tract. These include herpes simplex virus, *Haemophilus ducreyi*, and *T. pallidum*. *C. inguinale* is recovered from biopsy material taken from beneath the characteristic lesion. Collection of specimens from lesions will be discussed in a separate section below.

19.2. Collection and Transport of Specimens from the Urethra and Vagina

Urethral discharge may occur in both males and females infected with certain pathogens, such as *N. gonorrhoeae* and *T. vaginalis*. Because the discharge is usually less profuse and may be masked more easily in the female by vaginal secretions, the presence of infection is more likely to be asymptomatic in females. *U. urealyticum* and *C. trachomatis* can also be isolated from male urethral discharge.

A urogenital swab designed expressly for collection of such specimens should be used. These swabs are made of cotton that has been treated with charcoal to adsorb material toxic to gonococci, wrapped tightly over one end of a thin wooden stick that has also been treated to remove resins and toxic chemicals (Chapter 6). Certain wooden sticks may be toxic to mycoplasma and chlamydiae; plastic sticks are generally less toxic. Rayon-tipped swabs on thin wire may also be used for collection of specimens for isolation of mycoplasma and chlamydiae. Calcium alginate swabs are generally more toxic for herpes virus, gonococci, and mycoplasma than are treated cotton swabs. Rare lots of calcium alginate swabs have been toxic for chlamydiae.

The swab is inserted approximately 2 cm into the urethra and rotated gently before withdrawing. Since chlamydiae are intracellular pathogens, it is important to remove epithelial cells from the urethral mucosa. Separate samples for cultivation of gonococci and chlamydiae or ureaplasma are required. In cases where there is profuse urethral discharge, particularly in males, the discharge may be collected externally without inserting a sampling device into the urethra.

Since *T. vaginalis* may be present in urethral discharge, material for culture should be collected by swab as above, but a swab should also be placed into a tube containing 0.5 ml of sterile physiological saline and hand-delivered to the laboratory immediately. Direct wet mounts and cultures can be performed from this specimen. Commercial media for culture of trichomonas are available. The first few drops of voided urine may also be a suitable specimen for recovery of trichomonas from infected males, if it is inoculated into culture media immediately.

Organisms that cause purulent vaginal discharge (vaginitis) include *T. vaginalis*, yeast, gonococci, and, rarely, beta hemolytic streptococci. The same organisms that cause purulent infections in the urethra may also infect the epithelial cells in the cervical opening. Mucus is removed by gently rubbing the area with a cotton ball. A special swab (the urethral swab described above) is inserted into the cervical canal, rotated and moved from side to side for 30 seconds before removal. Swabs are handled as urethral swabs for isolation of *Trichomonas* and gonococci. Chlamydiae cause a mucopurulent cervicitis with much discharge. Endocervical specimens are obtained after the vagina has been exposed by insertion of a speculum, which allows visualization of vaginal architecture. The speculum is moistened with warm water, since many lubricants contain antibacterial agents. Because the normal vaginal secretions contain great quantities of bacteria, care must be exercised to avoid contaminating swabs for culture by contact with these secretions. Swabs of Bartholin gland exudate may also be obtained for culture. Care must be exercised to avoid contamination with vaginal secretions.

In addition to cervical specimens, which are particularly useful for isolation of gonococci, *Mycoplasma*, and chlamydiae, vaginal discharge specimens may be collected. Organisms likely to cause vaginal discharge include *Trichomonas*, yeast, and the agents of **bacterial vaginosis** (presumably *G. vaginalis* and various anaerobic bacteria). The absence of inflammatory cells in the vaginal discharge is suggestive of bacterial vaginosis (formerly called nonspecific vaginitis). Swabs are dipped into the fluid that collects in the posterior fornix of the vagina.

Swabs collected for isolation of gonococci may be transported to the laboratory in modified Stuart's or Amies charcoal transport media, held at room temperature until inoculated to culture media. Good recovery of gonococci is possible if swabs are cultured within 24 h of collection. Material that must be held longer

PROCEDURE 19.1. PREPARATION OF SUCROSE BUFFER (2-SP) FOR TRANSPORT OF *CHLAMYDIA* AND *MYCOPLASMA* SPECIMENS

A. Preparation of stock sucrose buffer.
   1. Dissolve 68.5 g sucrose in 100 ml distilled water.
   2. Dissolve 2.1 g K_2HPO_4 in 60 ml distilled water.
   3. Dissolve 1.1 g KH_2PO_4 in 40 ml distilled water.
   4. Mix all three solutions and add distilled water to 1 liter total volume.
   5. Boil the solution for 30 min.
   6. Cool to room temperature before preparing transport medium.
B. Preparation of 2-SP.
   7. To 100 ml stock sucrose buffer, add 10 ml fetal calf serum (commercially available), 2 mg gentamicin powder, 0.5 mg amphotericin powder, and 10 mg vancomycin powder (suppliers listed in Chapter 13).
   8. Dispense in 1 ml amounts into sterile, screw-topped plastic disposable test tubes, 16 × 150 mm.
   9. Store at −20° C for up to 6 months.

Modified from Mårdh. 1984. In Holmes, Mårdh, Sparling, and Wiesner, editors. Sexually transmitted diseases. McGraw-Hill Book Co., New York; and Gordon, Harper, Quan, et al. 1969. J. Infect. Dis. 120:451.

than 24 h should be inoculated directly to one of the commercial systems designed for recovery of gonococci, described below. Swabs for isolation of chlamydiae and *Mycoplasma* are best transported in sucrose buffer with antibiotics (2-SP), as described in Procedure 19.1. If the specimens are not going to be inoculated to cell culture within several hours, they should be refrigerated but **never frozen.**

19.3. Direct Microscopic Examination

In addition to culture, urethral discharge may be examined by Gram stain for the presence of gram-negative intracellular diplococci (Plate 19.1), usually indicative of gonorrhea in males. After inoculation to culture media, the swab is rolled over the surface of a glass slide, covering an area of at least 1 cm.[2] If the Gram stain is diagnostic, cultures of urethral discharge need not be performed. In homosexual males, however, *N. meningitidis* has been increasingly isolated from such specimens, so that the assumption that gram-negative diplococci are gonococci may no longer be valid for that patient population. Urethral smears from females may also be examined, but presumptive diagnosis of gonorrhea from vaginal smears is only reliable if the microscopist is experienced, since normal vaginal flora such as *Veillonella* or occasional gram-negative coccobacilli may resemble gonococci. If extracellular organisms resembling *N. gonorrhoeae* are seen, the microscopist should continue to examine the smear for intracellular diplococci for a longer time period than if no suspicious bacteria are seen. Cultures should always be performed on specimens from females. Some strains of *N. gonorrhoeae* are sensitive to the amount of vancomycin present in selective media. If suspicious organisms seen on smear fail to grow in culture, reculture on chocolate agar without antibiotics may be warranted.

FIGURE 19.3
The commercial collection and monoclonal antibody stain test system for chlamydiae (MicroTrak, Syva Co.).

FIGURE 19.4
"Clue cells" in vaginal discharge, suggestive of bacterial vaginosis.

Within the last several years, very sensitive fluorescein-conjugated monoclonal antibody reagents have been developed for visualization of the inclusions of *C. trachomatis* in cell cultures and elementary bodies in urethral and cervical cell specimens (further discussed in Chapter 38). The reagents are available commercially in a complete collection and test system (Figure 19.3 MicroTrak, Syva Co.). The swab is rolled over the surface of a special glass slide and the material is fixed with acetone. In some studies, the sensitivity of visual detection of chlamydiae with these newer reagents has been similar to that of culture, although such comparative results are obtained only by technologists who are experienced in fluorescent techniques and when the slides are examined quite thoroughly. False positive results should not occur if at least 10 morphologically compatible fluorescing organisms are seen on the entire smear. Use of this and other rapid antigen detection techniques (described below) should greatly facilitate diagnosis and increase our knowledge of the prevalence and epidemiology of genital chlamydial infections. Further discussion can be found in Chapter 38. No direct visual methods exist for detection of myco-

plasma at this time, but it is likely that a nucleic acid probe (Chapter 10) will be available soon.

Examination of a wet preparation of vaginal discharge is the most useful rapid diagnostic test for such specimens. Motile trophozoites of *Trichomonas* can be visualized in 80% of cases and budding cells and pseudohyphae of yeast can also be easily identified. The addition of 10% KOH serves two functions: by dissolving host cell protein, it enhances the visibility of fungal elements, and by causing the discharge to become alkaline, it elicits the fishy, amine-like odor associated with bacterial vaginosis.

Bacterial vaginosis is characterized by a profuse, homogeneous discharge with a disagreeable odor. The discharge is primarily sloughed epithelial cells, many of which are completely covered by tiny, gram-variable rods and coccobacilli. These cells are called **clue cells** (Figure 19.4). *G. vaginalis* has been associated with the syndrome historically, but the synergistic activity of a number of anaerobic organisms, including non–*Bacteroides fragilis*, *Bacteroides* species, anaerobic streptococci, and perhaps *Mobiluncus* species (curved, motile rods) seems to contribute to the pathology.

Although *G. vaginalis* can be cultured on a human blood bilayer plate and identified within 1 h (Chapter 39), diagnosis of bacterial vaginosis is best made using the following criteria. Three of four of the following characteristics are diagnostic for this syndrome: homogeneous, gray discharge; clue cells seen on wet mount or Gram stain; amine or fishy odor elicited by the addition of a drop of 10% KOH to the discharge on a slide or on the speculum; and pH greater than 4.5. The absence of a predominance of lactobacilli on Gram stain, present in the normal vagina (Figure 19.2), is another sign of bacterial vaginosis.

PROCEDURE 19.2. PREPARATION OF HENDERSON GC MEDIUM

1. Prepare lysed horse blood by adding 10% saponin (Fisher Scientific Co.) to defibrinated horse blood to a final concentration of 0.2%.
2. Prepare yeast dialysate by mixing 900 g active dry bakers' yeast (Fleischmann's, available at a grocery store) with 2.5 liters of distilled water. Autoclave for 10 min at 110° C and cool. Fill 4.8 mm diameter dialysis tubing (Fisher Scientific Co.) with the yeast suspension after softening the tubing in distilled water. Dialyse the yeast suspension against 2 liters of distilled water for 48 h at 4° C. Filter the dialysate through Whatman number 2 filter paper and dispense in 25 ml volumes. Autoclave the final yeast suspension for 10 min at 115° C and store at 4° C. The suspension remains usable for several months.
3. Prepare a stock 50% (vol/vol) glucose solution by adding 500 g glucose (Sigma Chemical Co.) to 680 ml distilled water. Dispense into 16 × 125 mm glass screw-capped tubes, autoclave for 10 min at 115° C, and store at 4° C until used.
4. Prepare the final agar as follows:

GC medium base (Difco Laboratories)	36 g
Yeast dialysate	25 ml
Stock glucose	10 ml
Horse serum	30 ml
Lysed horse blood	20 ml
Colistin	7.5 mg
Lincomycin hydrochloride	4 mg
Amphotericin B	2.5 mg
Trimethoprim lactate	5 mg
Distilled water	1,000 ml

Antibacterial agents are available from suppliers listed in Chapter 13. Concentrated solutions of antibacterial drugs may be prepared in distilled water and stored at −20° C until used. Autoclave the GC agar base in the distilled water according to manufacturer's instructions. Cool to 56° C and add the other ingredients aseptically. Pour plates, approximately 20 ml per plate.

Modified from Anstey, Gun-Munro, Rennie, et al. 1984. J. Clin Microbiol 20:905.

19.4. Direct Inoculation and Laboratory Handling of Urethral and Vaginal Specimens

Samples for isolation of gonococci may be inoculated directly to culture media, obviating the need for transport. Several commercially produced systems have been developed for this purpose (Appendix), and many clinicians inoculate standard plates directly if convenient access to an incubator is available. Modified Thayer-Martin medium is most commonly used, although New York City (NYC) medium has the added advantage of supporting the growth of mycoplasma as well as gonococci. These media are discussed in Chapter 26. A modification of NYC medium (Procedure 19.2) yields comparable results for growth of *N. gonorrhoeae* but costs as much as 70% less and is easier to prepare. Excellent recovery of gonococci is the rule when specimens are inoculated directly to these media or their modifications in Transgrow bottles or onto the surface of Jembec plates (Figure 19.5). Both media are commercially available. The swab containing material is rolled across the agar with constant turning to expose all surfaces to the medium. Transgrow bottles are filled with an atmosphere of increased CO_2, so they must be held upright during inoculation, a procedure often forgotten by busy clinicians. The Jembec plate, which generates its own increased CO_2 atmosphere by means of a tablet of sodium bicarbonate, is inoculated in a W pattern. It may be cross-streaked with a sterile loop in the laboratory (Figure 19.6).

FIGURE 19.5
Transgrow bottle, a self-contained agar medium and CO_2 atmosphere for culture and transport of *Neisseria gonorrhoeae*. The physician holds the bottle upright while rolling a swab across the agar surface to inoculate the medium. CO_2, which is heavier than air, thus remains in the bottle to enhance growth of the organism.

FIGURE 19.6
Method of cross-streaking Jembec plate after original specimen has been inoculated by rolling the swab over the surface of the agar in a W pattern.

T. vaginalis may be cultured from discharge material (Chapter 44) or direct wet preparations may be examined for the presence of motile trophozoites, as mentioned above and in Chapter 7. Specimens must be inoculated to other media in addition to gonococcal selective agar for isolation of yeast, streptococci, and *G. vaginalis*. Yeast will grow well on Columbia agar base with 5% sheep blood and colistin and nalidixic acid (CNA), as will most strains of *Gardnerella*, although more selective media are available (mentioned below). Most yeast and the streptococci will also grow on standard blood agar; thus, the addition of special fungal media such as SABHI or brain heart infusion agar (Chapter 8) seems unwarranted.

19.5. Infections of the Female Pelvis and Male Internal Genital Organs

Pelvic inflammatory disease is often caused by the same organisms that cause cervicitis or by organisms that comprise normal flora of the vaginal mucosa. Because of the profuse normal flora of the vaginal tract, species of which may be involved in peritoneal infection, specimens must be collected in such a way as to prevent vaginal flora contamination. Aspirated material collected by needle and syringe represents the best specimen. If this cannot be obtained at the time of surgery or laparoscopy, culdocentesis, following decontamination of the vagina by povidone-iodine, is satisfactory. Aspirated material should be placed into an anaerobic transport container. The presence of either mixed anaerobic flora, gonococci, or both can be rapidly detected from a Gram stain. Direct examination with fluorescent monoclonal antibody stain may also detect chlamydiae. All such specimens should be inoculated to media that allow the recovery of anaerobic, facultative, and aerobic bacteria, gonococci, fungi, mycoplasma, and chlamydiae. All material collected from normally sterile body sites in the genital tract should be inoculated to chocolate agar and placed into a suitable broth such as chopped meat medium or thioglycolate, in addition to the other types of media noted above.

Infections of the male prostate, epididymis, and testes are usually bacterial. In younger men, chlamydiae predominate as the cause of epididymitis and possibly of prostatitis. Urine or discharge collected via the urethra is the specimen of choice unless an abscess is drained surgically or by needle and syringe. Urine (the first few milliliters of voided urine) may be collected before and after prostatic massage to try to pinpoint the anatomic site of the infection. Cultures are inoculated to support the growth of anaerobic, facultative, and aerobic bacteria, as well as gonococci. In patients with suspected AIDS or other immunosuppression-related systemic cytomegalovirus disease, semen or urine can be cultured for the virus. The specimen is transported immediately to the virology laboratory for culture. Refrigeration may preserve the virus for several hours; specimens that must be held longer should be placed into viral transport media, as discussed in Chapter 42.

19.6. Specimens Obtained from Skin and Mucous Membrane Lesions

External genital lesions are usually either vesicular or ulcerative in nature. Causes of lesions can be determined by physical examination, histologic examination, or by microscopic examination or culture of exudate. **Since any genital lesion may be highly contagious, all manipulations of lesion material should be carried out by clinicians wearing gloves.**

19.6.a. Examination of vesicular lesions. Vesicles are almost always attributable to viruses, and herpes simplex is the most common cause. Material from the base of a vesicle may be spread onto the surface of a slide and examined for the typical multinucleated giant cells of herpes or stained by immunofluorescent antibody stains for viral antigens. Additionally or alternatively, the material is transported for culture of the virus, as outlined in Procedure 19.3.

PROCEDURE 19.3. COLLECTION OF MATERIAL FROM SUSPECTED HERPETIC LESIONS

1. Vesicles should be opened with a small gauge needle or Dacron-tipped swab.
2. Rub the base of the lesion vigorously with a small cotton- or Dacron-tipped swab to recover infected cells.
3. Place the swab into viral transport medium (described in Chapter 42) and refrigerate until inoculated to culture media. Specimens may be stored at −70° C for extended periods without loss of viral yield.
4. If large vesicles are present, material for culture may be aspirated directly by needle and syringe.
5. Material from another lesion can be applied directly to a glass slide for a Tzanck preparation (histology) with Wright-Giemsa or fluorescent antibody stain for detection of multinucleated giant cells.

There are several commercial fluorescein-conjugated monoclonal and polyclonal antibodies directed against herpetic antigens of either type 1 or 2. When fluorescent-antibody-stained lesion material containing enough cells is viewed under ultraviolet light, the diagnosis can be made in 70%-90% of cases. Laboratories that routinely process genital material for herpes should be using immunofluorescent staining reagents in emergency situations; otherwise, culture, which is generally positive in 2-3 days, is the method of choice. Nonfluorescent markers such as biotin-avidin-horseradish peroxidase or alkaline phosphatase have also been conjugated to these specific antibodies, often allowing earlier detection of herpes-infected cells in tissue culture monolayers. Such reagents are being perfected for use directly on clinical material. Use of this technique is described in Chapter 10.

19.6.b. Examination of ulcerative lesions. Ulcerative lesions are usually one of the following: a syphilitic chancre (caused by *T. pallidum*), the chancroid of *H. ducreyi*, later stages of herpetic vesicles, the ulcer of granuloma inguinale (also known as donovanosis, caused by *C. granulomatis*), or the result of some other rare infectious disease or even a noninfectious process. Macroscopically, lesions of syphilis are usually clean, with an even, indurated edge. Only 30% of syphilitic chancres are tender. Lesions of chancroid are usually ragged, necrotic, painful, and are often found in pairs where material from the first lesion autoinoculated a second area in close contact ("kissing lesions"). The beefy red nonpainful lesion of donovanosis is characterized by a white border. These lesions can usually be differentiated from the painful, erythematous-bordered lesions of herpes, which usually begin as vesicles and occur in groups. Lesions suggestive of syphilis should be examined by darkfield microscopy, as described in Chapter 7. Collection of material for darkfield is outlined in Procedure 19.4.

All slides and materials should be handled as infectious, since syphilitic lesions may contain large numbers of infectious treponemes.

All lesions suspected of infectious etiology may be Gram stained in addition to the procedures described above. The smear of lesion material from a chancroid patient may show

---

PROCEDURE 19.4. COLLECTION OF MATERIAL FOR DARKFIELD EXAMINATION FOR SYPHILIS (GLOVES SHOULD ALWAYS BE WORN)

1. Cleanse the area around the lesion with a sterile gauze pad moistened with sterile saline.
2. Abrade the surface of the ulcer with a sterile, dry gauze pad until some blood is expressed.
3. Continue to blot the blood until it stops bleeding, and then squeeze the area until serous fluid is expressed.
4. Touch the surface of a very clean glass slide or coverslip to the exudate and immediately cover the material on the slide with a coverslip or place the inoculated coverslip face-down onto a slide. If there was only very little material expressed, a drop of sterile physiologic saline may be added.
5. Immediately examine the material under darkfield microscopy (400 ×, high dry magnification) for the presence of motile spirochetes. Treponemes are very long (8-10 μm), slightly longer than a red blood cell, and consist of 8-14 tightly coiled, even spirals (Plate 19.2). They may bend slightly in the middle as they slowly move about. Once characteristic forms are seen, they should be verified by examination under oil immersion magnification (1,000 ×).

---

many small, pleomorphic gram-negative rods and cocccobacilli arranged in chains and groups, characteristic of *H. ducreyi* (Plate 19.3). Culture has been shown to be more sensitive for diagnosis of this agent, however. Material collected on cotton or Dacron swabs may be transported in modified Stuart's medium until it is inoculated to culture media. A special agar, consisting of chocolate agar enriched with 1% IsoVitaleX (BBL Microbiology Systems) and 3 μg vancomycin per milliliter, has yielded good isolation if cultures are incubated in 5%-7% CO_2 in a very moist atmosphere, such as a candle jar. Inoculation of a duplicate sample from each patient to a second agar, fetal bovine serum agar with vancomycin, mentioned in Chapter 29, has been suggested by Greenwood and Robertson to increase chances for recovery.[3]

Diagnosis of granuloma inguinale is achieved by staining a crushed preparation of a small piece of tissue biopsied from the edge of the base of the ulcer with Wright's or Giemsa stain and finding characteristic Donovan bodies (bipolar staining rods intracellularly within macrophages). Cytologists or pathologists usually examine such specimens, rather than microbiologists. No acceptable media for isolation of *C. granulomatis* are available.

19.7. Examination of Material from Buboes

Buboes, swollen lymph glands that occur in the inguinal region, are often evidence of a genital tract infection. Buboes are common in patients with primary syphilis, genital herpes, lymphogranuloma venereum, and chancroid. Patients suffering from AIDS may show generalized lymphadenopathy. Other diseases that are not sexually transmitted, such as plague, tularemia, and lymphoma, can also produce buboes. Those diseases will not be discussed further here. Material from buboes may be aspirated for microscopic examination and culture as described in Procedure 19.5.

PROCEDURE 19.5. ASPIRATION OF BUBO MATERIAL (TO BE DONE BY PHYSICIAN)

1. Wipe overlying skin with an iodophore, allowing it to remain on the skin for at least 1 min.
2. Vigorously wash off the iodophore with 70% alcohol, allowing it to dry.
3. Introduce a 21 gauge needle with an attached 5 ml syringe through the skin into the node.
4. If the node is nonfluctuant, such as those of syphilis, the needle is plunged gently in various directions within the node while continuous suction is applied to the syringe.
5. Material aspirated from nonfluctuant nodes is examined under darkfield microscopy for spirochetes.
6. Material from fluctuant nodes is obtained by applying suction. If no pus is aspirated, the needle is left in place and a syringe containing at least 1 ml of nonbacteriostatic physiologic sterile saline is exchanged for the initial empty syringe. This saline is injected into the node and withdrawn. Rigorous aseptic technique is important.
7. Pus is cultured on chocolate and 5% sheep blood agars, special media for *H. ducreyi* (described above), and in broth such as thioglycolate, and Gram stained.
8. Lesion material is also placed into sucrose buffer for chlamydial culture and examined by fluorescein-conjugated monoclonal chlamydial antibody stain.

19.8. Infections of Human Products of Conception

Certain infectious agents are known to cause fetal infection and even abortion. *Listeria monocytogenes*, although usually causing only mild flulike symptoms in the mother, can cause extensive disease and abortion of the fetus if infection occurs late in the pregnancy, as discussed in Chapter 33. The organism can be isolated from the placenta and tissues of the fetus. Methods for isolation of *Listeria* from tissue are discussed in Chapter 21. Other agents that cross the placental barrier to infect a developing fetus include *Toxoplasma gondii*, rubella, cytomegalovirus, herpes simplex virus, and *T. pallidum*. Infections that can be acquired by infants as they pass through an infected birth canal include herpes, cytomegalovirus (CMV), gonorrhea, group B streptococcal sepsis, chlamydial conjunctivitis and pneumonia, and *Escherichia coli* or other neonatal meningitis. Laboratory diagnosis of these infections is accomplished by culturing for the agents where possible and by performing serologic tests, especially for the presence of specific IgM directed against the agent in question. Specific IgM tests are commercially available for the "TORCH" agents (*Toxoplasma*, rubella, cytomegalovirus, and herpes) as discussed in Chapter 12. Unless serum IgM is separated from IgG (discussed in Chapter 12), the IgM tests for neonatal rubella, CMV, and herpes are unreliable. Cytomegalovirus infection is best diagnosed by culture of the virus from urine. The most reliable diagnostic tests for neonatal herpes infection are demonstration of the antigen in clinical specimens by direct fluorescent antibody stain or recovery of the virus in tissue culture.

19.9. Nonculture Methods for Diagnosis of Diseases of the Genital Tract

19.9.a. Serologic tests for syphilis. Since *T. pallidum* cannot be cultured in routine laboratories, diagnosis of syphilis must rest on demonstration of the organism in a lesion, a difficult and insensitive test, or demonstration of specific antibodies to the treponemes. Although a complete discussion of diagnosis of syphilis is beyond the scope of this text, certain tests will be mentioned here. The classic serologic tests for syphilis measure the presence of two types of antibodies: **treponemal** and **nontreponemal.** Treponemal antibodies are specifically produced against the antigens of the organisms themselves, whereas nontreponemal antibodies, often called **reaginic antibodies,** are produced by infected patients against components of their own or other mammalian bodies. These antibodies, although almost always produced by patients with syphilis, are also produced by patients with a number of other infectious diseases such as leprosy, tuberculosis, chancroid, leptospirosis, malaria, rickettsial disease, trypanosomiasis, lymphogranuloma venereum (LGV), measles, chickenpox, hepatitis, and infectious mononucleosis; noninfectious conditions such as drug addiction; autoimmune disorders including rheumatoid disease; and such nondiseases as old age, pregnancy, and recent immunization. When a positive serologic test for syphilis occurs in a patient without syphilis, it is called a **biologic false positive (BFP).**

The two most widely used nontreponemal serologic tests are the **VDRL (Venereal Disease Research Laboratory)** test and the **RPR (rapid plasma reagin)** test. Each of these tests is a flocculation (or agglutination) test, in which soluble antigen particles are coalesced to form larger particles that are visible as clumps when they are aggregated by antibody. The principles of these tests were discussed in Chapter 12.

Specific treponemal serologic tests include the **FTA-ABS (fluorescent treponemal antibody absorption)** test and the **MHA (microhemagglutination)** test. Another test, the **TPI (*Treponema pallidum* immobilization)** test, is rarely performed these days, since it requires the maintenance of viable treponemes by passage in rabbit testicles.

The FTA-ABS test is performed by overlaying whole treponemes fixed to a slide with serum from patients suspected of having syphilis because of a previous positive VDRL or RPR test. The patient's serum is first absorbed with non–*T. pallidum* treponemal antigens to reduce nonspecific cross reactivity. Fluorescein-conjugated anti–human antibody reagent is then applied as a marker for specific antitreponemal antibodies in the patient's serum. This test should not be used as a primary screening procedure. The MHA test utilizes treated erythrocytes from a turkey or other animal that are coated with treponemal antigens. The presence of specific antibody causes the red cells to agglutinate and form a flat mat across the bottom of the microdilution well in which the test is performed. The serologic tests for syphilis can be used to determine quantitative titers of antibody, which are useful for following response to therapy. The relative sensitivity of each test is shown in Table 19.1. To confirm that a positive nontreponemal test result is due to syphilis rather than one of the other infections mentioned above, a specific treponemal test should be performed. Enzyme-linked immunosorbent assay (ELISA) tests for syphilis antibodies are available. Although not widely used yet, they should offer a sensitive and specific alternative to existing methods.

19.9.b. Other serologic tests for genital pathogens. As mentioned in the chapters that deal with individual pathogens, many conventional serologic tests for antibodies to genital pathogens are in use. Complement fixation and microimmunofluorescence are both used with excellent sensitivity for detection of antibodies

TABLE 19.1
Sensitivity of Commonly Used Serologic
Tests for Syphilis

TEST*	STAGE		
	1°	2°	LATE
Nontreponemal (reaginic tests)			
Venereal Disease Research Laboratory (reaginic) test (VDRL)	70%	99%	1%[†]
Rapid plasma-reagin card test (RPR)	80%	99%	
Automated reagin test (ART)			0%
Specific treponemal tests			
Fluorescent treponemal antibody absorption test (FTA-abs)	85%	100%	98%
T. pallidum hemagglutination assay (TPHA-TP)	65%	100%	95%
Treponemal immobilization test (TPI)	50%	97%	95%

Reproduced from Tramont, E. 1985. *Treponema pallidum*
(syphilis). In Mandell, G.L., Douglas, R.G. Jr., and
Bennett, J.E., editors: Principles and practice of
infectious diseases, ed. 2. John Wiley & Sons, New York.
*Percentage of patients with positive serologic tests in
treated or untreated primary or secondary syphilis.
†Treated late syphilis.

to chlamydiae and mycoplasma, and complement fixation tests can detect antibodies to herpes and cytomegaloviruses, although newer tests such as indirect hemagglutination (Cetus Corp.) and latex particle agglutination (Hynson, Westcott & Dunning) are more sensitive and simpler. Commercially produced ELISA tests are also available for detection of herpes and CMV antibodies. Serologic tests for gonorrhea by antibody detection are not satisfactory in that they do not distinguish between past and current infection, nor between gonococcal and meningococcal infection.

19.9.c. Antigen detection tests for genital tract pathogens. In addition to the fluorescent microscopic methods mentioned above and described in more detail in the chapters relating to individual pathogens, several ELISA systems are currently available for detection of antigens of etiologic agents involved in sexually transmitted diseases without culture. For patients whose serum contains antibody to HTLV III, as detected by ELISA tests (Chapter 23), a Western blot nucleic acid hybridization test is used to confirm the diagnosis.

Welcome new test systems are an ELISA for antigens of *C. trachomatis* and of *N. gonorrhoeae* (Chlamydiazyme and Gonozyme, Abbott Laboratories). The Gonozyme test has been shown to be similar to culture for detection of gonococcal urethritis and especially useful for screening asymptomatic females (although less sensitive than culture). It is not useful for detection of pharyngeal or rectal infection. Early experience with Chlamydiazyme has shown sensitivity equal to the direct examination of material using a fluorescent monoclonal antibody stain (MicroTrak, described above), but false positive results may occur with this test (and not with culture). Systems are also being perfected for direct detection of herpes antigen with latex agglutination, an ELISA test, or by staining clinical material with polyclonal and monoclonal antibodies conjugated to either a fluorescent stain or to a biotin-avidin-enzyme marker (Chapter 10). Several commercial kits are available.

19.9.d. Other tests. As mentioned in Chapter 10, the *Limulus* amebocyte lysate assay has been used to detect gram-negative endotoxin in male and female genital exudates as a presumptive screening test for gonorrhea. The test has been quite successful, although it is not widely used.[6,7]

A presumptive diagnostic test for gonococcal urethritis in men was recently made available (Gonodecten, U.S. Packaging Corp.). Urethral discharge collected on a Dacron swab is exposed to oxidase reagent. The presence of large numbers of oxidase positive gonococci turns the swab purple. The test cannot distinguish between *N. gonorrhoeae* and *N. meningitidis,* and false positive and false negative results are possible. As evaluated by Janda and Jackson,[4] the Gram stain was a more reliable test than was Gonodecten. Clinical laboratories with culture and Gram stain facilities should not rely on such rapid screening tests.

We expect that rapid, reliable, nonculture antigen-detection methods will soon be available for diagnosis of all significant sexually transmitted diseases so that patients can be diagnosed and treated within minutes of being examined. The rapid specific therapeutic intervention thus made possible will contribute greatly to minimizing spread of sexually transmitted diseases and to a decrease in the morbidity that those infections currently produce.

REFERENCES

1. Anstey, R.J., Gun-Munro, J., Rennie, R.P., et al. 1984. Laboratory and clinical evaluation of modified New York City medium (Henderson formulation) for the isolation of *Neisseria gonorrhoeae*. J. Clin. Microbiol. 20:905.
2. Gordon, F.B., Harper, I.A., Quan, A.L., et al. 1969. Detection of chlamydiae (*Bedsonia*) in certain infections in man: I. Laboratory procedures: comparison of yolk-sac and cell culture for detection and isolation. J. Infect. Dis. 120:451.
3. Greenwood, J.R., and Robertson, C.A. 1983. *Haemophilus ducreyi*. Microbiol. No. MB 83-8. Check sample. Am. Soc. Clin. Pathol. vol. 26, no. 8. Chicago, Ill.
4. Janda, W.M., and Jackson, T. 1985. Evaluation of Gonodecten for the presumptive diagnosis of gonococcal urethritis in men. J. Clin. Microbiol. 21:143.
5. Mårdh, P.-A. 1984. Laboratory diagnosis of sexually transmitted diseases. In Holmes, K.K., Mårdh, P.-A., Sparling, P.F., and Wiesner, P.J., editors: Sexually transmitted diseases. McGraw-Hill Book Co., New York.
6. Prior, R.B., and Spagna, V.A. 1981. Application of a *Limulus* test device in rapid evaluation of gonococcal and non-gonococcal urethritis in males. J. Clin. Microbiol. 14:256.
7. Prior, R.B., and Spagna, V.A. 1982. Rapid evaluation of female patients exposed to gonorrhea by the use of the *Limulus* lysate test. J. Clin. Microbiol. 16:57.
8. Tramont, E. 1985. *Treponema pallidum* (syphilis). In Mandell, G.L., Douglas, R.G., Jr., and Bennett, J.E., editors: Principles and practice of infectious diseases, ed. 2. John Wiley & Sons, New York.

BIBLIOGRAPHY

Kramer, D.G., and Brown, S.T. 1984. Sexually transmitted diseases and infertility. Int. J. Gynaecol. Obstet. 22:19.

Krieger, J.N. 1985. Prostatitis, epididymitis, and orchitis. In Mandell, G.L., Douglas, R.G., Jr., and Bennett, J.E., editors: Principles and practice of infectious diseases, ed. 2. John Wiley & Sons, New York.

Ledger, W.J. 1985. Infections of the female pelvis. In Mandell, G.L., Douglas, R.G., Jr., and Bennett, J.E., editors: Principles and practice of infectious diseases, ed. 2. John Wiley & Sons, New York.

Rein, M.F. 1985. Skin and mucous membrane lesions. In Mandell, G.L., Douglas, R.G., Jr., and Bennett, J.E., editors: Principles and practice of infectious diseases, ed. 2. John Wiley & Sons, New York.

Rein, M.F. 1985. Inguinal adenopathy. In Mandell, G.L., Douglas, R.G., Jr., and Bennett, J.E., editors: Principles and practice of infectious diseases, ed. 2. John Wiley & Sons, New York.

Rein, M.F. 1985. Urethritis, In Mandell, G.L., Douglas, R.G., Jr., and Bennett, J.E., editors: Principles and practice of infectious diseases, ed. 2. John Wiley & Sons, New York.

Rein, M.F. 1985. Vulvovaginitis and cervicitis. In Mandell, G.L., Douglas, R.G., Jr., and Bennett, J.E., editors: Principles and practice of infectious diseases, ed. 2. John Wiley & Sons, New York.

20 Microorganisms Encountered in Wounds, Abscesses, Skin, and Soft Tissue Lesions

20.1. Introduction

Infections in the categories covered in this chapter are those most commonly encountered clinically and therefore those most commonly cultured. A wide variety of organisms may be involved, chiefly bacteria, fungi, and viruses. Parasites (*Trichinella, Taenia solium,* and *Toxoplasma*) may be involved in myositis but are not sought in the usual processing of specimens in the clinical laboratory; biopsy and serologic procedures are typically employed (see Chapter 44). Bite infections and clenched fist injuries, in a sense, might have been considered in this chapter but it was elected to discuss them in the chapter on infections of the head and neck (Chapter 22) since the bacterial flora involved originates in the oral cavity. Tissue obtained by debridement or biopsy may be an important source of information on the infections discussed in this chapter; see Chapter 21 for a discussion of this type of specimen. Venereal diseases of certain types produce skin and soft-tissue lesions; these are discussed in Chapter 19. Other agents are also discussed elsewhere in the book (*Bacillus anthracis* in Chapter 32, *Corynebacterium diphtheriae* in Chapter 33, mycobacteria in Chapter 41, viruses in Chapter 42, and fungi in Chapter 43). A number of the agents involved in the infections covered in this chapter are fastidious; accordingly, careful attention to specimen transport and culture techniques, including the use of specialized media, will be important to keep in mind. The potential for introduction of indigenous and transient skin flora into the specimen is great; particular attention to specimen collection is of great importance for laboratory diagnosis of these infections. In some cases, the amount of material available for direct examination and culture will be very small. The use of more than one swab (swabs will be the only practical collection device in such cases) and careful specimen transport will help insure reliable bacteriological results. Discussion between the microbiologist and the clinician will result in better specimen collection and transport and should provide the microbiologist with important information that will be of great assistance in selecting optimum culturing and processing procedures. For example, information on exposure of the patient to sea water or ingestion by the patient of raw shellfish would alert the laboratory to look for *Vibrio vulnificus*. Information that the specimen is from a necrotic palatal lesion in a patient with diabetic ketoacidosis would indicate the need to look carefully for *Aspergillus, Mucor, Rhizopus, Rhizomucor,* and *Absidia*. Clinical evidence of a necrotizing fasciitis would indicate the likely presence of group A streptococcus, *Staphylococcus aureus*, or various anaerobic bacteria.

20.2. Wound Infections, Abscesses

Wound infections and abscesses occur as complications of surgery, trauma or disease that may interrupt a mucosal or skin surface. The nature of the infecting flora will depend on the underlying problem and the location of the process. In the case of perforated appendix, the flora will be that of the indigenous flora of the lower gastrointestinal tract—*Escherichia coli, Streptococcus faecalis, Bacteroides* (*B. fragilis* group and others), *Peptostreptococcus* sp. and *Clostridium* sp. for the most part. In the case of postoperative wound infection following perforated peptic ulcer in a patient who has been

hospitalized for 2 weeks prior to the perforation and who has been receiving antimicrobial therapy for an unrelated process (e.g., pneumonia), nosocomial pathogens such as *Staphylococcus aureus, Klebsiella, Enterobacter,* and *Pseudomonas aeruginosa* are likely to be involved in addition to oral flora (streptococci of the viridans group, oral anaerobes) and flora related to the underlying peptic ulcer disease (in the presence of obstruction or bleeding, there is often colonization of the stomach with *E. coli* and other elements typical of the colonic flora, including the *B. fragilis* group). Thus, knowledge of the indigenous flora of a viscus or an area, of the way in which this flora may be modified by disease or antimicrobial agents, and of the environmental flora permits one to make an educated guess as to the likely etiologic agents. The clinician, of course, uses this approach (along with certain clinical features that may indicate the presence of one organism or another) to choose empirical therapy prior to availability of microbiologic data; naturally, information from Gram stain or other direct examination is taken into account as well. The microbiologist uses this type of information to be certain that appropriate media, culture conditions, etc. are employed. In general, the organisms encountered are as follows:

Staphylococcus aureus
Streptococcus pyogenes
Escherichia coli
Bacteroides sp.
Fusobacterium sp.
Proteus, Morganella, Providencia
Other Enterobacteriaceae
Pseudomonas sp.
Clostridium sp.
Peptostreptococcus sp.
Microaerophilic streptococci
Enterococci
Non-spore-forming anaerobic gram-positive rods
Candida sp.

Since anaerobic bacteria are involved in many

or most infections of this type, collection of specimens so as to avoid indigenous flora and specimen transport under good anaerobic conditions (which will not interfere with recovery of even obligate aerobes) are particularly important. Blood cultures, including special fungal blood cultures (Chapter 14), should be taken since bacteremia is encountered in a number of patients with wound infection or abscess.

Quantitative or semiquantitative reporting of culture results is desirable. This provides some information on the relative importance of the various organisms present in a mixed infection (the typical situation with wounds and abscesses). It may also provide information on the response of the infection to therapy.

20.3. Extremity Infections Related to Vascular and Neurologic Problems

These infections are very common. The classic patient is one with diabetes mellitus, poor arterial circulation (often there is both large- and small-vessel disease), and peripheral neuropathy. Such individuals traumatize their feet readily (often just by virtue of wearing a new pair of shoes) without being aware of it (loss of sensation because of the neuropathy). The traumatized area develops into an ulcer that does not heal readily because of the poor vascular supply and often becomes infected. The infections tend to be chronic and difficult to clear up, manifesting primarily as purulent discharge in the base of the ulcer, often with a foul odor. Extension to the underlying bone to produce a difficult-to-manage osteomyelitis is very common. Periodically, there may be an acute cellulitis and lymphangitis engrafted on the chronic low-grade infection. This infection may make control of the patient's diabetes difficult. Peripheral vascular disease unrelated to diabetes mellitus may also predispose to this problem but is usually less difficult to manage because there is no associated neuropathy. Venous insufficiency, particularly when it leads

to stasis ulcers, also predisposes to infection, again primarily on the lower extremities (in this case, often in the area of the calf or lower leg, rather than the foot).

Infections related to poor blood supply often involve S. aureus and S. pyogenes. Those with open ulcers often become colonized with Enterobacteriaceae and P. aeruginosa which may or may not play a role in the infection. Less well appreciated is the fact that anaerobes are commonly involved in the infectious process, particularly in diabetics or others with peripheral vascular disease. The poor blood supply, of course, contributes to anaerobic conditions. Various anaerobes may be recovered, including the B. fragilis group (commonly) and pigmented Bacteroides, Peptostreptococcus sp. and, less frequently, Clostridium sp.

Another common type of infection in this general category, especially with the elderly or very ill bedridden patient, is infected **decubitus ulcer** (pressure sore) (Plate 20.1). Anaerobic conditions are present in such lesions because of the necrosis of tissue. Because the majority of these lesions are located in proximity to the anus and because so many of these patients are relatively helpless, the ulcers become contaminated with bowel flora, which leads to chronic infection. This contributes to further death of tissue and enlargement of the decubitus ulcer. Furthermore, bacteremia is not an uncommon complication; the B. fragilis group is often involved in bacteremia, along with clostridia and enteric bacteria. The ulcers themselves yield a variety of anaerobes and non-anaerobes characteristic of the colonic flora; nosocomial pathogens such as S. aureus and P. aeruginosa may also be recovered.

Collection and transport of specimens are important considerations for laboratory diagnosis of this type of infection. Specimen collection is particularly difficult because many of these lesions are open and therefore readily colonized by nosocomial pathogens that may or may not be involved in the infection. In the event of an underlying osteomyelitis or a collection of pus in the subcutaneous tissues, attempts should be made to obtain a bone biopsy (for histology as well as smear and culture) or to drain the abscess by needle and syringe aspiration, in both cases traversing only normal skin to get to the underlying infected area, if possible. Bacteremia does not usually accompany this type of infection unless there is an acute lymphangitis as part of the picture, with the major exception of infected decubitus ulcers.

20.4. Pyoderma, Cellulitis

Included in this category are such infections of the skin and subcutaneous tissue as impetigo, folliculitis, furuncles, carbuncles, paronychia, cellulitis, erysipelas (Plate 20.2), and similar lesions. *Staphylococcus aureus* and group A streptococci are the most common infecting organisms, with *Candida* and *P. aeruginosa* seen less frequently. Various non-spore-forming anaerobes are encountered more often than had been realized in the past. Bacteremia is not a common accompaniment with this type of infection.

20.5. Vesicles, Bullae

This type of fluid-filled lesion characteristically involves certain predictable organisms so that if the laboratory is aware of the nature of the lesion the microbiologist can anticipate the flora and use appropriate techniques to insure recovery of the agent(s). Following is a list of the organisms seen in these lesions:

>   *Staphylococcus aureus*
>   Group A streptococci
>   *Pseudomonas aeruginosa*
>   Other gram-negative bacilli
>   *Clostridium* sp.
>   Varicella-zoster virus
>   Herpes simplex virus
>   Other viruses

The material in the blisterlike lesion varies

from serous fluid to serosanguineous or hemorrhagic fluid. Large bullae permit withdrawal of 0.5-1 ml of fluid by needle and syringe aspiration. Some vesicles are quite tiny so that one must use a swab for specimen collection. The clinical nature of the lesion is usually such that the clinician can readily anticipate whether the lesion is viral or bacterial in nature; recovery of the agent will be facilitated if this information is imparted to the microbiologist. Bullous lesions are caused by bacteria and are often associated with sepsis so that blood cultures are mandatory. With this type of lesion as well, the clinician may often be able to suspect a particular type of organism based on the clinical picture. In the case of an immunosuppressed patient with acute leukemia, for example, *P. aeruginosa* would be a common cause of bullous lesions (a type of ecthyma gangrenosum, Plate 20.3). One may see bronzed skin with bullous lesions in gas gangrene (Plate 20.4), an entity with a very distinctive clinical picture; *Clostridium perfringens* and other clostridia are the key pathogens. Gram stain of the fluid from such lesions typically reveals the etiologic agent and provides the clinician with additional valuable information on which to base initial therapy.

20.6. Draining Sinuses, Fistulas

The most common situation in which one finds draining sinuses is a deep-seated infection which spontaneously drains itself externally; the deep lesion is most often a chronic osteomyelitis. Unfortunately, this type of drainage does not usually cure the underlying process, so that such sinuses themselves tend to be chronic. The organisms most often involved in sinuses with an underlying osteomyelitis are *S. aureus*, various Enterobacteriaceae, *P. aeruginosa*, anaerobic gram-negative bacilli, anaerobic gram-positive cocci and occasionally other anaerobes. In the case of actinomycotic bone involvement, of course, one would expect to recover *Actinomyces* sp., *Arachnia*, pigmented

Bacteroides and other non-spore-forming anaerobes and perhaps *Actinobacillus actinomycetemcomitans*. In the case of other types of draining sinuses, such as that associated with recurrent breast abscess of the periareolar type, the organisms involved will depend on the nature of the underlying process; in the example of the breast abscess cited, non-spore-forming anaerobic bacteria are most commonly isolated.

Other situations in which chronic draining sinuses are found typically include actinomycosis (cervicofacial [Plates 20.5 and 20.6], thoracic, abdominal or pelvic), tuberculosis and atypical mycobacterial infection, *Nocardia* infection, and certain infections associated with implanted foreign bodies.

Fistulas (abnormal communications between two surfaces or between a hollow viscus and the exterior) may be seen under certain circumstances and are difficult management problems. They also pose problems that are often insurmountable in terms of collection of meaningful specimens since the viscus (such as the bowel) which has the abnormal communication to the skin surface often has its own profuse indigenous flora. Examples are perirectal fistulas and enterocutaneous fistulas from the small bowel to the skin in association with Crohn's disease or chronic intraabdominal infection. When the bowel is involved, only cultures for specific key organisms such as mycobacteria or *Actinomyces* are meaningful.

One should always attempt to rule out specific underlying causes such as tuberculosis, actinomycosis, and malignancy; biopsy is most useful.

20.7. Suppurative Lymphadenitis

Lymphadenopathy may be seen in a variety of infectious processes, but the clinical microbiology laboratory is not usually involved directly in diagnosis of the underlying problem except for serologic testing (e.g., in infectious mononucleosis syndromes). In the case of suppurative breakdown of a lymph node, material aspirated from the node will be submitted for direct examination and culture. Agents that may cause suppuration in a lymph node include group A streptococci, *S. aureus*, *M. tuberculosis*, *M. scrofulaceum*, *Yersinia pestis*, *Francisella tularensis*, *Pseudomonas pseudomallei*, *P. mallei*, *Sporothrix*, *Coccidioides*, *Chlamydia trachomatis* and the agent of cat scratch disease.

20.8. Myositis

Involvement of muscle occurs with a wide variety of infectious agents. The nature of the pathologic process is variable, sometimes involving extensive necrosis of muscle, as in gas gangrene or clostridial myonecrosis, **necrotizing cutaneous myositis** or **synergistic nonclostridial anaerobic myonecrosis,** anaerobic streptococcal myonecrosis, myonecrosis due to *Bacillus* sp., or myonecrosis due to *Aeromonas*, and sometimes presenting with focal collections of suppuration in muscle (staphylococcal pyomyositis). Muscle involvement may also manifest as a vasculitis in muscle tissue (*Vibrio vulnificus*), and sometimes as an inflammatory myositis presenting clinically as a benign myalgia (but occasionally with myoglobinuria secondary to muscle breakdown, as occurs in influenza and other viral infections, rickettsial infections, infective endocarditis, bacteremia, *Legionella* infection [perhaps related to sepsis], toxoplasmosis, trichinosis, and cysticercosis). Abscess in the psoas muscles may involve *M. tuberculosis*, *S. aureus* or various facultative gram-negative bacilli. Serious vascular problems may lead to death of muscle due to loss of blood supply; such muscle may become secondarily infected (infected vascular gangrene) but this is usually a low-grade process. Blood cultures should always be drawn from patients with significant myonecrosis. Transport of material (tissue is always better than pus, which is, in turn, better than a swab) should be under anaerobic conditions. In the course of setting up anaerobic cultures, consideration should be given to setting up a Nagler plate (Chapter 34) directly from the clinical specimen in order to rapidly detect *Clostridium perfringens* presumptively (in 12-18 h). Similarly, *Bacteroides* bile esculin agar plates (Chapter 34) should be set up in the case of synergistic nonclostridial anaerobic myonecrosis; this permits rapid presumptive identification of the *B. fragilis* group (18-24 h). Obviously, very early presumptive identification requires examination of plates at frequent intervals and much sooner than the usual 48 h interval used conventionally. This may be accomplished readily if the laboratory has an anaerobic chamber that contains an incubator or by use of the Gas Pak pouch (BBL Microbiology Systems) or the BioBag (Marion Laboratories); these approaches avoid exposing the plates to air before it is determined that there is adequate growth. Organisms producing myositis or other muscle pathology are as follows:

> *Clostridium perfringens*
> *C. novyii*
> *C. septicum*
> *C. bifermentans*
> *C. histolyticum*
> *C. sordellii*
> *C. sporogenes*
> *Bacillus* sp.
> *Aeromonas* sp.
> *Peptostreptococcus* sp.
> Microaerophilic streptococci
> *Bacteroides* sp.
> Enterobacteriaceae
> *Staphylococcus aureus*
> Group A streptococci
> *Pseudomonas mallei*
> *P. pseudomallei*
> *Vibrio vulnificus*
> *Mycobacterium tuberculosis*
> *Salmonella typhi*
> *Legionella* sp.
> *Rickettsia*
> Viruses
> *Trichinella*
> *Taenia solium*
> *Toxoplasma*

20.9. Serious Soft Tissue and Skin Infections

This category is used for a miscellaneous collection of infections, some extensive and some localized, but all serious or potentially serious. Anthrax and cutaneous diphtheria are discussed elsewhere, as noted previously. An often fatal, but fortunately rare, infection known as mucormycosis is found in patients with diabetes, acidosis, or with hematologic neoplasms or other conditions requiring corticosteroid or cytotoxic therapy. Necrotic lesions of the palate or nasal mucous membranes are often noted first, but lesions may also spread to the brain or involve other deep organs early in the illness. The fungi most commonly involved are *Mucor*, *Rhizopus*, *Absidia*, and *Rhizomucor*, but occasionally other fungi of the order Mucorales may be involved; *Aspergillus* species and *Pseudallescheria boydii* may produce similar clinical pictures. Material should be obtained by biopsy of the necrotic tissue for direct examination (Chapter 7) and culture.

Necrotizing fasciitis is a serious infection that is more common than mucormycosis, but still relatively uncommon. The basic pathology is infection involving the fascia overlying muscle groups, often with concomitant involvement of the overlying soft tissue. At the fascial level there is no barrier to spread of infection so that fasciitis may extend widely and rapidly to involve huge areas of the body in short periods. This process, once known as hospital gangrene, commonly involves group A streptococci or *S. aureus*. It is not recognized as widely as it should be, but necrotizing fasciitis also commonly involves anaerobic bacteria, especially anaerobic gram-negative bacilli of the genera *Bacteroides* and *Clostridium*. Many or most cases of perineal gangrene or phlegmon (Fournier's gangrene) and of necrotizing dermogenital infection are forms of necrotizing fasciitis, although some involve only the more superficial soft tissues (and thus are not as dangerous).

Progressive bacterial synergistic gangrene is usually a chronic gangrenous condition of the skin most often encountered as a postoperative complication, particularly after abdominal surgery requiring retention sutures or after thoracic surgery. The lesions may be extensive and, in the case of involvement of the abdominal wall, may lead to evisceration. As the name suggests, this is typically a mixed infection with microaerophilic streptococci and S. aureus. At times, the streptococci are obligate anaerobes and at times there may be any of a number of organisms other than S. aureus (most commonly Proteus). If only the purulent or necrotic material from the central portion of the wound is cultured, the microaerophilic streptococcus will be missed and the nature of the lesion may not be appreciated. This may happen since this infection is very uncommon and the clinician may not recognize the usually distinctive clinical features. Cultures should be taken from the advancing outer edge of the lesion.

Chronic undermining ulcer or **Meleney's ulcer** is a slowly progressive infection of the subcutaneous tissue with associated ulceration of the overlying skin. The causative organism is classically a microaerophilic streptococcus, but anaerobic streptococci, and occasionally other organisms, may be involved.

Anaerobic cellulitis is an acute anaerobic infection of soft tissue that is much more common than the other infections in this category. It is most often found in the extremities and is particularly common in diabetics. It may involve the neck, the abdominal wall, the perineum or connective tissue in other areas. Anaerobic cellulitis also may occur as a postoperative problem. Although the onset and spread of this lesion are not usually rapid and the patients do not show impressive systemic effects at first, it is not an illness to be taken lightly. The bacteriology is almost always that of a mixed aerobic-anaerobic infection. The aerobes include E. coli, alpha hemolytic or nonhemolytic streptococci and S. aureus predominantly, but group A streptococci and other Enterobacteriaceae are encountered as well. The anaerobes are typically found in greater numbers and in more variety than the aerobes; prominent among the anaerobes present are Peptostreptococcus sp., B. fragilis group strains, pigmented Bacteroides, other Bacteroides and clostridia; Fusobacterium sp. are encountered occasionally. Bacteremia is not usually present. Good anaerobic transport and culture techniques are important.

20.10. Burn Infections

Infection of burn wounds is essentially universal, not uncommonly is associated with bacteremia, may carry a significant mortality and interferes with the acceptance of skin grafts. Many organisms are capable of infecting the eschar of a burn. Those most commonly encountered are various streptococci, S. aureus, S. epidermidis, Enterobacteriaceae, Pseudomonas species, other gram-negative bacilli, Candida, and Aspergillus. The setting would seem to be ideal for anaerobic bacteria, and clostridia and Bacteroides have been recovered occasionally; very likely a carefully done study would reveal that anaerobes are more commonly involved than has been appreciated to date.

20.11. Uncommon But Important Causes of Skin and Soft Tissue Infection

There are a number of organisms that may cause infection with serious consequences that are encountered uncommonly or rarely. Included are Clostridium tetani (tetanus), C. botulinum (wound botulism), Francisella tularensis (tularemia), various mycobacteria, Erysipelothrix insidiosa (erysipeloid), Actinomyces, Nocardia, Vibrio alginolyticus (cellulitis in marine wound infection), V. vulnificus (wound infection), Sporothrix schenckii (sporotrichosis), and dematiaceous fungal agents of chromoblastomycosis and mycetoma. Various other systemic fungi, such as Coccidioides immitis, Blastomyces dermatitidis, etc., may involve skin and subcutaneous tissue either as a primary inoculation infection or as part of the process of dissemination.

20.12. Miscellaneous Skin and Soft Tissue Infections of Mild to Moderate Severity

Erythrasma is a very mild and superficial skin infection; the causative organism is *Corynebacterium minutissimum*. The clinical picture is distinctive, but if cultures are desired skin scrapings may be submitted. There are numerous superficial mycoses involving skin, nails, and hair. They are discussed in Chapter 43, but it is well to be aware that on rare occasions under unusual circumstances, organisms such as *Pityrosporum orbiculare* (formerly *Malassezia furfur*) or *Trichosporon* can cause systemic infection. *Mycobacterium marinum* causes "swimming pool" or "fishbowl" granuloma. Hidradenitis suppurativa is a chronic, troublesome, annoying infection of the obstructed apocrine glands in the axillae and genital and perianal areas with intermittent discharge of pus (often foul smelling), draining sinuses at times, and scarring. Secondary infection involves anaerobic gram-negative rods, anaerobic cocci, staphylococci, streptococci, and various aerobic and facultative gram-negative rods. Infected pilonidal cysts almost invariably yield anaerobic bacteria, sometimes to the exclusion of other types of bacteria. The anaerobes involved include the *B. fragilis* group, other *Bacteroides*, *Fusobacterium*, anaerobic gram-positive cocci, and clostridia. Various nonanaerobes, especially Enterobacteriaceae, enterococci, and other streptococci, may also be recovered. Infected **inclusion** or **sebaceous cysts** often yield anaerobic cocci or *Bacteroides;* staphylococci and streptococci are also found commonly in such cysts.

20.13. Skin Lesions as Part of Systemic Infection

Cutaneous manifestations of systemic infection such as bacteremia or endocarditis are not uncommon; they may be important clues for the clinician and they may present an opportunity for direct or cultural demonstration of the presence of a particular organism. For example, one may be able to scrape petechiae in cases of meningococcemia and demonstrate gram-negative diplococci. In other cases, the skin lesion represents a more impressive type of metastatic infection. The lesions of ecthyma gangrenosum in *Pseudomonas aeruginosa* sepsis are prominent. In *Vibrio vulnificus* sepsis, dramatic appearing cutaneous ulcers with necrotizing vasculitis may be found. In some cases, skin lesions in the course of a systemic infection may actually represent a noninfectious complication of the illness. An example would be the rash of toxic shock syndrome.

Various organisms that may be involved in systemic infection with cutaneous lesions are as follows:

Viridans streptococci
Staphylococcus aureus
Enterococci
Group A and other beta hemolytic streptococci
Neisseria gonorrhoeae
N. meningitidis
Haemophilus influenzae
Pseudomonas aeruginosa
P. mallei
P. pseudomallei
Listeria monocytogenes
Vibrio vulnificus
Salmonella typhi
Mycobacterium tuberculosis
M. leprae
Treponema pallidum
Leptospira
Streptobacillus moniliformis
Spirillum minus
Bartonella bacilliformis
Rickettsia
Candida sp.
Cryptococcus neoformans
Blastomyces dermatitidis
Coccidioides immitis
Histoplasma capsulatum

BIBLIOGRAPHY

Bonner, J.R., Coker, A.S., Berryman, C.R., et al. 1983. Spectrum of *Vibrio* infections in a gulf coast community. Ann. Intern. Med. 99:464.

Chow, A.W., Galpin, J.E., and Guze, L.B. 1975. Clinical experience with clindamycin in sepsis caused by decubitus ulcers. J. Infect. Dis. 135:S65.

Churchill, M.A., Geraci, J.E., and Hunder, G.G. 1977. Musculoskeletal manifestations of bacterial endocarditis. Ann. Intern. Med. 87:754.

Finegold, S.M. 1977. Anaerobic bacteria in human disease. Academic Press, New York.

Louie, T.J., Bartlett, J.G., Tally, F.P., and Gorbach, S.L. 1976. Aerobic and anaerobic bacteria in diabetic foot ulcers. Ann. Intern. Med. 85:461.

Meislin, H.W., Lerner, S.A., Graves, M.H., et al. 1977. Cutaneous abscesses. Anaerobic and aerobic bacteriology and outpatient management. Ann. Intern. Med. 87:145.

Sapico, F.L., Canawati, H.N., Witte, J.L., et al. 1980. Quantitative aerobic and anaerobic bacteriology of infected diabetic feet. J. Clin. Microbiol. 12:413.

Swartz, M.N. 1985. Skin and soft tissue infections. In Mandell, G.L., Douglas, R.G. Jr., and Bennett, J.E., editors. Principles and practice of infectious diseases, ed. 2. John Wiley & Sons, New York.

21

Microorganisms Encountered in Solid Tissue, Bone, Bone Marrow, and Body Fluids

21.1. Introduction

Etiologic agents of disease from all four categories (bacteria, fungi, viruses, and parasites) may be found within the tissues of the body and in body fluids. This chapter will discuss the types of microorganisms likely to be recovered from specimens of tissue, bone marrow, bone, and "sterile" body fluids. Bacteria, fungi, and viruses can be identified by microbiologic techniques practiced in routine clinical laboratories, and the discussion that follows will focus on those agents. Because even one colony of a potential pathogenic microorganism could be significant, all of the specimen types discussed in this chapter must be handled with extreme care. We recommend that all manipulations of the specimens, transferring material, and inoculating media, be performed by a technologist wearing gloves and working within a **biological safety cabinet** (Chapter 2).

In most cases, the detection of parasites in tissue is accomplished by observing characteristic morphologic structures in stained histologic sections; examination of tissue for parasites is usually done by pathologists. *Pneumocystis carinii*, however, is often diagnosed in lung biopsy material by microbiologists, as outlined in Chapters 16, 23, and 44. Occasionally, a wet preparation of pleural fluid may reveal *Entamoeba histolytica*. *E. histolytica* may also be identified in material from the wall of an amebic liver abscess. Other

314

tissues may be cultured for parasites such as *Leishmania* and trypanosomes (Chapter 44).

21.2. Sterile Body Fluids

In response to infection, fluid may accumulate in any body cavity. Infected solid tissue often presents as a phlegmon or cellulitis or with abscess formation (Chapter 20). Areas of the body from which fluids are commonly sent for microbiologic studies (in addition to blood and cerebrospinal fluids, covered in Chapters 14 and 15) include the thorax (thoracentesis fluid or pleural fluid), abdominal cavity (paracentesis fluid [ascitic fluid or peritoneal fluid]), joints, and pericardium (pericardial fluid). Techniques for laboratory processing of all sterile body fluids are somewhat similar. Clear fluids may be concentrated by centrifugation or filtration, while purulent material can be inoculated directly to media. Any body fluid that is received in the laboratory already clotted must be homogenized to release trapped bacteria and minced or cut to release fungal cells. Either processing such specimens in a tissue homogenizer (Stomacher Lab-blender 80, Tekmar Co.; Figure 21.1) or grinding them manually in a mortar and pestle or glass tissue grinder will allow better recovery of bacteria. Grinding may lyse fungal elements, therefore it is not recommended for specimens for fungi. Small amounts of whole material from a clot should be aseptically cut with a scalpel and placed directly onto media for isolation of fungi.

21.2.a. Pleural fluid. Pleural fluid or pleural effusion is a collection of fluid from the pleural space, extending between the lung and the chest wall. The fluid may contain few or no cells and be of a consistency similar to that of serum (but with a lower protein content). This type of effusion, called a **transudate,** is often the result of cardiac, hepatic, or renal disease. Pleural effusion that contains numerous white blood cells and other evidence of an inflammatory response is usually due to infection, but malignancy, pulmonary infarction, or autoim-

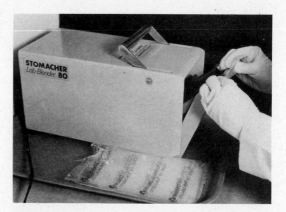

FIGURE 21.1

A mechanical tissue grinder (Stomacher Lab-blender 80, Tekmar Co.) Tissue is placed in 2 ml sterile broth in plastic bags. The action of two paddles serves to homogenize the tissue or drive the bacteria from the tissue into the broth.

mune diseases in which an antigen-antibody reaction initiates an inflammatory response, may also be responsible. Such an effusion, called an **exudate,** is the usual specimen submitted to microbiology laboratories. This fluid, called **pleural effusion,** is collected from the patient by needle aspiration (thoracentesis) and submitted to the laboratory as "pleural fluid," "thoracentesis fluid," or "empyema fluid." Exudative pleural effusions that contain numerous polymorphonuclear neutrophils, particularly those that are grossly purulent, are called **empyema fluids.** Empyema usually occurs secondary to pneumonia, but other infectious sites near the lung (e.g., subdiaphragmatic infection) may seed microorganisms into the pleural cavity.

The bacteria that may be recovered from pleural fluid include those that are associated with pneumonia, such as *Streptococcus pneumoniae, Staphylococcus aureus, Haemophilus influenzae,* Enterobacteriaceae, pseudomonads, and anaerobes. Anaerobic organisms in pleural fluid or empyema occur secondary to aspiration pneumonia or its complications such as lung abscess. Less commonly, other streptococci, *Mycobacterium tuberculosis* or nontuberculous mycobacteria, *Actinomyces* species, *Nocardia* species, fungi, and rarely mycoplasma or viruses may be recovered from empyema cultures.

Pleural fluid, as with other body fluids from sterile sites, should be transported to the laboratory in a sterile tube or vial that excludes oxygen. From 1-5 ml of specimen is adequate for isolation of most bacteria, but the larger the specimen the better, particularly for isolation of *M. tuberculosis* and fungi. Anaerobic transport vials are available from several sources, as mentioned in Chapter 6 and the Appendix. These vials are prepared in an oxygen-free atmosphere and are sealed with a rubber septum or short stopper through which the fluid is injected. Fluid may be transported quickly to the laboratory in a syringe capped with a sterile rubber stopper, but this method is a less desirable alternative to proper containers. Most clinically significant anaerobic bacteria survive adequately in nonanaerobic transport containers (such as syringes and sterile screw-capped tubes) for short periods if the specimen is frankly purulent and of some volume.

Specimens that are received in anaerobic transport vials or syringes should be inoculated to routine aerobic and anaerobic media as quickly as possible, as outlined in Chapters 8 and 34. Gram stains should be examined. If long, thin, gram-positive branching rods are seen, a second smear should be prepared and stained with the modified acid fast stain (Chapter 33) for *Nocardia*. Non–acid fast branching rods are usually *Actinomyces* species; other possibilities are discussed in Chapter 33.

Specimens for recovery of only fungi or mycobacteria may be transported in sterile, screw-capped tubes. At least 10-15 ml of fluid is required for adequate recovery of small numbers of organisms. Those specimens that are thin enough are concentrated by centrifugation at $1500 \times g$ for at least 15 min. The supernatant is aseptically decanted or aspirated with a sterile pipette, leaving approximately 1 ml liquid in which to thoroughly mix the sediment. Vigorous vortexing or drawing the sediment up and down into a pipette several times will adequately resuspend the sediment. This procedure should be done in a biological safety cabinet, of course. The suspension is used to inoculate media and prepare smears. Specimens for fungi should be examined by direct wet preparation in addition to Gram stain. Either 10% KOH or calcofluor white (Chapters 7 and 43) are recommended for visualization of fungal elements. In addition to hyphal forms, material from the thoracic cavity may contain spherules of *Coccidioides* or budding yeast cells. Specimens are inoculated to the primary media that support the growth of fungi, including brain heart infusion agar supplemented with sheep blood and inhibitory mold agars (Chapters 8 and 43). Although *Legionella* species are seldom recovered from pleural fluid, special media for isolation of these organisms may be inoculated if clinically indicated. The physician should notify the laboratory to culture the specimen for *Legionella*.

21.2.b. Peritoneal fluid. The peritoneal cavity surrounds the liver, pancreas, spleen, stomach and intestinal tract, bladder, and Fallopian tubes and ovaries. The kidneys occupy a retroperitoneal position. Within the healthy human peritoneal cavity is a small amount of fluid that maintains moistness of the surface of the internal organs and the peritoneum itself. Normal peritoneal fluid may contain as many as 300 white blood cells per milliliter, but the protein content and specific gravity of the fluid are low. Agents of infection gain access to the peritoneum either through a perforation of the bowel, infection within abdominal viscera, by way of the bloodstream, or by external inoculation (as in surgery or trauma). On occasion, as in pelvic inflammatory disease (PID), organisms travel through the natural channels of the Fallopian tubes into the peritoneal cavity. In

primary peritonitis, no apparent focus of infection is evident. **Secondary peritonitis** involves a rupture of a viscus or other known source of infection. During an infectious or inflammatory process, increased amounts of fluid accumulate in the peritoneal cavity. The fluid, often called **ascites** or ascitic fluid, contains an increased number of inflammatory cells and an elevated protein level.

The organisms likely to be recovered from specimens from patients suffering from primary peritonitis vary with the age of the patient. The most common etiologic agents in children are *Streptococcus pneumoniae* and group A streptococci. Enterobacteriaceae, other gram-negative bacilli, and staphylococci may also be isolated. In adults, *E. coli* is the most common bacterium recovered, followed by *S. pneumoniae* and group A streptococci. Polymicrobic peritonitis is unusual when only aerobic bacteria are associated with disease. Among sexually active young women, *Neisseria gonorrhoeae* and *Chlamydia trachomatis* are common etiologic agents of peritoneal infection, often in the form of a perihepatitis (inflammation of the surface of the liver, called **Fitz-Hugh-Curtis syndrome**). Tuberculous peritonitis is uncommon in the United States today. It is a more likely etiology for recent arrivals from South America, Southeast Asia, or less developed areas of the world. Fungal causes of peritonitis are rare, but *Candida* species may be recovered from immunosuppressed patients and patients on prolonged antibacterial therapy. *Coccidioides immitis* is an uncommon cause of peritonitis found in patients who live in or have visited endemic areas such as the southwestern United States.

Secondary peritonitis is a sequel to a perforated viscus, surgery, traumatic injury, or loss of integrity of bowel mucosa due to destructive disease (e.g., ulcerative colitis, carcinoma), obstruction, or a preceding infection (liver abscess, salpingitis, septicemia, etc.). The nature and etiology of the underlying process govern the agents that will be recovered from peritoneal fluid. For pelvic inflammatory disease, therefore, gonococci, anaerobes, or chlamydia will be isolated. In the case of peritonitis or intraabdominal abscess, anaerobes will usually be found in peritoneal fluid, usually together with Enterobacteriaceae and enterococci or other streptococci. In patients whose bowel flora has been altered by antimicrobial agents, of course, more resistant gram-negative bacilli and *Staphylococcus aureus* may be encountered. Since anaerobes outnumber aerobes in the bowel by 1000 fold, it is not surprising that anaerobic organisms play a prominent role in intraabdominal infection, perhaps acting synergistically with facultative bacteria. The organisms likely to be recovered include *E. coli*, the *Bacteroides fragilis* group, enterococci and other streptococci, other *Bacteroides* species, other anaerobic gram-negative bacilli, anaerobic gram-positive cocci, and clostridia.

Specimens are collected by percutaneous needle aspiration (**paracentesis**) or at the time of surgery and sent to the laboratory for smears and appropriate cultures. Transport should be in an anaerobic vial, as discussed above for pleural fluid. Usually 1-5 ml of fluid is sufficient for the diagnosis of peritonitis but, again, a larger volume is desirable. Material should be inoculated as soon as possible, as should all specimens that may contain anaerobes. If a large volume of clear or serosanguineous fluid is received, it may be concentrated by centrifugation, as described above. Procedures for isolation of fungi, *Chlamydia*, viruses, and bacteria are as previously described and in Chapter 38 (*Chlamydia*).

21.2.c. Peritoneal dialysis fluid. Over 5,000 patients with end-stage renal disease are maintained on **chronic ambulatory peritoneal dialysis (CAPD);** fluid injected into the abdomen allows exchange of salts and water and removal of various wastes in the absence of kidney function. The average incidence of peritonitis in these patients is approximately two episodes per year per patient. Although white blood cells are usually plentiful, the number of organisms is usually too low for detection on Gram stain of the peritoneal fluid sediment; fungi are more readily detected. Most infections originate from the patient's own skin flora; *Staphylococcus epidermidis* and *S. aureus* are the most common etiologic agents, followed by streptococci, aerobic or facultative gram-negative bacilli, *Candida* species, *Corynebacterium* species, and others. The oxygen content of peritoneal dialysate is usually too high for development of anaerobic infection. Among the gram-negative bacilli isolated, *Pseudomonas* species, *Acinetobacter* species, and the Enterobacteriaceae are common. Contaminated dialysis machinery may also contribute to peritoneal dialysis infections.

Fluid is usually received in the laboratory in a sterile tube or urine cup. Almost all patients with peritonitis have cloudy peritoneal dialysis fluid, with over 100 white cells/mm^3. Fluid received in a container other than the original dialysis bag should be concentrated, either by centrifugation, as for other clear, sterile body fluids or by filtration. Filtration through a 0.45 µm pore size membrane filter allows a greater volume of fluid to be processed and will usually yield better results. Since the numbers of infecting organisms may be quite low (<1/10 ml fluid), a large quantity of fluid must be processed. Sediment obtained from at least 50 ml fluid is recommended. Gram stains or acridine orange stains should be performed, even though the yield may be low. If the specimen is filtered, the filter should be cut aseptically into three pieces, one of which is placed on chocolate agar for incubation in 5% CO_2, one of which is placed on MacConkey agar, and the other of which is placed on a blood agar plate for anaerobic incubation. Sediment should be inoculated to similar media. Other plates and a broth may be included. Incubating peritoneal dialysis fluid in blood culture media is acceptable, but the volume of specimen cultured is

thus quite low and therefore may be inadequate for diagnosis.

A recent study by Dawson and others[1] documented the sensitivity of culturing the entire contents of a patient's dialysis exchange bag (1, 1.5, or 2 liters). A 300 ml blood transfer bag containing 50 ml of fivefold concentrated sterile thioglycolate broth and a second 300 ml blood transfer bag containing 100 ml of tenfold concentrated sterile brain heart infusion broth are prepared by the laboratory. The patient's dialysis bag is mixed thoroughly and 250 ml of its contents are allowed to fill the thioglycolate bag by decontaminating the connection sites with povidone-iodine and connecting the two bags together. The thioglycolate bag with added dialysate is disconnected and incubated at 35° C for growth of anaerobic bacteria. The 100 ml of brain heart infusion is allowed to flow into the patient's dialysis bag via a similar connection. These two bags remain connected and are incubated in the same way. Bags are observed for up to 7 days; as soon as turbidity is visible, material for Gram stain and subculture can be withdrawn through the injection port with a sterile needle and syringe. Processing dialysis fluid in this way yields more positive cultures than does processing small amounts of dialysate.

21.2.d. Pericardial fluid. The heart and contiguous major blood vessels are surrounded by a protective tissue, the pericardium. The area between the heart muscle and the pericardium, the pericardial space, normally contains 15-20 ml clear fluid. If an infectious agent is present within the fluid, the pericardium may become distended and tight, and eventually interference with cardiac function and circulation can ensue. Agents of **pericarditis** (inflammation of the pericardium) are usually viruses. Parasites, bacteria, or certain fungi are also associated with this disease, and pericarditis may be due to noninfectious causes as well. Inflammation of the heart muscle itself, **myocarditis,** may accompany pericarditis. The pathogenesis

of disease involves the host inflammatory response contributing to fluid buildup and cell
and tissue damage. The most common etiologic
agents of peri- and myocarditis are enteroviruses, primarily coxsackieviruses A and B.
Echoviruses, adenoviruses, influenza viruses,
and other viruses play a lesser role. Among
nonviral agents, *Mycoplasma pneumoniae*,
Chlamydia, *M. tuberculosis*, *S. aureus*, *S.
pneumoniae*, Enterobacteriaceae, other aerobic
gram-negative bacilli, anaerobic bacteria, *Coccidioides immitis*, *Aspergillus* species, *Candida*
species, *Cryptococcus neoformans*, *Histoplasma capsulatum*, *Entamoeba histolytica*,
and *Toxoplasma gondii* may be found. Other
bacteria, fungi, and parasitic agents have been
recovered from pericardial effusions, however,
and all agents should be sought. Patients who
develop pericarditis due to agents other than
viruses are often compromised in some way.

Collection of pericardial effusion is performed by needle aspiration with electrocardi-
ographic monitoring or as a surgical procedure.
The laboratory personnel should be alerted in
advance so that the appropriate media, tissue
culture media, and stain procedures are available immediately. Fluid should be processed in
the same way as other sterile body fluids, as
discussed above.

21.2.e. Joint fluid. Infectious arthritis may
involve any joint in the body. It usually occurs
secondary to hematogenous spread of bacteria
or, rarely, fungi, and less commonly occurs as
a direct extension of infection of the bone. It
may also occur following injection of material
(especially corticosteroids) into joints or after
insertion of prosthetic material (e.g., total hip
replacement). Although infectious arthritis usually occurs at only one site (**monoarticular**), a
preexisting bacteremia or fungemia may seed
more than one joint to establish **polyarticular**
infection. Knees and hips are the most commonly affected joints.

In addition to active infections associated
with viable microorganisms within the joint,

sterile, self-limited arthritis due to antigen-antibody interactions may follow an episode of infection, such as meningococcal meningitis.
When an etiologic agent cannot be isolated
from an inflamed joint fluid specimen, either
the absence of viable agents or inadequate
transport or culturing procedures can be
blamed. Nonspecific test results such as increased white blood cell count, decreased glucose, or elevated protein may seem to implicate an infectious etiology, but are not
conclusive. A role has been postulated for the
persistence of bacterial L-forms (cell wall deficient forms) in joint fluid after systemic infection, but such organisms have not generally
been recovered.

Staphylococcus aureus is the most common
etiologic agent of septic arthritis, accounting for
approximately 70% of all such infections. In
adults less than 30 years old, however, *N. gonorrhoeae* is isolated most frequently. *H. influenzae* is the most common agent of bacteremia
in children less than 2 years of age, and consequently it is the most common cause of infectious arthritis, followed by *S. aureus*. Streptococci, including groups A and B, pneumococci,
and viridans streptococci are prominent among
bacterial agents associated with infectious arthritis in patients of all ages. *Bacteroides*, including *B. fragilis*, may be recovered as may
Fusobacterium necrophorum, which commonly
involves more than one joint in the course of
sepsis. Among people living in certain endemic
areas of the United States and Europe, infectious arthritis is a prominent feature of Lyme
disease (Chapter 31). The Lyme disease spirochete, *Borrelia burgdorferi*, has not been cultured from joint fluid. It is unclear whether
this arthritis is due to an active infection or to
a host immune response, as is the case for certain other arthritides, mentioned below. Some
of the more commonly encountered etiologic
agents of infectious arthritis are as follows:

Bacterial
Staphylococcus aureus

Beta hemolytic streptococci
Streptococci (other)
Haemophilus influenzae
Haemophilus sp. (other)
Bacteroides sp.
Fusobacterium sp.
Neisseria gonorrhoeae
Pseudomonas sp.
Salmonella sp.
Pasteurella multocida
Moraxella osloensis
Kingella kingae
Branhamella catarrhalis
Capnocytophaga sp.
Corynebacterium sp.
Clostridium sp.
Peptostreptococcus sp.
Eikenella corrodens
Actinomyces sp.
Mycobacterium sp.
Mycoplasma sp.
Ureaplasma urealyticum
Borrelia burgdorferi
Fungal
  Candida sp.
  Cryptococcus neoformans
  Coccidioides immitis
  Sporothrix schenckii
Viral
  Hepatitis B
  Mumps
  Rubella
  Other viruses (rarely)

Most of these agents act to stimulate a host inflammatory response, and it is this response that is ultimately responsible for the pathology of the infection. Arthritis is also a symptom associated with infectious diseases caused by certain agents, such as *Neisseria meningitidis* and *Streptobacillus moniliformis*, in which the agent cannot be recovered from joint fluid. Presumably, antigen-antibody complexes formed during active infection accumulate in a joint, initiating an inflammatory response which is responsible for the ensuing damage. Other agents, such as viruses, yeasts, and mycoplasmas, are unusual causes of infectious arthritis, but they must be considered.

Infections in prosthetic joints are usually associated with different etiologic agents than those in natural joints. Following insertion of the prosthesis, organisms that gained access during the surgical procedure slowly multiply until they reach a critical mass and produce a host response. This may occur long after the initial surgery; approximately one half of all prosthetic joint infections occur more than 1 year after surgery. Skin flora are the most common etiologic agents, with *Staphylococcus epidermidis*, other coagulase negative staphylococci, *Corynebacterium* species, and *Propionibacterium* species predominating.

Specimens are collected by aspiration with a sterile needle and syringe, as are most other "sterile" body fluids. The specimen should be injected into an anaerobic transport vial to preserve viability of anaerobes, which are probably present more often than has been appreciated. It may also prove beneficial to inoculate one bottle of blood culture medium with some of the initial specimen, particularly if the specimen cannot be delivered to the laboratory immediately. This culture is processed as a blood culture, facilitating the recovery of small numbers of organisms and diluting out the effects of antibiotics. Gonococci may be recovered from joint fluids that have been incubated in hyperosmotic medium, such as sucrose-containing broth (Chapter 14). Very purulent specimens are plated directly to several agars, including one which supports the growth of fastidious organisms, such as chocolate agar, and an enriched broth such as thioglycolate. Material should also be inoculated onto primary anaerobic media as discussed in Chapter 34. If fungi or mycobacteria are suspected, appropriate media for their isolation should also be inoculated. Methods for isolation of viruses and mycoplasma are described in Chapters 42 and 38.

Direct Gram stains, KOH or calcofluor white preparations for fungi, and acid fast stain for mycobacteria are also performed.

21.3. Bone Marrow Aspiration or Biopsy

Diagnosis of certain diseases, including brucellosis, histoplasmosis, and leishmaniasis, can sometimes be made only by detection of the organism in the bone marrow. *Brucella* species can be isolated on culture, as can fungi, but parasitic agents must be visualized in smears made from bone marrow material. Bone marrow is aspirated from the interstitium of the iliac crest or the sternum in a small, cylindrical plug. Some of the material may be inoculated directly into blood culture media for recovery of bacteria. Some laboratories report good recovery from bone marrow material that has been injected into a Pediatric Isolator tube (DuPont Co.; described in Chapter 14) as a collection and transport device. The lytic agents within the Isolator tube are thought to lyse cellular components, presumably freeing intracellular bacteria for enhanced recovery. A special medium for enhancement of growth of *Brucella* species may be used (Chapter 29). Other material may be inoculated directly to fungal media, as described in Chapter 43. Smears are made for fixation, staining, and examination (usually by pathologists) for the presence of fungal or parasitic agents.

21.4. Bone Biopsy

A small piece of infected bone is occasionally sent to the microbiology laboratory for determination of the etiologic agent of **osteomyelitis** (infection of bone). It has been shown that cultures taken from open wound sites above infected bone or material taken from a draining sinus leading to an area of osteomyelitis may not reflect the actual etiologic agent of the underlying osteomyelitis. Patients develop osteomyelitis from hematogenous spread of an infectious agent, invasion of bone tissue from an adjacent site of infection, such as joint infection

or dental infection, or by breakdown of tissue due to trauma or surgery or lack of adequate circulation followed by colonization with microorganisms. Parasites are rarely, if ever, etiologic agents of osteomyelitis. Once established, infections in bone may tend to progress toward chronicity, particularly if there is a lack of effective blood supply to the affected area.

Staphylococcus aureus, seeded during bacteremia, is the most common etiologic agent of osteomyelitis among people of all age groups. The toxins and enzymes produced by this bacterium, as well as its ability to adhere to smooth surfaces and produce a protective glycocalyx coating, seem to contribute to its pathogenicity (Chapter 24). Among young persons, osteomyelitis is usually associated with a single agent, *S. aureus*. Such infections are usually of hematogenous origin. Other organisms that have been recovered from hematogenously acquired osteomyelitis include *Salmonella* species, *Haemophilus* species, Enterobacteriaceae, *Pseudomonas* species, *Fusobacterium necrophorum*, and yeast species. *Pseudomonas aeruginosa*, as well as *S. aureus* and other gram-negative bacilli including *Eikenella corrodens*, is often recovered from drug addicts, whereas a preceding animal bite may lead to *Pasteurella multocida* infection. Bone biopsies from infections that have spread to a bone from a contiguous source or that are associated with poor circulation (especially in diabetics) are more likely to yield multiple isolates. *Mycobacterium tuberculosis* is presently an uncommon cause of osteomyelitis. Gram-negative bacilli are increasingly common among hospitalized patients; a break in the skin (surgery or intravenous line) may precede establishment of gram negative osteomyelitis. Breaks in skin from other causes (bite wound, trauma) also may be the initial event that leads to underlying bone infection. Poor oral hygiene may lead to osteomyelitis of the jaw with *Actinomyces* species, *Capnocytophaga* species, and other oral flora, particularly anaerobes. Pigmented

Bacteroides, other *Bacteroides, Fusobacterium,* and *Peptostreptococcus* species are commonly involved. Pelvic infection in the female may lead to mixed aerobic and anaerobic osteomyelitis of the pubic bone.

Patients with poor circulation to the extremities, notably diabetics who commonly have neuropathy as well and therefore are subjected to trauma that they cannot feel, will develop ulcers on the toes and feet that do not heal, become infected, and eventually progress to involve underlying bone. These infections are usually polymicrobial, involving anaerobic and aerobic bacteria. Commonly encountered are the *B. fragilis* group, the pigmented *Bacteroides,* other gram-negative anaerobes, *Peptostreptococcus* species, *S. aureus,* and group A and other streptococci.

Bone removed at surgery or by percutaneous biopsy is sent to the laboratory in a sterile container. It is very difficult to break up bones; grinding them in a mortar and pestle may help to break off some pieces. It is sometimes possible to aseptically scrape off small shavings from the most necrotic-looking areas, which can be inoculated to media. Pieces should be placed directly into fungal media for recovery of fungi. Small bits of bone can be ground with sterile broth to form a suspension for bacteriologic and mycobacterial cultures. If anaerobes are to be recovered, all manipulations should ideally be performed in an anaerobic chamber. If such an environment is unavailable, microbiologists should work quickly to inoculate anaerobic plates and broth with material from the bone.

21.5. Tissue

Pieces of tissue are removed from patients during surgical or needle biopsy procedures or are collected at autopsy. Any etiologic agent of infection may cause disease in tissue and laboratory practices should be adequate to recover bacteria, fungi, and viruses, and to detect the presence of parasites. Fastidious organisms, such as *Brucella* species, and agents of chronic disease such as systemic fungi and mycobacteria, may require special media and long incubation periods for isolation. Some agents that require special supportive or selective media are as follows:

    Actinomyces sp.
    Brucella sp.
    Legionella sp.
    Listeria monocytogenes (not fastidious)
    Systemic fungi
    Mycobacteria
    Viruses

The conditions required for their isolation are discussed in the appropriate chapters. This chapter will not attempt to delineate all of the possible etiologic agents that can be recovered from tissue specimens, but will discuss general techniques for laboratory handling of such material. It is the responsibility of the clinician or pathologist to inform the microbiologist of any suspected etiology, since the appropriate procedures can then be initiated once the specimen reaches the laboratory. Often, the physician will consult the microbiologist about possible agents to search for in advance of removing the tissue. The optimal diagnostic services are rendered when such dialogue is a constant and important part of the practice of clinical medicine and laboratory microbiology.

Tissue specimens are obtained after careful preparation of the skin site (Chapter 6). It is critical that biopsies be collected aseptically. The best specimen is that collected aseptically at the time of surgery and submitted to the microbiology laboratory in a sterile container. A wide-mouthed, screw-capped bottle or plastic container is recommended. Anaerobic organisms will survive within infected tissue long enough to be recovered from culture. A small amount of sterile nonbacteriostatic saline may be added to keep the specimen moist. If anaerobic organisms are a particular concern, a small amount of tissue can be placed into a Bio-Bag (Marion Laboratories), Gas Pak Pouch (BBL), or other anaerobic transport device (available from Marion Laboratories, Anaerobe Systems, BBL Microbiology Systems, Scott Laboratories, and other suppliers). The surgeon should take responsibility for seeing that a second specimen is submitted to pathology for histologic studies. Formaldehyde-fixed tissue is not very useful for recovery of viable microorganisms, although some organisms can be recovered at times so that an attempt should be made to subculture from formalin if that is the only specimen available. Material from draining sinus tracts should include a portion of the wall of the tract, obtained by deep curettage. Material from infective endocarditis should contain a portion of the valve and vegetation if the patient is undergoing valve replacement or comes to autopsy.

In some instances, **contaminated** material may be submitted for microbiologic examination. Such specimens as tonsils, autopsy tissue, or similar material may be surface cauterized with an electric soldering iron or heated spatula or blanched by immersing in boiling water for 5-10 seconds to reduce surface contamination. The specimen may then be dissected with sterile instruments to permit culturing of the **center** of the specimen, which will not be affected by the heating.

Because surgical specimens are obtained at great risk and expense to the patient and because supplementary specimens cannot be obtained easily, it is important that the laboratory save a portion of the original tissue (if enough material is available) in a small amount of sterile broth in the refrigerator and at $-70°$ C (or if necessary, at $-20°$ C), for at least 4 weeks in case additional studies are indicated. If the entire tissue must be ground up for culture, then a small amount of the suspension should be placed into a sterile tube and refrigerated. Refrigeration is also used to recover *Listeria monocytogenes* from tissue (cold enrichment), as described below.

Tissue should be manipulated within a lam-

inar flow biological safety cabinet by an operator wearing gloves. Processing tissue within an anaerobic chamber is best. The microbiologist should cut through the infected area (often discolored) with a sterile scalpel blade. The pathologist or clinician can help select a good area to sample. One half of the specimen can then be used for fungal cultures and the other for bacterial cultures. Both types of agents should be sought in all tissue specimens. Some sample should be saved for histology, if this has not already been done. Specimens should be cultured for viruses or acid fast bacilli when such tests are requested. If material is to be cultured for parasites, it is finely minced or teased before inoculation into broth (Chapter 44). Direct examination of stained tissue for parasites is performed by pathologists. As described by Fung et al.,[3] imprint cultures of tissues yielded bacteriological results identical to homogenates. The procedure followed in one of our laboratories (EJB) for culturing tissue is outlined in Procedure 21.1.

Additional media may be inoculated for incubation at lower temperatures, which may facilitate recovery of certain systemic fungi and mycobacteria (Chapters 41 and 43). It is possible to obtain reliable microbiologic information from tissues after a body has been embalmed. Bacteria and fungi can survive the embalming fluids for a period of time.

Occasionally it is important to ascertain the number of organisms present per gram of tissue. Particularly for burn patients, greater than 10^5 colony forming units (CFU)/g of tissue is considered to be indicative of infection, whereas less than that number probably indicates only colonization. Although rarely required, a laboratory should be able to perform quantitative cultures of tissue. Procedure 21.2 describes one method.

Tissue may be inoculated to virus tissue culture media for isolation of viruses. Brain, lung, and blood are most useful. Other specimens, such as a fecal swab or a nasopharyngeal

---

**PROCEDURE 21.1. PREPARATION AND INOCULATION OF TISSUE
FOR MICROBIOLOGICAL CULTURE**

1. Hold the tissue in a sterile Petri dish with sterile forceps and slice through it with a sterile scalpel blade.
2. Make an imprint of the sliced edge on two areas of each of the agar plates to be inoculated, usually including blood agar, chocolate agar, Columbia base colistin-nalidixic acid agar, MacConkey agar, anaerobic blood agar, selective anaerobic agar, brain heart infusion agar, and inhibitory mold agar. For lung, buffered charcoal yeast extract agar with alpha-ketoglutarate (Chapter 39) should be inoculated for *Legionella*. It is recommended that a small piece of tissue sliced from the specimen be embedded in the center of each of the fungal agar media inoculated. Inoculate the most inhibitory media last. Special agars are inoculated if requested. By holding the tissue with the forceps, the microbiologist can exert pressure to help express any microorganisms from the cut surface onto the agar. If the tissue stops making a visible imprint before all media are inoculated, a fresh slice should be made from the surface to expose new tissue.
3. Streak the inoculum from one of the two imprints for isolated colonies.
4. Grind one of the halves of tissue with sterile broth (we use *Brucella* broth) in a tissue grinder, mortar and pestle, or homogenizer, unless the tissue is lung. Lung tissue must be ground or finely minced, since homogenization fails to release bacteria from within alveolar spaces. The suspension should be about 10%-20% tissue.
5. Use portions of the ground tissue to inoculate viral and mycobacterial media and supportive broths, as well as to prepare smears for acid fast and Gram stains.
6. Small portions of remaining tissue may be examined with 10% KOH or calco-fluor white for fungal elements, if indicated.
7. A cut edge of tissue can be used to prepare a Gram stain after all inoculations have been made. This is especially useful for sections of the valve or vegetations from cases of endocarditis; the distribution and quantity of bacteria in the tissue can be ascertained, which is of value in diagnosis.

---

swab, are handled in the usual way (Chapter 42).

Tissue may be examined by immunofluorescence for the presence of herpes, cytomegalovirus, or rabies viral particles, as mentioned in Chapters 10, 12, and 42. Lung tissue may be examined by direct fluorescent antibody test for *Legionella* species. Fluorescent reagents are also available for detection of agents of plague, anthrax, and certain *Bacteroides* species, although most laboratories do not routinely per-

form such procedures. Detection of other etiologic agents of disease is usually performed by pathologists.

The tissues of all fetuses, premature infants, and young babies who have died from an infectious process should be cultured for listeriae (Procedure 21.3) for reasons given previously (see discussion of blood cultures). Specimens of the brain, liver, and spleen are most likely to contain the organism. The isolation procedure is given in detail by Seeliger and Cherry.[5]

PROCEDURE 21.2. QUANTITATIVE BACTERIOLOGIC CULTURE OF TISSUE

1. Cut a small piece of tissue, several millimeters cubed, aseptically in a sterile Petri dish.
2. Weigh a second empty sterile Petri dish.
3. Add the tissue and reweigh the dish.
4. Place the specimen and 1 ml sterile nutrient broth in a glass tissue grinder and macerate the specimen.
5. Prepare six serial dilution tubes of 4.5 ml sterile physiological saline. make 1:10 serial dilutions of the macerated specimen by adding 0.5 ml of the original suspension to the first dilution tube, vortexing vigorously, and then adding 0.5 ml of this dilution to the second tube of saline. Repeat this procedure until all six dilutions have been made. Discard 0.5 ml from the last tube. This process can be done in an anaerobic chamber.
6. Inoculate 0.1 ml from each of the six dilutions onto a blood agar plate, a Columbia colistin-nalidixic acid agar plate, an anaerobic blood agar plate (if indicated) and into thioglycolate broth. Spread the inoculum on the plates with a sterile glass spreading rod or a loop. Additional plates may be inoculated after the results of the Gram stain are known, but not all dilutions need to be plated on selective media.
7. Incubate plates in 5%-10% CO_2 overnight and count the colonies of bacteria on the plate that contains between 30 and 300 CFU.
8. Calculate the number of CFU per gram of tissue with the formula: Number of CFU × Reciprocal of dilution (10^{-3} or 10^{-4}, etc.) × 10 (the inoculation of only 0.1 ml per plate) divided by the weight of the tissue.

For example, for tissue that weighed 0.02 g, 68 CFU were observed on the plate that received the 10^{-3} dilution of suspension.

$$\frac{68 \times 10^3 \times 10}{0.02} = \frac{6.8 \times 10^5}{0.02} = 3.4 \times 10^7 \text{ CFU/g}$$

Modified from Loebl et al. 1974. Am. J. Clin. Pathol. 61:20.

PROCEDURE 21.3. ISOLATION OF *LISTERIA* SPECIES FROM TISSUE

1. Add 5-10 ml of ground tissue to each of two flasks of infusion broth.
2. Incubate one flask at 35° C for 24 h, and inoculate a drop of this to a blood agar plate and a tellurite blood agar plate. Incubate these in a candle jar or CO_2 incubator for at least 48 h, along with the original broth flask.
3. Store the second flask in a refrigerator at 4° C. If the 35° C subcultures (step 2) are unsuccessful, subculture material from the refrigerated flask at weekly intervals for at least 1 month.
4. Identify isolates as detailed in Chapter 33.

21.6. Autopsy Cultures

Several concepts about the microbiology of autopsy specimens are important. Most internal organs of previously uninfected patients remain sterile for approximately 20 h after death. A significant portion of positive necropsy cultures, therefore, are due to contamination from the autopsy room or autopsy personnel. It is estimated that only half of all autopsies should yield positive cultures and that 75% of all tissues obtained at necropsy should be sterile. Procedures modified from studies by De Jongh et al.[2] and Silver and Sonnenwirth[6] are used by the pathologists at our institution (EJB) with good success. These are outlined in Procedure 21.4.

PROCEDURE 21.4. COLLECTION OF POSTMORTEM SPECIMENS FOR MICROBIOLOGICAL STUDIES

A. General tenets.
   1. Use fresh sterile instruments for each tissue sample collected.
   2. Change to fresh sterile gloves if the current gloves become wet.
   3. Sear outside of tissue to dryness before tissue is resected with sterile scalpel or scissors.
   4. Bring material for culture to microbiology laboratory as soon as possible after collection.
B. Preparation of body (critical if microbiological data are significant for determination of cause of death or adequacy of treatment prior to death).
   1. Shave anterior trunk
   2. Thoroughly scrub body with povidone-iodine (5 min) followed by 70% alcohol (5 min).
   3. Autopsy technicians and pathologists scrub for 10 min with hexachlorophene-containing soap. Personnel don sterile masks, gowns, gloves, and boots, just as for surgery.
   4. Drape body in sterile plastic drapes and cover skin with adhesive plastic sterile drape.
C. Blood cultures.
      Make usual Y-shape incision, but draw blood cultures first before any additional manipulation. Reflect skin over thorax and sear third intercostal space next to the sternum on the left side with a red-hot spatula. If seared tissue is not completely moisture-free, it must be seared a second time. Insert a sterile, 18 gauge needle with attached 30 ml syringe into the heart (right ventricle). Withdraw as much blood as possible, up to 20 ml. Thoroughly and vigorously wipe the rubber septa of the blood culture containers with 70% alcohol. Change

PROCEDURE 21.4. COLLECTION OF POSTMORTEM SPECIMENS FOR MICROBIOLOGICAL STUDIES—cont'd

needles on the syringe, and inject 3-5 ml blood into each of two Bactec bottles (aerobic and anaerobic) for bacterial cultures and 10 ml into Isolator tube for fungal and acid fast bacterial cultures (See Chapter 14).

D. Collection of material from the peritoneal cavity.

Peritoneal fluid from the base of the mesentery should be collected on a swab (Culturette, Marion Scientific) immediately after entering the peritoneal cavity. If intraabdominal or other abscess is suspected, the outside of the abscess should be seared to dryness with a red-hot spatula and a sterile needle and syringe should be used to collect pus through intact cavity walls. Vigorously scrub the rubber top of an anaerobic transport vial with 70% alcohol, change needles, and inject aspirated material suspected of harboring anaerobes through the rubber septum into the anaerobic transport vial. All other fluid may be collected on Culturette swabs, with the exception of urine. If there is a significant amount of peritoneal fluid, it should be collected in a 20 ml syringe. For collection of urine, sear the bladder surface and collect bladder urine with a needle and syringe. Remove the needle and expel the urine into a sterile urine cup.

E. Collection of tissue specimens for culture.

Avoid sectioning any large vessels before adequate tissue specimens for culture are obtained. Be certain that the gloves of the prosector are dry and cannot drip onto the tissue. Sear a large area of the surface of the tissue to complete dryness, using a 5 cm by 5 cm red-hot bent spatula tip. Using fresh sterile scissors and forceps for each tissue specimen obtained, cut a 1 cm^3 block of tissue from the center of the seared area and place it immediately into a sterile Petri dish or sterile screw-cap urine cup, which is quickly covered up again.

F. Abscesses—special considerations.

In addition to the aspirated material, the abscess wall may be the only site from which certain organisms, like *Nocardia* and *Actinomyces*, may be recovered. In such cases, submit a small (1 cm^2) section of the abscess wall.

G. Collection of material from thoracic cavity.

Change to fresh, dry, sterile gloves and collect fluid from the pericardium, pleural cavity, etc. by needle and syringe or on Culturette swabs if necessary. Collect purulent or necrotic material with a needle and syringe, as described for abdominal abscess. Submit such material in an anaerobic transport vial. Tissue specimens are collected as described above.

REFERENCES

1. Dawson, M.S., Harford, A.M., Garner, B.K., et al. 1985. Total volume culture technique for the isolation of microorganisms from continuous ambulatory peritoneal dialysis patients with peritonitis. J. Clin. Microbiol. 22:391.
2. De Jongh, D.S., Loftis, J.W., Green, G.S., et al. 1968. Postmortem bacteriology: a practical method for routine use. Am. J. Clin. Pathol. 49:424.
3. Fung, J.C., Sun, T., Kilius, I., and Gross, S. 1983. Printcultures for postmortem microbiology. Ann. Clin. Lab. Sci. 13:83.
4. Loebl, E.C., Marvin, J.A., Heck, E.L., et al. 1974. The method of quantitative burn wound biopsy cultures and its routine use in the care of the burned patient. Am. J. Clin. Pathol. 61:20.
5. Seeliger, H.P.R., and Cherry, W.B. 1957. Human listeriosis: its nature and diagnosis. U.S. Government Printing Office, Washington, D.C.
6. Silver, H., and Sonnenwirth, A.C. 1969. A practical and efficacious method for obtaining significant postmortem blood cultures. Am. J. Clin. Pathol. 52:433.

BIBLIOGRAPHY

Brewer, N.S., and Weed, L.A. 1976. Diagnostic tissue microbiology methods. Human Pathol. 7:141.

Levison, M.E., and Pontzer, R.E. 1985. Peritonitis and other intra-abdominal infections. In Mandell, G.L., Douglas, R.G. Jr., and Bennett, J.E., editors. Principles and practice of infectious diseases, ed. 2. John Wiley & Sons, New York.

Minshew, B.H. 1983. Are quantitative wound cultures worthwhile? Clin. Microbiol. Newsletter 5:51.

O'Toole, W.F., Saxena, H.M., Golden, A., and Ritts, R.E. 1965. Studies of postmortem microbiology using sterile autopsy technique. Arch. Pathol. 80:540.

Quinn, E.L. 1985. Pleural effusion and empyema. In Mandell, G.L., Douglas, R.G. Jr., and Bennett, J.E., editors. Principles and practice of infectious diseases, ed. 2. John Wiley & Sons, New York.

Rubin, S.J. 1984. Continuous ambulatory peritoneal dialysis: dialysate fluid cultures. Clin. Microbiol. Newsletter 6:3.

Steigbiegel, R.T., and Cross, A.S. 1984. Infections associated with hemodialysis and chronic peritoneal dialysis. In Remington, J.S., and Swartz, M.N., editors. Current clinical topics in infectious diseases 5. McGraw-Hill Book Co., New York.

22 Infections of the Head and Neck

22.1. Introduction

22.1.a. General considerations, anatomy (Figure 22.1). The delicate intraocular structures are enveloped in a tough collagenous coat. The eyes themselves are enclosed within the bony orbits, four-sided pyramids. Three of the four walls of the orbit are contiguous with the paranasal (facial) sinuses. The roof of the orbit is contiguous with the frontal sinus, the floor of the orbit forms the top wall of the maxillary sinus, and the ethmoid sinus runs along the medial aspect of the orbit. Thus, sinus infections may extend directly to the periocular orbital structures. The conjunctival membranes line the eyelids and extend onto the surface of the eye itself. The eyelashes tend to prevent entry of foreign material into the eye. The lids blink 15-20 times per minute during which time secretions of the lacrimal glands and goblet cells wash away bacteria and foreign matter. Lysozyme and IgA are secreted locally and serve as part of the natural defense mechanisms of the eye.

The head and neck have a rich vascular supply that promotes rapid healing after trauma or surgery and permits rapid mobilization of host defenses. Conversely, the rich venous drainage permits the spread of embolic infection throughout the body, in particular to the central nervous system. The mastoids and sinuses are unique air-filled cavities within the head.

329

FIGURE 22.1
Location of the paranasal sinuses. (From Milliken, M.E., and Campbell, G. 1985. Essential competencies for patient care. The C.V. Mosby Co. St. Louis.)

These structures, as well as the Eustachian tube, the middle ear, and the respiratory portion of the pharynx are lined by respiratory epithelium. The clearance of secretions and contaminants depends on normal ciliary activity and mucus flow. The maxillary sinuses are close to the roots of the upper teeth so that dental infections can extend into these sinuses. The fascias (firm, fibrous covering of muscles) of the neck behave like cylinders surrounding the important muscles, and other, deeper fascias surround the important viscera of the neck (pharynx, trachea, and major salivary glands). These fascias communicate; they create neck spaces which tend to confine infection to specific areas within the neck. Unfortunately, spread to the mediastinum is not prevented. Collection and transport of specimens from the sites discussed here is covered in section 22.6.

22.1.b. Microbial flora of the head and neck. There is a rather sparse indigenous flora

in the conjunctival sac. *Staphylococcus epidermidis* and *Lactobacillus* sp. are the most commonly encountered organisms. *Staphylococcus aureus* is found in from 0%-30% of people and *Haemophilus influenzae* in from 0.4%-25%. *Branhamella catarrhalis*, various Enterobacteriaceae and various streptococci (*Streptococcus pyogenes*, *S. pneumoniae* and alpha- and gamma-hemolytic forms) are found in a very small percent of subjects. The normal flora of the external ear canal is also rather sparse. It is very much like that of the conjunctival sac qualitatively except that pneumococci, *S. aureus* and Enterobacteriaceae are encountered somewhat more often and *Pseudomonas aeruginosa* is found on occasion. *Candida* sp. (non-*albicans*) are common. The normal respiratory tract flora is discussed in Chapter 16. In addition to the organisms listed there, the oral flora may contain *Leptotrichia buccalis*, *Selenomonas*, *Wolinella*, *Campylobacter*, and the following organisms which would be more apt to be involved in infection—*Clostridium perfringens* (found irregularly), *Eikenella corrodens*, *Capnocytophaga*, *Actinobacillus*, and *Haemophilus aphrophilus* and closely related species. Two protozoa, *Entamoeba gingivalis* and *Trichomonas tenax*, are found as normal flora but are rarely involved in infectious processes. We must also be concerned with indigenous flora of animals in the case of bite infections. *Pasteurella multocida* is commonly involved in infection following dog and cat bites. A particularly virulent organism encountered in relation to dog bites is a fastidious gram-negative bacillus designated by The Centers for Disease Control (CDC) as DF-2.

22.1.c. Pathogenic mechanisms. Much of the discussion of pathogenic mechanisms in Chapter 16 is pertinent to this chapter as well. *Capnocytophaga* (which includes organisms formerly called *Bacteroides ochraceus* and DF-1) has been shown to release lysosomal enzymes from human polymorphonuclear leukocytes. A sonic extract of these bacteria inhibits migration of phagocytes and suppresses the proliferation of human fibroblasts. One species of *Capnocytophaga* (*C. sputigena*) shows relatively weak endotoxin activity. Cell envelopes of *Capnocytophaga* exhibit several types of immunomodulating activity and evoke dermatoxic reactions on rabbit skin. The pathogenicity of *Clostridium perfringens* is discussed in Chapter 35.

22.2. Eye Infections

22.2.a. Conjunctivitis. *Chlamydia trachomatis* is responsible for one of the most important types of conjunctivitis, trachoma. This disease is one of the leading causes of blindness in the world. *C. trachomatis* is also one of the causes of acute conjunctivitis in the newborn.

Bacterial conjunctivitis is the most common type of infectious conjunctivitis. In adults, the most common organisms cultured are *Streptococcus pneumoniae*, *Staphylococcus aureus*, and *S. epidermidis*. However, there is dispute as to the significance of isolates of the latter two organisms. In children, the most common causes of conjunctivitis are *Haemophilus influenzae*, *S. pneumoniae*, and perhaps *S. aureus*. *S. pneumoniae* and *H. influenzae* have been responsible for epidemics of conjunctivitis. Gonococcal conjunctivitis may be quite destructive. Diphtheritic conjunctivitis occurs in conjunction with diphtheria elsewhere in the body. *Moraxella lacunata* produces a localized angular conjunctivitis with little discharge from the eye. Distinctive clinical pictures may also occur with conjunctivitis due to *Mycobacterium tuberculosis*, *Francisella tularensis*, *Treponema pallidum* and *Yersinia enterocolitica*. A number of other bacteria and many different types of viruses have been isolated from cases of conjunctivitis. Fungi and parasites may also be responsible for this type of infection.

22.2.b. Keratitis. Keratitis, or inflammation of the cornea, may be caused by a wide variety of infectious agents, usually only after some type of trauma produces a defect in the ocular surface. Keratitis should be regarded as an emergency situation since corneal perforation and loss of the eye can occur within 24 h when organisms such as *Pseudomonas aeruginosa* or *Staphylococcus aureus* are involved. The most common symptom of keratitis is pain, usually accompanied by some decrease in vision, but typically with no discharge from the eye. Bacteria account for 65%-90% of corneal infections. In the United States, the most common infecting organisms are *S. aureus*, *Streptococcus pneumoniae*, *P. aeruginosa*, and *Moraxella*. The first three organisms listed account for over 80% of all bacterial corneal ulcers. A toxic factor known as exopeptidase has been implicated in the pathogenesis of corneal ulcer produced by *S. pneumoniae*. In the case of *P. aeruginosa*, proteolytic enzymes are responsible for the corneal destruction. The gonococcus may cause keratitis in the course of inadequately treated conjunctivitis. *Acinetobacter*, which may look identical microscopically to the gonococcus and is penicillin resistant, can cause corneal perforation. Many other organisms, including mycobacteria, *Treponema pallidum*, *Nocardia*, *Chlamydia trachomatis*, several viruses and parasites, and a large number of fungi may cause keratitis.

22.2.c. Endophthalmitis. Surgical trauma, non-surgical trauma (uncommonly) and hematogenous spread from distant sites of infection are the background factors in endophthalmitis. The infection may be limited to specific tissues within the eye or may involve all of the intraocular contents. Pain, especially on movement of the eye, is a prominent aspect of the clinical picture. Bacteria are the most common infectious agents responsible for endophthalmitis. Bacterial endophthalmitis develops suddenly and progresses rapidly. Following surgery or trauma, evidence of the disease is found within 24-48 h. Postoperative infection involves primarily bacteria from the ocular surface microflora. *Staphylococcus aureus* is responsible for 50% of cases of endophthalmitis following cataract extraction. *S. aureus* and *Pseudomonas* usually lead to fulminating infection early in the postoperative period. Any bacterium, including those considered to be primarily saprophytic, may cause endophthalmitis. In hematogenous endophthalmitis, a septic focus elsewhere is usually evident before onset of the intraocular infection. *Bacillus cereus* has caused endophthalmitis following transfusion with contaminated blood and in narcotic addicts. Endophthalmitis associated with meningitis may involve various organisms including *H. influenzae*, streptococci, and *Neisseria meningitidis*. *Nocardia* endophthalmitis follows pulmonary infection with this organism. Endophthalmitis may be seen in the course of miliary tuberculosis and in syphilis.

Mycotic infection of the eye has increased significantly over the past three decades because of increased use of antibiotics, corticosteroids, antineoplastic chemotherapy, addictive drugs and hyperalimentation. Fungi generally considered to be saphrophytic are important causes of endophthalmitis. Fungi recovered from postoperative infection include *Volutella* sp., *Neurospora sitophila*, *Monosporium apiospermum*, *Candida parapsilosis*, *Trichosporon cutaneum*, *Paecilomyces lilacinus*, *Cephalosporium*, and *Torulopsis glabrata*. Endogenous mycotic endophthalmitis is most commonly due to *Candida albicans*. Other causes of hematogenous ocular infection include *Aspergillus*, *Cryptococcus*, *Coccidioides*, *Sporothrix*, and *Blastomyces*; *Histoplasma* is rarely involved.

Viral causes of endophthalmitis include herpes simplex I, herpes zoster, cytomegalovirus and measles viruses. The most common parasitic cause is *Toxocara*. *Toxoplasma gondii* is a well-known cause of chorioretinitis. Thirteen percent of patients with cysticercosis have ocular involvement. *Onchocerca* usually produces keratitis, but intraocular infection also occurs.

22.2.d. Periocular infections. Included in this category are infections of the eyelids, of the lacrimal apparatus and of the orbit. Lid infections include blepharitis (inflammation of the lid margins), hordeolum or the common sty, and chalazion. Most eyelid infections are due to bacteria, especially *S. aureus* and *S. epidermidis*. Other organisms that may be encountered include molluscum contagiosum and herpes simplex viruses, *Proteus mirabilis* and *Moraxella*.

The three infections of the lacrimal apparatus are canaliculitis (chronic inflammation of the lacrimal canals), dacryocystitis (inflammation of the lacrimal sac) and dacryoadenitis (inflammation of the main lacrimal gland). Canaliculitis is usually due to *Actinomyces* or *Arachnia*, *Pityrosporum pachydermatis* or *Fusobacterium*. Infection of the lacrimal sac may involve *Aspergillus*, *Candida albicans*, or *Actinomyces*. Other causes are *S. pneumoniae*; mixed infection with *Staphylococcus*, *Streptococcus* and *P. aeruginosa*; and *Chlamydia trachomatis*. Dacryoadenitis often involves pyogenic bacteria such as *S. aureus* and streptococci, but gonococci and *Cysticercus cellulosae* have been reported. Chronic infections of the lacrimal gland occur in tuberculosis, syphilis, leprosy, and schistosomiasis. Acute inflammation of the gland may occur in the course of mumps and infectious mononucleosis.

Orbital cellulitis is an acute infection of the orbital contents that is most commonly caused by bacteria. It is a serious infection because it may spread posteriorly to produce cavernous sinus thrombosis. Most cases involve spread from contiguous sources such as the paranasal sinuses. In children, blood-borne bacteria, notably *H. influenzae*, may lead to orbital cellulitis. Intrauterine infections may be a background factor in newborns. *Staphylococcus aureus* is the most common etiologic agent; *S. pyogenes* and *S. pneumoniae* are also common. Anaerobes may be involved secondary to chronic sinusitis. Mucormycosis of the orbit is a serious, invasive infection seen particularly in diabetics with poor control of their disease, patients with acidosis due to other causes, and patients with malignant disease receiving cytotoxic and immunosuppressive therapy. *Aspergillus* may produce a similar infection in the same settings, but also can cause mild, chronic infections of the orbit.

22.3. Ear, Nose, and Throat Infections

22.3.a. Pharyngitis, tonsillitis, peritonsillar abscess. The various forms of pharyngitis and tonsillitis, including diphtheria, are discussed in Chapter 16. The predominant organisms in peritonsillar abscess are non-spore-forming anaerobes including *Fusobacterium*, *Bacteroides* (including the *B. fragilis* group), and anaerobic cocci. *Streptococcus pyogenes* and viridans streptococci may also be involved.

22.3.b. Dental and oral infections. Oral infection with herpes simplex virus, gonococci and *Candida* has been discussed in Chapter 16. Oral lesions may be encountered in secondary syphilis (see Chapter 19 for a discussion of darkfield preparations and syphilis serology). A large spirochete seems to be a key pathogen in acute necrotizing ulcerative gingivitis (Vincent's gingivitis); clinical microbiology laboratories are not asked to do bacteriologic studies for diagnosis of this condition. The three dental problems in which help may be requested from clinical laboratories are root canal infections, with or without periapical abscess; orofacial odontogenic infections, with or without osteomyelitis of the jaw; and perimandibular space infections. The bacteriology is similar in all of these situations, involving only anaerobic bacteria and streptococci except for perimandibular space infections, which may also involve staphylococci and *Eikenella corrodens* in about 15% of cases. The streptococci are microaerophilic or facultative and are usually alpha-hemolytic; they are usually found in 20%-30% of infections of the above type. Members of the *Bacteroides fragilis* group are found in root canal infections, orofacial odontogenic infections and in bacteremia secondary to dental

extraction in 5%-10% of cases. Anaerobic cocci (both *Peptostreptococcus* and *Veillonella*), pigmented *Bacteroides*, the *Bacteroides oralis* group and *Fusobacterium* are found in about 20%-50% of the three conditions mentioned above, as well as in postextraction bacteremia. Bacterial stomatitis is rarely seen now in the United States. It is characterized by superficial (and sometimes deep) tissue necrosis with pseudomembrane formation and a fetid odor. Anaerobes are clearly involved, but bacteriologic studies are unsatisfactory; spirochetes are likely important. Oral bacteria are clearly important in other dental processes such as caries, periodontal disease (pyorrhea) and localized juvenile periodontitis, but there is no indication for routine culturing in such cases.

22.3.c. Salivary gland infections. Acute suppurative parotitis is seen in very ill patients, especially those that are dehydrated, malnourished, elderly, or recovering from surgery. It is associated with painful, tender swelling of the parotid gland; there may be purulent drainage evident at the opening of the duct of the gland in the mouth. *Staphylococcus aureus* is the major pathogen, but on occasion viridans streptococci and oral anaerobes may play a role. A chronic bacterial parotitis has been described which usually involves *S. aureus*. Less commonly, other salivary glands may be involved with a bacterial infection; this is usually due to ductal obstruction. The mumps virus is the major viral agent involved in parotitis, but the influenza virus and enteroviruses may also cause this. Uncommonly, *Mycobacterium tuberculosis* may involve the parotid gland in conjunction with pulmonary tuberculosis.

22.3.d. Sinusitis. Acute sinusitis is usually due to bacterial infection; it tends to be self-limited, usually lasting 1 to 3 weeks. Most often it follows a common cold or other viral upper respiratory infection. Complications include local extension into the orbit, skull, meninges, or brain and development of chronic sinusitis. Most studies of the microbiology of acute sinusitis have dealt with maxillary sinusitis because this is the most common type and the one most accessible for puncture and aspiration. Bacterial cultures are positive in about two-thirds of patients. About half of the bacterial isolates are accounted for by S. *pneumoniae* and *H. influenzae*. Next in order of frequency are various anaerobes (found in 10% of cases), aerobic or facultative gram-negative rods (9%), S. *aureus* (4%), and S. *pyogenes* and B. *catarrhalis* (2% each). Rhinovirus is found in 15% of patients, influenza virus in 5%, parainfluenza virus in 3%, and adenovirus in <1%. Bacteria, particularly anaerobes, are essentially always present in chronic sinusitis, but their pathogenic role is uncertain. The primary problems are inadequate drainage, impaired mucociliary clearance, and mucosal damage. Ordinarily, surgery is required for successful management.

22.3.e. External ear infections. Otitis externa is similar to skin and soft-tissue infections elsewhere but there is the unique problem of a narrow, tortuous ear canal. There are several types of external otitis. Acute localized disease occurs in the form of a pustule or furuncle and is due to S. *aureus*. Erysipelas caused by group A streptococci may involve the external ear canal and the soft tissue of the ear itself. Acute diffuse otitis externa (swimmer's ear) is related to maceration of the ear from swimming or hot, humid weather. Gram-negative bacilli, particularly *P. aeruginosa*, play an important role. A severe, hemorrhagic external otitis due to *P. aeruginosa* has been related to hot tub use. Chronic otitis externa is due to the irritation of drainage from the middle ear in patients with chronic, suppurative otitis media and a perforated ear drum. Rarely, this condition may be caused by tuberculosis, syphilis, yaws, or leprosy. Malignant otitis externa is a necrotizing infection that spreads to adjacent areas of soft tissue, cartilage, and bone. It may progress to a life-threatening situation by spreading into the central nervous system or vascular chan-

nels. *P. aeruginosa* and anaerobes may be frequently associated with this process. This process is seen in diabetics with small blood vessel disease of the skin overlying the temporal bone; the poor local perfusion of tissues results in a milieu for invasion by bacteria. On occasion, external otitis will extend into the cartilage of the ear; this usually leads to a requirement for surgical intervention. Certain viruses may infect the external auditory canal, the soft tissue of the ear, or the tympanic membrane; influenza A virus is a suspected, but not an established cause. *Mycoplasma pneumoniae* is definitely implicated as a cause of bullous myringitis (a painful infection of the ear drum with hemorrhagic bullae or blisters); the ear canal itself may be involved. Varicella-zoster virus may cause painful vesicles or blisters within the soft tissue of the ear and the ear canal.

22.3.f. Middle ear infection (otitis media) and mastoiditis. Acute otitis media may begin as a viral infection, but bacterial infection typically supervenes. In children (and most acute otitis media is in children), the two most commonly encountered pathogens are the pneumococcus and *H. influenzae;* in third place in terms of frequency of occurrence is group A streptococcus. Other organisms, encountered in only 1%-3% of cases, include B. *catarrhalis*, S. *aureus*, gram-negative enteric bacilli, and anaerobes. S. *pneumoniae* is found in about 33% of patients, *H. influenzae* in about 20%, and S. *pyogenes* in 8%. Viruses, chiefly respiratory syncytial virus and influenza virus, have been recovered from middle ear fluid of 4% of children with acute or chronic otitis media. *Chlamydia trachomatis* has been isolated from middle ear aspirates occasionally and *M. pneumoniae* rarely.

Chronic otitis media and its complication, mastoiditis, yield a predominantly anaerobic flora with *Peptostreptococcus* sp., B. *fragilis* group, pigmented *Bacteroides* group, other *Bacteroides* sp., and *F. nucleatum* as the principal pathogens; less commonly present are S.

19.1

19.2

PLATE 19.1.   Gram-negative intracellular diplococci; diagnostic for gonorrhea in urethral discharge.
PLATE 19.2.   Appearance of fluorescent antibody–stained *Treponema pallidum*. Organisms appear to bend only near the center.

19.3

PLATE 19.3. Gram stain of genital lesion showing typical "school-of-fish" formation of pleomorphic gram-negative bacilli characteristic of *Haemophilus ducreyi* infection.

20.1

20.2

20.3

20.4

PLATE 20.1.   Sacral decubitus ulcer.
PLATE 20.2.   Erysipelas caused by *Streptococcus pyogenes*.
PLATE 20.3.   Ecthyma gangrenosum caused by *P. aeruginosa*.
PLATE 20.4.   Gas gangrene, abdominal wall. Note bronze discoloration and fluid-filled blisters (bullae).

20.5

20.6

PLATE 20.5.   Actinomycosis. Note "lumpy" jaw.
PLATE 20.6.   Actinomycosis, side view. Note sinuses in skin of face and neck.

22.1

22.2

PLATE 22.1.   Ludwig's angina.
PLATE 22.2.   Human bite infection.

22.3

PLATE 22.3. Animal bite infection caused by *Pasteurella multocida*.

aureus, *P. aeruginosa*, *Proteus* sp. and other gram-negative facultative bacilli. *M. tuberculosis* may also cause a chronic otitis media and mastoiditis.

22.4. Neck Space Infections

Infections of the deep spaces of the neck are potentially serious because they may spread to critical structures such as major vessels of the neck or to the mediastinum leading to mediastinitis, purulent pericarditis, and pleural empyema. One of these infections, Ludwig's angina (Plate 22.1), may lead to airway obstruction. The oral flora is responsible for these infections. Accordingly, the predominant organisms are anaerobes—*Peptostreptococcus*, various *Bacteroides* and *Fusobacterium* species, and *Actinomyces* for the most part. Streptococci, chiefly of the viridans variety, are also important and *S. aureus* and various gram-negative non-anaerobic bacilli may also be recovered, particularly from patients developing these problems in the hospital setting.

22.5. Bite Infections

Human bites (Plate 22.2), including clenched fist injuries, yield, among the aerobic or facultative flora, alpha hemolytic streptococci, *S. aureus*, group A streptococcus, and *Eikenella corrodens*, in that order of frequency. Anaerobes recovered include, in order of frequency, *Peptostreptococcus*, pigmented *Bacteroides*, *Bacteroides oris-buccae*, and *Fusobacterium nucleatum*. In infected animal bite wounds (Plate 22.3), the most commonly encountered aerobic and facultative bacteria are alpha hemolytic streptococci, *S. aureus*, *Pasteurella multocida* and *Enterobacter cloacae*. Predominant anaerobes in the animal bites are anaerobic gram-positive cocci, *Fusobacterium* sp. and *Bacteroides* sp.

Oral and nasal fluids from dogs yield IIj, EF-4, *P. multocida*, and *S. aureus*. *Simonsiella* is found in the oral cavity of most dogs and is also found in the oral cavity of humans, cats, and other animals. The oral flora of snakes contains various gram-negative bacilli including *Pseudomonas*, *Klebsiella*, *Proteus*, and *E. coli*. Clostridia may also be recovered from snakebite wounds.

A fastidious gram-negative bacillus designated as DF-2 by CDC has been responsible for a number of serious infections, including bacteremia, endocarditis, and meningitis. Most of these patients had a history of dog bite and most had underlying diseases that impair host defense mechanisms. This organism is typically resistant to aminoglycosides and is susceptible to penicillin G.

22.6. Collection and Transport of Specimens

For culture of purulent conjunctivitis, the purulent material is collected on a sterile swab from the surface of the lower conjunctival sac and inner canthus of the eye. Both eyes should be cultured separately. Chlamydial cultures are taken with a dry calcium alginate swab; this is placed in chlamydial culture medium (Chapter 38). In the case of keratitis, an ophthalmologist should obtain scrapings of the ulcer with a heat-sterilized platinum spatula. Multiple inoculations with the spatula are made to blood agar, chocolate agar, an agar for fungi, thioglycolate broth, and an anaerobic blood agar plate. Other special media may be used if indicated. For culture of herpes simplex virus and adenovirus, corneal material is transferred to viral transport media. In the case of endophthalmitis, cultures should be made from material obtained by the ophthalmologist from the anterior chamber of the eye, the vitreous, wound abscesses, and wound dehiscenses. Lid infections are cultured by obtaining material on a swab in a conventional manner. In canaliculitis, concretions from the lacrimal canal should be transported under anaerobic conditions (Chapter 6). In the case of orbital cellulitis, aspiration of fluid from the orbit is contraindicated. Since sinusitis is the most common background factor, the assistance of an otolaryngologist in obtaining material from the sinuses by antral puncture is helpful. Blood cultures should be obtained. In mucormycosis, tissue biopsy is essential; cultures are usually negative, the diagnosis being made by histologic examination.

For laboratory diagnosis of external otitis, the external ear should be cleansed with a mild germicide such as 1:1000 aqueous solution of benzalkonium chloride to reduce the contaminating skin flora before obtaining the culture. Material from the ear, especially that obtained after perforation of the eardrum or by needle aspiration of middle ear fluid (tympanocentesis), should be collected by an otolaryngologist, using sterile equipment and a sterile cotton or polyester swab. Cultures from the mastoid are generally taken on swabs during surgery; they should be transported anaerobically.

In the case of oral and dental infections, the problem is to avoid or minimize contamination with oral flora. For collection of material from root canal infection, the tooth is isolated by means of a rubber dam. A sterile field is established, the tooth is swabbed with 70% alcohol, and after the root canal is exposed, a sterile paper point is inserted, removed, and placed into semisolid, nonnutritive anaerobic transport medium.

Specimens from neck space infections can usually be obtained with a syringe and needle by the surgeon. Transport must be under anaerobic conditions. Bite wound infections usually involve relatively small lesions and minimal exudate. Accordingly, a swab technique with anaerobic transport will usually be needed. Surrounding skin should be thoroughly cleansed before the specimen is obtained (Chapter 6).

22.7. Direct Visual Examination

All material submitted for culture should always be smeared and examined directly by Gram stain and/or other appropriate technique. In bacterial conjunctivitis, polymorphonuclear leukocytes will predominate; in viral infection, the host cells will be primarily lymphocytes and monocytes. Multinucleated epithelial cells may be seen in herpes infections; one may seek intranuclear inclusion bodies by the Tzanck technique (Chapter 42). In chlamydial infection, basophilic intracytoplasmic inclusion bodies are seen in epithelial cells; a fluorescent antibody technique using a monoclonal antibody is available (Chapter 38). Immunoelectron-microscopy and immunofluorescent techniques may aid in diagnosing viral conjunctivitis. In the case of keratitis, scrapings are examined by Gram, Giemsa, PAS, and methenamine silver stains. Transmission electron microscopy may establish viral etiology. In the case of endophthalmitis, material is also examined by Gram, Giemsa, PAS, and methenamine silver stains. Material aspirated from the maxillary sinus, from middle ear or mastoid infections, from neck space infections, and from bite infections is also examined directly for bacteria and fungi.

22.8. Culturing

Because of the constant washing action of the tears, the number of organisms recovered from cultures of certain eye infections may be relatively low. Unless the clinical specimen is obviously purulent, it is recommended that a relatively large inoculum and a variety of media be used to ensure recovery of an etiologic agent. At a minimum, one should use blood agar and chocolate agar plates incubated under increased carbon dioxide tension. Since potential pathogens may be present in an eye without causing infection, it may be very helpful to the clinician, when only one eye is infected, to culture both eyes. When *Moraxella lacunata* (the Morax-Axenfeld bacillus) is suspected, Loeffler medium (Chapter 45) may prove useful; the growth of the organism often leads to proteolysis and pitting of the medium, although there are non-proteolytic strains. If diphtheritic conjunctivitis is suspected, Loeffler or cystine-tellurite medium should be used. For more serious eye infections such as keratitis, endophthalmitis, and orbital cellulitis, one should always include, in addition to the media noted above, a reduced anaerobic blood agar plate, a medium for fungi, and a broth such as thioglycolate broth. Blood cultures are also essential in the case of serious eye infections.

A number of the other infections discussed in this chapter, such as peritonsillar abscess, oral and dental infections, chronic sinusitis, chronic otitis media and mastoiditis, neck space infections, and bite wound infections, commonly involve anaerobic bacteria. The anaerobes involved typically originate in the oral cavity and are more delicate than anaerobes isolated from other clinical material. Very careful attention must be paid to providing optimum techniques of anaerobic cultivation, as well as transport (Chapters 6 and 34).

One study compared results of middle ear cultures obtained by tympanocentesis with simultaneous semiquantitative culture of the nasopharynx. The latter cultures were reasonably predictive (72%) if the material was plated immediately on appropriate solid media and if semiquantitative reading of growth was used.

The DF-2 organism which produces such serious infection after dog bite is a gram-negative rod that grows slowly on blood or chocolate agar (it does best with a heart infusion base). The growth of this fastidious organism is enhanced by cultivation under increased carbon dioxide tension; rabbit serum also enhances growth. Identification of this organism is discussed in Chapter 28.

22.9. Noncultural Detection Methods

Although acute and convalescent serologic tests for viral agents might be used in the event of epidemic conjunctivitis, these are not generally done since the infections are self-limited. A microimmunofluorescent test for *Chlamydia trachomatis* inclusion conjunctivitis is available (Chapter 38). In more serious eye infections, some workers have used a *Limulus* lysate test (Chapter 10) on corneal scrapings or aqueous or vitreous humor for rapid detection of gramnegative infection. An ELISA test of aqueous humor is available for diagnosis of *Toxocara* infection. One may look for antigens such as pneumococcal and *H. influenzae* antigen in middle ear exudates using latex agglutination, coagglutination, CIE, or RIA, but it is doubtful that this would be more useful than Gram stain except, perhaps, in patients who had already received antimicrobial therapy.

BIBLIOGRAPHY

Bartlett, J.G., and Gorbach, S.L. 1976. Anaerobic infections of the head and neck. Otolaryngol. Clin. North Am. 9:655.

Baum, J.L. 1978. Ocular infections. N. Engl. J. Med. 299:28.

Brook, I., and Finegold, S.M. 1979. Bacteriology of chronic otitis media. J.A.M.A. 241:488.

Butler, T., Weaver, R.E., Ramani, T.K.V., et al. 1977. Unidentified gram-negative rod infection: a new disease of man. Ann. Intern. Med. 86:1.

Farr, B., and Gwaltney, J.M., Jr. 1983. Acute and chronic sinusitis. In Pennington, J.E., editor, Respiratory infections: diagnosis and management. Raven Press, New York.

Finegold, S.M. 1977. Anaerobic bacteria in human disease. Academic Press, New York.

Goldstein, E.J.C., Citron, D.M., Wield, B., et al. 1978. Bacteriology of human and animal bite wounds. J. Clin. Microbiol. 8:667.

Hirst, L.W., Thomas, J.V., and Green, W.R. 1985. Conjunctivitis; Keratitis; Endophthalmitis; and Periocular infections. In Mandell, G.L., Douglas, R.G. Jr., and Bennett, J.E., editors, Principles and practice of infectious diseases. John Wiley & Sons, New York.

Klein, J.O. 1983. Otitis media. In Pennington, J.E., editor, Respiratory infections: diagnosis and management. Raven Press, New York.

Newman, M.G., and Goodman, A.D., editors. 1984. Guide to antibiotic use in dental practice. Quintessence Publishing Co., Chicago.

Sutter, V.L., Citron, D.M., Edelstein, M.A.C., and Finegold, S.M. 1985. Wadsworth anaerobic bacteriology manual, ed. 4. Star Publishing Co., Belmont, Calif.

23

Infections in the Compromised Host

23.1. Introduction

An individual may be at increased risk of acquiring an infectious disease either because of inherent host factors, such as age or disease, environmental factors, manipulations performed as part of medical practice, or combinations of these factors (see p. 339). One of the ironies of modern medicine is that as treatments are improved to prolong the survival of patients suffering from many types of disease, these patients become more vulnerable to infectious diseases. Exposure to certain agents, such as viruses, may be related to occupation or life-style. This chapter focuses on some of the categories of patients who are at a greater risk of acquiring infections than are normal hosts and on some likely etiologic agents of these infections. In most cases, diagnosis of infectious disease is handled in the same way for compromised patients as for any infected host, as described in the preceding chapters. When special considerations are appropriate, they will be mentioned in this chapter. A discussion of all conditions that predispose a person to acquiring an infectious disease is beyond the scope of this text.

23.2. Infections Related to Age

23.2.a. Infections in neonates. As a fetus develops within the uterus, it is effectively protected from most environmental influences, in-

338

**FACTORS CONTRIBUTING TO
INCREASED RISK OF ACQUIRING
INFECTIOUS DISEASE**

Host factors
   Age—very young or very old
   Anatomical defects, congenital or ac-
      quired (meningocele, benign pros-
      tatic hypertrophy, etc.)
   Disease (cystic fibrosis, diabetes, can-
      cer, sickle cell anemia, viral or
      other concomitant infections, etc.)
   Immune system abnormalities
   Poor nutritional state
Environmental factors
   Iatrogenic (antibiotic or myelosup-
      pressive therapy, foreign implants,
      surgery, access conduits such as
      catheters, etc.)
   Tissue damage (trauma or surgery)
   Life-style (sexual behavior, travel,
      eating habits, alcohol, drugs, etc.)
   Occupation
   Proximity to other infected hosts, an-
      imal and human

---

cluding infectious agents, by the placenta and
the amniotic fluid. The human immune system
does not become wholly competent until several months after birth. Immunoglobulins that
cross the placental barrier, primarily IgG,
serve to protect the newborn from many agents
until the infant begins to produce immunoglobulins of his or her own in response to antigenic
stimuli. This unique environmental niche,
however, does expose the vulnerable fetus to
pathogens present in the mother. Infections in
infants are of two types: **congenital,** acquired
by the fetus as a result of a maternal infectious
agent that crosses the placenta; and **neonatal,**
acquired during passage through the birth
canal or immediately postpartum.

The most common agents of **congenital infection** in the United States are *Toxoplasma
gondii,* rubella, cytomegalovirus, and herpes
simplex virus, the so-called **TORCH** agents.
Congenital disease may also be caused by a
number of other agents (see p. 340). Of these,
Treponema pallidum (syphilis) and *Listeria
monocytogenes* (neonatal listeriosis or abortion)
are probably the most common.

Suspected congenital infection can be diagnosed culturally or serologically. Because maternal IgG crosses the placenta, serologic tests
are often difficult to interpret. If the presence
of IgG is the only available test, serum samples
from both mother and baby must be tested simultaneously and the baby's titers must be observed to rise over several weeks, indicating
that antigenic stimulation of active antibody
production occurred as a result of infection.
For culturable agents, the most definitive diagnoses involve recovery of the pathogen in
culture. Rubella, herpes simplex, varicella-
zoster, enteroviruses, and cytomegalovirus can
be cultured easily (Chapter 42), as can most
bacterial agents. Nasal and urine specimens offer the greatest yield for viral isolation, while
blood, cerebrospinal fluid, and lesion material
can also be productive. Bacteria and fungi can
be isolated from lesion sites, blood, and occasionally from other sources.

Determination of the presence of fetal IgM
directed against the agent in question establishes the serologic diagnosis of congenital infection. Until recently, ultracentrifugation was
required for separation of IgM from IgG, the
only definitive means of preventing false positive results due to maternal IgG or fetal rheumatoid factor. A column that separates IgM
from IgG by ion-exchange chromatography is
now commercially available (Chapter 12). By
using column eluate for serologic tests, the microbiologist can better differentiate maternal
and fetal antibody. Serologic procedures are
described in Chapter 12. Indirect fluorescent
antibody test systems are commercially avail-

ETIOLOGIC AGENTS OF CONGENITAL AND NEONATAL INFECTIONS

Viruses
  *Cytomegalovirus
  Enteroviruses
  Hepatitis B virus
  *Herpes simplex virus
  Measles virus
  *Rubella virus
  Vaccinia virus
  Varicella-zoster virus

Bacteria
  Borrelia
  Brucella
  Campylobacter
  **Chlamydia*
  Francisella
  Gardnerella
  Leptospira
  **Listeria*
  Mycobacterium
  Mycoplasma
  Salmonella
  Staphylococcus
  **Streptococcus*, group B
  **Treponema*

Fungi
  **Candida*
  Coccidioides

Parasites
  Leishmania
  Plasmodium
  **Toxoplasma*
  Trypanosoma

Modified from Peter, Cherry, and Bryson. 1982. Diagn. Med. 5:61.
*More commonly recognized agents of infection.

able for detection of IgM against *Toxoplasma gondii*, rubella, cytomegalovirus (CMV), herpes simplex, and varicella-zoster. Interference by rheumatoid factor is still a consideration in most of the commercial IgM test systems. Commercially produced ELISA systems showing excellent specificity and sensitivity for diagnosis of toxoplasmosis, rubella, CMV, and herpes may also be used. Our ability to detect viral inclusions in tissue, conjunctival scrapings, and vesicular lesions, traditionally performed with Giemsa stain, has been improved by availability of monoclonal and polyclonal fluorescent antibody reagents, described in the chapters that discuss individual agents.

If an infant is born to a mother with both a positive VDRL and FTA-ABS, the diagnosis of congenital syphilis is presumptive and treatment is begun. With VDRL positive mothers who were adequately treated for their disease in the past, diagnosis of a congenitally infected baby due to maternal reinfection may be more difficult. Congenital syphilis may be diagnosed by either darkfield examination of lesions or serologically. Since antitreponemal IgM tests may be unreliable, infants should be tested sequentially over several months.

Although the Sabin-Feldman dye test is the standard against which all other serologic tests for toxoplasmosis are measured, it is performed in only a few specialized laboratories. A commercially available latex agglutination test (Hynson, Wescott & Dunning) has been shown to be adequate for detection of IgG against *Toxoplasma*, a useful screening test for women before they become pregnant. A fourfold rise in titer during pregnancy is indicative of a newly acquired infection. Laboratory diagnosis of congenital disease, however, requires demonstration of specific IgM in fetal serum by either conventional ELISA, indirect immunofluorescent stain, or a recently described IgM immunosorbent assay developed by Remington and others.[8] This test is recommended as the most sensitive and specific test available.

Hepatitis B can be transmitted to fetuses of chronically infected mothers, and a significant number of such infected infants will themselves become chronic carriers of hepatitis B. Laboratory diagnosis of congenital hepatitis requires demonstration of HBsAg in fetal serum, usually accomplished by performing an ELISA or a radioimmunoassay test. For the parasitic agents of congenital infection other than *T. gondii*, visual evidence of the agent in fetal circulation is diagnostic.

Demonstration of the presence of bacterial capsular antigen is the most rapid method for diagnosis of group B streptococcal infection. Latex and coagglutination reagents are commercially available (Chapters 12, 15, and 25), and counterimmunoelectrophoresis has been used with good results. Unfortunately, rapid antigen detection reagents are not yet available for the other bacterial agents of congenital infections.

Neonatal infections are often related to a difficult labor, premature birth, premature rupture of membranes, maternal genital infection, or other event. Meningitis with Enterobacteriaceae, usually *Escherichia coli*, sepsis with group B streptococci or *Listeria*, or herpes infections (often systemic) are the most common types encountered. Infections with *Haemophilus influenzae*, *Gardnerella vaginalis*, *Bacteroides fragilis* or other anaerobic bacteria, sepsis due to mycoplasma that infect the genital tract, ophthalmia neonatorum caused by *Neisseria gonorrhoeae*, and inclusion conjunctivitis and pneumonia caused by *Chlamydia trachomatis* also occur, although less often.

Diagnosis of these infections is usually based on recovery of the agent, but direct examination of conjunctival smears by Giemsa, fluorescent antibody stain, or Gram stain can allow a much more rapid determination of the etiology of purulent discharge from the infant's eye. Direct antigen detection tests are available for gonococci, herpes, cytomegalovirus, *Chlamydia*, and group B streptococci. The appropriate specimens (cerebrospinal fluid, serum, pus, tracheal aspirate, etc.) should be examined immediately with these reagents. For all other agents, culture of blood, nasopharyngeal secretions, or stool will produce the greatest yield. As reviewed by Miller,[6] the results obtained by culturing placental membranes and gastric aspirates do not correlate well with identification of an etiologic agent of neonatal infection.

23.2.b. Infections in the elderly. Pneumonia is the most common infection in aged patients; it is the fourth leading cause of death in patients older than 75 years in the United States. Factors such as decreased mucociliary function, decreased cough reflex, periodontal disease, and decreased general mobility probably contribute to a greater incidence of pneumonia in aged patients. Such patients have been found to be more frequently colonized with gram-negative bacilli than are younger people, perhaps due to poor oral hygiene, decreased saliva, or decreased epithelial cell turnover. When these patients are institutionalized, their oral colonization rate is higher and their chances of acquiring gram-negative bacterial pneumonia are enhanced. Mortality due to bacterial pneumonia following respiratory viral infections, influenza in particular, is greater in elderly patients. The bacteria associated with pneumonia in the elderly are *Streptococcus pneumoniae*, *Legionella* species, oral anaerobes, *Staphylococcus aureus*, the Enterobacteriaceae, and *Pseudomonas* species (especially in hospitalized patients). Reactivation tuberculosis and lung disease caused by nontuberculous mycobacteria occur relatively often in elderly patients. The incidence of atypical mycobacterial disease is low, and the species of organisms involved may vary depending on the locality. Diagnosis of these infections is performed as described in Chapter 16.

Urinary tract infections pose significant problems for elderly patients. Women may suffer from cystocele, loss of pelvic muscle tone, and changes in urinary tract mucosa, which predispose them to infection, whereas prostatic disease in males is the most common condition contributing to urinary tract infection in that group. It is possible that due to loss of somatic tissue integrity and poorer immune response associated with age, urinary tract infections in elderly patients are more likely to lead to sepsis. Important factors include obstructive uropathy and manipulation of the urinary tract (e.g., catheterization). Gram-negative bacteremia, as a result of another focus of infection (often in the urinary tract), is an important problem infection seen in the elderly. Other infections likely to be encountered among older patients include peritonitis or intraabdominal abscess, often initiated by gastrointestinal tract disorders such as cholecystitis, obstruction, diverticulosis, ulcer, or malignancy. Circulating bacteria may colonize heart valves, leading to endocarditis. The loss of some immune functions and of vascular integrity with age may predispose older patients to serious varicella-zoster infections (including pneumonia), infectious arthritis, meningitis, and skin and soft tissue infections. The specimens required for diagnosis and the handling of those specimens are no different from those used to diagnose infections in any patient, as described in previous chapters.

23.3. Infections in Patients with Underlying Disease

Diseases that alter the body's normal metabolism can affect the "steady-state" of the host, rendering the patient more vulnerable to infection. In addition, a number of diseases affect the immune system itself, preventing functional activity that serves to protect a normal host from many etiologic agents. A few of the more notable diseases that predispose the sufferer to infection are mentioned here.

23.3.a. Cystic fibrosis. Patients with cystic fibrosis may present as young adults with chronic respiratory tract disease, as well as the more common presentation in children that may also include gastrointestinal problems and stunted growth. A very mucoid *Pseudomonas* species, characterized by production of copious amounts of extracellular capsular polysaccharide (see Chapter 28, Figure 28.3), can be isolated from the sputum of almost all cystic fibrosis patients older than 18 years, becoming more prevalent with increased age of the patient after the age of 5 years. Even if cystic fibrosis has not been diagnosed, isolation of a mucoid *P. aeruginosa* of this type from sputum should alert the clinician to the possibility of such an underlying disease. Microbiologists should always report this unusual morphologic feature if it is encountered. In addition to the mucoid *Pseudomonas*, cystic fibrosis patients are likely to harbor *Staphylococcus aureus*, *Haemophilus influenzae*, and *Pseudomonas cepacia*. Sputum specimens from patients known to have cystic fibrosis should be inoculated to selective agar, such as mannitol salt for recovery of *S. aureus* and selective horse blood-bacitracin (Chapter 45), incubated anaerobically and aerobically, for recovery of *H. influenzae* which may be obscured by the mucoid *Pseudomonas* on general supplemented media.

23.3.b. Diabetes mellitus. Diabetes mellitus, especially in older patients, seems to predispose sufferers to several infectious diseases. Lack of adequate peripheral circulation (via both small and large vessels) and peripheral neuropathy lead to tissue necrosis and the commonly encountered "diabetic foot ulcer" (Chapter 20). Chronic soft tissue infections, often of mixed bacterial etiology, including anaerobic and facultative bacteria (including *S. aureus*), can lead to osteomyelitis (Chapter 21). Diabetics are also at risk of developing synergistic necrotizing cellulitis caused by mixed aerobic and anaerobic bacteria, various other forms of anaerobic cellulitis and fasciitis (Chapter 20), malignant otitis externa, and streptococcal cellulitis. Acidosis predisposes patients to fungal infection. Rhinocerebral mucormycosis and candidiasis are relatively frequent in patients with diabetes.

23.3.c. Sickle cell disease. Circulating antibodies of patients with sickle cell disease seem to display impaired ability to opsonize certain bacteria, particularly *S. pneumoniae* and *Salmonella* species. These patients suffer from defective complement activity and lack of a functional spleen, which may also contribute to their increased risk for infection. Primary pneumococcal sepsis, peritonitis, and meningitis are common in patients with sickle cell disease. *Salmonella* is the cause of 80% of osteomyelitis cases in patients with sickle cell disease; this is usually secondary to sepsis. Other gram-negative bacilli account for the other 20%.

23.3.d. Congenital immune deficiency diseases. A number of children are born with defects of the immune system, either cellular or humoral, or combined immunodeficiency syndromes that involve components of each of the immune effector systems. Additional defects include lack of certain complement components. In all of these cases, infections that are easily handled by the normal host become problems in the immunodeficient host. For example, patients with antibody deficiencies are often plagued by infections caused by encapsulated bacteria such as pneumococci, meningococci, and *H. influenzae*. Patients who lack certain elements of the complement cascade are more likely to contract infections with meningococci and gonococci. Children with chronic granulomatous disease, a disease with polymorphonuclear neutrophil (PMN) dysfunction, have gram-negative bacterial and staphylococcal infections. A complete discussion of the infectious consequences of inherited immunologic defects is beyond the scope of this book.

23.3.e. Neoplastic diseases. Patients with cancer are more likely to become infected, and the nature of the malignancy often determines the etiologic agent(s). Table 23.1 contains a list of etiologic agents associated with certain malignancies. Hodgkin's disease affects the cell-mediated immune response which normally helps to protect the body from intracellular

TABLE 23.1
Infectious Agents Commonly Associated with Certain Malignancies

MALIGNANCY (SITES AND TYPES OF INFECTIONS)	PATHOGENS
Acute nonlymphocytic leukemia (pneumonia, oral lesions, cutaneous lesions, urinary tract infections, hepatitis, most commonly sepsis without obvious focus)	Enterobacteriaceae *Pseudomonas* Staphylococci *Corynebacterium JK* *Candida* *Aspergillus* *Mucor* Hepatitis (non-A, non-B)
Acute lymphocytic leukemia (pneumonia, cutaneous lesions, pharyngitis, disseminated disease)	Streptococci (all types) *Pneumocystis carinii* Herpes simplex Cytomegalovirus Varicella-zoster
Lymphoma (disseminated disease, pneumonia, urinary tract, sepsis, cutaneous lesions)	*Brucella* *Candida* (mucocutaneous) *Cryptococcus neoformans* Herpes simplex (cutaneous) Herpes zoster Cytomegalovirus *Pneumocystis carinii* *Toxoplasma gondii* *Listeria monocytogenes* Mycobacteria *Nocardia* *Salmonella* Staphylococci Enterobacteriaceae *Pseudomonas* *Strongyloides stercoralis*
Multiple myeloma (pneumonia, cutaneous lesions, sepsis)	*Haemophilus influenzae* *Streptococcus pneumoniae* *Neisseria meningitidis* Enterobacteriaceae *Pseudomonas* Herpes varicella-zoster *Candida* *Aspergillus*

pathogens such as herpes, mycobacteria, *Salmonella, Brucella, Nocardia,* and *Listeria.* Even before chemotherapy, patients with Hodgkin's-type lymphoma are likely to become infected with these and other agents normally handled by the cellular immune system. Treatment with certain chemotherapeutic agents and with corticosteroids also impairs cellular immunity. Other malignancies may affect the humoral immune response, which contributes to protection against agents such as viruses, *Pneumocystis, Giardia,* staphylococci, and encapsulated bacteria. Cancer patients are likely to be undergoing treatment for their disorder, and a discussion of infection in such hosts must consider the effects of therapy as a necessary consequence of the disease. Although a few infectious agents are associated with certain carcinomas irrespective of therapy, such as *Streptococcus bovis* and *Clostridium septicum* bacteremia in patients with bowel malignancy, most infections in cancer patients are at least partially a result of the loss of immunological effector cells, either as a part of the disease process or as a consequence of chemotherapy.

The most important factor that determines whether an immunosuppressed patient will suffer increased risk of infection is the number of circulating granulocytes, primarily PMNs. Patients with severe **granulocytopenia** (markedly decreased numbers of circulating granulocytes, less than $500/mm^3$ PMNs and particularly those with less than $100/mm^3$ PMNs) are the most likely to develop infections. Gram-negative facultative organisms and staphylococci are the most common etiologic agents. Gram-negative anaerobic organisms and fungi are encountered less often. The authors of one major study found that routine surveillance cultures of nose, throat, urine, and stool were not helpful for predicting those patients at risk for septicemia or for determining empiric therapy once the patients became febrile.[5] Follow-up daily blood cultures drawn on febrile patients after they had been started on empiric therapy, however, were helpful for identifying an etiologic agent and ultimately for guiding therapy. By drawing such blood cultures into resin-containing media to remove antibiotics from the milieu or into the Isolator system (both described in Chapter 14), microbiologists should increase the chances of recovering an organism from a patient receiving antibiotics. Persistent fever in the granulocytopenic patient on antibiotics suggests the presence of a fungal infection, particularly *Candida* or *Aspergillus* and less often *Mucor.* Diagnosis of such fungal infections is difficult, and empiric antifungal therapy with amphotericin B is often necessary.

23.3.f. Patients with acquired immune deficiency syndrome (AIDS). See Section 23.8.

23.4. Infections in Hospitalized Patients (Nosocomial Infections)

Patients are at increased risk for acquiring infections merely by being hospitalized. Approximately 2 million people (5% or greater of all hospitalized patients) acquire a **nosocomial infection** (an infection that occurs at least 72 h after admission and was not present at the time of admission) each year. The cost of increased antibiotics, increased length of hospital stay, and loss of work due to nosocomial infections is staggering; it has been estimated to exceed $4 billion annually. Factors that contribute to the risk of acquiring a nosocomial infection include the poor state of health of many patients, the use of immunosuppressive therapy, extensive surgery, invasive diagnostic tests, uses of indwelling catheters in veins, arteries, and the bladder, infusion of contaminated intravenous fluids, contaminated respiratory therapy equipment, and the widespread use of broad-spectrum antibiotics which leads to the prevalence of antibiotic-resistant strains of bacteria in the hospital environment.

Pneumonia is the leading cause of death among nosocomial infections (as high as 50% mortality in intensive care unit patients), although urinary tract infections are the most prevalent type of nosocomial infection. Etiologic agents recovered from nosocomial urinary tract infections include *Escherichia coli*, enterococci, *Pseudomonas aeruginosa*, *Klebsiella* species, and *Proteus* species. Urinary tract, surgical wound, and lower respiratory tract infections account for more than 70% of all nosocomial infections. Hospitalized patients are often colonized in the respiratory tract, gastrointestinal tract, and the skin by endemic hospital strains of bacteria within several days of admission. The nosocomial infection rate is highest among patients admitted to the surgery service (where most patients experience a breakdown of skin barriers), and the lowest rates are found among neonates and pediatric patients. Surgical wound infections are most commonly caused by *Staphylococcus aureus*, *E. coli*, other Enterobacteriaceae, anaerobes, *P. aeruginosa*, and enterococci. Intraabdominal and burn infections often lead to bacteremia secondary to the primary infection. The most common isolates are *Bacteroides* species, *Serratia* species, *S. aureus*, *Acinetobacter* species, *Streptococcus agalactiae*, and *Providencia* species.

Nosocomial pneumonia is a risk for any hospitalized patient, and in particular for intubated patients. Organisms associated with these infections include *Klebsiella* species, other Enterobacteriaceae, *S. aureus*, anaerobes, *Streptococcus pneumoniae*, *Legionella*, and *P. aeruginosa*. Other agents have been associated with nosocomial outbreaks. Recently at the Wadsworth VA Hospital, outbreaks of influenza with complicating pneumonia and Legionnaires' disease have occurred. Viruses such as respiratory syncytial virus, adenovirus, and influenza A are often implicated as causes of nosocomial pneumonia among hospitalized children. Material introduced into the lungs of patients via contaminated fluids or equipment during respiratory therapy has led to infections with *P. aeruginosa*, *Acinetobacter* species, *Serratia* species, and other gram-negative bacteria. In addition to breathing in aerosolized infectious agents, hospitalized patients are at increased risk of aspirating upper respiratory

flora into the lungs (anesthesia, stroke, depressed sensorium, etc.). **Aspiration pneumonia,** as it is called, is usually caused by mixed anaerobic oral bacteria and aerobic streptococci. In the hospital setting, *S. aureus* and various gram-negative bacteria may also be involved. Transtracheal aspiration and perhaps thin needle biopsy (Chapter 16) may be the only reliable means of obtaining a specimen for culture.

Antibiotic treatment, by altering normal flora and thus removing the protective effect of such flora, can select for multiply resistant strains of bacteria or allow fungal agents to multiply within the susceptible host. Such colonizing organisms may become involved in a variety of hospital-acquired infections. Alteration of the gastrointestinal flora may allow overgrowth of toxin-producing *Clostridium difficile*. This may lead to a syndrome called **antibiotic-associated pseudomembranous colitis (PMC),** definitively diagnosed by visualizing (by sigmoidoscopy or colonoscopy) typical pseudomembranous plaques made up of necrotic epithelial cells and pus cells on the mucosal surface of the lower gastrointestinal tract (Plate 17.1). Patients experience cramps and diarrhea which is sometimes bloody. Chapter 17 contains further information about this syndrome and its diagnosis.

23.5. Infections in Patients with Grafts, Shunts, or Prosthetic Devices

Production of an artificial opening in the surface epithelium and then insertion of a plastic catheter into a blood vessel of a patient compromises the skin's ability to exclude pathogens and allows such agents direct access to the bloodstream. Devices such as intravenous catheters, heparin locks, hemodialysis shunts, total parenteral nutrition catheters, and arterial catheter lines expose patients to increased risk of infection. The agents present on the skin surface near the site of access are the most prevalent isolates from nosocomial infections; included are *Staphylococcus aureus* and coagulase negative staphylococci, gram-negative bacilli, *Candida albicans*, other *Candida* species, *Torulopsis glabrata*, and *Corynebacterium* JK. *S. aureus* is the most common etiologic agent of infected hemodialysis shunts, and *Staphylococcus epidermidis* is most commonly associated with peritonitis in patients undergoing ambulatory peritoneal dialysis. *S. epidermidis* is the most common etiologic agent of infected intravenous catheters, heparin locks, and cerebrospinal fluid shunts. Other skin flora, including diphtheroids, micrococci, and colonizing gram-negative bacilli, are common causes of infection associated with catheters and shunts. Patients receiving parenteral nutrition via a Broviac, Hickman, or other catheter are at risk of developing infections due to *Candida* species, *T. glabrata*, staphylococci, or gram-negative bacilli. It is important to culture the blood and the catheter tip to document catheter-associated septicemia (described in Chapter 14). Contaminated intravenous fluids have been documented as a cause of serious nosocomial sepsis. The most common agents have been gram-negative rods, including *Citrobacter freundii*, *Enterobacter agglomerans*, *Pseudomonas aeruginosa*, *Pseudomonas cepacia*, *Klebsiella* species, and *Serratia* species.

Prosthetic devices often present a surface on which bacteria and fungi can adhere and multiply. Accordingly, a small percentage of patients receiving vascular grafts, prosthetic heart valves, cardiac pacemaker devices, and joint prostheses become infected with bacteria or fungi. The time until presentation of infection may vary from 1 week to 2 years. Staphylococci again dominate as the most important etiologic agents of such infections. It is postulated that coagulase negative staphylococci possess an adherence mechanism that allows them to attach to intravenous devices. The "slime" produced by certain strains of staphylococci may enhance their ability to adhere to intravascular prostheses, contributing to their predominance in many such infections. Prosthetic heart valve infections may also be caused by diphtheroids, gram-negative bacilli, *C. albicans*, and *Aspergillus* species, particularly in the early postoperative period. In addition enterococci and viridans streptococci can cause late-appearing (after 60 days) infections in patients with prosthetic valves. *Mycobacterium chelonei* and fungi have been rare causes of porcine valve infection.

23.6. Infections in Drug Abusers

Drug abusers are at increased risk of acquiring infectious disease for several reasons: they may inject contaminated foreign material or their own cutaneous or oral flora into their bloodstreams along with the drug; they may be malnourished or inattentive to proper hygiene; they may suffer from lapses of consciousness and thus be at risk of aspirating oral secretions into their lungs; and they may contract viral infections (such as hepatitis and AIDS) via contaminated needles.

Sites of injection of drugs are often infected, most commonly with *Staphylococcus aureus*, which is carried on the skin of most drug abusers. Streptococci are also common etiologic agents of cutaneous and subcutaneous infections, and severe necrotizing fasciitis and pyomyositis following introduction of mixed aerobic and anaerobic oropharyngeal flora have been seen occasionally in "skin poppers." Injection of microorganisms directly into the bloodstream often results in endocarditis among drug abusers. The most common agents include *S. aureus*, streptococci, enterococci, *Pseudomonas aeruginosa*, *Serratia marcescens*, other gram-negative bacilli including *Eikenella corrodens*, and *Candida* species. Staphylococcal involvement of the tricuspid valve is particularly common.

Drug addicts, due to drug-induced stupor and depressed cough reflex, may aspirate oropharyngeal flora into the lungs, causing lung abscess, aspiration pneumonia, and empyema. Organisms associated with these syndromes are black-pigmented and other *Bacteroides* species, *Peptostreptococcus* species, microaerophilic and facultative streptococci, fusobacteria, and other bacteria. General poor health and depressed respiratory defense mechanisms predispose such patients to the more common agents of pneumonia, including *Streptococcus pneumoniae*, *Haemophilus influenzae*, viruses, and mycoplasma. As mentioned above, most addicts are positive for hepatitis B surface antigen and many will suffer from hepatitis (either hepatitis B or non-A, non-B) at least once. Sexually transmitted diseases are common among drug abusers, particularly women, who may to turn to prostitution to support their habit. Those drug abusers who are homosexual, bisexual, or who develop AIDS are at even greater risk of acquiring infections, as outlined below.

23.7. Infections in Homosexual Males

Homosexuality per se does not predispose a person to infectious disease, and homosexual women are at no greater risk than heterosexual women of becoming infected. Many common practices among some homosexual men, however, including oral-genital, anal-genital, and oral-anal activities, as well as interacting with multiple partners over a relatively short time period, predispose these men to a number of infectious diseases. As might be suspected, acquisition of the standard sexually transmitted diseases (Chapter 19) is facilitated by participating in sexual activity with increased numbers of partners. Gonorrhea, syphilis, and herpes are more prevalent among homosexuals than heterosexuals of similar demographic groups. In addition to the usual genital sites of infection, gonococci and herpes are often isolated from oropharyngeal lesions and as causes of proctitis. Oral-genital practices may predispose some patients to unusual oral presentation of sexually transmitted diseases. Frequent isolation of *Neisseria meningitidis* from the oropharynx, anus, and urethra of homosexual men

is probably also a consequence of oral-genital contact.

Anal-genital and anal-oral practices predispose participants to a number of infections that are usually transmitted by the fecal-oral route. Non-B hepatitis (as well as type B) is prevalent among homosexual males. A group of agents has been found to comprise the most common causes of inflammatory, diarrheal, or ulcerative bowel disease in homosexual men, collectively called the **gay bowel syndrome.** Diarrhea is usually caused by *Entamoeba histolytica*, *Giardia lamblia*, *Cryptosporidium*, *Salmonella* species, *Shigella* species, or *Campylobacter jejuni*. Painful lesions may be caused by herpes, gonococci, meningococci, *Chlamydia* (both LGV and non-LGV strains), *Haemophilus ducreyi*, *Calymmatobacterium granulomatis*, or *Candida* species. The primary chancre of syphilis may go undiagnosed within the rectum. In addition to hepatitis virus, cytomegalovirus and human T-cell lymphotropic virus (HTLV III) or lymphadenopathy associated virus (LAV) may be transmitted sexually. Homosexual males are the largest risk group in the United States for contracting acquired immune deficiency syndrome (AIDS), a devastating disease of the cell-mediated immune system marked by destruction of a subclass of T lymphocytes by the HTLV III virus. This entity is discussed below.

23.8. Infections in Patients with AIDS

Since 1981, when the first cluster of cases of pneumonia caused by the rare pathogen *Pneumocystis carinii* was reported among young homosexuals, an ever-increasing number of patients have developed diseases that were previously recognized only in compromised hosts. Patients suffering from this disorder were said to have the acquired immune deficiency syndrome (AIDS). Until the etiologic agent (HTLV III) was isolated, the Centers for Disease Control defined a case of AIDS as any person diagnosed as having a disease at least moderately indicative of an underlying cellular immune deficiency but who has no known underlying cause of immune deficiency or decreased resistance. The diseases included as moderately indicative of an immune disorder are listed in the boxed material. Other infectious organisms reported in AIDS patients include pneumococci, *Mycobacterium tuberculosis, Legionella* species, *Campylobacter jejuni, Salmonella* species, *Isospora belli,* varicella-zoster virus, *Histoplasma* species, and other fungi.

23.8.a. Epidemiology of AIDS. Over 14,000 cases of AIDS have been recognized,

---

DISEASES AT LEAST MODERATELY INDICATIVE OF AN UNDERLYING CELLULAR IMMUNE DEFICIENCY

Bacterial
    Mycobacteria other than *M. tuberculosis*
Fungal
    Esophageal candidiasis
    Disseminated aspergillosis
    Cryptococcosis
Parasitic
    Cryptosporidiosis, longer than 1 month duration
    Pneumocystis carinii pneumonia
    Strongyloidosis, other than intestinal
    Toxoplasmosis, pneumonia or central nervous system infection
Viral
    Disseminated cytomegalovirus infection
    Chronic (>1 month) or disseminated herpes simplex infection
    Progressive multifocal leukoencephalopathy (JC virus)
Neoplastic
    Kaposi's sarcoma
    Lymphoma of the brain

---

with an overall long-term mortality of approximately 70%. Patients with Kaposi's sarcoma alone have the best prognosis for survival; those with only an opportunistic infection have the worst prognosis. Forty percent of all AIDS cases reported to CDC occur in New York City, and 25% occur in California. Although homosexual and bisexual men comprise the largest single risk group (approximately three-fourths of all cases), other groups at risk included intravenous drug abusers (approximately one-fifth of all cases), Haitians (approximately 5% of all cases), recipients of transfused blood and blood products, and hemophiliacs who receive factor VIII concentrate (1% of cases). Sexual contacts and children of people within risk groups are also at risk of acquiring AIDS. Recently, increasing numbers of patients with only heterosexual exposure are developing AIDS. Although cases have occurred in health care workers, occupational transmission has been documented only rarely (see below).

In addition to patients with infectious diseases or neoplasms suggestive of an underlying immune disorder, there are a number of patients whose only symptom is lymphadenopathy. These patients, usually homosexual or bisexual men, may also complain of malaise, weight loss, and fever. These symptoms are indicative of the **AIDS-related complex, ARC,** and may signify a prodrome to definitive AIDS in some cases. It appears that most of the patients with ARC do possess antibody to HTLV III, indicating prior contact with that agent. In addition, the HTLV III virus has been cultured from peripheral blood and saliva of patients with ARC. Now that ELISA and Western blot tests have been developed to allow for detection of the HTLV III antibody (Abbott Laboratories; DuPont Company; Electro-Nucleonics; Litton Bionetics; and Travenol-Genentech), prospective blood donors can be screened. Screening has introduced a disturbing new group of patients to the medical community: those HTLV III antibody positive patients with no signs or symptoms of disease. It is unknown whether such patients are protected from infection, in a prodrome stage, or comprise a group of patients who will carry the agent without ever becoming ill. The virus has been cultured from semen, saliva, and blood of healthy homosexual men, suggesting a possible asymptomatic carrier state which may be important in dissemination of the disease.[3,4]

23.8.b. Infection-control guidelines for patients with AIDS. A task force composed of specialists from the University of California, San Francisco, published guidelines for infection control for patients with AIDS.[2] These guidelines are primarily concerned with practices involved in caring for the patient and collecting and transporting laboratory specimens. In general, precautions similar to those taken with patients suspected of having hepatitis B are suggested. Gloves should be worn by persons who must contact body secretions, blood or blood products, stool, tissue, or any articles that may be contaminated by these products. If there is danger of splatter of body secretions or fluids, protective eyewear and gowns should be worn. Masks should be worn by coughing patients and by persons expected to have prolonged contact with such patients, although the majority of respiratory infections in such patients will not be contagious. All laboratory specimens should be double-bagged and labeled as to possible infectious agent, as they are for suspected hepatitis. Some workers use a yellow tape with AIDS prominently written in large letters to identify specimens from such patients, but some code such as "blood precautions" would be better. All precautions normally taken for presumptive hepatitis-infected material are suggested. The use of a 1:10 dilution of 5.25% sodium hypochlorite solution (household bleach) to clean all contaminated surfaces is recommended. It must be remembered that chlorine and formalin can combine to form a carcinogenic substance, so that areas or objects with wet formalin should be washed with soap and water prior to disinfection with chlorine solutions.

Precautions for clinical and laboratory staffs were published in *Morbidity and Mortality Weekly Report* in 1982.[1] Recommendations for handling patient specimens and decontaminating surfaces are as stated above. In addition, a few additional safety precautions for laboratories are listed. Briefly, they state that extraordinary care must be taken to avoid accidental wounds from sharp instruments contaminated with material from AIDS patients. Gowns should be worn if there is a chance that contaminated material may soil clothing. Needles should be placed directly into a puncture-resistant container and autoclaved before disposal. All other precautions are those practiced by most clinical laboratories handling potentially infectious material, as stated in Chapter 2. As always, hand washing is strongly advised after performing any procedure.

Additional precautions for workers performing autopsies on AIDS patients have been outlined by CDC and the College of American Pathologists. All persons performing or viewing autopsies should wear double gloves, mask, protective eye coverings, cap, gown, and waterproof apron and shoe coverings. Personnel should label and bag all contaminated articles, including the cadaver. Efforts should be made to minimize aerosol production, for instance by using hand saws instead of electric saws for bone. Workers must decontaminate all surfaces with bleach solution (being careful not to combine formalin and bleach) and fix tissues thoroughly in 10% buffered formalin before trimming or cutting.

Although hundreds of people have sustained a needle-puncture injury with needles contaminated with blood from AIDS patients, to date, only two health-care persons have been infected via this route. *California Morbidity* reported in December 1984 that 326 health care workers in the United States have sustained documented percutaneous or per-mucosal exposure to potentially infectious material from patients with AIDS.[9] There has been little evidence of infection in health care workers. One nurse caring for an AIDS patient in England has been reported to have seroconverted 49 days after a needle puncture injury. At 3 months after the injury, she had developed no symptoms. The risk of acquiring AIDS by person-to-person contact of a nonintimate nature has not been assessed entirely, but it appears to be extremely low.

23.8.c. Laboratory diagnosis. In addition to routine procedures, the following measures have been useful in diagnosing opportunistic infections in AIDS patients. Patients with bacteremia due to *Mycobacterium avium-intracellulare* complex often have large numbers of circulating bacteria, and blood cultures are often positive, particularly with a lysis-centrifugation system (DuPont Isolator System, Chapter 14). Blood is drawn directly into the Isolator tube, which is allowed to remain at room temperature for approximately 1 h before centrifugation and plating. Presumably this time period allows the white cells to be lysed, releasing viable mycobacteria that would not have been detected if the white cells were to remain intact. Additionally, numbers of circulating organisms can be quantitated by using the Pediatric 1.5 ml Isolator tube in a manner similar to that used for the standard Isolator. Quantitation of this sort can help to monitor the patient's response to therapy.

A number of procedures including open lung biopsy, transbronchial biopsy, and bronchoalveolar lavage are useful in diagnosing *P. carinii* pneumonia, although even bronchial washings may often be positive in AIDS patients. A rapid stain such as toluidine blue O (Chapter 16) for detection of *P. carinii* can be used on open lung biopsy material or bronchial washings. In our institution, we perform the toluidine O as a stat procedure and follow up with a semirapid modified Gomori methenamine silver stain performed at 80° C (Chapter 16), which takes approximately 1 h to perform.

In addition to *Pneumocystis*, the silver stain will reveal fungal elements. Other agents of pulmonary infection can be detected by standard methods. Acid fast stains of stool, as well as sputum, may be helpful in detecting mycobacteria and also *Cryptosporidium*. One must carefully examine all specimens from AIDS patients with an open mind since unusual pathogens and unusual presentations of infectious diseases are not uncommon.

REFERENCES

1. Centers for Disease Control. 1982. Acquired immune deficiency syndrome (AIDS): precautions for clinical and laboratory staffs. M.M.W.R. 31:577.
2. Conte, J.E., Hadley, W.K., Sande, M., and the UCSF Task Force on AIDS. 1983. Infection-control guidelines for patients with the acquired immune deficiency syndrome (AIDS). N. Engl. J. Med. 309:740.
3. Groopman, J., Salahuddin, S.Z., Sarngadharan, M.G., et al. 1984. HTLV-III in saliva of people with AIDS-related complex and healthy homosexual men at risk for AIDS. Science 226:447.
4. Ho, D.D., Schooley, R.T., Rota, T.R., et al. 1984. HTLV-III in the semen and blood of a healthy homosexual man. Science 226:451.
5. Kramer, B.S., Pizzo, P.A., Robichaud, K.J., Witebsky, F., and Wesley, R. 1982. Role of serial microbiologic surveillance and clinical evaluation in the management of cancer patients with fever and granulocytopenia. Am. J. Med. 72:561.
6. Miller, J.M. 1984. Predictive value of culturing placental membranes and gastric aspirates of newborns. Clin. Microbiol. Newsletter 6:125.
7. Peter, J.B., Cherry, J.D., and Bryson, Y.J. 1982. Improving diagnosis of congenital infections. Diagn. Med. 5:61.
8. Remington, J.S., Eimstad, W.M., and Araujo, F.G. 1983. Detection of immunoglobulin M antibodies with antigen-tagged latex particles in an immunosorbent assay. J. Clin. Microbiol. 17:939.
9. State Department of Health Services. Assessment of risk to healthcare workers with parenteral exposure to blood from AIDS patients. California Morbidity. Dec. 21, 1984. No. 50.

BIBLIOGRAPHY

Centers for Disease Control. 1984. Nosocomial infection surveillance, 1983. In CDC Surveillance Summaries 33 (no. 2SS):9SS.

Janda, W.M. 1984. Update on the acquired immune deficiency syndrome. Clin. Microbiol. Newsletter 6:9.

Mandell, G., Douglas, R.G. Jr., and Bennett, J.E., editors. 1985. Principles and practice of infectious diseases, ed. 2. Part IV: Special problems. Section A: Nosocomial infections and Section B: Infections in special hosts. John Wiley & Sons. New York.

Marx, J.L. 1985. More progress on the HTLV family. Science 227:156.

Murray, J.F., Felton, C.P., Garay, S.M., et al. 1984. Pulmonary complications of the acquired immune deficiency syndrome. N. Engl. J. Med. 310:1682.

Ostrow, D.G. 1984. Homosexuality and sexually transmitted diseases. In Holmes, K.K., Mårdh, P.-A., Sparling, P.F., and Wiesner, P.J., editors. Sexually transmitted diseases. McGraw-Hill Book Co., New York.

Quinn, T.C., and Holmes, K.K. 1984. Proctitis, proctocolitis, and enteritis in homosexual men. In Holmes, K.K., Mårdh, P.-A., Sparling, P.F., and Wiesner, P.J., editors. Sexually transmitted diseases. McGraw-Hill Book Co., New York.

Remington, J.S., and Klein, J.O., editors. 1983. Infectious diseases of the fetus and newborn infant. W. B. Saunders Co., Philadelphia.

Rivin, B.E., Monroe, J.M., Hubschman, B.P., and Thomas, P.A. 1984. AIDS outcome: a first follow-up. N. Engl. J. Med. 311:857.

Sen, P., Kapila, R., Chmel, H., Armstrong, D.A., and Louria, D.B. 1982. Superinfection: another look. Am. J. Med. 73:706.

Steigbigel, R.T., and Cross, A.S. 1984. Infections associated with hemodialysis and chronic peritoneal dialysis. In Remington, J.S., and Swartz, M.N., editors. Current clinical topics in infectious diseases. McGraw-Hill Book Co., New York.

Sun, T., and Kaplan, M. 1983. Opportunistic infections related to AIDS. ASCP Teleconference S-529. American Society of Clinical Pathologists, Chicago.

Yoshikawa, T.T. 1983. Geriatric infectious diseases: an emerging problem. J. Am. Geriatr. Soc. 31:34.

Part Four

Methods for
Identification of
Etiologic Agents
of Infectious Disease

24 Micrococcaceae: Staphylococci and Micrococci

24.1. Introduction

The genera *Staphylococcus*, *Micrococcus*, and *Planococcus* are members of the family Micrococcaceae. The majority of planococci and micrococci are free-living saprophytes, but the natural habitat of staphylococci is the surface of primates and other mammals. Their presence as endogenous flora allows many species of staphylococci the opportunity to cause infection under certain circumstances. Both staphylococci and micrococci have been isolated from clinically significant sources.

Staphylococcus aureus (usually coagulase positive staphylococci, described below in 24.1.a) has been recognized historically as a virulent and important human pathogen; its capacity to produce human disease has not diminished with the introduction of antibiotics. Recent reviews by Sheagren[18] and by Kaplan and Tenenbaum[9] are excellent sources of information about this ubiquitous pathogen. *Staphylococcus intermedius* and *Staphylococcus hyicus* are also coagulase positive, but they have not yet been implicated as human pathogens. During the last several years, coagulase negative staphylococci have surfaced as important pathogens, preying primarily on compromised hosts, including patients with some sort of prosthetic device. Archer[1] and Kloos[10] have each effectively discussed current thought on these organisms.

355

Specimens that may harbor clinically important Micrococcaceae include those from almost any source. The organisms are hardy and do not require special collection procedures other than those outlined in Chapter 6. *S. aureus* is recovered from a variety of infections including skin lesions such as furuncles and carbuncles, various abscesses, wound infections, pneumonia, and endocarditis. From these sites, organisms can invade the bloodstream and seed metastatically, appearing in the urine or forming abscesses in various body organs, or producing septic shock (Chapter 14). The organism can also be recovered from the anterior nares, perineum, and other skin sites from as many as 10%-15% of healthy people. This **carrier state** can serve as a reservoir of infection of hospitalized patients, especially if the carrier is a health care provider such as a doctor or nurse, but most carriers do not disseminate the organism and are not a risk to patients. Although it is also an important source of food poisoning, *S. aureus* is usually not isolated from the patient suffering from this intoxication, and clinical laboratories usually do not attempt to culture pathogens from food. Coagulase negative staphylococci are a common cause of bacteremia in neutropenic patients; of infections related to indwelling catheters, shunts, and prosthetic devices; and of urinary tract infections in young, sexually active women. Micrococci become pathogens during accidental introduction into a susceptible host. They may cause endocarditis and other diverse syndromes. It appears that they are less virulent than the staphylococci.

24.1.a. Morphology and general characteristics. Micrococcaceae are spherical cocci with gram-positive cell walls; they are nonmotile, aerobic or facultatively anaerobic, and catalase positive (Chapter 9). During binary fission, Micrococcaceae divide along both longitudinal and horizontal planes, forming pairs, tetrads, and ultimately irregular clusters (Figure 24.1). The Greek word *staphyle*, mean-

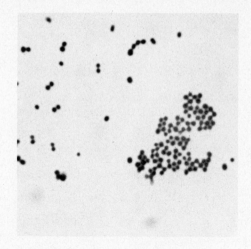

FIGURE 24.1
Appearance of Micrococcaceae in Gram stain.

ing a 'bunch of grapes,' is the descriptive stem for the genus name. Very old cells may lose their ability to retain crystal violet, and thus may be more easily decolorized in a Gram stain than young cells.

Staphylococci and micrococci will grow on most laboratory media that support gram-positive organisms, yielding circular, opaque, smooth colonies. The growth is usually **butyrous** (like butter) and colonies can be emulsified in water easily to form a smooth suspension. Hemolysis on blood agar and color of the colony are variable characteristics. Since yeast colonies can resemble Micrococcaceae and yeast may be catalase positive, all colonies should be examined microscopically by wet mount or Gram stain (Chapter 7) before further tests are performed. Mannitol salt agar, which is both selective and differential (Chapter 8), is commonly used to isolate staphyloccoci from clinical material. This medium contains high salt concentration, mannitol, and phenol red pH indicator (Chapter 8). Because it ferments mannitol, *S. aureus* will yield colonies surrounded by a yellow halo. Other staphylococci (particularly *S. saprophyticus*) may resemble *S. aureus* on mannitol salt agar.

PROCEDURE 24.1. TUBE COAGULASE TEST

1. Prepare coagulase reagent, rabbit plasma with EDTA (Difco Laboratories and BBL Microbiology Systems) in 0.5 ml amounts in 13 × 100 mm glass or plastic tubes. The tubes can be prepared in large numbers and refrigerated for 10 days, or frozen at −20° C for several months.
2. Emulsify a visible portion of growth from isolated colonies in the plasma by rubbing the material on the side of the tube while holding the tube at an angle. Straighten the tube, causing the plasma level to cover the site of inoculation.
3. Incubate the suspension for 1-4 h at 35°-37° C and observe for the presence of a gel or clot that cannot be resuspended by gentle shaking (Figure 24.2). If no clot forms after 4 h, the tube should be incubated at room temperature overnight. Rare isolates require such extended incubation.
4. Organisms that fail to clot the plasma within 24 h are considered coagulase negative, and must be identified by other methods.

Once an organism isolated from a clinical specimen has been characterized as a gram-positive, catalase positive coccoid bacterium, it is further identified in a series of steps, the first of which involves the **coagulase test.** S. *aureus* is identified on the basis of presence of the enzyme **coagulase,** which binds plasma fibrinogen, causing the organisms to agglutinate or plasma to clot. A rapid screening slide test for the production of **clumping factor** (cell-bound coagulase) that is positive with over 95% of strains of S. *aureus* is described in Chapter 9. A positive coagulase test is sufficient for naming an isolate S. *aureus* in most cases. Isolates that do not produce clumping factor must be tested for the ability to produce extracellular coagulase (**free coagulase**). This enzyme will cause clotting of plasma after 1-4 h of incubation at 37° C. The **tube coagulase test** for free coagulase is described in Procedure 24.1. Coagulase plasma with citrate is not suitable for use in this test because citrate-utilizing organisms may yield false positive results.

24.1.b. Differentiation of coagulase negative staphylococci from micrococci. Coagulase

FIGURE 24.2
Tube coagulase test. Presence of clot (tube on top) indicates a positive coagulase result.

negative organisms may be either staphylococci or micrococci. The micrococci are resistant to lysostaphin (an enzyme produced by certain staphylococci), are benzidine positive, and contain cytochrome C, as determined by a positive modified oxidase test (Procedure 24.3). In ad-

TABLE 24.1
Differences Between *Staphylococcus* and *Micrococcus* Genera

GENUS	RESISTANT TO LYSOSTAPHIN (200 μg/ml)	MODIFIED OXIDASE AND BENZIDINE	RESISTANT TO BACITRACIN (0.04 U)
Micrococcus	+	+	−
Staphylococcus	−	−	+

PROCEDURE 24.2. BACITRACIN SUSCEPTIBILITY

1. Growth from the colony to be tested is inoculated into 1 ml of trypticase soy broth to a turbidity equal to that of a McFarland 0.5 standard.
2. Using a cotton swab saturated with the test suspension, the microbiologist must streak a small (90 mm diameter) Mueller-Hinton agar plate in three directions, exactly as if preparing the inoculum for agar disk diffusion susceptibility testing.
3. Place a 0.04 U bacitracin impregnated filter paper disk (Taxo A, BBL Microbiology Systems, or Bacto Group A Differential Disk, Difco) on the surface of the plate.
4. Incubate the plate at 35° C in air for 18 h and observe for any zone of inhibition around the disk. Micrococci will yield zones of inhibition, and staphylococci will be resistant, showing growth up to the disk. If an organism fails to grow, it is probably a micrococcus.

Modified from Falk and Guering. 1983. J. Clin. Microbiol. 18:719.

PROCEDURE 24.3. MODIFIED OXIDASE TEST

1. A visible amount of a colony from a 15-24 h old 5% sheep blood agar plate is smeared onto a piece of filter paper as for the standard oxidase test (Chapter 9). Colonies from other media or colonies older than 24 h will give aberrant results.
2. A drop of modified oxidase reagent (6% tetramethylphenylenediamine hydrochloride [Eastman Kodak Co.] in dimethyl sulfoxide [DMSO, Sigma Chemical Co.]) is added to the bacteria on the filter paper. Disks impregnated with this reagent are available from Remel Laboratories.
3. Oxidase positive organisms turn dark blue within 2 min. All oxidase positive organisms are micrococci, with the exception of the rare *Staphylococcus sciuri* (which has been isolated only from animals).

Modified from Faller and Schleifer. 1981. J. Clin. Microbiol. 13:1031.

dition, they are susceptible to the antibiotic bacitracin (Procedure 24.2), as described by Falk and Guering.[5] Differentiation of coagulase negative staphylococci from micrococci (considered to be less virulent) is based on characteristics delineated by Schleifer and Kloos[16] and Faller and Schleifer,[6] as well as the bacitracin test, as shown in Table 24.1. Two methods recommended for routine laboratories are detailed in Procedures 24.2 and 24.3. Using a combination of these two tests, microbiologists should easily be able to differentiate staphylococci and micrococci likely to be found in clinical material.

24.2. Staphylococcus aureus

24.2.a. Structure and extracellular products. Because of its structure, S. aureus is uniquely suited to be a human pathogen. The cell wall is composed of tightly cross-linked peptidoglycan and teichoic acid moieties that protect the organism from lysis under harsh osmotic conditions and probably aid in attachment of the bacteria to mucosal cell receptor sites. Certain strains produce a polysaccharide capsule that helps to protect them from phagocytosis by polymorphonuclear neutrophils (PMNs). In addition, most strains possess a cell wall protein, protein A, that binds the F_c segment of IgG, preventing antibody-mediated phagocytosis by PMNs, which usually depends on recognition of the F_c portion of antibody specifically bound to other antigens via the antigen-binding sites. In the bloodstream, aggregates of IgG bound to protein A on staphylococcal surfaces will fix complement, causing complement-mediated tissue damage to the host. The ability of protein A to bind IgG has been exploited by using staphylococci as particles for specific in vitro immunologic reagents (described in Chapter 12).

S. aureus produces a number of enzymes and toxins that contribute substantially to its ability to cause disease. In addition to coagulase, S. aureus produces the enzymes phosphatase, thermostable deoxyribonuclease, lipase, gelatinase, protease, and fibrinolysin. Another enzyme, hyaluronidase, may contribute to the spread of infection involving S. aureus. Among the toxins elaborated by S. aureus are alpha, beta, gamma, and delta toxins and leukocidin, which act on the red and white blood cell membranes of some species. The role of these toxins in the pathogenesis of disease is unclear.

Toxins that have been clearly shown to contribute to certain disease syndromes are enterotoxins, exfoliative toxin, and the toxin associated with toxic shock syndrome. S. aureus produces at least six different enterotoxins, some of which are implicated in gastroenteritis. The toxins are elaborated by the organisms growing in food and then are ingested by the patient. Staphylococcal scalded skin syndrome, often affecting newborns, is caused by an exfoliative toxin called **exfoliatin** (which cleaves the middle layers of the epidermis, allowing the surface skin to peel). The most recently described toxin-mediated staphylococcal disease is **toxic shock syndrome,** a systemic disease characterized by fever, hypotension, and multiorgan involvement. The article by Broome and Reingold[2] summarizes current knowledge. The disease is caused by a toxin called toxic shock syndrome toxin-1 (TSST-1), which is elaborated by certain S. aureus strains growing in a localized focus of infection or colonization. Most cases have occurred in menstruating young females who were vaginal carriers of S. aureus and who used tampons. Any site, however, such as an abscess or wound, may harbor the toxin-producing organisms. Although the clinical laboratory may be asked to isolate S. aureus from suspected sites of infection, performance of tests for toxin production is beyond the scope of hospital laboratories.

24.2.b. Identification. S. aureus is coagulase positive, which is its most distinguishing characteristic. For the rare isolate suspected of being S. aureus that fails to produce coagulase, an even more specific test for thermostable

PROCEDURE 24.4. THERMOSTABLE NUCLEASE TEST

1. Prepare toluidine blue DNA agar (Chapter 45 or available from Edge Diagnostics) plates by preincubating them at 35° C for 1 h before performing the test.
2. Remove a plug of 5% sheep blood agar containing the colony to be tested by vertically inserting a glass microcapillary tube into the agar directly over the colony. Colonies 18-24 h old are suitable.
3. Move the agar plug to the center of the capillary tube with a cool sterile straight wire.
4. Seal both ends of the capillary tube in the flame of a Bunsen burner and label the tube with autoclave tape.
5. Heat the tube in a boiling water bath for 15 min.
6. After it cools, score both ends of the capillary tube with a file and break them off.
7. Push the agar plug and bacterial growth out of the tube with a straight wire and onto the surface of the DNA agar plate.
8. Incubate the test agar at 37° C for 1-4 h and observe for a halo of pink surrounding the inoculum. Organisms showing this pink zone produce thermostable nuclease and can be identified as *S. aureus*.

Modified from Menzies. 1977. J. Clin. Pathol. 30:606.

deoxyribonuclease can be performed. Procedure 24.4 describes a thermostable nuclease test that is performed on colonies from a primary culture plate. Other methods for testing thermostable nuclease, such as that of Zarzour and Belle,[21] require that wells be punched in the DNA test agar and boiled suspensions of overnight broth cultures of the organisms be placed in the wells, a more cumbersome procedure, but necessary for laboratories that do not have access to gas burners.

Madison and Baselski[13] used 1 ml of the culture supernatant from blood culture bottles showing positive cocci in clusters for a rapid modification of the thermostable nuclease test described above. The supernatant was boiled for 15 min and placed into 3 mm diameter wells cut into the surface of DNA agar plates. Correlation with standard methods was 100% and only 2 h incubation was needed before re-

sults could be interpreted. Another very similar rapid method for performing a thermostable nuclease test directly from blood culture broth was described in Chapter 9. The source of the DNAse test agar was critical for reliable results. Another rapid method for determining that gram-positive cocci in clusters visualized in blood culture broths are *S. aureus*, a modification of the lysostaphin test of Severance et al.,[17] has been described by Knight and Shlaes[12] (Procedure 24.5). Polymyxin susceptibility has also been reported to distinguish between coagulase positive and coagulase negative strains of *S. aureus*. Heltberg and Bruun[8] found that *S. aureus*, including rare coagulase negative strains, is resistant to polymyxin, whereas other species of *Staphylococcus* are susceptible.

Several commercial particle agglutination tests (discussed in Chapter 12) are available for

PROCEDURE 24.5. LYSOSTAPHIN TEST FROM BLOOD CULTURE MEDIA

1. Add 0.5 ml of blood culture supernatant (with or without evenly dispersing the sediment throughout the medium) to each of two tubes containing 4.5 ml brain heart infusion broth.
2. Add 0.05 ml of lysostaphin (Sigma Chemical Co.; 57.4 U/ml prepared in phosphate buffered saline, pH 7.3, stored at −20° C for 30 days or at −70° C for 1 year) to one tube, for a final lysostaphin concentration of 0.574 U/ml or 2 μg/ml. The other tube serves as a control.
3. Vortex both tubes and incubate them at 35°-37° C with agitation on a shaker or rotating platform for 30 min.
4. Centrifuge both tubes for 10 min at 1,000 × g and discard the supernatant.
5. Resuspend both sediments and place a drop of each onto a glass slide. Allow the slide to air dry, heat fix, and Gram stain the two smears.
6. Observe the smears for lysis of cocci. The test is positive for *S. aureus* (lysostaphin susceptible) if more than 90% of the cells present in the control smear are absent in the smear prepared from lysostaphin-containing broth.

Modified from Knight and Shlaes. 1983. J. Clin. Microbiol. 17:97.

rapid differentiation of *S. aureus* from other staphylococci. Staphylatex (American Scientific Products), Sero-STAT (Scott Laboratories), Staph Latex (Difco Laboratories), and Accu-Staph (Carr-Scarborough Microbiologicals) use latex particles, and Staphyloslide (BBL Microbiology Systems) uses sensitized sheep erythrocytes as particles. Although these systems are quite accurate, there may be a small percentage of false negative results with methicillin-resistant strains, as reported by Woolfrey and others.[20] Methicillin-resistant strains of *S. aureus* are often slide coagulase negative as well, suggesting that a common cell wall structure contributes to both clumping factor expression and methicillin resistance. The rapid commercial tests mentioned above can be used in most institutions with confidence if microbiologists confirm the identify of methicillin-resistant strains (mentioned below) by tube coagulase.

Strains of *S. aureus* may be identified for epidemiologic purposes by phage typing (Chapter 5). Characterizing strains by phage type, biotype, plasmid profile, and slime production may help to delineate the path of spread of strains among hospitalized patients, the environment, and the attending medical staff. Used primarily for investigation of nosocomial outbreaks of *S. aureus* infection, phage typing schemes have also been developed for coagulase negative staphylococci. In some cases, possession of virulence factors can be traced to particular phage types. This time-consuming procedure is performed by a small number of laboratories in the United States, Canada, and England.

24.2.c. Susceptibility. Most strains (85%-90%) of *S. aureus*, even those acquired in the community, are penicillin resistant. In most cases, this resistance is attributable to beta-lactamase production and is effected by extrachromosomal plasmids. Staphylococci that are penicillin resistant may also be resistant to the newer beta-lactamase-resistant semisynthetic penicillins such as methicillin, oxacillin, and nafcillin. Clinically significant methicillin-resistant *S. aureus* are being isolated with greater frequency in the United States, often posing problems as causes of nosocomial infections. It has been shown that these strains, although they may exhibit susceptibility to cephalosporins in vitro, may not be treated effectively with either cephalosporins or beta-lactamase resistant penicillins. Strategies for susceptibility testing and reporting of *S. aureus* are described in Chapter 13. In particular, the addition of 2% or 4% NaCl to cation-supplemented Mueller-Hinton broth (2%) or Mueller-Hinton agar (4%), incubation at temperatures ≤35° C (preferably 30° C), and incubation for a full 48 h before reading results have been shown to increase the chances of detecting methicillin-resistant *S. aureus.* Collopy and others[4] have suggested that methicillin-resistant strains are less likely to be associated with severe infections, but once established, they are more difficult to eradicate. All staphylococci are still susceptible to vancomycin, and many or most strains are susceptible to rifampin. Certain *S. aureus* strains exhibit in vitro tolerance (MBC at least 32 times greater than MIC) to some antimicrobial agents due to clones of bacteria that are killed more slowly than the majority of cells in the population. There is no definitive evidence that tolerance is of clinical significance.

24.2.d. Nonculture methods for diagnosing *Staphylococcus aureus* infections. Tests for staphylococcal antigen have not been shown to aid in diagnosis of disease. However, some workers feel that detection of circulating antibodies to the teichoic acid component of the *S. aureus* cell wall is useful for monitoring the course of infection and for differentiating long-standing or deep-seated infections from lesser infections. Although radioimmunoassay, ELISA, crossed immunoelectrophoresis, agar-gel diffusion, and immunoprecipitation methods (described in Chapters 11 and 12) have all been used to successfully detect such antibodies, many of these methods are too sensitive to differentiate between patients with more serious or less serious infections. Almost all human sera can be found to contain antibodies against staphylococcal teichoic acid if a sensitive enough assay is used for detection. White and co-workers[19] reported that finding elevated titers of antibody (>1:4) as detected with a commercial kit (Endo-Staph, Meridian Medical Diagnostics) was quite accurate in identifying those patients with complicated bacteremias who required prolonged therapy.

24.3. Coagulase Negative Staphylococci

According to Kloos,[10] coagulase negative staphylococci vary in pathogenic potential. As is true for many other resident human flora of relatively low virulence, these organisms are more likely to cause infection in compromised hosts, particularly cancer patients. *Staphylococcus epidermidis* is known to cause infections of native heart valves and intravascular prostheses, including intravenous catheters and artificial heart valves. It can cause peritonitis in patients receiving peritoneal dialysis. *S. epidermidis*, usually introduced via a break in the patient's skin, also causes infections in prosthetic joints, central nervous system shunts, and has been isolated from subcutaneous infections. *S. saprophyticus* is isolated most frequently from uncomplicated urinary tract infections in nonhospitalized patients, notably sexually active young women. The incidence of *S. saprophyticus* urinary tract infection varies considerably among the patient populations served by institutions and in different geographic areas. Species that are less commonly implicated as pathogens include *S. cohnii*, *S. haemolyticus*, *S. hominis*, *S. saccharolyticus*, *S. simulans*, and *S. warneri*. Those species rarely isolated from patients are *S. auricularis*, *S. capitis*, *S. carnosus*, *S. lentus*, *S. sciuri*, and *S. xylosus*.

24.3.a. Morphology and extracellular products. Morphologically similar to *S. aureus*, coagulase negative staphylococci may possess many of the same virulence properties. Although they do not produce the number of extracellular products that S. *aureus* does, many species produce hemolysins and some seem to possess an antiphagocytic capsule. In addition, the production of slime may correlate with pathogenicity, particularly in prosthesis-associated infection where slime may mediate bacterial adherence. Christensen and others[3] have begun to study coagulase negative staphylococci in relation to virulence.

24.3.b. Identification. The majority of coagulase negative staphylococci isolated from clinically significant sources are S. *epidermidis*. Since S. *epidermidis* is the most common coagulase negative staphylococcus organism on human skin, these isolations may merely reflect prevalence. Since any of the other species can cause disease, coagulase negative staphylococci cannot arbitrarily be reported as S. *epidermidis* without further biochemical tests. For those laboratories that do not identify this group to species, a report of "coagulase negative staphylococci" is sufficient.

Isolates obtained from the urinary tract of nonhospitalized patients are usually S. *saprophyticus*. It may be involved in recurrent infection and in stone formation. This species is resistant to the antibiotic novobiocin, as are S. *cohnii*, S. *lentus*, S. *sciuri*, and S. *xylosus*. The latter four species, however, are rarely isolated from patients. We recommend that for coagulase negative staphylococcal isolates from sources other than blood, body fluids, or other sterile sites, a **presumptive** identification of S. *saprophyticus* should be reported based on the broth disk elution novobiocin test (Procedure 24.6) or novobiocin resistance, as indicated by a zone of inhibition of ≤16 mm diameter surrounding a 5 μg novobiocin disk, in an agar disk diffusion test performed in the same way as the procedure of Bauer, Kirby, et al. (Chapter 13). Phosphatase production, as described by Pickett and Welch,[15] can also be used to distinguish between S. *saprophyticus* (negative) and S. *epidermidis* (positive).

Table 24.2 shows some of the biochemical reactions used to differentiate coagulase negative staphylococci. Many other reactions may be used to identify these organisms, but the

---

PROCEDURE 24.6. RAPID NOVOBIOCIN TEST

1. Inoculate growth from isolated colonies into two tubes of 3 ml each of trypticase soy broth. The inoculum should be extremely light, such that there is no visible turbidity.
2. Immediately add one 5 μg novobiocin filter paper disk, such as those used for agar diffusion susceptibility testing, to one of the tubes and shake the tube gently for 10 seconds to disperse the antibiotic.
3. Incubate both tubes at 37° C for up to 5 h, or until the control tube (without novobiocin) reaches the turbidity of a McFarland 0.5 standard.
4. Observe the tube containing the novobiocin disk for turbidity. Novobiocin resistant organisms, presumptively identified as S. *saphrophyticus*, yield turbidity equal to that of the control tube. Most other coagulase negative staphylococci are novobiocin susceptible and show no visible turbidity after 5 h of incubation.

Modified from Harrington and Gaydos. 1984. J. Clin. Microbiol. 19:279.

TABLE 24.2
Abridged Identification of Coagulase Negative *Staphylococcus* Species

| SPECIES | ARGININE UTILIZATION | UREASE | ACID FROM | | | NOVOBIOCIN RESISTANCE |
			MANNITOL	SUCROSE	TREHALOSE	
S. epidermidis	+	+	−	+	−	−
S. saprophyticus	−	+	+/−	+	+	+
S. haemolyticus	+	−	+/−	+	+	−
S. hominis	−/+	+	−	+	+/−	−
S. warneri	−/+	+	+/−	+	+	−
S. cohnii	−	−	+/−	−	+	+
S. simulans	+	+	+	+	+/−	−
S. saccharolyticus	+	NT	−	−	−	−

+ = >90% of strains positive.
− = >90% of strains negative.
+/− = Variable results; results more often positive.
−/+ = Variable results; results more often negative.
NT = Not tested.

tests require specialized media and may be difficult to perform. A commercial identification kit, the API STAPH-IDENT system (Analytab Products) has been shown by Kloos and Wolfshohl[11] to correlate very well with the conventional scheme developed by Kloos and Schleifer and can be interpreted after 5 h incubation. None of the fully automated systems for identification of coagulase negative staphylococci have been shown to be as reliable as standard or rapid conventional biochemicals.

24.3.c. Susceptibility. Unlike *S. aureus*, coagulase negative staphylococci have no predictable patterns of susceptibility. Strains associated with nosocomial infections are likely to be multiply resistant and may carry resistance plasmids that serve to spread antimicrobial resistance among other bacterial strains. Like *S. aureus*, coagulase negative staphylococci resistant to penicillinase-resistant penicillins in vitro may also fail to respond in infections treated with cephalosporins. Strains exhibiting oxacillin resistance should be reported as cephalosporin resistant regardless of in vitro susceptibilities to cephalosporins. Unlike the other coagulase negative staphylococci, *S. saprophyticus* is usually susceptible to most antimicrobial agents with the exception of the urinary tract agent nalidixic acid (which is only active against gram-negative bacilli). There are presently no diagnostic methods for disease caused by coagulase negative staphylococci that do not require isolation of the bacteria.

24.4. Micrococci

Rarely identified as causes of infection, micrococci are saprophytic, often pigmented members of the Micrococcaceae. Species include *M. agilis*, *M. kristinae*, *M. luteus*, *M. lylae*, *M. nishinomiyaensis*, *M. roseus*, *M. sedentarius*, and *M. varians*. Hospital microbiology laboratories should not attempt identification of species of these bacteria. Isolates of micrococci that are unequivocally implicated as causes of infection should be sent to a reference laboratory for further studies.

REFERENCES

1. Archer, G.L. 1984. *Staphylococcus epidermidis:* the organism, its diseases, and treatment. In Remington, J.S., and Swartz, M.N., editors. Current clinical topics in infectious diseases 5. McGraw-Hill Book Co., New York.

2. Broome, C.V., and Reingold, A.L. 1984. Current issues in toxic shock syndrome. In Remington, J.S., and Swartz, M.N., editors. Current clinical topics in infectious diseases 5. McGraw-Hill Book Co., New York.

3. Christensen, G.D., Parisi, J.T., Bisno, A.L., et al. 1983. Characterization of clinically significant strains of coagulase negative staphylococci. J. Clin. Microbiol. 18:258.

4. Collopy, B.T., Dalton, M.F., Wright, C., and Mullany, C. 1984. Comparison of the clinical significance of methicillin-resistant and methicillin-sensitive *Staphylococcus aureus* isolations. Med. J. Aust. 140:211.

5. Falk, D., and Guering, S.J. 1983. Differentiation of *Staphylococcus* and *Micrococcus* spp. with the Taxo A bacitracin disk. J. Clin. Microbiol. 18:719.

6. Faller, A., and Schleifer, K.H. 1981. Modified oxidase and benzidine tests for separation of staphylococci and micrococci. J. Clin. Microbiol. 13:1031.

7. Harrington, B.J., and Gaydos, J.M. 1984. Five-hour novobiocin test for differentiation of coagulase negative staphylococci. J. Clin. Microbiol. 19:279.

8. Heltberg, O., and Bruun, B. 1984. Recognition of coagulase-negative *Staphylococcus aureus* strains by primary polymyxin susceptibility testing. Acta Pathol. Microbiol. Immunol. Scand. [B] 92:115.

9. Kaplan, M.H., and Tenenbaum, M.J. 1982. *Staphylococcus aureus:* cellular biology and clinical application. Am. J. Med. 72:248.

10. Kloos, W.E. 1982. Coagulase negative staphylococci. Clin. Microbiol. Newsletter 4:75.

11. Kloos, W.E., and Wolfshohl, J.F. 1982. Identification of *Staphylococcus* species with the API STAPH-IDENT system. J. Clin. Microbiol. 16:509.

12. Knight, R.G., and Shlaes, D.M. 1983. Rapid identification of *Staphylococcus aureus* and *Streptococcus pneumoniae* from blood cultures. J. Clin. Microbiol. 17:97.

13. Madison, B.M., and Baselski, V.S. 1983. Rapid identification of *Staphylococcus aureus* in blood cultures by thermonuclease testing. J. Clin. Microbiol. 18:722.

14. Menzies, R.E. 1977. Comparison of coagulase, deoxyribonuclease (DNase), and heat-stable nuclease tests for identification of *Staphylococcus aureus*. J. Clin. Pathol. 30:606.

15. Pickett, D.A., and Welch, D.F. 1985. Recognition of *Staphylococcus saprophyticus* in urine cultures by screening colonies for production of phosphatase. J. Clin. Microbiol. 21:310.

16. Schleifer, K.H., and Kloos, W.E. 1975. A simple test system for the separation of staphylococci from micrococci. J. Clin. Microbiol. 1:337.

17. Severance, P.J., Kauffman, C.A., and Sheagren, J.N. 1980. Rapid identification of *Staphylococcus aureus* by using lysostaphin sensitivity. J. Clin. Microbiol. 11:724.

18. Sheagren, J.N. 1984. *Staphylococcus aureus*, the persistent pathogen. N. Engl. J. Med. 309:1368; 310:1437.

19. White, A., Wheat, L.J., and Kohler, R.B. 1983. Diagnostic and therapeutic significance of staphylococcal teichoic acid antibodies. Scand. J. Infect. Dis. Suppl. 41:105.

20. Woolfrey, B.F., Lally, R.T., and Ederer, M.N. 1984. An evaluation of three rapid coagglutination tests: Sero-STAT, Accu-Staph, and Staphyloslide, for differentiating *Staphylococcus aureus* from other species of staphylococci. Am. J. Clin. Pathol. 81:345.

21. Zarzour, J.Y., and Belle, E.A. 1978. Evaluation of three test procedures for identification of *Staphylococcus aureus* from clinical sources. J. Clin. Microbiol. 7:133.

BIBLIOGRAPHY

Hindler, J.A., and Inderlied, C.B. 1985. Effect of the source of Mueller-Hinton agar and resistance frequency on the detection of methicillin-resistant *Staphylococcus aureus*. J. Clin. Microbiol. 21:205.

Scand. J. Infect. Dis. [Suppl. 41], 1983. Entire issue devoted to *S. aureus* organisms and disease.

Selepak, S.T., and Witebsky, F.G. 1984. Beta-lactamase detection in nine staphylococcal species. J. Clin. Microbiol. 20:1200.

25

Streptococci, Including Enterococci and Pneumococci, and *Aerococcus*

Members of the genus *Streptococcus* are catalase negative gram-positive cocci that tend to grow in chains in liquid media. Streptococci form large quantities of lactic acid as the end-product of carbohydrate metabolism, and they are facultatively anaerobic. They are not only normal flora of humans, but some species are the etiologic agents of several devastating diseases, including pneumococcal pneumonia, meningitis, sepsis, bacterial endocarditis and streptococcal exudative pharyngitis, cellulitis, wound infection, and visceral abscesses. **Acute rheumatic fever** and **poststreptococcal glomerulonephritis** are secondary sequelae of infection caused by *Streptococcus pyogenes.*

The single species of *Aerococcus*, *A. viridans*, is included in the family Streptococcaceae, but it is rarely isolated from humans. *Aerococcus* is an opportunistic pathogen, probably occurring naturally in the environment. It has been isolated from cases of bacteremia, endocarditis, meningitis, and osteomyelitis. It will be briefly mentioned below in the section about laboratory identification of streptococci, since it may be confused with streptococci because of similar colony morphology.

The streptococci can be identified in the laboratory by several different processes. The methods most universally used in clinical microbiology laboratories involve preliminary grouping of isolates based on the hemolytic pattern of colonies growing on blood agar. In the United States, 5% sheep blood agar is commonly used. Originally used primarily for cultures of inflamed throats because it inhibits growth of hemolytic *Haemophilus* species, considered to be nonpathogenic oral flora, and thus allows recognition of beta hemolytic colonies that might be streptococci without the conflicting presence of other similar-appearing beta hemolytic colonies, 5% sheep blood agar is now used routinely for initial cultivation of almost all types of clinical specimens (Chapter 8). Horse blood is commonly used for initial processing in Europe; hemolytic patterns of streptococci are virtually the same as on sheep blood agar. In discussions about epidemiology and pathogenesis in this chapter, clinically important streptococci are grouped according to hemolytic patterns or species. Beta hemolytic streptococci include S. *pyogenes*, S. *agalactiae*, and a number of other species. Alpha hemolytic streptococci include S. *pneumoniae*. Another group of variably hemolytic streptococci, primarily alpha or nonhemolytic (and occasionally beta hemolytic), are the "enterococci," so-called because they are part of the normal fecal flora. These organisms share several characteristics that differ from other streptococci, including resistance to salt and broader antibiotic resistance. Several authors, including Schleifer and Killper-Balz,[12] have recently proposed moving organisms of the "enterococcus" group from the genus *Streptococcus* to a new genus, *Enterococcus*. Because of the clinical importance and biochemical differences between enterococci and other streptococci, this new genus designation seems likely to be accepted.

25.1. Epidemiology and Pathogenic Mechanisms

25.1.a. *Streptococcus pneumoniae.* S. *pneumoniae*, bile sensitive alpha hemolytic streptococci, are found as normal nasopharyngeal and oropharyngeal flora in as many as 15% of children and approximately 5% of adults. They are also found in the upper respiratory tract of animals, but not in the inanimate environment. Organisms are presumably passed from person to person via respiratory secretions and aerosols. The organisms are surrounded by an antiphagocytic capsule composed of polysaccharide antigens, of which more than 80 have been characterized. S. *pneumoniae*, also called **pneumococci,** are etiologic agents of the second most common cause of bacterial meningitis, often preceded by pneumonia. Pneumococcal pneumonia is the most common type of community-acquired pneumonia; the fatality rate of uncomplicated pneumococcal pneumonia is still relatively high (5%-7%), even with prompt institution of appropriate therapy. In addition to pneumonia and meningitis, S. *pneumoniae* is an etiologic agent of otitis media, purulent sinusitis, and occasionally peritonitis, especially in young patients with nephrotic syndrome.

Pneumococci cause disease in the presence of a predisposing host condition, often a viral respiratory tract infection. Individuals with other compromising conditions of the respiratory tract, such as chronic obstructive pulmonary disease, silicosis, anthracosis, treatment with anesthetic agents, and alcoholism, are at increased risk. The pathogenesis of pneumonia was discussed in depth in Chapter 16. For S. *pneumoniae*, the capsular polysaccharide plays a key role in allowing the establishment of infection. The organisms enter the alveoli via the bronchial tree in the face of impaired host defenses that normally include the cough reflex, ciliary movement, and secretory immunoglobulin. Once within alveoli, they resist phagocytosis by macrophages, multiply, and induce an inflammatory response that impairs lung function. Patients usually experience an abrupt onset of fever following a shaking chill. Sputum is often purulent and may appear rusty colored. The best evidence that capsular polysaccharide is the primary virulence factor is that antibody to the capsular antigen is protective. Recovery from pneumococcal pneumonia in a nonimmune individual is accompanied by a rise in antibody titer, whereas presence of circulating antibodies prevents establishment of the disease. This fact has spurred development of a pneumococcal vaccine, containing antigens of 23 serotypes, the most commonly recognized etiologic serotypes in the United States and Europe. Patients with chronic respiratory tract disease, those without spleens, immunosuppressed patients, elderly patients, and others deemed to be at increased risk have all been cited as those for whom vaccine is warranted, although not all will respond optimally to it. *S. pneumoniae* produces other factors that may play a role in virulence, including pneumolysin O, an oxygen-sensitive toxin that is cytolytic for cells, and a neuraminidase, an enzyme that degrades surface structures of host tissue. The cell wall of pneumococci contains C-substance, a teichoic acid that reacts with a certain serum protein (C-reactive protein, CRP), resulting in the activation of some nonspecific host immune responses.

25.1.b. *Streptococcus pyogenes.* Most streptococci that contain cell wall antigens of Lancefield group A (discussed below) are known as *S. pyogenes.* Members of this species are almost always beta hemolytic. They are found in the respiratory tract of humans, and are always considered to be potential pathogens. A number of persons, particularly children, however, do carry the organism without signs of illness. The numbers of organisms isolated from such asymptomatic carriers are usually low. Because numbers of colony forming units seen on primary culture plates is dependent on many factors, including the presence of competing normal oral flora, the skill with which the specimen was obtained, the way in which the culture medium was inoculated, culture medium incubation conditions, and the culture medium itself, the likely presence or absence of streptococcal infection should not be assessed entirely on the numbers of colonies recovered. Infection is spread by aerosols and

respiratory secretions, although food-borne and milk-borne epidemics do occur. Members of this species are among the etiologic agents of pharyngitis, cellulitis, scarlet fever, erysipelas, pyoderma (a purulent skin infection), puerperal fever (uncommonly seen today), and other purulent (or **suppurative**) infections. *S. pyogenes* may also be involved with other bacteria in impetigo (a form of pyoderma). Infections which extend from the pharynx into the paranasal sinuses, tonsils, and other parts of the respiratory tract can lead to abscesses, pneumonia, otitis media, and other suppurative processes. With the decline of rheumatic fever in the United States, treatment of streptococcal pharyngitis is often initiated for prevention of these other sequelae.

In terms of human morbidity and mortality worldwide, however, the role of *S. pyogenes* in the subsequent development of acute rheumatic fever and poststreptococcal glomerulonephritis is more important. Both diseases are most prevalent among children. Rheumatic fever and subsequent valvular heart disease are syndromes of major importance in developing nations throughout the world. In the United States, rheumatic fever is uncommon today, occurring primarily in the rural South and in areas of crowding and lower socioeconomic status. Acute rheumatic fever and poststreptococcal glomerulonephritis are considered to be **nonsuppurative,** because the organism itself and a purulent inflammatory response are not present in the affected organs (heart, joints, blood vessels, kidneys). Although the pathogenesis of these diseases has not been entirely clarified, it seems certain that they are autoimmune phenomena. It is believed that cross-reactive antibodies, originally directed against streptococcal cell membranes, specifically bind to myosin in human heart muscle cells; other cross-reactive antibodies bind to components of the glomerular basement membrane, forming immune complexes at the affected site. These antigen-antibody complexes attract host reactive cells and enzymes that ultimately cause the damage. Patients with previous rheumatic heart disease (as a result of rheumatic fever) are at significantly increased risk of developing cardiac malfunction and endocarditis at a later time. Patients who develop streptococcal glomerulonephritis are also at risk of developing later renal failure.

Not all infections with *S. pyogenes* lead to nonsuppurative sequelae. Acute rheumatic fever occurs only after upper respiratory tract infection. The development of this disease is dependent on host factors, such as HLA (chromosome constituent) type, immunoglobulin secretory status, and immune responsiveness; and organism factors, such as adherence mechanisms and cell wall carbohydrate components. Glomerulonephritis, on the other hand, occurs after pharyngitis or after suppurative skin infection (**pyoderma**). Acute glomerulonephritis is associated with a limited number of serotypes. These serotypes are defined by antisera against a protein component of the cell wall, the M protein, which is also mentioned below in connection with virulence.

S. pyogenes produces a number of extracellular products and toxins that probably enhance virulence (see Figure 12.1). **Erythrogenic toxin,** elaborated by scarlet fever associated strains, is responsible for the characteristic rash. Group A streptococci also produce **DNase, hyaluronidase** (also known as **spreading factor**) which breaks down host cell connective tissue, and **streptokinase,** an enzyme that dissolves clots. NADase, proteinases, and other enzymes are secreted. The two hemolysins, **streptolysin O,** an oxygen-labile enzyme, and **streptolysin S,** oxygen-stable, can lyse human and other erythrocytes, as well as the cell membranes of polymorphonuclear neutrophils, platelets, and other cells. There are pathogenic strains of *S. pyogenes* that do not produce hemolysins, which makes them extremely difficult to recognize on primary blood agar culture plates. The cell wall **lipoteichoic acids** serve to

effect adherence of the organism to host cell respiratory epithelium, an essential first step in the development of infection (Chapter 16). In association with the **hyaluronic acid capsule,** cell wall **M protein** serves to prevent phagocytosis, another essential virulence mechanism. The M protein is the major virulence factor of the bacteria since strains of *S. pyogenes* that lack M protein cannot cause disease.

25.1.c. *Streptococcus agalactiae.* These beta hemolytic streptococci, also known as Lancefield group B streptococci, are normal flora in the genitourinary tract of humans and other mammals. They are an important etiologic agent of bovine mastitis, from which they can be transmitted in milk. They are destroyed by pasteurization. From their carriage site in the human vagina, they can colonize neonates; *S. agalactiae* is currently the most common etiologic agent of neonatal sepsis and meningitis (Chapter 15), accounting for over one third of all cases (*Escherichia coli* still accounts for another third). Postpartum fever and sepsis, not surprisingly, are also commonly associated with *S. agalactiae.* This organism has been found to be the etiologic agent in cases of sepsis in nonparturient women and in men, in joint infection, osteomyelitis, urinary tract infection, and wound infection. *S. agalactiae* is associated with endocarditis, pneumonia, and pyelonephritis in immunosuppressed patients.

25.1.d. Other Lancefield groupable beta hemolytic streptococci. Streptococci of serologic group C (*S. equisimilis, S. zooepidemicus, S. dysgalactiae,* and *S. equi*), group F (*S. anginosus*), group G (*S. canis*), and a few strains not containing group antigens are occasional etiologic agents of human disease. Streptococci possessing other group antigens have been isolated only from animals or environmental sources. They are carried as normal flora of the pharynx, vagina, or skin of wild and domestic animals. Species of group C and G may additionally colonize the human gastrointestinal tract and vagina. Group C and G streptococci may cause suppurative infection in humans, including postpartum sepsis, erysipelas, pharyngitis, and bacteremia. Endocarditis is rare. Group C, in particular, may cause a severe pharyngitis, often followed by bacteremia and metastatic infection. Unusual for bacteria other than group A streptococci, one species of group C (*S. zooepidemicus*) has been associated with post-streptococcal glomerulonephritis, acquired after drinking milk from a cow with mastitis. Persons such as dairy farmers, because of their close contact with infected animals, are at increased risk.

Beta hemolytic streptococci with cell wall carbohydrates of groups A, C, and G may form tiny pinpoint colonies, called **minute** colonies. The Centers for Disease Control in Atlanta calls these organisms *S. anginosus* while the British nomenclature includes them in the *S. milleri* classification. These organisms are part of the normal flora of the human gastrointestinal tract, oral mucosa, and female genital tract. Such minute streptococci have also been associated with suppurative infections, including abscesses of the brain, the oral cavity, intraabdominal sites, perirectal sites, cellulitis, lower respiratory tract infection, and facial infections.

25.1.e. Viridans streptococci. Species of streptococci that are not beta hemolytic (with rare exceptions) do not possess Lancefield group B or D cell wall antigens, are not *S. pneumoniae* (which are bile soluble and inhibited by the antipneumococcal agent **optochin**), and cannot grow in broth containing 6.5% sodium chloride are considered to belong to the general category of **viridans streptococci.** Viridans was derived from the Latin word *viridis*, meaning 'green.' Most species in this group are alpha hemolytic and produce a "green" discoloration in blood agar (Chapter 8), probably due to the action of extracellular enzymes. Many characteristics of this group of streptococcal species are variable, including cell wall carbohydrates and biochemical and morphological characteristics. There are ten viridans strepto-

coccal species included in the current American taxonomic scheme delineated by Facklam[4] and eight species currently recognized by British taxonomists Colman and Ball,[2] as shown in Table 25.1.

The viridans streptococci are normal inhabitants of the oral, respiratory and gastrointestinal mucosa of humans and animals. They are opportunistic pathogens of low virulence. Viridans streptococci are, however, the major etiologic agents of bacterial endocarditis in the United States and are important in various suppurative infections. Patients who develop streptococcal endocarditis usually possess a previously damaged heart valve (from previous rheumatic fever or other cause). Gingival disease or dental manipulations, including dental prophylaxis, are often predisposing factors in the development of endocarditis. Viridans streptococci are able to adhere to epithelial and endothelial cells, and adherence is probably a key factor in their ability to cause disease. *Streptococcus mutans* has been definitively established as a major etiologic agent of dental caries in addition to being a cause of endocarditis. The production of extracellular sugars,

TABLE 25.1
Species of Viridans Streptococci Recognized by the Two Primary Identification Schemes

AMERICAN (FACKLAM)	BRITISH (COLMAN)
S. acidominimus	S. acidominimus
S. mutans	S. mutans
S. salivarius	S. salivarius
S. sanguis I	S. sanguis
S. sanguis II	S. mitior (dextran positive)
S. mitis	S. mitior
S. intermedius	S. milleri
S. constellatus	S. milleri
S. morbillorum	None
S. uberis	S. uberis

Modified from Facklam, R.R. 1984. The major differences in the American and British *Streptococcus* taxonomy schemes with special reference to *Streptococcus milleri*. Eur. J. Clin. Microbiol. 3:91.

called **dextrans,** which serve as attachment mediators, undoubtedly allows these organisms to establish niches on tooth surfaces as well as heart valves. The viridans streptococci have also been implicated as etiologic agents (often in combination with anaerobic or other bacterial species) of brain abscess, perioral abscess, aspiration pneumonia, liver abscess, and other suppurative infections. Some species of viridans streptococci produce extracellular enzymes and toxins similar to those produced by beta hemolytic streptococci. The role of these products in virulence is not known. There are many published reports of an association of a particular species, called *S. milleri* in the British scheme, with more serious infection, particularly abscesses. Until the nomenclature of these organisms is better defined, this association is open to question. It is possible that beta hemolytic *S. milleri* are more likely to cause pyogenic abscesses than are the non-beta hemolytic organisms called *S. milleri* by some workers and *S. intermedius* (formerly *MG-intermedius*) by others. In all series, *S. sanguis* I and *S. sanguis* II, *S. mutans*, and the *S. milleri-intermedius* species are the most common etiologic agents of endocarditis. Since the organisms are normal oral flora, isolation of viridans streptococci from a single blood culture may not be indicative of an ongoing infectious process, although it usually is. Cultivation of the same organism from more than one blood culture is highly suggestive of endocarditis, liver abscess, or other serious infection. We have found several instances of polymicrobial endocarditis caused by more than one species of viridans streptococcus or by one species with two distinct morphotypes and biotypes.

25.1.f. Nutritionally variant streptococci. A group of streptococci, first described in the early 1960s have been found to be significant etiologic agents of endocarditis. These organisms, also called "nutritionally deficient," "pyridoxal-dependent," "satelliting streptococci," or "thiol-requiring," are presumably normal flora. As reported by Roberts et al.[10] at one

major medical center, New York Hospital, 5%-6% of all cases of endocarditis were caused by such streptococci. Nutritionally variant streptococci require vitamin B_6, or **pyridoxal,** for growth. Consequently, standard 5% sheep blood agar plates do not support growth of these organisms. As reported by Reimer and Reller,[8] commercial lots of chocolate agar vary with respect to their ability to support growth. Accordingly, many cases of endocarditis due to nutritionally deficient streptococci have probably not been diagnosed bacteriologically. Subcultures from blood culture broth media (which usually support growth because the human erythrocytes provide the necessary growth factor) must be made to plates containing 0.001% pyridoxal (obtainable from Sigma Chemical Co. and other chemical supply houses) or to chocolate plates known to support growth of such organisms. The same authors later showed that addition of pyridoxal to all blood agar plates would inhibit growth of other commonly encountered bacteria.[9]

The radiometric blood culture system or routine visual examination of stained smears, as described in Chapter 14, may be necessary for detection of nutritionally variant streptococci in the blood of patients with endocarditis. If the chocolate agar is supportive of growth of such strains, as determined by testing a known nutritionally variant strain as part of ongoing quality control, subculture from the lysis-centrifugation tube will be adequate. Alternatively, blood culture media can be subcultured to a blood agar plate cross-streaked with a *Staphylococcus aureus* strain (Plate 25.1). *S. aureus* provides the necessary growth factor, just as it does for *Haemophilus influenzae* (which requires NAD), allowing development of **satelliting** colonies of the streptococci in a zone surrounding the staphylococcus. It is for this reason that the nutritionally variant streptococci have also been called the satelliting streptococci.

25.1.g. Group D streptococci. The cell wall group D antigen, unlike the carbohydrate antigens of groups A, B, C, F, and G, is composed of glycerol-teichoic acid, requiring lysozyme or hot acid treatment for extraction. Two physiologically and genetically (by DNA homology studies) different groups of organisms are included in those streptococci isolated from humans that possess antigens of Lancefield group D: (1) the enterococcal group, S. *(Enterococcus) faecalis*, S. *(Enterococcus) faecium*, and S. *(Enterococcus) durans;* and (2) the nonenterococci S. *equinus* and S. *bovis*. Other enterococci, S. *(Enterococcus) gallinarum*, S. *(Enterococcus) avium*, S. *(Enterococcus) casseliflavus*, S. *(Enterococcus) malodoratus*, and *Enterococcus hirae* have rarely been shown to be clinically significant for humans. Group N (sometimes included with the enterococci) represent yet another group of streptococci, unrelated genetically to other Lancefield groups. Many of the group D streptococci are found as normal flora in the human gastrointestinal tract and that of other animals and birds. S. *faecalis*, in addition, is found in human oral flora. The nonenterococcal group D species are morphologically (and in terms of penicillin G susceptibility) more related to viridans streptococci than to the other group D streptococci. They are also similar in the spectrum of disease with which they are associated, endocarditis being most common. S. *faecalis* and S. *bovis* together account for as many as one fifth of all cases of bacterial endocarditis. Although S. *equinus* is rarely encountered, S. *bovis* may be responsible for as many as one third of all cases of viridans streptococcal endocarditis. The presence of S. *bovis* bacteremia, associated with endocarditis or not, is almost always indicative of a loss of integrity of the gastrointestinal mucosa. A strong correlation exists between isolation of S. *bovis* from blood and colon cancer. Since detection of this organism may be the first evidence of such a malignancy, this may be an impelling reason for identification of the streptococci to species.

The enterococci (the genus *Enterococcus*)

are able to grow in 6.5% sodium chloride. These organisms are commonly encountered as etiologic agents of urinary tract infections, wound infections, and, next to *E. coli* and *Bacteroides fragilis*, are the most common isolates from intraabdominal abscesses. They must possess some virulence factors, but these have not been characterized. Superinfection with enterococci, including bacteremia, is a relatively common occurrence in patients being treated with a third generation cephalosporin, as they are resistant to these agents as well as to penicillin.

25.2. Laboratory Identification of Streptococci

Streptococci grow on standard laboratory media containing blood or blood products, such as tryptic soy agar with 5% sheep blood and chocolate agar, as well as the selective agars Columbia agar with colistin and nalidixic acid (CNA) and phenylethyl alcohol agar (PEA; Chapter 8). Blood culture media support the growth of streptococci (Chapter 14). For those streptococci that require pyridoxal, subculture may require a staphylococcal cross-streak or media containing the necessary growth factors, as discussed above. The identification strategy we recommend is that of the Centers for Disease Control, since it divides the streptococci into a number of morphologically discrete groups. Differences between the scheme outlined below and the British taxonomic scheme, first presented by Colman and Williams,[3] will be discussed further. Only until the definitive DNA homology studies have been performed and a uniform set of physiologic tests have been agreed upon can taxonomic confusion be eliminated. Until then, it is important that a standard format be followed, and that reported identifications be accompanied by the criteria used for identification so that clinicians can use the data to determine whether a given species is associated with a particular prognosis or demands a particular therapy.

25.2.a. Initial characterization of streptococci and *Aerococcus*. Because most laboratories incubate all blood agar plates (except the anaerobic plates) in 5%-10% CO_2, colony morphology of streptococci from that environment will be described. The streptococci are facultative anaerobes and will grow very well anaerobically (often better than they will aerobically). Those organisms that grow better in reduced oxygen tension are sometimes called **microaerophilic** streptococci; they are usually identified as members of the viridans streptococci. Those streptococci that grow as obligate anaerobes, *Peptostreptococcus* species, are covered in Chapters 34 and 37. Visualization of beta hemolytic streptococcal colonies from throat specimens, as well as recovery of group A beta hemolytic streptococci, is enhanced by anaerobic incubation. Detection of group A beta hemolytic streptococci in pharyngeal cultures will be discussed separately below.

Identification of streptococci should be initiated by careful examination of colony morphology and hemolytic pattern on 5% sheep blood agar. Visualization of hemolysis is enhanced by stabbing the inoculating loop into the agar several times (Figure 25.1). Colonies can then grow throughout the depth of the agar, producing subsurface oxygen-sensitive hemolysins (streptolysin O) if they are able to. Streptococci grow on the agar surface as translucent to milky, circular, small (approximately 1 mm diameter) colonies with a shiny surface. Colony variants are common, however, including rough, umbonate, dull matte, and spreading morphologies. *Aerococcus* colonies are gray-white, convex, and circular. All streptococci should be catalase negative, but occasional enterococci and *Aerococcus* species produce a pseudocatalase that yields a very weak positive test (test performed as described in Chapter 9). *S. pneumoniae*, *Aerococcus viridans*, and many species of viridans streptococci, enterococci, and other group D streptococci will show a zone of alpha hemolysis surrounding the colony. Alpha hemolysis, macroscopically appearing as a green discoloration

Side view

FIGURE 25.1
Stabbing the inoculating loop vertically into the agar after streaking the blood agar plate allows subsurface colonies to display hemolysis due to streptolysin O.

of the medium surrounding the colony, is characterized by the presence of intact erythrocytes, visible by observing the medium surrounding the colony through the low power of a microscope (Plate 25.2). If the presence of hemolysis is uncertain, it may be detected by moving the colony aside with a loop and examining the area of medium directly beneath the original colony site. Plates are always examined by holding them in front of a light source (Figure 25.2).

Microscopically, streptococci are gram-positive, round or oval-shaped, occasionally forming elongated forms that resemble pleomorphic corynebacteria or lactobacilli. Streptococci may occasionally appear gram-negative if cultures are old or if there has been treatment with antibiotics. Differentiation between streptococci and lactobacilli may be difficult, especially if the lactobacilli are catalase negative strains. Plating a lawn of growth on a blood agar plate, much as for a disk diffusion test, placing a 10

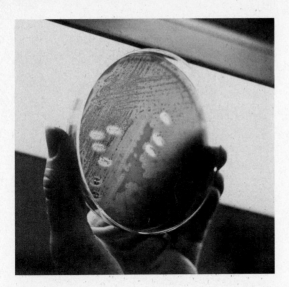

FIGURE 25.2
Observing hemolysis on sheep blood agar plates by viewing the plates in front of a light source.

FIGURE 25.3
Chains of streptococci seen in Gram stain prepared from broth culture.

U penicillin susceptibility disk in the center, and incubating the culture overnight may be useful. A Gram stain of growth just outside the zone of inhibition will reveal long bacilli if the organism is a *Lactobacillus* and spherical forms if it is a *Streptococcus*. Additionally, growth in thioglycolate broth usually induces streptococci to form long chains of cocci (Figure 25.3). *Aerococcus* species will grow in thioglycolate as large, spherical cocci arranged in tetrads and pairs, rather than chains. This morphology is the most important feature for identification of aerococci. Nearly all streptococci are susceptible to vancomycin, whereas most lactobacilli are typically resistant. An unusual type of alpha hemolysis produced by some viridans streptococci is called **"wide-zone alpha hemolysis."** Colonies are surrounded by a zone of incomplete hemolysis of erythrocytes, but a wider zone further out consists of completely lysed red cells, as seen in true beta hemolysis (Plate 25.3). Wide-zone alpha hemolysis macroscopically resembles beta hemolysis.

Nonhemolytic (sometimes called **gamma** hemolytic) colonies are usually enterococci or viridans streptococci. Beta hemolytic colonies may rarely be S. *(Enterococcus) faecalis*, S. *(Enterococcus) durans*, or S. *mutans*, but they are almost always groupable with Lancefield antisera to cell wall carbohydrates of groups A, B, C, F, or G. Colonies of group A streptococci (*S. pyogenes*) are small, transparent to translucent, convex, entire, circular, shiny, and surrounded by a rather wide zone of beta hemolysis.

Beta hemolysis is characterized by complete lysis of erythrocytes, as determined by examining the medium microscopically (Plate 25.4). Group B streptococci, S. *agalactiae*, yield larger, more translucent to opaque, whitish gray, soft, smooth colonies surrounded by a much smaller zone of beta hemolysis. The colonies of S. *agalactiae* resemble those of *Listeria* species (Chapter 33), which are catalase positive. Group C, F, and G colonies are usually small (approximately 0.5-1 mm diameter) and surrounded by a very wide zone of complete hemolysis. The minute colony variants produce pinpoint colonies surrounded by a zone of beta hemolysis. Although the British taxonomic schemes classify these minute streptococci within the genus *S. milleri,* the American scheme (promulgated primarily by Facklam at the CDC) considers these organisms to be included within the species *S. anginosus,* which also includes group F beta hemolytic streptococci, which normally produce tiny colonies. For all practical purposes, the great majority of beta hemolytic streptococci isolated from clinical material can be identified serologically, as outlined below. Beta hemolytic streptococcal colonies are rather distinctive and should not easily be confused with those of other beta hemolytic bacteria, with the exception of *Listeria.*

25.2.b. Serologic identification of beta hemolytic streptococci. Beta hemolytic streptococci are definitively identified by detection of group specific cell wall carbohydrate antigens. Rebecca Lancefield first characterized beta hemolytic streptococci by developing antisera to specific cell wall carbohydrate moieties that were distinctive for each species. Species often could be distinguished biochemically as well. For performance of the test developed by Lancefield, the **Lancefield precipitin test,** cell wall antigens must be extracted, either physically by heating, by chemically treating a suspension of the bacterial cells, or by enzymatic extraction. Cells are grown overnight in Todd-Hewitt broth in order to provide a pure suspension with sufficient antigen for the test. Because routine laboratories seldom perform the classic procedure any more, it is described only briefly. A small amount of the antiserum (previously produced by hyperimmunizing rabbits with fixed cells of the appropriate serogroup, available from Difco Laboratories, Burroughs Wellcome Co. and other suppliers) is drawn up into a microcapillary tube (1.5 mm diameter) and the extract is drawn into the tube below the antiserum. After approximately 10 min, a positive reaction is visible as a diffuse white precipitate that forms at the juncture of the two

materials. The precipitin line may vanish quickly, so tubes should be inspected often. A separate tube is needed for each serogroup being tested. The extraction procedures and performance of the precipitin test are described by Facklam and Carey in the American Society for Microbiology *Manual of Clinical Microbiology,* fourth edition.[5] Modifications of the precipitin test include counterimmunoelectrophoresis or gel diffusion detection of antigen-antibody reactions. For unusual group antigens, those other than A, B, C, F, and G, and for group D antigens, the Lancefield test in some form is still used in reference laboratories.

An additional method for identifying the cell wall carbohydrate of groups A and B streptococci is fluorescent antibody staining. Antisera, directed against the specific cell wall carbohydrate antigens, conjugated with fluorescein, are layered over an area on a slide that contains a dried suspension of bacteria from the colony to be tested. A positive test is identified by bright apple-green fluorescence of the streptococcal cells, showing a very bright ring of fluorescence outlining each cell and dark centers (Plate 25.5). Even this method, also described by Facklam and Carey,[5] is infrequently used in routine clinical laboratories today, due to the availability of commercially produced reagents for rapid serogrouping of beta hemolytic streptococci.

The use of highly sensitive polyclonal antibody reagents and monoclonal antibodies, conjugated to carrier particles, latex beads or staphylococci (described in Chapter 10), has greatly facilitated the ability of microbiologists to rapidly and specifically identify beta hemolytic streptococcal colonies by latex agglutination or coagglutination methods (Chapter 10). Some of these methods require an extraction step, which may take an hour or longer, whereas others do not. Identification can usually be accomplished with one or two isolated colonies, shortening the laboratory turnaround

TABLE 25.2

Some of the Commercial Products Available for Serologic Identification
of Beta Hemolytic Streptococci

PRODUCT	STREPTOCOCCAL GROUP	MANUFACTURER
A. Coagglutination		
1. Phadebact	Groups A, B, C, F, and G	Pharmacia Diagnostics
2. Strepto-Sec	Groups A, B, C, and G	Organon Diagnostics
3. Microstrep	Groups A, B, C, and G	American MicroScan
4. MERITEC-Strep	Groups A, B, C, F, and G	Meridian Diagnostics
B. Latex agglutination		
1. Streptex	Groups A, B, C, D, F, and G	Wellcome Diagnostics
2. Serostat	Groups A, B, C, and G	Scott Laboratories
3. BBL Strep Kit	Groups A, B, C, F, and G	BBL Microbiology Systems

FIGURE 25.4
Flow chart for initial identification of beta hemolytic streptococci.

time by at least 24 h. Table 25.2 lists some of the commercial products available for streptococcal serogrouping. As with all commercial systems, manufacturers' instructions should be followed exactly, and substitutions of reagents or specified equipment are not acceptable. All of the commercial products listed yield satisfactory serogroup identifications as compared with the Lancefield precipitin standard. Choices of which antisera to test against a given isolate are determined by the clinical setting from which the organism was recovered and by colony morphology.

25.2.c. Biochemical identification of beta hemolytic streptococci. In addition to serogrouping, which is expensive and somewhat laborious intensive, there are a few presumptive tests commonly used by clinical laboratories for identification of beta hemolytic streptococci. As outlined in Figure 25.4, initial identification can be achieved with just a few simple tests. Group A streptococci are susceptible to bacitracin >99% of the time when the test is performed properly (Procedure 25.1). A pure culture is necessary because as many as 50% false negative results will be obtained if the test is performed with a mixed culture, as on a primary inoculation plate. Some alpha hemolytic streptococci and all aerococci are also bacitracin susceptible, so the test is valid only for truly beta hemolytic organisms.

A recently described test, the hydrolysis of

PROCEDURE 25.1. BACITRACIN SUSCEPTIBILITY TEST

1. Inoculate one quadrant or one half of a 5% sheep blood agar plate with a pure culture of the organism to be tested by heavily streaking the entire surface.
2. Place a 0.04 U bacitracin disk (Taxo A, BBL Microbiology Systems or Bacto Bacitracin Differentiation disk, Difco Laboratories) in the center of the inoculum.
3. Incubate overnight in air or 5%-10% CO_2 at 35° C and examine for a zone of inhibition of growth around the bacitracin disk.
4. Any zone of inhibition is indicative of bacitracin susceptibility. In addition to *S. pyogenes*, essentially all of which are susceptible, a small percentage of group B (*S. agalactiae*) and 10%-20% of group C and G are susceptible. Since group B streptococci can be differentiated morphologically and biochemically, and since isolates of groups C and G occur infrequently, bacitracin serves as an adequate presumptive test for group A streptococci.

L-pyrrolidonyl-beta-naphthylamide (**PYR test**), has been found by Facklam and others[6] to more accurately presumptively identify group A streptococci (and enterococci) than bacitracin does. An agar medium containing the PYR substrate (available as triplates from Remel Laboratories and Carr-Scarborough Microbiologicals) is inoculated with a pure culture of the organism to be tested. The triplates also contain 5% sheep blood agar and modified bile esculin agar (for testing esculin hydrolysis by enterococci, described below). After overnight incubation at 35° C in air, the presence of the free beta-naphthylamine released by hydrolysis of the substrate is detected by adding a drop of PYR reagent (*N,N*-dimethylaminocinnamaldehyde plus detergent) directly onto the growth on the agar. Colonies of organisms positive for PYR hydrolysis develop a bright cherry red color within 2 min. A light orange color reaction is considered negative. All group A streptococci and almost all enterococci (>99%) are PYR positive. Because this test is more specific than bacitracin, we recommend its use. Modifications of the PYR test, including a broth test

that can be read within 4 h of incubation and even more rapid chromogenic substrates and fluorescent systems are commercially available (Carr-Scarborough Microbiologicals, Strep-A-Chek from E-Y Laboratories, Strep-A-Fluor from Bio-Spec Laboratories division of Wampole Laboratories, and others). A colony of a PYR positive organism that is rubbed on a substrate-impregnated filter paper exhibits a red color after addition of the color indicator (Plate 25.6).

Group B streptococci are able to hydrolyze hippurate (Procedure 25.2). Although a few strains of group D streptococci and *Aerococcus* species can also hydrolyze hippurate, they are rarely beta hemolytic. The rapid hippurate hydrolysis test takes advantage of the fact that one of the products of hydrolysis, serine, can be deaminated by ninhydrin, which is reduced to a purple-colored product in the process. A hippurate disk (Chapter 9) is commercially available (Remel Laboratories).

Group B streptococci produce a proteinlike compound called the **CAMP factor** that is able to act synergistically with the beta toxin pro-

PROCEDURE 25.2. RAPID HIPPURATE HYDROLYSIS TEST

1. Prepare 1% sodium hippurate substrate as follows:

   Sodium hippurate (Sigma Chemical Co.)   1 g
   Distilled water   100 ml

   Mix together and dispense into small (12 × 75 mm) plastic disposable test tubes with snap top caps, 0.4 ml per tube. Store frozen for a maximum of 6 months.
2. Prepare ninhydrin reagent as follows:

   Ninhydrin (Sigma)   3.5 g
   Acetone   50 ml
   Butanol   50 ml

   Mix the acetone and butanol together and then add the ninhydrin. Store at room temperature in a brown bottle with a tight seal for a maximum of 6 months.
3. Defrost the sodium hippurate substrate and heavily inoculate a tube with a pure culture of the organism to be tested. The suspension should be milky. Inoculate a positive control (group B streptococcus) and a negative control (hippurate negative enterococcus) at the same time.
4. Incubate the capped tubes for 2 h in a 35° C waterbath.
5. Add 0.2 ml ninhydrin reagent and reincubate for an additional 15 min. Observe for a deep purple color change, indicating that the hippurate has been hydrolyzed. This test can also be used to identify other organisms, as mentioned throughout the book.

Modified from Hwang and Ederer. 1975. J. Clin. Microbiol. 1:114.

PROCEDURE 25.3. CAMP TEST

1. Inoculate a streak of beta toxin-producing *Staphylococcus aureus* down the center of a 5% sheep blood agar plate.
2. Inoculate straight lines of the isolates to be tested, along with a group B positive control and a group A negative control strain, at right angles to the staphylococcal streak, stopping just before the staphylococcal line is reached. Several different isolates can be tested on one plate.
3. Incubate plates at 35°-37° C overnight in air or for 6 h in 5%-10% CO_2. Air incubation will increase the specificity of the test, since fewer non–group B streptococci will be positive in an air atmosphere. Observe for an arrowhead-shaped zone of enhanced hemolysis at the juncture between positive streptococci and the staphylococcus (Plate 25.7). Approximately 95% of group B streptococci, as well as rare strains of other groups, are CAMP positive.

Modified from Washington. 1981. In Washington, J.A. II, editor. Laboratory procedures in clinical microbiology. Springer-Verlag, New York.

FIGURE 25.5
Flow chart for preliminary identification of alpha hemolytic streptococci.

FIGURE 25.6
Colony morphology of pneumococci after 24 h incubation (20×).

duced by some strains of *Staphylococcus aureus* to produce even more potent hemolysis (Plate 25.7). This principle is utilized in the CAMP test (Procedure 25.3), named for the originators, Christie, Atkins, and Munch-Peterson.[1] The CAMP test requires overnight incubation, but it is much less expensive than serological typing for identification of group B streptococci. If an appropriate staphylococcus is unavailable, a commercial CAMP factor impregnated filter paper disk can be used (Remel Laboratories).

25.2.d. Identification of alpha and nonhemolytic streptococci and aerococci. Alpha hemolytic streptococci are preliminarily identified as shown in Figure 25.5. The colony morphology of *S. pneumoniae* is usually distinctive, with very mucoid and glistening colonies that tend to dip down in the center and resemble a doughnut after increased incubation time due to the action of autolytic enzymes (Figure 25.6). Suspicious colonies must be tested for either bile solubility (test described in Chapter 9) or susceptibility to **ethylhydroxycupreine**

hydrochloride, also called **optochin** (Procedure 25.4).

Once it has been determined that an alpha hemolytic streptococcus is not *S. pneumoniae*, it is tested for its ability to hydrolyze esculin in the presence of bile. This test, **bile esculin,** is performed by inoculating a slant or plate of bile esculin agar (commercially available), incubating in air for as long as 4 days, and observing for a blackening of the agar, indicating the presence of the endproduct of esculin hydrolysis combined with iron in the medium. All group D streptococci are bile esculin positive, as are some strains of *S. intermedius*, *S. mutans*, *S. uberis*, *S. sanguis* I, and *S. constellatus*. Additionally, all enterococci can grow in the presence of 6.5% NaCl in tryptic soy broth, a characteristic shared by rare strains of viridans streptococci. Of the three clinically important enterococcus species, only *S. (Enterococcus) faecium* can ferment arabinose. *E. faecalis* is able to ferment sucrose and sorbitol, while *E. durans* does not ferment arabinose, sucrose, or sorbitol. *S. bovis* possesses cell wall group D antigens, is able to hydrolyze esculin in the presence of bile (bile esculin positive), but cannot grow in 6.5% NaCl, and cannot hydrolyze PYR. Because some strains of viridans streptococci may also share these characteris-

TABLE 25.3

Selected Biochemical Reactions of Viridans Streptococci and S. *bovis*

	MANNITOL	INULIN	SUCROSE BROTH GEL	ARGININE DIHYDROLASE	ESCULIN HYDROLYSIS
S. *acidominimus*	0	0	0	33	0
S. *bovis**	91	50	57	0	100
S. *constellatus*	0	0	0	24	73
S. *intermedius*	0	0	10	26	100
S. *mitis*	0	0	10	16	0
S. *morbillorum*	0	0	0	0	0
S. *mutans*	100	99	88	1	90
S. *salivarius*	0	100	0	0	91
S. *sanguis* I	0	100	72	64	77
S. *sanguis* II	0	0	43	21	0
S. *uberis*	100	71	0	40	86

Modified from Rubin, S.J. 1984. Species identification and clinical significance of viridans streptococci. Lab. Med. 15:171. (Percent positive of 1187 clinical isolates.)
Data from Facklam, R.R. 1977. Physiological differentiation of viridans streptococci. J. Clin. Microbiol. 5:184.
*Data from Facklam, R.R. 1972. Recognition of group D streptococcal species of human origin by biochemical and physiological tests. Appl. Microbiol. 23:1131. (Only 44 strains studied.)

PROCEDURE 25.4. OPTOCHIN SUSCEPTIBILITY TEST

1. Streak one quadrant or one half of a 5% sheep blood agar plate with an inoculum from a pure isolate of the organism to be tested.

2. Place an optochin disk (Taxo P, BBL Microbiology Systems, or Bacto Optochin disk, Difco Laboratories) in the center of the inoculum.

3. Incubate overnight at 35° C in 5%-10% CO_2 or a candle jar. Observe for zones of inhibition surrounding the disk. Zones of equal to or greater than 14 mm surrounding a 6 mm diameter disk and zones equal to or greater than 16 mm surrounding a 10 mm diameter disk are considered positive, presumptive identification of S. *pneumoniae*. Zone sizes between 6 and 14 mm (6 mm disk) and 10 and 16 mm (10 mm disk) are equivocal, and those isolates should be tested for bile solubility.

Modified from Facklam and Carey. 1985. In Lennette, E.H., Balows, A., Hausler, W.J. Jr., and Shadomy, H.J., editors. Manual of clinical microbiology, ed. 4. American Society for Microbiology, Washington, D.C.

HIPPURATE HYDROLYSIS	LACTOSE	RAFFINOSE	SUCROSE AGAR		
			ADHERENT	NON-ADHERENT GUMMY	NON-ADHERENT MUCOID
99	0	0	0	0	100
0	100	98	ND	ND	84
0	0	9	0	0	100
0	100	18	12	1	87
0	100	0	13	0	87
0	0	0	0	0	100
0	99	85	96	0	4
0	89	95	11	55	34
0	94	45	84	0	16
0	100	100	49	0	51
57	100	86	0	0	100

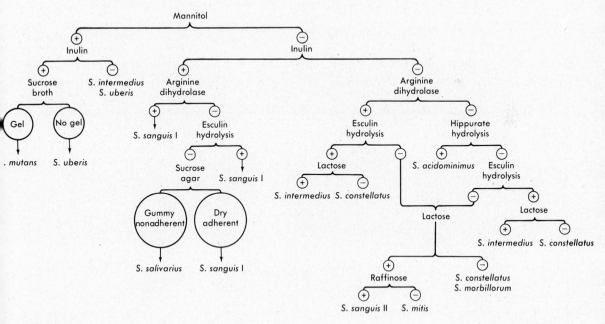

FIGURE 25.7
Flow chart for identification of viridans streptococci.

PROCEDURE 25.5. PREPARATION AND USE OF MEDIA FOR IDENTIFICATION OF VIRIDANS STREPTOCOCCI

A. Carbohydrate fermentation media
  1. Prepare carbohydrate utilization broths as follows:

Brain heart infusion broth	900 ml
10% carbohydrate in H_2O	100 ml
Bromcresol purple (1.6% in 95% ethanol)	1 ml

  Carbohydrates include inulin, mannitol, lactose, raffinose, and sorbitol. Dispense 3 ml each into 12 × 75 mm glass screw cap tubes, and autoclave at 121° C for 10 min. Unlike other carbohydrate broths, these carbohydrate media are autoclaved containing the carbohydrates. Certain carbohydrates, such as inulin and starch, will not completely dissolve in the water. Gentle heating may help but will not entirely clear the solutions. Do not boil them to try to clear them, but merely agitate them thoroughly immediately before adding to the brain heart infusion broth.
  2. Inoculate broths with pure isolates and incubate in air for up to 4 days. Positive results (acid production) are visualized by a change in the indicator to yellow.

B. Production of extracellular polysaccharide (glucan)
  1. Prepare 5% sucrose broth by mixing together two separate solutions, autoclaved before mixing, as follows:

Thioglycolate broth base (Difco)	28.5 g
K_2HPO_4	10 g
Sodium acetate	12 g
Distilled water	500 ml

  Mix together in a 1000 ml flask.

Sucrose	50 g
Distilled water	500 ml

  Mix together in a separate 1,000 ml flask. Autoclave the two solutions at 121° C for 15 min. Cool both to 55° C and aseptically mix them by pouring the contents of one flask into the other. Dispense aseptically in 5 ml amounts into 16 × 125 mm sterile glass test tubes with screw caps. Store refrigerated.
  2. Inoculate a pure culture of the organism, incubate in air at 35° C for up to 1 week, and observe for gelation of the medium. Glucan production is indicated by formation of complete or partial gel in the broth (observed by gently tipping the tube back and forth). If the broth is merely thickened, this is not glucan production, but may suggest slime produced by *S. bovis*.

Modified from Rubin. 1984. Lab. Med. 15:171, using data from original work by Facklam.

PROCEDURE 25.5. PREPARATION AND USE OF MEDIA FOR IDENTIFICATION OF VIRIDANS STREPTOCOCCI—cont'd

C. Colony morphology on sucrose agar.
  1. Prepare 5% sucrose agar as follows:

Brain heart infusion agar (Difco)	40 g
Sucrose	50 g
Distilled water	1,000 ml

Mix together, autoclave for 15 min at 121° C, cool to 55° C, and pour into 90 mm diameter Petri plates, at least 20 ml per plate. Allow to set, and store tightly wrapped in polyethylene bags in the refrigerator. Plates are good for several weeks.
  2. Inoculate plates with pure cultures of the organisms to be tested. Incubate in air for a maximum of 4 days. Examine for colony morphology. *S. sanguis* and *S. mutans*, both glucan producers, form very dry, adherent, refractile colonies that are difficult to move with a loop. Levan producers, such as *S. salivarius*, yield opaque, very gummy (gumdrop-like), but nonadherent colonies. Growth can be scraped up and lifted (in a glob) from the agar surface. Organisms that produce no extracellular polysaccharides, such as *S. uberis*, *S. constellatus*, *S. mitis*, *S. acidominimus*, most *S. intermedius*, and *S. morbillorum*, produce mucoid, nonadherent colonies.

tics, an identification of *S. bovis* using only the criteria stated here must be considered presumptive. Definitive identification is accomplished by using the tests that are shown in Table 25.3.

Nonenterococcal streptococci must be identified using the scheme shown in Figure 25.7 and Table 25.3. It is critical that biochemical reagents be prepared according to Facklam's methods for the identifications to match those of the CDC (described below, Procedure 25.5). Different pH indicators and different broth bases will lead to different results and ultimately to different species designations. Only bromcresol purple broths, prepared as below, should be used for carbohydrate utilization tests. Although commercial biochemical systems and rapid kits are available (mentioned below), we have not found any of them to reliably differentiate the viridans streptococci without additional tests. If definitive biochemicals are not cost-effective for a laboratory, then important isolates of viridans streptococci should be sent to a reference laboratory for identification. It is important to inquire as to the scheme and the reagents being used by the reference laboratory, as they are not alike in their performance of identification tests for viridans streptococci. Tests other than those delineated in Procedure 25.5 are performed as previously described. Esculin hydrolysis is performed on slants of esculin medium without bile, which are available commercially (dry powder is also available commercially). The arginine dihydrolase test is performed as described in Chapter 27.

25.3. Rapid Methods and Commercial Systems for Identification of Streptococci

For diagnosis of neonatal sepsis and meningitis due to group B streptococci, several commercial antigen detection kits are available that have good sensitivity and specificity. Developed for use on serum, urine, or cerebrospinal fluid, the best results have been achieved with cerebrospinal fluid so far. Latex agglutination procedures appear to be the most sensitive. Use of these tests is covered in Chapter 15.

Identification of *S. pneumoniae* can be made rapidly with the quellung test (Chapter 12). Addition of specific capsular antibody to a wet preparation of sample containing the organism, either from an isolated colony or in the actual clinical material (sputum or cerebrospinal fluid), results in an antigen-antibody response, visible as apparent capsular swelling (Figure 25.8). The capsules become more visible and refractile due to antibody attachment. Omniserum (available from Statens Serum Institute or DAN-Serum Inc.) will react with the most common serotypes of pneumococci. Counterimmunoelectrophoresis for detection of

FIGURE 25.8
Quellung reaction with *Streptococcus pneumoniae*, showing apparent capsular swelling.

pneumococcal capsular antigens in body fluids and specimens has not yielded results within a range of sensitivity useful for diagnosis. Latex reagents are available for pneumococci, as described for detection of pneumococcal meningitis (Chapter 15). A coagglutination reagent (Pneumoslide, Phadebact by Pharmacia Diagnostics) is also available.

A modification of conventional biochemical identification procedures for viridans streptococci, described above, involves the use of reagent-impregnated filter paper disks, the Minitek system (BBL Microbiology Systems, described in Chapter 9). Plastic trays with wells containing the inocula are incubated anaerobically for 48 h, and 2 or 3 drops of 0.025% phenol red indicator solution is added to each well before reading results. Certain biochemicals, such as inulin, are not available on disks and other tests may require longer incubation. This approach was thoroughly described by Setterstrom and others.[13] Several other systems for biochemical or enzymatic identification of the viridans streptococci are currently available, produced by API and Innovative Diagnostics, and for instruments such as the Vitek and the Abbott MS-2. Although the systems work well for presumptive identification of beta hemolytic streptococci and differentiation of the group D streptococcal species, they are unable to differentiate the viridans streptococci with reliability at this time. These systems are constantly being improved, however, and they will eventually achieve acceptable performance.

25.4. Detection of Group A Streptococci in Throat Swab Specimens

Detection of group A streptococci or their group specific antigen in throat cultures is important for clinicians. If group A are present, therapy can be initiated to prevent sequelae and the spread of infection to others. In addition, prompt initiation of therapy can significantly shorten the duration of symptoms of pharyngitis. Since pharyngitis caused by streptococci cannot always be distinguished from that due to viruses (the most common etiologic agents) on clinical grounds, microbiologic procedures are necessary. A large number of commercial kits for rapid detection of group A streptococcal antigen, utilizing latex agglutination, coagglutination, or ELISA technologies, are currently available. As discussed in Chapter 16, these reagents have been reported to be very specific. Sensitivity, however, is dependent on a number of variables, and reports have ranged from approximately 60% sensitivity to greater than 95%. Strict adherence to manufacturers' recommendations, including close monitoring of incubation temperatures by using a water bath or heat block, are necessary for proper results. It has been found that personnel must be carefully trained in the correct interpretation of these tests. We recommend that a blood agar or selective streptococcal blood agar plate be inoculated with each throat swab tested before the rapid antigen test is performed. For those tests that yield negative results, the plate can then be incubated and read on the following day. Plates inoculated with swabs that were positive for direct antigen could be discarded without further manipulation.

The direct group A antigen detection tests are probably most effective when they are performed immediately after collection of the specimen in a doctor's office and when the physician, believing in the results of the test, bases immediate treatment on the test outcome. The argument that follows (proposed by Richard Facklam of the CDC) suggests that much overuse of antibiotic therapy may be prevented by proper use of rapid antigen detection tests by clinic-based physicians. The initial assumption is that 30% of all cases of pharyngitis are due to group A streptococci. If the direct antigen detection test correctly identifies 75% of those patients infected with group A streptococci (and correctly identifies almost all patients without group A streptococcal infection), then physicians will correctly treat 75% of 30%

of the patients seen (based on a positive test result) and will fail to treat only 25% of the 30%, or 7.5%, of patients with true streptococcal infections. The laboratory will incubate the plates inoculated with those swabs that yielded negative direct antigen tests and the remaining 7.5% of infected patients will be identified by culture on the following day, at which time treatment can be started. If it is assumed that at least 40 million throat cultures are taken annually and that physicians, diagnosing group A streptococcal infection based on clinical grounds, treat all 40 million patients without waiting for culture results, then reliance on the rapid test results will alleviate improper antibiotic therapy in approximately 28 million patients. An additional 3 million patients will have treatment delayed by one day, which does not alter the ability of treatment to prevent development of sequelae. The schema outlined above is, in fact, being practiced by some physicians. However, the sequential testing described above is probably cost effective only for physicians' office laboratories; hospital laboratories usually batch such tests, performing them once or twice daily.

Selective media for isolation of group A streptococci have been used for several years. The newest medium, Strep Selective Agar (SSA, BBL Microbiology Systems), has allowed greater recovery of group A streptococci from throat specimens than has conventional culture on 5% sheep blood. Other selective media are available from other manufacturers. SSA contains concentrations of colistin, crystal violet, and trimethoprim-sulfamethoxazole that inhibit growth of most beta streptococci except A and B. Placing a bacitracin disk on the initial inoculum can allow presumptive identification of group A streptococci after overnight incubation (Plate 16.1). The use of selective media is not universally accepted; many clinicians feel that it distorts the true picture of the relative numbers of different bacterial species present in the throat culture. For laboratories wishing to use only one blood agar plate, placing a bacitracin disk contiguous to a trimethoprim-sulfamethoxazole susceptibility disk (Chapter 13) on the heavily inoculated area of a 5% sheep blood agar plate allows presumptive identification of the majority of group A streptococci after overnight incubation in CO_2 (Plate 25.8). The sulfa agent inhibits most normal flora, allowing growth of groups A and B streptococci, whereas the bacitracin inhibits only group A. Beta hemolytic colonies in numbers too small to evaluate must be subcultured for further studies, as outlined above.

Other considerations for identification of *S. pyogenes* from throats are collection and transport of the specimen. Unlike most bacteria, streptococci are very resistant to drying. Swabs may be placed in paper, or material may even be transferred to filter paper for transport without significant loss of recovery. Specimen collection and handling is discussed in Chapters 6 and 16. Since introduction of newer methods, pour plates, limited growth in broth followed by visual detection by fluorescent antibody stains, and other more cumbersome methods for dealing with throat specimens are rarely performed in clinical laboratories in the United States.

25.5. Serologic Diagnosis of Group A Streptococcal Infection

Individuals with disease due to *S. pyogenes* produce antibodies against many of the extracellular products mentioned at the beginning of this chapter. For determining whether a patient has recently suffered streptococcal infection, several tests are usually performed. The diagnostic usefulness of such tests is extremely limited, especially with the decline of rheumatic fever in the United States. They should be used only for diagnosis of nonsuppurative sequelae of streptococcal infection. The most common of these is the **ASO,** determination of presence and titers of antistreptolysin O antibodies. Anti-DNAse B, antistreptokinase, and antihyaluronidase have all been used to retrospectively diagnose streptococcal infection.

TABLE 25.4
Products Available for Determining Antistreptococcal Antibody Titers

TEST	MANUFACTURER
ASO Latex Test	ICL Scientific
ASO Quantum	Sclavo
ASO Test	American Dade
LEAP Strep test	Cooper Biomedical
Rapitex ASO Kit	Behring Diagnostics
SerImmSure	Analytab Products
Strep-phile	BioDiagnostics Systems
Streptonase	Wampole Laboratories
Streptozyme	Wampole Laboratories

Pharyngitis seems to be followed by rises in antibody titers against all three antigens, whereas the ASO titers of patients with pyoderma are frequently not above normal. Anti-DNAse B titers, however, do increase after pyoderma, and thus this test is the most sensitive. Commercial products are available for detection of these antibodies, using latex agglutination or whole red blood cell agglutination methodologies (Table 25.4). Serum obtained as long as 2 months after infection will usually demonstrate increased antibodies. As with other serologic tests, an increasing titer over time is most useful for diagnosing previous streptococcal infection.

25.6. Treatment of Streptococcal Infections

Penicillin is still the drug of choice for most streptococcal infections. With the exception of rare *S. pneumoniae* and the enterococci, most streptococci (including nonenterococcal group D organisms) are susceptible to penicillins, which can be given in high dosage. For penicillin-allergic patients, erythromycin or vancomycin may be used. Erythromycin resistance has been reported.

The enterococci are uniquely antibiotic resistant. They are resistant to penicillin, aminoglycosides, cephalosporins, clindamycin, and numerous other agents. Synergism between a penicillin and an aminoglycoside (usually gentamicin) has been repeatedly demonstrated, however, and this combination is the therapy of choice. Vancomycin is also typically effective. High level resistance to streptomycin, indicating in vivo resistance to the combination of penicillin and streptomycin, can be detected by testing the enterococcus isolate against 2,000 µg of streptomycin (Chapter 13). Growth in the presence of this quantity of antibiotic indicates that synergism with a beta-lactam agent may be absent.

REFERENCES

1. Christie, R., Atkins, N.E., Munch-Peterson, E. 1944. A note on the lytic phenomenon shown by group B streptococci. Aust. J. Exp. Biol. 22:193.
2. Colman, G., and Ball, L.C. 1984. Identification of streptococci in a medical laboratory. J. Appl. Bacteriol. 57:1.
3. Colman, G., and Williams, R.E.O. 1972. Taxonomy of some human viridans streptococci. In Wannamaker, L.W., and Matsen, J.M., editors. Streptococci and streptococcal diseases, recognition, understanding, and management. Academic Press, New York.
4. Facklam, R.R. 1984. The major differences in the American and British *Streptococcus* taxonomy schemes with special reference to *Streptococcus milleri*. Eur. J. Clin. Microbiol. 3:91.
5. Facklam, R.R., and Carey, R.B. 1985. Streptococci and aerococci. In Lennette, E.H., Balows, A., Hausler, W.J. Jr., and Shadomy, H.J., editors. Manual of clinical microbiology, ed. 4. American Society for Microbiology, Washington, D.C.
6. Facklam, R.R., Thacker, L.G., Fox, B., and Eriquez, L. 1982. Presumptive identification of streptococci with a new test system. J. Clin. Microbiol. 15:987.
7. Hwang, M., and Ederer, G.M. 1975. Rapid hippurate hydrolysis method for presumptive identification of group B streptococci. J. Clin. Microbiol. 1:114.
8. Reimer, L.G., and Reller, L.B. 1981. Growth of nutritionally variant streptococci on common laboratory and 10 commercial blood culture media. J. Clin. Microbiol. 14:329.
9. Reimer, L.G., and Reller, L.B. 1983. Effect of pyridoxal on growth of nutritionally variant streptococci and other bacteria on sheep blood agar. Diagn. Microbiol. Infect. Dis. 1:273.
10. Roberts, R.B., Krieger, A.G., Schiller, N.L., and Gross, K.C. 1979. Viridans streptococcal endocarditis: the role of various species, including pyridoxal-dependent streptococci. Rev. Infect. Dis. 1:955.
11. Rubin, S.J. 1984. Species identification and clinical significance of viridans streptococci. Lab. Med. 15:171.
12. Schleifer, K.H., and Killper-Balz, R. 1984. Transfer of *Streptococcus faecalis* and *Streptococcus faecium* to the genus *Enterococcus* nom. rev. as *Enterococcus faecalis* comb. nov. and *Enterococcus faecium* comb. nov. 1984. Int. J. Syst. Bacteriol. 34:31.
13. Setterstrom, J.A., Gross, A., and Stanko, R.S. 1979. Comparison of Minitek and conventional methods for biochemical characterization of oral streptococci. J. Clin. Microbiol. 10:409.
14. Washington, J.A. II. 1981. General classification of bacteria. In Washington, J.A. Jr., editor. Laboratory procedures in clinical microbiology. Springer-Verlag, New York.

BIBLIOGRAPHY

Auckenthaler, R., Hermans, P.E., and Washington, J.A. II. 1983. Group G streptococcal bacteremia: clinical study and review of the literature. Rev. Infect. Dis. 5:196.

Barnham, M., Thornton, T.J., and Lange, K. 1983. Nephritis caused by *Streptococcus zooepidemicus* (Lancefield group C). Lancet 1:945.

Bisno, A.L. 1985. Classification of streptococci. In Mandell, G.L., Douglas, R.G. Jr., and Bennett, J.E., editors. Principles and practice of infectious diseases, ed. 2. John Wiley & Sons, New York.

Bisno, A.L. 1985. Nonsuppurative poststreptococcal sequelae: rheumatic fever and glomerulonephritis. In Mandell, G.L., Douglas, R.G. Jr., and Bennett, J.E., editors. Principles and practice of infectious diseases, ed. 2. John Wiley & Sons, New York.

Brennan, R.O., and Durack, D.T. 1984. The viridans streptococci in perspective. In Remington, J.S., and Swartz, M.N., editors. Current clinical topics in infectious diseases. McGraw-Hill Book Co., New York.

Carey, R.B. 1984. Handling the nutritionally deficient streptococci in the diagnostic laboratory. Clin. Microbiol. Newsletter 6:131.

Fernandez, C., Daasch, V.N., and Folds, J.D. 1983. Streptococcal serology. Clin. Microbiol. Newsletter 5:73.

Klein, J.O., Dashefsky, B., Norton, C.R., and Mayer, J. 1983. Selection of antimicrobial agents for treatment of neonatal sepsis. Rev. Infect. Dis. 5(Suppl 1):S55.

Krisher, K., and Cunningham, M.W. 1985. Myosin: a link between streptococci and heart. Science 227:413.

Roberts, R.B. 1985. Viridans and beta hemolytic (nongroup A, B, and D) streptococci. In Mandell, G.L., Douglas, R.G. Jr., and Bennett, J.E., editors. Principles and practice of infectious diseases, ed. 2. John Wiley & Sons, New York.

Senitzer, D., and Freimer, E.H. 1984. Autoimmune mechanisms in the pathogenesis of rheumatic fever. Rev. Infect. Dis. 6:832.

Shlaes, D.M. 1985. Demystifying the streptococci; their clinical relevance and identification. Diagn. Med. 7:40.

26 Aerobic Gram-Negative Cocci (*Neisseria* and *Branhamella*)

26.1. Introduction

The family Neisseriaceae contains several genera; those to be discussed in this chapter include *Neisseria* and *Branhamella*. Other genera within the family are *Moraxella* and *Acinetobacter*, which are discussed in Chapter 28. Although the latest edition of *Bergey's Manual of Systematic Bacteriology* has classified *Branhamella* as a subgenus of *Moraxella*, we chose to discuss the *Branhamella* species in this chapter, because their morphology and biochemical identification parameters most closely resemble those of *Neisseria*. These organisms are gram-negative cocci, grow as strict aerobes, and are oxidase positive (see Chapter 9). They are normal flora of the respiratory, alimentary, and genitourinary mucosal surfaces of humans. Although any of the normally commensal *Neisseria* species can cause disease in a debilitated host, the organisms most commonly responsible for disease in this group are *N. gonorrhoeae* (gonococcus), the agent of gonorrhea, and *N. meningitidis* (meningococcus), the agent of meningococcal meningitis and septicemia. The pathogenesis of infections due to the *Neisseria* species is discussed in the sections that relate to the diseases they cause, particularly Chapters 15 and 19. Recently, *Branhamella catarrhalis* has been recognized more frequently as a cause of lower respiratory tract disease.

    26.1.a. Morphology. These organisms all appear as kidney bean–shaped diplococci on

Gram stain. In smears made from clinical material, groups of *Neisseria* and *Branhamella* are often seen within polymorphonuclear neutrophils, sometimes in large numbers (Figure 26.1). This morphological appearance is known as **GNID (gram-negative intracellular diplococci)** and helps the microbiologist to identify a true infection.

26.1.b. General growth characteristics. Although these cocci are strict aerobes, they grow best on enriched media in a humid atmosphere of 2%-8% CO_2. *N. gonorrhoeae* requires the added nutrients of chocolate agar or special enrichments, while *N. meningitidis*, other *Neisseria* species and *Branhamella catarrhalis* can grow on blood agar. The commensal *Neisseria* species and *Branhamella* are able to grow at room temperature, but some strains of the pathogenic *Neisseria* are very sensitive to temperature variations; for this reason, clinical specimens sent to the laboratory for recovery of these organisms must be guarded from the cold and inoculated to growth media as soon as

FIGURE 26.1
Gram-negative intracellular diplococci, typical of *Neisseria* or *Branhamella* species, within polymorphonuclear neutrophils.

possible after collection. Although it is not necessary, culturing *Neisseria* on room temperature media will facilitate luxuriant growth.

26.2. *Neisseria gonorrhoeae*

26.2.a. Specimen collection. Specimens to be collected for the isolation of *N. gonorrhoeae* include material from genital sources such as the urethra, cervix, and anal canal, as well as specimens from sites of extragenital infection such as the oropharynx, skin lesions, inflamed joints, blood, and pelvic inflammatory disease. Neonates may become infected during passage through the birth canal of an infected mother; a particularly virulent conjunctivitis, **gonococcal ophthalmia neonatorum,** is often the result. With the requirement that silver nitrate or penicillin drops be instilled in the eyes of all infants at birth, this disease has become quite uncommon. Swabs of discharge from the eye may be collected for culture. The use of nontoxic cotton swabs (treated with charcoal to absorb toxic fatty acids) or calcium alginate swabs (available from several commercial suppliers, discussed in Chapter 6, and listed in the Appendix) will allow the best recovery of organisms. Specimens that are not inoculated immediately to culture media should be transported and held at room temperature in a protective carrying medium that prevents or minimizes overgrowth of nonpathogens, preferably Amie's charcoal transport medium (Chapter 45). It is better to refrigerate genital specimen swabs in transport media for a maximum of 3 h than to incubate the swabs. The best method for culture and transport of *N. gonorrhoeae* is to inoculate agar immediately after specimen collection and to place the medium in an atmosphere of increased CO_2 for transport, discussed in Chapters 6 and 19. Specimens can be inoculated to selective or nonselective agar plates (depending on the source of the specimen) and then placed immediately into a candle extinction jar (see below). Specialized packaged media consisting of selective agar in plastic trays that contain a CO_2 generating system (Jembec plates, Neigon plates, and Transgrow bottles) are also available.

26.2.b. Culture media and methods. Since gonococci must often be recovered from sites that contain large numbers of organisms from the commensal flora, such as the genital tract, and even from sites that may harbor nonpathogenic *Neisseria* species, such as the oropharynx, special selective media have been developed to aid in the detection of *N. gonorrhoeae*. The first of these was Thayer-Martin medium (Chapter 45), chocolate agar with an enrichment supplement and the antibiotics colistin (to inhibit gram-negative bacilli), nystatin (to inhibit yeast), and vancomycin (to inhibit gram-positive bacteria). Modifications of this medium include the addition of trimethoprim lactate to inhibit swarming *Proteus* species (modified Thayer-Martin medium, MTM) and the substitution of anisomycin, an antifungal agent with a longer half-life, for nystatin (Martin-Lewis medium). A transparent medium containing buffered proteose-peptone with many supplements and the same antibiotics as Thayer-Martin medium (New York City medium, NYC) has been employed with good success for the recovery of gonococci (Chapter 45). As many as 5% of gonococci are inhibited by the concentrations of antibiotics (particularly vancomycin) in the selective media commonly used, so the use of nonselective media is warranted in suspect cases that are culture negative and for specimens not contaminated with normal flora. The increased CO_2 necessary for the growth of gonococci can be attained by incubating inoculated media in an incubator that regulates the flow of extraneously provided gas from a commercially purchased gas cylinder or by incubating inoculated media in a closed glass jar (such as a commercial mayonnaise jar) in which a small white candle has been allowed to burn to extinction, called a **candle jar** (see Chapter 6,

Figure 6.2), thus removing atmospheric oxygen (to approximately 3%) and creating a bit of extra water vapor.

Sites to culture and techniques to apply for maximum recovery of *N. gonorrhoeae* from genital sites are discussed in Chapter 19. Chapter 16 mentions methods of obtaining material for recovery of gonococci from the oropharynx. Special methods for recovery of gonococci from blood in cases of disseminated disease are mentioned in Chapter 14. The recovery of *N. gonorrhoeae* from normally sterile body fluids does not require any special methods other than those routinely used for such specimens, except that they should be plated onto enriched chocolate agar (in addition to other media) and incubated for 48 h at 36°-37° C in a humidified atmosphere of 5%-10% CO_2.

26.2.c. Preliminary identification. After 24-48 h incubation, colonies of *N. gonorrhoeae* appear as small (0.5-2 mm), translucent, grayish, convex, shiny colonies with entire margins. They will often lift off the agar surface as whole colonies, and may appear to be mucoid or sticky. Since the organisms produce an active autolytic enzyme, they must not be exposed to room air for too long.

Colonies on chocolate or selective agar that resemble those of *N. gonorrhoeae* can be screened for the presence of the enzyme indophenol oxidase either by removing a portion of a colony to a piece of filter paper for the Kovac's test (as described in Chapter 9) or by dropping the fresh reagent (tetramethyl-*p*-phenylenediamine dihydrochloride) directly onto the colony on the agar surface. Oxidase positive colonies will turn purple, darkening with time (Plate 26.1). These colonies must be subcultured immediately, since the oxidase reagent will rapidly render them nonviable. A Gram stain of the oxidase positive organism will show typical gram-negative diplococci, with adjacent sides flattened. It has been recommended that the isolation of oxidase positive, gram-negative diplococci on selective agar such as Thayer-Martin medium from genital sites of infection may be reported presumptively as *N. gonorrhoeae.* However, several recent reports have documented the increasing incidence of gonorrhea-like infections in genital sites caused by *N. meningitidis,* indicating that the reporting of gonococcal disease based on presumptive criteria is no longer valid. Definitive biochemical identification methods and newer identification techniques are discussed in Sections 26.5 and 26.6.

26.2.d. Colony morphology variation. On translucent agar, at least five distinct types of colony morphology can be distinguished, as first reported by Kellogg and co-workers in 1963.[5] Types T1 and T2, small, bright reflective colonies typical of fresh isolates from cases of gonorrhea, differed from the larger, flatter, nonreflecting colonies of Types T3, T4, and T5, that developed from fresh isolates after in vitro passage (Figure 26.2). Further study revealed that the T1 and T2 colony types were virulent

FIGURE 26.2
Colony morphology variants of *Neisseria gonorrhoeae.* The large colonies (type T3 or T4) represent nonpiliated organisms, whereas the small colonies (T1 or T2) indicate that the organisms possess pili and are more virulent. (Courtesy D.S. Kellogg, Jr., Centers for Disease Control.)

for human volunteers, while the T3, T4, and T5 organisms failed to cause infection in human urethras. Microscopic study showed that the virulent organisms T1 and T2 possess multiple hairlike projections extending from the cell membrane, called fimbriae or pili. These proteinaceous structures are thinner and shorter than flagella, which they resemble (Figure 26.3). The pili function in adherence of bacteria to mucosal cell surfaces, as well as for the conjugal transfer of genetic material between bacteria. It seems likely that virulence, ability to adhere to host surfaces by virtue of possession of pili, and colony morphology of the gonococci are all interrelated.

26.2.e. Nutritionally variant gonococci. Another feature of *N. gonorrhoeae* that deserves mention is the phenomenon of "auxotypes." Certain strains, or auxotypes, of gonococci require the addition of particular defined nutrients to grow on artificial media. Those strains that require arginine, hypoxanthine, and uracil (AHU-dependent auxotypes) are usually sensitive to penicillin, resistant to the bactericidal activity of human serum, and are more likely to cause asymptomatic urethritis in males and disseminated gonococcal disease in females. Although at least 30 auxotypes have been described, the methods are not yet readily available for routine epidemiologic studies.

26.2.f. Antibiotic resistance. Penicillin-resistant *N. gonorrhoeae* have been causing disease in the United States for more than 30 years, but the incidence of such strains has increased in certain areas. The ability to hydrolyze the beta-lactam ring of penicillin-like antibiotics is mediated by a bacterial plasmid harboring the gene for the enzyme beta-lactamase. **PPNG, penicillinase-producing *N. gonorrhoeae,*** can be easily detected using a rapid test for hydrolysis of a chromogenic cephalosporin, nitrocefin, as described in Chapter 13. We recommend that all isolates of *N. gonor-*

FIGURE 26.3
Neisseria gonorrhoeae with pili extending from their surfaces. (Courtesy Chuen-mo To and C.C. Brinton, Jr., University of Pittsburgh.)

rhoeae be tested by this method and reported as "beta-lactamase positive" or "beta-lactamase negative."

26.3. *Neisseria meningitidis*

26.3.a. Specimen collection. *N. meningitidis* is a normal inhabitant of the human nasopharynx, with carriage rates as high as 44% in some populations during certain times. The presence of meningococci in the upper respiratory tract of a normal host has not been shown to predispose the host to meningococcal disease; thus isolation of the organism from nasopharyngeal cultures has no clinical significance. However, close contacts (persons who eat and sleep together) of a patient with known meningococcal meningitis have as much as 1,000 times greater risk of developing meningococcal disease than others; therefore, carriage of *N. meningitidis* by a close contact of a

patient has significance—this carrier should be given prophylaxis, often rifampin. Since the organism is not normal oropharyngeal flora, it may be significant if recovered with polymorphonuclear neutrophils in the absence of other pathogens (especially if found intracellularly) from sputum in large numbers. It is definitely significant if recovered from a transtracheal aspirate or material from percutaneous needle biopsy of lung infiltrates from a patient with pneumonia. Definitive diagnosis of meningococcal bacteremia, meningitis, or other serious disease is usually accomplished by isolation of the organism from a normally sterile body fluid, such as blood, cerebrospinal fluid, synovial fluid or pleural fluid, or from petechial aspirates. Other specimens may also yield meningococci; included are material from eyes, the genital tract, and the anus. Methods for isolation of the *Neisseria* species from blood are discussed in Chapter 14. Handling of other specimens for recovery of meningococci must minimize exposure to air and cool temperatures, as well as prevent dehydration.

26.3.b. Culture media and methods. Body fluids for isolation of any organisms are treated identically, as outlined in Chapter 21. Any volumes of clear fluid greater than 1 ml are centrifuged at room temperature at $1500 \times g$ for 15 min. The supernatant is removed to a sterile tube (and may be utilized for direct antigen detection studies for soluble antigens) and the sediment is vigorously vortexed, inoculated onto an enriched supportive medium, such as enriched chocolate agar, into a supportive broth medium, such as thioglycolate, and a direct Gram stain is prepared from the last drop of sediment. Purulent fluids may be handled directly without concentrating. All media are immediately incubated in a moist atmosphere of 5%-10% CO_2 at 36°-37° C for at least 5 days before discarding as negative.

N. meningitidis strains are able to grow on blood agar as well as on chocolate agar, unlike the gonococcus, although both organisms grow better in increased CO_2 concentration. Specimens from sites with contaminating normal flora may be inoculated to Thayer-Martin or NYC media for selective isolation.

26.3.c. Preliminary identification. The same techniques that are used for preliminary identification of gonococci are useful for the meningococci. A positive oxidase test combined with typical gram-negative diplococcal morphology defines those isolates that require further identification, either with the biochemical tests described below or with the use of one of the new techniques to be discussed.

26.3.d. Serologic classification. Nine serogroups of *N. meningitidis* (A, B, C, D, X, Y, Z, 29E, and W135) have been defined on the basis of differing capsular polysaccharides. The most important serogroups in the United States are A, B, C, and Y. Interestingly, group B polysaccharide is a very poor immunogen for humans and animals, leading to difficulty in developing an effective vaccine against this strain and limiting the development of serologic reagents prepared in animals for laboratory diagnostic tests. Only since the development of techniques for the preparation of monoclonal antibodies, described in Chapter 10, has a consistently good immunologic reagent for identification of group B meningococci become widely available.

26.3.e. Rapid detection of *N. meningitidis* antigen in body fluids. The sometimes rapidly fulminant course of meningococcal meningitis has spurred the development of several rapid methods for the detection of capsular polysaccharide antigen in body fluids (urine, serum, and cerebrospinal fluid) before culture results are available. Although counterimmunoelectrophoresis (CIE) was the first of these methods to be developed, it has been shown to be less sensitive (and more time consuming) than particle agglutination techniques such as latex and coagglutination. Basic principles of these tests are discussed in Chapter 12, and their application to the diagnosis of meningitis is further discussed in Chapter 15. Briefly, antibodies to the capsular polysaccharide, either produced in animals and processed to remove most cross-reacting factors or produced artificially as monoclonal antibodies (serogroup B), are adsorbed to the surface of latex particles or protein A–containing staphylococci. In the presence of antigen, the particles show visible agglutination. These reagents are able to detect minute amounts of antigen, often in the absence of viable organisms due to previous treatment or dilution. The latex particles have been the most sensitive in direct assays for antigen, although a thoroughly studied Gram stain is still the most definitive rapid diagnostic method. The methods used in direct detection of antigens are outlined in Chapter 12.

26.4. *Branhamella catarrhalis* and *Neisseria cinerea*

26.4.a. *Branhamella catarrhalis*. Although classified as a member of the *Moraxella* genus on the basis of DNA homology studies, *Branhamella* morphologically and biochemically resembles the *Neisseria* species (Table 26.1). It is normal flora of the upper respiratory tract, but has been isolated as the causative agent of disease, including septicemia, meningitis, endocarditis, otitis media, conjunctivitis, laryngitis, pneumonia, and bronchitis. Any gram-negative diplococci recovered in large numbers from the lower respiratory tract of a patient with pneumonia should be identified. *Branhamella* is commonly beta-lactamase positive.

26.4.b. *Neisseria cinerea*. This organism has recently been recognized as a pathogen associated with nosocomial pneumonia[1] and proctitis.[3] Although part of the normal oropharyngeal and genital tract flora, *N. cinerea* has rarely been reported from infection. The recognition of this strain is largely due to its biochemical resemblance to, and consequent confusion with, *N. gonorrhoeae*. Rare strains of *N. cinerea* have been found to metabolize glucose when tested by more than one system. To prevent misidentification, all strains of glucose and oxidase-positive gram-negative diplococci recovered from noninhibitory media (such as chocolate agar) should be plated to tryptic soy or Mueller-Hinton agar, which support growth of *N. cinerea* but not *N. gonorrhoeae*, and to selective agar such as modified Thayer-Martin, on which growth of *N. cinerea* is inhibited.

26.5. Definitive Biochemical Identification

Isolated bacterial colonies on inhibitory media to be characterized by biochemical confirmatory tests must be subcultured to nonselective agar, such as chocolate, for purification and amplification. Subcultures are incubated for a maximum of 48 h before inoculation to carbohydrates. Cystine trypticase soy agar (CTA) base, pH 7.6, with the addition of 1% filter-sterilized carbohydrate solutions, has been shown to yield the most consistent results. Morello, Janda, and Bohnhoff present an excellent discussion of the test and its ambiguities.[6] The use of an extremely heavy inoculum in a small volume of substrate, as described by Kellogg, Holmes, and Hill,[4] may also yield acceptable results. Table 26.1 shows the reactions used to differentiate members of the Neisseriaceae.

Several commercial identification systems that employ biochemical substrates are available for identification of the *Neisseria* species and *Branhamella* (RapID NH, Innovative Diagnostic Systems; RIM-Neisseria kit, Austin Biological Laboratories; Minitek, BBL Microbiology Systems; GONOCHEK II, DuPont Co.; QuadFERM +, Analytab Products; and RINTEST, Winfield Laboratories). These products usually use the ability of preformed enzymes to act on substrates (conventional or chromogenic) to form a colored endproduct as the indicator system. A heavy inoculum of the organism is necessary for proper reactions, although viable organisms may not be necessary. Rapid identification systems such as these are described in Chapter 9.

26.6. Nonbiochemical Identification Methods

26.6.a. Fluorescent antibody stains. Fluorescent antibody stains are commercially available (Difco Laboratories) for *N. gonorrhoeae*. Because of a large number of cross-reacting organisms in urethral or other discharge, these stains are not particularly useful for direct examination of such specimens. Once an oxidase-positive organism morphologically consistent with gonococci has been isolated on selective media, however, fluorescent stain may provide a rapid identification; equivocal reactions must be confirmed by some other method. Good fluorescent reagents are not available for other members of the Neisseriaceae.

26.6.b. Radiometric method. The measurement of radioactive endproducts of metabolism

TABLE 26.1
Characteristics of *Neisseria* Species and *Branhamella*

| | NEISSERIA SPECIES | | | | | | | | BRANHAMELLA |
	GONORRHOEAE	*MENINGITIDIS*	*CINEREA*	*LACTAMICA*	*SICCA*	*SUBFLAVA*	*FLAVESCENS*	*MUCOSA*	*CATARRHALIS*
Acid from									
Glucose	+	+	−	+	+	+	−	+	−
Maltose	−	+	−	+	+	+	−	+	−
Fructose	−	−	−	−	+	V	−	+	−
Sucrose	−	−	−	−	+	V	−	+	−
Lactose (ONPG)	−	−	−	+	−	−	−	−	−
Growth at 22° C	−	−	V	V	V	V	+	+	V
Growth on nutrient agar, 35° C	−	−	+	V	V	V	+	+	+
Pigment*	−	−	−/gray	Y/V	sl Y	Y	Y	Y/V	gray
NO$_3$ reduced	−	−	−	−	−	−	−	+	+
DNase	−	−	−	−	−	−	−	−	+

+ = > 90% of strains positive.
− = > 90% of strains negative.
V = variable.
Y = yellow.
*On Loeffler's agar slant (see Chapter 45).

from labeled substrates in fluid medium has also been used as a method for identification of *Neisseria* species. Specially formulated media containing carbohydrates labeled with ^{14}C are inoculated with pure cultures of the organism to be identified. The cultures are incubated for a short time, and the gas that collects in the bottle above the liquid medium is sampled for the presence of radioactive $^{14}CO_2$, indicating the ability of the organism to metabolize the carbohydrate. *N. gonorrhoeae* and *N. meningitidis* can be identified with the Bactec instrument (Chapter 11) in this way.

26.6.c. *Limulus* amebocyte lysate (LAL) assay. The lysate fluid obtained from amebocytes (motile, phagocytic cells) that circulate through the hemolymph of the horseshoe crab, *Limulus polyphemus*, will form a gel in the presence of minute amounts of endotoxin (lipopolysaccharide found in gram-negative bacterial cell walls, discussed in Chapter 14). This test is useful for detection of meningitis caused by meningococci, especially if organisms are present at $>10^3/cm^3$. The gel formation of the lysate is nonspecific, however, and will occur in the presence of endotoxin from any organism, such as gram-negative bacteria and *Listeria monocytogenes* (Chapter 10). Surprisingly, this assay has also been found to be useful as a diagnostic test for gonococcal infection in females. Material collected on swabs from the endocervical canal of women with gonorrhea, including early cases and asymptomatic cases, may yield positive *Limulus* amebocyte lysate tests.

26.6.d. Enzyme-linked immunosorbent assay (ELISA). The ELISA tests used in clinical microbiology today consist of specific antibody bound to a solid matrix, such as the wells of a microdilution plate (Chapter 10).

A commercial ELISA system (Gonozyme, Abbott Laboratories) has been shown to be very sensitive and specific for the detection of gonococcal antigen in the urethral and endocervical discharge from suspected cases of gonorrhea, although no more sensitive than a Gram stain of male urethral discharge. The test is much more rapid than culture and is suitable for large-scale screening programs among sexually active people.[2]

The ELISA tests have not been particularly useful for rapid diagnosis of meningitis, perhaps due to the time required to perform the assays (often 4-6 h). Studies are exploring ways to speed up the endpoint determination, which may allow the ELISA systems to better serve as diagnostic tests for antigen in CSF.

REFERENCES

1. Boyce, J.M., Taylor, M.R., Mitchell, E.B. Jr., and Knapp, J.S. 1985. Nosocomial pneumonia caused by a glucose-metabolizing strain of *Neisseria cinerea*. J. Clin. Microbiol. 21:1.
2. Demetriou, E., Sackett, R., Welch, D.F., and Kaplan, D.W. 1984. Evaluation of an enzyme immunoassay for detection of *Neisseria gonorrhoeae* in an adolescent population. J.A.M.A. 252:247.
3. Dossett, J.H., Appelbaum, P.C., Knapp, J.S., and Totten, P.A. 1985. Proctitis associated with *Neisseria cinerea* misidentified as *Neisseria gonorrhoeae* in a child. J. Clin. Microbiol. 21:575.
4. Kellogg, D.S., Jr., Holmes, K.K., and Hill, G.A. 1976. Cumitech 4, Laboratory diagnosis of gonorrhea. American Society for Microbiology, Washington, D.C.
5. Kellogg, D.S. Jr., Peacock, W.L. Jr., Deacon, W.E., et al. 1963. *Neisseria gonorrhoeae*. I. Virulence genetically linked to clonal variation. J. Bacteriol. 85:1274.
6. Morello, J.A., Janda, W.M., and Bohnhoff, M. 1985. *Neisseria* and *Branhamella*. In Lennette, E.H., Balows, A., Hausler, W.J. Jr., and Shadomy, H.J. editors. Manual of clinical microbiology, ed. 4. American Society for Microbiology, Washington, D.C.

BIBLIOGRAPHY

Apicella, M.A. 1985. *Neisseria meningitidis*. In Mandell, G.L., Douglas, R.G. Jr., and Bennett, J.E., editors. Principles and practice of infectious diseases, ed. 2. John Wiley & Sons, New York.
Black, J.R., and Sparling, P.F. 1985. *Neisseria gonorrhoeae*. In Mandell, G.L., Douglas, R.G. Jr., and Bennett, J.E., editors. Principles and practice of infectious diseases, ed. 2. John Wiley & Sons, New York.
Gröschel, D.H.M. 1985. Other gram negative cocci. In Mandell, G.L., Douglas, R.G. Jr., and Bennett, J.E., editors. Principles and practice of infectious diseases, ed. 2. John Wiley & Sons, New York.
Philip, A., and Bentsen, C. 1984. *Branhamella catarrhalis*: effects and identification. Lab. Management 22:49.

27 Enterobacteriaceae

rebrospinal fluid, respiratory tract, gastrointestinal tract, urinary tract, soft tissue infections, sterile body fluid infections, and infections in immunocompromised hosts. The only major category of infectious diseases with which Enterobacteriaceae have not yet been definitively associated is that of sexually transmitted disease.

Identification of the Enterobacteriaceae to species level is of importance epidemiologically as well as clinically. The susceptibility patterns of many species are predictable, allowing the clinician to choose therapy based on an isolate's identification. The association of certain species with known disease syndromes can aid a clinician to establish an etiology under circumstances when such an isolate has been detected. The presence of an epidemic or small outbreak, due to a particularly virulent strain of Enterobacteriaceae or due to a breakdown in technique among health care workers, is often first detected by microbiologists who have noticed a cluster of isolates of an unusual biotype. The discovery of an extremely rare biotype in a cluster of blood cultures led a Milwaukee microbiologist to discover the source of a nationwide outbreak of septicemia associated with contaminated intravenous fluids. The importance of species differentiation for epidemiologic purposes is discussed in Chapter 5.

Within the last several years, the number of recognized species of Enterobacteriaceae has grown from 26 to over 100 (approximately 70 species have been named), and more species are being validated monthly. This rapid expansion is somewhat overwhelming to clinical microbiologists, who are not taxonomists and generally wish only to convey some meaningful information to clinicians concerning bacterial species isolated from clinical material. It is primarily due to the availability of commercially produced multibiochemical and enzymatic parameter test systems (Chapter 9) that most microbiology laboratories are able to identify the newly recognized species of Enterobacteri-

27.1. Introduction

Bacteria belonging to the family Enterobacteriaceae are the most commonly encountered organisms isolated from clinical specimens. They are gram-negative bacilli, able to grow readily on all supportive media (blood and chocolate agars), and they form distinctive colonies on selective agars depending on their metabolic capabilities and the components of the media, as discussed in Chapter 8. Some species are classical pathogens, assumed to be the etiologic agents of disease when they are encountered in clinical specimens, independent of the numbers of colony forming units detected (such as *Salmonella, Shigella,* and *Yersinia pestis*). Other species can colonize humans without evoking any pathologic response, such as those Enterobacteriaceae that colonize the human intestinal tract. These "commensal" organisms, if they are introduced into a susceptible site (peritoneal cavity, lung of an immunosuppressed host, cerebrospinal fluid, etc.) are able to cause disease. Still others, such as *Escherichia coli,* are associated with certain syndromes based on the presence of virulence factors that are not possessed by all strains or even by the same strain at all times. Members of this ubiquitous family of similar organisms have been mentioned in association with each of the anatomic sites of infectious disease covered in previous chapters, including blood, ceaceae. This chapter will focus on the 13 genera of Enterobacteriaceae that are most likely to be encountered in clinical specimens. Although we advocate the definitive identification of isolates that can be causally related to disease, particularly from systemic sites of infection such as blood, cerebrospinal fluid, tissue, or other sterile body fluids, it is not practical for routine clinical laboratories to maintain all of the unusual, rarely used, or technically demanding media or test reagents necessary for thorough studies of rarely isolated organisms. Such isolates should be forwarded to a reference laboratory for further studies.

27.2. Epidemiology and Pathogenesis of Infections Due to the Enterobacteriaceae

Enterobacteriaceae are the predominant facultative flora in the human bowel, a site from which they can easily be disseminated. Lapses in personal hygiene, especially during periods of diarrheal disease, can contribute to the fecal-oral route of transmission of the agents of gastroenteritis and related diseases. Countries with poor sanitation systems are more likely to have environmental reservoirs of the Enterobacteriaceae, from which disease is maintained in the population. Hospitalized patients quickly become colonized on the skin or in the respiratory tract with strains endemic to the hospital, allowing these organisms easy access to the host under any compromising situation.

In addition to their presence as normal human fecal flora, Enterobacteriaceae are found in natural habitats worldwide, including soil, water, plants of all types, fish, insects, and other animals. Their importance in human disease is at least equalled by their importance as causes of disease in poultry, domestic livestock, fish, and several vegetable and plant crops, with major economic consequences. Although the genera that have not been associated with human disease will be listed here (Table 27.1), they will not be discussed in detail. It is possible that any species of Enterobacteriaceae may

be isolated from clinical specimens, especially as more immunocompromised patients survive long enough to become infected. Only by identifying unusual clinical isolates can microbiologists discover previously unrecognized agents of human disease.

27.2.a. Enterobacteriaceae associated with gastroenteritis and enteric fevers. As discussed in Chapter 17, several Enterobacteriaceae have been associated with gastroenteritis and food-borne disease. *Salmonella* species are the etiologic agents of the majority of food-borne gastroenteritis in the United States. Over 44,000 cases were reported to the Centers for Disease Control (CDC) in 1983. For some reason, the incidence of salmonellosis has increased steadily since 1955, particularly among elderly patients. The organism is naturally found in poultry, but disease can be transmitted in a wide variety of foods. The most recent major outbreak occurred in Chicago in spring 1985, when several truckloads of contaminated milk were inadvertently dumped into local drainage systems. More than 5,000 individuals contracted culture-positive *Salmonella* gastroenteritis, resulting in several fatalities. Because *Salmonella* are susceptible to gastric acid, a large inoculum (approximately 10^5 organisms) must be ingested. As discussed in Chapter 17, *Salmonella* are able to invade the intestinal mucosa. Some strains produce an enterotoxin. *S. typhi* and *S. cholerae-suis* are more likely to invade systemically, entering the bloodstream and causing serious febrile disease (typhoid or enteric fever). These strains are usually carried only in human hosts, passed among individuals by fecal contamination of food or water. Very young, very old, and other compromised hosts are most likely to become seriously ill. Forty percent of all cases of salmonellosis reported in 1982 occurred in children less than 5 years old. The incidence of typhoid fever in the United States is quite low (507 cases reported in 1983), and approximately half of these were acquired during foreign

TABLE 27.1
Genera and Species of Enterobacteriaceae

GENUS	SPECIES	COMMENTS
Buttiauxella	*agrestis*	Found in water, not associated with human disease.
Cedecea	*davisae*	Isolated from humans, primarily respiratory tract and wounds.
	lapagei	
	neteri	
	(others)	
Citrobacter	*amalonaticus*	Isolated from humans, wound infections, urine, sepsis; fecal flora. Also isolated from environment.
	diversus	
	freundii	
	(others)	
Edwardsiella	*hoshinae*	Isolated from humans and animals; associated with diarrhea, wound infections, sepsis.
	ictaluri	
	tarda	
	(others)	
Enterobacter	*aerogenes*	Very common, normal fecal flora; isolated from wounds, respiratory tract, urine, blood. *E. agglomerans* also in animals, others found in environment. *E. cloacae* most clinically significant. *E. agglomerans* and *E. sakazakii* yellow pigmented.
	agglomerans	
	amnigenus	
	cloacae	
	gergoviae	
	intermedium	
	sakazakii	
	taylorae	
	(others)	
Escherichia	*blattae*	Isolated from humans and animals, *E. coli* most common human pathogen. *E. blattae* found only in cockroaches. *E. hermannii* and *E. vulneris* isolated from wounds. Others normal stool flora.
	coli	
	fergusonii	
	hermannii	
	vulneris	
Ewingella	*americana*	Isolated from humans, respiratory tract, blood. No environmental source known.
Hafnia	*alvei*	Isolated from humans, respiratory tract, other sources. No environmental source known.
	(others)	
Klebsiella	*oxytoca*	Normal stool flora, some strains found in environment. Isolated from respiratory tract, urine, wounds, blood. *K. terrigena* only found in water.
	ozaenae	
	planticola	
	pneumoniae	
	rhinoscleromatis	
	terrigena	
Kluyvera	*ascorbata*	Probably normal stool flora. Isolated from human infections, respiratory tract, blood, urine.
	cryocrescens	
Koserella	*trabulsii*	Isolated from human feces, wounds, respiratory tract, knee joint.
Leminorella	*grimontii*	Isolated from human feces. H_2S positive, not known to be pathogenic for humans.
	richardii	
Moellerella	*wisconsinsis*	Isolated from human stool and natural water. Not known to be pathogenic for humans.
Morganella	*morganii*	Normal stool flora. Isolated from human infections (urine, blood, others).
	(others)	
Obesumbacterium	*proteus*	Isolated from brewery yeast. Not known to be pathogenic for humans.

TABLE 27.1

Genera and Species of Enterobacteriaceae—cont'd

GENUS	SPECIES	COMMENTS
Proteus	*mirabilis* *myxofaciens* *penneri* *vulgaris*	Most species normal fecal flora. Isolated from human infections, urine, wounds, blood, others, *P. myxofaciens* isolated from moths only.
Providencia	*alcalifaciens* *rettgeri* *rustigianii* *stuartii*	Most species are normal fecal flora. Isolated from human infections, urine, wounds, blood. *P. rustigianii* not known to be pathogenic for humans.
Rhanella	*aquatilis*	Isolated from water. Only one human isolate reported. Not known to be pathogenic for humans.
Salmonella	I (*cholerae-suis*) II (*salamae*) III (*arizonae*) IV (*houtenae*) V (*bongori*) (others)	Widely distributed in humans and animals. Cause of gastroenteritis and enteric fever. Genus *Arizona* now included in *Salmonella*. Nomenclature still undecided.
Serratia	*ficaria* "*fonticola*" *liquefaciens* *marcescens* *odorifera* *plymuthica* *rubidaea* (others)	Isolated from humans, water, rarely animals. Some species important human pathogens. Isolated from respiratory tract, wounds, blood, urine, others. *S. ficaria, odorifera, plymuthica, rubidaea* not known to be human pathogens. *S. fonticola* probably not true member of *Serratia* genus.
Shigella	*boydii* *dysenteriae* *flexneri* *sonnei*	Human reservoir only, not normal flora. Cause of gastroenteritis and bacterial dysentery. Genetically identical to *E. coli*.
Tatumella	*ptyseos*	Isolated from humans, respiratory tract, urine, blood. Unlike other Enterobacteriaceae, *Tatumella* has polar flagella; susceptible to penicillin; poor grower, better at 25° C.
Xenorhabdus	*luminescens* *nematophilus*	Isolated from nematodes only. Grow only at 25° C, not at 35° C. No human isolates.
Yersinia	*enterocolitica* *frederiksenii* *intermedia* *kristensenii* *pestis* *pseudotuberculosis* *ruckerii*	Isolated from humans, animals, environment. Some important human pathogens. Agents of plague, gastroenteritis, other infections. Isolated from stool, blood, urine, wounds. *Y. ruckerii* not found in humans, cause of "red mouth" disease of fish. *Y. ruckerii* probably not true member of genus *Yersinia*.

travel. Domestically acquired typhoid, however, is often transmitted by a chronic carrier of *S. typhi*. After recovering from typhoid fever, some individuals carry the bacteria asymptomatically for long periods of time. Another set of individuals will be asymptomatic carriers without ever suffering from disease. The silent carriers contribute to continued episodes of infections.

Shigella species are carried primarily by humans and are not disseminated in nature. The organism is able to resist gastric acidity, allowing a very small inoculum (as few as 10 organisms) to cause disease. Shigellosis also occurs primarily in children, although the incidence is not as high as that of salmonellosis. In 1983, approximately 20,000 cases of shigellosis were reported to the CDC. *Shigella* produce an enterotoxin, but it is not as important to virulence as is their invasiveness. The organisms invade the epithelial cells of the large bowel, causing a dysentery-like syndrome, as discussed in Chapter 17. *Shigella* rarely invade systemically.

Escherichia coli is also an important cause of Enterobacteriaceae-mediated gastrointestinal disease. It can be associated with nursery outbreaks of diarrhea as well as with travelers' diarrhea (turista, Delhi belly, and other amusing epithets), a major source of morbidity to Americans traveling to other countries. Virulence mechanisms of *E. coli* include production of an enterotoxin similar to that of *Vibrio cholerae*, invasiveness, production of cytotoxins, and adherence (Chapter 17). In previous years, nursery outbreaks of *E. coli*–mediated gastroenteritis were associated with particular serotypes of the organism, called **enteropathogenic E. coli.** Serotypes may still be associated with epidemics or geographic regions, but the serotype is not the only significant factor; it does serve as a marker for a particular strain. Toxin production is carried on a plasmid, a transmissible genetic element that can be easily transferred from strain to strain among and between species. For this reason, serotyping of isolates of *E. coli* from patients with diarrhea is not recommended except for epidemiologic reasons. Tests for toxin production and tests utilizing genetic probes to detect the toxin gene sequences (Chapter 10) more accurately identify etiologic agents (**enterotoxigenic E. coli**), but these tests have not been simplified for routine laboratory use yet (Chapter 17). The gastrointestinal disease mediated by invasive or cytotoxic *E. coli* can resemble shigellosis, and the disease mediated by enterotoxigenic *E. coli*

can resemble cholera. Other mechanisms of pathogenicity also occur in still other types of *E. coli.*

The fourth genus of Enterobacteriaceae containing organisms that are major etiologic agents of diarrheal disease is *Yersinia,* which also includes the etiologic agent of human plague. *Y. enterocolitica* and, less commonly, *Y. pseudotuberculosis* have only recently been implicated as significant causes of gastroenteritis. The organisms possess the ability to invade the intestinal mucosa, as well as to produce a heat-stable enterotoxin similar to that of some strains of *E. coli.* Virulence factors shared among other members of *Yersinia* species, such as the ability to survive intracellularly, may also contribute to pathogenesis. Symptoms that accompany *Y. pseudotuberculosis,* and occasionally *Y. enterocolitica* infections, may mimic those of appendicitis (although the symptoms are actually due to mesenteric lymphadenitis). The organisms can invade the epithelium to cause systemic disease. *Y. enterocolitica* has also been associated with exudative pharyngitis.

Although the incidence of diarrheal disease associated with *Yersinia* is much higher in Europe and Canada than in the United States, more isolations are occurring in the United States over time, aided by increased awareness of the organism and better laboratory techniques designed especially for its detection (Chapter 17). Certain serotypes (primarily 03 and 09) have been recovered from patients with diarrhea in Europe and Scandinavia. These serotypes are less common in the United States, where 08 predominates. The incidence of 03 isolations, however, seems to be increasing, at least in the New York area, with an accompanying greater risk of acquiring disease via human-to-human transmission.

Gastroenteritis has also been associated with *Edwardsiella tarda,* a member of the Enterobacteriaceae that resembles salmonellae in its pathogenic mechanisms, as well as morphologically. The organism has also been known to invade through the intestinal epithelium, causing systemic disease. Reported cases of *Edwardsiella*-associated gastroenteritis are uncommon.

27.2.b. *Yersinia pestis*. The agent of human plague, *Y. pestis*, is found as a zoonosis among many wild animal species, including prairie dogs, squirrels, rabbits, chipmunks, and others. The organism is transmitted among these animals by fleas, which also spread the organism to carnivores that prey upon the smaller rodents. Humans acquire the disease when bitten by an infected flea or handling the carcass of an infected animal. Rarely, infection can be spread from person to person via infected aerosol droplets from respiratory secretions of patients who have plague pneumonia. Most cases occur among young individuals in the southwestern and western United States; Navajos are at higher risk because of intense rodent plague in areas of the reservation in Arizona. The incidence has increased since 1965, with 19 cases reported in 1982 and 40 cases reported in 1983. This probably reflects a natural cycle of increased plague within the wild rodent population.

Once the organisms penetrate the skin, through small breaks or via flea bites, or are breathed in, they are taken up by macrophages and polymorphonuclear neutrophils, within which they can multiply. During this first intracellular phase, the bacteria are stimulated by their immediate environment (lack of Ca^{++}, temperature, ionic concentration) to produce a protein and a lipoprotein antigen, called **V** and **W antigens,** that render the organism less susceptible to intracellular killing by other reticuloendothelial cells once they escape the original cell through lysis of that cell. *Y. pestis* also possesses an envelope antigen (F-1) that may contribute to resistance to phagocytosis. Virulent *Y. pestis* produce three factors, a bacteriocin (Chapter 5) called **pesticin I,** coagulase, and fibrinolysin. These three factors, produced together, are probably plasmid-mediated and seem to contribute to virulence. Other factors that are correlated to virulence include the ability of virulent strains to absorb hemin and basic aromatic dyes to form colored colonies, the ability to synthesize purines, and production of a toxin.

Primary disease is usually of the **bubonic** variety, characterized by infected and swollen lymph nodes and fever. Sepsis and sometimes pneumonia follow within several days. Septicemic and pneumonic plague may also occur without the lymphadenopathy stage. Untreated human plague is 50%-60% fatal. Streptomycin and tetracycline are the antimicrobial agents of choice. If meningitis develops, chloramphenicol should be added to the regimen.

27.2.c. Other infections associated with members of the family Enterobacteriaceae. Enterobacteriaceae, particularly *E. coli*, are the most common cause of urinary tract infections (Chapter 18). Urinary tract infections are the largest cause of nosocomial infections; they may lead to secondary sepsis, shock, and death. Factors contributing to the development of nosocomial infections are discussed in Chapter 23. In addition to urinary tract infections, nosocomial infections include pneumonia, surgical wound infections, and catheter-related sepsis. In all of these infections, Enterobacteriaceae play a major role. The species that are most likely to be recovered from urine of infected individuals are those that are able to adhere to urinary epithelium. Attachment-mediating, fingerlike projections composed of protein, called **fimbriae,** are often found on strains that are able to adhere, not only to urinary tract, but to many other human and animal epithelial cell types (Figure 16.1). Fimbriae are also found among gastroenteritis-producing strains, especially in animals. The ability to colonize the gastrointestinal tract, resisting the action of peristalsis and other factors (Chapter 17), is mediated at least in part by fimbriae.

Most of the Enterobacteriaceae may be involved in bacterial pneumonia, but *Klebsiella pneumoniae* seems especially suited to this role. The copious polysaccharide capsular material produced by this species probably aids the organism to escape phagocytosis. Chapter 16 contains a discussion of those factors that contribute to the pathogenesis of pneumonia. Elderly patients and those compromised by alcoholism and other chronic diseases are most likely to contract community-acquired *Klebsiella* pneumonia. It is a significant cause of hospital-acquired pneumonia as well (Chapter 23).

Neonatal meningitis has been associated with certain strains of *E. coli*, most of which possess the K1 capsular antigen (shared by group B streptococci, the other principal cause of neonatal meningitis). Capsular polysaccharide may also contribute to the pathogenesis of this disease. *Citrobacter* species, also encapsulated, have been associated with neonatal meningitis as well. It is postulated that the organisms can somehow invade through infant intestinal epithelium to cause systemic disease. *E. coli* is no more likely to be the etiologic agent of adult meningitis than are any other members of the Enterobacteriaceae. The role of capsular polysaccharide as a factor in the development of meningitis is mentioned in Chapter 15.

Serratia species are sometimes associated with especially severe hospital-acquired infections, including pneumonia and surgical wound infections. The organisms recovered from blood may be resistant to the bactericidal activity of serum and complement. Nosocomially derived *Serratia* strains are often resistant to multiple antibiotics. Rarely, strains of *S. marcescens* will display a red, non-water-soluble pigment (Plate 27.1). These pigmented strains are less likely to be resistant and are more likely to be community acquired.

All members of the Enterobacteriaceae have been associated with various infections, particularly among hospitalized and otherwise compromised hosts. The *Proteus, Providencia,* and *Morganella* species are most often recovered from urine of patients with urinary tract infections, although they can also be found associated with pneumonia, wound infections, and other syndromes. Those strains that are able to hydrolyze urea have been associated with the development of renal calculi in infected patients.

A virulence factor possessed by all Enterobacteriaceae (as well as all gram-negative bacteria) is the cell wall lipopolysaccharide, **endotoxin.** Biological activity of this component, released during growth and breakdown of gram-negative bacterial cells, was discussed in Chapter 14. The major pathologic consequence of gram-negative septicemia, that of shock, is mediated by endotoxin. Patients may experience disseminated intravascular coagulopathy, respiratory tract problems, cellular and tissue injury, fever, and other debilitating problems. Although species of Enterobacteriaceae possess flagella, and species other than those mentioned above possess polysaccharide capsules and fimbriae, the effect of these factors on the virulence of a particular strain has not been completely elucidated.

27.3. Taxonomy of Enterobacteriaceae

The confusion that arose when the eighth edition of *Bergey's Manual* was published, creating a dichotomy between the classification scheme used by the major reference publication in the United States (Bergey's) and the major reference laboratory in the United States, Centers for Disease Control, has been resolved with the recent publication of the ninth edition of *Bergey's Manual of Systematic Bacteriology*, containing the chapter on Enterobacteriaceae written by Don J. Brenner of the CDC.[1] The reader is referred to publications by Farmer and others,[2] Russell and Henke,[6] and the previous edition of this text (1982) by Finegold and Martin for an explanation of some of the nomenclature changes that have occurred among the Enterobacteriaceae since 1974. The application of deoxyribonucleic acid (DNA) homology technology to the study of the relatedness of two bacterial clones has been the major factor leading to the ability to definitively assign morphologically or biochemically distinct strains of bacteria to species. As described and illustrated in Chapter 10, the more closely related two strains of bacteria are, the greater the chromosomal homology shared between them, as demonstrated by the extent to which single strands of DNA from one strain will realign with single strands of DNA from the other strain under carefully controlled experimental conditions (called **stringent** conditions). The recombined DNA, possessing one strand from each of two test strains, is called a **hybrid**, and the analysis to determine relatedness is called **DNA-DNA hybridization**. Arbitrarily, clones of bacteria that share 70% or more of their chromosomal sequences are considered to belong to the same species. Definition of genera is not so easily determined. In addition to DNA-DNA hybridization studies, relatedness of bacteria can be determined by differences in the melting temperature of DNA, which is directly related to the number of guanine and cytosine bonds compared to the number of adenine and thymine bonds. The guanine and cytosine content (%G + C) can be used to begin to characterize strains of bacteria, but DNA-DNA hybridization is the most definitive arbitrator.

Table 27.1 lists the genera and species of Enterobacteriaceae that have been validly published as of this writing. Species that were included in Enterobacteriaceae in the past, such as *Erwinia*, a plant pathogen, have been deleted or included with other genera. The *Erwinia* have been encompassed by *Enterobacter agglomerans*. A number of the newer species have not yet been isolated from humans, although in the future they may be associated with human disease. The identification of these species is possible with many of the commer-

cial identification systems (Chapter 9). Those laboratories that do not use such systems should refer to the publication by Farmer et al.[2] and subsequent descriptions of newly characterized species for biochemical tests used to identify these isolates, if they do not choose to send the isolates to a suitable reference laboratory. Tests described in this chapter as well as in Chapter 9 will often be used to characterize the new species as well. The bulk of discussion in this chapter, however, will focus on the 13 genera most likely to be encountered in clinical specimens. The basic differential characteristics of the most commonly isolated Enterobacteriaceae are given in Table 27.2.

27.4. Laboratory Identification of Enterobacteriaceae

27.4.a. Isolation of Enterobacteriaceae from clinical material. Material from any site can harbor members of the family Enterobacteriaceae. Specimens of fecal material, in which these organisms are normal flora, are inoculated to selective and differential agars for detection of those organisms known to be the etiologic agents of gastroenteritis to the exclusion of the nonpathogenic commensal fecal Enterobacteriaceae. Strategies for cultivation of stool are discussed in Chapter 17, and an overview of culture media to initially inoculate is presented in Chapter 6. Most other clinical specimens, including material from wounds, respiratory tract secretions, aspirations from abscesses, sterile body fluids, urines, tissues, and blood cultures, are inoculated to at least one supportive medium, such as blood or chocolate agar, that will support the growth of all Enterobacteriaceae, as well as to one selective agar for gram-negative bacilli, usually MacConkey agar. Discussion of initial selection of media for isolation of etiologic agents of disease from each of these sites is found in the appropriate chapters of this text, and initial inoculation of specimens is summarized in Chapter 6. Descriptions of colony morphologies of isolates

TABLE 27.2
Identification of Clinically Important Enterobacteriaceae*

SPECIES	INDOLE PRODUCTION	METHYL RED	VOGES-PROSKAUER	CITRATE (SIMMONS)	HYDROGEN SULFIDE (TSI)	UREA HYDROLYSIS	PHENYLALANINE DEAMINASE	LYSINE DECARBOXYLASE	ARGININE DIHYDROLASE	ORNITHINE DECARBOXYLASE	MOTILITY (36° C)	GELATIN HYDROLYSIS (22° C)	D-GLUCOSE, GAS	LACTOSE FERMENTATION	SUCROSE FERMENTATION	D-MANNITOL FERMENTATION	DULCITOL FERMENTATION	ADONITOL FERMENTATION	D-SORBITOL FERMENTATION	L-ARABINOSE FERMENTATION	RAFFINOSE FERMENTATION	L-RHAMNOSE FERMENTATION	D-XYLOSE FERMENTATION	MELIBIOSE FERMENTATION	DNase, 25° C	ONPG†
Escherichia coli	98	99	0	0	1	1	0	90	17	65	95	0	95	95	50	98	60	5	94	99	50	80	95	75	0	95
Shigella serogroups A, B, and C	50	100	0	0	0	0	0	0	5	1	0	0	2	0	0	93	2	0	30	60	50	5	2	50	0	2
Shigella sonnei	0	100	0	0	0	0	0	0	2	98	0	0	0	2	1	99	0	0	2	95	3	75	2	25	0	90
Salmonella, most serotypes	1	100	0	95	95	1	0	98	70	97	95	0	96	1	1	100	96	0	95	99	2	95	97	95	2	2
Salmonella typhi	0	100	0	0	97	0	0	98	3	0	97	0	0	1	0	100	0	0	99	2	0	0	82	100	0	0
Salmonella paraty-phi A	0	100	0	0	10	0	0	0	15	95	95	0	99	0	0	100	90	0	95	100	0	100	0	95	0	0
Citrobacter freundii	5	100	0	95	80	70	0	0	65	20	95	0	95	50	30	99	55	0	98	100	30	99	99	50	0	95

Klebsiella pneumoniae	0	10	98	98		0	95	0	0	98		0	0	97	0	0	0	98	99	99	99	90	99	99	99	99	99	99	99	99	99	99	0	0	99
Klebsiella oxytoca	99	20	95	95	90	2	0	1	100	6	0	0	85	0	55	0	2	10	99	0	100	0	5	2	95	1	97	98	2	0	99	0	0	0	100
Enterobacter aerogenes	0	5	98	95	2	0	0	0	99	0	98	97	98	90	55	2	2	99	99	0	100	99	40	99	0	0	0	7	0	98	99	0	98	0	100
Enterobacter cloacae	0	5	100	100	65	0	0	97	96	96	0	95	98	93	15	2	1	15	100	0	99	92	25	97	0	1	1	98	0	90	99	50	7	0	99
Hafnia alvei	0	40	85	10	4	0	0	6	98	95	0	85	98	0	0	2	97	15	99	0	95	97	0	2	0	5	5	98	0	0	0	50	80	0	90
Serratia marcescens	1	20	98	98	15	0	0	0	99	0	99	97	99	90	0	2	0	99	99	0	99	0	40	0	99	2	0	7	0	0	0	98	98	95	0
Proteus mirabilis	2	97	50	65	98	98	98	0	0	0	90	95	0	91	2	97	15	0	1	0	0	1	0	0	0	1	98	0	50	80	1
Proteus vulgaris	98	95	0	15	95	95	98	0	0	0	90	95	0	85	15	2	15	0	0	0	5	1	0	0	0	5	95	0	80	0	5
Providencia rettgeri	99	93	0	95	98	98	0	0	0	0	0	94	10	0	100	5	100	1	1	5	70	5	100	10	5	0	0	10	1	5	5
Providencia stuartii	98	100	0	93	30	95	0	0	0	0	0	85	0	0	10	1	50	1	7	5	0	7	10	0	10	5
Providencia alcalifaciens	99	99	0	98	0	98	0	0	0	1	0	1	85	0	2	0	15	1	98	1	1	0	1	0	1	0	1
Morganella morganii	98	97	0	0	5	95	98	0	0	98	90	0	0	1	0	0	0	0	0	0	0	0	0	0	0	0	5
Yersinia enterocolitica	50	97	2	0	75	0	0	0	0	95	5	5	95	98	0	0	98	5	1	70	1	5	95
Yersinia pestis	0	80	0	0	5	0	0	0	0	0	0	0	0	97	0	0	50	100	0	1	90	20	1	0	50
Yersinia pseudotuberculosis	0	100	0	0	95	0	0	0	0	0	0	0	0	100	0	0	0	50	15	100	70	70	0	0	70

From Farmer, J.J. III, Davis, B.R., Hickman-Brenner, F.W., et al. 1985. Biochemical identification of the new species and biogroups of Enterobacteriaceae isolated from clinical specimens. J. Clin. Microbiol. 21:46.

*Each number gives the percentage of positive reactions after 2 days of incubation at 36° C. The vast majority of these positive reactions occur within 24 h. Reactions that become positive after 2 days are not considered.

†ONPG, orthonitrophenyl-beta-D-galactopyranoside.

on various selective and differential media commonly used for cultivation of Enterobacteriaceae are found in Chapter 8. Except for the most fastidious or biologically damaged strains, all Enterobacteriaceae will grow on Mac-Conkey agar, yielding pink or reddish colonies if they are able to ferment lactose, and colorless, translucent colonies if they are slow or nonlactose fermenters (Plate 27.2). Growth on MacConkey agar is one of the first criteria used to establish the identification of an unknown gram-negative bacillus. Except for a few *Bacillus* species and tiny pinpoint colonies of enterococci, staphylococci, and an occasional yeast, gram-positive organisms do not grow on MacConkey agar.

27.4.b. General phenotypic features shared by all or most Enterobacteriaceae. The Enterobacteriaceae are straight-sided gram-negative bacilli that grow well on most laboratory media. Many selective and differential media, as well as enrichment broths, have been developed for cultivation of selected Enterobacteriaceae from specific sites; these media were discussed in Chapters 8 and 17 and other appropriate chapters. The Enterobacteriaceae are facultative anaerobes—all will grow in air or anaerobically; CO_2 does not appreciably enhance growth. If they are motile, with the exception of *Tatumella ptyseos*, they possess peritrichous flagella. *T. ptyseos* has polar flagella. All species of *Klebsiella* and *Shigella* are nonmotile. Some species of *Escherichia*, *Salmonella*, and *Yersinia*, among clinically important Enterobacteriaceae, are nonmotile as well. Selected strains within other species may also be nonmotile. All Enterobacteriaceae ferment glucose and are oxidase negative, and almost all are able to reduce nitrates to nitrites. Performance of the nitrate test was outlined in Chapter 9. Except for one group of *Shigella* species and a species of *Xenorhabdus*, all Enterobacteriaceae are catalase positive. An additional clue to the identification of an unknown organism as an Enterobacteriaceae is luxuriant

growth on most routine media incubated at 35° C in air within 24 h. Colonies on blood agar are usually gray, shiny, entire, convex, and opaque. Hemolysis may be present. Strains of some *Proteus* species display a recognizable "swarming" pattern that resembles waves of growth spreading from the original inoculum (Figure 27.1) due to their active motility. Most Enterobacteriaceae will yield large (at least 1–2 mm diameter after 24 h) colonies on blood agar and MacConkey agar plates. A few strains of Enterobacteriaceae isolated from clinical specimens, however, may not grow well on MacConkey agar, especially if the organisms have been previously damaged by antibiotic treatment.

The first test that should be performed on a gram-negative bacillus isolated from clinical material is the oxidase test, as described in Chapter 9. The oxidase test must be performed with colonies growing on plates that do not contain dyes which may obscure the results. Plates yielding mixed cultures from clinical material may often contain colonies of more than one species of Enterobacteriaceae. If several colony morphologies can be differentiated only on MacConkey agar, each morphotype should

FIGURE 27.1
Appearance of swarming *Proteus* species on blood agar. Note successive waves of growth extending from a central inoculum.

be subcultured to a portion of a blood agar plate for performance of an oxidase test. Oxidase negative, luxuriantly growing, facultatively anaerobic bacilli (initially isolated aerobically, in most cases) are likely to be members of the Enterobacteriaceae. The ability to ferment glucose anaerobically is the next criterion to be met. Organisms are tested for glucose metabolism by inoculating portions of a colony to a Kligler's iron agar (KIA) or triple sugar iron agar (TSIA) slant. Fermentation is detected by a change in the indicator phenol red from red to yellow in the butt of the tube. Descriptions of inoculation and interpretation of KIA and TSIA are found in Chapter 9. The preliminary tests mentioned above will place the unknown

Alk/A gas	Alk/A no gas	A/A gas	Alk/A H₂S	A/A H₂S	Possible species
+	+	+	−	−	Escherichia coli Hafnia alvei
+	+	−	−	−	Morganella morganii Providencia alcalifaciens P. rettgeri P. stuartii Serratia sp.
+	−	+	−	−	Enterobacter aerogenes E. cloacae
+	−	+	+	+	Citrobacter sp.
+	+	−	+	−	Salmonella sp.
−	+	−	−	−	Shigella sp.
−	+	+	−	−	Yersinia sp.
−	−	+	−	−	Klebsiella sp.
−	−	−	+	+	Proteus mirabilis P. vulgaris
−	−	−	+	−	Edwardsiella tarda

*Some species show slight gas.

FIGURE 27.2
Chart showing basic reactions of Enterobacteriaceae on Kligler's iron agar.

organism into one of several categories, helping to determine which tests are necessary for further identification. Enterobacteriaceae are fermentative, oxidase negative, MacConkey positive bacilli. Those organisms that are grouped as nonfermentative gram-negative bacilli or other non-Enterobacteriaceae are further identified, as described in Chapters 28, 29, and 30. More rarely, isolates will fall into categories as described in Chapter 39. Initial reactions in KIA (or TSIA) agar can be used to guide identification of the 13 more commonly isolated genera of Enterobacteriaceae, as suggested in Figure 27.2.

Many laboratories no longer rely on KIA for initial testing of gram-negative bacilli, but instead inoculate a commercial identification system (Chapter 9) with an emulsion made from one isolated colony. Depending on the system, results are available within 4 h or after overnight incubation, at which time the oxidase reaction can be correlated with the biochemical reactions for definitive identification. Because these systems usually include a larger number of differential parameters than can be utilized cost-effectively as individual components, the identifications that result are more specific. The immense data bases used by the commercial systems, as discussed in Chapter 9, contribute to the detection of unusual and new biotypes.

There are a few basic biochemical parameters, however, that have classically been employed by microbiologists to categorize the Enterobacteriaceae (and other bacteria) into species groups. Even if laboratories are using commercial identification systems, with the exception of the totally automated instruments (such as Vitek and Abbott MS-2 or Avantage, outlined in Chapter 11), technologists can still observe visual changes in indicators that correlate to individual biochemical reactions. Technologists are urged to try to identify isolates based on manually observed biochemical patterns before the organisms are identified by comparing the numerical code generated by

the pattern of results with the company-furnished list of profile numbers and their related species identifications. Trying to identify species by recognizing their biochemical patterns is challenging and contributes to the continued maintenance of cognitive abilities.

Toward this end, the performance of some of the classical biochemical tests used to identify Enterobacteriaceae will be outlined in this chapter. These reactions are not only used to identify Enterobacteriaceae but are often necessary for identification of more fastidious, unusual, or relatively metabolically inactive microorganisms (not only bacteria) that cannot be identified with commercially available systems. A rudimentary flow chart that begins to differentiate commonly isolated Enterobacteriaceae on the basis of a few biochemical reactions is shown in **Figure 27.3**. Excellent commentaries on the biochemical bases of these tests and their performance are found in the *ASM Manual of Clinical Microbiology*,[4] Washington's laboratory manual,[7] and in the books by MacFaddin[5] and by Koneman, Allen, Dowell, and Sommers.[3] Media for performing these tests are all available from commercial suppliers, either already prepared or in dry powder form for in-house preparation. The results listed in Table 27.2 are based on conventional tests such as those described below. Results of individual tests performed as part of a miniaturized or automated biochemical identification system cannot be compared with the results obtained with conventional methods. Identifications that result from miniature systems are based on patterns generated from the entire system and not on results of individual tests.

27.4.c. Urease test. The ability of an organism to hydrolyze urea to ammonia and water, as described in Chapter 9, is determined classically by heavily inoculating a urea-containing agar slant (Christensen urea agar, available commercially) or a urea-containing, weakly buffered broth (Rustigian and Stuart urea broth, described in Chapter 45 and also available commercially). Organisms should be well

FIGURE 27.3
Flow chart for initial identification of Enterobacteriaceae based on basic biochemical reactions.

dispersed in broth for best results. The media are incubated at 37° C, preferably in a water bath or small incubator. Strongly urease positive organisms will begin to produce alkaline products, which turn the phenol red indicator red to purple within minutes. The heavier the inoculum, the more rapid the positive result. Tubes or broths should be examined at 10 min, 30 min, 1 h, and several hours after inoculation. Several suppliers (including Key Scientific Products, E-Y Laboratories, and Difco Laboratories) produce a rapid urease test reagent containing substrates impregnated on filter paper or in tablets, as mentioned in Chapter 9. Of particular utility for identification of *Proteus* and *Providencia* species are the filter paper disks produced by Remel Laboratories, which test for urease and phenylalanine deaminase. In addition to differentiation of Enterobacteriaceae, the classical urease test is also used to differentiate between certain *Brucella* species, to aid in identification of encapsulated yeasts, and as an additional test for identification of certain gram-negative coccobacilli.

27.4.d. Decarboxylation and dihydrolation of amino acids. Differentiation among many species of Enterobacteriaceae requires determining the ability of the organism to break down the amino acids **lysine, arginine,** and **ornithine,** forming an amine endproduct and CO_2. Lysine and ornithine are decarboxylated, whereas arginine is broken down first by dihydrolation and then by decarboxylation. The amine endproduct of these reactions is alkaline, causing a shift in the pH indicator bromcresol purple to purple (also discussed in Chapter 9). The ability to decarboxylate lysine is a prominent feature of most species of *Salmonella, Klebsiella, Enterobacter aerogenes, Hafnia alvei,* and *Serratia marcescens.*

Definitive tests for lysine and ornithine decarboxylases and arginine dihydrolase are carried out in broth media developed by Moeller, called **Moeller's decarboxylase medium** (also discussed in Chapter 9). Performance of the test entails inoculation of Moeller's medium, which contains glucose, bromcresol purple, a protein source, cresol red indicator, the enzyme activator pyridoxal, and the amino acid to be tested. In addition to tubes containing each amino acid, a control tube containing only the basal medium must be inoculated each time the test is performed, to ascertain that the organism does not form alkaline endproducts in the absence of an available amino acid. The tubes are inoculated with a small amount of growth from isolated colonies, being certain that the inoculum is emulsified in the broth below its surface. All tubes are overlayed with sterile mineral oil or vaspar to a depth of 1 cm to prevent introduction of oxygen. Tubes are incubated at 35°-37° C for up to 14 days, although results can usually be read in 4 days. A change in the color of the medium to purple indicates a positive test and the ability of the organism to utilize the amino acid to form alkaline endproducts (purple = positive). A yellow color indicates that only the glucose was utilized, with the formation of acid. The control tube, of course, should remain its original color (pale purple). A gray color may indicate reduction of the indicator, rather than alkaline endproducts. If the test is critical, the addition of more bromcresol purple solution (0.01% aqueous solution) to the broth below the seal may allow detection of a pH shift. Additional incubation of tubes displaying intermediate results after 4 days often allows interpretation of results later. Other bacteria in addition to those within the Enterobacteriaceae may be inoculated to Moeller's broths for detection of decarboxylase and dihydrolase enzymes. The test is particularly useful in the identification of viridans streptococci (Chapter 25) and some nonfermentative gram-negative bacilli (Chapter 28).

Lysine iron agar (LIA), a medium that detects hydrogen sulfide (H_2S) formation, lysine decarboxylation, and phenylalanine deamination (positive for *Proteus*, *Providencia*, and *Morganella*), is often used to differentiate H_2S-producing nonpathogens isolated on selective agar such as Hektoen and xylose-lysine-deoxycholate (XLD; Chapter 8) from etiologic agents of gastroenteritis. *Citrobacter* species, often confused with *Salmonella* on initial isolation, are lysine negative. LIA contains glucose, lysine, ferric ammonium citrate and sodium thiosulfate for H_2S detection, and bromcresol purple pH indicator. Organisms are inoculated in the same manner as for KIA, except that it is helpful to stab the butt of LIA several times to ensure an adequate inoculum. After 18 h incubation at 35° C with a **loose cap,** the tube is examined. The formation of a black precipitate in the butt is indicative of H_2S production. Organisms that are able to decarboxylate lysine (a reaction that takes place anaerobically in the butt), will produce alkaline endproducts that result in a purple color. Those bacteria that do not decarboxylate lysine will ferment the small amount of glucose, yielding acid byproducts and causing the bromcresol purple to turn the butt yellow. Even in the presence of a large amount of black precipitate, the yellow colored butt can be seen by observing the tube with light behind it. Deamination of phenylalanine is detected by a change in the color of the slant from purple to reddish. LIA is often used as a basic preliminary screening medium to detect fecal pathogens because it incorporates several parameters into one medium. With the exception of *Salmonella paratyphi A*, most of the salmonellae and *Edwardsiella tarda* are lysine decarboxylase positive.

27.4.e. Methyl red and Voges-Proskauer tests. Organisms that utilize glucose may do so by producing abundant acidic endproducts such as formate and acetate from the intermediate pyruvate metabolite, or they may metabolize the carbon compounds to acetoin and butanediol, which are more neutral in pH. The methyl red and Voges-Proskauer (MR and VP) tests detect the presence of the endproducts of these two divergent metabolic pathways. The same substrate broth, MR/VP broth, is used for both tests. Tubes of broth (5 ml per tube), containing peptones, glucose, and buffer, are avail-

PROCEDURE 27.1. METHYL RED AND VOGES-PROSKAUER TESTS

1. Prepare methyl red (MR) reagent as follows:

Methyl red (Mallinckrodt)	0.1 g
Ethyl alcohol (95%)	300 ml
Distilled water	200 ml

   Dissolve the methyl red in the alcohol before adding the distilled water. Store in a brown bottle in the refrigerator.

2. Prepare Voges-Proskauer (VP) reagent A as follows:

Alpha naphthol (Sigma Chemical Co.)	5 g
Ethyl alcohol (absolute)	100 ml

   Dissolve the alpha naphthol in a small amount of ethyl alcohol and bring the volume to 100 ml in a volumetric flask or cylinder. Store in a brown bottle in the refrigerator.

3. Prepare (VP) reagent B as follows:

Potassium hydroxide (KOH)	40 g
Distilled water	100 ml

   Weigh out the KOH very quickly, as it is hygroscopic and will become caustic when moist. Add less than 100 ml water to the pellets in a flask in a cold water bath to prevent overheating. Bring the volume to 100 ml in a volumetric flask or cylinder. Store this reagent in the refrigerator in a polyethylene bottle or one that has been specially treated for storage of caustic chemicals.

4. From a tube of inoculated MR/VP broth base that has been incubated for at least 48 h, remove 2.5 ml to another tube for the VP test.

5. To the 2.5 ml of organism suspension, add 0.6 ml (6 drops) of VP reagent A (alpha naphthol). Second, add 0.2 ml (2 drops) of VP reagent B (40% KOH). Gently shake the tube and allow it to sit for as long as 15 min.

6. Observe for the formation of a pink to red color, indicating the presence of acetoin (acetylmethylcarbinol). A pink color in the medium is indicative of a positive test. A negative test will appear colorless or yellow.

7. While the VP reaction is developing, the remaining 2.5 ml of substrate is tested for acidity by adding 0.5 ml (5 drops) of the methyl red reagent and observing the color. If the indicator remains red, the methyl red test result is positive. A change to yellow indicates that the pH of the medium is greater than 6.0, a negative MR test. If the reagent remains orange, the test must be repeated after a longer incubation period.

Modified from MacFaddin. 1980. Biochemical tests for identification of medical bacteria, ed. 2. Williams & Wilkins, Baltimore.

PROCEDURE 27.2. INDOLE TEST

1. Prepare Kovac's reagent as follows:

p-Dimethylaminobenzaldehyde (Sigma Chemical Co.)	10 g
Isoamyl or butyl alcohol (absolute)	150 ml
Concentrated hydrochloric acid	50 ml

   Dissolve the p-dimethylaminobenzaldehyde in the alcohol and slowly add the acid while constantly stirring the mixture. The reagent should be pale colored and should be stored refrigerated in a brown bottle. If it turns brown or if quality control organisms fail to give correct reactions, discard the reagent and make a fresh lot. The aldehyde may require gentle heating in order to go into solution.
2. Inoculate the organism to a broth that contains tryptophan and incubate for at least 24 h. Most commercial peptone, casein hydrolysate, or tryptone broths will contain enough tryptophan for use in this test.
3. To perform the test, remove 2 ml of the broth suspension to a second tube. Add 0.5 ml (5 drops) of the Kovac's reagent to the broth. Gently shake the tube and observe for a pink color in a ring around the interface between the broth and the alcoholic reagent, which rises to the surface (Plate 27.3).
4. If the test is negative, the remaining broth may be reincubated for an additional 24 h and the test may be repeated.

able commercially or can be prepared in the laboratory from powder base. The organism is inoculated below the surface of the medium in the tube, and the tube is incubated with a loose cap at 35°-37° C for at least 48 h. A longer incubation period may be necessary, especially for the demonstration of a positive VP reaction. To perform the test, the substrate broth is divided into two equal aliquots, one of which is used for the MR test and the other for the VP test (Procedure 27.1). The subtle nature of this reaction demands that all reagents and substrates are controlled. Quality control strains, such as E. coli (MR positive, VP negative) and Klebsiella pneumoniae (MR negative, VP positive), must be used to test each batch of reagents and media prepared before they are used, as discussed in Chapter 3. As for all of the tests described in this section, the MR/VP test is sometimes used in the identification of organisms other than Enterobacteriaceae.

27.4.f. Indole test. The ability of an organism to degrade the amino acid tryptophan can be detected by testing for the product of tryptophan deamination, indole. Reaction of indole with an aldehyde will result in a colored end-product. The rapid indole test described in Chapter 9 is performed with dimethylaminocinnamaldehyde reagent, which turns blue or blue-green in the presence of indole. The classic test described here (Procedure 27.2) calls for p-dimethylaminobenzaldehyde as the indicator substrate. Quality control organisms as listed in Chapter 3 are used to test each batch of media and reagents. When the indole test is used to test bacteria other than Enterobacteriaceae, the more sensitive Ehrlich's reagent (described in Chapter 28) should be used to detect indole.

27.4.g. Citrate utilization test. Certain organisms are able to utilize a single substrate as a sole carbon source. The ability to use citrate can be used to differentiate among members of the Enterobacteriaceae. The medium, Simmons' citrate agar, contains buffers, salts, cations, citrate, and bromthymol blue as the pH indicator. The medium can be purchased prepared or as dry powder. Since the reaction requires oxygen, the organism is inoculated to the surface of an agar slant of the medium. A very light inoculum (usually picked with a straight wire) is necessary to prevent false positive reactions due to carryover of substrates from previous media. The tube is incubated for 24 h or up to 4 days at 35°-37° C with a **loose cap.** Growth of the organism on the slant, with reversion of the color indicator from green to blue or turquoise blue (Plate 27.4) is evidence of a positive test, indicating that the organism was able to grow and produce acetate and other alkaline carbonate endproducts. There may be a rare citrate positive organism that can utilize the substrate without producing enough alkaline reaction to change the pH indicator. Luxuriant growth on the slant without a blue color may indicate a positive test, but the test should be repeated with a minimal inoculum.

27.4.h. Motility test. Another important differential test among Enterobacteriaceae and many other bacteria is motility. The fastest and most direct method to detect motility is to microscopically examine a wet preparation of the organism from the initial isolation plates or broth incubated at room temperature for 2-4 h under oil immersion (1,000 ×), as described in Chapter 7. After the organisms have settled, the directed and purposeful movement of a single bacterium or several bacteria, as opposed to the flowing movement of all bacteria within a field, is indicative of motility. Motility must be distinguished from Brownian motion, which usually involves all visible organisms equally.

Motility can be encouraged by growing bacteria in semisolid media. Good commercial motility semisolid media are available from Difco Laboratories and BBL Microbiology Systems, as well as from other commercial media suppliers. The media are prepared as butt tubes with a depth of 5 cm or greater. The organism is inoculated by stabbing a straight wire carrying the inoculum once vertically into the center of the agar butt to a depth of approximately 2 cm. After overnight incubation, motility will be evident as a haze of growth extending into the agar from the stab line. It is not recommended to include a colored growth indicator in motility medium, such as tetrazolium salts, since it may be inhibitory to some bacteria. Because a much larger sample of a bacterial population can be tested with the semisolid motility agar than can be visualized microscopically, these media are probably more sensitive for detection of motility. Solid and semisolid motility detection media are read after overnight incubation at the temperature preferred by the organism being tested. For example, *Yersinia enterocolitica* are motile at room temperature but not at 37° C. Organisms other than Enterobacteriaceae for which semisolid motility media are commonly used include *Listeria monocytogenes* and nonfermentative gram-negative bacilli.

27.4.i. Phenylalanine deaminase test. Of the well-characterized Enterobacteriaceae, only *Enterobacter agglomerans, Enterobacter sakazakii, Morganella* species, *Proteus* species, *Providencia* species, *Rhanella aquatilis,* and *Tatumella ptyseos* are able to deaminate the amino acid phenylalanine. The organism to be tested is grown overnight on an agar slant containing phenylalanine, salts, yeast extract, and buffers. Phenylalanine agar is available prepared or in dry powder form. The product of phenylalanine deamination, phenylpyruvic acid, is detected by a colored endproduct that forms when phenylpyruvic acid combines with ferric chloride solution. Procedure 27.3 describes performance of the test. As listed in Chapter 3, appropriate quality control organisms should be tested regularly with the medium and reagents.

27.4.j. Substrate fermentation tests. A large proportion of the tests used to differen-

PROCEDURE 27.3. PHENYLALANINE DEAMINASE TEST

1. Prepare ferric chloride reagent as follows:

Ferric chloride ($FeCl_3$) (Sigma Chemical Co.)	12 g
Distilled water	94.6 ml
Concentrated HCl (37%)	5.4 ml

   Dissolve $FeCl_3$ in water and slowly add the hydrochloric acid while working under a fume hood. Store the reagent in a brown bottle in the refrigerator.

2. After overnight incubation of the test organism on an agar slant containing phenylalanine, add 0.5 ml (5 drops) of the reagent to the growth on the surface of the slant and gently rotate the tube so that the reagent covers the entire surface. Observe for an immediate development of a green color, indicating the presence of phenylpyruvic acid and a positive test result. Certain species may deaminate phenylalanine so rapidly that the test will be positive within 4 h of incubation. Within 10 min, the color will fade, so observation must take place immediately after the reagent has been added.

Modified from MacFaddin. 1980. Biochemical tests for identification of medical bacteria, ed. 2. Williams & Wilkins, Baltimore.

tiate among members of the Enterobacteriaceae (as well as among other microorganisms) determine the ability of the organism to utilize a carbohydrate with the production of acid metabolic endproducts. In addition to detecting acid, carbohydrate fermentation media can be modified to detect the formation of gas by placing a very small, inverted glass tube (called a **Durham** tube) into the broth. If gas is produced during fermentation of the carbohydrate, it will be collected in the inverted tube and will be visible as a bubble (Plate 27.5). Most Enterobacteriaceae produce gas during glucose fermentation, but *Shigella, Salmonella typhi, Providencia stuartii*, most *Yersinia* species, and certain *E. coli* species do not produce gas (called **anaerogenic**). The carbohydrates are usually prepared as individual aqueous solutions and filter sterilized to prevent their destruction by the heat of the autoclave. The heart infusion or other broth base containing a pH indicator, which may be 0.0018% (wt/vol)

phenol red, 1% Andrade's acid fuchsin, or 0.0016% (wt/vol) bromcresol purple (originally dissolved in 95% ethanol, 1.6 g/100 ml ethanol), is made up, autoclaved, and allowed to cool before the sterile carbohydrate solutions are aseptically added to a final concentration of 1% carbohydrate. For most applications, bromcresol purple yields satisfactory and consistent results. A variety of sugars, including lactose, sucrose, maltose, glucose, and others, and a variety of alcohols, including mannitol, erythritol, dulcitol, and others, can be added to carbohydrate broth base for fermentation tests. All generally used carbohydrate broths are available commercially from several media suppliers.

27.4.k. ONPG test. Enterobacteriaceae are preliminarily grouped according to their ability to ferment lactose. *Salmonella, Shigella, Proteus, Providencia*, and *Morganella* are usually considered to be nonlactose fermenters. Other organisms, including certain *E. coli, Shigella*

PROCEDURE 27.4. ONPG (O-NITROPHENYL-BETA-GALACTOPYRANOSIDE) TEST FOR BETA-GALACTOSIDASE

1. Prepare peptone water as follows:

Peptone (Difco)	1 g
NaCl	0.5 g
Distilled water	100 ml

   Autoclave at 121° C for 15 min.

2. Prepare sodium phosphate buffer as follows:

Na_2HPO_4	13.8 g
Distilled water	90 ml

   Add the sodium phosphate to the distilled water in a 100 ml volumetric flask. Dissolve it by warming at 37° C. Slowly add approximately 15 ml of 5 N NaOH (or approximately 6 g) until the pH stabilizes at 7.0. Bring the volume to 100 ml with distilled water. Because of its causticity, NaOH should be handled carefully, and manipulations should be performed in a fume hood.

3. Prepare ONPG solution as follows:

ONPG (Sigma)	0.6 g
Sodium phosphate buffer (step 2)	100 ml

   Add the ONPG to the buffer, sterilize this by filtration, and store solution in a sterile brown glass bottle, refrigerated at 4°-10° C.

4. Prepare ONPG broth as follows:

   Aseptically add 25 ml of ONPG solution to 75 ml peptone water. Aseptically dispense this solution into sterile 13 × 100 mm plastic snap capped tubes, 0.5 ml per tube. Store refrigerated for 1 month or frozen at −20° C for up to 6 months. If the solution appears yellow, discard it.

5. Inoculate one tube of ONPG broth with a heavy suspension of the organism to be tested (taken from a KIA or TSIA slant or from the surface of a fresh subculture plate). Control organisms, such as *Escherichia coli* and *Proteus mirabilis*, should be inoculated to separate tubes at the same time. Incubate the tubes for a minimum of 1 h (preferably overnight) at 37° C.

6. Examine tubes for color change. A change to yellow indicates a positive result (presence of beta-galactosidase), and no color change indicates a negative result (absence of the enzyme). The *E. coli* should be positive, and the *Proteus* sp. should be negative. If the test organism has not changed color after 1 h incubation, incubation should be continued for additional time up to the full 24 h. Tubes may be checked at hourly intervals. If the organism produces yellow pigment, the test cannot be performed, and the longer test for utilization of lactose must be substituted.

Modified from MacFaddin. 1980. Biochemical tests for identification of medical bacteria, ed. 2. Williams & Wilkins, Baltimore; and from Hendrickson. 1985. Reagents and stains. In Lennette, Balows, Hausler, and Shadomy, editors. Manual of clinical microbiology, ed. 4. American Society for Microbiology, Washington, D.C.

sonnei, Hafnia alvei, Serratia marcescens, and some *Yersinia* species, may appear to be non-lactose fermenters because they lack the enzyme (permease) that actively transports lactose across the cell membrane, making it available to intracellular beta-galactosidase. True nonlactose fermenters do not possess beta-galactosidase. If beta-galactosidase but not permease is produced by a species, strains will eventually be able to ferment lactose that slowly diffuses across the cell membrane, although this process may be too slow to detect with carbohydrate fermentation broths. A rapid test for the presence of beta-galactosidase is the ONPG test (Procedure 27.4). Beta-galactosidase acts on the substrate orthonitrophenyl-beta-D-galactopyranoside (**ONPG**) in the same way as the enzyme hydrolyzes lactose to form galactose and glucose, although the endproduct of ONPG hydrolysis is a visible (yellow) product, orthonitrophenol. The ONPG test is actually a rapid method for determining whether an organism has the capability of utilizing lactose. Organisms other than Enterobacteriaceae, including *Neisseria* and streptococci, can also be differentiated with the ONPG test. Because the reagents are difficult to prepare, we recommend that laboratories purchase ONPG-impregnated filter paper disks from Difco Laboratories or Remel Laboratories or the tablets produced by Key Scientific Products. To perform the tests, an **extremely heavy** inoculum of the organism to be tested is emulsified in a small volume of buffer and the reagents are eluted from the disk or tablet into the liquid. After several hours of incubation, a yellow color is indicative of hydrolysis of the substrate by beta-galactosidase, or a positive test. The medium remains colorless when the test is negative. Manufacturers' recommendations and strict quality control practices should be followed.

27.4.l. Gelatin hydrolysis test. Enzymes that degrade proteins, often important virulence factors, are produced by relatively few members of the Enterobacteriaceae. *Serratia, Proteus, Xenorhabdus,* and several of the unnamed groups produce proteinases. Gelatinase production can be detected by observing whether an organism can remove the gelatin coating from exposed x-ray film. A small piece of exposed but not developed x-ray film (obtained from the hospital radiology department) is dropped into a tube containing a very heavy suspension of the organism in tryptic soy or other nutrient broth. After 1-48 h of incubation, the film is observed for removal of the gelatin layer, leaving behind the pale blue clear plastic film. A commercially purchased gelatin broth medium may also be used. Duplicate tubes of media are inoculated with the culture. One tube is incubated at 37° C, and the other is incubated at room temperature. At the same time, an uninoculated tube is incubated at 37° C to serve as a control. All media will be liquid at incubator temperatures. After sufficient growth (which may take as long as 30 days) the tubes are placed in the refrigerator for 30 min, or until the uninoculated control tube resolidifies. If the test organism made gelatinase, either one or both of the inoculated tubes will remain liquid, indicating breakdown of the gelatin present in the medium. A positive control should always be tested with each assay. The gelatinase test is also used in identification schemes for many other organisms in addition to Enterobacteriaceae.

27.4.m. DNase test. Extracellular nucleases are produced primarily by the same species that produce the protease gelatinase. The detection of these enzymes is most sensitive at room temperature. Tests for DNase detection were outlined in Chapter 9. Commercially produced agars, either prepared as plates or as slants, are available from several sources, as are dry powder media. In addition to toluidine blue O agar, described in Chapters 9 and 24, other agar formulas are available commercially (Plate 27.6).

27.5. Serologic Characterization of Enterobacteriaceae

27.5.a. General antigenic features of Enterobacteriaceae. In addition to biochemical and morphologic features, the Enterobacteriaceae can also be differentiated serologically, based on their possession of at least three classes of antigenic determinants. The cell wall structure of a typical Enterobacteriaceae was illustrated in Chapter 14 (Figure 14.2). Not all species have been antigenically characterized yet, but those that have been intensely studied include *E. coli*, *Klebsiella*, *Shigella*, and most extensively, *Salmonella*. The first category of antigens is associated with the lipopolysaccharide, or endotoxin moiety of the cell wall, called **O** antigens or **somatic (body)** antigens. These antigens are heat stable. Among *E. coli*, certain O antigens are associated with specific virulent phenotypes, such that *E. coli* 0111 and 0125, for example, are often found as etiologic agents of infantile diarrhea, and *E. coli* 0112 is often an invasive strain that causes a dysentery-like syndrome. *Shigella* species have classically been grouped according to O serotypes. Since the *Shigella* have now been shown to be identical to *Escherichia* by DNA hybridization studies, no new serotypes will be added. For the convenience of clinicians and microbiologists, the name *Shigella* will continue to be used for those organisms that can be distinguished biochemically from the *E. coli* group (Table 27.2). Classically, the serotypes of *Shigella* correspond to species as follows: *S. dysenteriae*, serotype A; *S. flexneri*, serotype B; *S. boydii*, serotype C; and *S. sonnei*, serotype D.

The second category of antigens are the capsular polysaccharide antigens, called **K** antigens. These antigens are heat labile, and they are known to be produced by organisms that include *Klebsiella*, *Salmonella*, and *E. coli*. The K antigens of some strains of *Salmonella* are called **Vi** antigens. Certain *Citrobacter* species may also possess Vi antigens, although they can

be differentiated from the salmonellae biochemically. The presence of capsular antigens may inhibit the ability of antiserum to detect the underlying O antigen. By heating the organism suspension to boiling for 30 min or longer (described below), technologists may be able to detect the masked O antigens. Nomenclature for *E. coli* antigens associated with virulence became confused when certain antigens, important to adherence of the organisms to intestinal epithelium, were named K antigens before their composition was known. These antigens, called K88 and K99, are now known to be protein, analogous to fimbriae; they are not capsular polysaccharide and should not be called "K." Under new classification schemes, fimbriae-associated K antigens have been renamed as F antigens.

The third category of antigens possessed by Enterobacteriaceae are flagellar, or **H** antigens. These antigens are protein in nature and heat labile. *Salmonella* species often will produce two different antigenic types of flagella, or H antigens, called **phase 1** and **phase 2.** Obviously, only motile strains will display H antigens, but certain salmonellae may express only one of their two phases of antigens at a given time. These strains can be encouraged to express the second phase of their H antigens by cultivation in special media.

27.5.b. Serological characterization of *Salmonella* species. *Salmonella* species of epidemiologic importance are characterized according to their O and H antigens in a scheme called the **Kauffmann-White scheme.** There are many more than 2,000 different serovars of *Salmonella*, based on the combined O, Vi, and H antigens that each serovar expresses. Most human pathogens are found in subgenus I (species I, Table 27.1, which can be differentiated biochemically from the other species). In addition to their serotypes, the salmonellae are also named. The names usually represent the town in which they were first isolated or some other factor with which they are associated. For practical purposes, these organisms will be treated as if the name is a species; e.g., *Salmonella* subgroup I 1,4,5,12:i:1,2, representing the O:phase 1:phase 2 antigens, will be called *Salmonella typhimurium*. Serotyping of isolates of Enterobacteriaceae is important for epidemiologic purposes (Chapter 5). The unabridged list of all currently accepted serovars can be found in *Bergey's Manual of Systematic Bacteriology*. Clinical laboratories often perform a very abbreviated preliminary serologic grouping on isolates of *Salmonella*, using commercially available polyvalent antisera designated A, B, C_1, C_2, D, E, F, G, H, and Vi. Some of the more common etiologic agents of gastrointestinal disease and enteric fever can be classified by their agglutination in antisera belonging to one of the pools. For example, *S. paratyphi* A is agglutinated by antiserum A, *S. typhimurium* is agglutinated by antiserum B, and *S. typhi* is agglutinated by antiserum D. The slide agglutination test is performed as described in Chapter 12. A suspension of the organism in physiologic saline must be tested for autoagglutination before antiserum is added. As mentioned above, those biochemically suspicious organism isolates that fail to agglutinate in the polyvalent antisera should be boiled by placing a heavy suspension of the organisms, in 0.5 ml sterile physiologic saline in a small screw-capped glass tube, into a beaker of boiling water for 15-30 min. Some isolates may require prolonged (up to 1 h) boiling. After cooling, the suspension is retested for specific agglutination. All isolates that biochemically resemble *Salmonella* but fail to agglutinate in any typing sera should be sent to a reference laboratory for definitive identification. The widespread use of commercial biotyping systems with many parameters (discussed in Chapter 9) has allowed almost every laboratory, no matter how small, to definitively identify (by biotype) isolates that resemble stool pathogens recovered from patients with gastroenteritis. It is important to notify both the physician caring for the patient and public health workers (or the hospital epidemiologist) so that the patient may be appropriately isolated if he or she is in the hospital, or so that the patient may be instructed as to hygienic practices if at home, to prevent spread of the disease.

27.6. Treatment of Infections Caused by Enterobacteriaceae

The great diversity among species of Enterobacteriaceae, as well as their propensity to indiscriminately pass genetic elements containing resistance factors among each other, makes it difficult to make specific statements about antimicrobial resistance. Multiple resistance is common among hospital strains of Enterobacteriaceae, those most involved in serious nosocomial infections. A few generalizations can be made, however. Several genera of Enterobacteriaceae display patterns of resistance that aid in their identification. Technologists can check the biochemically derived identification with the known susceptibility pattern as a form of quality assurance. *Klebsiella pneumoniae* and *Citrobacter diversus* are resistant to ampicillin and carbenicillin; most *Enterobacter* species and *Hafnia* are resistant to ampicillin and cephalothin, although newer cephalosporins are more active against *Enterobacter*. Swarming *Proteus* species are usually resistant to nitrofurantoin, and *Proteus* and *Morganella* are resistant to colistin. *Providencia* and *Serratia* are multiply resistant, and *E. coli* (particularly community-acquired strains), in contrast, are often susceptible to all antibiotics tested. Treatment of nosocomial infections associated with any of the Enterobacteriaceae usually consists of an aminoglycoside, alone or in combination with another agent such as a beta lactam. Some of the newer agents, such as cefoperazone, ceftazidime, or mezlocillin, may be effective against *Proteus*, *Citrobacter*, *E. coli*, and *Klebsiella*. For nosocomially acquired infections, the best policy is to start empiric therapy based on the prevailing susceptibility patterns for known isolates in the institution, changing therapy if results of in vitro susceptibility tests indicate the necessity for change. For this reason, it is very important that the laboratory have available statistics concerning the percentage of susceptible isolates, categorized by species and antimicrobial agent. These statistics should be distributed to all clinicians and updated regularly. In the case of seriously ill patients, the best agents should be used in combination until data are available regarding the specific susceptibility pattern of the etiologic agent in question.

Treatment of Enterobacteriaceae-associated gastroenteritis varies with the severity of disease. Many infections, particularly with *Salmonella*, are self-limiting and should not be treated. Treatment may encourage development of the carrier state. If treatment is warranted, ampicillin or trimethoprim-sulfamethoxazole is the drug of choice. Chloramphenicol may be necessary for life-threatening illness. Susceptibility tests are important, however, since ampicillin and multiply-resistant strains of *Salmonella* are being reported more frequently. *Shigella* are usually ampicillin resistant. Trimethoprim-sulfamethoxazole and furazolidone may be useful agents for treatment of bacillary dysentery. *Yersinia* are susceptible to chloramphenicol, aminoglycosides, tetracycline, and trimethoprim-sulfamethoxazole. *Yersinia enterocolitica* and *Y. pseudotuberculosis* septicemia have high fatality rates despite therapy; these syndromes require aggressive treatment with an aminoglycoside, ampicillin, or both. As stated previously, tetracycline or streptomycin is the preferred agent for treatment of plague. For severe disease, chloramphenicol can be added.

REFERENCES

1. Brenner, D.J. 1984. Enterobacteriaceae Rahn 1937. In Krieg, N.R., and Holt, J.G., editors: Bergey's manual of systematic bacteriology, ed. 9. Williams & Wilkins, Baltimore.
2. Farmer, J.J. III, Davis, B.R., Hickman-Brenner, F.W., et al. 1985. Biochemical identification of the new species and biogroups of Enterobacteriaceae isolated from clinical specimens. J. Clin. Microbiol. **21**:46.
3. Koneman, E.W., Allen, S.D., Dowell, V.R. Jr., and Sommers, H.M. 1983. Color atlas and textbook of diagnostic microbiology. J.B. Lippincott Co., Philadelphia.
4. Lennette, E.H., Balows, A., Hausler, W.J. Jr., and Shadomy, H.J., editors. 1985. Manual of clinical microbiology, ed. 4. American Society for Microbiology, Washington, D.C.
5. MacFaddin, J.F. 1980. Biochemical tests for identification of medical bacteria, ed. 2. Williams & Wilkins, Baltimore.
6. Russell, R.L., and Henke, R.P. 1983. An update on the taxonomy and clinical significance of the family Enterobacteriaceae. Check Sample Microbiology **26**:1. American Society of Clinical Pathologists.
7. Washington, J.A. II, editor. 1985. Laboratory procedures in clinical microbiology, ed. 2. Springer-Verlag, New York.

BIBLIOGRAPHY

Boyce, J.M. 1985. *Yersinia* species. In Mandell, G.L., Douglas, R.G. Jr., and Bennett, J.E., editors. Principles and practice of infectious diseases, ed. 2. John Wiley & Sons, New York.

Centers for Disease Control. 1983. Annual summary 1982: reported morbidity and mortality in the United States. M.M.W.R. **31**:1.

Farmer, J.J. III., Brenner, D.J., and Morris, G.K. 1984. The *Salmonella-Arizona* group of Enterobacteriaceae: nomenclature, classification, and reporting. Clin. Microbiol. Newsletter **6**:63.

Hickman-Brenner, F.W., Vohra, M.P., Huntley-Carter, G.P., et al. 1985. *Leminorella*, a new genus of Enterobacteriaceae: identification of *Leminorella grimontii* sp. nov. and *Leminorella richardii* sp. nov. found in clinical specimens. J. Clin. Microbiol. **21**:234.

Silverblatt, F.J., and Weinstein, R. 1985. Enterobacteriaceae. In Mandell, G.L., Douglas, R.G. Jr., and Bennett, J.E., editors: Principles and practice of infectious diseases, ed. 2. John Wiley & Sons, New York.

28 Nonfermentative Gram-Negative Bacilli and Coccobacilli

The nonfermentative gram-negative bacilli are found in nature as inhabitants of soil and water and as harmless parasites on the mucous membranes of humans and animals. These bacteria can cause disease by colonizing and subsequently infecting immunocompromised individuals or by gaining access to normally sterile body sites through trauma. Less than one-fifth of all gram-negative bacilli isolated from clinical specimens received in a routine clinical microbiology laboratory are likely to be nonfermentative bacilli, and the predominant species among those strains is *Pseudomonas aeruginosa*. Of the nonfermentative strains received by the University of California at Los Angeles (UCLA) clinical laboratory in 1976, 66% were *P. aeruginosa*, as described by Pickett and Pedersen.[6] Although nonfermenters comprise a small percentage of the total isolates recovered, they generally require more effort for their identification because microbiologists are less familiar with these bacteria, which often require specialized tests. *Pseudomonas*, the second most common etiologic agent of nosocomial infections (after *Escherichia coli*) in many hospitals, will be discussed here. The other bacteria covered in this chapter include two of the five genera included in the family Neisseriaceae, *Moraxella* and *Acinetobacter*. Two other genera within that family, *Neisseria* and *Branhamella*, were covered in Chapter 26 because of their unique diplococcal morphology and because of the importance of the Neisseriae as etiologic agents of human disease. The fifth genus, *Kingella*, will be discussed in Chapter 29, since it is able to ferment glucose, a property shared by none of the bacteria discussed in this chapter. *Eikenella*, *Flavobacterium*, *Alcaligenes*, and *Agrobacterium* are also included in this chapter. The genus *Achromobacter*, formerly a valid taxon, has not been included in the *Approved Lists of Bacterial Names*, published in 1980.[9] Organisms that would have been called *"Achromobacter"* are included in the genus *Alcaligenes*. In addition to the bacteria covered in this chapter, there are several unnamed species, including Centers for Disease Control (CDC) Groups Ve-1, Ve-2, IVc-2, IVe, EO-1, and others (often similar to *Alcaligenes* or *Pseudomonas*) that have been recovered from clinical specimens but will not be mentioned further. The definitive identification of all of the various nonfermentative gram-negative bacilli that might be encountered in a clinical laboratory is beyond the scope of this text. Readers are referred to the excellent references by Gilardi,[1,2] Rubin, Granato, and Wasilauskas,[8] Pickett and Pedersen,[6] and King et al.[4] for detailed information and identification schemes.

28.1. Epidemiology and Pathogenesis of Infections Due to Nonfermenters

28.1.a. *Pseudomonas aeruginosa*.
The most frequently isolated nonfermentative bacillus found in clinical specimens, *P. aeruginosa*, has one of the broadest ranges of infectivity among all pathogenic microorganisms. This species can cause disease in plants, insects, fish, amphibians, reptiles, birds, and mammals. It is a significant cause of burn wound infections and nosocomial infections, and an unusual mucoid variant is almost universally found to colonize the respiratory tract of patients with cystic fibrosis (Chapters 16 and 23). A particularly destructive infection of the eye (keratitis and en-

dophthalmitis) is associated with *P. aeruginosa;* contact lens wearers are one group at increased risk for such infections. *P. aeruginosa* is the third most frequently isolated etiologic agent in hospital-acquired pneumonia (Chapter 23). The organisms are so well adapted to survival in harsh environments that they can exist on the minimal organic nutrients present in distilled water. Under-chlorinated water used to fill hot tubs was thought to be the vehicle of a widespread epidemic of *P. aeruginosa*–associated folliculitis that initially appeared across the United States during the late 1970s. Strains of *P. aeruginosa* have even been isolated from the disinfectant soap solutions used by nurses and physicians to wash their hands. When hospital environments are sampled, *P. aeruginosa* is found in drains, water faucets, sinks, cleaning solutions, medicines, and other sites, including the flowers in patients' rooms. It appears that the incidence of nosocomial infection associated with this organism is increasing.

Although *P. aeruginosa* possesses many possible virulence factors, it must be remembered that it is a significant human pathogen only in compromised patients. Those strains that cause pneumonia appear to possess fimbriae that mediate adherence to respiratory epithelial cells. The mucoid polysaccharide, particularly pronounced in strains isolated from patients with cystic fibrosis, seems to protect the bacteria from phagocytosis. The ability of *P. aeruginosa* strains to destroy tissue may be related to the production of a number of extracellular enzymes, including proteases, elastase, pigments that may inhibit growth of other bacteria (called **pyocins**), and hemolysins. In addition, virulent strains produce an exotoxin, called **exotoxin A,** which inhibits protein synthesis much as does the toxin of *Corynebacterium diphtheriae* (Chapters 16 and 33). Exotoxin A also seems to promote tissue destruction and aggravate the host's inflammatory response, further contributing to tissue damage. As do all other nonanaerobic gram-negative bacteria, *P. aeruginosa* possesses endotoxin.

28.1.b. Other pseudomonads. Other pseudomonads that have been isolated from human clinical sources include a number of species that are saprophytic inhabitants of the soil and water, infecting humans as opportunistic pathogens. The number of isolations of *P. cepacia* in association with *P. aeruginosa* in respiratory secretions from cystic fibrosis patients has recently increased dramatically. The presence of this organism seems to be associated with decreased pulmonary function. Many strains of *P. cepacia* produce protease and lipase, and a number of strains also produce biologically active endotoxin. Most of the other pseudomonads and many other nonfermenters are isolated more frequently from respiratory specimens from cystic fibrosis patients than from patients with other types of pneumonia. These patients are particularly at risk for pulmonary infection due to these agents.

There are at least 24 species of *Pseudomonas* that have been implicated as the etiologic agents of human disease. Many more species can be recovered from the environment, including soil, water, and plants. Most of these species probably do not possess any particular virulence properties but infect humans opportunistically.

Specific syndromes, however, can be attributed to *P. mallei*, the agent of **glanders,** and *P. pseudomallei*, the agent of **melioidosis,** both considered to be "true" pathogens. Glanders, a disease of horses and occasionally other animals such as goats, sheep, donkeys, and dogs, is transmitted to humans by contact with infected animals. The disease, rarely seen in the United States, may present as a systemic septicemic infection, a local suppurative infection with lymphadenopathy, acute pneumonia, or chronic disease. Melioidosis, found primarily among returning Vietnam veterans and Southeast Asian immigrants, is usually a pneumonia-like illness, although it may be a systemic, febrile illness or an acute or chronic suppurative infection. Although *P. pseudomallei* can be found in the soil, *P. mallei* has been isolated only from animals that are susceptible to infection with this agent. The etiologic *Pseudomonas* species can be recovered from blood, aspirated lesion material, or respiratory secretions from patients suffering from glanders or melioidosis. *P. pseudomallei* and *P. mallei* both produce extracellular toxins, and *P. mallei* has an endotoxin-like material that may contribute to pathogenesis.

28.1.c. *Acinetobacter, Agrobacterium, Alcaligenes,* and *Flavobacterium* species. These four genera of nonfermenters are found in soil and water. They infect humans when they have been introduced into a traumatic wound or by opportunistic colonization and infection of compromised hosts. In addition, *Acinetobacter* species have been isolated as the etiologic agent of pneumonia and urinary tract infections in healthy individuals. Although no definite virulence factors have been elucidated for these organisms, *Flavobacterium* species, in particular *F. meningosepticum*, is associated with outbreaks and sporadic cases of neonatal meningitis and septicemia. These bacteria must possess some mechanism such as neurotropism that allows them to produce such a syndrome. The flavobacteria also produce proteases and gelatinase, which may contribute to virulence.

28.1.d. *Eikenella* and *Moraxella* species. Both of these genera are normal inhabitants of human mucous membranes of the mouth and upper respiratory tract. From this site, they can cause disease in immunosuppressed hosts. As with the other nonfermenters, infection may follow deposition in normally sterile tissues. *E. corrodens* is a commonly recovered etiologic agent of human bite wound infections and is an important pathogen in many other types of infection on occasion. The virulence factors that contribute to pathogenesis of disease due to these nonfermentative bacteria are not well characterized.

28.2. Laboratory Identification

28.2.a. General considerations. Once it has been determined that a gram-negative bacillus isolated from clinical material is not a member of the Enterobacteriaceae by criteria listed in Chapter 27 (Enterobacteriaceae are oxidase negative, able to ferment glucose, as detected by production of a yellow butt in triple sugar iron agar [TSIA] or Kligler's iron agar [KIA], and grow well on MacConkey and other media) and that the isolate is not *Pseudomonas aeruginosa* (as detailed below), a set of preliminary tests must be performed to categorize the isolate so that it can be identified by the most expedient method. These tests include determining the ability of the organism to grow on MacConkey agar (Chapter 8), performing the oxidase reaction, and determining whether the organism is able to metabolize carbohydrates or the circumstances under which the organism produces acid from the carbohydrates glucose and maltose (Chapter 9). The ability of an isolate to utilize carbohydrates and whether it does so oxidatively (in the presence of air) or fermentatively (in the absence of air) or both is one of the most important characteristics needed to separate the nonfermenters from Enterobacteriaceae. It was first realized by Hugh and Leifson that organisms that were able to utilize carbohydrates only very minimally would produce tiny amounts of acid. In media containing large amounts of peptones and other protein sources, these organisms would utilize the peptones preferentially, producing enough alkaline endproducts to overshadow any pH indicator changes that might occur due to acid production. They developed a **low peptone** medium, called **oxidative-fermentative** medium (**O-F medium**), that would allow detection of acid production by weak metabolizers. Preparation, inoculation, and interpretation of O-F medium test results is described in Procedure 28.1.

Oxidative-fermentative reactions are interpreted as shown in Figure 28.1. Fermentation takes place in the medium without oxygen (the overlaid tubes). Organisms that are able to ferment a carbohydrate are also able to oxidize it (the open tubes). These organisms are still called "fermenters." Organisms that produce acid products and yellow reactions only in open tubes are "oxidizers," and organisms that do not utilize glucose, either fermentatively or oxidatively, are called "nonoxidizers." Some nonoxidizers may actually produce such a large volume of alkaline endproducts that the indicator turns blue; this is called an "alkaline" O-F result. O-F media may be purchased from most media manufacturers. Flow Laboratories produces a single tube that can be inoculated for determination of both oxidative and fermentative glucose utilization (Plate 28.1).

Based on their reaction in oxidative-fermentative (O-F) glucose, ability to grow on MacConkey agar, and oxidase reaction, all unusual non-Enterobacteriaceae may be placed preliminarily into a category requiring particular additional tests for identification (Figure 28.2). The ability of these organisms to utilize carbohydrates other than glucose is also usually tested in O-F medium; standard methods (Chapter 9) are used for performance of most of the other biochemical tests required to identify these organisms. Since indole production may be an important characteristic, a more sensitive method for extracting indole is often used for the nonfermenters (Procedure 28.2). For most other biochemical tests, methods discussed in previous chapters (particularly Chapters 9 and 27) are satisfactory. Key differential features of commonly recovered nonfermenters are discussed in this chapter (Table 28.1). Enterobacteriaceae were covered in Chapter 27. Other clinically significant gram-negative bacilli that grow on conventional media, other than the nonfermenters mentioned in this chapter, are discussed in Chapters 29, 30, and 39.

In addition to biochemical metabolism, another important taxonomic feature of organisms classified as nonfermenters is the arrangement

PROCEDURE 28.1. OXIDATIVE-FERMENTATIVE (O-F) TEST
FOR CARBOHYDRATE UTILIZATION

1. Prepare O-F base medium as follows:

Peptone or tryptone	2 g
Sodium chloride	5 g
Agar	2.5 g
Dipotassium phosphate	0.3 g
Bromthymol blue	0.03 g
Distilled waterg	1,000 ml

    Combine all ingredients, which are available from Difco Laboratories and standard chemical supply companies, or purchase O-F base from commercial suppliers of media (Appendix). Adjust pH to 7.1 and divide the solution into several smaller flasks with known volume, one flask for each carbohydrate being prepared. For example, if O-F glucose, maltose, sucrose, lactose, and mannitol are to be made, divide the O-F base into five flasks containing 200 ml each. Autoclave the flasks at 121° C for 15 min.

2. Prepare 10% aqueous carbohydrate solutions by adding 2 g carbohydrate (glucose, lactose, etc.) to 20 ml distilled water. Immediately sterilize the carbohydrate solutions by passing them through a 0.2 μm membrane filter. Autoclave sterilization will destroy some of the carbohydrates. These solutions can be refrigerated for several months, although they may require redissolving before use.

3. When the O-F base has cooled to 55° C after autoclaving, aseptically add 20 ml of the sterile 10% carbohydrate solution to the 200 ml flask of O-F base, for a final concentration of 1% carbohydrate. The correctly prepared medium is green, but it appears somewhat bluish while it is still hot.

4. Dispense the 1% carbohydrate O-F media into 16 × 125 mm screw cap test tubes, 5 ml per tube. Allow the tubes to solidify upright (forming a semisoft butt), tighten caps, and refrigerate. The medium should be usable for several months. If desired, the base can be dispensed without carbohydrates, which can then be added to melted and cooled tubes of base as needed (0.5 ml 10% carbohydrate to 5 ml base).

5. For testing the nature of glucose utilization, two tubes of 1% O-F glucose are inoculated. Material from isolated colonies is picked up with a straight wire and stabbed at least four times into each medium. Stabs should extend approximately 5 mm deep into the surface layer of the butt.

6. The medium in one of each of the two identical tubes is overlayed with sterile melted petrolatum or melted paraffin combined with an equal volume of petroleum jelly (called **vaspar**) approximately 1 cm deep to prevent oxygen from reaching the inoculum. Sterile mineral oil is not recommended for overlaying the medium, probably because some lots are acidic and can contribute to false positive results.

7. The tubes are incubated at 35° C for as long as 4 days and examined daily for production of acid, as indicated by a change in the bromthymol blue indicator from green to yellow.

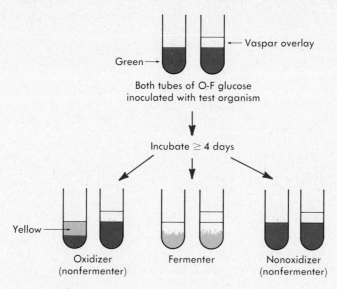

FIGURE 28.1
Interpretation of oxidative-fermentative (O-F) utilization of glucose test.

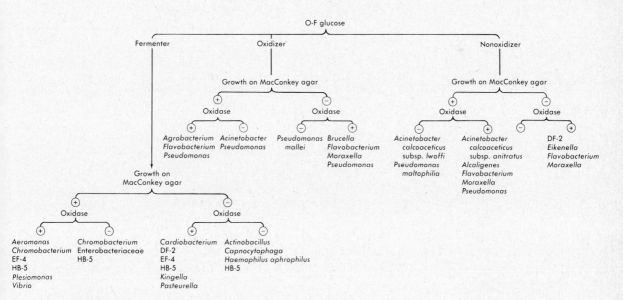

FIGURE 28.2
Initial characterization of gram-negative bacilli based on utilization of glucose in oxidative-fermentative (O-F) media, growth on MacConkey agar, and oxidase reaction.

PROCEDURE 28.2. XYLENE EXTRACTION FOR DEMONSTRATION OF INDOLE PRODUCTION

1. Prepare Ehrlich's reagent as follows:

   Paradimethylaminobenzaldehyde (Sigma Chemical Co.)　　　2 g
   Ethyl alcohol (95%)　　　190 ml
   Hydrochloric acid (concentrated)　　　40 ml
   Store refrigerated in a brown bottle.
2. Add 1 ml of xylene to a 48 h culture of organisms in tryptone or trypticase broth or other appropriate medium. Shake the tube well, and allow it to stand for a few minutes until the solvent rises to the surface.
3. Gently add about 0.5 ml of the reagent down the sides of the tube, so that it forms a ring between the medium and the solvent. If indole has been produced by the organisms, it will, being soluble in solvent, be concentrated in the solvent layer, and on addition of the reagent, a brilliant **red ring** will develop just below the solvent layer. If no indole is produced, no color will develop.

Modified from Bohme. 1906. Zentralbl. Bakt., Orig. 40:129.

TABLE 28.1
Key Characteristics of Nonfermentative and Slowly Fermentative Gram-Negative Bacilli

GENUS	OXIDASE	CATALASE	GLUCOSE OXIDIZER	INDOLE	MOTILITY	FLAGELLAR ARRANGEMENT	PIGMENT
Acinetobacter	−	+	+/−	−	Twitching	⊖	−
Agrobacterium	+	+	+	−	+	Peritrichous	−
Alcaligenes	+	+	−	−	+	Peritrichous	−
Eikenella	+	−	−	−	Twitching	⊖	−
Flavobacterium	+	+	+/−	+/−	−	⊖	Yellow
Kingella	+	−	+	+/−	Twitching	⊖	−
Moraxella	+	+	−	−	Twitching	⊖	−
Pseudomonas	+	+	+/−	−	+	Polar	Variable
Pasteurella	+	+	+	+*	−	⊖	−

+ = >90% strains positive; − = >90% strains negative; ⊖ = none; +/− = variable results.
*Some species do not produce indole.

of their flagella. Performance of a flagella stain is not easy; it is an art that must be developed with experience. Flagella are fragile and tend to break off from the surface of bacteria during manipulation. Many individual bacteria within a culture will not produce flagella, and the stain sometimes fails to work. Procedure 28.3 outlines a flagella stain that should yield excellent results if all of the steps are followed carefully.

28.2.b. Identification of *P. aeruginosa*. As noted earlier, by far the most commonly encountered nonfermenter is *P. aeruginosa*. These organisms can grow on most routine laboratory media, including MacConkey agar. On 5% sheep blood agar, colonies are flat with a

PROCEDURE 28.3. FLAGELLA STAIN

1. Prepare solution A as follows:

Basic fuchsin (certified for flagella stain; Aldrich Chemical Co.)	0.6 g
Ethyl alcohol (95%)	50 ml

   Add the fuchsin to the alcohol and allow to stir overnight on a magnetic stirring plate to dissolve the fuchsin.
2. Prepare solution B as follows:

Sodium chloride	0.37 g
Tannic acid (Sigma Chemical Co.)	0.75 g
Distilled water	50 ml

3. Combine solutions A and B and mix thoroughly. Adjust the pH to 5.0 with 1.0 N NaOH. Place the stain into a tightly capped brown bottle and let it remain for 3 days in the refrigerator (4° C) before using it, to allow it to cure. It is stable in the refrigerator for 1 month and in the freezer for at least 1 year. The stain deteriorates rapidly at room temperature. Use only the clear supernatant for the staining procedure; do not disturb the sediment that settles in the bottom of the bottle. Before performing each staining procedure, draw a small amount of the stain from the bottle and allow it to warm to room temperature. Discard the stain that is left over after the procedure.
4. Clean slides by soaking them in 3% concentrated hydrochloric acid in 95% ethanol for 4 days. Rinse thoroughly in tap water (by allowing tap water to run through the slides in a beaker for 10 min), and then rinse with several changes of distilled water. Lean the slides against an upright surface to drain and air dry.
5. Flame a clean slide in a gas burner. Enclose a rectangular area with a thick wax pencil line.
6. Place a large drop of distilled water at one end of the slide, within the wax-penciled area.
7. Pick up a small amount of growth from the tops of several young colonies on an agar plate or from a freshly inoculated slant on the end of an inoculating needle. Touch the needle to the drop of water on the slide in several places, allowing a small amount of the organism to disperse in the water. Tip the slide slightly to allow the drop of water to run toward the opposite end of the slide. Allow the suspension to air dry and do not heat fix before staining.
8. Apply 1 ml of the stain to the dry slide and observe the slide for the formation of a fine, metallic red precipitate (which will take 5-15 min).
9. Rinse the slide gently in tap water, holding the slide horizontal. Do not tilt to drain the water, and allow the slide to air dry.
10. Examine under oil immersion (1,000 ×) for flagella (Plate 28.2). It is possible that only a few of the bacteria in the suspension retained intact flagella; thorough examination is often required.

Modified from Clark. 1976. J. Clin. Microbiol. 3:632.

feathered edge, rough or "ground-glass" appearing, and beta hemolytic (Plate 28.3). Colonies can grow to 3-5 mm in diameter within 48 h incubation at 35°-37° C in air, and growth is equally good at room temperature. The mucoid (alginate-producing) strains isolated primarily from patients with cystic fibrosis may be blue-green or pale yellow-green, and they are extremely mucoid. This mucoid material may be produced in such quantities that it slides across the surface of the plate when the plate is tipped (Figure 28.3). *P. aeruginosa* exhibits a particularly striking characteristic odor, which resembles overripe grapes (or corn tortillas). Most strains of *P. aeruginosa* produce **pyocyanin,** a turquoise-blue or blue water-soluble and chloroform-extractable pigment, visible on uncolored media, such as Mueller-Hinton agar (Plate 28.4), and especially visible on *Pseudomonas* P agar (Difco Laboratories) and Tech agar (BBL Microbiology Systems). No other bacteria produce this pigment, so its detection is sufficient for identification of an isolate as *P. aeruginosa*. Some strains of *P. aeruginosa* produce other pigments, pyoverdins (yellow), pyorubin (red), and pyomelanin (brown), which may mask the pyocyanin. Such strains, which

appear yellow-green, blue-green, red, purple, or brown, must be further characterized. Occasional strains of *P. aeruginosa* fail to produce pyocyanin. These strains, however, are able to grow at 42° C, are able to dihydrolyze arginine, are motile by means of polar flagella, and are unable to produce acid in O-F lactose or sucrose. *P. aeruginosa* and other pseudomonads isolated from humans often produce water-soluble fluorescent pigments; pyoverdin is also one of these. Fluorescent-pigment-producing strains fluoresce under *short wave* ultraviolet light (Plate 28.5). A standard Woods' lamp emits light at 365 nm; the fluorescence of pseudomonads is best observed at 254 nm.

Several selective agars have been developed for isolation of *P. aeruginosa* from "contaminated" specimens, such as stool. It has been shown that development of nosocomial infection with *P. aeruginosa* is often preceded by gastrointestinal colonization; thus detection of colonized persons at risk of developing *Pseudomonas* infection may aid in prevention of subsequent morbidity. Agar containing **cetrimide** (cetrimethylammonium bromide), available as Pseudosel agar (BBL Microbiology Systems); **irgasan** (2,2,2-trichloro-2-hydroxydiphenyl ether), available as Irgasan agar (Difco Laboratories); and noncommercially available agar containing 30 μg/ml **C-390** (9-chloro-9-[diethylaminophenyl]-10-phenylacridan), available from Norwich-Eaton Pharmaceuticals (Norwich, N.Y.), have been used successfully, as reported by Robin and Janda.[7] Since C-390 inhibits the growth of all other bacteria, it may be used in an identification scheme. Isolates that are able to grow on trypticase soy agar containing 30 μg/ml C-390 can be presumptively identified as *P. aeruginosa*.

For practical purposes, isolates on blood agar that exhibit the characteristic colonial morphology and odor, that are beta hemolytic, and that are oxidase positive can be presumptively identified as *P. aeruginosa*. When the susceptibility pattern also agrees with that generally exhibited by *P. aeruginosa*, that of resis-

FIGURE 28.3
Abundant mucoid material produced by a strain of *Pseudomonas aeruginosa* isolated from a patient with cystic fibrosis.

tance to most antimicrobial agents except for aminoglycosides and colistin (polymyxin B), the identification is more assured. All *P. aeruginosa* strains are oxidase positive, motile by means of polar flagella, able to oxidize glucose in O-F carbohydrate base, unable to oxidize maltose, unable to decarboxylate lysine or ornithine (Chapters 9 and 27), and able to dihydrolyze arginine. As are all pseudomonads, they are catalase positive. In addition to growth on C-390, all *P. aeruginosa* are able to grow at 42° C, an ability shared by several of the other *Pseudomonas* species but none that produce fluorescent pigment. Fluorescent pigment may be enhanced by growth on *Pseudomonas* F agar (Difco Laboratories), GNF agar (Flow Laboratories), or Flo agar (BBL). In KIA or TSIA, *P. aeruginosa* yields an alkaline slant over a red or unchanged butt. Growth on the slant surface often appears metallic. Table 28.2 lists key characteristics used to differentiate some species of clinically important pseudomonads.

28.2.c. Identification of other *Pseudomonas* species. *P. maltophilia* is second to *P. aeruginosa* in frequency of isolation. As the name implies, this species is able to oxidize maltose as well as glucose. Because *P. maltophilia* lacks certain key traits of the genus *Pseudomonas* (*P. maltophilia* possesses multitrichous polar flagella and is usually oxidase negative), some workers have proposed moving it to the genus *Xanthomonas*, a group of yellow-pigment-producing plant pathogens. *Xanthomonas*, on the other hand, possesses a single polar flagellum, unlike *P. maltophilia*. The taxonomic status of *P. maltophilia* is uncertain at this time.

Colonies of *P. maltophilia* on blood agar are rough, lavender-green, and have an ammonia-like odor (Plate 28.6). They may be slightly alpha hemolytic. The organism is oxidase negative, arginine dihydrolase negative, ornithine decarboxylase negative, but lysine decarboxylase positive. It does not produce pyoverdin and, according to Palleroni,[5] it cannot grow at 42° C. *Pseudomonas maltophilia*, rare strains of *P. cepacia* and *P. paucimobilis*, and some

strains of *P. mallei* are the only oxidase negative pseudomonads named (several unnamed strains are oxidase negative).

The pseudomallei group includes organisms that grow on a wide variety of organic compounds as single sources of carbon and energy. Several species in the group are not human pathogens, but *P. pseudomallei*, *P. mallei*, *P. cepacia*, *P. pickettii*, and *P. gladioli* have been isolated from clinical specimens. *P. pseudomallei* grows slowly on blood agar, forming colonies that may be wrinkled at first, becoming umbonate with time (Plate 28.7). Colonies exhibit varying degrees of hemolysis. Growth is characterized by a putrid odor followed by an aromatic, pungent odor. The organisms possess multitrichous polar flagella and are able to grow at 42° C and on MacConkey agar. Of course, the clinical history of the patient is usually suggestive for melioidosis, which aids the microbiologist in identifying the etiologic agent.

P. mallei is the only nonmotile species in the genus *Pseudomonas*. This species, which may be suspected because of a clinical picture suggestive of glanders, is unable to grow at 42° C and may not grow on blood agar. Colonies on brain-heart infusion agar (with added glycerol) are grayish white and translucent after 48 h incubation, later becoming yellowish and opaque. A Gram stain will reveal coccal forms and occasional filaments and pleomorphic forms that may branch.

The third species in the pseudomallei group is *P. cepacia*. Next to *P. aeruginosa*, *P. cepacia* is the pseudomonad most commonly isolated from cystic fibrosis patients and is an important nosocomial pathogen. *P. cepacia* often produces diffusible pigments, appearing as yellow or yellow-green, rough, serrate-edged colonies. It does not fluoresce. Strains are motile and able to oxidize glucose, lactose, maltose, and mannitol. It is resistant to polymyxin B.

In addition to *P. aeruginosa*, there are two other species that may produce fluorescent pigments, *P. fluorescens* and *P. putida*. Whereas

TABLE 28.2
Some Characteristics of Commonly Encountered *Pseudomonas* Species (Given as Percent Positive Reactions)

SPECIES (NUMBER OF STRAINS)	OXIDASE	GROWTH AT 42°C	GAS FROM NITRATE	ACID IN O-F† GLUCOSE	ACID IN O-F LACTOSE	ACID IN O-F FRUCTOSE	LYSINE DECARBOXYLASE	ARGININE DIHYDROLASE	ORNITHINE DECARBOXYLASE	GELATIN HYDROLYSIS
*P. aeruginosa** (84)	100	100	61	98	0	89	0	100	0	50
P. maltophilia (527)	2	48	0	100	88	99	99	0	0	100
P. cepacia (201)	92	58	0	100	98	100	90	0	65	74
P. fluorescens (194)	100	0	5	100	12	99	0	99	0	100
P. putida (273)	100	0	0	100	14	99	0	99	0	0
P. stutzeri (168)	100	89	100	100	0	94	0	5	0	1
P. putrefaciens (72)	100	65	0	100	3	53	0	0	99	97
P. paucimobilis (110)	90	0	0	100	100	100	0	0	0	0
P. acidovorans (95)	100	10	0	0	0	100	0	0	0	2
P. alcaligenes (51)	100	59	16	0	0	0	0	10	0	2

Data from Gilardi, G.L. 1984. Identification of glucose-nonfermenting gram-negative bacilli. Clin. Microbiol. Newsletter 6:111, 127.
*Apyocyanogenic strains.
†O-F, oxidative-fermentative.

P. aeruginosa has one polar flagellum, these two species have polar tufts of flagella. Many strains grow best at 30° C, and none grow at 42° C. They are both resistant to carbenicillin. *P. stutzeri* is distinguished by production of yellow to tan, flat, dry, and wrinkled colonies that resemble those of *P. pseudomallei* (Plate 28.8). *P. putrefaciens* is the only nonfermenter known to produce hydrogen sulfide (H_2S) in the butt of a TSIA or KIA slant. For this reason, an isolate may be mistaken for an H_2S-producing Enterobacteriaceae unless the oxidase result is checked. *P. putrefaciens* is oxidase positive. A number of other pseudomonads have been isolated from clinical material, including *P. acidovorans*, *P. alcaligenes*, *P. diminuta*, *P. extorquens*, *P. marginata*, *P. mendocina*, *P. mesophilica*, *P. paucimobilis*, *P. pickettii*, *P. pseudoalcaligenes*, *P. testosteroni*, *P. thomasii*, and *P. vesicularis*. The reader is referred to references by Gilardi[1,2] and King et al.[4] for methods for definitive identification of these organisms. If a clinically significant isolate must be identified, it should be sent to an appropriate reference laboratory.

28.2.d. Genus *Alcaligenes* (including organisms formerly called *Achromobacter* species). The *Alcaligenes* species of clinical importance have been isolated from blood, respiratory secretions, infected wounds, urine, and several other sources. They are usually opportunistic pathogens, infecting patients with suppressed host defenses. According to Kersters and De Ley,[3] the genus *Alcaligenes* consists of two authentic species, *A. faecalis* and *A. denitrificans* (one subspecies of which was fomerly called *Achromobacter xylosoxidans*), and eight other species that have not been formally recognized. None of the eight unrecognized species has been isolated from human material. A species known to clinical microbiologists as *Alcaligenes odorans* has now been found to belong with the *A. faecalis* species. All *Alcaligenes* are oxidase positive and catalase positive, possess peritrichous flagella (which distinguishes them from

pseudomonads), and are able to utilize acetate as a sole source of carbon. On blood agar, the colonies are flat, spreading, and rough with a feathery edge. *Alcaligenes* does grow on MacConkey agar. *Alcaligenes faecalis* is biochemically quite inert, whereas *A. denitrificans* is nitrate positive. The strain of *A. faecalis* previously called *A. odorans* produces a distinctive sweet odor, reminiscent of fresh apple cider; colonies may be slightly alpha hemolytic on sheep blood agar. *A. denitrificans* subsp. *xylosoxidans* oxidizes glucose and xylose.

28.2.e. Genus *Acinetobacter*. Found as a major constituent of the flora of soil, water, and sewage and within the hospital environment, *Acinetobacter* is also found to colonize the skin of hospitalized patients. It is additionally involved in wound infections, particularly if there has been soil or water contamination of the wound. After *P. aeruginosa* and *P. maltophilia*, *A. calcoaceticus* var. *anitratus* is the most commonly isolated nonfermenter in clinical laboratories. It is possible that *Acinetobacter* species is actually normal flora of the skin and mucous membranes of humans. It has been implicated as an etiologic agent of pneumonia (both community and hospital acquired) and urinary tract infection. It may also be involved in sepsis and other infections. Colonies on blood agar are convex, gray to white, 2-3 mm in diameter, and variably hemolytic (Plate 28.9). Some strains produce a tan to yellow pigment. It is oxidase negative and catalase positive and may initially be confused with Enterobacteriaceae, since it resembles non-lactose-fermenting Enterobacteriaceae on MacConkey agar. It cannot, however, grow in the butt of a TSIA or KIA, and it cannot reduce nitrate. Differentiation from *P. maltophilia*, which is also oxidase negative, may be based on arginine dihydrolase and lysine and ornithine decarboxylase reactions. *Acinetobacter* cannot utilize any of the three amino acids in Moeller's decarboxylase media, whereas *P. maltophilia* is arginine dihydrolase and lysine and ornithine decarboxylase positive. Two variants of the one species, *A. calcoaceticus,* are clinically important. *Acinetobacter calcoaceticus* var. *anitratus* (formerly known as *Herellea vaginicola*) is able to oxidize glucose, xylose, and some other sugars in oxidative-fermentative (O-F) carbohydrate base; whereas *A. calcoaceticus* var. *lwoffi* (formerly known as *Mima polymorpha*) is inactive biochemically. On Gram stain, the cells of *Acinetobacter* are very plump, almost coccoid rods that tend to resist alcohol decolorization; they may be mistaken for *Neisseria* sp. Similar to most gram-negative bacilli but unlike other *Moraxella*-like organisms, *Acinetobacter* species are resistant to penicillin in vitro.

28.2.f. Genus *Moraxella*. Six species of *Moraxella* have been cultivated from human clinical material. All are normal flora of the mucous membranes of humans and other animals. They have been isolated as the etiologic agents of nosocomial infections, wound infections, pneumonia, and other types of opportunistic infections. *Moraxella* species are gram-negative coccobacilli, and in the case of *Moraxella (Branhamella) catarrhalis,* the cells are true cocci. For this reason and because all *Moraxella* are oxidase positive, *M. (B.) catarrhalis* will always be initially identified as a *Neisseria* species. The complete discussion of this organism has been included, therefore, in Chapter 26 with the *Neisseria* species, although *M. (B.)*

catarrhalis is, by DNA homology studies, a true subgenus of the genus *Moraxella.* The other five clinically relevant species in the genus *Moraxella* are *M. lacunata, M. nonliquefaciens, M. atlantae, M. phenylpyruvica,* and *M. osloensis.* These organisms are nonpigmented and are unable to utilize carbohydrates. The organisms are nonmotile and susceptible to penicillin. Most strains grow slowly on MacConkey agar, resembling nonlactose fermenting Enterobacteriaceae. *M. lacunata,* isolated most frequently from eye infections, fails to grow on MacConkey but may produce pitting of blood agar. The organism is able to liquefy serum, so that depressions are formed on the surface of Loeffler's serum agar slants (Chapter 45) due to digestion of the medium inoculated with strains of this species. Strains of *M. nonliquefaciens* may be very mucoid. *M. phenylpyruvica* is able to hydrolyze urea and deaminate phenylalanine. Other characteristics are shown in Table 28.3.

28.2.g. Genus *Eikenella*. *Eikenella corrodens,* the only species within the genus, is usually characterized by the ability to pit ("corrode") the agar. The organisms are found as normal flora in the human mouth and gastrointestinal tract, and they are common etiologic agents of human bite wounds and clenched fist wounds. They have also been isolated from cases of meningitis, endocarditis, aspiration

TABLE 28.3
Characteristics of *Moraxella* Species

	GROWTH ON MacCONKEY AGAR	UREASE	PHENYL-ALANINE DEAMINASE	NITRATE→ NITRITE	NITRITE→ GAS	SODIUM ACETATE UTILIZATION
M. atlantae	+/−	−	−	−	+/−	+/−
M. lacunata	−	−	+/−	+	ND	−
M. nonliquefaciens	−	−	−	+	ND	−
M. osloensis	+/−	−	+/−	+/−	−	+
M. phenylpyruvica	+/−	+	+	+/−	−	+/−
M. urethralis	+	−	+	−	+	+/−

+, ≥90% positive; −, ≥90% negative; +/−, variable results; ND, not done.

pneumonia, osteomyelitis, brain and intraabdominal abscess, and periodontitis. Because some isolates will initially grow only anaerobically, the organism was first thought to be an anaerobe and named "*Bacteroides corrodens.*" An obligately anaerobic organism that greatly resembles *Eikenella* has been named *Bacteroides corrodens* and later *Bacteroides ureolyticus;* further taxonomic changes are discussed in Chapter 36. *Eikenella* is facultatively anaerobic. *E. corrodens* is oxidase positive but is unable to utilize carbohydrates. It is catalase, urease, indole, and arginine dihydrolase negative, but lysine decarboxylase and nitrate positive. Blood is required for growth, and chocolate agar is the most supportive medium. Colonies are yellowish, opaque, and consist of three distinct zones of growth: a moist, shiny central zone; a refractile circle of growth with a pearly sheen, resembling a mercury drop; and an outer flat, rougher spreading zone. The colonies are quite tiny, however, and because they often are sunk into small craters in the agar (pitting), they must be viewed under magnification. The colonies produce a bleachlike odor. In broth, the organisms grow in discrete granules, often adherent to the sides of the tube. Noncorroding colonies may also be seen, either as morphologic variants among the initial colonies of an isolate or as a homogeneous strain. Fresh isolates require hemin for growth. Gram stains reveal a small, even, straight-sided gram-negative bacillus. Because they are so resistant to clindamycin, a clindamycin-impregnated filter paper disk (5 μg clindamycin) may be used to help isolate the organism in mixed culture.

28.2.h. Genus *Flavobacterium.* So named because of their typical yellow pigment (Plate 28.10), the flavobacteria are ubiquitous inhabitants of soil and water, and have been found in food as well as from sources within the hospital. Although the flavobacteria grow best at 25°-30° C, clinical isolates will grow at 35° C on initial isolation. The most clinically significant species is *F. meningosepticum*, an etiologic agent of neonatal meningitis and sepsis. Episodes of this syndrome are likely to occur as small epidemics, affecting a number of babies in the same nursery. Although many infants are asymptomatically colonized with the organism, mortality can be 50% among those that contract disease. Other species, *F. aquatile*, *F. breve*, *F. odoratum*, *F. multivorum*, and *F. spiritovorum*, have only rarely been isolated from humans. All species have been implicated as the etiologic agents of sepsis, wound infections, endocarditis, and pneumonia. Flavobacteria, in addition to producing yellow pigmentation, usually grow on MacConkey agar (except for *F. aquatile*), are catalase and oxidase positive and nonmotile, and (except for *F. odoratum*) are able to produce acid from glucose in O-F carbohydrate medium. *F. odoratum* produces a sweet, fruity odor similar to that of *Alcaligenes odorans*, by which it can be recognized. All flavobacteria are resistant to penicillin. Due to extensive proteolytic enzyme production, colonies on blood agar are usually surrounded by a lavender-green discoloration. Gram stains of colonies reveal long, thin, filamentous gram-negative bacilli with occasional swollen ends. According to King et al.[4] and Gilardi,[2] *Flavobacterium* species are nonfermentative. Gelatinase is produced by most strains, except for *F. aquatile*. The extracellular proteins and gelatinase may account in part for the virulence of some species.

28.2.i. Genus *Agrobacterium.* Only one species of *Agrobacterium*, *A. radiobacter* (from the Greek *radius*, meaning "ray"; star-shaped aggregates of bacteria are observed occasionally), has been recovered from human clinical material. Normally an invasive plant pathogen, *A. radiobacter*, has been isolated from wound infections, sputum, urine, and blood. Whether this organism is a true pathogen or only a saprophytic contaminant has not been determined. *Agrobacterium* is oxidase variable (by Kovac's method), rapidly urease positive, able to hydrolyze esculin, motile by means of peritrichous flagella, and able to use sucrose as a sole carbon source, unlike *Alcaligenes* and certain *Pseudomonas* species with which it may be confused.

28.3. Nonconventional Methods for Identification of Nonfermentative Bacilli

Numerous identification package systems, rapid methods, and automated methods are available for identification of nonfermenters. Because of the complexity and diversity of this group of organisms, no one system has proven to accurately identify all nonfermenters. New products are in developmental stages, so that eventually microbiologists will be able to obtain definitive identifications more easily.

Several manufacturers produce miniature biochemical identification systems (Chapter 9). The Uni N/F Tek (Flow Laboratories), Oxiferm (Roche Diagnostics), Minitek (BBL Microbiology Systems), and two API systems, API Rapid NFT and the API 20E (Analytab Products), have all been used to identify nonfermenters. With those species that comprise the great majority of the isolates seen in routine clinical microbiology laboratories, each of the systems performs adequately. The unusual or rare species are identified with difficulty even in reference laboratories; the commercial systems should not be relied on for definitive identifications of such organisms.

The makers of automated identification and identification/susceptibility testing systems have incorporated substrates and data bases for identification of nonfermenters. The AMS AutoMicrobic System (Vitek Systems, Inc.), the Avantage (Abbott Diagnostics), the Autobac IDX (General Diagnostics), and several manufacturers of MIC/ID systems in the microdilution tray format (Sceptor, BBL Microbiology Systems; MicroScan, American Scientific Products; and Fox, Micro-Media Systems) each include gram-negative nonfermenter identification capability. For all of these systems,

approximately 90% of the clinically relevant nonfermenters tested will be identified accurately. Microbiologists should retain a slight skepticism, however, and correlate the results of the identification system of choice with the morphological characteristics, both cellular and colonial, growth characteristics, and other traits (smell, hemolysis, speed of growth) of the organism being examined.

28.4. Treatment of Infections Caused by Nonfermentative Gram-Negative Bacilli

Pseudomonads, particularly *P. aeruginosa*, are notoriously resistant to a large number of commonly used antimicrobial agents; they are usually susceptible to aminoglycosides, the drugs of choice. There is a tremendous amount of literature concerning treatment of *Pseudomonas* infections; treatment choices vary with the clinical situation and the site of infection. Certain medical centers experience a high rate of aminoglycoside-resistant *P. aeruginosa* isolates. New beta-lactam antimicrobials, including cefsulodin, ceftazidime, imipenem, and others, have shown promise, although resistance can occur during a course of therapy. If the organism is susceptible, piperacillin, mezlocillin, carbenicillin, or moxalactam may be chosen. For serious infections, combination therapy is recommended. It is beyond the scope of this text to discuss the many ramifications of therapy for treatment of *Pseudomonas* infections.

Most strains of *Alcaligenes* are susceptible to some aminoglycosides, carbenicillin, rifampin, piperacillin, cefoperazone, cefamandole, trimethoprim-sulfamethoxazole, and colistin. For *Alcaligenes* species, in vitro susceptibility test results should be used to guide therapy. *Acinetobacter* species are usually susceptible to trimethoprim-sulfamethoxazole, carbenicillin, cefotaxime, and ceftizoxime. Aminoglycosides are also usually effective. For serious infections, combinations of an aminoglycoside and a beta lactam drug are recommended. *Moraxella* species are susceptible to penicillin, ampicillin, chloramphenicol, and aminoglycosides in vitro. *Eikenella corrodens* has been successfully treated with penicillin, ampicillin, carbenicillin, and tetracycline. Newer agents such as moxalactam and third generation cephalosporins are also active against *Eikenella* in vitro.

Flavobacteria are multiply resistant, although most isolates are susceptible to trimethoprim-sulfamethoxazole, rifampin, moxalactam, cefotaxime, and clindamycin. In vitro susceptibility bactericidal tests should be used to guide therapy of serious infections. Treatment with erythromycin has not been generally successful, although in vitro test results indicate susceptibility. Most strains are resistant to aminoglycosides, penicillins, and chloramphenicol. Susceptibility data for *Agrobacterium* species are not available.

REFERENCES

1. Gilardi, G.L. 1984. Identification of glucose-nonfermenting gram-negative bacilli. Clin. Microbiol. Newsletter 6:111, 127.
2. Gilardi, G.L. 1985. *Pseudomonas*. In Lennette, E.H., Balows, A., Hausler, W.J. Jr., and Shadomy, H.J., editors. Manual of clinical microbiology, ed. 4. American Society for Microbiology, Washington, D.C.
3. Kersters, K., and De Ley, J. 1984. Genus *Alcaligenes Castellani* and *Chalmers 1919*. In Krieg, N.R., and Holt, J.G., editors. Bergey's manual of systematic bacteriology, ed. 9. Williams & Wilkins, Baltimore.
4. King, E.O., Weaver, R.E., Hollis, D.G., Clark, W.A., and Riley, P. 1983. The identification of unusual pathogenic gram-negative bacilli. Centers for Disease Control, Department of Health and Human Services, Public Health Service, Atlanta.
5. Palleroni, N.J. 1984. Genus *Pseudomonas Migula 1894*. In Krieg, N.R., and Holt, J.G., editors. Bergey's manual of systematic bacteriology, ed. 9. Williams & Wilkins, Baltimore.
6. Pickett, M.J., and Pedersen, M.M. 1978. New methodology for identification of nonfermenters: rapid methods. In Gilardi, G.L., editor. Glucose nonfermenting gram-negative bacteria in clinical microbiology. CRC Press. West Palm Beach, Fla.
7. Robin, T., and Janda, J.M. 1984. Enhanced recovery of *Pseudomonas aeruginosa* from diverse clinical specimens on a new selective agar. Diagn. Microbiol. Infect. Dis. 2:207.
8. Rubin, S.J., Granato, P.A., and Wasilauskas, B.L. 1985. Glucose-nonfermenting gram-negative bacteria. In Lennette, E.H., Balows, A., Hausler, W.J. Jr., and Shadomy, H.J., editors. Manual of clinical microbiology, ed. 4. American Society for Microbiology, Washington, D.C.
9. Skerman, V.D.B., McGowan, V., and Sneath, P.H.A. 1980. Approved lists of bacterial names. Int. J. Syst. Bacteriol. 30:225.

BIBLIOGRAPHY

Hugh, R., and Gilardi, G.L. 1980. *Pseudomonas*. In Lennette, E.H., Balows, A., Hausler, W.J. Jr., and Truant, J.P., editors. Manual of clinical microbiology, ed. 3. American Society for Microbiology, Washington, D.C.

Lyons, R.W. 1983. *Acinetobacter calcoaceticus*. J. Clin. Microbiol. 5:87.

Symposium on *Pseudomonas aeruginosa* infections. 1983. Rev. Infect. Dis. 5 (suppl. 5):S833.

29 Gram-Negative Facultatively Anaerobic Bacilli and Aerobic Coccobacilli

Seven named genera and two unnamed species of gram-negative organisms are discussed in this chapter. Three genera, *Pasteurella*, *Brucella*, and *Francisella*, are agents of zoonoses and infect humans only by accident, when the humans come into close contact with the preferred animal hosts or with insects that have acquired the organisms from the animals. DF-2, named **dysgonic fermenter** by the Centers for Disease Control (CDC) because the organism grew poorly in standard microbiological media, is also carried by animals as normal oral flora, particularly in dogs and rarely in cats. Four other genera, *Haemophilus*, *Bordetella*, *Kingella*, and *Actinobacillus*, are found among the normal flora of the human respiratory tract and occasionally other mucosal surfaces. Organisms designated by the CDC as HB-5 seem to be normal flora of the human genitourinary mucosa. All of the organisms discussed in this chapter are morphologically **pleomorphic**, occurring as short bacilli, coccobacilli, or exhibiting chains or filamentous forms. *Pasteurella*, HB-5, *Kingella*, and *Actinobacillus* species will grow on routine laboratory media, but the other genera usually require specialized growth factors.

29.1. Genus *Francisella*

29.1.a. Epidemiology and pathogenesis of *Francisella* infection. *Francisella* contains two species, *F. novicida*, an animal pathogen, and *F. tularensis*, the agent of human and animal tularemia. Since *F. novicida* is not involved in human disease, it will not be discussed further. *F. tularensis* is carried by many species of wild rodents, rabbits, beavers, and muskrats in North America. Humans become infected by handling the carcasses or skin of infected animals, through insect vectors (chiefly deerflies and ticks in the United States), by being bitten by carnivores that have themselves eaten infected animals, or by inhalation. The capsule of *F. tularensis* may be a factor in virulence, allowing the organism to avoid immediate destruction by polymorphonuclear neutrophils. The organism is extremely invasive, being one of only a few infectious agents reported to penetrate intact skin, still a debatable property. In addition to invasiveness, the organisms are intracellular parasites, able to survive in the cells of the reticuloendothelial system, where they reside after a bacteremic phase. Granulomatous lesions may develop in various organs. Patients experience high fevers, headache, lymphadenopathy, and an ulcerative lesion at the site of inoculation. Pneumonia is a common complication. Tularemia is primarily a disease of adult men who hunt since they have the most contact with wild animals and are most likely to be exposed to the insect vectors.

29.1.b. Laboratory diagnosis. *F. tularensis* is a Biosafety level 2 pathogen (Chapter 2), a designation that requires technologists to wear gloves and to work within a biological safety cabinet when handling material that potentially harbors this agent. Because tularemia is one of the most common laboratory-acquired infections, however, most microbiologists do not attempt to work with infectious material from suspected cases. We recommend that specimens be sent to reference laboratories or state or other health laboratories that are equipped to handle *Francisella*. The CDC has fluorescent antibody stains available for direct detection of the organism in lesion smears, but such procedures are best performed by reference laboratories.

F. tularensis is strictly aerobic and requires enriched media for primary isolation. Commercial media for cultivation of the organism are available (glucose cystine agar, BBL Microbiology Systems, and cystine heart agar, Difco Laboratories); both require the addition of 5% sheep or rabbit blood. *F. tularensis* may also grow on chocolate agar and rarely on Thayer-Martin agar with prolonged incubation. It does not grow on MacConkey agar, and growth is not enhanced by carbon dioxide. The organisms, which grow slowly, requiring 2-4 days for maximum colony formation, are weakly catalase positive and oxidase negative. Some strains may require up to 2 weeks to develop visible colonies. Colonies are transparent, mucoid, and easily emulsified. Although carbohydrates are fermented, isolates should be identified serologically (by agglutination) or by a fluorescent antibody stain. They should ideally be sent to a reference laboratory for characterization. Diagnosis of disease in patients is usually accomplished serologically by whole cell agglutination (febrile agglutinins, Chapter 12) or by newer enzyme-linked immunosorbent assay (ELISA) techniques.

29.1.c. Treatment. The organism is susceptible to aminoglycosides, and streptomycin is the drug of choice. Gentamicin is a possible alternative; tetracycline and chloramphenicol have also been used, although the latter two agents have been associated with a higher rate of relapses following treatment.

29.2. Genus *Brucella*

29.2.a. Epidemiology and pathogenesis of *Brucella* infection. The agents of brucellosis, *Brucella* species, are normal flora of the genital and urinary tract of many animals including goats, pigs, cows, and dogs. Most humans acquire disease through ingestion of contaminated milk or through occupational exposure; the disease is particularly common among abat-

toir workers. Farmers and veterinarians are also at increased risk. The primary virulence factor for *Brucella* seems to be the organism's ability to survive intracellularly. It is probably this characteristic, as well as granuloma and abscess formation, that accounts for the chronic and relapsing nature of the febrile disease. Patients often present with a gradual onset of nonspecific systemic symptoms including malaise, chills, sweats, fatigue, and mental changes. Localized lesions can occur in most any organ or bone; they may be granulomatous or suppurative and destructive. Pulmonary, cardiovascular, skeletal, genitourinary, and central nervous system localization are also possible complications.

29.2.b. Collection and transport of specimens. *Brucella* species are usually isolated from blood cultures or bone marrow cultures during the acute illness. Organisms may also be recovered from joint fluid of patients with arthritis. Blood cultures may require prolonged incubation times, as mentioned in Chapter 14. Bone marrow cultures are handled as discussed in Chapter 21. Material from infected lymph nodes, other tissue, cerebrospinal fluid, and urine may also yield *Brucella*. The laboratory should be notified that brucellosis is suspected so that supplemented media that better support growth of the organism can be inoculated. Although most strains will grow on chocolate and blood agar and some strains will grow on MacConkey agar, *Brucella* agar (Gibco Laboratories and BBL) or some type of infusion base agar is recommended. The addition of 5% heated horse or rabbit serum will enhance growth on all media. Cultures should be incubated in 5%-10% CO_2 in a humidified atmosphere, such as a candle extinction jar (Chapter 8). Blood cultures are held for 4 weeks, and inoculated plates are incubated for 3 weeks before being discarded as negative. It has been found that organisms may be present in blood culture broths without visible evidence and without an increase in the growth index as measured on the Bactec radiometric blood culture instrument (Chapters 11 and 14). For this reason, weekly blind subcultures to *Brucella* broth are recommended for optimal recovery of *Brucella* species from blood cultures. *Brucella* is also considered to be a type 2 biohazard and should be handled with all appropriate precautions. Many laboratory-acquired cases of brucellosis have been documented; it is one of the most prevalent laboratory-acquired infections.

29.2.c. Laboratory diagnosis. Colonies appear small, convex, smooth, translucent, slightly yellow and opalescent after at least 48 h incubation. The colonies may become brownish with age. The organisms are catalase positive and most strains are oxidase positive. None of the *Brucella* species ferment carbohydrates; other nonfermentative gram-negative coccobacilli that may be confused with *Brucella* are *Bordetella, Moraxella, Kingella, Acinetobacter* species, and others (Chapter 28). *Brucella*, however, is nonmotile, nonhemolytic and strictly aerobic. The most rapid test for presumptive identification of *Brucella* is the particle agglutination test with antismooth *Brucella* serum, available from Difco Laboratories. Agglutination is carried out as described in Chap-

ter 12. This test cannot be performed on rough colony variants. Six species of *Brucella* may be isolated from humans: *B. melitensis, B. abortus, B. suis, B. canis, B. ovis,* and *B. neotomae*. The species are differentiated by the rapidity with which they hydrolyze urea, their relative ability to produce hydrogen sulfide (H_2S) gas, their requirements for CO_2, and their susceptibility to the aniline dyes thionine and basic fuchsin, as briefly described in Procedure 29.1. Performance of the urease and H_2S detection tests is also described in Procedure 29.1. Differential characteristics are listed in Table 29.1. For determination of CO_2 requirement, identical plates of *Brucella* agar or brain heart infusion agar should be given equal inocula (with a calibrated loop, for example) of a broth suspension of the organism to be tested. One plate should be incubated in a candle jar and the other plate should be incubated in air, both in the same incubator. Most strains of *B. abortus* and all strains of *B. ovis* will not grow in air, but will show growth in the candle jar. Isolates of *Brucella* should be sent to state reference laboratories for confirmation or definitive identification since most clinical laboratories lack the necessary media and containment facilities and since the tests are variable enough

TABLE 29.1

Characteristics of *Brucella* Species*

SPECIES	CO₂ REQUIRED FOR GROWTH	TIME TO POSITIVE UREASE	H₂S PRODUCED	GROWTH ON MEDIA CONTAINING	
				THIONINE†	FUCHSIN†
B. abortus	+/−	2 h (rare 24 h)	+ (most strains)	+/−	+/− (most strains +)
B. melitensis	−	2 h (rare 24 h)	−	+	+
B. suis	−	15 min	+/−	+	− (most)
B. ovis	+	≥7 days	−	+	− (most)
B. neotomae	−	15 min	+	−	−
B. canis	−	15 min	−	+	− (most)

*+ = >90% of strains positive; − = >90% of strains negative; +/− = variable results.
†1:50,000 wt/vol, as described in text.

to necessitate very stringent quality control measures employing known strains of *Brucella*. Because of the difficulty of isolating the organism, many cases of brucellosis are diagnosed serologically by the *Brucella* **febrile agglutinin**

test, as mentioned in Chapter 12. An ELISA procedure has also been described.

29.2.d. Treatment of brucellosis. For initial therapy, tetracycline combined with an aminoglycoside, streptomycin or gentamicin, is

---

PROCEDURE 29.1. SPECIAL TESTS FOR SPECIES DIFFERENTIATION AMONG *BRUCELLA*

1. Urease activity is determined by inoculating a large loopful of growth from a broth suspension made from isolated colonies to the surface of a Christensen's urea agar slant (Chapter 9).
2. Examine the slant immediately and incubate the slant at 37° C, examining at 15 min, 1 h, 2 h, and 24 h.
3. Urease activity is evidenced by a change in color on the slant surface from yellow to pink to bright pinkish-purple.
4. Production of hydrogen sulfide is determined by placing a strip of lead acetate–impregnated filter paper (available from Remel Laboratories and other suppliers) suspended in the air above an agar slant culture (tryptic soy agar or serum-supplemented agar) of the organism being tested. The paper must not contact the agar or the sides of the tube. This can be accomplished by bending the paper over the edge of the tube mouth before lightly screwing on the cap, leaving a length of the strip inside the tube.
5. The tube is incubated at 37° C in air or CO_2, as required, and the paper strip is examined and changed daily. A complete blackening of the entire strip after the first day, or slight blackening of the strip on subsequent days, is indicative of hydrogen sulfide production.
6. Growth on media containing aniline dyes is determined by incorporating the dyes thionine and basic fuchsin (available from National Aniline Division, Allied Chemical and Dye Co.) in tryptic soy agar plates. Dyes are prepared by boiling 0.1 g of each dye in 100 ml distilled water and adding 2 ml dye solution to 100 ml molten agar before pouring plates of 20 ml agar per plate to yield a final dye concentration of 1:50,000 (wt/vol). Different lots of dye may vary, so testing plates with quality control strains is necessary.
7. Equal quantities of the organisms are inoculated to plates without dyes and plates with each dye, and the inocula are streaked for isolation in four quadrants. The plates are incubated at 37° C in the appropriate atmosphere for up to 4 days and examined for growth. Growth in at least three quadrants is considered positive.

Modified from Corbel and Brinley-Morgan. 1984. Genus *Brucella Meyer and Shaw 1920.* In Krieg and Holt, editors. Bergey's manual of systematic bacteriology, ed. 9. Williams & Wilkins, Baltimore.

probably best. Trimethoprim-sulfamethoxazole has also been effective for treatment of brucellosis in adults.

29.3. Genus *Bordetella*

29.3.a. Epidemiology and pathogenesis of *Bordetella* infection. *Bordetella* species are obligate parasites of animals and humans, residing on the mucous membranes of the respiratory tract. The organisms colonize the ciliated epithelial cells, adhering closely to the surface; the adherence may be mediated by fimbriae. Mechanisms of pathogenesis of etiologic agents of respiratory tract infections were discussed in Chapter 16. Bordetellae seem to be the only bacteria that adhere only to ciliated mucosal cells. Other virulence factors associated with Bordetellae, particularly *B. pertussis*, include a capsule that surrounds the cells of virulent strains, production of dermonecrotic toxins, production of hemagglutinins, production of extracellular enzymes (adenylate cyclase), and production of other biologically active substances including endotoxin (Chapter 14) and an exotoxin (pertussis toxin) that acts on various cells of the immune system and other tissues.

Of the three species, *B. pertussis*, *B. bronchiseptica*, and *B. parapertussis*, only *B. bronchiseptica* is found naturally in animals such as rabbits, dogs, swine, and many other wild and domestic animals. All three species can, however, cause disease in humans that resembles **pertussis,** or **whooping cough** (Chapter 16), although the disease associated with *B. pertussis* is most severe. *B. bronchiseptica* has been isolated from infected wounds as well as from the respiratory tract of humans. Incidence of whooping cough in the United States has steadily declined since 1950 when vaccine became widely used, leveling at approximately 1,900 cases reported annually. Fatalities still occur, however, and it seems plausible that the incidence of pertussis will increase as public fear of the disease and consequent vaccine usage decline. Recent epidemiologic studies in New York and Wisconsin have shown recovery of *B.*

pertussis from children and adults with respiratory tract disease that does not resemble classical whooping cough. The organism may be more prevalent than is currently assumed, since very few laboratories use methods that allow its detection unless instructed to do so by a clinician who suspects the disease.

29.3.b. Collection and transport of specimens. Specimens are collected either as nasopharyngeal washings or on a nasopharyngeal swab (calcium alginate on a wire handle [Chapter 6], available commercially from several suppliers [Appendix]). The swab is bent to conform to the nasal passage and held against the posterior nasopharynx. If coughing does not occur, another swab is inserted into the other nostril to initiate the cough. The swab is left in place during the entire cough, removed, and immediately inoculated onto a selective medium such as Bordet-Gengou agar containing 20% sheep blood cells and 2.5 μg/ml methicillin instead of penicillin (Chapter 45) or the recently evaluated Jones-Kendrick charcoal agar containing 40 μg/ml cephalexin (Chapter 16). Stauffer and others[7] have found cephalexin to be superior to methicillin for inhibition of normal respiratory flora and Jones-Kendrick agar to be acceptable for transport and cultivation of *Bordetella* species from respiratory tract specimens. This agar will remain effective even after 2 months storage in tightly wrapped plastic bags in the refrigerator. A fluid transport medium may be used for swabs (it must be held for less than 2 h). Cold casein hydrolysate medium or casamino acid broth (available commercially) has been found to be an effective transport medium, particularly for preparation of slides for direct fluorescent antibody staining (Chapter 16).

29.3.c. Laboratory diagnosis of *Bordetella*. Plates are incubated at 35°-37° C in a humidified atmosphere; they do not require increased CO_2. If grown on Bordet-Gengou agar with 20% blood, colonies will show a diffuse zone of hemolysis. Colonies will grow within 7 days, appearing small, smooth, convex, with a pearly

TABLE 29.2
Characteristics of *Bordetella* Species*

SPECIES	GROWTH ON HEART INFUSION AGAR	UREASE	NITRATE REDUCTION	MOTILITY
B. pertussis	−	−	−	−
B. parapertussis	+	+ (18 h)	−	−
B. bronchiseptica	+	+ (4 h)	+	+

*+ = All strains positive; − = all strains negative.

luster, resembling mercury drops (Plate 29.1). The colonies are mucoid and tenacious. A Gram stain of the organism will reveal minute, faintly staining coccobacilli singly or in pairs. The use of a 2 min safranin O counterstain or the carbol-fuchsin counterstain (Chapter 7) will enhance their visibility. *B. bronchiseptica* and *B. parapertussis* will grow on MacConkey agar; *B. pertussis* will not.

A direct fluorescent antibody stain is available for detection of *B. pertussis* in smears made from nasopharyngeal material. The procedure is described in Chapter 16. In experienced hands, this reagent has been very efficient for early diagnosis of cases of whooping cough. Slides may be prepared, heat fixed, and mailed to a reference laboratory for evaluation. This reagent may also be used to presumptively identify organisms growing on agar. The fluorescent antibody identification method is much faster than conventional biochemicals. Whole cell agglutination reactions in specific antiserum may also be used for species identification (Chapter 12). Abbreviated biochemical reactions of the three known species of *Bordetella* are shown in Table 29.2. A fourth organism, designated *Bordetella*-like, has been isolated from domestic poultry but has not been well characterized. An enzyme immunoassay for detection of antibody to *B. pertussis* (Labsystems) has recently become available. Preliminary trials have yielded promising results for early diagnosis of pertussis.

29.3.d. Treatment of pertussis. Adequate microbiological therapy may not alter the course of the disease. Erythromycin does eradicate organisms from the respiratory tract, however, and should be given to all patients with pertussis.

29.4. Genus *Haemophilus*

The following three genera, *Haemophilus*, *Actinobacillus*, and *Pasteurella*, are all members of the family Pasteurellaceae, a group of organisms that are pleomorphic, gram-negative, nonmotile bacilli and coccobacilli and that are able to reduce nitrates and utilize carbohydrates either fermentatively or with oxygen as the terminal electron acceptor. All three genera live on animals, including humans, primarily on mucosal surfaces. They may be differentiated by their requirements for nicotinamide adenine dinucleotide (NAD), as well as by other criteria, as outlined below.

29.4.a. Epidemiology and pathogenesis of *Haemophilus* infection. Carried in the normal respiratory tract (and occasionally genital tract) of humans, pigs, sheep, and most other vertebrates, the organisms cause upper respiratory tract infections, suppurative infections, primarily in areas adjacent to the respiratory tract, and systemic infections, particularly meningitis. In humans, *Haemophilus influenzae* is the most common etiologic agent of acute bacterial meningitis in children (Chapter 15). *H. influenzae*, the most important human pathogen among the species of *Haemophilus*, is also associated with acute, contagious conjunctivitis ("pinkeye" [*H. aegyptius*]), acute and chronic otitis media, epiglottitis, cellulitis, and other

TABLE 29.3

Biotypes of *Haemophilus influenzae*

BIOTYPE	SYNDROME (SITE OF INFECTION)	INDOLE	UREASE	ORNITHINE
I	Sepsis, meningitis	+	+	+
II	Eye (United States), bacteremia, ear, lower respiratory tract	+	+	−
III	Eye (Europe), respiratory tract	−	+	−
IV	Ear (rare), respiratory tract	−	+	+
V	Ear, lower respiratory tract	+	−	+
VI	Upper respiratory tract (rare)	+	−	−

Modified from Kilian, M., and Biberstein, E.L. 1984. Genus *Haemophilus Winslow, Broadhurst, Buchanan, Krumwiede, Rogers and Smith* 1917. In Krieg, N.R., and Holt, J.G., editors. Bergey's manual of systematic bacteriology, ed. 9. Williams & Wilkins, Baltimore.

infections. *H. influenzae* has even been isolated by Gabre-Kidan and others[3] from the urine of patients with urinary tract infections. *H. ducreyi*, not found as part of normal genital flora of humans or known to be harbored by any animals, is associated with chancroid, a widespread venereal disease, found most commonly in tropical parts of the world. Other species of *Haemophilus*, which include *H. parainfluenzae*, *H. haemolyticus*, *H. aphrophilus*, *H. paraphrophilus*, and *H. segnis*, are normal flora of humans only, occasionally causing upper and lower respiratory tract infections. These organisms may also occasionally enter the bloodstream from a mucosal focus, disseminating to cause systemic disease, including endocarditis, metastatic abscesses, septic arthritis, and osteomyelitis. They have also been known to infect tissue adjacent to the mucosa, causing jaw infections, dental abscesses, and, when they are traumatically inoculated into healthy tissue, bite wound infections. *H. influenzae* and *H. parainfluenzae* are associated with invasive disease in humans more often than are the other species. *H. parainfluenzae* tends to grow in tangled clumps or strands of filamentous bacterial forms; these may easily break off the main colony. Particularly in cases of sepsis or endocarditis, there may be metastatic abscess formation.

The polysaccharide capsule is clearly a virulence factor for *H. influenzae*, since anticapsular antibody is protective against acquisition of meningitis. A number of immunologic reagents have been developed for the rapid identification of *H. influenzae* capsular polysaccharide type b (the most common pathogenic agent), as described below and in Chapter 15. Unencapsulated strains, however, are often recovered from specimens taken from patients with infections other than meningitis, including pneumonia, cellulitis, otitis media, and soft tissue infections. Pathogenic mechanisms of the *Haemophilus* species are not well understood. Since the organisms enter the bloodstream so readily after colonization of the respiratory epithelium, they may possess some invasive properties. Their ability to multiply in host tissues and evoke an inflammatory response contributes to the pathology of pyogenic *Haemophilus* disease.

Recent studies on identification of *H. influenzae*, primarily initiated and reported by Kilian,[4] and Kilian and Biberstein,[5] have shown that certain biotypes of that organism are more commonly associated with particular syndromes, as outlined in Table 29.3. Biotyping can be easily accomplished, as discussed below, and microbiologists should routinely identify significant *H. influenzae* isolates to biotype.

As more laboratories procure such definitive identifications, our understanding of the epidemiology and pathogenesis of infection with this prevalent microorganism will expand.

29.4.b. Specimen collection and transport. Most any specimen may harbor *Haemophilus* species, and it is primarily for isolation of this organism that most clinical material received for routine culture in microbiology laboratories is inoculated to chocolate agar and incubated in 5%-10% CO_2. Blood, cerebrospinal fluid, middle ear exudate collected by tympanocentesis, joint fluids, respiratory tract specimens, swabs from inflamed conjunctivae, and abscess drainage are a few of the many types of specimens that are likely to yield *Haemophilus* species.

Most swabs routinely used for collection of material for culture, including calcium alginate, cotton, and Dacron, are suitable for collection of specimens for detection of most species of *Haemophilus*. Modified Stuart's transport medium or Amie's charcoal transport medium (Chapters 6 and 45) will adequately maintain viability of the organism until the specimen is inoculated to growth media. For recovery of *H. ducreyi* from genital ulcers, however, special measures are necessary due to the fastidious nature of the bacterium. The ulcer should be cleansed with sterile gauze moistened with sterile saline. A physician uses a cotton swab premoistened with phosphate buffered saline to collect material from the ulcer base. This swab must be plated to media (described in Chapter 19 and mentioned below) within 10 min of collection for maximum yield.

29.4.c. Media and incubation conditions for isolation of *Haemophilus* species. Chocolate agar supplies the factors necessary for growth of most *Haemophilus* species. These factors are **hemin** (called **X factor**) and **nicotine adenine dinucleotide** (**NAD**; called **V factor**). *H. influenzae*, *H. haemolyticus*, and *H. ducreyi* require X factor, whereas *H. aphrophilus* requires X factor only for initial isolation. All clinically significant species except for *H.*

aphrophilus and *H. ducreyi* require V factor. Chocolate agar, horse blood agar, and rabbit blood agar all contain adequate quantities of both growth factors and support the growth of *Haemophilus* species that require both factors. Either rabbit blood or horse blood are used for visualization of hemolysis. Sheep blood that has not been chocolatized (Chapter 8) contains enough NADase (produced by the sheep blood cells) to destroy the NAD normally present, although sheep blood agar does contain adequate hemin for growth of *Haemophilus* that require hemin. *Haemophilus* species that require both X and V factors can grow on sheep blood agar if the V factor is exogenously provided. Several other bacterial species produce V factor as a metabolic byproduct. Therefore, tiny colonies of *Haemophilus* may be seen growing very close to colonies of bacteria on sheep blood agar that produce V factor. This phenomenon, known as **satelliting** (Plate 29.2), often occurs around hemolytic staphylococci because they produce sufficient V factor. Pneumococci, neisseriae, and many other organisms also produce enough NAD to allow satellite colonies of *Haemophilus* species to form in their vicinity. With the exceptions of *H. aphrophilus* and *H. ducreyi*, all clinically significant *Haemophilus* species require V factor.

Media that adequately support growth of *H. ducreyi* are Mueller-Hinton base chocolate agar supplemented with 1% IsoVitaleX (BBL Microbiology Systems) and 3 µg/ml vancomycin, and heart infusion base agar with 10% fetal bovine serum and 3 µg/ml vancomycin. For best recovery, material from suspected chancroid lesions should be inoculated to two plates, one of each different agar formula, both of which are incubated in a candle jar at 35°-37° C for a maximum of 7 days.

H. influenzae is a significant etiologic agent of lower respiratory tract infection, particularly among elderly patients and young individuals with cystic fibrosis (Chapter 23). The number of isolates of *Haemophilus* species is increased when selective media such as horse blood–bacitracin developed by Klein and Blazevic (Chapter 45) are employed for recovery of these organisms. Such media are particularly important for isolating *Haemophilus* from respiratory secretions of patients with cystic fibrosis, where the organisms may be etiologic agents of disease, but they are overgrown and their presence obscured by the coexisting mucoid *Pseudomonas aeruginosa* (Chapter 23).

Most strains of *Haemophilus* are able to grow aerobically and anaerobically. Growth is usually stimulated by 5%-10% CO_2 so that incubation in a candle extinction jar or carbon dioxide incubator is recommended. The organisms usually grow within 24 h, but some strains, particularly *H. ducreyi*, may require as long as 7 days.

29.4.d. Laboratory identification of clinically significant *Haemophilus* species. *Haemophilus* species are often not visible in broth, especially in blood culture media, since they do not grow to turbidity. For this reason, blind subcultures to chocolate agar or examination of smears (acridine orange is recommended, Chapters 7 and 14) is necessary for their detection. *H. parainfluenzae* may appear as filamentous, intertwining strands of gram-negative bacilli, whereas the other species usually are seen as coccobacilli with long filamentous forms occasionally interspersed (Plate 29.3). Gram stains from colonies growing on solid agar are more typical, showing pleomorphic coccobacilli.

Colonies on chocolate agar are transparent, moist, smooth, convex, with a distinct odor,

---

PROCEDURE 29.2. PORPHYRIN TEST FOR X FACTOR REQUIREMENT

1. Prepare delta-aminolevulinic acid substrate as follows:

   δ-aminolevulinic acid (Sigma Chemical Co.) (2 mM)   0.34 g
   $MgSO_4$ (0.08 mM)   0.0096 g
   Phosphate buffer (0.1 M, pH 6.9)   1,000 ml

   The $MgSO_4$ may be prepared in a more concentrated solution and diluted to reach the desired final concentration.

   Mix thoroughly, dispense into small plastic snap top tubes (12 × 75 mm) 0.5 ml per tube, and freeze at −20° C until use.

2. Thaw the substrate and add a very heavy loopful of the organism to be tested, making a heavy suspension. Also inoculate a known positive control strain and include an uninoculated tube as a negative control.

3. Incubate the tubes at 37° C for 4 h and then take the tubes into a darkroom and shine an ultraviolet light source of 360 nm wavelength (long wave) on the contents of the tube.

4. Presence of a brick red to orange fluorescence indicates that porphyrins were produced, and that the organism does not require hemin (X factor). The negative control should display no fluorescence.

Modified from Kilian and Biberstein. 1984. Genus *Haemophilus Winslow, Broadhurst, Buchanan, Krumwiede, Rogers and Smith 1917.* In Krieg and Holt, editors. Bergey's manual of systematic bacteriology, ed. 9. Williams & Wilkins, Baltimore.

variously described as "mousy" or "bleachlike." X and V factor requirements are carried out using the **porphyrin test** (Procedure 29.2). This test detects the presence of enzymes that convert delta-aminolevulinic acid (ALA) into porphyrins or protoporphyrins. The more traditional method for detection of X and V factor requirements, that of inoculating the organism to media without blood and placing X and V factor-impregnated filter paper strips on the plate, incubating overnight, and examining for growth around the appropriate strip, cannot be recommended. Many X factor–requiring organisms are able to carry over enough X factor from the primary medium to yield false negative tests with the filter paper method.

A commercial ALA reagent impregnated on a filter paper disk is available from Remel Laboratories. The test is performed according to the manufacturer's instructions. The technologist must be careful not to overmoisten the disk, as false negative results can occur due to dilution of the endproduct.

In addition to the porphyrin test, *Haemophilus* isolates may be identified using biochemical parameters (Table 29.4). Although conventional media are acceptable for performance of these tests, several new rapid enzymatic biochemical systems (Chapter 9) have been developed for identification of *Haemophilus*, including the Minitek System (BBL Microbiology Systems), the RapID-NH (Innovative Diagnostics), Micro-ID (General Diagnostics), and others.

Those species that require V factor have been grouped into biotypes but the biotypes have not yet been associated with particular clinical syndromes. *H. segnis* is the only oxidase negative species among this group. *H. aphrophilus* can be confused with a closely related organism, *Actinobacillus actinomycetemcomitans*, another agent of endocarditis acquired during transient bacteremia with normal oral flora related to oral manipulation or disease. As discussed below, *A. actinomyce-*temcomitans is catalase positive, does not require V factor, and cannot ferment lactose or sucrose. *H. aphrophilus* yields the opposite reactions in those tests. Colony morphology of *H. aphrophilus* on a clear medium can be used to aid in differentiating it from *A. actinomycetemcomitans*. The colony of *H. aphrophilus* is round and convex and displays an opaque zone near the center (Plate 29.4), whereas *A. actinomycetemcomitans* colonies appear to have a central star-shaped structure (Plate 29.5).

29.4.e. Rapid identification of *H. influenzae* type b. The clinical significance of *H. influenzae* type b has prompted workers to develop rapid immunologic methods for detection of its capsular polysaccharide directly in clinical specimens, such as cerebrospinal fluid (Chapter 15), serum, and urine. The organism, once isolated, can also be rapidly identified with the same reagents. The classical quellung procedure (Chapter 12), can be used with specific antibody to presumptively identify the organisms in respiratory secretions and cerebrospinal fluid. Specific antisera are available from Difco Laboratories, Hyland Diagnostics, and Wellcome Diagnostics. Coagglutination reagents produced by Pharmacia Biotechnology and latex agglutination reagents (Hynson, Westcott & Dunning, Wellcome Diagnostics, Wampole Laboratories) have been shown to be very sensitive and specific for detecting the presence of *H. influenzae* type b in cerebrospinal fluid and slightly less sensitive when used with other body fluids (Chapter 15).

In addition to rapid detection and identification of the organism, the increasing incidence of ampicillin resistance necessitates that microbiologists perform a rapid test for detection of beta lactamase. Because of widespread chloramphenicol resistance found in other parts of the world (and occasional chloramphenicol-resistant isolates seen in the United States), microbiologists may wish to perform a rapid test for detection of chloramphenicol resistance as well. These tests, produced commercially as

TABLE 29.4

Characteristics of *Haemophilus* Species Isolated from Humans*

SPECIES	REQUIRES V FACTOR FOR GROWTH	ALA → PORPHYRINS	UREASE	INDOLE	ACID FROM GLUCOSE	ACID FROM LACTOSE	BETA HEMOLYTIC†	CATALASE
H. influenzae	+	−	+/−	+/−	+	−	−	+
H. parainfluenzae	+	+	+/−	−	+ (some gas)	−	−	+/− (slow)
H. haemolyticus	+	−	+	+/−	+	−	+	+
H. aphrophilus	−	+ (weak)	−	−	+ (gas)	+	−	−
H. paraphrophilus	+	+	−	−	+ (gas)	+	−	−
H. segnis	+	+	−	−	+	−	−	+/− (slow)
H. aegyptius	+	+	+	−	+	−	−	+
H. ducreyi	−	−	−	−	+/−	−	−	−

Modified from Kilian, M., and Biberstein, E.L. 1984. *Genus Haemophilus Winslow, Broadhurst, Buchanan, Krumwiede, Rogers and Smith 1917*. In Krieg, N.R., and Holt, J.G., editors. Bergey's manual of systematic bacteriology, ed. 9. Williams & Wilkins, Baltimore.

* + = >90% of strains positive; − = >90% of strains negative; +/− = variable results.

†Rabbit or horse blood agar.

reagent-impregnated filter paper disks by Remel Laboratories and other suppliers, are discussed fully in Chapter 13.

29.4.f. Treatment of *Haemophilus* infections. During meningitis, certain antimicrobial agents that would normally be unable to do so can penetrate the blood-brain barrier, allowing agents such as ampicillin to be used for treatment of this disease. However, due to the recent increase in ampicillin resistance among *H. influenzae* and the possibility of chloramphenicol resistance, the current recommended initial therapy for meningitis is a combination of ampicillin and chloramphenicol pending the results of in vitro susceptibility tests. Chloramphenicol achieves excellent levels in most tissues, including bone, and is the drug of choice for serious infections caused by susceptible *Haemophilus* species, alone or in combination with ampicillin. Once an isolate has been shown to be susceptible to ampicillin, this agent may be used alone to continue treatment. Newer cephalosporins, such as cefotaxime, are effective as single drug regimens for treatment of meningitis. Patients with less severe disease caused by *H. influenzae* being treated as outpatients are usually given oral amoxicillin, ampicillin, or trimethoprim-sulfamethoxazole. Other species of *Haemophilus* may often be successfully treated with tetracycline in addition to the agents mentioned above. Treatment for chancroid involves either oral erythromycin or trimethoprim-sulfamethoxazole. Rifampin is the antimicrobial agent of choice for prophylaxis of close contacts of a patient with *H. influenzae* meningitis.

29.5. Genus *Actinobacillus*

29.5.a. Epidemiology and pathogenesis of *Actinobacillus* infection. *A. lignieresii*, *A. equuli*, *A. suis*, and *A. capsulatus* are found as pathogens and as part of the normal oral flora of many domestic animals, including cows, horses, sheep, and pigs. *A. actinomycetemcomitans* is normal flora of human oral mucosa and is not found in other animals. Humans are infected with the animal species through traumatic inoculation of the organism, such as via a bite wound or other wound. Infections associated with *A. actinomycetemcomitans* are probably all of endogenous origin. This species is often isolated along with *Actinomyces* or *Arachnia* (Chapter 35) from actinomycotic lesions of the jaw (Plates 20.4 and 20.5) or abscesses within the thoracic cavity. Failure to eradicate the *Actinobacillus* may account for persistence of actinomycosis, even after the *Actinomyces* or *Arachnia* has been cleared. *Actinobacillus actinomycetemcomitans* has recently been associated with a destructive periodontitis that occurs in adolescents. This species, as well as the closely related *Haemophilus aphrophilus*, is occasionally isolated as the etiologic agent of endocarditis. The organism probably possesses very low virulence, acting as a pathogen only opportunistically.

29.5.b. Laboratory identification. *A. actinomycetemcomitans*, the clinically important species, grows on blood and chocolate agars; unlike the other species of *Actinobacillus*, it does not grow on MacConkey agar. Growth is enhanced in a candle jar or a CO_2 incubator, but colonies may require up to 7 days to achieve maximum size. Growth in broth media is often barely visible, with no turbidity produced. Microcolonies may be seen as tiny puffballs growing on the blood cell layer in blood culture bottles, or alternatively, growth may appear as a film or as tiny puffs on the sides of a bottle or tube. On blood agar, the medium surrounding the colonies exhibits a slight greenish tinge. The colonies themselves are rough and sticky. A very characteristic finding is the presence of a four- to six-pointed starlike configuration in the center of a mature colony growing on clear medium (such as brain heart infusion agar); this star pattern can be easily visualized by examining the colony under low power (100 ×) with a standard microscope (Plate 29.5). On Gram stain, the organisms are gram-negative bacilli, often displaying coccoid forms. The coccoid shapes may be found at the end of bacilli, giving the overall appearance of the dots and dashes of Morse code. *Actinobacillus* species may resemble *Haemophilus* species and *Pasteurella* species; their differentiation is outlined in Table 29.5. Key characteristics of the five *Actinobacillus* species are shown in Table 29.6

29.5.c. Treatment of *Actinobacillus* infections. All members of the genera are susceptible to tetracycline and chloramphenicol. Penicillin resistance has been reported, and the organisms are all resistant to aminoglycosides and clindamycin.

29.6. Genus *Pasteurella*

29.6.a. Epidemiology and pathogenesis of *Pasteurella* infection. *Pasteurella* species are normal flora of the respiratory and gastrointestinal tract of many species of domestic and wild animals and birds. They are the etiologic agents of hemorrhagic septicemia, gastrointestinal infections, and respiratory tract infections in many animals. Humans acquire *Pasteurella* primarily through animal exposure. The majority of human infections are associated with animal bites, but a large number of respiratory tract and intraabdominal infections are associated with possible inhalation of the organism or with no known source of acquisition. *Pasteu-*

TABLE 29.5
Differential Characteristics of Some Similar Fermentative Gram-Negative Coccobacilli*

GENUS/SPECIES	CATALASE	INDOLE	NITRATE TO NITRITE	ORNITHINE DECARBOXYLASE	FERMENTATION OF	
					LACTOSE	SUCROSE
Actinobacillus actinomycetemcomitans	+	−	+	−	−	−
Cardiobacterium hominis	−	+	−	−	−	+†
DF-2	+	−	−	−	+	−
Haemophilus aphrophilus (also *paraphrophilus*)	−	−	+	−	+	+
HB-5	−	+‡	−	−	−	−
Kingella denitrificans	−	−	+	−	−	−
Kingella kingae	−	−	−	−	−	−
Pasteurella multocida	+	+	+	+	−	+

*+ = >90% of strains positive within 2 days; − = >90% of strains negative.
†Positive results may require extended incubation period.
‡Xylene extraction required.

TABLE 29.6
Characteristics of *Actinobacillus* Species*

SPECIES	OXIDASE	UREASE	ESCULIN HYDROLYSIS	FERMENTATION OF		SODIUM HIPPURATE HYDROLYSIS
				TREHALOSE	SALICIN	
A. actinomycetemcomitans	+	−	−	−	−	ND
A. lignieresii	+	+	−	−	−	−
A. equuli	+/−	+	−	+	−	+
A. suis	+/−	+	+	+	+	+

*+ = >90% of strains positive; − = >90% of strains negative; +/− = variable results; ND = not done.

rella multocida, the most common human pathogen among the Pasteurellae, can be isolated from animal bite wounds, respiratory secretions from patients with pneumonia, cerebrospinal fluid, abscesses, biopsy specimens from patients with osteomyelitis, blood, joint fluid from septic arthritis, and many other sites. Other species of *Pasteurella, P. pneumotropica, P. haemolytica, P. ureae, P. aerogenes,* and *P. gallinarum,* are more commonly associated with animal disease, although they have been reported from human cases of endocarditis, pneumonia, septicemia, and primarily from infected wounds, occasionally involving osteomyelitis.

Virulence of *Pasteurella* is related to the polysaccharide capsule that allows the organism to resist phagocytosis. Although some strains produce a cytotoxin, its role in the pathogenesis of disease has not been elucidated. *P. multocida* appears to be the most virulent of the species. Virulence may be enhanced by the ability of the organism to utilize free iron, a factor in the pathogenicity of several bacterial strains.

29.6.b. Laboratory identification. Since *Pasteurella* species grow well on routinely inoculated laboratory media including blood agar, they are easily isolated from all sites in which they may be present. Growth is not appreciably enhanced by increased concentrations of carbon dioxide. Colonies are small and translucent and may be smooth or rough. Only colonies of *P. haemolytica* are beta hemolytic on blood agar, although a brown discoloration of the medium may develop around colonies of *P. multocida.* The colonies on blood agar have a musty or "mushroom" sort of smell, which is recognizable to experienced microbiologists. All species are oxidase positive by the Kovac's test (Chapter 9). A quick screening procedure used for presumptive identification of *Pasteurella* species takes advantage of their penicillin susceptibility, unusual for gram-negative bacteria. The surface of a Mueller-Hinton blood

agar plate is inoculated with a suspension of the organism equal to a McFarland 0.5 turbidity, using a cotton swab and streaking in three directions, as for the disk-diffusion susceptibility test. A filter paper disk containing 2 U of penicillin (used for susceptibility testing) is placed in the center of the plate, which is then incubated overnight in air. A zone of inhibition around the disk is indicative of susceptibility; most other gram-negative bacilli are resistant to penicillin (Plate 29.6).

The organism is a small, coccoid or rod-shaped bacillus that often exhibits bipolar staining. All species are nonmotile and catalase positive and able to reduce nitrates to nitrites. Differentiation among species can be achieved using biochemical parameters listed in Table 29.7. Only two species produce gas from carbohydrates, *P. aerogenes* and *Pasteurella* n. sp. I, called *Pasteurella* "gas" by King, as discussed by Weaver and Hollis.[8] The "gas" species is considered by Carter to be a biovar of *P. pneumotropica,* as stated in the new edition of *Bergey's Manual.*[1] Isolates of this biovar are often associated with dog and cat bites and may go on to cause systemic disease. Other biovars have been identified, but they have not been fully characterized or named yet. As more DNA homology studies are completed, definition of the genus *Pasteurella* may change.

Most of the biochemical identification systems available commercially (Chapter 9) will identify *Pasteurella,* at least to genus. *Pasteurella* should be suspected when any isolate is associated with an animal bite. Again, it is important for clinicians to inform the laboratory of the source of a wound specimen and pertinent clinical information so that the microbiologists can perform the appropriate tests early in the identification protocol.

29.6.c. Treatment of infections due to *Pasteurella* species. Penicillin is the antimicrobial agent of choice for all *Pasteurella* infections. Tetracycline and chloramphenicol may also be effective, but aminoglycosides, erythromycin,

TABLE 29.7

Differentiation of Species of *Pasteurella**

SPECIES	BETA HEMOLYSIS	GROWTH ON MacCONKEY AGAR	INDOLE	UREASE	GAS FROM GLUCOSE
P. multocida	−	−	+	−	−
P. pneumotropica	−	−	+	+	+/−
P. haemolyticus	+	+	−	−	−
P. ureae	−	−	−	+	−
P. aerogenes	−	+	−	+	+
P. gallinarum	−	−	−	−	−

Modified from Carter, G.R. 1984. Genus *Pasteurella Trevisan 1887*. In Krieg, N.R., and Holt, J.G., editors. Bergey's manual of systematic bacteriology, ed. 9. Williams & Wilkins, Baltimore.

* + = >90% of strains positive; − = >90% of strains negative; +/− = variable results.

and clindamycin are not recommended. Cephalothin has also been found to be effective for therapy of wound infections due to *Pasteurella*.

29.7. Genus *Kingella*

29.7.a. Epidemiology and pathogenesis of *Kingella* infection. The three species of *Kingella*, *K. kingae*, *K. denitrificans*, and *K. indologenes*, are normal oropharyngeal flora of humans. Although the pathogenicity of *K. denitrificans* is unknown, *K. indologenes* has been isolated (rarely) from eye infections. *K. kingae*, on the other hand, has been associated with infection more often. The organism has been found as the etiologic agent of bacteremia and skin lesions, and it seems to be particularly associated with septic arthritis. Pathogenic mechanisms have not been well characterized.

29.7.b. Laboratory diagnosis. Colonies of *K. kingae* on 5% sheep blood agar are small with a clear zone of hemolysis. Initial growth may require several days of incubation. Increased CO_2 seems to enhance growth. Colony morphology may vary; one morphotype pits the agar and assumes a "fried egg" appearance with a thin, spreading haze of growth surrounding the central colony. Gram stain reveals short, plump bacilli with squared-off ends that may form chains.

K. denitrificans produces nonhemolytic colonies resembling those of *K. kingae*. One distinguishing feature is the ability of *K. denitrificans* to grow on Thayer-Martin medium (Chapters 8, 19, and 26). Because it is also oxidase positive and able to produce acid from glucose, *K. denitrificans* may be confused with *Neisseria gonorrhoeae*. Differential tests include nitrate reduction (*N. gonorrhoeae* is unable to reduce nitrate, whereas most *K. denitrificans* are nitrate positive) and inhibition of growth of *N. gonorrhoeae* by amylase. All of 52 *K. denitrificans* isolates tested by Odugbemi and Arko[6] were not inhibited from growing up to a 13 mm diameter filter paper disk impregnated with 0.05 ml diluted human saliva or alpha-amylase (Sigma Chemical Co.) when inoculated to the surface of plates made from GC agar base with IsoVitaleX (BBL Microbiology Systems).

All *Kingella* species are oxidase positive and nonmotile and able to ferment glucose. Almost all *Kingella* are catalase negative, which helps to differentiate them from *Moraxella* species and *Neisseria* species. In contrast to the other two species, *K. indologenes* is indole positive, as the name suggests. None of the species will produce acid in the butt of a triple sugar iron agar tube; they may not grow at all in that medium. Oxidative-fermentative carbohydrate media (Chapter 28) may need to be supplemented with 5% horse serum to allow sufficient growth.

29.7.c. Treatment of infections due to *Kingella*. Penicillin appears to be the drug of choice for treatment of infections due to *K. kingae*. The organism is also susceptible to gentamicin and chloramphenicol, both of which have been used to successfully treat septic arthritis. There is limited information on susceptibilities of the other two species.

29.8. DF-2

These organisms, probably normal oral flora in dogs and possibly cats, have been isolated from more than 20 cases of severe infection, often following a dog bite. Patients with underlying disorders are more likely to develop infection. The organism is usually isolated from blood or cerebrospinal fluid, but may be missed in other specimens because of its fastidious nature and slow growth rate. After 4 days or longer of incubation at 37° C in 5%-10% CO_2, pinpoint colonies appear on chocolate agar. Heart infusion agar with 5% rabbit blood may yield better growth. The organisms display a characteristic morphology of long, thin, pleomorphic gram-negative bacilli with occasional curved forms. Spindle- and cigar-shaped rods, some with tapered ends, may also be seen. The organism is catalase and oxidase positive and indole, nitrate, and urease negative. Some strains may hydrolyze esculin or produce arginine dihydrolase. The addition of 3% rabbit serum may be necessary for growth of the organism in carbohydrate broths. Alternatively, the rapid enzymatic carbohydrate tests described in Chapter 9 may be used. DF-2 is susceptible to penicillin, cephalothin, chloramphenicol, and carbenicillin but resistant to gentamicin and kanamycin.

29.9. HB-5

HB-5 is isolated from the genitourinary tract of men and women. The organism has been associated with skin infections and abscesses. It is a gram-negative coccobacillus. Growth occurs as nonhemolytic colonies on blood agar after 24 h of incubation at 37° C in 5%-10% CO_2. Oxidase is variable and catalase is not produced. The organisms are nitrate positive and weakly indole positive. A triple sugar iron agar slant inoculated with HB-5 will be uniformly yellow after overnight incubation; glucose but not sucrose or lactose is fermented.

REFERENCES

1. Carter, G.R. 1984. Genus *Pasteurella Trevisan 1887*. In Krieg, N.R., and Holt, J.G., editors. Bergey's manual of systematic bacteriology, ed. 9. Williams & Wilkins, Baltimore.
2. Corbel, M.J., and Brinley-Morgan, W.J. 1984. Genus *Brucella Meyer and Shaw 1920*. In Krieg, N.R., and Holt, J.G., editors. Bergey's manual of systematic bacteriology, ed. 9. Williams & Wilkins, Baltimore.
3. Gabre-Kidan, T., Lipsky, B., and Plorde, J.J. 1984. *Hemophilus influenzae* as a cause of urinary tract infections in men. Arch. Intern. Med. 144:1623.
4. Kilian, M. 1980. A taxonomic study of the genus *Haemophilus*, with the proposal of a new species. J. Gen. Microbiol. 93:9.
5. Kilian, M., and Biberstein, E.L. 1984. Genus *Haemophilus Winslow, Broadhurst, Buchanan, Krumwiede, Rogers and Smith 1917*. In Krieg, N.R., and Holt, J.G., editors. Bergey's manual of systematic bacteriology, ed. 9. Williams & Wilkins, Baltimore.
6. Odugbemi, T., and Arko, R.J. 1983. Differentiation of *Kingella denitrificans* from *Neisseria gonorrhoeae* by growth on a semisolid medium and sensitivity to amylase. J. Clin. Microbiol. 17:389.
7. Stauffer, L.R., Brown, D.R., and Sandstrom, R.E. 1983. Cephalexin-supplemented Jones-Kendrick charcoal agar for selective isolation of *Bordetella pertussis*: comparison with previously described media. J. Clin. Microbiol. 17:60.
8. Weaver, R.E., and Hollis, D.G. 1980. Gram-negative fermentative bacteria and *Francisella tularensis*. In Lennette, E.H., Balows, A., Hausler, W.J. Jr., and Truant, J.P., editors: Manual of clinical microbiology, ed. 3. American Society for Microbiology, Washington, D.C.

BIBLIOGRAPHY

Franklin, G.W., and Shafi, N.A. 1983. Spontaneous septic arthritis due to *Kingella kingae*. Clin. Microbiol. Newsletter 5:53.

Gay, R.M., Lane, T.W., and Keller, D.C. 1983. Septic arthritis caused by *Kingella kingae*. J. Clin. Microbiol. 17:168.

McCarthy, L.R. 1983. Identification and taxonomy of the genus *Haemophilus*. Clin. Microbiol. Newsletter 5:1.

Phillips, J.E. 1984. Genus *Actinobacillus Brumpt 1910*. In Krieg, N.R., and Holt, J.G., editors. Bergey's manual of systematic bacteriology, ed. 9. Williams & Wilkins, Baltimore.

Pittman, M. 1984. Genus *Bordetella Moreno-Lopez 1952*. In Krieg, N.R., and Holt, J.G., editors. Bergey's manual of systematic bacteriology, ed. 9. Williams & Wilkins, Baltimore.

Smith, C., and Rubin, S.J. 1983. DF-2 septicemia. Clin. Microbiol. Newsletter 5:90.

Weaver, R.E., Hollis, D.G., and Bottone, E.J. 1985. Gram-negative fermentative bacteria and *Francisella tularensis*. In Lennette, E.H., Balows, A., Hausler, W.J. Jr., and Shadomy, H.J., editors. Manual of clinical microbiology, ed. 4. American Society for Microbiology, Washington, D.C.

30

Vibrionaceae Family (*Vibrio, Aeromonas,* and *Plesiomonas*) and *Campylobacter* Species

Members of the genera *Vibrio, Campylobacter, Aeromonas,* and *Plesiomonas* have a few features in common: most of them are oxidase positive gram-negative rods, some with curved cellular morphology, and some species from each genus are the etiologic agents of diarrheal disease in humans. Species in all genera are motile by means of polar flagella, although the types of flagella and their arrangements vary. The Vibrionaceae are found in freshwater and seawater, where they are pathogenic for aquatic animals. Recovery of *Vibrio* species as the etiologic agents of diarrheal disease may require the use of special media, and for some *Campylobacter,* special atmosphere and temperature of incubation as well.

30.1. *Vibrio* Species

30.1.a. Epidemiology and pathogenesis of *Vibrio* infection. Members of the genus *Vibrio* are natural inhabitants of seawater. They are also found as normal flora on and in many aquatic animals. All organisms in this group are able to grow in media containing increased salt concentrations, and with the exception of *V. cholerae* and *V. mimicus* (the so-called **nonhalophilic vibrios**), they require sodium chloride for growth. The chloride ion–requiring members are called **halophilic vibrios.** There are nine species of clinical importance among the *Vibrio* species. Agents associated with gastroenteritis or diarrheal disease include *V. cholerae, V. parahaemolyticus, V. fluvialis, V. furnissii, V. mimicus,* and *V. hollisae. V. cholerae, V. vulnificus, V. alginolyticus, V. parahaemolyticus,* and *V. damsela* have been isolated from wound cultures or blood. *V. parahaemolyticus* and *V. alginolyticus* have also been implicated as etiologic agents of ear infections. *V. metschnikovii* has been reported from one human infection; it is not likely to be seen in a routine clinical laboratory. In the United States, in almost every case in which a *Vibrio* has been isolated from an infectious process, there has been some association with water or seafood. Although selective media are helpful for recovery of *Vibrio* from stool, the organisms grow well on routine bacteriologic media (sheep blood agar) and should not be overlooked when isolated from blood, wound cultures, or other sources as long as all gram-negative colonies are screened for oxidase production.

The enterotoxin of *V. cholerae* is one of the best characterized among bacteria (Chapter 17). It consists of three subunits, one of which serves to bind the toxin to a receptor site on the surface of the mucosal cells of the intestinal tract. The action of the toxin is to activate adenylate cyclase, which in turn raises the intracellular level of cyclic AMP, ultimately causing an active secretion of electrolytes into the intestinal lumen. The outpouring of ions is followed by a release of water. Patients with cholera have been known to secrete fluid volumes equal to their body weight within 4 days. More importantly, the loss of water can dehydrate the patient so quickly that death occurs within 12 h of onset of disease. In addition to the toxin, adherence to intestinal epithelium and motility are important factors in the pathogenicity of *V. cholerae.*

Other species of *Vibrio* produce a number of extracellular cytolytic toxins or cytotoxins and enzymes that probably contribute to their virulence. Pathogenesis of *V. vulnificus* and *V.*

parahaemolyticus infections is probably related to invasiveness. *V. parahaemolyticus* can invade colonic epithelium and produce disease that resembles dysentery. It appears that *V. parahaemolyticus* may also produce an enterotoxin, since it will produce fluid in the ligated rabbit ileal loop (described in Chapter 17).

V. vulnificus, the lactose positive halophilic vibrio, appears to have a remarkable invasive potential. Primarily in patients with underlying hepatic disease, but also in healthy patients, this organism produces a primary septicemia with 50% mortality. The organisms are assumed to enter the bloodstream via the gastrointestinal tract, usually within 24 h after ingestion of raw shellfish, particularly oysters. *V. vulnificus* also produces a cytotoxin, which may contribute to its virulence. Wound infections with *V. vulnificus* may also lead to septicemia. Infections caused by *V. vulnificus* have been reported primarily from coastal states.

30.1.b. Isolation of *Vibrio* species from feces. Fecal specimens received in microbiology laboratories in the United States are not routinely inoculated to media selective for vibrios due to the low incidence of *Vibrio*-related gastroenteritis in the U.S. If a patient with diarrheal disease has a history of having consumed shellfish or had other contact with seawater, vibrios should be considered. Stool should be transported in Cary-Blair transport media (Chapters 6 and 17) if it cannot be plated to selective agar immediately. Plating onto 5% sheep blood agar will also adequately support the growth of *Vibrio* species. The most commonly used selective agar is thiosulfate citrate–bile salts–sucrose agar (TCBS; Chapter 45), which can be heavily inoculated. An evaluation of dry powder TCBS from four different commercial manufacturers by West, et al.[9] showed media produced by Oxoid Ltd. in England to perform consistently better for isolation and typical colony morphology formation than three other media tested. (Oxoid distributes in the United States under Oxoid USA, Inc.) Conventional selective enteric agars (Chapter 8) should be inoculated, of course, for isolation of other possible etiologic agents (Chapter 17). All vibrios will grow on nonselective media, but their colonies will not be distinctive enough to ensure their detection in mixed flora containing large numbers of other bacteria unless some screening procedure (such as oxidase) is used. In very dilute, typical "rice water" stools of cholera, vibrios are present in large numbers, often to the exclusion of much of the normal flora. An enrichment broth particularly useful for detection of small numbers of *V. cholerae* is alkaline peptone water (pH 8.4, Chapter 45). This broth should be subcultured to selective media (TCBS) as soon as possible after 8 h incubation (at 35° C) to prevent overgrowth of other bacteria. For optimal isolation of the halophilic vibrios, selective enteric media, except for TCBS, should be supplemented with 3% NaCl; this is not necessary, however, since these organisms do grow in brain heart infusion broth and on blood agar without added salt. If colonies are tested for oxidase positivity, vibrios will be detected.

30.1.c. Laboratory identification of vibrios. After 18-24 h incubation at 35° C in air, sucrose-fermenting vibrios (*V. cholerae, V. alginolyticus,* and *V. fluvialis*) will appear as medium-sized, smooth, opaque, thin-edged yellow colonies on TCBS agar (Plate 30.1). The other clinically important vibrios do not ferment sucrose and will appear olive-green (Plate 30.2). When *V. cholerae* is suspected, the enrichment broth may be examined under phase or darkfield microscopy (Chapter 7) for the presence of small rods with characteristic darting motility. If the motility is inhibited by adding one drop of polyvalent *V. cholerae* 01 typing sera, the organism can be presumptively identified.

On Gram stain, vibrios are small gram-negative bacilli that may occasionally exhibit slightly curved forms (Figure 30.1). Morphol-

FIGURE 30.1
Gram stain of smear made from *Vibrio cholerae* colony on TCBS agar.

ogy cannot be used for identification. Oxidase positive fermentative organisms isolated from wound cultures, blood, and other sources may be vibrios, and biochemical tests should be performed. Most of the commercially produced biotyping systems will identify *Vibrio* species. Except for *V. metschnikovii*, all vibrios are oxidase positive. The halophilic vibrios may require the addition of increased (up to 3%) NaCl to all identification media and prepackaged commercial systems (Chapter 9) in order to display proper reactions. Systems that utilize a saline suspension of the inoculum are likely to support the growth of some of the clinically important vibrios without added salt. Identification procedures are no different than those used for other gram-negative bacilli. Key differential characteristics of the more commonly isolated clinically relevant vibrios are listed in Table 30.1.

V. cholerae of serotypes 01 and non-01 both cause cholera-like disease, although only serotype 01 is associated with epidemic disease. These two serotypes are biochemically identical but differ in their ability to agglutinate in *V. cholerae* 01 antiserum. Non-01 vibrios have been associated with large outbreaks, however, often characterized by septicemic disease. In the United States, the occasional isolate of *V. cholerae* is likely to be nontypable (nonagglutinable in 01 typing serum). Almost all *V. cholerae* and many other *Vibrio* species (with the exceptions of *V. parahaemolyticus* and *V. alginolyticus*) will release DNA in the presence of 0.5% sodium deoxycholate in water. This test is similar to the potassium hydroxide (KOH) test for identification of gram-negative organisms (described in Chapter 9). A suspension of the organism is emulsified in a drop of the deoxycholate reagent on a slide. When the loop is gently lifted, a mucuslike string of material is formed. This "string test" helps to presumptively identify vibrio isolates. Although there is no genetic basis for a division, *V. cholerae* have been divided into two biovars or bio-

types, **classical** and **eltor** (formerly El Tor). The eltor biovar is Voges-Proskauer positive, will agglutinate chicken red blood cells, and is resistant to a 300 U disk of polymyxin B; whereas the classical biovar yields the opposite reactions. Many recently isolated eltor biovars are nonhemolytic on sheep blood agar, in contrast to the typical beta hemolysis displayed by organisms of this biovar that were isolated several years ago.

Oxidase positive organisms that may be confused with vibrios include *Aeromonas* species, *Plesiomonas* species, and *Pseudomonas* species. Key differential characteristics are outlined in Table 30.2. One important test to differentiate vibrios from *Aeromonas* species (discussed below), which they closely resemble, is susceptibility to the vibriostatic agent 2,4-diamino-6,7-diisopropylpteridine phosphate (0/129). This agent, available as 10 μg and 150 μg disks (or powder) from Oxoid USA inhibits the growth of all vibrios at a concentration of 150 μg/ml or greater. *Aeromonas*, Enterobacteriaceae, and *Pseudomonas* species are resistant. Differential susceptibilities of *Vibrio* species to 0/129 and other key features aiding in the identification of *Vibrio* species and phenotypically related organisms are shown in Table 30.2. Of organisms likely to be confused with vibrios, essentially all *Plesiomonas* species are susceptible to 0/129 at 10 μg and all are susceptible to 0/129 at 150 μg. *Plesiomonas* fail to grow in 6% salt; all the vibrios except certain *V. mimicus* and *V. cholerae* strains are able to grow in media containing 6% salt.

30.1.d Treatment of vibrio disease. Cholera is best treated with fluid and electrolyte replacement, although tetracycline or furazolidone will shorten the course of disease and may decrease bacterial excretion. In areas of the world where cholera is endemic, such as Bangladesh, tetracycline resistance is common. The decision whether to treat a patient with antimicrobial agents depends on demographic, economic, and clinical factors, including the

TABLE 30.1
Differential Characteristics of Some Vibrios Likely to be Recovered from Clinical Specimens*

SPECIES	GROWTH IN NaCl					VOGES-PROSKAUER	LYSINE DECAR-BOXYLASE	ORNITHINE DECAR-BOXYLASE	LACTOSE	SUCROSE	SALICIN
	0%	3%	6%	8%	10%						
V. alginolyticus	-	+	+	+	+	+	+	+/-	-	+	-
V. cholerae	+	+	+/-	-	-	+/-	+	+	-	+	-
V. damsela	-	+	+	-	-	+	+/-	-	-	-	-
V. fluvialis	-	+	+	+/-	+/-	-	-	-	-	+	+
V. furnissii	-	+	+	+/-	-	-	-	-	-	+	-
V. hollisae	-	+	+	-	-	-	-	-	-	-	-
V. mimicus	+	+	+/-	-	-	-	+	+	-	-	-
V. parahaemolyticus	-	+	+	+	-	-	+	+/-	-	-	-
V. vulnificus	-	+	+	-	-	-	+	+/-	+	-	+

*+ = ≥90% positive; - = ≥90% negative; +/- = variable results; ND = test not done.

TABLE 30.2
Key Characteristics of Oxidase Positive Fermentative Gram-Negative Bacilli*

CHARACTERISTIC	AEROMONAS	PLESIOMONAS	VIBRIO
Susceptible to 0/129			
10 μg	−	+/−	+/−
150 μg	−	+	+
Acid from			
Inositol	−	+	−
Mannitol	+	−	+
Sucrose	+	−	+/−
Gelatin liquefaction	+	−	+
Requires or stimulated by Na$^+$	−	−	+

*+ = most strains positive; − = most strains negative; +/− = variable results.

nutritional status of the patient. There have been ampicillin-, trimethoprim-sulfamethoxazole-, and tetracycline-resistant isolates reported from the developed world as well, so a susceptibility test should be performed. The agar disk diffusion test is adequate; Mueller-Hinton agar will support the growth of halophilic and nonhalophilic vibrios; salt should not be added, as it alters the activity of certain antimicrobial agents. Most strains of *V. parahaemolyticus, V. alginolyticus, V. damsela, V. vulnificus,* and *V. hollisae* are susceptible to gentamicin, tetracycline, and chloramphenicol. Ampicillin and sulfonamide susceptibilities vary.

30.2. *Campylobacter* Species

30.2.a. Epidemiology and pathogenesis of *Campylobacter* infection. *Campylobacter* species are microaerophilic inhabitants of the gastrointestinal tracts of a number of animals, including poultry, dogs, cats, sheep, and cattle, as well as the reproductive organs of several animal species. *Campylobacter venerealis* is found only in cattle, *C. fetus* subsp. *fetus* is found in cattle and sheep (occasional infections have occurred through secondary human transmission), *C. coli* is found in pigs, *C. laridis* is normal flora in seagulls, and *C. jejuni* is found extensively in warm-blooded animals (primarily birds). When fecal samples from chicken carcasses chosen at random from butcher shops in the New York City area were tested for *Campylobacter,* 83% of the samples yielded over 10^6 colony forming units per gram of feces. The *Campylobacter* species associated with most human infections are usually transmitted via contaminated food, milk, or water. Outbreaks have been associated with contaminated drinking water and consumption of improperly pasteurized milk, among other sources. In contrast to other agents of foodborne gastroenteritis, including *Salmonella* and staphylococci, *Campylobacter* does not multiply in food. Among homosexual populations, *Campylobacter* is thought to be transmitted sexually, as are other agents of gastroenteritis (Chapter 23). Quinn et al.[6] have reported a number of isolates of *Campylobacter*-like organisms from stool of homosexual men with gastroenteritis; their etiologic significance is unknown. The names *Campylobacter cinaedi* and *Campylobacter fennelliae* have been proposed for these organisms.[7]

Species of *Campylobacter* produce two primary syndromes in humans: (1) systemic disease characterized by fever and (2) gastroenteritis. There are four species that are likely to be recovered as the etiologic agents of human disease. *C. jejuni, C. laridis,* and *C. coli* are associated with gastroenteritis. *C. fetus* subsp.

fetus has been isolated from blood of patients with septicemia, as a cause of meningitis, abscesses, other infections, and occasionally from feces of patients with gastroenteritis. *Campylobacter pyloridis* has also been implicated in upper gastrointestinal disease. Catalase negative species, *C. sputorum* subsp. *sputorum* and *C. concisus*, have been isolated from animals and from human gingival crevices, but they have not been implicated in human disease. *C. sputorum* subsp. *mucosalis* and *bubulus* and catalase positive *C. fetus* subsp. *venerealis*, *C. hyointestinalis*, and others have been found only in animals.

Since most laboratories in the United States have begun to process stools from patients with diarrhea specifically for isolation of *Campylobacter* species, it has been recognized as the most common etiologic agent of gastroenteritis. In the laboratory of one of us (EJB), *C. jejuni* is isolated from 17% of all stools submitted for culture. *Salmonella* species, the next most common isolate, is found in 10% of all positive stool cultures.

Campylobacter species seem to possess several virulence factors (Chapter 17). The production of bloody diarrhea, characterized by the presence of numerous polymorphonuclear neutrophils, in patients with gastroenteritis and the appearance of certain strains of *Campylobacter* in the blood of patients after ingestion of contaminated material, are indicative of the invasive capacity of the organism. *Campylobacter* species are known to produce a cytotoxin and an enterotoxin, which may account for those cases characterized by watery diarrhea. The actual importance of toxin production in development of disease is not known.

Although 97% of patients with diarrhea due to *C. jejuni* cease excreting the organism within 4-7 weeks even without treatment, the remaining patients continue to carry the organism for long periods of time (1 to several years). Therefore, *C. jejuni* may be recovered from stool specimens in which it is not the etiologic agent of diarrhea. Carriers of *C. jejuni* are far more common in tropical countries than in the United States. Increased prevalence of infection in tropical countries results in an endemic level of mild disease, probably due to herd immunity.

30.2.b. Laboratory isolation of *Campylobacter fetus* subsp. *fetus*. *C. fetus* subsp. *fetus* will grow in most blood culture media, although it may require as long as 2 weeks for growth to be detected. Subcultures from broths must be incubated in a microaerophilic atmosphere or the organisms will not multiply. There is often no visible turbidity in blood culture media, therefore blind subcultures or visual examination using acridine orange stain (detailed in Chapter 14) is necessary. The presence of *Campylobacter* species in blood cultures is detected effectively by radiometric monitoring (Bactec system, Chapters 11 and 14). Isolation from sources other than blood or feces (extremely rare) is ideally accomplished by inoculating the material (tissue, wound exudate, etc.) to a blood agar plate and incubating the plate at 37° C in a CO_2-enriched, microaerophilic atmosphere, as described below. Isolation of *C. fetus* subsp. *fetus* from stool may be attempted by inoculating a selective medium without cephalosporins and incubating for 48 h at 37° C microaerophilically. Skirrow's medium, containing blood agar base, 5% lysed horse blood, vancomycin (10 mg/liter), polymyxin (2,500 U/liter) and trimethoprim (5 mg/liter) would adequately support growth of *C. fetus* from stool. *C. fetus* subsp. *fetus* is inhibited by cephalosporins; they should not be included in selective media used for isolation of this species.

30.2.c. Isolation of *C. jejuni*, *C. coli*, and *C. laridis* from feces. The three agents of gastroenteritis are able to grow well at 42° C, a characteristic which is useful for their initial isolation. There is not an increased number of colonies at this temperature, but the colonies are larger and the growth of most normal fecal

25.1

25.2

25.3

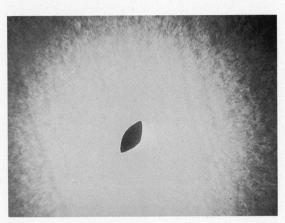

25.4

PLATE 25.1. Nutritionally variant streptococci growing as satelliting colonies surrounding growth of *Staphylococcus aureus.*

PLATE 25.2. Alpha hemolysis surrounding the elliptical subsurface colony of an isolate of viridans streptococcus growing in a pour plate of 5% sheep blood agar, as seen by examining the colony microscopically under low power (100 × magnification). Notice that the red blood cells are intact.

PLATE 25.3. Wide zone alpha hemolysis surrounding the elliptical subsurface colony of a streptococcus growing in a pour plate of 5% sheep blood agar, as seen by observing the colony microscopically under low power (100 × magnification). Notice that there is a narrow zone of intact red blood cells, seen as a red haze, immediately surrounding the colony and a wider zone containing no intact red cells extending further out from the colony.

PLATE 25.4. Beta hemolysis surrounding the elliptical subsurface colony of a beta hemolytic streptococcus growing in a pour plate of 5% sheep blood agar, as seen by observing the colony microscopically under low power (100 × magnification). Notice that there are no intact red blood cells in the vicinity of the colony.

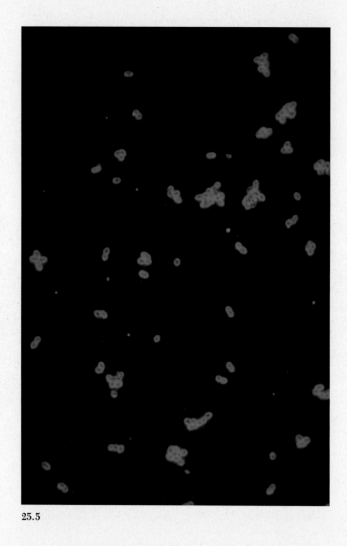

25.5

PLATE 25.5. Group A streptococci stained with fluorescein-conjugated anti-group A antibody, examined with ultraviolet light under oil immersion (1,000 × magnification). Notice that the organisms stain as rings, with dark centers.

25.6

25.7

POSITIVE FOR GROUP A BETA STREP

25.8

PLATE 25.6. The PYR test (E-Y Laboratories). A portion of a colony is rubbed onto the substrate-impregnated filter paper strip and a drop of the color reagent is added. The development of a red color (strip on the right) indicates a positive test; only group A streptococci and enterococci possess the enzyme, pyroglutamyl aminopeptidase.

PLATE 25.7. The CAMP test for presumptive identification of group B streptococci. The S. *agalactiae* (group B streptococcus) streaked down the right side of the plate exhibits the enhanced zone of hemolysis in an "arrow" shape near the S. *aureus* streak. The beta hemolytic streptococcal isolates streaked down the left and center of the test plate are not group B.

PLATE 25.8. Placement of a bacitracin disk and a trimethoprim-sulfamethoxazole disk next to each other in the primary inoculated area of a throat culture plated to 5% sheep blood agar. The sulfa drug inhibits most normal flora and the bacitracin inhibits group A beta streptococci.

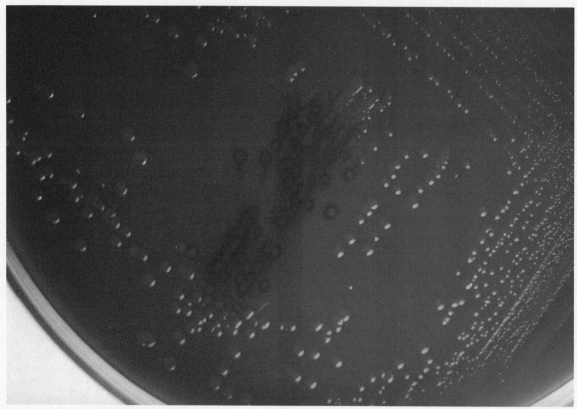

26.1

PLATE 26.1.   Colonies of *Neisseria* species on Thayer-Martin agar after addition of oxidase reagent. Oxidase positive organisms turn purple within several seconds.

27.1

27.2

PLATE 27.1. A pigmented *Serratia marcescens* species.
PLATE 27.2. Colonies of lactose-fermenting (pink) and non-lactose-fermenting (colorless) gram-negative bacilli on MacConkey agar.

27.3

27.4

27.5

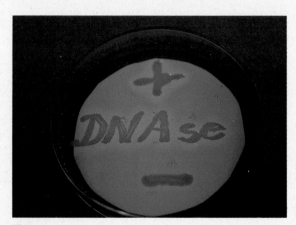

27.6

PLATE 27.3. Indole test; positive result is visible as a red to pink ring around the top of the tube where the reagents float. A negative test is seen as no change in color of the reagents.

PLATE 27.4. Citrate utilization as shown by color change from green to blue on Simmon's citrate agar.

PLATE 27.5. Fermentation of glucose with the production of gas, as seen by the bubble that has collected in the inverted Durham tube in the tube on the right. The organism in the tube on the left does not ferment glucose at all, as evidenced by a lack of change of the pH indicator to yellow.

PLATE 27.6. DNAse test agar containing methyl green indicator. Organisms that produce DNAse are identified by production of a clear zone (hydrolysis of DNA and subsequent breakdown of the indicator) surrounding growth of the organism after overnight incubation.

28.1

28.2

PLATE 28.1. Commercially produced O-F media that incorporates both tests into one tube (Flow Diagnostics).

PLATE 28.2. Bacteria stained with the flagella stain demonstrating peritrichous flagella.

28.3

28.4

PLATE 28.3. Strong beta hemolysis exhibited by most strains of *Pseudomonas aeruginosa*.
PLATE 28.4. Two different pyocyanin-producing strains of *Pseudomonas aeruginosa* and a control plate with no growth.

28.5

28.6

PLATE 28.5. The two outer tubes were inoculated with fluorescing strains of pseudomonads; the central tube is the uninoculated control. Photograph taken under ultraviolet light.

PLATE 28.6. *Pseudomonas maltophilia* growing on 5% sheep blood and MacConkey agars.

28.7

28.8

PLATE 28.7. Colonies of *Pseudomonas pseudomallei* after 96 h of incubation on blood agar.
PLATE 28.8. Dry, wrinkled colonies of *Pseudomonas stutzeri* on blood agar after 48 h of incubation.

28.9

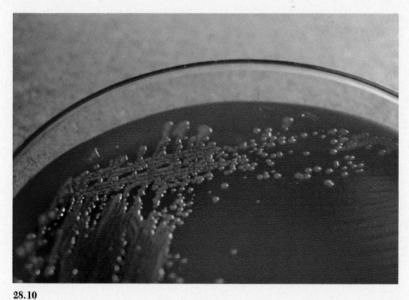

28.10

PLATE 28.9.   Colonies of *Acinetobacter calcoaceticus* on blood and MacConkey agars.
PLATE 28.10.   Yellow-pigmented colonies of *Flavobacterium* species on blood agar.

29.1

29.2

PLATE 29.1. Colonies of *Bordetella pertussis* resembling mercury drops on Bordet-Gengou agar after 48 h incubation.

PLATE 29.2. Satelliting colonies of *Haemophilus influenzae*. The chocolate agar plate on the right and the sheep blood agar plate on the left were both streaked with a similar inoculum. Colonies of the *Haemophilus* are visible as satelliting colonies surrounding the *Staphylococcus aureus* streaked across several quadrants of the sheep blood agar plate.

29.3

29.4

PLATE 29.3. Gram stain of cerebrospinal fluid containing many polymorphonuclear leukocytes and *Haemophilus influenzae*. Note both coccobacilli and long filamentous forms.

PLATE 29.4. Colony of *Haemophilus aphrophilus* on heart infusion agar. Note opaque central area.

29.5

29.6

PLATE 29.5. Colony of *Actinobacillus actinomycetemcomitans* on heart infusion agar. Note the central star-shaped structure.
PLATE 29.6. Susceptibility of *Pasteurella multocida* to a 2-unit penicillin disk.

30.1

30.2

PLATE 30.1.   Colonies of *Vibrio cholerae* on TCBS agar.
PLATE 30.2.   Colonies of *Vibrio parahaemolyticus* on TCBS agar.

31.1

PLATE 31.1. Appearance of *Treponema pallidum* in darkfield preparation.

flora is inhibited. Feces may be transported to the laboratory directly for inoculation onto media. If a delay of longer than 2 h is anticipated, material should be placed either in Cary-Blair transport medium (Chapter 17) or in Campythio—a thioglycolate broth base with 0.16% agar and vancomycin (10 mg/liter), trimethoprim (5 mg/liter), cephalothin (15 mg/liter), polymyxin B (2,500 U/liter), and amphotericin B (2 mg/liter). The same antimicrobial agents are incorporated into *Brucella* agar base with 10% sheep blood to produce Campy-BAP, one of the selective agars that is useful for cultivation of these strains. A number of media manufacturers produce commercial plates for *Campylobacter* isolation.

The stool should be plated onto a selective agar. All plates are incubated at 42° C in a microaerophilic atmosphere. The atmosphere can be generated in several ways. One of the least expensive and most ingenious has been recommended by Kaplan and others.[3] The inoculated plates are placed in a plastic bag (Poly Bag, Levine Brothers Paper Co., Chicago), taking up half the volume. The technologist holds his or her breath for 10 seconds and then exhales through a 10 ml pipette (around which the opening of the bag is tightly wrapped) until the bag is full. The pipette is pulled out, and the bag is sealed with a rubber band. This method is useful especially if no other methods are available (approximately 15% of possible isolates will not be recovered). Another inexpensive method for generating a microaerophilic atmosphere was reported by Pennie and others,[4] described in Procedure 30.1.

Other methods for creating the atmosphere necessary for optimum growth of *Campylobacter* species include evacuation and replacement of the atmosphere in a plastic bag with commercially purchased gas (85% nitrogen, 10% CO_2, and 5% O_2); use of the Campy Bio-Bag Cfj system (Marion Scientific); or the Campy Pak, a gas generator and catalyst system used in a sealed plastic jar, similar to the anaerobic atmosphere system (GasPak) marketed by BBL Microbiology Systems.

Plates should be examined at 24 and 48 h for characteristic colonies, which are gray to pinkish or yellowish gray, slightly mucoid-look-

---

PROCEDURE 30.1 CREATION OF MICROAEROPHILIC ATMOSPHERE FOR ISOLATION OF *CAMPYLOBACTER* SPECIES FROM FECES

1. Prepare a solution of 2.5% copper sulfate ($CuSO_4$) in water. Keep this solution in a wide-mouth bottle.
2. Place four inoculated plates into a plastic bag (21 × 38 cm; Poly Bags, Levine Brothers Paper Co., Chicago).
3. Place two plastic or paper medicine cups into the bag.
4. Into one cup, place a 1.5 g wad of fine steel wool (grade 0) that was briefly soaked in the copper sulfate solution and allowed to drain on a facial tissue.
5. Into the other cup, place 10 ml of water, and right before the bag is closed, drop one Alka-Seltzer tablet (Miles Laboratories) into the water.
6. Quickly squeeze excess air from the bag and close it by twisting the opening and securing it.

Modified from Pennie, et al. 1984. J. Clin. Microbiol. **20**:320.

ing colonies; some colonies may exhibit a tailing effect along the streak line (Figure 30.2).

30.2.d. Laboratory identification of *Campylobacter* species. Suspicious-looking colonies seen on selective media incubated at 42° C may be presumptively identified with a few simple tests. A wet preparation of the organism may be examined under phase or darkfield microscopy (Chapter 7) for characteristic darting motility and curved forms. On Gram stain, the organisms are small, curved, or seagull-winged gram-negative rods (Figure 30.3). All *C. jejuni* and *C. coli* are oxidase and catalase positive, whereas *C. laridis* may be oxidase negative. *C. laridis* has been isolated from humans only rarely, however.

The most common isolate is *C. jejuni;* an organism may be presumptively designated as "*C. jejuni* group" if it meets the minimal criteria: isolation from feces on selective agar incubated at 42° C, oxidase and catalase positive, typical Gram morphology, and darting motility. *C. laridis* may be differentiated from the other two species by its resistance to nalidixic acid. Nalidixic acid susceptibility can be tested by inoculating a 5% sheep blood agar plate or a Mueller-Hinton agar plate with a suspension of the organism, as is done for performance of

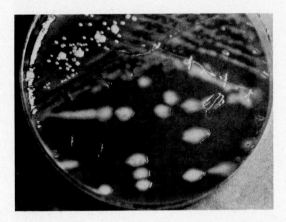

FIGURE 30.2
Campylobacter jejuni growing on a Campy blood agar plate after 48 h of incubation.

FIGURE 30.3
Gram stain appearance of *Campylobacter jejuni* smeared from primary isolation plate. Note seagull-shaped and curved forms.

agar disk diffusion susceptibility testing (Chapter 13), and placing a 30 μg disk on the agar surface. *C. jejuni* and *C. coli* are susceptible to nalidixic acid, yielding a zone of inhibition around the disk after overnight incubation at 37° C. Once these organisms have been isolated, they may be incubated at 37° C for further testing. *C. coli* and *C. jejuni* can be differentiated with the rapid hippurate hydrolysis test described in Chapter 25. A commercial rapid hippurate disk test (Chapter 9) is also available (Remel Laboratories). Tests useful in identifying the species of *Campylobacter* commonly isolated from clinical specimens are summarized in Table 30.3.

30.2.e. Treatment of campylobacterial disease. Erythromycin is the drug of choice for those patients with complicated gastroenteritis (hyperpyrexia, dehydration, or bacteremia). For patients with bacteremia, therapy is continued for 4 weeks. Gastroenteritis is usually treated for 10 days. Tetracycline is an alternative choice in the United States, although 15%-20% of strains are resistant; children under 7 years should be given clindamycin. The organisms are susceptible to gentamicin, other aminoglycosides, chloramphenicol, cefotaxime, and ciprofloxacin.

30.3. *Aeromonas* Species

30.3.a. Epidemiology and pathogenesis of *Aeromonas* infection. *Aeromonas* are ubiquitous inhabitants of natural waters, both fresh and salt, where they infect animals, including amphibians, reptiles, and fish. In humans, they are most commonly associated with infections of wounds acquired near or in water, or with diarrheal disease. *A. salmonicida* is not associated with disease in humans, in contrast to the three other species, *A. hydrophila, A. sobria,* and *A. caviae. Aeromonas* species have been recovered from blood, cerebrospinal fluid, exudate from otitis media, urine, peritoneal fluid, necrotic muscle, infected heart valves, and bone. *A. hydrophila* and *A. sobria* are more likely to be associated with gastrointestinal disease, whereas *A. caviae* usually is associated with wound infections. *A. caviae* is rarely isolated from blood, suggesting that it is less virulent.

It has been shown that *A. hydrophila* produces a heat-labile enterotoxin and a cytotoxin. Some species have been found to adhere to intestinal epithelial cells. *Aeromonas* also produce a large number of extracellular enzymes, including protease, amylase, lipase, nuclease, and others. The role of these enzymes in the pathogenesis of *Aeromonas* infections, if any, has not been defined.

30.3.b. Laboratory identification. The *Aeromonas* species grow on standard laboratory media, including blood agar and MacConkey agar. They would be identified as would any other gram-negative bacillus isolated from a

TABLE 30.3
Differential Characteristics of Clinically Relevant *Campylobacter* Species*

SPECIES	GROWTH AT			HIPPURATE HYDROLYSIS	SUSCEPTIBLE TO NALIDIXIC ACID	SUSCEPTIBLE TO CEPHALOTHIN
	25° C	37° C	42° C			
C. jejuni	−	+	+	+	+	−
C. coli	−	+	+	−	+	−
C. laridis	−	+	+	−	−	ND
C. fetus						
subsp. *fetus*	+	+	−	−	−	+

Modified from Buck, G.E. 1984. Recent taxonomic changes in the genus *Campylobacter.* Clin. Microbiol. Newsletter 6:119.

*+ = most strains positive; − = most strains negative; ND = not done.

source such as a sterile body fluid, tissue, or wound. On Gram stain, the cells are straight-sided, medium-sized, nonpleomorphic gram-negative bacilli (Figure 30.4). Recognition of *Aeromonas* species as etiologic agents of diarrhea, however, is more difficult, since many strains ferment lactose and sucrose and would not be distinctive enough to recognize on MacConkey agar. The selective media commonly used to detect *Salmonella*, *Shigella*, and *Campylobacter* species are inhibitory to some *Aeromonas*. Many *Aeromonas* are beta hemolytic on 5% sheep blood agar, allowing one to choose colonies to screen for the presence of oxidase by the Kovac's method (Chapter 9). Nonhemolytic colonies should be screened as well. All members of the Vibrionaceae family are oxidase positive, and they can be differentiated from oxidase-positive pseudomonads by the spot indole test (Chapter 9). *Pseudomonas* species are all indole negative, whereas most Vibrionaceae are indole positive. In our laboratory (EJB) we test a sweep loopful of organisms on the primary blood agar plate for oxidase production. If a predominance of non-pseudomonas-appearing oxidase positive colonies are found on the blood agar plate inoculated with diarrheal stool, the possibility of *Aeromonas* should be further explored. Von Graevenitz and Bucher[8] discussed the value of several selective media that have been used for isolation of *Aeromonas* and *Plesiomonas*. None of the commercially available media was satisfactory. Recently, however, we and others have noticed that CIN agar, used to select for *Yersinia enterocolitica* (Chapter 45), supports the growth of many strains of *Aeromonas*, while it inhibits growth of most nonpathogenic fecal flora. Further studies on the use of this medium for isolation of *Aeromonas* from feces are in progress. Media containing ampicillin are also useful for selective isolation of *Aeromonas*.

Aeromonas are distinguished from the Enterobacteriaceae, which they closely resemble both morphologically and biochemically, by the oxidase test; Enterobacteriaceae are oxidase negative. *Aeromonas* are differentiated from oxidase positive vibrios by their resistance to the vibriostatic agent 0/129 (Table 30.2). Table 30.4 outlines differentiation of the three *Aeromonas* species pathogenic for humans, as well as the closely related *Plesiomonas shigelloides*. The commercial biochemical and enzymatic identification systems routinely used for characterization of Enterobacteriaceae (Chapter 9) will identify *Aeromonas* and *Plesiomonas*, at least to genus, with the addition of the oxidase test result to the profile number generated. We have found, however, that at least one widely used system (API 20E, Analytab Products) does not distinguish between *Aeromonas* and certain *Vibrio* species and that the performance of the 0/129 test is critical.

30.3.c. Treatment of *Aeromonas* infections. *Aeromonas*-associated diarrhea is usually self-limited and normally does not require treatment. For protracted diarrhea and more severe infections, several antimicrobial agents are effective. The organisms are susceptible to gentamicin, trimethoprim-sulfamethoxazole, third generation cephalosporins, and chloramphenicol. They are resistant to streptomycin and penicillins.

30.4. *Plesiomonas* Species

There is only one species of *Plesiomonas*, *P. shigelloides*. The species resembles *Aeromonas*, although it is not beta hemolytic. *Plesiomonas* also maintains a water habitat and is carried asymptomatically by a large number of aquatic and other animals. The organism causes wound infections and has been isolated as the etiologic agent of meningitis, septic arthritis, cholecystitis and, most commonly, diarrhea. The pathogenesis of diarrhea associated with *Plesiomonas* has not been conclusively established. It is possible that the organism produces an enterotoxin.

Gram-stained colonies may reveal long filamentous forms as well as regular bacilli. Al-

FIGURE 30.4
Gram stain appearance of *Aeromonas hydrophila* smeared from blood agar. Note the even, straight-sided rods, compared with the more pleomorphic, slightly curved *Vibrio* species in Figure 30.1.

TABLE 30.4
Key Differential Characteristics of *Aeromonas* Species (Isolated from Humans) and *Plesiomonas shigelloides**

SPECIES	ESCULIN HYDROLYSIS	LYSINE DECARBOXYLASE	VOGES-PROSKAUER	GAS FROM GLUCOSE
A. hydrophila	+	+	+	+
A. caviae	+	−	−	−
A. sobria	−	+	+	+
P. shigelloides	−	+	−	−

*Data from Janda[2] and Popoff.[5]

though the colonies are not distinctive from Enterobacteriaceae on MacConkey agar, they are oxidase positive and may be detected in the same manner as *Aeromonas* colonies. Both lactose-fermenting and non-lactose-fermenting strains exist, exhibiting lactose positive and lactose negative colonies on MacConkey agar. *P. shigelloides* is identified biochemically, as outlined in Table 30.4.

As with *Aeromonas*, only patients with underlying disease or very severe infections should be treated. Patients treated with tetracycline or trimethoprim-sulfamethoxazole have recovered from *Plesiomonas* infection. Chloramphenicol and aminoglycosides are active against *Plesiomonas* in vitro. All isolates have been resistant to penicillin, ampicillin, and carbenicillin.

REFERENCES

1. Buck, G.E. 1984. Recent taxonomic changes in the genus *Campylobacter*. Clin. Microbiol. Newsletter 6:119.
2. Janda, J.M. 1985. Biochemical and exoenzymatic properties of *Aeromonas* spp. Diagn. Microbiol. Infect. Dis. 3:223.
3. Kaplan, R.L., Barrett, J.E., and Goodman, L.J. 1983. Monograph: *Campylobacter*, supplement. Marion Scientific, Kansas City, Mo.
4. Pennie, R.A., Zunino, J.N., Rose, C.E., Jr., and Guerrant, R.L. 1984. Economical, simple method for production of the gaseous environment required for cultivation of *Campylobacter jejuni*. J. Clin. Microbiol. 20:320.
5. Popoff, M. 1984. Genus *Aeromonas Kluyver and Van Niels 1936*. In Krieg, N.R., and Holt, J.G., editors. Bergey's manual of systematic bacteriology. ed. 9. Williams & Wilkins, Baltimore.
6. Quinn, T.C., Goodell, S.E., Fennell, C., et al. 1984. Infections with *Campylobacter jejuni* and *Campylobacter*-like organisms in homosexual men. Ann. Intern. Med. 101:187.
7. Totten, P.A., Fennell, C.L., Tenover, F.C., et al. 1985. *Campylobacter cinaedi* (sp. nov.) and *Campylobacter fennelliae* (sp. nov.): two new *Campylobacter* species associated with enteric disease in homosexual men. J. Infect. Dis. 151:131.
8. von Graevenitz, A., and Bucher, C. 1983. Evaluation of differential and selective media for isolation of *Aeromonas* and *Plesiomonas* spp. from human feces. J. Clin. Microbiol. 17:16.
9. West, P.A., Russek, E., Brayton, P.R., and Colwell, R.R. 1982. Statistical evaluation of a quality control method for isolation of pathogenic *Vibrio* species on selected thiosulfate-citrate-bile salts-sucrose agars. J. Clin. Microbiol. 16:1110.

BIBLIOGRAPHY

Baumann, P., and Schubert, R.H.W. 1984. Vibrionaceae. In Krieg, N.R., and Holt, J.G., editors. Bergey's manual of systematic bacteriology. ed. 9. Williams & Wilkins, Baltimore.

Blake, P.A., Merson, M.H., Weaver, R.E., Hollis, D.G., and Heublein, P.C. 1979. Disease caused by a marine vibrio: clinical characteristics and epidemiology. N. Engl. J. Med. 300:1.

Claesson, B.E., Holmlund, D.E., Lindhagen, C.A., and Matzsch, T.W. 1984. *Plesiomonas shigelloides* in acute cholecystitis: a case report. J. Clin. Microbiol. 20:985.

Clarridge, J.E., and Zighelboim-Daum, S. 1985. Isolation and characterization of two hemolytic phenotypes of *Vibrio damsela* associated with a fatal wound infection. J. Clin. Microbiol. 21:302.

Desmond, E.P., Janda, J.M., Adams, F.I., and Bottone, E.J. 1984. Comparative studies and laboratory diagnosis of *Vibrio vulnificus* and invasive *Vibrio* species. J. Clin. Microbiol. 19:122.

Fekety, R. 1983. Recent advances in management of bacterial diarrhea. Rev. Infect. Dis. 5:246.

Fliegelman, R.M., Petrak, R.M., Goodman, L.J., et al. 1985. Comparative in vitro activities of twelve antimicrobial agents against *Campylobacter* species. Antimicrob. Ag. Chemother. 27:429.

Gilardi, G.L. 1983. *Aeromonas* and *Plesiomonas*. Clin. Microbiol. Newsletter 5:49.

Holmberg, S.D., and Farmer, J.J. III. 1984. *Aeromonas hydrophila* and *Plesiomonas shigelloides* as causes of intestinal infections. Rev. Infect. Dis. 6:633.

Janda, J.M., Reitano, M., and Bottone, E.J. 1984. Biotyping of *Aeromonas* isolates as a correlate to delineating species-associated disease spectrum. J. Clin. Microbiol. 19:44.

Karnaugh, L. 1984. *Vibrio vulnificus:* Neptune's revenge? Diagn. Med. 7:21.

Kelly, M.T. 1982. *Vibrio vulnificus*. Check sample Microbiology No. MB 82-5 (MB-120). American Society of Clinical Pathologists, North Chicago.

Popoff, M., and Veron, M. 1976. A taxonomic study of the *Aeromonas hydrophila-Aeromonas punctata* group. J. Gen. Microbiol. 94:11.

Rennels, M.B., Levine, M.M., Daya, V., Angle, P., and Young, C. 1980. Selective vs. nonselective media and direct plating vs. enrichment technique in isolation of *Vibrio cholerae*: recommendations for clinical laboratories. J. Infect. Dis. 142:328.

Rolston, K.V., and Hopfer, R.L. 1984. Diarrhea due to *Plesiomonas shigelloides* in cancer patients. J. Clin. Microbiol. 20:597.

Roop, R.M. II, Smibert, R., and Krieg, N.R. 1984. Improved biotyping schemes for *Campylobacter jejuni* and *Campylobacter coli*. J. Clin. Microbiol. 20:990.

Smibert, R.M. 1984. *Campylobacter*. In Krieg, N.R., and Holt, J.G., editors. Bergey's manual of systematic bacteriology, ed. 9. Williams & Wilkins, Baltimore.

Taux, R.V., Patton, C.M., Edmonds, P., et al. 1985. Illness associated with *Campylobacter laridis*, a newly recognized *Campylobacter* species. J. Clin. Microbiol. 21:222.

von Graevenitz, A. 1983. Clinical microbiology of *Vibrio* species. Clin. Microbiol. Newsletter 5:41.

31 Spirochetes

31.1. Introduction

The Spirochaetaceae family includes organisms that have been known to cause human disease since prehistoric times, such as *Treponema carateum*, the agent of pinta, as well as organisms that have been discovered and associated with disease as recently as 1975, such as *Borrelia burgdorferi*, the newly named agent of Lyme disease. Most of the spirochetes multiply within a living host, having no natural reservoir in the inanimate environment. Treponemes pathogenic for humans are transmitted from person to person through direct contact, either sexual or otherwise. *Borrelia* species pass through an arthropod vector, and *Leptospira* species are contracted accidentally by humans who come into contact with water contaminated by animal urine or who are bitten by an infected animal. Although the spirochete *Treponema hyodysenteriae* has been unequivocally established as an agent of swine dysentery, the role of intestinal spirochetes in human gastroenteritis is still largely unknown. Intestinal spirochetosis will be briefly mentioned in this chapter.

31.1.a. Morphology. The spirochetes are all long, slender, helically curved gram-negative bacilli, with the unusual morphologic features of axial fibrils and an outer coating, the sheath. These fibrils, or axial filaments, are flagellalike organelles that wrap around the cell wall of the bacteria, are enclosed within the outer sheath, and facilitate motility of the organisms. The fibrils are attached within the cell wall by plate-like structures located near the ends of the cells, called insertion disks. The protoplasmic cylinder gyrates around the fibrils, causing bacterial movement to appear as a corkscrewlike winding. Differentiation of genera within the Spirochaetaceae is based on the number of axial fibrils, the number of insertion disks present (Table 31.1), as well as on biochemical and metabolic features. The spirochetes, in general, also fall into genera based loosely on their gross morphology (Figure 31.1). Treponemes are slender with tight coils, *Borrelia* are somewhat thicker with looser coils of fewer number, and the *Leptospira* resemble the *Borrelia* except for their hooked ends.

TABLE 31.1
Spirochetes Pathogenic for Humans

GENUS	AXIAL FIBRILS	INSERTION DISKS
Treponema	6-10	1
Leptospira	2	3-5
Borrelia	30-40	2
Brachyspira*	4	2

*Proposed name.

FIGURE 31.1
Species designation of spirochetes based on general morphology.

31.1.b. Taxonomical considerations. The genera that contain organisms pathogenic for humans are *Treponema*, including the causative agents of syphilis, pinta, yaws, and bejel; *Borrelia*, including vector-borne agents of relapsing fever and Lyme disease; *Leptospira*, which includes the agents of leptospirosis; and the newly proposed genus *Brachyspira*, the type species of which, *B. aalborgi*, may cause intestinal spirochetosis. The current state of spirochete taxonomy is less than perfect. The standard practice has been to name fastidious spirochetes that are transmitted by vectors as *Borrelia* species and all others as *Treponema* species. *Leptospira* species, in contrast to the other spirochetes, contain diaminopimelic acid in their cell walls instead of ornithine. *Leptospira* organisms can be cultivated more easily in vitro than the other genera.

31.2. *Treponema* Species

Virulent strains of these spirochetes, the agents of syphilis and several other diseases, had not been cultivated in the laboratory except by animal passage in rabbit testicles or mouse footpads until 1981. At that time, Fieldsteel and others, using a very complex tissue culture system of fibroblast cell monolayers, reported in vitro growth of *T. pallidum* biotype *pallidum*, the causative agent of syphilis.[2] The organisms were microaerophilic, in contrast to the anaerobic non-syphilis-associated treponemes that had been cultivated before.

31.2.a. Laboratory diagnosis of syphilis— serology and darkfield examination. Cultivation of this organism is still not possible for clinical laboratories, so for the most part the diagnosis of syphilis must rest on serologic methods and clinical acumen. Serologic diagnosis of syphilis is discussed in Chapters 12 and 19.

The microbiology laboratory can, however, examine the primary lesion of syphilis, the chancre, for the presence of motile spirochetes under darkfield illumination, as described in

Chapter 7. Although the darkfield examination is very much dependent on technical expertise and the numbers of organisms in the lesion, it can be highly specific when performed on genital lesions. Since the normal oral cavity contains spirochetes that are usually nonpathogenic but can mimic *T. pallidum* in appearance, one should not perform darkfield microscopy on material from lesions within the oral cavity. The method for collection of the specimen is described in Chapter 19. Treponemes, if present in material from the lesion, will be long (5-20 μm), slender, tightly coiled spirochetes, moving very slowly (rarely spiraling) and perhaps bending in the middle (Plate 31.1). It is best to examine the darkfield preparation under the oil immersion lens (1000 ×) to substantiate the morphology. Since positive lesions may be teeming with viable spirochetes that are highly infectious, all supplies and patient specimens must be handled with extreme caution and carefully discarded as required for contaminated materials. Although a fluorescent antibody reagent for *T. pallidum* is available, its use on exudate material from lesions has not yielded consistently reliable results. Recent development of a monoclonal antibody directed against the treponeme outer membrane protein should allow production of much more sensitive and specific immunologic reagents, such as fluorescent or immunoperoxidase-conjugated stains, that will greatly enhance the reliability of direct examination of lesion material.

31.2.b. Other treponemes. The other species of treponemes associated with human disease include *T. pallidum* biotype *pertenue*, the agent of yaws; *T. pallidum* biotype *endemicus*, the agent of endemic syphilis (bejel); and *T. carateum*, the agent of pinta. These diseases are primarily found in tropical or subtropical regions and are usually spread by human contact. Poor personal hygiene plays a role in their transmission. The serologic tests and the microscopic morphologies of all of these organisms, including *T. pallidum* biotype *pallidum*, are indistinguishable from each other; only manifestations of the disease vary.

Another group of treponemes are normal inhabitants of the oral cavity or the human genital tract; these include *T. vincentii*, *T. denticola*, *T. refringens*, *T. macrodentium*, and *T. oralis*. These organisms are cultivable anaerobically on artificial media. Patients with acute necrotizing ulcerative gingivitis (also known as Vincent's gingivitis), a destructive lesion of the gums, show combinations of morphological types of bacteria on methylene blue stained material from the lesions, which include spirochetes and fusiforms. It appears that oral spirochetes, particularly an unusually large one, may be important in this disease, along with other anaerobes. Further discussion of oral infections is found in Chapter 22. Penicillin G (or tetracycline in penicillin-allergic patients) is effective in all treponematoses.

31.3. *Borrelia* Species

31.3.a. Relapsing fever. Human relapsing fever is caused by more than 15 species of *Borrelia* and is transmitted to humans by the bite of a louse or a tick. Those carried by lice are called *B. recurrentis*. All others that cause disease in the United States are transmitted via tick bites and are named after the species of tick (usually of the genus *Ornithodoros*) from which they are recovered. Common species in the United States include *B. hermsii*, *B. turicatae*, *B. parkeri*, and *B. bergmanni*.

Although the organisms can be cultured in nutritionally rich media under microaerophilic conditions, the procedures are cumbersome and unreliable and are used primarily as research tools. Clinical laboratories rely on direct observation of the organism in peripheral blood from patients for diagnosis. Organisms can be found in 70% of cases when blood specimens from febrile patients are examined. The organisms can be seen either directly in wet preparations of peripheral blood (mixed with equal parts of sterile nonbacteriostatic saline) under darkfield illumination, in which the spirochetes move rapidly, often pushing the red blood cells around, or by staining thick and thin films with Wright's or Giemsa stains, by procedures similar to those used to detect malaria (Chapter 44).

Serological tests for *Borrelia*-caused relapsing fever have not proven to be reliable for diagnosis due to the many antigenic shifts undergone by the *Borrelia* organisms during the course of disease. Patients may exhibit increased titers to *Proteus* OX K antigens (up to 1:80), but other cross-reacting antibodies are rare. Certain reference laboratories, such as those at the Centers for Disease Control in Atlanta, may perform special serologic procedures on sera from selected cases. Several antibiotics, including tetracycline, are effective therapeutically.

31.3.b. Lyme disease. The agent of Lyme disease, named after its discovery as the cause of an epidemic of "pseudojuvenile rheumatoid arthritis" among young boys living in Lyme, Connecticut, has been named *B. burgdorferi*. The spirochete has been recovered from the blood, cerebrospinal fluid, and skin lesions (erythema chronicum migrans) of patients, but not yet from joint fluid. The bacteria are transmitted by the bite of a tick. Several genera of ticks act as vectors in the United States, including *Ixodes pacificus* in California and in other areas *I. dammini*. Endemic areas of disease that have been identified at this time include 14 states (including Massachusetts, Connecticut, Maryland, Wisconsin, Minnesota, Oregon, and California) as well as Europe and Australia. Approximately 1,500 cases of Lyme disease were reported in the United States during 1984; Lyme disease is thus the most prevalent tick-borne disease in the United States.

Culture of the spirochete may be attempted, although the yield is low. The periphery of the annular lesion of erythema chronicum migrans, blood, or cerebrospinal fluid are the best specimens to culture. The re-

suspended plasma from blood, spinal fluid sediment, or macerated tissue biopsy is inoculated into a tube of modified Kelly's medium (described in Chapter 45) and incubated at 33° C for 1 month. Blind subcultures (0.1 ml) are performed weekly to fresh media, and the cultures are examined by darkfield microscopy for the presence of spirochetes. Serological diagnosis is more reliable than culture at this time. Patients show a rise in titer of IgM against the spirochete within 2-3 weeks of onset of symptoms and a concomitant rise in IgG very early in disease. These specific antibodies both last for at least several years. The antigens are not yet available commercially. Penicillin and tetracycline are useful therapeutically, particularly early in the illness.

31.4. Leptospirosis

The leptospires include both free-living and parasitic forms. All pathogenic species are called *Leptospira interrogans*, and all saprophytic leptospires are called *L. biflexa*. The pathogens include over 180 different serologically defined types, which used to be designated as species and are now known as serovars or serotypes of *L. interrogans*. Physiologically, the saprophytes can be differentiated from pathogens by their ability to grow at 10° C and lower, or at least 5° C lower than the growth temperature of pathogenic leptospires.

The organisms are too small to be seen in wet preparations made from fresh blood and they do not push the erythrocytes around as the *Borrelia* do. Currently, the most reliable method for laboratory diagnosis of leptospirosis is to culture the organisms from blood or cerebrospinal fluid during the first week of illness or from urine thereafter for several months. A few drops of heparinized or sodium-oxalate anticoagulated blood are inoculated into tubes of Fletcher's or Ellinghausen, McCullough, Johnson, and Harris (EMJH) media (both described in Chapter 45). Urine should be inoculated soon after collection, as acidity (diluted out in the broth medium) may harm the spirochetes. One or two drops of undiluted and a 1:10 dilution of urine are added to 5 ml medium. The addition of 200 μg/ml of 5-fluorouracil (an anticancer drug) may prevent contamination by other bacteria without harming the leptospires. Tissue specimens (especially liver and kidney) may be aseptically triturated (macerated) and inoculated in dilutions of 1:1, 1:10, and 1:100 as for urine cultures. All cultures are incubated at room temperature or 30° C in the dark for up to 6 weeks. The organisms grow below the surface. Material collected from a few centimeters below the surface of broth cultures should be examined weekly for the presence of growth using a direct wet preparation under darkfield illumination. Leptospires will exhibit corkscrew like motility. A more complete discussion of these methods can be found in Alexander.[1]

Serological diagnosis of leptospirosis is best performed using pools of bacterial antigens containing many serotypes in each pool. Positive results are visualized by examining for the presence of agglutination under darkfield. A macroscopic agglutination procedure is more readily accessible to routine clinical laboratories. Reagents are available commercially. Indirect hemagglutination and an enzyme-linked immunosorbent assay (ELISA) test for IgM antibody are also available. Penicillin or tetracycline may modify the course of the illness, but only if started not later than the fourth day of illness.

31.5. Intestinal Spirochetosis

The normal gastrointestinal tract of humans is colonized with spirochetes, most of which cause no harm to the host. Since 1981, however, several groups have reported patients with diarrhea, inflammatory cellular responses, and numerous spirochetes found to be invading the intestinal epithelium (into the lamina propria), as well as within macrophages. Many of these patients also suffered from other illnesses

such as Crohn's disease. Hovind-Hougen and others were able to culture the spirochetes from five patients in vitro and found that they differed from other known genera morphologically.[3] Since growth characteristics and morphology differed from previously named spirochetes, they designated this organism *Brachyspira aalborgi*. Whether intestinal spirochetosis is a more common syndrome than has been appreciated until now remains to be elucidated. The ability to recognize an agent associated with a particular syndrome will stimulate the study of this disease, ultimately resulting in definition of the agent's role.

REFERENCES

1. Alexander, A.D. 1980. *Leptospira*. In Lennette, E.H., Balows, A., Hausler, W.J. Jr., and Truant, J.P., editors. Manual of clinical microbiology, ed. 3. American Society for Microbiology. Washington, D.C.
2. Fieldsteel, A.H., Cox, D.L., and Moeckii, R.A. 1981. Cultivation of virulent *Treponema pallidum* in tissue culture. Infect. Immun. 32:908.
3. Hovind-Hougen, K., Birch-Anderson, A., Henrik-Nielsen, R., et al. 1982. Intestinal spirochetosis: morphological characterization and cultivation of the spirochete *Brachyspira aalborgi* gen. nov., sp. nov. J. Clin. Microbiol. 16:1127.

BIBLIOGRAPHY

Alexander, A.D. 1980. Serological diagnosis of leptospirosis. In Rose, N.R., and Friedman, J., editors. Manual of clinical immunology, ed. 2. American Society for Microbiology, Washington, D.C.

Antonakopoulos, G., Newman, J., and Wilkinson, M. 1982. Intestinal spirochetosis; an electron microscopic study of an unusual case. Histopathology 6:477.

Berger, B.W., Clemmensen, O.J., and Ackerman, A.B. 1983. Lyme disease is a spirochetosis. Am. J. Dermatopathol. 5:111.

Burgdorfer, W. 1985. Spirochetes. In Lennette, E.H., Balows, A., Hausler, W.J., Jr., and Shadomy, H.J., editors. Manual of clinical microbiology, ed. 4. American Society for Microbiology, Washington, D.C.

Burgdorfer, W., Barbour, A.G., Hayes, S.F., et al. 1982. Lyme disease—a tick-borne spirochetosis? Science 216:1317.

Johnson, R.C., and Harris, V.G. 1967. Differentiation of pathogenic and saprophytic leptospires. I. Growth at low temperatures. J. Bacteriol. 94:27.

Johnson, S.E., Klein, G.C., Schmid, G.P., et al. 1984. Lyme disease: a selective medium for isolation of the suspected etiological agent, a spirochete. J. Clin. Microbiol. 19:81.

Norris, S.J. 1982. In vitro cultivation of *Treponema pallidum;* independent confirmation. Infect. Immun. 36:437.

Steere, A.C., Broderick, T.F., and Malawista, S.E. 1978. Erythema chronicum migrans and Lyme arthritis: epidemiologic evidence for a tick vector. Am. J. Epidemiol. 108:312.

Steere, A.C., Grodzicki, R.L., Kornblatt, A.N., et al. 1983. The spirochetal etiology of Lyme disease. N. Engl. J. Med. 308:733.

Steere, A.C., Hardin, J.A., Ruddy, S., et al. 1979. Lyme arthritis: correlation of serum and cryoglobulin IgM with activity, and serum IgG with remission. Arthritis Rheum. 22:471.

Steere, A.C., and Malawista, S.E. 1979. Cases of Lyme disease in the United States: locations correlated with distribution of *Ixodes dammini.* Ann. Intern. Med. 91:730.

32

Aerobic or Facultative Spore-Forming Rods (*Bacillus* Species)

32.1. Introduction

The genus *Bacillus* contains a large number of species that are aerobic or facultative, usually gram-positive and spore-forming; several of these species have been involved in clinically significant infections of a variety of types. *Bacillus* species are widely distributed in nature and are therefore frequent contaminants in laboratory cultures from clinical specimens. Contamination of radiometric blood culture apparatus and of alcohol swabs has also led to clusters of pseudobacteremia. Species identification within the genus is not important for clinical purposes, but identification of *Bacillus anthracis* (the agent of anthrax) is a major exception. Reference laboratories may be used for this purpose.

32.1.a. Morphology and general characteristics. *Bacillus* species may or may not grow on eosin-methylene blue (EMB) agar. Because they may vary in Gram stain and oxidase and other reactions and spores may not be evident, they may resemble nonfermentative gram-negative bacilli. Such organisms cannot be classified in any known gram-negative species or Centers for Disease Control (CDC) taxon. Since some *Bacillus* strains are strict aerobes, they may appear as nonfermentative gram-negative bacilli on Kligler's or triple sugar iron (TSI) agar. Most do not grow on enteric agars (Chapter 8), but some show limited growth.

However, several gram-negative nonfermenters also fail to grow on such media. The colonial morphology of the *Bacillus* strains that simulate gram-negative rods is not typical of the usual *Bacillus* species (large, flat colonies and frequent beta hemolysis). Some of these strains even have minute colonies. Spore formation often fails to occur within the time required to report a clinical isolate. Sporulation (Figure 32.1) is often stimulated on esculin agar and may be facilitated on acidified media such as TSI agar. Two other tests may be useful. One is susceptibility to vancomycin; with the exception of *Flavobacterium* species, no gram-negative nonfermenter is known to be susceptible to vancomycin by the Bauer-Kirby technique (Chapter 13), whereas most *Bacillus* species are susceptible. However, there are strains of *Bacillus* species that are vancomycin resistant, so only vancomycin susceptibility can be used diagnostically. The second procedure that may be helpful is the KOH test (described in Chapter 7) in which gram-negative organisms show a viscous thread. Some *Bacillus* strains, particularly from older cultures that have also lost their gram-positivity, may give a "gram-negative" reaction by this test. Accordingly, the test is of value for identification of *Bacillus* species only if no viscous thread is formed.

Treatment of specimens or mixed cultures that may contain *Bacillus* species with 50% ethanol for 1 h is effective for selecting *Bacillus* species, just as it is for selecting spore-forming anaerobes (Chapter 34).

32.1.b. Differentiation of *Bacillus* species. Species differentiation within the genus *Bacillus* is based on size and location of spores, whether the organism is obligately aerobic or facultative, action on xylose and arabinose, starch hydrolysis, indole production, nitrite production from nitrate, presence of protein bodies, susceptibility to gamma phage, capsule production, the "string of pearls" test (see below) and animal pathogenicity.

FIGURE 32.1
Gram stain of *Bacillus* species visualized under oil immersion (1,000 ×) showing the clear intracellular (subterminal) spores that fail to pick up the stain.

32.2. *Bacillus anthracis*

B. anthracis is the primary human pathogen in the genus. Anthrax is a rare disease in the United States so the organism is seldom encountered in the average hospital or public health laboratory. Cases in the United States are most often related to handling of imported wool or goat hair, animal hides, shaving brushes, etc. originating principally in Asia, the Middle East, and Africa. Cases may also result from contact with diseased animals, primarily cattle, swine, and horses and from inadvertent self-inoculation of veterinary anthrax vaccine. Between 1970 and 1980 there were only an average of 2.5 cases of anthrax per year in the United States.

Anthrax is manifested in humans in three forms:

1. **Cutaneous anthrax** (malignant pustule) is the most common form in the United States. Infection is initiated by the entrance of bacilli through an abrasion of the skin. A pustule usually appears on the hands or forearms. The bacilli are readily recognized in the serosanguineous discharge.
2. **Pulmonary anthrax** is also known as woolsorter's disease. The bacilli may be found in large numbers in the sputum. Spores are inhaled during shearing, sorting, or handling of animal hair. If not properly treated, this form progresses to fatal septicemia.
3. **Gastrointestinal anthrax** is the most severe and rarest form of anthrax. The bacilli or spores are swallowed, thus initiating intestinal infection. The organisms may be isolated from the patient's stools. This form is also usually fatal if not treated.

32.2.a. Structure, extracellular products. The organism is a facultative, large, square-ended, nonmotile rod, with an ellipsoidal to cylindrical centrally located spore. The sporangium is not swollen as a rule. The cells frequently occur in long chains, giving a bamboo appearance, especially on primary isolation from infected tissue or discharge. The chains of virulent forms are usually surrounded by a capsule. Encapsulation occurs also in enriched media and when grown on sodium bicarbonate agar under 5% CO_2. Avirulent forms are usually unencapsulated. Sporulation occurs in the soil and on culture media, but not in living tissue.

The colonies of *B. anthracis* are normally large (4-5 mm), opaque, raised, and irregular, with a curled margin. When the margin of the colony is pushed inward and then lifted gently with an inoculating needle, the disturbed portion of the colony stands up like beaten egg whites. Comma-shaped colony outgrowths are common. On sheep blood agar, the colonies are invariably nonhemolytic. Smooth and rough colony forms may be observed, and both of these may be virulent. In broth, the bacillus produces a heavy pellicle, with little if any subsurface growth.

Two potent exotoxins are produced. Both toxin molecules are dependent on a third protein, called protective antigen (PA), for their biologic activity. The two exotoxins are known as lethal factor (LF) and edema factor (EF). It appears that PA is essential for the toxins to enter into the target cells. The combination of EF and PA increases host susceptibility to infection by suppressing polymorphonuclear neutrophil function.

32.2.b. Identification methods. When working with suspected *B. anthracis*, one should use extreme caution, work in a bacteriologic safety hood, avoid creating aerosols, and decontaminate all areas thoroughly with a sporicidal germicide such as Alcide.

The optimal growth temperature for the organism is 35° C; when grown at 42° or 43° C, it becomes attenuated or avirulent. This is due to the loss of the capsule.

Biochemically, the organism is characterized as follows:

Carbohydrate fermentation—glucose, fructose, maltose, sucrose and trehalose are fermented with acid only; arabinose, xylose, galactose, lactose, mannose, raffinose, rhamnose, adonitol, dulcitol, inositol, inulin, mannitol and sorbitol are not fermented.

Gelatin—inverted pine-tree growth; slow liquefaction.

Nitrates—reduced to nitrites.

Starch—hydrolyzed.

Voges-Proskauer—positive.

A simple presumptive test for identification of *B. anthracis* has been proposed. It is a modification of the string of pearls test, which reflects the susceptibility of a strain to penicillin. Single streaks of the suspect organism, as well as positive and negative controls, are made on a Mueller-Hinton agar plate. Ten unit penicillin disks are placed on each streak, and a coverslip is placed over the streak. After incubation for 3-6 h at 37° C, growth beneath the coverslip is examined microscopically for the presence of strings of spherical cellular forms of the organism. The presence of such cells resembling strings of pearls is considered a positive test.

Specific identification may be made by use of a gamma bacteriophage (at CDC or state health department laboratories).

The pathogenicity of *B. anthracis* may be determined by injecting each of 10 white mice (2 to 3 weeks of age) subcutaneously with 0.2 ml of a saline suspension of the organism. Rabbits or guinea pigs may also be used. Animals usually die 2 to 5 days after inoculation from septicemia; the organism is readily recovered from the heart, blood, spleen, liver, and lungs of the animal. Animal inoculation is not generally done in clinical laboratories.

32.2.c. Susceptibility to antimicrobial agents. Penicillin is the drug of choice for treatment. Alternative drugs for the penicillin-sensitive patient are tetracycline, erythromycin, and chloramphenicol.

32.2.d. Noncultural methods of identification. Encapsulated strains may be used for fluorescent antibody staining; this is available through CDC. Both the cell wall and the capsule fluoresce simultaneously. This test would presumably work well directly on clinical specimens, if it were feasible to get it done promptly.

Antibodies to the organism may be detected by an indirect hemagglutination or enzyme-linked immunosorbent test (using the PA component of the toxin as the capture antigen). These tests are available through state health department laboratories.

32.3. *Bacillus cereus*

This organism is the cause of serious infections of various types, usually, but not always, in immunocompromised hosts. Other patient background factors include surgery and other trauma, burns, intravenous drug abuse, implantation of catheters and various prosthetic devices (including heart valves), and use of hemodialysis and peritoneal dialysis. Types of infections described include septicemia, endocarditis, necrotizing pneumonia with or without empyema, meningitis, rapidly destructive ophthalmitis, peritonitis, wound infection, myonecrosis, and osteomyelitis. Myonecrosis has followed surgery and trauma and may simulate clostridial myonecrosis (gas gangrene).

B. cereus has long been known as an important cause of food-poisoning. The short incubation type of food-poisoning due to *B. cereus* is most often associated with fried rice that has been cooked and held warm for extended periods; it is due to preformed toxin. Long incubation food poisoning due to *B. cereus* is frequently associated with meat or vegetable dishes; in these cases, toxin is formed in vivo. These entities are discussed in greater detail in Chapter 17.

32.3.a. Structure, extracellular products. *B. cereus* colonies vary from small, shiny and compact to the large, feathery, spreading type.

A lavender colored colony with beta hemolysis is seen on sheep blood agar.

Injection of *B. cereus* exotoxin into the skin of rabbits causes increased vascular permeability and necrosis; production of this toxin seems to correlate with the severity of clinical infection. Rabbit skin necrosis is attributed to two factors—an enterotoxin and a hemolysin. Phospholipase C (lecithinase) is produced by almost all strains of *B. cereus;* its pathogenic role is doubtful. The toxin can also be demonstrated to cause fluid accumulation in the rabbit ileal loop model. *B. cereus* produces beta lactamase.

32.3.b. Identification methods. Unlike *B. anthracis, B. cereus* is resistant to gamma phage, is usually resistant to penicillin, does not encapsulate on bicarbonate agar, and on fluorescent antibody-stained smears does not exhibit fluorescence of both cell wall and capsule. Lecithinase and hemolysin production are very useful in the provisional identification of *B. cereus.*

32.3.c. Susceptibility to antimicrobial agents. Because of beta lactamase production, *B. cereus* is usually not susceptible to penicillin and many other beta lactam antimicrobial agents. It is also resistant to trimethoprim. It is susceptible to gentamicin, clindamycin, erythromycin, vancomycin, and probably to chloramphenicol. Most strains are inhibited by sulfonamides and tetracycline.

32.4. Other *Bacillus* Species

Several other of the 60 or so species in this genus have been encountered in significant infections, especially *B. subtilis* and *B. licheniformis.* The latter two species have been implicated in food-poisoning and in a number of infections including septicemia, panophthalmitis, pneumonia, wound infection, and peritonitis. Ocular infection has been produced by a biological insecticide made up of *Bacillus thuringiensis;* the material was inadvertently splashed into the patient's eye. Other *Bacillus* species incriminated in infection of one type or another on at least one occasion include *B. brevis, B. circulans, B. coagulans, B. macerans, B. megaterium, B. pumilus,* and *B. sphaericus.* Allergic reactions in workers manufacturing laundry detergent containing derivatives of *B. subtilis* have been described. Also, hypersensitivity pneumonitis related to exposure to wood dust contaminated with *B. subtilis* has been described.

32.4.a. Morphology and extracellular products. *B. subtilis* colonies are usually large, flat and dull, with a ground glass appearance (Plate 32.1). Several species produce collagenases. *B. megaterium* produces a filterable hemolysin, and *Bacillus mycoides* produces potent toxins that can be lethal to experimental animals.

32.4.b. Susceptibility to antimicrobial agents. Susceptibility to penicillin G and other older beta lactam antibiotics is variable and may be species related, tending to be high for *B. subtilis* and intermediate for *B. pumilus.* Although clindamycin is generally considered to be an effective drug for treating *Bacillus* infections, there is a report of one strain of *B. licheniformis* that was resistant to clindamycin and susceptible to penicillin. Vancomycin should be one of the more dependable drugs for therapy of serious infections due to *Bacillus* species. Obviously, the type and the location of the infection will influence the choice of therapy.

BIBLIOGRAPHY

Bekemeyer, W.B., and Zimmerman, G.A. 1985. Life-threatening complications associated with *Bacillus cereus* pneumonia. Am. Rev. Respir. Dis. 131:466.

Blachman, U., Gilardi, G.L., Pickett, M.J., Slotnick, I.J., and von Graevenitz, A. 1980. *Bacillus* spp. strains posing as nonfermentative gram-negative rods. Clin. Microbiol. Newsletter 2:8.

Brachman, P.S. 1983. Anthrax. In Hoeprich, P.D., editor. Infectious diseases, ed. 3., Philadelphia, Harper & Row, Publishers.

Editorial. 1983. *Bacillus cereus* as a systemic pathogen. Lancet 2:1469.

Parry, J.M., Turnbull, P.C.B., and Gibson, J.R. 1983. A colour atlas of *Bacillus* species. Wolfe Medical Atlases—19. Ipswich, England. Wolfe Medical Publications, Ltd.

Pennington, J.E., Gibbons, N.D., Strobeck, J.E., et al. 1976. *Bacillus* species infection in patients with hematologic neoplasia. JAMA 235:1473.

Tuazon, C.V., Murray, H.W., Levy, C., et al. 1979. Serious infections from *Bacillus* sp. JAMA 241:1137.

Turnbull, P.C.B., and Kramer, J.M. 1983. Non-gastrointestinal *Bacillus cereus* infections: an analysis of exotoxin production by strains isolated over a two-year period. J. Clin. Pathol. 36:1091.

33 Aerobic, Non-Spore-Forming, Gram-Positive Bacilli

33.1. Introduction

Gram-positive, aerobic, non-spore-forming rods are ubiquitous inhabitants of the natural environment, becoming human pathogens only by accident. Although they may rarely stain gram-negative due to breakdown of the cell wall, especially in older cultures, they usually appear gram-positive. Most of the bacteria in this group are pleomorphic, exhibiting various morphologies that include branching, clubbing, coccoid forms, and palisading. These organisms all grow well on commonly used nonselective media, including 5% sheep blood agar. Other bacteria that may grow aerobically on such media and resemble aerobic, non-spore-forming, gram-positive bacilli in one or more respects include mycobacteria, *Bacillus* species, *Propionibacterium* species, *Actinomyces* and *Arachnia* species, and *Gardnerella vaginalis* (which has been found to possess a cell wall structure more closely resembling that of gram-negative bacteria). Mycobacteria are differentiated by being acid fast, and *Bacillus* species will usually fail to grow on MacConkey agar and can be induced to produce spores. *Propionibacterium, Arachnia,* and *Actinomyces* species grow better under anaerobic conditions, and *Gardnerella* is usually gram-variable and exhibits slight beta hemolysis on human blood agar. As outlined by Clarridge and Weissfeld[2] and Hollis and Weaver,[6] the organ-

481

isms are divided into groups on the basis of the catalase test (Chapter 9). Figure 33.1 illustrates a basic strategy for preliminary identification of aerobic, gram-positive, non-spore-forming bacilli.

Two genera, *Nocardia* and *Corynebacterium,* are closely related to mycobacteria. All three groups of organisms contain unusual cell wall structural components called **mycolic acids,** branched, long-chain fatty acids. The length of the chain differs among the three genera, and it is the mycolic acid that contributes to the "acid fast" property of the cell wall (acid fast stain is discussed in Chapter 7). Corynebacteria, usually non-acid fast, contain mycolic acids of 28 to 40 carbon atoms; *Nocardia* mycolic acids are 40 to 60 carbon atoms in length, and the *Nocardia* are partially acid fast; the true mycobacteria contain mycolic acid chains of 60 to 90 carbon atoms and all *Mycobacterium* species (Chapter 41) are acid fast.

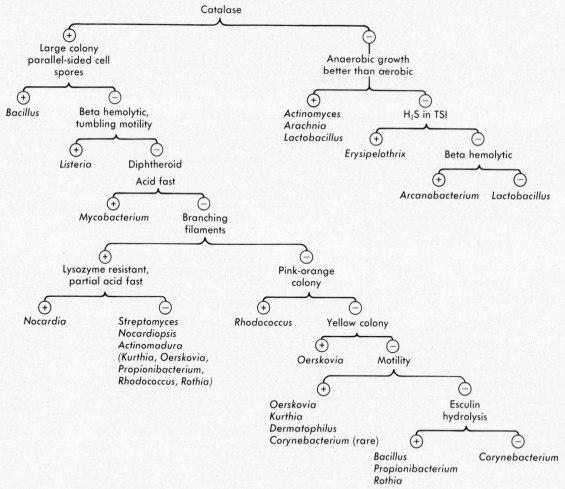

FIGURE 33.1

Flow chart for preliminary identification of aerobic, gram-positive non-spore-forming bacilli.

33.2. *Listeria* Species

33.2.a. Epidemiology and pathogenesis of listeriosis.

Among the aerobic gram-positive pathogenic bacilli, *Listeria* species is one of the most commonly isolated etiologic agents of disease today, since the advent of widespread immunization against diphtheria has significantly decreased the incidence of diphtheria in the United States. The incidence of *Listeria* infection is dependent on geographical factors as well as the patient population being considered. *Listeria* species, found in soil, on vegetation, in silage, and carried by many domestic and wild animals in their feces and on their mucous membranes, can also be found in the feces of healthy humans. The carriage rate varies with the population. Pathogenic *Listeria* species are differentiated from nonpathogenic environmental strains on the basis of several factors, one of which is production of a hemolysin that is particularly enhanced by factors elaborated by strains of *Rhodococcus equi* (mentioned below). *Listeria* has been studied intensely over the years as a classic example of an intracellular pathogen. The organism possesses antiphagocytic components on the cell surface as well as a lipopolysaccharide complex within the cell wall that is indistinguishable from gram-negative endotoxin (Chapter 14). Pathogenic strains of *Listeria* produce enzymes that act lipolytically to destroy cell membranes. After being taken up by cells of the host reticuloendothelial system, the organisms destroy internal membranes, preventing lysosomal fusion. It appears that virulence is mediated by action of at least three components: the phospholipase, the hemolysin, and the lipopolysaccharide.

Listeria causes sepsis and meningitis in immunocompromised hosts; it has been the most common cause of meningitis among patients at Memorial Sloan-Kettering Cancer Hospital. In pregnant women, for whom the organism seems to have an increased tropism, infection results in malaise, fever, and generalized symptoms similar to those of influenza. Because the organism can cross the placenta, however, the effects on the fetus can be much more serious. Abortion, systemic disease, and meningitis are manifestations of listeriosis in the newborn. Infection of the mother postpartum may cause puerperal sepsis similar to that caused by beta hemolytic streptococci. A recent (spring, 1985) outbreak of listeriosis in Los Angeles County, resulting in at least 28 deaths (primarily in infants, pregnant women, and the elderly), was traced to cheese made from improperly pasteurized milk.

33.2.b. Laboratory identification.

The genus *Listeria* contains six species, *L. monocytogenes*, *L. denitrificans*, *L. grayi*, *L. innocua*, *L. ivanovii*, and *L. murrayi*. Some workers may place certain of these species in other genera and others recognize other species of *Listeria*. Only *L. monocytogenes* and the newly proposed *L. ivanovii* are pathogenic for humans. Because species other than *L. monocytogenes* are rarely encountered in clinical specimens, they will not be discussed here. Studies by Skalka and co-workers[11,12] have described methods by which pathogenic *Listeria* species can be differentiated from nonpathogenic species. The nonpathogenic species differ from *L. monocytogenes* and *L. ivanovii* in failing to demonstrate slight beta hemolysis on sheep blood agar. For this reason, they will probably be presumptively identified as "diphtheroids," or contaminating nonpathogenic *Corynebacterium* species. *Listeria*, however, are able to hydrolyze esculin (Chapter 9) and most (although not all) *Corynebacterium* species are not.

L. monocytogenes grows well on most laboratory media, yielding smooth, translucent gray colonies 1-2 mm in diameter. On blood agar (irrespective of the animal from which the erythrocytes were obtained) the colonies exhibit a small zone of diffuse beta hemolysis (Plate 33.1). The colony morphology closely resembles that of group B beta hemolytic streptococci, with which it is often confused. Like *Streptococcus agalactiae*, *Listeria* hydrolyzes esculin and sodium hippurate. *L. monocytogenes* also yields a positive reaction in the CAMP test (Chapter 25). A catalase test (Chapter 9) will differentiate between streptococci (catalase negative) and *Listeria* (catalase positive). Colonies grown on clear media, such as nutrient agar, will display a **blue-green** color when they are observed with an oblique (45-degree angle) light source. *Listeria* can also be presumptively identified by observation of motility under direct wet preparation. *Listeria* exhibits a characteristic end-over-end tumbling motility when incubated in nutrient broth for 1-2 h at room temperature. An identical broth culture incubated at 37° C will show very little, if any, motility. This motility pattern will also be illustrated by the "umbrella-shaped" pattern that develops after overnight incubation at room temperature of a culture that has been stabbed into a tube of semisolid agar (Plate 33.2). The cellular morphology can vary widely, from very straight-sided gram-positive bacilli to almost coccoid forms. Table 33.1 shows the basic biochemical and enzymatic tests used to differentiate *Listeria* from organisms with which it might be confused.

Although *L. monocytogenes* grows readily from cerebrospinal fluid, blood, and most other specimens, it may be difficult to isolate from placenta and other tissue. Placing the specimen in the refrigerator (4° C) for several weeks to months and then plating may serve to enhance recovery. This procedure, called **cold enrichment**, is particularly useful for epidemiologic studies when specimens are contaminated with other flora. A procedure for handling tissue suspected of containing *Listeria* is given in Chapter 21.

33.2.c. Therapy. *Listeria* demonstrates susceptibility to penicillin, ampicillin, tetracycline, erythromycin, aminoglycosides, rifampin, and chloramphenicol in vitro. Choramphenicol may not be clinically effective, however, and ampicillin seems to be more active than penicillin in human infections. Current recommendations for therapy are for combinations of ampicillin or penicillin with an aminoglycoside. If meningitis is being treated, intrathecal administration of the aminoglycoside may be necessary to achieve effective levels.

33.3. *Corynebacterium* and Related Species, Including *Rhodococcus*, *Arcanobacterium*, and *Actinomyces pyogenes*

33.3.a. General considerations, epidemiology, and pathogenesis of infection due to these organisms. The corynebacteria are pleomorphic, primarily nonmotile, aerobic, or facultative, gram-positive bacilli. These organisms are found throughout nature, acting as pathogens and parasites of plants and animals. Pref-

TABLE 33.1
Differentiation of *L. monocytogenes* from Other Bacteria It Resembles*

ORGANISM	CATALASE	ESCULIN HYDROLYSIS	MOTILITY	BETA HEMOLYSIS	GROWTH IN 6.5% NaCl
L. monocytogenes	+	+	+	+	+
Corynebacterium sp.	+	−	−/+	−/+	+/−
Propionibacterium sp.	+	+/−	−	+/−	+
Arcanobacterium	−	+/−	−	+	−
S. agalactiae (group B streptococci)	−	−	−	+	−
Enterococci	−	+	−	−/+	+

*+ = >90% of strains positive; − = >90% of strains negative; +/− = variable (most strains positive); −/+ = variable (most strains negative).

erential synthesis of cell wall components at one end of the cell wall often results in clubbing and uneven division during binary fission, seen as "Chinese letter forms" (Figure 33.2). The genus name comes from the Greek word for "club," *koryne.* Although most species are harmless saprophytes and many are part of the normal human skin and mucous membrane flora, *Corynebacterium diphtheriae,* the agent of diphtheria, and *Corynebacterium* group JK, a relatively common cause of infection in compromised hosts, are major pathogens of humans. Other *Corynebacterium* species have been called "diphtheroids" because they resemble *C. diphtheriae* morphologically. There are numerous species of *Corynebacterium,* most of which are rarely isolated from clinical specimens and will not be discussed here. Species other than *C. diphtheriae* and group JK have also been associated with human infection, however, as outlined in Table 33.2 and by Hollis and Weaver.[6] Certain strains have been placed in new genera that were formerly within *Corynebacterium,* such as *Rhodococcus equi* (formerly *C. equi*), *Arcanobacterium haemolyticum* (formerly *C. haemolyticum*), and *Actinomyces pyogenes* (formerly *C. pyogenes*). *C. xerosis,* *C. pseudodiphtheriticum,* "*C. minutissimum,*" *C. ulcerans,* *C. bovis,* group D2, and others have also been reported to cause human disease rarely. Coral red fluorescence under a Wood's lamp is characteristic of erythrasma skin lesions caused by a number of corynebacteria, called "*C. minutissimum*" by dermatologists. Laboratory cultures are unnecessary for diagnosis. A newly described group of corynebacteria, closely related to each other genetically and closely related immunologically to *Mycobacterium leprae,* are the **leprosy-derived corynebacteria,** reviewed by Cocito and Delville.[3] These organisms can be cultivated from lesions of leprosy and may contribute synergistically with *M. leprae* in development of disease. Corynebacteria of groups JK and D2 are noteworthy for exhibiting resistance to multiple antimicrobial agents.

FIGURE 33.2
Pleomorphic forms of *Corynebacterium* species seen on Gram stain.

TABLE 33.2
Corynebacteria Associated with Human Infection

SPECIES	INFECTION(S)
C. diphtheriae	Pharyngeal, nasal, cutaneous*
Group JK	Systemic, endocarditis, pneumonia, cutaneous
Group D2	Systemic, cutaneous, catheter
pseudotuberculosis	Lymphadenitis, pneumonia
Leprosy-derived	Associated with leprosy
minutissimum	Associated with erythrasma
Rhodococcus equi	Systemic, pneumonia, osteomyelitis
Arcanobacterium haemolyticum	Wound, pharyngitis, abscess, cutaneous
Actinomyces pyogenes	Cutaneous, endocarditis (rare)

*Although the infection is localized, the effects of toxin are systemic.

Pathogenesis of infection due to nontoxigenic strains of *Corynebacterium* species is not well understood. It is possible that the hemolysins produced by certain species contribute to disease. *C. ulcerans* and *C. pseudotuberculosis* may be infected with a lysogenic phage that produces toxin identical to that of toxigenic *C. diphtheriae*, but these strains are rare.

One of the most well-studied bacterial toxins is that of *C. diphtheriae*. The gene for toxin production is carried into the bacteria by a bacteriophage, which then produces a nonlytic infection within the bacteria, replicating with the bacterial genome. Such an infection that does not lyse the host cell is called **lysogenic.** Although *C. diphtheriae* that are not infected with toxin-producing phage can cause diphtheria-like disease, the disease is usually not as severe. The diphtheria toxin acts to inhibit protein synthesis, particularly in heart muscle and neural cells.

33.3.b. Isolation of *C. diphtheriae* from suspected cases of diphtheria. Although the corynebacteria will grow well on most routinely used laboratory media, there are media that

are selective and differential for *C. diphtheriae* which should be used if diphtheria is suspected. Cystine tellurite blood agar (Chapter 45) will reliably support growth of *C. diphtheriae*. The organisms appear black or gray with a characteristic garliclike odor, usually after 24 h incubation in air. Colony morphology differences on cystine tellurite agar have been used to differentiate the three subspecies of *C. diphtheriae*: *mitis*, *intermedius*, and *gravis*. They may occasionally require 48 h incubation for initial isolation. Modified Tinsdale agar (Chapter 45) has been used for isolation of *C. diphtheriae*; colonies are black with dark brown halos. The halos develop particularly around colonies that have grown into stabbed areas of the agar. This medium must be used within 4 days of preparation and does not support growth of many strains. When small numbers of organisms must be isolated, primary inoculation to a Loeffler agar slant and overnight incubation at 35° C in air before subculturing to cystine tellurite blood agar may improve recovery. Gram-stained colonies that exhibit coryneform morphology should be streaked to a sheep blood agar plate for purity before biochemical tests are performed. Identification of subspecies of diphtheria isolates is best accomplished biochemically.

33.3.c. Laboratory identification of corynebacteria. These organisms usually grow as opaque, white or gray colonies. They may, however, resemble nonhemolytic or alpha hemolytic streptococci, yeast, staphylococci, and commensal *Neisseria* species. The organisms grow well on most commonly used media. Gram-stain morphology is typical of the genus, and no true branching should be observed. Most corynebacteria are catalase positive. Aerotolerant *Actinomyces* and *Arachnia* are thin bacilli with even sides and branching morphology. They grow better anaerobically and are primarily catalase negative. Problems are more commonly encountered in identifying members of the *Corynebacterium* species. Two

PROCEDURE 33.1. PYRAZINAMIDASE TEST FOR CORYNEBACTERIA

1. Prepare substrate medium as follows:

Agar (Bacto agar, Difco Laboratories)	2 g
Pyrazinamide (Sigma Chemical Co.)	0.1 g
Pyruvic acid, sodium salt (Sigma)	2 g
Distilled water	1,000 ml

   Mix thoroughly, heat to dissolve, and dispense in 5 ml amounts in 16 × 125 mm screw cap test tubes. Autoclave for 15 min at 121° C. Allow the medium to harden upright to form a butt. Medium will keep 6 months at 4° C.
2. Inoculate a **heavy** suspension of the test organism into the top half of the substrate medium tube by scraping up growth from a 24-72 h culture on blood or chocolate agar with a cotton swab and gently rotating the swab in the medium. The suspension should be milky. Inoculate identical tubes of medium with a negative control *(C. ulcerans)* and a positive control *(C. xerosis).*
3. Incubate the tubes for 2 h at 37° C in a water bath or a dry bath.
4. To the tube of each test organism, add 1 ml of freshly prepared 1% ferrous ammonium sulfate (0.1 g ferrous ammonium sulfate [Sigma] in 10 ml sterile distilled water).
5. Examine tubes after 1-5 min at room temperature for a rusty pink band in the agar, indicating hydrolysis of pyrazinamide and presence of pyrazinamidase. An additional incubation of 4 h in the refrigerator may enhance color formation.
6. Only *C. diphtheriae, C. ulcerans,* and *C. pseudotuberculosis* lack pyrazinamidase.

Modified from Coyle, Harborview Medical Center, Seattle, Wash., and from Sulea et al. 1980. J. Clin. Microbiol. 30:466.

new tests, that of pyrazinamidase activity[13] (Procedure 33.1) and production of the enzyme phospholipase D^1 (Procedure 33.2), can be used to differentiate among corynebacteria.

Selected biochemical reactions of some clinically relevant species are shown in Table 33.3. Fermentation broths should be supplemented with 2 drops of rabbit serum per tube. *R. equi* is further differentiated due to production of a pale pink or salmon-colored pigment. The *Rhodococcus* associated with human infection has been reported to stain variably acid fast. A number of other corynebacteria have been isolated from human clinical specimens, but their significance has not yet been determined. As described by Thompson, Gates-Davis, and Yong,[14] rapid biochemical tests are reliable for identification of several groups of corynebacteria. Performance of these rapid tests is described in Procedure 33.3. The chapter by Coyle, Hollis, and Groman in the American Society for Microbiology manual,[4] contains definitive schemes for species identification within the genus. Besides *C. diphtheriae,* it is important to identify the group JK and group D2 corynebacteria, as they are commonly seen with multiple antibiotic resistance.

PROCEDURE 33.2. DETECTION OF PHOSPHOLIPASE D BY INHIBITION OF CAMP TEST

1. Fresh cultures of each organism needed for performance of the test are incubated overnight on blood agar plates
   a. *Staphylococcus aureus*, beta-toxin-positive strain
   b. *Streptococcus agalactiae*, known to be positive in the CAMP test (Chapter 25)
   c. *Corynebacterium ulcerans* as positive control
   d. Unknown strain of *Corynebacterium*
2. A 5% sheep blood agar plate is inoculated with the test organisms by swabbing the colonies with a cotton-tipped swab and rubbing the swab on the surface of the test plate in the pattern shown in Figure 33.3.
3. The plate is incubated 48 h at 37° C. Inhibition of the enhanced zone of hemolysis formed at the junction of the staphylococcal hemolysin and the streptococcal hemolysin is caused by phospholipase D.

Modified from Barksdale et al. 1981. J. Clin. Microbiol. 13:335.

TABLE 33.3
Differentiation of *Corynebacterium* Species*

SPECIES	NITRATE	UREASE	DEXTROSE	MALTOSE
C. diphtheriae (mitis)	+†	−	+	+
C. diphtheriae (gravis)	+	−	+	+
C. diphtheriae (intermedius)	+	−	+	+
C. ulcerans	−	+	+	+
C. pseudodiphtheriticum	+	+	−	−
C. pseudotuberculosis	+/−	+	+	+
C. xerosis	+	−	+	+/−
C. group JK	−	−	+/−	+/−
Actinomyces pyogenes	−	−	+	+
Arcanobacterium haemolyticum	−	−	+	+

Compiled from material presented by Coyle, Harborview Medical Center, Seattle, Wash., and from Thompson, J.S., Gates-important corynebacteria. J. Clin. Microbiol. 18:926.
*+ = >90% of strains positive; − = >90% of strains negative; +/− = variable (most strains positive); −/+, variable (most
†*C. diphtheriae (mitis, belfanti* strain) is nitrate negative.

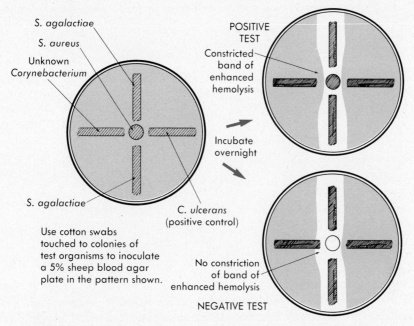

FIGURE 33.3
Pattern of inoculation of plate for test for phospholipase D (inhibition of CAMP test).

SUCROSE	STARCH	TREHALOSE	GLYCOGEN	PYRAZINAMIDASE	PHOSPHOLIPASE
−	−	−	−	−	−
−	+	−	+	−	−
−	−	−	−	−	−
−	+	+	−/+	−	+
−	−	−	−	+	−
−	−	−	−	−	+
+	−	−	−	+	−
−	+/−	+/−	+/−	+	−
+/−	+/−	+/−	NT	+	+
+/−	+/−	+/−	NT	+	+

Davis, D.R., and Yong, D.C. 1983. Rapid microbiochemical identification of *Corynebacterium diphtheriae* and other medically

strains negative); NT = not tested.

PROCEDURE 33.3. RAPID BIOCHEMICAL TESTS FOR IDENTIFICATION OF *CORYNEBACTERIUM* SPECIES

1. Prepare biochemicals as follows:
   Biochemical medium base

Casamino acids (Difco Laboratories)	20 g
L-cysteine HCl (Sigma Chemical Co.)	0.3 g
Sodium sulfate (J.T. Baker Chemical Co.)	0.3 g
Neopeptone (Difco Laboratories)	25 g
Phenol red (Difco Laboratories)	0.1 g
Distilled water	1 liter

   Dispense in 50 ml quantities into six 100 ml screw-cap flasks.
   To one flask, add:

Starch (Difco Laboratories)	1 g

   To another flask, add:

Glycogen (Difco Laboratories)	1 g

   Autoclave all of the flasks for 10 min at 121° C.
   Prepare 20% carbohydrate solutions of dextrose, maltose, sucrose, and trehalose in distilled water (4 g carbohydrate in 20 ml distilled water). Filter sterilize through a 0.45 μm membrane filter. Add 5 ml of each carbohydrate solution to one each of the four remaining flasks of autoclaved broth base.
   Also prepare nitrate broth and urea broth (Chapter 45) or purchase such media commercially (Appendix).
   Store all media in sterile dropper bottles.
2. Just before use, dispense 1 drop (approximately 0.025 ml) of each medium into a sterile microtube (6 × 50 mm borosilicate disposable glass, Kimble Division of Owens-Illinois) held upright in a microdilution plate (Appendix).
3. Inoculate each medium with one third of a large loopful of a colony from overnight growth on blood agar. Be certain that the inoculum is very evenly dispersed in the medium. Complete emulsification is required for rapid reactions.
4. Overlay the inoculated urea tube with mineral oil.
5. Incubate the tubes for 1 h in a shallow water bath at 37° C. Results are interpreted as for conventional tests: positive carbohydrate utilization is shown by yellow, negative is red; urea hydrolysis turns the indicator pink, and the nitrate test requires addition of standard reagents (Chapter 9), after which a positive test is red.

Modified from Thompson, et al. 1983. J. Clin. Microbiol. 18:926.

Interestingly, the groups D2 and JK corynebacteria can be identified with a commercial biochemical kit developed for species identification of viridans streptococci, the API 20S (Analytab Products). As described by Kelly et al.[7] the biochemical strip is inoculated with a very heavy inoculum of the organism, prepared by removing the entire growth from a pure subculture plate with a cotton swab and emulsifying the growth in 5 ml of sterile saline to approximately the turbidity of skim milk. After 4 h incubation at 37° C, reagents are added to the strip according to the manufacturer's recommendations and a profile number is generated. The JK group yield profile numbers of 0044010 or 0044012. Group D2 yield profiles of 0244010, 0244012, or 4244010. Although this system has not proven to be adequate for identifying many of the viridans streptococci, it seems to be very reliable for identifying the multiply resistant strains of corynebacteria. *Corynebacterium* group JK can also be differentiated from *C. bovis*, the other fastidious corynebacterium it resembles, by the ONPG test (Chapter 27). *C. bovis* is ONPG positive, and group JK is ONPG negative.

33.3.d. In vitro toxigenicity test. Definitive identification of a strain of *C. diphtheriae* as a true pathogen requires demonstration of toxin production. A patient may be infected with several strains at once, so that performance of a test that utilizes a pooled inoculum will enhance chances of detecting toxin activity. The most useful test is that described originally by Elek,[5] the **in vitro toxigenicity test,** or **Elek plate.** The test should be performed only in reference laboratories today, since the incidence of diphtheria is quite low and the test poses numerous technical problems due to variability of reagents. Briefly, a filter paper strip impregnated with diphtheria antitoxin is buried just below the surface of a special agar plate before the agar hardens. Strains to be tested and known positive and negative toxigenic strains are streaked on the surface of the

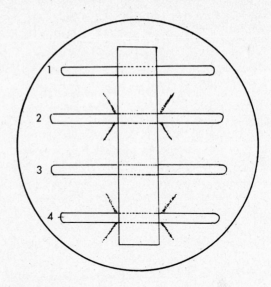

FIGURE 33.4
Diagram of an Elek plate for demonstration of toxin production by *Corynebacterium diphtheriae.*

agar in a line across the plate, at a right angle to the antitoxin paper strip (Figure 33.4). After 24 h incubation at 37° C, plates are examined with transmitted light for the presence of fine precipitin lines at a 45-degree angle to the streaks. The presence of precipitin lines indicates that the strain produced toxin that reacted with the homologous antitoxin. Under some circumstances, precipitin lines may take up to 72 h to develop.

33.3.e. Therapy of infections caused by corynebacteria. *C. diphtheriae* are usually susceptible to penicillin, erythromycin, and most other antimicrobial agents useful against gram-positive bacteria. In all cases of diphtheria, antibiotic therapy should be initiated. Antitoxin therapy is given to patients from whom toxigenic strains are isolated or if the clinical picture dictates such therapy. The isolates should be tested for susceptibility, however, since erythromycin and tetracycline resistance has been observed. The other corynebacteria, except for JK and D2, are variable in susceptibility. All corynebacteria are resistant to oxacillin, methicillin, and nafcillin. Groups JK and D2, additionally, exhibit multiple resistance, usually being susceptible only to vancomycin, which is the drug of choice for treatment of infections with those strains.

33.4. *Nocardia* Species

33.4.a. General considerations, epidemiology, and pathogenesis of *Nocardia* infection. *Nocardia* are members of the group of aerobic actinomycetes, which include *Streptomyces*, *Nocardiopsis*, *Actinomadura*, *Dermatophilus*, and other species that rarely cause human infection. Some of these organisms are discussed briefly below. *Dermatophilus* is discussed in Chapter 39. The *Nocardia* are inhabitants of the soil and water. They infect humans after inhalation of the organisms and primary establishment of growth in the lungs or by inoculation through breaks in the skin. The infection is usually chronic, but occasionally is fulminant, and is usually seen in immunosuppressed patients. The clinical syndrome of a chronic disease with both respiratory and central nervous system components, particularly if abscess formation is apparent, is suggestive of nocardiosis.

Infections caused by *Nocardia* are primarily suppurative, with necrosis and abscess formation. The incidence is higher in males than females. Although pneumonic processes are often seen, a lymphocutaneous infection resembling sporotrichosis (Chapter 43) can occur. Spread to other tissues from the primary pulmonary lesions occurs by advancing growth (to produce empyema, chest wall involvement, and draining sinuses) or hematogenously. The organism seems to be able to resist phagocytosis and therefore persists in the host. Definitive determinants of pathogenicity are not known, but the filamentous stage of growth seems to be more virulent than the stationary coccoid phase.

33.4.b. Laboratory identification. Cells of *Nocardia* are pleomorphic, exhibiting branching and coccoid forms. The most distinguishing characteristic of *Nocardia* is its tendency to retain carbol-fuchsin stain with mild acid decolorization, called **partial acid fastness.** The characteristic may be difficult to demonstrate. Growing the organism to be tested, along with a fresh subculture of a known positive control (*Nocardia asteroides*) and a known negative control (*Actinomadura madurae*), for approximately 4 days on Middlebrook 7H11 agar (Chapter 45) or in litmus milk broth (Chapter 45) will enhance the acid fast nature of an isolate. The partial acid fast stain is performed as outlined in Procedure 33.4. We (EJB) have had excellent results with this stain in our laboratory.

Nocardia may be first suspected when long, thin, branching gram-positive bacilli are seen in smears of lesion material or sputum. The organism also stains with Gomori methenamine silver stain (Chapters 16 and 46 and Plate 33.3). Since it grows slowly, *Nocardia* is often overgrown by normal flora and other bacteria on routine microbiological media. Insertion of a glass rod dipped in paraffin to a liquid culture of a contaminated specimen (sputum, for example) diluted 1:1 in buffered saline may aid in isolation of *Nocardia*, which can utilize paraffin as a sole carbon source.[9] Material from specimens that contain no other flora, such as tissue and abscess drainage, may be inoculated to brain heart infusion agar, which supports growth of *Nocardia*. The organism grows well on Sabouraud dextrose agar, but is inhibited by chloramphenicol. Occasional isolates will first be seen on mycobacterial culture media, since *Nocardia* can survive the usual decontamination procedures (Chapter 41). Incubating at least one primary isolation medium at 45° C may enhance recovery of *N. asteroides*. *Nocardia* grows better in 10% CO_2.

Colonies will appear from 3 to 30 days after inoculation, appearing as waxy, bumpy, or velvety rugose forms, usually with yellow to orange pigment (Figure 33.5). The presence of

PROCEDURE 33.4. PARTIAL ACID FAST STAIN
FOR IDENTIFICATION OF *NOCARDIA*

1. Emulsify a very small amount of the organisms to be stained in a drop of distilled water on the slide. A known positive control and a negative control should be stained along with the unknown strain.
2. Allow to air dry and heat fix.
3. Flood the stain with Kinyoun's carbol-fuchsin (Chapter 46) and allow the stain to remain on the slide 3 min.
4. Rinse with tap water, shake off excess water, and decolorize briefly with 3% acid alcohol (940 ml of 95% ethanol and 60 ml of concentrated HCl) until no more red color rinses off the slides.
5. Counterstain with Kinyoun's methylene blue (Chapter 46) for 30 seconds.
6. Rinse again with tap water. Allow the slide to air dry and examine the unknown strain compared to the controls. Partially acid fast organisms show reddish to purple filaments, compared to non–acid fast organisms that are blue only.

FIGURE 33.5
Colony of *Nocardia asteroides* after 10 days of incubation.

TABLE 33.4
Differentiation of Selected Aerobic Actinomycetes*

ORGANISM	ACID FROM CELLOBIOSE	HYDROLYSIS OF					LYSOZYME RESISTANCE
		CASEIN	HYPOXANTHINE	TYROSINE	UREA	XANTHINE	
Actinomadura madurae	+	+	+	+	-	-	-
A. pelletieri	-	+	+/-	+	-	-	-
Nocardia asteroides	-	-	-	-	+	-	+
N. brasiliensis	-	+	+	+	+	-	+
N. caviae	-	-	+	+/-	+	+	+
Nocardiopsis dassonvillei	+	+	+	+	+/-	+	-
Streptomyces griseus	+	+	+	+	+	+	-
S. somaliensis	-	+	-	+	-	-	-
Streptomyces species (other)	+/-	+	+	+	+/-	+/-	+/-

Modified from McGinnis et al. 1982. Pictorial handbook of medically important fungi and aerobic actinomycetes. Praeger Publishers, New York.

*+ = ≥90% of strains positive; - = ≥90% of strains negative; +/- = variable results.

branching filaments and partial acid fastness differentiates these isolates from mycobacteria. Differentiation from *Streptomyces* species is more difficult. Aerial hyphae of *Nocardia*, *Streptomyces*, *Nocardiopsis*, and *Actinomadura* are best displayed on the slightly acid Sabouraud dextrose agar made from Difco Laboratories' dry powder, according to Leonore Haley of the Centers for Disease Control (CDC). Mishra et al.[8] have developed a taxonomic scheme that divides these genera on the basis of biochemical characteristics. There are

numerous species of *Nocardia*, not all of which have been recovered from clinical specimens. A simplified scheme for identification of the most commonly isolated species, developed by McGinnis, D'Amato, and Land,[10] is shown in Table 33.4. Readers are referred to this publication for instructions on preparation of the media used to identify these organisms. The *Nocardia* are resistant to the action of lysozyme, while almost all *Streptomyces* are susceptible. Lysozyme resistance is tested according to Procedure 33.5. This test is subject to

---

PROCEDURE 33.5. LYSOZYME RESISTANCE FOR DIFFERENTIATING *NOCARDIA* FROM *STREPTOMYCES*

1. Prepare basal broth as follows:

Peptone (Difco Laboratories)	5 g
Beef extract (Difco)	3 g
Glycerol (Difco)	70 ml
Distilled water	1,000 ml

   Dispense 500 ml of this solution into 16 × 125 mm screw cap glass test tubes, 5 ml per tube. Autoclave the test tubes and the remaining solution for 15 min at 121° C. Tighten caps and store the tubes in the refrigerator for a maximum of 2 months.

2. Prepare lysozyme solution as follows:

Lysozyme (Sigma Chemical Co.)	100 mg
HCl (0.01 N)	100 ml

   Filter sterilize through a 0.45 μm membrane filter.

3. Add 5 ml lysozyme solution to 95 ml basal broth, mix gently, avoiding bubbles, and aseptically dispense in 5 ml amounts to sterile, screw cap tubes as above. Store refrigerated for a maximum of 2 weeks.

4. Place several bits of the colony of the isolate to be tested into a tube of the basal glycerol broth without lysozyme (control) and into a tube of broth containing lysozyme. Test a known negative control (*Streptomyces griseus*) and a known positive control (*N. asteroides*) in the same way.

5. Incubate at room temperature for up to 7 days. Observe for growth in the control tube. An organism that grows well in the control tube but not in the lysozyme tube is considered to be susceptible to lysozyme.

Modified from McGinnis, et al. 1982. Pictorial handbook of medically important fungi and aerobic actinomycetes. Praeger Publishers, New York.

variation, however, and occasionally does not yield useful results. Another helpful test for differentiating *Nocardia*, *Nocardiopsis*, and *Streptomyces* from the other aerobic actinomycetes is ONPG (*o*-nitrophenyl-beta-D-galacto-pyranoside), the test for beta galactosidase. The reagents are available commercially since they are usually used for identification of Enterobacteriaceae. The three genera mentioned are positive (able to utilize lactose), while other genera of actinomycetes are negative. In cases where definitive identification of a *Nocardia*-like organism is required, the isolate should be sent to a reference laboratory where cell wall analysis can be performed.

33.4.c. Therapy. Sulfonamides still appear to be the antimicrobial agents of choice for treatment of nocardiosis. Trimethoprim-sulfamethoxazole has not proven to be as active as sulfonamides alone against *Nocardia*. Minocycline seems to be a good alternative for sulfonamide-allergic patients, and newer aminoglycosides such as amikacin are very promising. In vitro susceptibility tests can be performed by reference laboratories, and they should be attempted with isolates from cases that appear resistant to treatment.

33.5. Miscellaneous Other Aerobic Actinomycetes

Human infections with strains of the genera *Nocardiopsis*, *Actinomadura*, *Dermatophilus*, and *Streptomyces* are usually chronic, granulomatous lesions of the skin and subcutaneous tissue, acquired by inoculation. **Mycetoma,** a chronic lesion of the extremities, usually the feet, characterized by swollen tissue and draining sinus tracts, although usually associated with fungal infection, can be caused by members of the actinomycetes. The infection is then called **actinomycetoma.** These organisms may become more common as causes of infection in immunocompromised hosts. All of the aerobic actinomycetes are soil saprophytes. With the exception of rare strains of *Streptomyces*, aerobic actinomycetes are susceptible to the action of lysozyme. Because the biochemical reactions that are used to identify these organisms are difficult to perform and because cell wall analysis is usually needed for ultimate species identification, clinically significant strains should be sent to a reference laboratory for testing. Table 33.4 illustrates a simplified scheme for differentiation among some medically important species.

33.6. *Erysipelothrix rhusiopathiae*

The only species in the genus, *E. rhusiopathiae* is primarily a pathogen of animals, including swine and mice. Veterinarians may be infected from animals. The organism causes a spreading, cellulitis-like lesion called **erysipeloid,** usually on the fingers or hand, but it may disseminate to cause septicemia with arthritis or endocarditis. The organism grows well on blood agar, showing hemolysis on horse blood. It is facultatively anaerobic or microaerophilic, growing best at 30°-35° C. Aspirated material should be inoculated into brain heart infusion broth with 1% dextrose for initial isolation. Subcultures of this broth, which is incubated at 35° C in air or CO_2, are made at 24 h intervals to blood agar. On primary isolation, the organism may yield two or more different morphologic colony types, each containing bacteria with different cellular morphologies, mimicking a polymicrobic infection. *E. rhusiopathiae* smeared from large, rough colonies is a slender, filamentous gram-positive bacillus with a tendency to overdecolorize and appear gram negative. A Gram stain made from the smaller, translucent colony yields small slender bacilli. The organism is nonmotile, but its primary distinguishing characteristic is that it is the only catalase-negative, gram-positive, aerobic bacillus that produces H_2S when inoculated into triple sugar iron or Kligler's iron agar slant tubes (Chapter 27).

33.7. Other Aerobic Non-Spore-Forming Bacilli: *Rothia*, *Kurthia*, *Oerskovia*, and *Lactobacillus*

33.7.a. *Rothia dentocariosa*. The genus *Rothia* was created in 1967 to accommodate an organism that resembled *Actinomyces* (but grew well aerobically) and resembled *Nocardia* (but did not contain the same cell wall constituents). The only species, *R. dentocariosa*, has caused abscesses and endocarditis and is part of normal human oral flora. It has also been recovered from gingival crevices of patients with periodontal disease and can cause periodontitis in germ-free rats. Unlike other filamentous, gram-positive organisms, *Rothia* contains fructose as a component of the cell wall. The organism grows well on nutrient agar, producing smooth colonies at 48 h that become rough or globose on prolonged incubation. Microscopically, the cells are coccoid, only becoming branched after several days of incubation in broth. The organism is catalase positive, lactose negative, and produces acetoin from glucose (exhibits a positive Voges-Proskauer test, as described in Chapter 27). *Rothia* is susceptible to most antimicrobial agents, including penicillin, erythromycin, aminoglycosides, and cephalosporins.

33.7.b. *Kurthia* and *Oerskovia* species. Both of these genera are soil saprophytes, being only rarely implicated in human infection. *Kurthia bessonii* has been isolated from endocarditis. The organism resembles *Bacillus cereus* by forming irregular colonies and by its cellular morphology (large, straight-sided, motile gram-positive bacilli). *Kurthia*, however, does not form spores and is strictly aerobic and nonsaccharolytic. At least two species of *Oerskovia*, *O. turbata*, and *O. xanthineolytica* can cause human infection. Isolates have been recovered from infected heart valves, blood, wounds, and other sites. Most strains of *Oerskovia* produce a yellow pigment. Microscopically, the organisms are branching, filamentous bacilli that fragment into coccoid forms after prolonged incubation. Differentiation from *Corynebacterium* species is extremely difficult. The ability of *Oerskovia* to hydrolyze esculin and motility may be helpful. Only very rare strains of corynebacteria (*C. aquaticum* and a few CDC groups) are motile.

33.7.c. *Lactobacillus* species. The lactobacilli are common inhabitants of the oral cavity, gastrointestinal tract, and female genital tract of humans. They have only rarely been reported to cause serious human infection. Lactobacilli have been isolated from blood, cerebrospinal fluid, abscess material, amniotic fluid, and pleural fluid. The organism is a facultative or strict anaerobe, usually preferring to grow microaerophilically; strains are usually identified using anaerobic media and methods (Chapters 34 and 35). The presence of large numbers of lactobacilli in the culture or Gram stain of vaginal contents is indicative of a healthy vagina. When the organism gains access to an unnatural site, it is able to cause suppurative infection. Large amounts of lactic acid are produced as byproducts of metabolism, which helps to maintain the acid pH that lactobacilli thrive in. It is possible that endocervical lactobacilli play a role in protecting human females from gonococcal infection.

The colonies can assume any morphology on blood agar, ranging from pinpoint, alpha hemolytic colonies resembling streptococci to large, rough, gray colonies. The microscopic morphology is highly variable as well, with the existence of forms similar to *Bacillus* species, possibly chaining, as well as coccobacilli, spiral forms, and others. All species are catalase negative. Differentiation from streptococci may be difficult, but the formation of chains of rods in thioglycolate broth and moderate vancomycin resistance (unusual for any gram-positive organism) help to characterize isolates as lactobacilli. Using prereduced, anaerobically sterilized carbohydrate media (Chapter 34),

TABLE 33.5
Selected Key Features of Lactobacilli Most Commonly Isolated from Clinical Specimens*

SPECIES	ARGININE TO AMMONIA	GROWTH AT 45° C	ACID FROM	
			MANNITOL	RAFFINOSE
Lactobacillus acidophilus	−	−	−	+/−
L. casei	−	+	+	−
L. leichmannii	+	−	−	+/−
L. plantarum	−	+/−	+/−	+

*+ = ≥90% of strains positive; − = ≥90% of strains negative; +/− = variable results.

microbiologists can identify some species of lactobacilli. Minimal characteristics of four of the more commonly isolated species that are able to grow aerobically are shown in Table 33.5.

Penicillin, ampicillin, clindamycin, and cephalothin are able to inhibit growth of lactobacilli, but bactericidal activity is not commonly seen. It is possible that the acid environment produced by the organisms contributes to the decreased activity of certain antimicrobial agents against lactobacilli. For treatment of endocarditis, it is recommended that combinations of penicillin and aminoglycosides be used, perhaps with addition of rifampin for increased bactericidal activity.

REFERENCES

1. Barksdale, L., Linder, R., Sulea, I.T., and Pollice, M. 1981. Phospholipase D activity of *Corynebacterium pseudotuberculosis (Corynebacterium ovis)* and *Corynebacterium ulcerans*, a distinctive marker within the genus *Corynebacterium*. J. Clin. Microbiol. 13:335.
2. Clarridge, J.E., and Weissfeld, A.S. 1984. Aerobic asporogenous gram-positive bacilli. Clin. Microbiol. Newsletter 6:115.
3. Cocito, C., and Delville, J. 1983. Properties of microorganisms isolated from human leprosy lesions. Rev. Infect. Dis. 4:649.
4. Coyle, M.B., Hollis, D.G., and Groman, N.B. 1985. *Corynebacterium* spp. and other coryneform organisms. In Lennette, E.H., Balows, A., Hausler, W.J.

Jr., and Shadomy, H.J., editors. Manual of clinical microbiology, ed. 4. American Society for Microbiology, Washington, D.C.
5. Elek, S.D. 1949. The plate virulence test for diphtheria. J. Clin. Pathol. 2:250.
6. Hollis, D.G., and Weaver, R.E. 1981. Gram-positive organisms: a guide to identification. Centers for Disease Control, Atlanta. May, 1981.
7. Kelly, M.C., Smith, I.D., Anstey, R.J., et al. 1984. Rapid identification of antibiotic-resistant corynebacteria with the API 20S system. J. Clin. Microbiol. 19:245.
8. Mishra, S.K., Gordon, R.E., and Barnett, D.A. 1980. Identification of nocardiae and streptomycetes of medical importance. J. Clin. Microbiol. 11:728.
9. Mishra, S.K., and Randhawa, H.S. 1969. Application of paraffin bait technique to the isolation of *Nocardia asteroides* from clinical specimens. Appl. Microbiol. 18:686.
10. McGinnis, M.R., D'Amato, R.F., and Land, G.A. 1982. Pictorial handbook of medically important fungi and aerobic actinomycetes. Praeger Publishers, New York.
11. Skalka, B., and Smola, J. 1983. Selective diagnostic medium for pathogenic *Listeria* spp. J. Clin. Microbiol. 18:1432.
12. Skalka, B., Smola, J., and Elischerova, K. 1982. Routine test for in vitro differentiation of pathogenic and apathogenic *Listeria monocytogenes* strains. J. Clin. Microbiol. 15:503.
13. Sulea, I.T., Pollice, M.C., and Barksdale, L. 1980. Pyrazine carboxylamidase activity in *Corynebacterium*. J. Clin. Microbiol. 30:466.
14. Thompson, J.S., Gates-Davis, D.R., and Yong, D.C. 1983. Rapid microbiochemical identification of *Corynebacterium diphtheriae* and other medically important corynebacteria. J. Clin. Microbiol. 18:926.

BIBLIOGRAPHY

Barresi, J. 1980. *Listeria monocytogenes:* a cause of premature labor and neonatal sepsis. Am. J. Obstet. Gynecol. 136:410.

Curry, W.A. 1980. Human nocardiosis: a clinical review with selected case reports. Arch. Intern. Med. 140:819.

Fagnant, J.E., Sanders, C.C., and Sanders, W.E. Jr. 1982. Development of and evaluation of a biochemical scheme for identification of endocervical lactobacilli. J. Clin. Microbiol. 16:926.

Goodfellow, M., Alderson, G., and Lacey, J. 1979. Numerical taxonomy of *Actinomadura* and related organisms. J. Gen. Microbiol. 112:95.

Haley, L.D., and Callaway, C.S. 1978. Isolation and identification of some aerobic actinomycetes. In Laboratory methods in medical mycology, ed. 4. U.S. Department of Health, Education, and Welfare Publication CDC 78-8361. Washington, D.C.

Middlebrook, J.L., and Dorland, R.B. 1984. Bacterial toxins: cellular mechanisms of action. Microbiol. Rev. 48:199.

Nieman, R.E., and Lorber, B. 1980. Listeriosis in adults: a changing pattern. Report of eight cases and review of the literature, 1968-1978. Rev. Infect. Dis. 2:207.

Philip, A., and Roberts, G.D. 1984. *Nocardiopsis dassonvillei* cellulitis of the arm. Clin. Microbiol. Newsletter 6:14.

Prauser, H., editor. 1970. The actinomycetales. VEB Gustav Fischer Verlag, Jena.

Slack, J.M., and Gerencser, M. 1975. Actinomyces, filamentous bacteria: biology and pathogenicity. Burgess Publishing Co., Minneapolis.

Smego, R.A., Jr., and Gallis, H.A. 1984. The clinical spectrum of *Nocardia brasiliensis* infection in the United States. Rev. Infect. Dis. 6:164.

Tisdall, P.A., and Roberts, G.D. 1979. Aerobic actinomycetes and the clinical laboratory. Clin. Microbiol. Newsletter 1:1.

Van Etta, L.L., Filice, G.A., Ferguson, R.M., and Gerding, D.N. 1983. *Corynebacterium equi:* a review of 12 cases of human infection. Rev. Infect. Dis. 5:1012.

34

Processing Clinical Specimens for Anaerobic Bacteria: Isolation and Identification Procedures

Martha A.C. Edelstein, B.A., MT(ASC

34.1. Initial Processing Procedure

Properly collected and transported specimens for anaerobic culture may be processed on the bench, in an anaerobic chamber, or with the roll tube system (Chapters 6 and 8). Initial processing includes direct examination and inoculation of the specimen onto appropriate media as represented in Figure 34.1.

34.1.a. Direct examination. Direct examination involves a gross and microscopic examination of the clinical material and may include endproduct analysis by gas liquid chromatography, darkfield or fluorescent-antibody screening techniques. The direct examination provides immediate semiquantitative information about the types of organisms present. This is important for initial therapy since culture results may not be available for several days.

The specimen is inspected for characteristics that include (1) foul odor, (2) brick red fluorescence under ultraviolet light (wavelength 366 nm) indicating pigmented *Bacteroides* sp., (3) black discharge due to pigmented *Bac-*

□This represents the approach of the Wadsworth Anaerobic Bacteriology Laboratory, Los Angeles. It is adapted from the *Wadsworth Anaerobic Bacteriology Manual*, ed. 4, of V.L. Sutter, D.M. Citron, M.A.C. Edelstein, and S.M. Finegold, Star Publishing Co., Belmont, Calif., 1985.

Specimen

Direct examination

Gross   Microscopic

Plate media

Liquid media

Thioglycolate
BHI-S
CMC

O₂ incubation

MacConkey
*Mannitol salt

10% CO₂ incubation

BA
*CA
PEA or CNA

Anaerobic incubation
BBE
KVLB
PEA
*EYA
BA

Isolated colony

EYA
Use for:
  Clostridia-like organisms
  Pigmenting *Bacteroides* sp.
  F. necrophorum-like organisms

BA
Add special
potency disks

Pure colony isolate
see Figure 34.2

Gram
stain

Aerotolerance
testing

CO₂-CA
O₂-BA

*Optional—according to specimen source or Gram stain results
Abbreviation: BA, 5% sheep blood agar
               CA, chocolate agar
               PEA, phenylethyl alcohol
               BHI-S, brain heart infusion, supplemented with 0.05%
                      yeast extract
               CMC, chopped meat carbohydrate
               BBE, *Bacteroides* bile esculin agar
               KVLB, kanamycin-vancomycin laked blood agar
               EYA, egg yolk agar

FIGURE 34.1
Initial specimen processing scheme. (From Sutter, V.L., Citron, D.M., Edelstein, M.A.C., and
Finegold, S.M. 1985. Wadsworth anaerobic bacteriology manual, ed. 4. Star Publishing Co., Belmont,
Calif.)

teroides sp., (4) sulfur granules associated with *Actinomyces* sp. or *Arachnia* sp. (and other organisms), (5) blood, and (6) purulence.

The microscopic examination always includes a Gram stain (Chapter 7). The Gram stain reveals the types and relative numbers of microorganisms and host cells present and is a quality control measure for the microbiologist. Results may also indicate the need for addi-

tional media such as egg yolk agar for clostridia.

Darkfield or phase-contrast microscopy may aid in detecting poorly staining organisms and spores and in observing motility directly. A 2 h direct fluorescent antibody strain (FA) for the *Bacteroides fragilis* group (Fluoretec-F) and some pigmented *Bacteroides* sp. (Fluoretec-M) is available (General Diagnostics).

34.1.b. Specimen preparation and inoculation. After direct visual examination, the prepared specimen is inoculated onto appropriate anaerobic and aerobic plating media, into a liquid medium, and onto a slide for Gram stain.

Grossly purulent material is mixed by vortexing in the gas-tight anaerobe transport vial to ensure even distribution of the organisms. Specimens transported in a syringe are injected into an anaerobic tube for vortexing. Pieces of tissue or bone fragments are homogenized with approximately 1 ml of liquid medium using a tissue grinder to make a thick mixture. Grinding should be done in an anaerobic chamber to minimize aeration. If a chamber is not available, process the specimen as rapidly as possible. Swab specimens are "wrung out" in about 0.5 ml of broth and treated as a liquid specimen. Using a Pasteur pipette, add the prepared specimen as follows: (1) 1 drop per plate for purulent material, (2) 2-3 drops per plate for nonpurulent material, (3) 0.5-1 ml to the middle or bottom of the tube of liquid medium, and (4) 1 drop evenly spread onto the slide. If the swab specimen is inoculated directly onto the media, inoculate the nonselective plates first (both aerobic and anaerobic plates), and then the selective and differential plates.

The direct smears are methanol fixed for 30 seconds in order to preserve red and white cell morphology. Standard Gram stain procedures and reagents are used except that dilute basic fuchsin is used for counterstain (Chapter 46).

The following media are used for the primary isolation of obligately anaerobic bacteria:

1. *Brucella* 5% sheep blood agar supplemented with vitamin K_1 and hemin (BA) for the isolation of all bacteria.
2. *Bacteroides* bile esculin (BBE) agar for the selection and presumptive identification of *B. fragilis* group organisms.
3. Kanamycin-vancomycin-laked blood (KVLB) agar for the selection of pig-

mented and other *Bacteroides* sp. BBE and KVLB are available as biplates from several prepared media manufacturers.

4. Phenylethyl alcohol sheep blood agar (PEA) for the inhibition of enteric and certain other nonanaerobic gram-negative bacilli which otherwise may overgrow the anaerobes.
5. Thioglycolate medium (BBL 135C) supplemented with vitamin K_1 (0.1 μg/ml), hemin (5 μg/ml), and a marble chip or sodium bicarbonate (1 mg/ml, add prior to use). This serves as a backup culture and an enrichment medium for small numbers of bacteria.

The primary plates are reduced in an anaerobic atmosphere for at least 24 h prior to use, unless freshly prepared media are used **within 4 h.** Prereduced anaerobically sterilized (PRAS) plate media are available (Anaerobe Systems). Subsequent BA plates used for subculturing usually do not need to be reduced. The liquid medium is boiled or steamed to drive off residual oxygen and is used on the day of steaming.

The blood agar plate may also be prepared with Columbia, Schaedler, or brain heart infusion base medium supplemented with 0.5% yeast extract. Unsupplemented tryptic soy and heart infusion or brain-heart infusion agar plates should not be used because these do not adequately support the growth of all anaerobes. The following supplements are added to the basal medium: (1) 5% sheep, horse, or rabbit blood for enrichment and for detecting hemolysis and pigment production (rabbit blood is best for the latter), (2) vitamin K_1 (final concentration 10 μg/ml) for growth of some pigmented *Bacteroides,* and (3) hemin (final concentration 5 μg/ml) for growth enhancement of the *B. fragilis* group and other *Bacteroides* sp.

The BBE agar is useful for the rapid isolation and presumptive identification of the *B. fragilis* group. It contains 100 μg/ml of gentamicin which inhibits most aerobic organisms,

20% bile, which inhibits most anaerobes except for the *B. fragilis* group and a few other species; and esculin, which aids in detecting the *B. fragilis* group which are usually esculin positive. Other non-*B. fragilis* group organisms that may rarely grow on this medium are *Fusobacterium mortiferum, Klebsiella pneumoniae,* enterococci, and yeast. However, unlike the *B. fragilis* group, their colony size is usually less than 1 mm in diameter.

The KVLB agar is useful for the rapid isolation of *Bacteroides* sp. The medium contains 75 μg/ml kanamycin, which inhibits most aerobic, facultative, and anaerobic gram-negative rods except for *Bacteroides,* and 7.5 μg/ml vancomycin, which inhibits most gram-positive organisms. The laked blood allows earlier pigmentation by the pigmented *Bacteroides* sp. However, many strains of the *Bacteroides asaccharolyticus* group will not grow on this medium because of their susceptibility to vancomycin. Yeast and other kanamycin-resistant organisms sometimes grow on this medium; therefore one should prepare a Gram stain and check the aerotolerance of all isolates.

The PEA agar inhibits nonanaerobic gram-negative rods. It prevents *Proteus* sp. from swarming and other enterics from overgrowing the anaerobes. Most gram-positive and gram-negative anaerobes will grow on the primary PEA plates, especially in mixed culture, and the colony morphology is similar to that on blood agar; however, it may take an additional 48 h incubation to detect the more slowly growing and pigmenting anaerobes.

The thioglycolate broth serves only as a backup source of culture material, which may be needed in the event of a jar failure or growth inhibition on plates due to antibiotic or bacteriostatic factors (e.g., penicillin or polymorphonuclear leukocytes) in the specimen; these factors will be diluted out in the broth.

If clostridia are suspected (because of clinical picture or if spores or large gram-positive rods are seen on initial Gram stain), an egg yolk agar (EYA) plate is also inoculated to check for the production of lecithinase and lipase. If boxcar shaped cells resembling *Clostridium perfringens* are seen on Gram stain (Plate 34.1), a direct Nagler test (Procedure 34.5) can also be set up along with the primary plates.

34.2. Incubation of Cultures

Inoculated plates are streaked for isolation, are immediately placed into an anaerobic environment (jars, chamber, GasPak pouch [BBL], or Bio-Bag type A [Marion Scientific] as described in Chapter 8), and are incubated at 35° C for 48 h. The cultures must not be exposed to oxygen until after 48 h of incubation, since anaerobes are most sensitive to oxygen during their log phase of growth. Plates incubated in a chamber or anaerobic bag can be inspected at 24 h or earlier without oxygen exposure for the presence of *B. fragilis* group on the BBE plate and *Clostridium* sp. on the BA or EYA plates. Isolates from the BBE and EYA may be further characterized when good growth is evident. The BA plate incubated in a bag should also be held 48 h prior to processing. Plates incubated and further processed inside a chamber may be handled at any time. Negative culture plates are held for 7 days before final examination.

The thioglycolate broth associated with plates showing no growth is inspected daily for 7 days and, when turbid or on day 7, subcultured to a BA plate (anaerobic incubation) and a chocolate agar plate (CO_2 incubation). A 24 h inspection for growth in the broth is important in the case of no growth on the primary aerobic plates. Growth in the broth, especially in the lower half of the tube, indicates that anaerobes may be present. A final report of a negative culture should be issued at 7 days, although the liquid medium is held for at least 1 more week before a final visual examination and discarding.

34.3. Examination of Primary Plates

Anaerobes are usually present in mixed culture with other anaerobes or with facultative bacteria; the combination of enrichment and selective agar plates yields information that will suggest the presence and perhaps the type of anaerobe(s). Primary anaerobic plates should be examined with a hand lens (8 ×) or a stereoscopic microscope. Colonies are described from the various media, as listed below, and semiquantitated (Chapter 8).

The BBE plate selects for the *B. fragilis* group; therefore only colonies growing on this plate that are greater than 1 mm in diameter should be described, enumerated, and subcultured. The *B. fragilis* group are greater than 1 mm in diameter, circular, entire, and raised, with three distinct morphotypes: (1) low convex, dark gray, friable, and surrounded by a dark gray zone and a precipitate; (2) glistening, convex, light to dark gray, and surrounded by a gray zone; and (3) similar to the second morphotype, but with no gray zone (Plate 34.2). Growth on the KVLB plate suggests the presence of *Bacteroides* sp. All colony types are subcultured from the KVLB plate and carefully checked for pigment (this may take more than 48 h to appear) and brick red fluorescence which is detected with UV light (BLAK-RAY, Ultra Violet Products, Inc.).

It is important to further characterize all colony morphotypes from the nonselective BA since facultative and anaerobic bacteria sometimes have similar colony appearances. Nevertheless, the distinct colonial morphologies of certain anaerobes are suggestive of their presence in a culture. Pitting colonies present on the anaerobic but not the CO_2 plate are suggestive of the *Bacteroides ureolyticus*-like group. Large colonies with a double zone of beta hemolysis (Plate 34.3) made up of large gram-positive rods are presumptively *C. perfringens*. These colonies may be subcultured additionally to an egg yolk agar plate for the Nagler test. Breadcrumblike or speckled colonies with greening of the agar around the colonies that subsequently are shown to be slender fusiform gram-negative bacilli (Plate 34.4) suggest *Fusobacterium nucleatum*. Dark pigmented (Plate 34.5) or brick red fluorescent colonies that are gram-negative coccobacilli are pigmented *Bacteroides* sp. A molar tooth colony (Plate 34.6) of gram-positive branching rods (Plate 34.7) may be *Actinomyces* sp.

Colonies on the PEA plate are further processed only if they are different from ones growing on the BA plate or if colonies on the BA plate are impossible to subculture because of overgrowth by swarming *Proteus*, clostridia, or other organisms.

34.4. Subculture of Isolates

Only one colony of each type described is Gram stained and subcultured to the following:

1. BA plate to be incubated anaerobically for isolation of the organism and subsequent testing.
2. Chocolate agar plate to be incubated in CO_2 for aerotolerance testing.
3. EYA plate for suspected lipase and lecithinase producers (*Clostridium* sp., *Fusobacterium necrophorum*, *Bacteroides intermedius*)—optional.
4. Rabbit blood (preferably laked) agar (RBA) plate for gram-negative bacilli in order to better detect pigment production.

We have found it useful to use a sterile wooden applicator stick to subculture colonies. Four to six isolates can be inoculated onto an EYA or RBA plate, and many can be inoculated onto a single CO_2 chocolate agar plate. The same colony subcultured to the purity plate must be used for aerotolerance testing and the Gram stain. If the original colony is not large enough to determine atmospheric requirements directly, then use growth from the purity plate for aerotolerance testing. An addi-

PROCEDURE 34.1. SPECIAL POTENTY ANTIBIOTIC DISK IDENTIFICATION

1. Streak the first quadrant of the purity BA several times in order to produce a heavy lawn of growth, and then streak the other quadrants for isolation.
2. Place the three disks in the first quadrant, well separated from each other (Plate 34.8).
3. Incubate anaerobically for 48 h at 35° C.
4. A zone size of 10 mm or less indicates resistance.

tional BA plate incubated in air will further define the atmospheric requirements of facultative organisms (e.g., microaerophilic streptococci).

The following special potency antibiotic disks are placed on the first quadrant of the purity BA (Procedure 34.1): kanamycin, 1 mg (BBL or Anaerobe Systems), colistin, 10 µg, and vancomycin, 5 µg (Plate 34.8). These disks aid in preliminary grouping of anaerobes and serve as a Gram stain check but do **not** imply susceptibility of an organism for antibiotic therapy. A sodium polyanethol-sulfonate (SPS) disk can be placed near the colistin disk for rapid identification of *Peptostreptococcus anaerobius*. A nitrate disk may be placed on the second quadrant for subsequent determination of nitrate reduction.

If the processing is performed on the open bench, all plates should be promptly incubated anaerobically since some clinical isolates may die after relatively short exposure to oxygen (e.g., *F. necrophorum* and pigmented *Bacteroides* sp.). The primary plates are reincubated along with the purity plates for an additional 48 h and are again inspected for new morphotypes of slow growers and pigmenters.

34.5. Identification of Isolates

34.5.a. General considerations. Pure culture isolates of anaerobes are further processed for identification as shown in Figure 34.2.

There are three levels at which laboratories can operate with regard to anaerobic workup. All laboratories should be capable of functioning at Level I: presumptive identification from primary plates and isolation and maintenance of an anaerobe in pure culture so that an isolate from important clinical cases can be sent to a reference laboratory for complete identification and susceptibility testing. Level II laboratories use simple tests to further group the anaerobes and identify certain ones to species level. Level III laboratories identify the anaerobes isolated as completely as possible using a variety of techniques that may include prereduced anaerobically sterilized (PRAS) biochemicals, miniaturized biochemical systems as described in Chapter 9 and below (e.g., API and Minitek), CDC thioglycolate biochemicals, rapid enzyme detection panels (Innovative Diagnostics Rapid ANA and API AnIdent), gas-liquid chromatography (Chapter 11), toxin assays, etc.

34.5.b. Level I identification. As described in Section 34.3, information from the primary plates in conjunction with the atmospheric requirements, Gram stain, and colonial morphology of a pure isolate provides presumptive identification of anaerobic organisms. Table 34.1 summarizes the extent to which isolates can be identified using this information.

34.5.c. Level II identification tests. Preliminary grouping of anaerobes and identification of some are based on colonial and cellular mor-

Pure colony isolate

Record:

Susceptibility to:
    Vancomycin (5 μg)
    Kanamycin (1 mg)
    Colistin (10 μg)
    *SPS
Colony morphology
Pigment
Hemolysis
Fluorescence
Pitting
*Lipase
*Lecithinase

Subculture to supplemented thioglycolate medium for:
1. Inoculation of biochemicals
2. Motility test
3. Susceptibility testing
Inoculate appropriate screening tests:
1. NO₃
2. SPS
3. EYA for lipase/lecithinase
4. Glutamic acid decarboxylase
5. Reverse CAMP test
6. Formate/fumarate stimulation test
7. Arginine stimulation test
8. 20% bile test
9. Urease
10. Ethanol spore test

Perform:

Gram stain
Spot indole
Catalase
*Nitrate test

*If available at this time
SPS—sodium polyanethol sulfonate

FIGURE 34.2
Pure culture isolate processing scheme. (From Sutter, V.L., Citron, D.M., Edelstein, M.A.C., and Finegold, S.M. 1985. Wadsworth anaerobic bacteriology manual, ed. 4. Star Publishing Co., Belmont, Calif.)

TABLE 34.1
Level I Identification*

ORGANISM	CELL SHAPE	GRAM REACTION	AEROTOLERANCE	DISTINGUISHING CHARACTERISTICS
B. fragilis group	B	−	−	Growth on BBE with colony size >1 mm in diameter
Pigmented Bacteroides sp.	CB B	−	−	Dark pigmenting or brick red fluorescing colony
B. ureolyticus-like group	B	−	−	Pitting colonies
F. nucleatum (presumptive)	B	−	−	Slender bacillus with pointed ends; breadcrumb, speckled colony
Anaerobic gram-negative bacillus	B CB	−	−	
Anaerobic gram-negative coccus	C	−	−	
Anaerobic gram-positive coccus	C	+	−	
C. perfringens (presumptive)	B	+	−	Double zone of beta hemolysis; boxcar shaped cells
Other Clostridium sp.	B	+	−⁺	Spores seen on Gram stain
Anaerobic gram-positive bacillus	B	+	−⁺	No boxcar shaped cells; no spores

From Sutter, V.L., Citron, D.M., Edelstein, M.A.C., and Finegold, S.M. 1985. Wadsworth anaerobic bacteriology manual, ed. 4. Star Publishing Co., Belmont, Calif.
*B = bacilli; CB = coccobacilli; C = cocci; + = most strains positive; − = most strains negative; superscripts indicate reactions of some strains.

phology, Gram reaction, susceptibility to special potency antibiotic disks, results of tests performed with nitrate disks, and results of indole, catalase, and other simple tests. The following characteristics are noted and tests are performed from the purity BA plate on **all** isolates as depicted schematically in Figure 34.2:

1. *Colony morphology.* It is standard procedure to describe the colonial features of the isolate from a 48 h pure BA culture. The description includes the shape, edge, elevation, opacity, color, and any other distinguishing characteristics (e.g., speckling).

2. *Hemolysis.* Use transmitted light to look for beta hemolysis, a double zone of beta hemolysis (clear zone of hemolysis extending just beyond the colonies and a zone of partial hemolysis extending well beyond the colony edge), and greening of the agar, which usually is more apparent after exposure to air.

3. *Pigment.* Few anaerobes produce pigment, but colors common among those that do vary from light tan to black (pigmented *Bacteroides* sp.) or pink to red (*Actinomyces odontolyticus*). Pigment production among the pigmented *Bacteroides* is due to either protohemin or protoporphyrin, depending on the species. Whole or hemolyzed laked rabbit blood is best for detecting pigment, and it is helpful to pick up several colonies on a white cotton swab to increase the contrast.

4. *Fluorescence.* Long wave UV light (366 nm) is used to detect fluorescing colonies. A variety of colors may be seen including brick red, pink, and chartreuse (Plate 34.9).

5. *Pitting.* The top of the colony usually appears just above the level of a crater-like depression in the agar; this depression has been created by an agarase en-

zyme produced by the organism. Hold the BA plate at an angle to the light source to better observe this phenomenon. This characteristic may be easier to detect after 4 days of incubation (Plate 34.10).

6. *Catalase.* See Section 9.2.a. and Procedure 9.1. Use 15% hydrogen peroxide in place of 3% hydrogen peroxide. Most anaerobes are catalase negative; some exceptions include several species in the *B. fragilis* group and a few of the anaerobic cocci.

7. *Indole.* See Section 9.2.d. and Procedure 9.4. (Plate 34.11).

8. *Special potency antibiotic disk susceptibility (Procedure 34.1).* Anaerobes vary in their susceptibility to colistin (10 µg), vancomycin (5 µg), and kanamycin 1 mg), and these reactions aid in determining the Gram reaction, in separating *Bacteroides* sp. and *Fusobacterium* sp., and in subdividing the *Bacteroides* (see Tables 34.2 and 34.3). Generally, gram-positive organisms are resistant to colistin and sensitive to vancomycin, whereas the gram-negative organisms are resistant to vancomycin. This is especially helpful with young cultures of pigmenting *Bacteroides* and clostridia which may appear gram-variable and those clostridia that consistently stain gram-negative. A few exceptions do occur, such as the pigmenting *Bacteroides asaccharolyticus* group, which is usually resistant to colistin and sensitive to vancomycin. *Fusobacterium* sp. are susceptible to both kanamycin and colistin and the *Bacteroides* are usually resistant to kanamycin but variable in susceptibility to colistin. The *Bacteroides ureolyticus* group is the exception as its pattern is the same as the fusobacteria. As with any disk

PROCEDURE 34.2. ETHANOL SPORE TEST

1. Use a 48 h broth culture such as chopped meat with carbohydrate that has incubated an additional 1-2 days at room temperature.
2. Add 1 ml of the broth culture to 1 ml of 95% ethanol.
3. Gently mix and allow to stand for 30-45 min.
4. Dip a swab into the alcohol mixture and spread onto a BA plate.
5. Dip a second swab into the original broth culture, spread this onto a BA, and streak for isolation. This plate serves as a control for purity and viability of the organism.
6. Incubate both plates in an anaerobic environment at 35° C for 48 h.
7. Growth on both plates indicates the presence of spores.

PROCEDURE 34.3. TWENTY PERCENT BILE TUBE TEST

1. Make a solution of 40% oxgall (Difco Laboratories). Sterilize by autoclaving.
2. Add 0.5 ml of oxgall to a freshly steamed or boiled 10 ml thioglycolate tube. This yields a concentration of 2% oxgall, equivalent to 20% bile.
3. Inoculate both the thioglycolate-bile tube and an unsupplemented thioglycolate control tube with 1-2 colonies from a pure BA culture plate.
4. Incubate 24-48 h.
5. Compare the growth in the bile-supplemented tube to the growth in the plain tube. Record as "bile inhibited" when there is no growth or significantly less growth in the bile tube.

PROCEDURE 34.4. LECITHINASE TEST

1. Inoculate a McClung Toabe egg yolk agar plate supplemented with egg yolk emulsion (commercially available from Difco Laboratories, Hana Biologics, and Oxoid USA) with a 24-72 h plate or broth culture of the test organism.
2. Incubate anaerobically for at least 24 h at 35° C.
3. Examine for a white opacity in the medium that surrounds the colony and extends beyond the edge of growth.

PROCEDURE 34.5. NAGLER TEST

1. Swab one-half of an egg yolk agar plate with antitoxin (available from Wellcome Animal Health as *Clostridium welchii* type A antitoxin).
2. Allow to dry.
3. Inoculate the test organism on the antitoxin-free half and then streak across to the antitoxin side of the plate.
4. Incubate anaerobically 24-48 h at 35° C.
5. Examine for disappearance of the turbidity on the antitoxin half of the plate, which denotes neutralization of the type A lecithinase and therefore a positive test (Plate 34.13).

---

diffusion test there are many variables that affect zone sizes, particularly the elapsed time between inoculation and streaking or between streaking and disk application. Therefore, in order to minimize misinterpretations, it may be necessary to inoculate the plates in batched groups of 5-10 plates.

The following additional tests are performed on certain isolates:

9. **Ethanol spore test (Procedure 34.2).** Spores are resistant to the effect of alcohol while vegetative cells are killed. Test gram-positive bacilli to separate *Clostridium* sp. from other gram-positive bacilli if spores are not seen on a gram-stained smear.

10. **Twenty percent bile test (Procedure 34.3).** This test is important to differentiate the bile resistant *B. fragilis* group from the other *Bacteroides* sp. and *F. mortiferum-varium* from most of the other fusobacteria. The test can be performed using bile-impregnated disks, bile-containing agar, or a bile tube test.

11. **Lecithinase reaction (Procedure 34.4).** The compound lecithin, a normal com-

ponent of egg yolk, is split by the enzyme lecithinase to release insoluble diglycerides. This results in an opaque halo in egg-yolk-containing medium that extends beyond the edge of colony growth (Plate 34.12). It is important to test all clostridia and clostridia-like organisms.

12. **Nagler test (Procedure 34.5).** *Clostridium perfringens*, *C. barati*, *C. bifermentans*, and *C. sordellii* produce an alpha lecithinase which is detected by a neutralization test using type A *C. perfringens* antitoxin. One should test *C. perfringens*-like and other lecithinase-positive clostridia with this test.

13. **Reverse CAMP test (Procedure 34.6).** This test is similar to the CAMP test for identifying group B beta hemolytic streptococci (Chapter 25), except that the "test" *Clostridium* sp. replaces the *Staphylococcus aureus* and a known group B beta hemolytic streptococcus is used. Although the group B streptococcus may exhibit some enhanced hemolysis with other clostridia, it is only with *C. perfringens* that the characteristic arrowhead form is demonstrated.

PROCEDURE 34.6. REVERSE CAMP TEST

1. Use growth from a fresh BA culture plate of the *Clostridium* sp. and the group B beta hemolytic streptococcus.
2. Inoculate the streptococcus in a single line at a 90-degree angle to a single line of the clostridium. Be sure there is a small gap between the lines.
3. Incubate anaerobically 24-48 h at 35° C.
4. Read using transmitted light; only the typical arrowhead of synergistic beta hemolysis (Plate 34.14) indicates a positive test.

PROCEDURE 34.7. UREASE BROTH TEST

1. Prepare a heavy suspension of the organism in sterile urea broth.
2. Incubate aerobically at 35° C for up to 24 h.
3. A bright pink to red color is positive. This color change may occur within 15-30 min.

PROCEDURE 34.8. NITRATE DISK TEST

1. After inoculating and streaking a BA plate with the test organism, place a nitrate disk in the first or second quadrant. Alternatively, place the disk on any area of growth on a 48 h plate culture of the test organism.
2. Incubate anaerobically for 48 h at 35° C.
3. Remove the disk to a glass slide or Petri dish and add to the disk 1 drop of reagent A followed with 1 drop of reagent B (Chapter 9, Section 9.3.d). (It is not necessary to remove the disk from the BA plate.)
4. Wait up to 5 min for the production of a red color which indicates the presence of nitrite and, therefore, a positive reaction.
5. If the test remains colorless then add zinc granules. The development of a red color indicates a negative reaction.

Test all *C. perfringens*-like gram-positive bacilli with this test.

14. **Lipase reaction.** Free fats present in egg yolk are broken down by the enzyme lipase to produce glycerol and fatty acids. The fatty acids appear either as a surface "oil on water" layer which covers the colony and may extend beyond the colony edge or as a zone of opacity directly beneath the colony (Plate 34.15). All clostridia, pigmented *Bacteroides* sp, and fusobacteria are tested for lipase production. Inoculate and incubate the egg yolk agar plate as described in the lecithinase test (Procedure 34.4). Hold the plate at an angle to the light source to more easily detect the "oil on water" phenomenon. It may be necessary to reincubate the plate for up to 2 weeks to detect slow lipase producers.

15. **Urease test (Procedure 34.7).** This test is useful for differentiating between the two indole positive, Nagler-positive clostridia (*C. sordellii* and *C. bifermentans*), among the *B. ureolyticus*-like group, and among the *Actinomyces* sp. See Section 9.2.f. of Chapter 9 for the principle and reagents.

16. **Nitrate disk test (Procedure 34.8).** The principle, reagents, and reactions are the same as those discussed in Section 9.3.d, Chapter 9. Test tiny indole negative gram-positive rods (*Eubacterium lentum*-like), *B. ureolyticus*-like organisms, and gram-negative cocci.

17. **SPS susceptibility test.** *P. anaerobius* is susceptible to a 1 mg SPS disk, whereas the other anaerobic gram-positive cocci are resistant. Follow the same procedure as for the special potency antibiotic disks. A zone size of greater than or equal to 12 mm is considered susceptible. Test all anaerobic gram-positive cocci that resemble *P. anaerobius* (large colony, sweetish foul odor, large cocci in chains).

18. **Formate and fumarate (F/F) growth stimulation test (Procedure 34.9).** The *B. ureolyticus*-like organisms grow poorly if at all in broth medium that is not supplemented with formate and fumarate. These organisms require formate or hydrogen as an electron donor and fumarate or nitrate as an electron acceptor in their metabolic processes. A simple test method is to supplement a thioglycolate broth with formate and fumarate and compare growth in that tube with growth in an unsupplemented broth culture. Test all gram-negative rods that form small transparent colonies or pit the agar.

19. **Arginine growth stimulation test.** *Eubacterium lentum* is one of the few anaerobes whose growth is enhanced by arginine; therefore, test all small gram-positive bacilli that do not resemble diphtheroids. This test is performed in a manner similar to the formate-fumarate growth test but with a filter-sterilized solution of arginine hydrochloride in a final concentration of 0.5% (wt/vol) instead of F/F.

20. **Motility.** Motility is occasionally helpful for identification of the anaerobes isolated from human clinical material, primarily with the gram-negative bacilli. Almost all the clinically isolated gram-negative bacilli belong to either the genus *Bacteroides* or the genus *Fusobacterium*. The species of these two genera are generally nonmotile with the rare exception of *B. praeacutus*. Test the *B. ureolyticus*-like group because it includes *Wolinella* and *Campylobacter* species, which are motile. Test any other gram-negative bacillus that does

PROCEDURE 34.9. FORMATE-FUMARATE (F/F) GROWTH STIMULATION TEST

1. Prepare a solution of formate-fumarate.
   a. Ingredients

Sodium formate (Fisher Scientific Co.)	3 g
Fumaric acid (Fisher Scientific Co.)	3 g
Distilled water	50 ml
Sodium hydroxide	20 pellets

   b. Preparation
      1. Combine ingredients, stirring until pellets are dissolved and fumaric acid is in solution.
      2. Adjust pH to 7.0 with 4 N sodium hydroxide.
      3. Sterilize by filtration through a 0.2 μm membrane filter.
2. Add 0.5 ml to a 10 ml thioglycolate broth tube.
3. Inoculate both an F/F-supplemented thioglycolate and an unsupplemented thioglycolate broth with several colonies from a 48-72 h BA plate culture.
4. Incubate 24-48 h at 35° C.
5. Compare the growth in the F/F-supplemented tube to that in the plain tubes. Record as "F/F stimulated" when there is growth in the supplemented tube and poor to no growth in the plain tube.

not key out otherwise according to Table 36.1. Motility is optimally performed on young broth cultures.

A few of the tests discussed above are incorporated in the Lombard-Dowell (LD) Presumpto 1 plate which is available from many sources, including Remel Laboratories. The more fastidious organisms (certain pigmenters, cocci, *Fusobacterium*) do not grow well on the LD basal medium and some manufacturers supplement it. Good growth on the basal medium is required to accurately interpret results.

34.5.d. Group identification. The gram-negative organisms are divided into the following major categories based on microscopic morphology, special potency antibiotic disk patterns, or other simple tests.

1. *B. fragilis* group. These gram-negative bacilli grow in 20% bile and are almost always resistant to all three special potency antibiotic disks.
2. Pigmented *Bacteroides* sp. Organisms that fluoresce brick red or produce brown to black colonies are placed in this group. Many are coccobacillary.
3. *B. ureolyticus*-like group. Members of this group require formate and fumarate for growth in broth culture and reduce nitrate. Their disk pattern is the same as the fusobacteria; however, the colony morphologies are different. *B. ureolyticus*, *B. gracilis*, *Wolinella*, and *Campylobacter concisus* form small translucent to transparent colonies which may corrode the agar, whereas the *Fusobacterium* colony is generally larger and more opaque.
4. Other *Bacteroides* sp. This term is applied to gram-negative bacilli that do not

fit the above categories or the *Fusobacterium* sp.

5. *Fusobacterium* sp. Gram-negative bacilli are placed in this group by their characteristic antibiotic disk pattern (sensitive to colistin and kanamycin and resistant to vancomycin) and colony and microscopic morphology.

6. Anaerobic gram-negative cocci. This category is based solely on Gram stain morphology and includes *Veillonella*, *Megasphaera*, and *Acidaminococcus*.

The gram-positive organisms are divided into three major categories based on microscopic morphology and the presence of spores.

1. Anaerobic gram-positive cocci. This group primarily includes *Peptostreptococcus* and *Streptococcus*. If a coccus is resistant to metronidazole, it probably is a *Streptococcus* or *Staphylococcus saccharolyticus*.

2. *Clostridium* sp. These are the endospore-forming anaerobic gram-positive bacilli. If spores are not present on Gram stain, then the ethanol or heat-spore test will separate this group from the non-spore-forming anaerobic bacilli.

3. Anaerobic non-spore-forming bacilli. This group includes the genera *Actinomyces*, *Arachnia*, *Bifidobacterium*, *Eubacterium*, anaerobic *Lactobacillus*, and *Propionibacterium*. It is impossible to differentiate this group accurately to the genus level without endproduct analysis. However, *Propionibacterium acnes* and *E. lentum* can be identified with a few additional tests, as discussed in the next section.

34.5.e. Level II identification. The readily speciated anaerobic organisms are shown in Tables 34.2 and 34.3. It is necessary that **all** stated characteristics are present in order to definitively identify them. If a characteristic is not present, only a group name can be applied, unless further biochemical testing is carried out.

B. ureolyticus, *B. gracilis*, and *Wolinella* sp. are thin gram-negative rods with round ends and are susceptible to colistin and kanamycin. The colonies are small, translucent or transparent, and may produce greening of the agar. Three colony morphotypes exist: smooth and convex, pitting, and spreading. All three can occur in the same culture. The organisms are asaccharolytic, nitrate or nitrite positive, and require formate and fumarate for growth in broth culture. The organisms can use hydrogen in place of formate. The *Wolinella* sp. and *Campylobacter concisus* are motile; *B. ureolyticus* is urease positive; and *B. gracilis* is nonmotile (although it does have gliding motility on agar) and urease negative.

An indole positive and lipase positive gram-negative coccobacillus that forms dark pigmented colonies or fluoresces brick red may be identified as *B. intermedius*. Lipase negative strains must be identified using other biochemical tests. A lipase positive, indole negative pigmented *Bacteroides* is identified as *B. loescheii*; however, lipase positive strains of *B. loescheii* are infrequently encountered.

F. nucleatum is an indole positive thin bacillus with pointed ends. It fluoresces chartreuse and produces greening of the agar upon exposure to air. There are three colony morphotypes of *F. nucleatum*: speckled, breadcrumblike, and smooth. The colony size varies from <0.5-2 mm in diameter. The breadcrumb colony is white; the speckled and smooth types are gray to gray-white. A lipase positive *Fusobacterium* is *F. necrophorum*. It is a pleomorphic rod with rounded ends and sometimes forms bizarre shapes. It is indole positive, fluoresces chartreuse, and produces greening of the agar. The colonies are umbonate and range in size from 0.5-2 mm in diameter. Lipase positive strains are often beta hemolytic. Lipase negative strains require further biochemical

TABLE 34.2
Level II Group and Species Identification of Anaerobic Gram-Negative Organisms*

	CELL SHAPE	SLENDER CELLS WITH POINTED ENDS	KANAMYCIN (1 mg)	VANCOMYCIN (5 µg)	COLISTIN (10 µg)	GROWTH IN 20% BILE	CATALASE	INDOLE PRODUCTION	LIPASE	GROWTH STIMULATED BY FORMATE-FUMARATE	NITRATE REDUCTION	UREASE	MOTILITY	PITTING	PIGMENT	BRICK-RED FLUORESCENCE
B. fragilis group	B		R	R	R	+	V	V	−		$-^{+}$					−
Other Bacteroides sp.	B		R	R	V	−	−	V	−							−
Pigmented Bacteroides sp.	CB/B		R	V	V	−	−	V	V						+	+
B. intermedius			R	R	S	−	−	+	+							−
B. loescheii			R	R	V	−	−	−	$-^{+}$							
B. ureolyticus-like group	B		S	R	S	−	−	−	−	+	+	V	V	V		
B. ureolyticus			S	R	S	−	−	−		+	+	+	−	V		
B. gracilis			S	R	S	−	−	−		+	+	−	−	V		
Wolinella sp.			S	R	S	−		−		+	+	−	+	V		
Fusobacterium sp.	B	V	S	R	S	V	−	V	V							−
F. nucleatum		+	S	R	S	−		+	−							
F. necrophorum		−	S	R	S	$-^{+}$		+	+							
F. mortiferum-varium		−	S	R	S	+		V	−							
Gram-negative coccus	C		S	R	S											
Veillonella sp.	C		S	R	S						V					+

From Sutter, V.L., Citron, D.M., Edelstein, M.A.C., and Finegold, S.M. 1985. Wadsworth anaerobic bacteriology manual, ed. 4. Star Publishing Co., Belmont, Calif.

*B = bacilli; C = cocci; CB = coccobacilli; R = resistant; S = sensitive; V = variable; + = most strains positive; − = most strains negative; superscripts indicate reactions of occasional strains.

TABLE 34.3
Level II Group and Species Identification of Anaerobic Gram-Positive Organisms*

Organism	CELLULAR MORPHOLOGY	SURVIVES ETHANOL SPORE TEST	KANAMYCIN (1 mg)	COLISTIN (10 µg)	VANCOMYCIN (5 µg)	SODIUM POLYANETHOL SULFONATE (SPS)	INDOLE PRODUCTION	NITRATE PRODUCTION	CATALASE	ARGININE STIMULATION	LECITHINASE	NAGLER TEST	REVERSE CAMP TEST	BOXCAR-SHAPED CELLS	DOUBLE ZONE BETA HEMOLYSIS	UREASE	COLONIES ON CCFA MEDIUM GROUND GLASS YELLOW
Anaerobic gram-positive coccus	C	–	V	R	S	V	V	$-^{+}$	V								
Peptostreptococcus anaerobius	C/CB	–	R	R	S	S	–										
Peptostreptococcus asaccharolyticus	C	–	S	R	S	R	+										
Clostridium species	B	+	V	R	S						V						
Nagler positive Clostridium sp.	B	+	S	R	S						+	+					
C. perfringens	B	+	S	R	S		–				+	+	+	+	+		
C. bifermentans	B	+	S	R	S		+				+	+	–	–	–	–	
C. sordellii	B	+	S	R	S		+				+	+	–	–	–	$+^{-}$	
Nagler negative Clostridium sp.	B	+	S	R	S						V	$-^{-}$					
C. difficile	B	+	S	R	S					+		–	–	–			+
Non-spore-forming bacilli	CB/B	–	S	R	S												
Propionibacterium acnes	B	–	S	R	S		$+^{-}$	$+^{-}$	$+^{-}$								
Eubacterium lentum	CB/B	–	S	R	S		–	+		+							

From Sutter, V.L., Citron, D.M., Edelstein, M.A.C., and Finegold, S.M. 1985. Wadsworth anaerobic bacteriology manual, ed. 4. Star Publishing Co., Belmont, Calif.

*B = bacilli; C = cocci; CB = coccobacilli; S = sensitive; R = resistant; V = variable; + = most strains positive; – = most strains negative; superscripts indicate reactions of occasional strains.

tests for identification. A bile resistant *Fusobacterium* may be identified tentatively as *F. mortiferum-varium* group. Other species of *Fusobacterium* (e.g., *F. necrophorum*) may grow in 20% bile; therefore further testing is required to confirm the presumptive identification.

A gram-negative coccus <0.5 μm in diameter that reduces nitrate or nitrite is *Veillonella* sp. The other gram-negative cocci do not reduce nitrate. Catalase is variable. The colonies are small and almost transparent.

A gram-positive coccus sensitive to sodium polyanetholsulfonate (SPS) is *P. anaerobius*. It is a large coccobacillus and often occurs in chains. The colonies vary in size from 0.5-2 mm in diameter (larger than most anaerobic cocci), and are gray-white and opaque. A sweet, fetid odor is associated with this organism. An indole positive, gram-positive coccus is *P. asaccharolyticus*. *P. indolicus*, another indole positive coccus, is rarely isolated from clinical specimens and, unlike *P. asaccharolyticus*, converts lactate to propionate and is usually nitrate positive and coagulase positive (Chapters 9 and 24).

C. perfringens is usually reverse CAMP test positive, whereas other clostridia have been reported to be negative. The reverse CAMP negative strains are identified with other biochemical tests. *C. perfringens* is a box-car-shaped gram-positive rod that is lecithinase and Nagler positive. Most strains show a typical double zone of beta hemolysis. *C. sordellii* and *C. bifermentans* are indole positive and Nagler positive. *C. sordellii* is usually urease positive and *C. bifermentans* is urease negative.

An indole positive, catalase positive, small pleomorphic (diphtheroid-like) gram-positive bacillus is *Propionibacterium acnes*. It usually reduces nitrate. The colonies are initially small and white, and become larger and more yellowish tan with age. Indole or catalase negative strains are identified with more extensive biochemical tests.

A nitrate positive, small, gram positive bacillus whose growth is stimulated by arginine is identified as *E. lentum*. The colonies are small, gray, and translucent.

34.5.f. Level III identification. In addition to tests performed in level II, species identification may require additional biochemical tests and metabolic endproduct analysis by gas-liquid chromatography (GLC). Differentiation of genera of anaerobes is shown in tables in succeeding chapters (Chapters 35-37). Level III identification tables and flow diagrams are based on reactions of organisms in prereduced anaerobically sterilized (PRAS) liquid media. Thioglycolate-based media with bromthymol blue indicator (CDC Laboratory Manual) give similar results. Results obtained in other systems may not agree with these tables. Gas chromatographic analysis may be performed from any carbohydrate-containing medium that supports good growth of the organism.

34.5.g. Level III identification systems. Several identification systems are currently available, including macrotube and microtube, agar plate, and enzyme substrate types. The PRAS system (macrotube) is still the standard method.

1. PRAS biochemicals are inoculated by either the open or closed technique. The open technique utilizes a special apparatus that allows for a continuous flow of anaerobic gas into the tube during manipulations, whereas the closed technique utilizes a needle and syringe to inject the inoculum into the tube through a rubber stopper. Scott Laboratories has further modified this latter system by replacing the rubber stopper with a rubber diaphragm in a Hungate type screw cap (PRAS II). Scott Laboratories has also developed several computer programs to aid in identification of the isolate at various levels of specificity.

Five to ten drops of a young broth culture (6-72 h, depending upon rapidity of growth) are inoculated into each tube of appropriate test medium. One to two drops are plated onto a BA plate (incubated anaerobically) to determine the purity and viability of the broth culture. The tubes are incubated at 35° C and read as soon as they show good growth or 1 day after no further increase in turbidity is seen. Growth is graded 1+ to 4+ after the tubes have been inverted several times to ensure resuspension of organisms that may have settled to the bottom. The pH is recorded for all carbohydrate, esculin, milk, and starch media. Esculin, gelatin, and starch hydrolysis, indole production, nitrate reduction, and growth in bile are determined. The milk tube is checked for clotting and for digestion. Appropriate biochemicals are processed for gas-liquid chromatography.

The PRAS system is expensive, labor intensive and not problem-free. The major problem is uninterpretable biochemical results which may be due to (1) an inadequate, nonviable or mixed inoculum, (2) partial oxidation of tubes, or (3) contamination.

2. The API 20A (Analytab Products, Inc.) and Minitek (BBL) are microtube biochemical systems that produce results in 24-48 h. The API 20A strip contains 16 carbohydrates and tests for indole, urea, gelatin, esculin, and catalase. The indicator is bromcresol purple, which turns yellow at a pH of 5.2. The Minitek system offers a wide choice of biochemical tests utilizing microtray plates and disks saturated with various substrates. The indicator is phenol red, which turns yellow at pH 6.8. The color reactions in both these systems are not always clearcut; shades of brown (API) and yellow-or-ange (Minitek) make interpretation of test results difficult. In this situation neither system should be relied upon for identification. Both systems are not useful for the identification of asaccharolytic organisms; supplemental tests, including GLC, are often necessary for definitive identification of isolates. Each system has a computerized data base to aid in identification.

3. The Centers for Disease Control (CDC) has developed three four-quadrant plates (Presumpto plates I, II, and III) that incorporate test substrates into Lombard-Dowell agar medium. The Anaerobe-Tek plate (Flow Laboratories) combines the tests from the three Presumpto plates into a single wheel containing individual agars that test glucose, mannitol, lactose, and trehalose fermentation; esculin, starch, and gelatin hydrolysis; casein hydrolysis; production of hydrogen sulfide, indole, catalase, deoxyribonuclease, lecithinase and lipase; and bile tolerance. A computerized data base is available. An unpublished study made in our laboratory has shown that the basal medium did not support the growth of approximately 50% of the anaerobes tested and that only 40% of evaluable isolates were correctly identified using PRAS biochemicals as the standard.

4. The RapID ANA panel (Innovative Diagnostics Systems) and the AnIDENT (Analytab Products) are both 4 h aerobically incubated test systems based on the degradation of conventional and chromogenic substrates by preformed enzymes. The inoculum consists of a suspension of the organism from a 24-48 h plate culture and must be equal to a No. 3 McFarland standard for the RapID ANA and a No. 5 McFarland standard for the AnIDENT. A color developer is added to 8 of the 10 wells in the RapID ANA panel for a total of 18 tests. Gradations in color reactions make interpretation somewhat difficult, but a color chart is provided to decrease the problem. The AnIDENT panel is a series of 20 substrate wells with a total of 21 tests. There are only limited reports on this system. Both systems offer a computerized data base with codebooks to facilitate identification. Preliminary trials suggest that these two systems without the use of gas liquid chromatography or supplemented tests **may** be, in certain instances, an alternative method for the rapid species identification of common clinical isolates.

BIBLIOGRAPHY

Beaucage, C.M., and Onderdonk, A.B. 1982. Evaluation of prereduced anaerobically sterilized medium (PRAS II) system for identification of anaerobic microorganisms. J. Clin. Microbiol. 16:570.

Dowell, V.R. Jr., and Hawkins, T.M. 1974. Laboratory methods in anaerobic bacteriology. In CDC laboratory manual, DHEW Publication No. (CDC) 74-8272, U.S. Government Printing Office, Washington, D.C.

Livingston, S.J., Kominos, S.D., and Yee, R.B. 1978. New medium for selection and presumptive identification of the *Bacteroides fragilis* group. J. Clin. Microbiol. 7:448.

Lombard, G.L., Whaley, D.N., and Dowell, V.R. Jr. 1982. Comparison of media in the Anaerobe-Tek and Presumpto plate systems and evaluation of the Anaerobe-Tek system for identification of commonly encountered anaerobes. J. Clin. Microbiol. 16:1066.

Sutter, V.L., Citron, D.M., Edelstein, M.A.C., and Finegold, S.M. 1985. Wadsworth anaerobic bacteriology manual, ed. 4. Star Publishing Co., Belmont, Calif.

35 Anaerobic Gram-Positive Bacilli

35.1. Introduction to Non-Spore-Forming Bacilli

Included here are the genera *Bifidobacterium*, *Propionibacterium*, *Eubacterium*, *Lactobacillus*, *Actinomyces* and *Arachnia*. These organisms, like other anaerobes, are found as normal flora in various sites, especially the upper respiratory tract and oral cavity, the bowel, the vagina, and, in the case of *Propionibacterium* in particular, the skin.

35.1.a. Role in infection and virulence factors. For the most part, this group of anaerobes is not very pathogenic except for the various species of *Actinomyces* and *Arachnia*. *Bifidobacterium eriksonii* has been isolated from serious pulmonary infections on occasion. Various *Propionibacterium* species, particularly *P. acnes*, have been implicated in infections related to implanted prosthetic devices and in endocarditis; these are usually relatively indolent infections. Other non-spore-forming, anaerobic, gram-positive rods may be isolated from time to time in clinical laboratories; at times, they are part of a mixed flora in which the other anaerobes and nonanaerobes are usually more important, and at times they simply represent contamination of a specimen with normal flora.

Although *Propionibacterium* species may take part in infection, as noted above, most isolates of these organisms represent contaminants. As the name suggests, *P. acnes* plays a role, although not the primary role, in acne. Relatively little work has been done on virulence factors and other mechanisms of pathogenicity in the non-spore-forming, gram-positive rods, no doubt reflecting the fact that these organisms are not major pathogens for the most part. *P. acnes* produces several enzymes, including hyaluronidase, chondroitin sulfatase, neuraminidase, acylneuraminic acid, lyase, and a lipase that hydrolyzes triglycerides but not phospholipids, cholesterol, linolenate, or the lipids in egg yolk. The lipase frees long chain fatty acids in the skin that may be irritating enough to contribute to formation of acne pustules, although other factors are almost certainly of importance as well. Many strains of anaerobic propionibacteria ("*Corynebacterium parvum*," for example) enhance cellular and humoral immunity in certain animals and in humans, under certain conditions.

Actinomyces species, particularly *A. israelii*, produce phosphatases and capsular material. Experimental animal pathogenicity is limited, for the most part, to minor inflammatory changes in response to intradermally injected organisms or their products; however, *Actinomyces* species, *Arachnia*, and *B. eriksonii* exhibit significant pathogenic potential when injected into certain animals by the intraperitoneal or intravenous routes.

35.1.b. Differentiation and identification of non-spore-forming, anaerobic, gram-positive bacilli. The definitive identification of this group of anaerobes requires the use of gas chromatography (Chapter 11) (or a substitute such as column chromatography), with rare exception. Comparative study of ultrastructure of *Actinomyces, Arachnia,* and certain nonanaerobic, gram-positive rods indicates that ultrastructural features of the cell wall are probably reliable criteria for identification purposes. This, of course, is beyond the scope of the usual clinical laboratory. In general, morphologic features are not adequate for distinguishing between different gram-positive non-spore-forming anaerobic bacilli. Moreover, there may be problems distinguishing this group of organisms from others, since they may look coccoid at times, may destain and appear gram-negative, and may be confused with clostridia that do not demonstrate spores. The use of egg yolk agar can be helpful in differentiating clostridia from these organisms. On this medium, none of the non-spore-forming bacilli produce lecithinase and only a few produce lipase.

The key feature that distinguishes among the various genera of non-spore-forming, anaerobic, gram-positive rods is the pattern of volatile and organic acids produced from carbohydrate fermentation (Table 35.1); as noted above, this is best studied by gas chromatography. The catalase-positive forms, *Propionibacterium acnes, P. granulosum, P. avidum,*

TABLE 35.1
Differentiation of Genera of Gram-Positive Anaerobic Bacilli

Spore-forming bacilli	*Clostridium*
Gram-positive non-spore-forming bacilli	
I. Produce propionic and acetic acids as major products	
A. Catalase usually positive	*Propionibacterium*
B. Catalase negative	*Arachnia*
II. No propionic acid produced	
A. Produce acetic and lactic acid (A > L)	*Bifidobacterium*
B. Produce lactic acid as sole major endproduct	*Lactobacillus*
C. Produce moderate acetic acid plus one of the following:	
1. Major succinic and lactic acids	
2. Major succinic acid	*Actinomyces*
D. Other: butyric ± others, acetic or no major acids	*Eubacterium*

Modified from Sutter, V.L., Citron, D.M., Edelstein, M.A.C., and Finegold, S.M. 1985. Wadsworth anaerobic bacteriology manual, ed. 4. Star Publishing Co., Belmont, Calif.

and *Actinomyces viscosus*, may be recognized without gas chromatography. For example, the disk identification procedure is helpful in identifying *P. acnes*, as noted in Chapter 34 (Plate 35.1). The interested reader is referred to Chapter 34 and other sources, such as the *Wadsworth Anaerobic Bacteriology Manual*, for details of gas chromatographic and other identification procedures. Table 35.2 outlines identifying characteristics. Laboratories not equipped for gas chromatography may send selected cultures to reference laboratories (e.g., the Centers for Disease Control [CDC], through the referring state laboratory).

Significant members of each genus are described in the material that follows.

35.1.c. *Bifidobacterium eriksonii*. *B. eriksonii* is part of the normal human oral and intestinal microflora and is usually isolated in clinical material from mixed-flora pulmonary infections, some of which may be severe. It grows as a white, convex, shiny colony with an irregular edge. In thioglycolate medium, growth is diffuse, and the Gram stain shows a diphtheroid to filamentous bacillus, branched or bifurcated. Catalase and indole are not produced; nitrate is not reduced; gelatin is not liquefied; but esculin is hydrolyzed. Carbohydrate fermentation reactions and metabolic end products are characteristic (Tables 35.1 and 35.2).

35.1.d. *Propionibacterium acnes*. The anaerobe (some strains are microaerophilic) *P. acnes* produces propionic acid by fermentation of glucose and is part of the resident flora of normal skin; it is the dominant flora of the anterior nose. It is a frequent contaminant of blood cultures and often contaminates other cultures as well. *Propionibacterium granulosum* and *P. avidum* may also represent contaminants from the skin. Accordingly, particular care must be exercised in the preparation of the skin before venipuncture, lumbar puncture, aspiration of pus from abscesses, and so on, as described in Chapters 6 and 14. *P. acnes* occasionally causes infection, especially endocarditis, ventricular shunt infections, and infection of other prostheses, including artificial joints. *P. acnes* characteristically grows as a small, white to pinkish, shiny to opaque colony with entire margins. A Gram stain of the colony shows slender, slightly curved rods, sometimes with false branching or a beaded appearance. Tests for catalase and indole production are usually positive. Nitrates are usually reduced. Gelatin is liquefied, but esculin is not hydrolyzed. Characteristic patterns of carbohydrate fermentation and organic acid endproducts are obtained. Fluorescent antibody reagents are available from CDC for direct detection of *P. acnes*, *P. granulosum*, and other *Propionibacterium* species in direct smears of clinical material and from cultures. *P. acnes* is very sensitive to penicillin G and most other antimicrobials, except aminoglycosides.

35.1.e. Genus *Eubacterium*. *Eubacterium* species are isolated from wound and other infections and are almost always associated with other anaerobes or facultative bacteria; they are part of the normal fecal microflora and are usually part of the indigenous oral flora as well. *Eubacterium* is not particularly pathogenic but it may be involved in bacteremia that is relatively mild in severity and also may cause endocarditis. Growing as raised to convex, translucent to opaque colonies, the organism appears microscopically as pleomorphic bacillary to coccobacillary forms, occurring in pairs and short chains (Plates 35.2 and 35.3). *Eubacterium lentum* is relatively inactive biochemically; its growth is stimulated by arginine. Characteristic metabolic endproducts are observed.

35.1.f. Genus *Lactobacillus*. The anaerobic members of the genus *Lactobacillus* produce primarily lactic acid from the fermentation of

TABLE 35.2
Characteristics of Gram-Positive Non-Spore-Forming Bacilli

	NITRATE REDUCTION	CATALASE	INDOLE PRODUCTION	ESCULIN HYDROLYSIS	UREASE	RED COLONY	OXYGEN TOLERANCE*	GLUCOSE	MANNITOL	RAFFINOSE	RIBOSE	TREHALOSE	ARABINOSE	ERYTHRITOL	MALTOSE	FATTY ACIDS FROM PEPTONE YEAST GLUCOSE BROTH
								FERMENTATION OF								
Actinomyces sp.	+	−	−	+⁻	V	−		+	+	+	+	+	−			A S (L)
A. israelii	+⁻	−	−	+	−	−	AM	+	+	+	+	+⁻	−	−	+	A L S
A. odontolyticus	+	−	−	+⁻	−	+⁻	AM	+	−	−	−ʷ	−⁺	−	−	V	A S
A. naeslundii	+⁻	−	−	+⁻	+	+	MF	+	−	+	V	+	−	−	+	A L S
A. viscosus	+⁻	V	−	V	+	−	AMF	+	−	+	−⁺	V	−	−	+	A L S
A. meyeri	−⁺	−	−	−	−	−	A	+	−	−	−ʷ	−	−	−	−	A S
Arachnia propionica	+	−	−	V	−	−	AM	+	V	V	+ʷ	+	+	−	+	A P S (L)
Propionibacterium sp.	V	V	V	V	−	−	AM	+								A P
P. acnes	+⁻	+	+	−	−	−	AM	+	−	−	−	−	−	−⁺	−	A p (iv L s)
P. granulosum	−	+	−	−				+						−	+⁻	A p (iv s)
P. avidum	−	+	−	+				+						+ʷ	+	A p (iv s)
Bifidobacterium sp.	−	−	−	+	−	−	AM	+	+	+	+	+	+	−	+	A L [A > L]
B. eriksonii	−	−	−	V			A	+⁻							+	A L [A > L]
Lactobacillus sp.	−⁺	−	−	V	−	−	AM	+⁻							−	L (a) [L > a]
Eubacterium sp.	V	−⁺	−⁺	+⁻	−	−	A	+⁻								
E. lentum	+	−	−	−	−	−	A	−	−	−	−	−	−	−	−	(a l s)

Modified from Sutter, V.L., Citron, D.M., Edelstein, M.A.C., and Finegold, S.M. 1985. Wadsworth anaerobic bacteriology manual, ed. 4. Star Publishing Co., Belmont, Calif.

*Oxygen tolerance: A = Anaerobic; M = microaerophilic; F = facultative.

Reactions: − = negative reaction; + = positive reaction for majority of strains; includes weak as well as strong acid production from carbohydrates in saccharolytic organisms; +⁻ = most strains positive, reaction helpful if positive; +ʷ = most strains positive, some weakly positive; −ʷ = most strains negative, some weakly positive; −⁺ = most strains negative, reaction helpful if negative; V = variable reaction.

PRAS carbohydrates: + pH <5.5; W pH 5.5-5.7; − pH >5.7.

Fatty acids; A = acetic; P = propionic; IB = isobutyric; B = butyric; IV = isovaleric; V = valeric; IC = isocaproic; C = caproic; C' = caprylic; L = lactic; S = succinic; PA = phenylacetic. NOTE: (1) Capital letters indicate major metabolic products. (2) Small letters indicate minor products. (3) Parentheses indicate a variable reaction. (4) Isoacids are primarily from carbohydrate-free media (such as PY) in the case of saccharolytic organisms.

glucose and are only occasionally involved in human infections, usually pleuropulmonary and as part of a mixed flora. They have, rarely, been isolated from urinary tract infection and from endocarditis. They are prominent as normal flora in the vagina and are also usually present in large numbers in the colon and in lesser numbers in the mouth. They may be confused with streptococci, as discussed in Chapter 33.

35.1.g. Genera *Actinomyces* and *Arachnia*. The etiologic agents of human actinomycosis include the most common and important organism, *Actinomyces israelii*, and several other species—*A. naeslundii*, *A. odontolyticus*, *A. viscosus*, *A. meyeri*, and *Arachnia propionica*. These organisms are a part of the normal microbiota of the mouth and female genital tract and produce infection primarily as endogenous opportunists. A large number of cases of pelvic actinomycosis caused by *A. israelii* have been described in association with the use of intrauterine contraceptive devices (IUDs). Although *A. israelii*, *A. odontolyticus*, and *Arachnia* grow best under anaerobic conditions (Plate 35.4), *A. naeslundii* and *A. viscosus* are either microaerophilic or facultative. *A. meyeri* is an obligate anaerobe. *A. israelii* produces a characteristically heaped, rough, lobate colony resembling a molar tooth (Plate 34.6); microscopically, it appears as long, filamentous, gram-positive bacilli, some of which may show branching. A Gram stain of "sulfur granules" (Plate 35.5) from actinomycotic pus reveals a similar morphology (Plates 35.6 and 35.7), often with diphtheroid and coccal forms (Plate 34.7). Colonies of the other organisms generally are smooth, flat to convex, whitish, and transparent, with entire margins. *A. odontolyticus* colonies may develop a red color on blood agar after several days. Microscopically, the other causes of actinomycosis are gram-positive bacilli consisting of diphtheroidal forms and branched elements; some filaments may show

clubbed ends. *Actinomyces* and *Arachnia* can be differentiated from *Nocardia* by the modified acid fast stain described in Chapter 33; *Nocardia* are weakly acid fast.

A. viscosus, being catalase positive, is often overlooked because it is assumed to be a *Propionibacterium* or diphtheroid and therefore not likely to be important. It differs from *P. acnes* by growing equally well aerobically and anaerobically, usually hydrolyzing esculin, not producing indole, not being proteolytic, not producing a pink sediment in thioglycolate broth, and fermenting melibiose, raffinose, sucrose, and salicin.

Kornman and Loesche[2] have described a highly efficient selective medium for isolation of *A. viscosus* and *A. naeslundii* from dental plaque that should be suitable for clinical specimens as well. This medium, containing metronidazole and cadmium sulfate, permits presumptive identification of the organisms based on the medium's selectivity and the characteristic cell morphology of the two organisms.

Direct identification of *Actinomyces* and *Arachnia* by immunofluorescent techniques has proved successful (available from CDC). Penicillin G remains the drug of choice in the treatment of actinomycosis. Tetracycline, clindamycin, and erythromycin also demonstrate activity against these organisms. Metronidazole is relatively poor in activity against *Actinomyces* and *Arachnia*, in sharp contrast to its excellent activity against virtually all other clinically important anaerobes (other non-spore-forming, anaerobic, gram-positive rods also tend to be resistant to metronidazole). It must be remembered that actinomycosis is typically a mixed infection involving, in addition to *Actinomyces* and *Arachnia*, pigmented and other *Bacteroides*, other anaerobes, and *Actinobacillus actinomycetemcomitans*. The latter organism is resistant to clindamycin and may account for less than optimum therapeutic results in actinomycosis when clindamycin is used.

35.2. Introduction to the Spore-Forming, Anaerobic, Gram-Positive Bacilli (*Clostridium*)

The genus *Clostridium* contains a large number of species, the majority of which are obligate anaerobes. Some species are aerotolerant, however, showing growth on enriched media on aerobic incubation. It is possible, then, to confuse these aerotolerant clostridia with certain facultative *Bacillus* species. Members of the genus *Clostridium* form spores under anaerobic conditions and are usually catalase positive. Also, aerotolerant clostridia form larger colonies under anaerobic conditions than under aerobic conditions, whereas the reverse is true for *Bacillus* species. The sporangia are often characteristically swollen, showing spindle, drumstrick, and "tennis racket" forms and containing central, subterminal or terminal spores. With rare exceptions in the aerotolerant forms, the enzymes catalase, cytochrome oxidase, and peroxidase are not produced. Many clostridia attack carbohydrates, and some are proteolytic.

35.2.a. Role in infection and virulence factors. Clostridia are widely distributed in soil, dust, and water and are common inhabitants of the intestinal tract, and to a much lesser extent the genital tract, of animals and humans. They are often found in unclean wounds and wound infections. Most clostridial infections are of endogenous origin, although clostridia from exogenous sources may be involved in certain conditions, such as botulism, tetanus, *Clostridium perfringens* food poisoning, and sometimes gas gangrene (clostridial myonecrosis). The classic infections involving *C. perfringens*, aside from gas gangrene, are gangrenous cholecystitis (with or without visceral gas gangrene) and postabortal sepsis with intravascular hemolysis. However, *C. perfringens* and a number of other species of clostridia are actually much more commonly involved in infections of diverse types throughout the body, of the sort caused by the non-spore-forming anaerobes. This includes such entities as brain abscess, aspiration pneumonia, thoracic empyema, intraabdominal infection, postoperative wound infection, infections related to gynecologic disease or surgery, and soft tissue infections. Bacteremia is found in about 15% of patients with clostridial myonecrosis and may be seen on occasion in the course of other clostridial infections as well.

Tetanus and botulism are classic toxin-related diseases. It is important to keep in mind that in botulism the disease may be related to wound infection as well as to ingestion of preformed toxin in contaminated food (Chapter 17). It should also be appreciated that infant botulism represents a different situation in that the organism colonizes the gastrointestinal tract of the infant (presumably because the infant's own flora is not yet fully developed) and produces toxin within the gastrointestinal tract, which is then absorbed to produce the disease (Chapter 17). It is speculated that in vivo toxin production and absorption may be a mechanism in certain cases of adult botulism as well.

Pseudomembranous colitis related to antimicrobial therapy (see Chapter 17, Plate 17.1) is now known to be caused primarily by *Clostridium difficile*. Rare cases may be due to type C *C. perfringens* and to other clostridia. *C. difficile* may also be involved in pseudomembranous colitis not related to the use of antimicrobial therapy, in disease following the use of methotrexate and other cytotoxic agents, in exacerbations of inflammatory bowel disease, and in complications of strangulation obstruction of the bowel. Most strains of *C. difficile* produce a toxin that is cytopathic for most tissue culture cell lines and also produce an enterotoxin. Diarrhea without colitis following antimicrobial therapy may involve *C. difficile* on occasion. There is evidence to implicate type A *C. perfringens* in some of these cases as well.

There is a definite association between

Clostridium septicum infection and malignancy, particularly in the colon. This underlines the importance of species identification.

The spores of some pathogenic species (*Clostridium botulinum*) may survive in improperly home-canned produce (in which they can develop vegetatively under normal domestic conditions), in inefficiently sterilized surgical dressings and bandages, in plaster of Paris for casts, and on the clothing and skin of humans (primarily *C. perfringens* in the latter three examples).

The toxins of *C. difficile* have already been mentioned. The exotoxins of *Clostridium tetani* and *C. botulinum* are among the most potent poisons known to man (estimated to be one million times as potent as rattlesnake poison). The toxin produced by *C. tetani*, tetanospasmin, becomes bound to gangliosides within the central nervous system; it acts very much like strychnine, suppressing the central inhibitory balancing influences on motor neuron activity, thus leading to intensified reflex response to afferent stimuli and to spasticity and convulsions. It also acts on the sympathetic nervous system and on the neurocirculatory and neuroendocrine systems. Botulinal toxin attaches to individual motor nerve terminals preventing acetylcholine release at the nerve endings. Numerous other toxins are produced by other species of clostridia. For example, *C. perfringens* produces an alpha toxin (a lecithinase, phospholipase C); it is a hemolysin, is also active against white blood cells and platelets, and has necrotizing activity. The lambda toxin of *C. perfringens* is a weak proteolytic enzyme. The nu toxin is an RNAse. The theta toxin is a hemolysin that is responsible for the zone of clear hemolysis that surrounds colonies of *C. perfringens* on blood agar plates. The kappa toxin is a collagenase that is also active in breakdown of gelatin. The mu toxin is a hyaluronidase. The epsilon and iota toxins lead to increased capillary permeability. There is also a neura-minidase and an enterotoxin, the latter acting very much like the enterotoxin of *Vibrio cholerae*. The beta toxin of type C (and B) *C. perfringens* is the key factor in necrotizing enterocolitis ("Darmbrand," pigbel). A number of other clostridia produce important toxins. The reader who is interested is referred to Smith's and Willis' excellent books cited in the bibliography.

35.2.b. Differentiation and identification of clostridia—rapid presumptive identification. The Gram stain may be very useful in helping the clinician or microbiologist to suspect the possibility of gas gangrene, although it should be emphasized that this must be a clinical diagnosis. The two findings of note are absence or distortion of white blood cells and other host cells in the stained smear of the exudate or aspirated material and the presence of large, relatively short, fat, gram-positive rods without evidence of spores (Plate 35.8). The ends of the rods are more or less squared off (Plates 34.1 and 35.9). The changes in the host cells are related to the alpha toxin produced by *C. perfringens*.

Clostridium ramosum, the second most commonly encountered *Clostridium* in clinical infections, is more slender and longer than *C. perfringens*, although also unlikely to reveal spores in direct smears, and the cells are often curved. *C. ramosum* often appears gram-negative in smears made from cultures. With other clostridia, spores may be apparent on Gram stain; phase contrast microscopy often reveals spores more readily however.

C. perfringens colonies on blood agar plates are often surrounded by a double zone of hemolysis (Plate 34.3) that is quite distinctive. The inner zone (which may be only immediately beneath the colony) shows complete hemolysis and the outer zone shows discoloration and incomplete hemolysis. *C. perfringens* is reverse CAMP positive (Chapter 34 and below). The Nagler reaction is recommended for

PROCEDURE 35.1. THE NAGLER REACTION

1. The medium for this reaction, 10% egg yolk in blood agar base (see Chapter 45), is placed in a Petri dish. After hardening, one half of the surface is smeared with a few drops of *C. perfringens* type A antitoxin (available from Wellcome Animal Health).
2. The culture is then streaked in a single line across the plate at a right angle to the antitoxin. The plate is incubated anaerobically for 24-48 h and examined.
3. The lecithinase toxin produces a precipitate (opalescence) about the growth in the line of streak (Plate 34.12) in the absence of antitoxin, but this precipitate is absent on the half of the plate with antitoxin (Plate 34.13).

the rapid identification of *C. perfringens* and other alpha toxin producers. This reaction is described in Procedure 35.1.

The Nagler plate may be used as a primary plate when *C. perfringens* is suspected. Three other clostridia are Nagler positive (see Table 35.3). One of these, *C. baratii*, is seldom encountered in clinical material. Another, *C. sordellii*, is almost always urease positive. The third Nagler positive strain is *C. bifermentans*, which is indole and gelatin positive and urease negative.

Gram stain of stool specimens from patients with *C. difficile* colitis may show polymorphonuclear leukocytes and a predominance of relatively thin, long, gram-positive rods with perfectly parallel sides (Plate 17.3), but these are not dependable criteria for presumptive identification. There is an excellent selective and differential medium for *C. difficile* (cycloserine cefoxitin fructose agar, CCFA [Chapter 45]) that permits early presumptive identification of the organism. *C. difficile* is the one anaerobe of clinical significance that may not grow by anaerobic jar technique. Accordingly, cultures for this organism should be set up in an anaerobic chamber (Plate 35.10). Plates may be placed in Bio-Bags (Marion Laboratories) or GasPak pouches (BBL) within the chamber after inoculation and then removed from the chamber for incubation in a standard incubator. In this manner, plates can be examined at frequent intervals. Colonies of *C. difficile* are usually 2 mm or more in diameter after 24 h of incubation (Plates 35.11 and 35.12). Relatively few organisms other than *C. difficile* grow on the CCFA medium, and most of those that do form much smaller colonies. The colonies fluoresce yellow under ultraviolet light. Such colonies, which on Gram stain show typical gram-positive rods, constitute good presumptive evidence of the presence of *C. difficile*.

The presence of swarming growth on the surface of only the anaerobically incubated blood agar plate and not on the aerobically incubated counterpart is suggestive of clostridia. Swarming growth on both the aerobic and the anaerobic plates may be due to *Proteus* sp. Gram stains of such colonies should show gram-positive rods, and spores may be noted as well.

35.2.c. General methods of isolation and cultivation of pathogenic clostridia. The procedures for specimen collection and transport and for anaerobic culture discussed in Chapters 6 and 8 are applicable to the clostridia. It should be reemphasized here that any material for anaerobic cultivation should be inoculated

32.1

PLATE 32.1. *Bacillus subtilis* on BAP.

33.1

33.2

33.3

PLATE 33.1. Colonies of *Listeria monocytogenes* on sheep blood agar after 48 h incubation, showing the diffuse zone of beta hemolysis surrounding the colonies.

PLATE 33.2. Characteristic umbrella-shaped motility pattern exhibited by colonies of *Listeria monocytogenes* after overnight incubation.

PLATE 33.3. *Nocardia* in lesion of lower leg, stained with Gomori methenamine silver stain.

34.1

34.2

PLATE 34.1. *Clostridium perfringens.* Box-car-shaped cells. (From Sutter et al. 1985.)
PLATE 34.2. *Bacteroides fragilis* growing on *Bacteroides* bile esculin agar (positive esculin reaction) in Bio-Bag.

34.3

34.4

PLATE 34.3. *C. perfringens.* Double zone of beta hemolysis on blood agar. (From Sutter et al. 1985.)

PLATE 34.4. *Fusobacterium nucleatum.* Thin bacillus with pointed ends.

34.5

34.6

PLATE 34.5. *Bacteroides intermedius.* Black pigmentation on sheep blood agar *(left)* vs. rabbit blood agar *(right).* (From Sutter et al. 1985.)
PLATE 34.6. *Actinomyces israelii.* "Molar tooth" colonies.

34.7

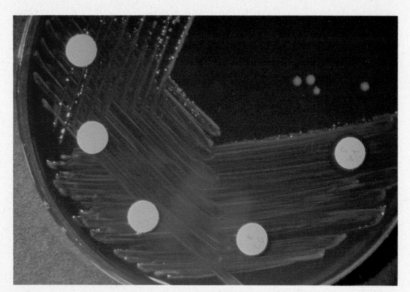

34.8

PLATE 34.7. *A. israelii.* A sulfur granule of gram-positive branching bacilli.
PLATE 34.8. *B. fragilis.* Special potency antibiotic disks.

34.9

34.10

PLATE 34.9.   Pigmented *Bacteroides* sp. Red fluorescence under ultraviolet light (366 nm).
PLATE 34.10.   *Bacteroides ureolyticus.* Pitting colonies on blood agar. (From Sutter et al. 1985.)

34.11

34.12

PLATE 34.11. Spot indole test using paradimethylaminocinnamaldehyde. Blue = positive; colorless or other than blue = negative. (From Sutter et al. 1985.)

PLATE 34.12. *C. perfringens.* Lecithinase reaction. (From Sutter et al. 1985.)

34.13

34.14

PLATE 34.13. *C. perfringens.* Positive Nagler test on egg yolk agar. Inhibition of lecithinase reaction by antitoxin *(left).*

PLATE 34.14. *C. perfringens.* Reverse CAMP test. (From Sutter et al. 1985.)

34.15

PLATE 34.15. *Clostridium*. Positive lipase reaction on egg yolk agar.

35.1

35.2

PLATE 35.1. *Propionibacterium acnes.* Disk identification tests. (From Sutter et al. 1985.)
PLATE 35.2. *Eubacterium* sp. Gram stain.

35.3

35.4

PLATE 35.3. *Eubacterium* sp. Gram stain. Anaerobes may be overdecolorized easily or they may lose their gram positivity.

PLATE 35.4. *Actinomycetes israelii* in thioglycolate broth (no growth near surface).

35.5

35.6

PLATE 35.5. Sulfur granules in thoracic empyema fluid. Actinomycosis.
PLATE 35.6. Sulfur granule, microscopic. Actinomycosis.

35.7

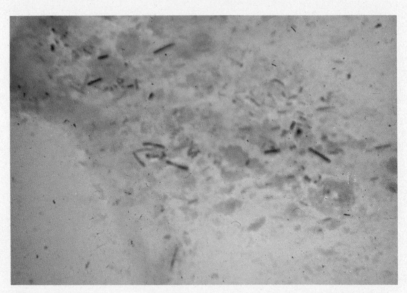

35.8

PLATE 35.7.   Edge of sulfur granule showing clubbing.
PLATE 35.8.   Perineal gas gangrene. *Clostridium perfringens* (large, broad gram-positive rods), coliforms, and white blood cells badly distorted by toxin of *C. perfringens*.

35.9

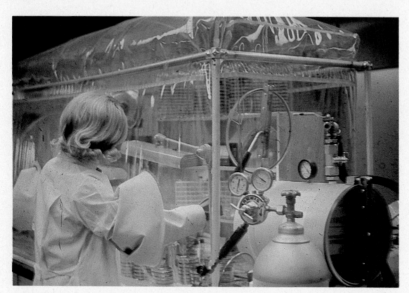

35.10

PLATE 35.9.   Intracellular *C. perfringens* in peripheral blood smear.
PLATE 35.10.   Anaerobic chamber.

35.11

35.12

PLATE 35.11. *Clostridium difficile* on BAP.
PLATE 35.12. *C. difficile* on cycloserine cefoxitin fructose agar.

35.13

35.14

PLATE 35.13. *Clostridium novyi* type A on egg yolk agar. Positive lecithinase and lipase reactions.
PLATE 35.14. *Clostridium septicum* on BAP.

35.15

35.16

PLATE 35.15. *C. septicum,* microscopic. Note spores.
PLATE 35.16. *Clostridium sordellii* on BAP.

35.17

35.18

PLATE 35.17. Tetanus. Patient exhibits opisthotonos (head and legs bent backward toward each other).

PLATE 35.18. *Clostridium tetani* on BAP.

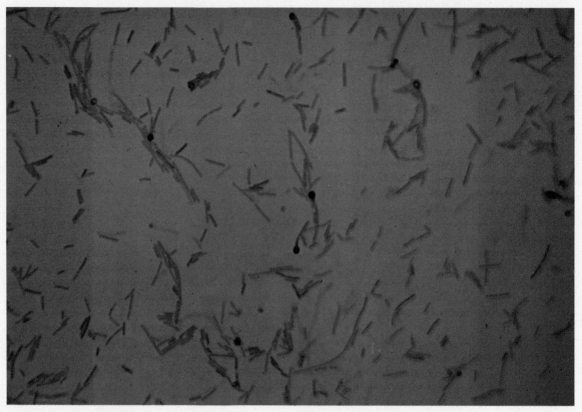

35.19

PLATE 35.19. *C. tetani,* microscopic.

36.1

36.2

PLATE 36.1.   Common sites of anaerobic infection.
PLATE 36.2.   Bile test. Left two tubes, *Bacteroides fragilis* control and bile (no inhibition). Right two tubes, *Fusobacterium nucleatum* control and bile (inhibition).

36.3

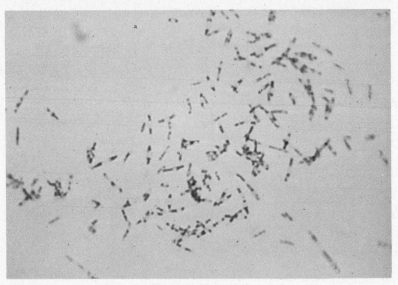

36.4

PLATE 36.3.   *Bacteroides fragilis* on BAP.
PLATE 36.4.   *B. fragilis*. Irregular staining.

36.5

36.6

PLATE 36.5. *B. fragilis.* Irregular staining and pleomorphism.
PLATE 36.6. Gram stain of intraabdominal abscess. Irregularly staining gram-negative rods are *B. fragilis.*

36.7

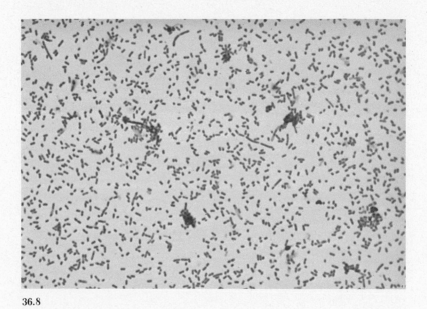

36.8

PLATE 36.7. Transtracheal aspirate. *Peptostreptococcus* and *Bacteroides*.
PLATE 36.8. Pigmented *Bacteroides* sp. Many coccobacillary forms as well as rods. (From Sutter et al. 1985.)

36.9

36.10

PLATE 36.9.   *Bacteroides oris-buccae* on BAP.
PLATE 36.10.   *Bacteroides ureolyticus* on BAP. Note spreading.

36.11

36.12

PLATE 36.11. *F. nucleatum*, microscopic (darkfield).
PLATE 36.12. *Fusobacterium mortiferum*. Very pleomorphic. (From Sutter et al. 1985.)

36.13

36.14

PLATE 36.13. *Fusobacterium necrophorum* on BAP.
PLATE 36.14. Positive blood culture. Note fluffy colonies at bottom of bottle *(F. necrophorum).*

36.15

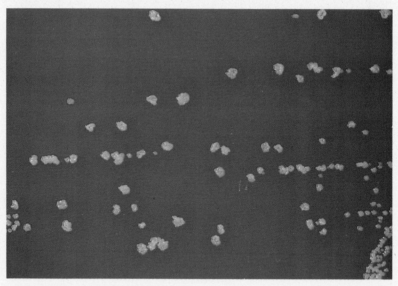

36.16

PLATE 36.15. *F. nucleatum.* Note internal speckling in colonies.
PLATE 36.16. *F. nucleatum.* "Bread crumb" colonies.

36.17

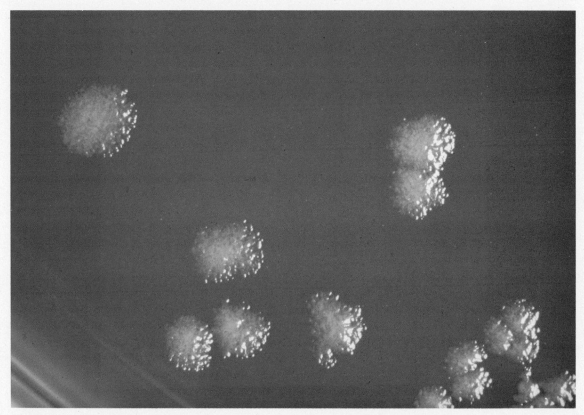

PLATE 36.17. *Leptotrichia buccalis* on BAP.

37.1

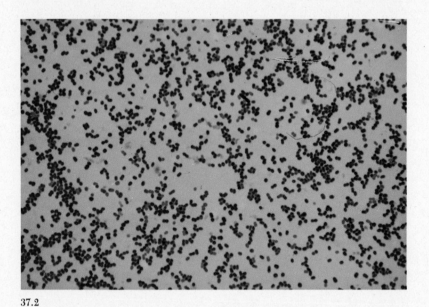

37.2

PLATE 37.1. *Peptostreptococcus asaccharolyticus* on BAP.
PLATE 37.2. *Peptostreptococcus anaerobius*. Large coccobacillary cells with chains. (From Sutter et al. 1985.)

37.3

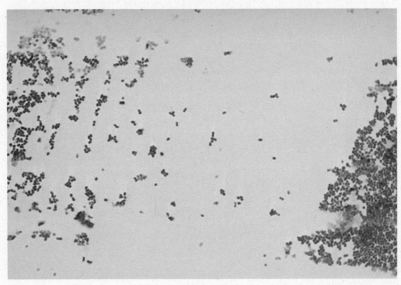

37.4

PLATE 37.3. *Peptostreptococcus magnus* in pus (appearance identical to that of staphylococci). (From Sutter et al. 1985.)

PLATE 37.4. *Peptostreptococcus micros*. Small cells, some chaining. (From Sutter et al. 1985.)

37.5

37.6

PLATE 37.5. *P. anaerobius* disk identification tests (resistant to kanamycin and colistin, sensitive to vancomycin and SPS).

PLATE 37.6. *Veillonella.* Small, gram-negative coccus. (From Sutter et al. 1985.)

TABLE 35.3
Characteristics of Nagler Positive *Clostridium* Species*

	INDOLE PRODUCTION	GELATIN HYDROLYSIS	UREASE	GROWTH ENHANCED BY 1% MANNOSE	PHENYLACETIC ACID PRODUCED	GLUTAMIC ACID DECARBOXYLASE	REVERSE CAMP TEST
C perfringens	−	+	−				+
C. baratii	−	−	−				−
C. bifermentans	+	+	−	−	−	−†	−
C. sordellii	+	+	+−	+	V	+	−

Modified from Sutter V.L., Citron, D.M., Edelstein, M.A.C., and Finegold, S.M. 1985. Wadsworth anaerobic bacteriology manual, ed. 4. Star Publishing Co., Belmont, Calif.
*− = negative reaction; + = positive reaction; V = variable reaction.
†Only a few strains have been tested.

TABLE 35.4

Characteristics of Clostridia*

	GELATIN HYDROLYSIS	GLUCOSE FERMENTATION	LECITHINASE	LIPASE	INDOLE	BUTYRIC ACID PRODUCED IN PYG	ISOACIDS PRODUCED IN PYG	AEROBIC GROWTH	UREASE	MILK REACTION
Saccharolytic-proteolytic										
C. bifermentans	+	+	+	−	+	+	−	−	−	d
C. sordellii	+	+	+	−	+	(+)	(+)	−	+	d
C. perfringens	+	+	+	−	−	+	−	−		d
C. novyi type A	+	+	+	+	−	+	−	−		c
C. sporogenes†	+	+	−	+	−	+	(+)	−		d
C. cadaveris	+	+	−	−	+	+	−	−		cd
C. septicum	+	+	−	−	−	+	−	−		cd
C. difficile	+	+	−	−	−	+	+	−		−
C. putrificum	+	+	−	−	−	+	+	−		d
Saccharolytic nonproteolytic										
C. baratii	−	+	+	−	−	+	−	−		c
C. tertium	−	+	−	−	−	+	−	+		c
C. butyricum	−	+	−	−	−	+	−	−		c
C. innocuum	−	+	−	−	−	+	−	−		−
C. ramosum	−	+	−	−	−	−	−	−		c
C. clostridiiforme‡	−	+	−	−	−⁺	−	−	−		c
Asaccharolytic-proteolytic										
C. tetani	+	−	−	−	V	+	−	−		d⁻
C. hastiforme	+	−	−⁺	−	−	+	+	−		−ᵈ
C. subterminale	+	−	−	−⁺	−	+	+	−		dᶜ
C. histolyticum	+	−	−	−	−	−	−	+⁻		d
C. limosum	+	−	+	−	−	−	−	−		d

Modified from Sutter, V.L., Citron, D.M., Edelstein, M.A.C., and Finegold, S.M. 1985. Wadsworth anaerobic

Reactions: − = negative reaction; + = positive reaction for majority of strains; includes weak as well as strong acid
most strains positive, some weakly positive; −ʷ = most strains negative, some weakly positive; −⁺ = most strains
positive, some negative; V = variable reaction.

PRAS carbohydrates; + = pH <5.5; W = pH 5.5-5.7; − = pH >5.7.

Milk reaction: d = digestion; c = clot. NOTE: Superscripts indicate reactions of some strains.

Spore shape and location: O = oval; R = round; S = subterminal; T = terminal.

Fatty acids: A = acetic; P = propionic; IB = isobutyric; B = butyric; IV = isovaleric; V = valeric; IC = isocaproic;
NOTE: (1) Capital letters indicate major metabolic products. (2) Small letters indicate minor products. (3) Parentheses
saccharolytic organisms.

*C. botulinum types vary in proteolytic, saccharolytic, and lipase reactions. Send suspected isolates or suspected C.

†C. botulinum types A, B, and F behave biochemically like C. sporogenes and can only be differentiated by toxin

‡C. clostridiiforme often appears gram-negative.

	FERMENTATION OF						NITRATE REDUCTION	SPORE SHAPE AND LOCATION	END-PRODUCTS FROM PYG
LACTOSE	MALTOSE	FRUCTOSE	CELLOBIOSE	ARABINOSE	MANNOSE	XYLOSE			
−	W⁻	V	−	−	−ʷ	−	−		A B L
−	W⁺	V	−	−	−ʷ	−	−		A (p ib b iv ic l)
+	+	+	−⁺	−	+	−	−		A B L (p s)
−	V	−ʷ	−	−	−	−	−	OS	A P B
−	−ʷ	−ʷ	−	−	−	−	−	OS	A B ib iv (p v l s)
−	−	V	−	−	−ʷ	−	−	OT	A b
+	+	+	+ʷ	−	+	−	V	OS	A B (p)
−	−	+	+ʷ	−	+⁻	−ʷ	−	OS	A ib B iv ic (v)
−	−ʷ	−ʷ	−	−	−	−	−		A ib B iv (p v l s)
+ʷ	+ʷ	+	+	−	+	−	V		
+	+	+	+	−	+	+⁻	+⁻	OT	A B L (s)
+	+	+	+	+⁻	+	+	−	OS	A B F (l s)
−	−	+	+	−	+	−ʷ	−	OT	A B L (s)
+	+	+	+	−	+	−ʷ	−	R/OT	a L (s)
+	+ʷ	+	+⁻	V	+	+	+⁻	OS	A (l s)
−	−	−	−	−	−	−	−	RT	A B (l s)
−	−	−	−	−	−	−	−⁺	S	A B iv ib (p ic)
−	−	−	−	−	−	−	−	OS	A B ib IV (p ic l s)
−	−	−	−	−	−	−	−⁺	OS	A (l s)
−	−	−	−	−	−	−	−	S	A (l s)

bacteriology manual, ed. 4. Star Publishing Co., Belmont, Calif.
production from carbohydrates in saccharolytic organisms; +⁻ = most strains positive, reaction helpful if positive; +ʷ =
negative, reaction helpful if negative; W⁺ = most strains weakly positive, some positive; W⁻ = most strains weakly

C = caproic, C' = caprylic; L = lactic; S = succinic; PA = phenylacetic.
indicate a variable reaction. (4) Isoacids are primarily from carbohydrate-free media (such as PY) in the case of

botulinum-containing material to the appropriate local or state agency.
neutralization studies.

PROCEDURE 35.2. ISOLATING CLOSTRIDIA FROM MIXED CULTURE

1. The original broth culture, shown to contain gram-positive sporulating rods, may be heat shocked at 80° C for 10 min and then streaked on blood agar and egg yolk agar plates for anaerobic cultivation. Alternatively, a fresh tube of enriched thioglycolate medium or starch broth may be inoculated from the original plate culture, heated immediately, and incubated for 24-48 h. Plates may be streaked from this.
2. Treat mixed cultures (a sweep inoculum from the surface of a plate) with 50% ethanol for 30-45 min to selectively isolate spore formers (see Chapter 8).
3. Incorporate 100 μg/ml of neomycin in blood agar or egg yolk agar plates. This compound can be autoclaved. Cycloserine, in a final concentration of 500 μg/ml, may also be useful; it should be added after autoclaving. Nonselective media should always be inoculated in parallel with selective media.

PROCEDURE 35.3. THE REVERSE CAMP TEST FOR C. PERFRINGENS

1. Inoculate a blood agar plate with a single streak of suspected *C. perfringens*. Then inoculate a group B streptococcus in a single streak at a 90-degree angle to within a few millimeters of the *Clostridium* (more than one test can be inoculated on each plate). Incubate anaerobically for 24-48 h.
2. Examine for an arrowhead of synergistic hemolysis (Plate 34.14) (a positive test).

immediately, using fresh media. Egg yolk medium should be used, in addition to the others mentioned in Chapter 8, when clostridia are anticipated to be present. Media with 5% agar may also be useful to minimize swarming of some species.

In most instances, the clostridia occur in mixed culture with gram-negative bacteria, such as coliforms, *Proteus*, or *Pseudomonas*, and with various non-spore-forming anaerobes. The anaerobic plates, therefore, may be overgrown with such organisms, and isolation of the clostridia becomes difficult or impossible. Procedure 35.2 may be used to combat this problem.

35.2.d. Identification of the pathogenic clostridia. By virtue of the disease syndromes they produce, the pathogenic species may be placed in five categories or groups:

Group I: the gas gangrene group, includes *C. perfringens* (type A), *C. novyi* (Plate 35.13), *C. septicum* (Plates 35.14 and 35.15), *C. bifermentans*, *C. histolyticum*, *C. sordellii* (Plate 35.16), *C. sporogenes*, and others. Of these, the three species first named are most important.

Group II: *C. tetani*, the etiologic agent of tetanus (Plates 35.17, 35.18, and 35.19).

Group III: the *C. botulinum* group, the etiologic agent of botulism.

Group IV: *C. difficile*, responsible for most cases of pseudomembranous colitis related to antimicrobial therapy.

Group V: the miscellaneous infection group (wound infection, abscesses, bacteremia, and so forth). This group includes *C. perfringens*, *C. ramosum*, *C. bifermentans*, *C. sphenoides*, *C. sporogenes*, and a number of others.

C. *perfringens* and C. *ramosum* are by far the most commonly isolated clostridia. Group V infections are the most commonly encountered. However, clostridia are found in such infections only about one tenth as often as nonspore-formers.

The Nagler reaction, recommended for the rapid identification of C. *perfringens* and other alpha toxin producers, has been discussed above. Buchanan[1] has evaluated the reverse CAMP test for presumptive identification of C. *perfringens*. C. *perfringens* is usually positive and other clostridia are negative. The method is presented in Procedure 35.3.

Details on examination of specimens for C. *difficile* and its cytopathic toxin are presented in Chapter 17. Details on identification of various other species of clostridia are presented in Table 35.4. Further information on test procedures can be found in the bibliography.

C. *ramosum*, although not as virulent as C. *perfringens*, takes on added importance by virtue of its resistance to antimicrobial agents. About 15% of strains are highly resistant to clindamycin, and many strains are resistant to tetracycline and erythromycin. Penicillin is the drug of choice against C. *ramosum* and clostridia in general, but minimal inhibitory concentrations of C. *ramosum* are as high as 8 U/ml. Occasional strains of C. *perfringens* and other clostridia are resistant to penicillin G. Some 20%-30% of certain clostridial species other than C. *perfringens* are also resistant to clindamycin. One third of clostridia other than C. *perfringens* are resistant to cefoxitin. Chloramphenicol and metronidazole are essentially universally active against clostridia. Surgical debridement and drainage are major aspects of the therapeutic approach to clostridial infections. Oral vancomycin and metronidazole are the drugs of choice for C. *difficile* colitis, and oral bacitracin is probably equally effective.

Most of the human pathogenic clostridia are pathogenic also for guinea pigs, mice, rabbits, and pigeons. To establish the toxigenicity of isolated strains, white mice, guinea pigs and hamsters are used in the laboratory. Susceptibility and rapidity of death may vary according to the virulence of the strain. This type of testing is beyond the scope of the clinical laboratory. Cultivation of C. *botulinum* should only be attempted by reference laboratories; personnel involved should be immunized. Determination of toxigenicity, where indicated, should be done by reference laboratories. An in vitro (enzyme-linked immunosorbent assay [ELISA]) procedure has recently been described for identification of C. *botulinum* toxins A and B.

REFERENCES

1. Buchanan, A.G. 1982. Clinical laboratory evaluation of a reverse CAMP test for presumptive identification of *Clostridium perfringens*. J. Clin. Microbiol. 16:761.
2. Kornman, K.S., and Loesche, W.J. 1978. New medium for isolation of *Actinomyces viscosus* and *Actinomyces naeslundii* from dental plaque. J. Clin. Microbiol. 7:514.

BIBLIOGRAPHY

Bartlett, J.G., Chang, T.W., Gurwith, M., et al. 1978. Antibiotic-associated pseudomembranous colitis due to toxin-producing clostridia. N. Engl. J. Med. 298:531.

Brock, D.W., Georg, L.K., Brown, J.M., and Hicklin, M.D. 1973. Actinomycosis caused by *Arachnia propionica*: report of 11 cases. Am. J. Clin. Pathol. 59:66.

Coleman, R.M., Georg, L.K., and Rozzell, A.R. 1969. *Actinomyces naeslundii* as an agent of human actinomycosis. Appl. Microbiol. 18:420.

Dowell, V.R. Jr., and Hawkins, T.M. 1968. Detection of clostridial toxins, toxin neutralization tests, and pathogenicity tests. Centers for Disease Control, Atlanta.

Finegold, S.M. 1977. Anaerobic bacteria in human disease. Academic Press, Inc., New York.

George, W.L. 1984. Antimicrobial agent-associated colitis and diarrhea: historical background and clinical aspects. Rev. Infect. Dis. 6(suppl.):S208.

George, W.L., Sutter, V.L., Citron, D., and Finegold, S.M. 1979. Selective and differential medium for isolation of *Clostridium difficile*. J. Clin. Microbiol. 9:214.

Gerencser, M.A., and Slack, J.M. 1969. Identification of human strains of *Actinomyces viscosus*. Appl. Microbiol. 18:80.

Gorbach, S.L., and Thadepalli, H. 1975. Isolation of *Clostridium* in human infections: evaluation of 114 cases. J. Infect. Dis. 131(suppl.):S81.

Holdeman, L.V., Cato, E.P., and Moore, W.E.C. 1977. Anaerobe laboratory manual, ed. 4. Virginia Polytechnic Institute and State University, Blacksburg, Va.

Lambert, R.F. Jr., Brown, J.M., and Georg, L.K. 1967. Identification of *Actinomyces israelii* and *Actinomyces naeslundii* by fluorescent antibody and agar-gel diffusion techniques. J. Bacteriol. 94:1287.

Midura, T.F., and Arnon, S.S. 1976. Infant botulism: identification of *C. botulinum* and its toxin in faeces. Lancet 2:934.

Pine, L., Malcolm, G.B., Curtis, E.M., and Brown, J.M. 1981. Demonstration of *Actinomyces* and *Arachnia* species in cervicovaginal smears by direct staining with species-specific fluorescent-antibody conjugate. J. Clin. Microbiol. 13:15.

Smith, L.DS. 1975. The pathogenic anaerobic bacteria, ed. 2. Charles C Thomas, Publisher, Springfield, Ill.

Sutter, V.L., Citron, D.M., Edelstein, M.A.C., and Finegold, S.M. 1985. Wadsworth anaerobic bacteriology manual, ed. 4. Star Publishing Co., Belmont, Calif.

Wang, W.L.L., Everett, E.D., Johnson, M., and Dean, E. 1977. Susceptibility of *Propionibacterium acnes* to seventeen antibiotics. Antimicrob. Agents Chemother. 11:171.

Willis, A.T. 1969. Clostridia of wound infection. Butterworth & Co. (Publishers) Ltd., London.

36.1. Introduction

The anaerobic gram-negative rods belong to the family Bacteroidaceae. They are obligately anaerobic, non-spore-forming rods that are straight, curved or helical and either motile or nonmotile. They metabolize carbohydrates, peptones or metabolic intermediates; most species produce organic acids. The Bacteroidaceae are prevalent among the indigenous flora of humans and animals, primarily on mucosal surfaces. In many locations they are the dominant members of the normal flora (e.g., the *Bacteroides fragilis* group outnumbers all other elements of the colonic flora in humans). Gram-negative anaerobic rods are the anaerobes most commonly involved in infections. These organisms constitute one third of the total anaerobic isolates from clinical specimens. Within the Bacteroidaceae, *Bacteroides fragilis* is the most commonly encountered pathogen. Other members of the *B. fragilis* group, especially *B. thetaiotaomicron*, *B. distasonis* and *B. vulgatus*, may also be involved. Other *Bacteroides* sp. often encountered in infection include the pigmented *Bacteroides* (especially *B. melaninogenicus*, *B. asaccharolyticus*, *B. intermedius* and *B. bivius*), *B. oris*, *B. buccae*, *B. disiens*, *B. oralis* group, and the *B. ureolyticus* group. Among the fusobacteria, *Fusobacterium nucleatum* and *F. necrophorum* are seen most often in infections. Surgery, trauma or disease disrupting a mucosal surface or introduction of anaerobes into a normally sterile site (as with aspiration of oropharyngeal contents or seeding of an organism in the course of bacteremia) may lead to an anaerobic or mixed infection. *Bacteroides* and *Fusobacterium* produce enzymes (collagenase, neuraminidase, DNase, heparinase, and proteinases) that may play a role in pathogenesis. Several gram-negative anaerobic rods have been demonstrated to inhibit phagocytic uptake and killing of aerobes by neutrophils. Infection with gram-negative anaerobic bacilli, as with anaerobic infection generally, is characterized by abscess formation and tissue destruction. The most common infections in which gram-negative anaerobic rods participate are pleuropulmonary, intraabdominal and female genital tract infections, but infections of any type anywhere in the body may involve these organisms (Plate 36.1).

Specimen collection and transport are of utmost importance in documenting the role of gram-negative anaerobic rods in an infectious process (see Chapter 6). Since these organisms are so prevalent on mucosal surfaces, it is important to avoid contaminating the specimen with normal flora when collecting a specimen. Transport must be carried out in an oxygen-free atmosphere.

36.1.a. Morphology and general characteristics. Colony morphology varies considerably from one member of the Bacteroidaceae to another. Some species are pigmented and some pit the agar by virtue of production of an agarase. Some colonies are flat, others umbonate; some have a "fried-egg" appearance and some produce spreading growth. In terms of microscopic morphology, there are also differences. *Bacteroides* have rounded ends; some are quite thin and delicate whereas others have broader cells. Filaments may be seen, and a certain degree of pleomorphism (in terms of both cell size and shape) is common. Vacuolization or irregular staining is common in *Bacteroides*. The pigmented *Bacteroides* tend to be coccobacillary. Many members of the genus *Fusobacte-*

rium are spindle shaped. Some of the Bacteroidaceae are spiral shaped and some are ovoid. Some gram-negative anaerobic rods are encapsulated and some are surrounded by less well-defined polysaccharide material. Motile forms may have polar or bipolar flagella and some forms have tufts of flagella on the concave side of curved cells.

36.1.b. Differentiation of anaerobic gram-negative rods. Genera of the Bacteroidaceae are differentiated by means of motility or nonmotility, location of flagella in motile forms, endproducts of metabolism, and shape of cells (Table 36.1). Within the major genus *Bacter-*

TABLE 36.1
Differentiation of Genera of Anaerobes

Gram-negative bacilli	
I. Nonmotile or peritrichous flagella	
A. Produce butyric acid (without isobutyric and isovaleric acid)	*Fusobacterium*
B. Produce major lactic acid	*Leptotrichia*
C. Produce acetic acid and hydrogen sulfide; reduce sulfate	*Desulfomonas*
D. Not as above (A,B,C)	*Bacteroides*
II. Polar flagella	
A. Fermentative	
1. Produce butyric acid	*Butyrivibrio*
2. Produce succinic acid	
a. Spiral-shaped cells	*Succinivibrio*
b. Ovoid cells	*Succinimonas*
3. Produce propionic and acetic acids	*Anaerovibrio*
B. Nonfermentative, produce succinic acid from fumarate	*Wolinella*
III. Tufts of flagella on concave side of curved cells	
A. Fermentative	*Selenomonas*
B. Nonfermentative	*Mobiluncus*
IV. Bipolar tufts of flagella	*Anaerobiospirillum*

From Sutter, V.L., Citron, D.M., Edelstein, M.A.C., and Finegold, S.M. 1985. Wadsworth anaerobic bacteriology manual, ed. 4. Star Publishing Co., Belmont, Calif.

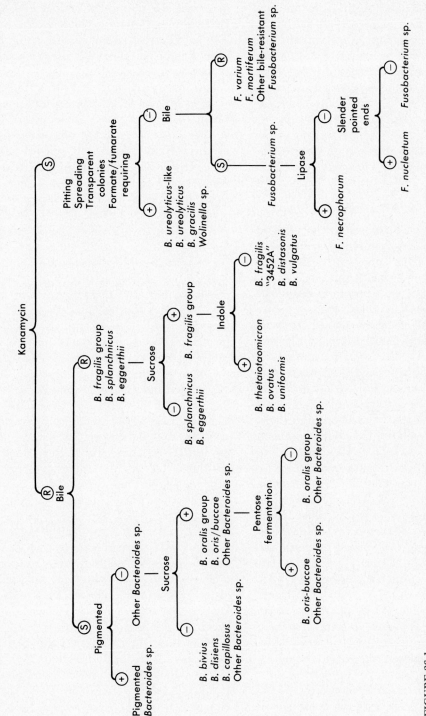

FIGURE 36.1

Identification of anaerobic gram-negative bacilli. (From Sutter, V.L., Citron, D.M., Edelstein, M.A.C., and Finegold, S.M. 1985. Wadsworth anaerobic bacteriology manual, ed. 4. Star Publishing Co., Belmont, Calif.)

oides, differentiation is initially based on resistance to bile (Plate 36.2), production of pigment, metabolic activity, susceptibility to certain antimicrobial agents (Plate 34.8), and miscellaneous biochemical tests. Figure 36.1 is a flow chart illustrating the major means for differentiating between various groups of *Bacteroides* and between certain *Bacteroides* and *Fusobacterium* groups. Further tests for differentiating these bacteria to the species level will be discussed under the various specific organism groups below.

36.2. Bile-Resistant *Bacteroides*

36.2.a. Structure and extracellular products. This group of *Bacteroides* includes the *B. fragilis* group and two other bile-resistant species not commonly encountered—*B. eggerthii* and *B. splanchnicus*. The key member of this group is *Bacteroides fragilis*, the most commonly encountered of all anaerobes in clinically significant infections and among the most resistant to antimicrobial agents. It possesses a distinctive capsule that can be demonstrated by ruthenium red staining, India ink staining, and electron microscopy. This capsule is an important virulence factor. The endotoxin of *B. fragilis* contains no lipid A, 2-ketodeoxyoctanate, heptose, or beta hydroxymyristic acid and is weak in biologic activity as compared to other gram-negative bacterial endotoxins. Nonetheless, it is clear that *B. fragilis* is a virulent organism by virtue of its capsule and production of certain enzymes such as neuraminidase, deoxyribonuclease, hyaluronidase, gelatinase, fibrinolysin, superoxide dismutase, and heparinase. *B. fragilis* group strains produce 1-3 mm diameter, smooth, white to gray, nonhemolytic, translucent colonies on blood agar (Plate 36.3). Microscopically, the organisms are pale-staining gram-negative bacilli with rounded ends, with some pleomorphism and irregularity of staining (Plates 36.4 to 36.7).

36.2.b. Identification methods. The *B. fragilis* group is distinguished from the other two species of bile-resistant *Bacteroides* by its ability to ferment sucrose (Table 36.2). Further data on differentiation of species within the *B. fragilis* group and the bile-resistant *Bacteroides* generally are noted in Table 36.2. A discussion of preliminary grouping and identification procedures for the various anaerobes appears in Chapter 34.

36.2.c. Susceptibility to antimicrobial agents. As noted earlier, *B. fragilis* is among the most resistant of the anaerobes. This resistance applies primarily to beta lactam drugs (such as penicillins and cephalosporins) and is mediated by production of beta lactamases which, though primarily cephalosporinases, also show significant ability to destroy penicillins. Certain beta lactam agents are largely resistant to these beta lactamases and thus retain activity against *B. fragilis*. In this group are the broad-spectrum penicillins such as ticarcillin, piperacillin and related drugs, cefoxitin and imipenem. However, resistance to the above drugs, except for imipenem, is seen in about 5% of strains and a few strains have demonstrated resistance to imipenem by destroying that compound. Resistance to tetracycline is common, and 5% of strains of *B. fragilis* are resistant to clindamycin. Metronidazole and chloramphenicol are active against essentially all strains of *B. fragilis*. Other members of the *B. fragilis* group, notably *B. thetaiotaomicron*, may also be quite resistant to antimicrobial agents.

36.2.d. Noncultural methods of identification. A fluorescent antibody reagent for the *B. fragilis* group is available commercially (General Diagnostics). The sensitivity and specificity of this reagent both approach 90%. False-negative results may occur with colonies of *B. ovatus*, *B. vulgatus*, and *B. distasonis*.

Direct gas liquid chromatographic analysis of clinical specimens for endproducts of anaerobic metabolism may provide rapid presumptive evidence for the presence of *B. fragilis* in an infectious process (also discussed in Chapter

TABLE 36.2
Characteristics of Bile-Resistant *Bacteroides* Species

	GROWTH IN 20% BILE	INDOLE PRODUCTION	CATALASE	ESCULIN HYDROLYSIS	SUCROSE	MALTOSE	RHAMNOSE	SALICIN	TREHALOSE	ARABINOSE	XYLAN	FATTY ACIDS FROM PEPTONE YEAST GLUCOSE BROTH
								FERMENTATION OF				
B. fragilis group												
B. distasonis	+	−	$+^{-}$	+	+		V	+	+	$-^{+}$		A p S (pa ib iv l)
3452A homology group												
B. fragilis	+	−	$-^{+}$	+	+		$-^{-}$	$+^{-}$	+	−		A p S pa
B. vulgatus	+	−	$+^{+}$	$-^{-}$	+		−	−	−	+		A p S
B. ovatus	+	+	$-^{-}$	+	+		+	$+^{-}$	+	+	+	A p S pa (ib iv l)
B. thetaiotaomicron	+	+	$+^{-}$	+	+		$+^{-}$	$-^{+}$	+	+		A p S pa
B. uniformis	W^{+}	+	$+^{-}$	+	+		$-^{-}$	$-^{+}$	−	+	−	a p l S (ib iv)
Other												
B. eggerthii	+	+	−		−	+	$+^{-}$		−	+		A p S (ib iv l)
B. splanchnicus	W^{+}	+	−	+	−	−	−		−	+		A P ib b iv S (l)

From Sutter, V.L., Citron, D.M., Edelstein, M.A.C., and Finegold, S.M. 1985. Wadsworth anaerobic bacteriology manual, ed. 4. Star Publishing Co., Belmont, Calif.

Reactions: − = negative reaction; + = positive reaction for majority of strains; includes weak as well as strong acid production from carbohydrates in saccharolytic organisms; $+^{-}$ = most strains positive; reaction helpful if positive; $-^{+}$ = most strains negative; reaction helpful if negative; W^{+} = most strains weakly positive, some positive; V = variable reaction.

PRAS carbohydrates: + = pH < 5.5; W = pH 5.5-5.7; − = pH > 5.7.

Fatty acids: A = acetic; P = propionic; IB = isobutyric; B = butyric; IV = isovaleric; V = valeric; IC = isocaproic; C = caproic; C' = caprylic; L = lactic; S = succinic; PA = phenylacetic. *Note:* (1) Capital letters indicate major metabolic products. (2) Small letters indicate minor products. (3) Parentheses indicate a variable reaction. (4) Isoacids are primarily from carbohydrate-free media (such as PY) in the case of saccharolytic organisms.

11). Other techniques under development for rapid identification of *B. fragilis* infection include an immunoperoxidase method, radioimmunoassay and a DNA probe; none of these is ready for routine clinical application as yet.

36.3. Pigmented *Bacteroides*

Initially, pigmented *Bacteroides* were combined in one species, *B. melaninogenicus*, with three subspecies. At present, there are 12 species in this group. Those most commonly encountered are *B. asaccharolyticus, B. bivius, B. gingivalis, B. intermedius* and *B. melaninogenicus*. The pigmented *Bacteroides* are found

as normal flora in the oropharynx and upper respiratory tract, the gastrointestinal tract, and the genitourinary tract. This group is not recovered from infections as frequently as the *B. fragilis* group but nonetheless plays an important role in infection. It is of particular importance in lower respiratory tract infections such as aspiration pneumonia and lung abscess.

36.3.a. Morphologic characteristics. These organisms are usually seen as pale-staining coccobacilli (Plate 36.8). Pigment production may not always be readily detected. The use of laked rabbit blood agar plates allows the earliest and most reliable pigment production (Plate

TABLE 36.3

Characteristics of More Common Pigmented *Bacteroides* Species*

	INDOLE PRODUCTION	LIPASE	FERMENTATION OF			ESCULIN HYDROLYSIS	PHENYLACETIC ACID PRODUCTION	FATTY ACIDS FROM PEPTONE YEAST GLUCOSE BROTH
			GLUCOSE	LACTOSE	CELLOBIOSE			
B. asaccharolyticus	+	−	−	−	−		−	A p ib B iv S
B. gingivalis	+	−	−	−	−		+	a p ib B IV s pa
B. intermedius	+	+	+	−	−			A iv S (p ib)
B. corporis	−	−	+	−	−			A ib iv S (b)
B. melaninogenicus	−	−	+	+	−	−		A S (ib iv l)
B. denticola	−	−	+	+	−	+		A S (ib iv l)
B. loescheii	−	−⁺	+	+	+	V		a S (l)

From Sutter, V.L., Citron, D.M., Edelstein, M.A.C., and Finegold, S.M. 1985. Wadsworth anaerobic bacteriology manual, ed. 4. Star Publishing Co., Belmont, Calif.

Reactions: − = negative reaction; + = positive reaction for majority of strains; includes weak as well as strong acid production from carbohydrates in saccharolytic organisms; − ⁺ = most strains negative; reaction helpful if negative; V = variable reaction.

PRAS carbohydrates: + pH <5.5; W pH 5.5-5.7; − pH >5.7.

Fatty acids: A = acetic; P = propionic; IB = isobutyric; B = butyric; IV = isovaleric; V = valeric; IC = isocaproic; C = caproic; C′ = caprylic; L = lactic; S = succinic; PA = phenylacetic.

NOTE: (1) Capital letters indicate major metabolic products. (2) Small letters indicate minor products. (3) Parentheses indicate a variable reaction. (4) Isoacids are primarily from carbohydrate-free media (such as PY) in the case of saccharolytic organisms.

B. endodontalis, a newly described pigmented *Bacteroides*, is phenotypically indistinguishable from *B. asaccharolyticus*. *B. bivius* forms black pigmented colonies on laked rabbit blood agar after prolonged incubation. See Table 36.4 for further characteristics.

34.5). Prior to development of pigment, colonies of these organisms may fluoresce brick red under ultraviolet light (Plate 34.9). At least one member of this group, *B. asaccharolyticus* (and probably *B. melaninogenicus* and *B. intermedius* as well) is encapsulated. *B. bivius*, in contrast to *B. fragilis*, has a potent endotoxin. Certain pigmented *Bacteroides* produce phospholipase A, collagenase, hyaluronidase, and fibrinolysin.

36.3.b. Identification methods. Key reactions for differentiation of species within the pigmented *Bacteroides* group are indole production (Plate 34.11), lipase, esculin hydrolysis, phenylacetic acid production, and fermentation of glucose, lactose, and cellobiose, as shown in Table 36.3 and Figure 36.2. All members of the pigmented *Bacteroides* are sensitive to bile.

36.3.c. Susceptibility to antimicrobial agents. This group was formerly quite susceptible to penicillin G, but, unfortunately, there is now a significant incidence of clinically significant resistance, mediated by beta lactamase production by these organisms. Thus, for example, penicillin G can no longer be considered the drug of choice for anaerobic coverage in seriously ill patients with aspiration pneumonia. Metronidazole and chloramphenicol are universally active against these organisms; clindamycin is also usually effective. The broad-spectrum penicillins related to carbenicillin are

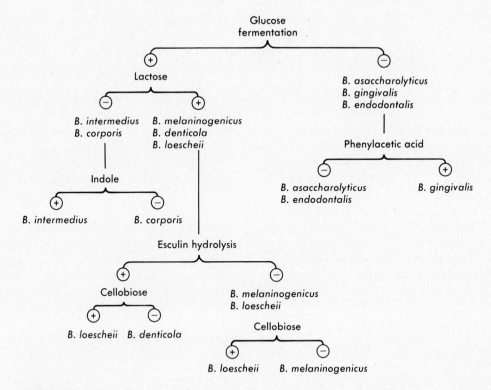

FIGURE 36.2
Identification of pigmented *Bacteroides* group organisms. (From Sutter, V.L., Citron, D.M., Edelstein, M.A.C., and Finegold, S.M. 1985. Wadsworth anaerobic bacteriology manual, ed. 4. Star Publishing Co., Belmont, Calif.)

active against about 95% of strains in this group, as is cefoxitin.

36.3.d. Noncultural methods of identification. There is a commercially produced fluorescent antibody reagent available for direct detection of some members of the pigmented *Bacteroides* group (General Diagnostics). Both sensitivity and specificity of this reagent are over 90%. Further study is required to know just what percent of which species of pigmented *Bacteroides* may be detected with this reagent, in view of recent taxonomic changes. Some strains of *B. disiens* cross-react with the reagent.

36.4. Bile-Sensitive, Nonpigmented *Bacteroides*

This remaining group of *Bacteroides* contains a number of organisms encountered with some frequency in various infections; included are *B. oris* and *B. buccae* (Plate 36.9) (both formerly known as *B. ruminicola*), the *B. oralis* group, *B. disiens* and *B. gracilis*. These organisms are found as normal flora in the oral cavity, gastrointestinal tract and genitourinary tract. They are involved in various infections, most commonly those of the lower respiratory and female genital tracts. *Bacteroides gracilis* is found primarily in serious, deep-seated infections.

36.4.a. Morphologic characteristics. For the most part, the organisms in this group are not distinctive morphologically. *B. gracilis* and *B. ureolyticus* colonies may pit the agar (Plate 34.10) or spread (Plate 36.10), but these characteristics are not consistent. *B. zoogleoformans* forms a zoogleal mass (the organisms are embedded in a jellylike matrix). There is some evidence that *B. oralis* and *B. oris-buccae* strains may be encapsulated.

36.4.b. Identification methods. As noted in Table 36.4, this group of organisms is further broken down into saccharolytic pentose fermenters, saccharolytic organisms that do not ferment pentose, a saccharolytic and proteo-

lytic group, and a nonsaccharolytic or weakly saccharolytic group. Other key features are the unique morphologic features referred to above, production of beta glucosidase, esculin hydrolysis, indole production, nitrate reduction, stimulation of growth by formate-fumarate, urease production, lack of motility, and endproducts of metabolism.

36.4.c. Antimicrobial susceptibility. As with the pigmented *Bacteroides*, some of the members of this group are displaying increasing resistance to antimicrobial agents on the basis of beta lactamase production. *Bacteroides gracilis* has a unique susceptibility pattern. It exhibits significant resistance (25%-35% of strains) to clindamycin, cefoxitin, penicillin G, and piperacillin and a small percent of strains are resistant to metronidazole and imipenem. All strains are susceptible to chloramphenicol. Surprisingly, all strains are also susceptible to tetracycline and erythromycin and almost all are susceptible to aminoglycosides. *B. ureolyticus*, which shares certain unique characteristics with *B. gracilis*, is quite different in other respects; it is found primarily in minor soft tissue infections and it is susceptible to a large variety of antimicrobial agents.

36.5. *Fusobacterium*

The two species of *Fusobacterium* most often identified in infections are *Fusobacterium nucleatum* and *F. necrophorum*. *F. nucleatum* is encountered much more commonly and is clearly an important pathogen, particularly in head and neck and lower respiratory infections, but *F. necrophorum* is much more virulent. *F. necrophorum* invades the bloodstream with some frequency, particularly as part of a syndrome that begins with membranous tonsillitis going on to septicemia and widespread metastatic infection that often includes lung abscesses, empyema, liver abscesses, osteomyelitis and purulent arthritis. Other species of fusobacteria that may play a role in infection include *F. gonidiaformans*, *F. mortiferum*, *F.*

Characteristics of Nonpigmented Bile-Sensitive *Bacteroides* Species*

	GLUCOSE	SUCROSE	LACTOSE	ARABINOSE	XYLOSE	SALICIN	XYLAN	ESCULIN HYDROLYSIS	BETA GLUCOSIDASE	ZOOGLEAL MASS	INDOLE PRODUCTION	GELATIN HYDROLYSIS	NITRATE REDUCTION	FATTY ACIDS FROM PEPTONE YEAST GLUCOSE BROTH	STIMULATION BY FORMATE-FUMARATE	UREASE	MOTILITY	AGAR PITTING
Saccharolytic																		
Pentose fermenters																		
B. oris	+	+	+	+	+	+		+	−	−	−			A S (p ib iv)				
B. buccae	+	+	+	+	+	+		+	+	−	−			A S (p ib b iv l)				
B. zoogleoformans	+	+	+	v	v	v		+		+	+⁻			A P S (ib iv)				
Pentose nonfermenters																		
B. oralis	+	+	+	−	−	+		+			−			A S (l)				
B. buccalis	+	+	+	−	−	−	+	−			−			a iv S				
B. veroralis	+	+	+	−	−	−	−	+			−			a S				
Saccharolytic and proteolytic																		
B. bivius*	+	−	+	−	−	−		−			−	+		A iv S (ib)				
B. disiens	+	−	−	−	−	−		−			−	+		A S (p ib iv)				
Nonsaccharolytic or weakly saccharolytic																		
B. capillosus	W⁻	−	−	−	−	−		+			−	−		a s (p l)				
B. praeacutus	−	−	−	−	−	−		−			−	+		A p ib B IV a (l)				
B. putredinis	−	−	−	−	−	−		−			+	+		a P ib b IV S (l)				
B. ureolyticus	−		−			−				−	−		+		+	+	−	+
B. gracilis	−		−			−				−	−		+		+	+	−	+

Modified from Sutter, V.L., Citron, D.M., Edelstein, M.A.C., and Finegold, S.M. 1985. Wadsworth anaerobic bacteriology manual, ed. 4. Star Publishing Co., Belmont, Calif.

Reactions: − = negative reaction; + = positive reaction for majority of strains; includes weak as well as strong acid production from carbohydrates in saccharolytic organisms; +⁻ = most strains positive; reaction helpful if positive; W⁻ = most strains weakly positive, some negative; V = variable reaction.

PRAS carbohydrates: + = pH < 5.5, W = pH 5.5-5.7; − = pH > 5.7.

Fatty acids: A = acetic; P = propionic; IB = isobutyric; B = butyric; IV = isovaleric; V = valeric; IC = isocaproic; C = caproic; C' = caprylic; L = lactic; S = succinic; PA = phenylacetic. NOTE: (1) Capital letters indicate major metabolic products. (2) Small letters indicate minor products. (3) Parentheses indicate a variable reaction. (4) Isoacids are primarily from carbohydrate-free media (such as PY) in the case of saccharolytic organisms.

*Most strains are black pigmented on laked rabbit blood agar after prolonged incubation.

naviforme, *F. russii*, and *F. varium*. The fuso-bacteria are found as indigenous flora in the upper respiratory tract in particular, but may also be found in the gastrointestinal and geni-tourinary tracts. They may be implicated in infection throughout the body, but with some predilection for the lower respiratory tract, head and neck, and central nervous system.

36.5.a. Morphologic characteristics. The members of this genus typically appear as long, slender, spear-shaped, pale-staining gram-negative rods with tapered ends. *F. nucleatum* often appears in pairs end-to-end (Plates 34.4 and 36.11). Some species, notably *F. mortiferum*, show a bizarre pleomorphism, with spheroid swellings along irregularly stained filaments and free round bodies (Plate 36.12). Colonies on blood agar are generally nonhemolytic but often show greening of the agar around the colonies after exposure to air. Colonies vary from flat to convex, with opaque centers and translucent irregular margins (e.g., the "fried-egg" appearance of *F. mortiferum* and *F. necrophorum*) (Plate 36.13); in broth, growth occurs in balls (Plate 36.14). Convex, glistening alpha hemolytic colonies with a flecked internal structure (Plate 36.15), or breadcrumblike colonies (Plate 36.16) are characteristic of *F. nucleatum*. The lipopolysaccharide of *Fusobacterium* strains resembles that of nonanaerobic gram-negative rods in structure. With most strains, biologic activity is strong. *F. necrophorum* produces a leukocidin and hemolyzes red blood cells of humans and a number of animal species. Phospholipase A and lysophospholipase are produced by *F. necrophorum*.

36.5.b. Identification methods. The genus *Fusobacterium* is characterized by the production of large amounts of butyric acid as a metabolic endproduct, without concomitant production of isobutyric or isovaleric acids. Aside from *F. varium* and *F. mortiferum*, bile is inhibitory to members of the genus. If the organism is definitely a fusobacterium, then lipase production is a key characteristic indicative of *F. necrophorum*. Other characteristics useful in identifying the pathogenic species of *Fusobacterium* are indicated in Table 36.5.

36.5.c. Antimicrobial susceptibility. In general, fusobacteria are more susceptible to antimicrobial agents than are the *Bacteroides*. Unfortunately, however, resistance is beginning to appear in certain species of *Fusobacterium*. *F. nucleatum*, *F. varium*, and *F. mortiferum* have recently been shown to produce beta lactamase and, as a result, are manifesting penicillin G resistance. Another phenomenon of interest with regard to fusobacteria is their production of L-form colonies upon exposure to cell wall active antimicrobial agents. The clinical significance, if any, of this ability is uncertain; but it has led to confusion in reading of susceptibility test results in the agar dilution test (Chapter 13). One can note a definite drop-off in the amount of growth at one point in this serial twofold dilution test, but the amount of persisting growth beyond this point (which is due to cell wall deficient forms) is clearly more than can be ignored (a faint haze or one colony). Consistency in reading is important, particularly in comparing data from one laboratory to another. We suggest, for now, that the endpoint be read at the point where there is a significant drop-off in the amount of growth; however, clinical studies correlating response to an agent such as penicillin with the in vitro test results are needed.

36.6. Miscellaneous Bacteroidaceae

The genera of Bacteroidaceae other than *Bacteroides* or *Fusobacterium* have been less well studied. They are uncommon causes of infection. *Leptotrichia buccalis* is part of the normal flora of the oral cavity and has been found, on occasion, in the intestine and the vagina. It has been recovered from dental infections, osteomyelitis of the mandible, bite wound infections, infections of the head and neck, and from the blood of a patient with a lung abscess. It is

TABLE 36.5

Characteristics of *Fusobacterium* Species

	DISTINCTIVE CELLULAR MORPHOLOGY	INDOLE PRODUCTION	GROWTH IN 20% BILE	LIPASE	GAS IN GLUCOSE AGAR	FERMENTATION OF GLUCOSE	FERMENTATION OF FRUCTOSE	FERMENTATION OF MANNOSE	ESCULIN HYDROLYSIS	LACTATE CONVERTED TO PROPIONATE	THREONINE CONVERTED TO PROPIONATE	FATTY ACIDS FROM PEPTONE YEAST GLUCOSE BROTH
F. nucleatum	Slender pointed ends	+	−	−	$-^2$	$-^w$	$-^w$	−	−	−	+	a p B (L s)
F. gonidiaformans	Gonidia forms	+	−	−	4^2	$-^w$	$-^w$	−	−	−	+	A p B (l s)
F. necrophorum	None	+	−	+	4^2	$-^w$	$-^w$	−	−	+	+	a p B (l s)
F. naviforme	Boat shape	+	−	−	4	W^-	−	−	−	−	−	a B L (p s)
F. varium	None	+	+	−	4	$+^w$	$+^w$	$+^w$	−	−	+	a p B L (s)
F. mortiferum	Bizarre, round bodies	−	+	−	4	$+^w$	$+^w$	$+^w$	+	−	+	a p B (v l a)
F. russii		−	+	−	2^-	−	−	−	−	−	−	a B L

From Sutter, V.L., Citron, D.M., Edelstein, M.A.C., and Finegold, S.M. 1985. Wadsworth anaerobic bacteriology manual, ed. 4. Star Publishing Co., Belmont, Calif.

Reactions: − = negative reaction; + = positive reaction for majority of strains; includes weak as well as strong acid production from carbohydrates in saccharolytic organisms; $+^w$ = most strains positive, some weakly positive; $-^w$ = most strains negative, some weakly positive; V = variable reaction.

PRAS carbohydrates: + = pH <5.5; W = pH 5.5-5.7; − = pH >5.7.

Gas in PYG agar deep: − = no gas detected; 2 = splits agar horizontally; 3 = agar displaced halfway to top of the tube; 4 = agar displaced to top of the tube.

NOTE: Superscripts indicate reactions of some strains.

Fatty acids: A = acetic; P = propionic; IB = isobutyric; B = butyric; IV = isovaleric; V = valeric; IC = isocaproic; C = caproic; C′ = caprylic; L = lactic; S = succinic; PA = phenylacetic. *Note:* (1) Capital letters indicate major metabolic products. (2) Small letters indicate minor products. (3) Parentheses indicate a variable reaction. (4) Isoacids are primarily from carbohydrate-free media (such as PY) in the case of saccharolytic organisms.

a long, plump, straight, or slightly curved gram-negative bacillus that grows end-to-end in pairs or chains. The ends that abut are flattened, whereas the other ends are often pointed. The colonies are 2-3 mm in diameter with a characteristic convoluted appearance (Plate 36.17). It is unique in producing lactic acid as its sole metabolic endproduct. *L. buccalis* is susceptible to virtually all antibacterial agents useful against anaerobes.

The various anaerobic vibrios and curved rods have been recovered, rarely, from infections such as bacteremia, central nervous system infection, pulmonary infection, intraabdominal infection, soft tissue infection and endophthalmitis.

BIBLIOGRAPHY

Felner, J.M., and Dowell, V.R. Jr. 1971. "Bacteroides" bacteremia. Am. J. Med. 50:787.

Finegold, S.M. 1977. Anaerobic bacteria in human disease. Academic Press, Inc., New York.

George, W.L., Kirby, B.D., Sutter, V.L., Citron, D.M., and Finegold, S.M. 1981. Gram-negative anaerobic bacilli: their role in infection and patterns of susceptibility to antimicrobial agents. II. Little-known *Fusobacterium* species and miscellaneous genera. Rev. Infect. Dis. 3:599.

Kasper, D.L., Fiddian, A.P., and Tabaqchali, S. 1979. Rapid diagnosis of *Bacteroides* infections by indirect immunofluorescence assay of clinical specimens. Lancet 1:239.

Kirby, B.D., George, W.L., Sutter, V.L., Citron, D.M., and Finegold, S.M. 1980. Gram-negative anaerobic bacilli: their role in infection and patterns of susceptibility to antimicrobial agents. I. Little-known *Bacteroides* species. Rev. Infect. Dis. 2:914.

Rotstein, O.D., Pruett, T.L., and Simmons, R.L. 1985. Mechanisms of microbial synergy in polymicrobial surgical infections. Rev. Infect. Dis. 7:151.

Sutter, V.L., Citron, D.M., Edelstein, M.A.C., and Finegold, S.M. 1985. Wadsworth anaerobic bacteriology manual, ed. 4. Star Publishing Co., Belmont, Calif.

Weissfeld, A.S., and Sonnenwirth, A.C. 1981. Rapid detection and identification of *Bacteroides fragilis* and *Bacteroides melaninogenicus* by immunofluorescence. J. Clin. Microbiol. 13:798.

37 Anaerobic Cocci

37.1. Introduction

There are several genera of anaerobic cocci. Gram-negative anaerobic cocci belong to the genera *Veillonella*, *Acidaminococcus*, and *Megasphaera*, whereas the gram-positive cocci of clinical significance belong to *Peptostreptococcus*, *Peptococcus*, or *Streptococcus*. There are two genera of gram-positive anaerobic cocci, *Coprococcus* and *Ruminococcus*, that are found in the normal flora of the colon but are nonpathogenic. Table 37.1 shows the basis for classification of the anaerobic cocci. Except for *Peptococcus niger*, all of the pathogenic species formerly in the genus *Peptococcus* have been transferred to the genus *Peptostreptococcus*. Few of the members of the genus *Streptococcus* are obligate anaerobes; strictly speaking, the term "anaerobic streptococci" would refer to these organisms. The **microaerophilic streptococci** are commonly considered together with obligately anaerobic cocci because good anaerobic transport and culture techniques are typically required to recover and identify these organisms. These organisms produce lactic acid as their sole metabolic endproduct and thus belong in the genus *Streptococcus*. They belong in the same group as the so-called "viridans streptococci" and are discussed in Chapter 25. The organism previously classified as *Peptococcus saccharolyticus* has been reclassified as *Staphylococcus saccharolyticus*.

TABLE 37.1
Anaerobic Cocci

Gram-negative cocci
  I. Produce propionic and *Veillonella*
     acetic acids
 II. Produce butyric and acetic *Acidaminococcus*
     acids
III. Produce isobutyric, butyric, *Megasphaera*
     isovaleric, valeric, and cap-
     roic acids
Gram-positive cocci
  I. Require a fermentable car-
     bohydrate
     A. Produce butyric acid *Coprococcus*
        (plus other acids)
     B. Do not produce butyric *Ruminococcus*
        acid
 II. Do not require a fermenta-
     ble carbohydrate
     A. Lactic acid sole major *Streptococcus*
        product
     B Not as above *Peptostreptococcus* or
                              Peptococcus

Modified from Sutter, V.L., Citron, D.M., Edelstein,
M.A.C., and Finegold, S.M. 1985. Wadsworth anaerobic
bacteriology manual, ed. 4. Star Publishing Co., Belmont,
Calif.

The anaerobic cocci are numerically important members of the indigenous flora in the
bowel, female genital tract, and oral cavity and
are found in other locations as well, including
the skin. Next to the anaerobic gram-negative
bacilli, the anaerobic gram-positive cocci are
the anaerobes most commonly encountered in
clinically significant infections. Reflecting differences in their presence as normal flora, the
gram-positive anaerobic cocci are relatively
more prevalent in respiratory tract and related
infections. They are seen commonly in female
genital tract infections; they are less often encountered in intraabdominal processes than are
the gram-negative anaerobic rods. As is true for
the gram-negative anaerobic bacilli, gram-positive anaerobic cocci may be found in virtually
all types of infection. At the Mayo Clinic, anaerobic cocci have been recovered from 31% of
all anaerobic cultures that yielded growth. The
anaerobic gram-negative cocci are much less

pathogenic. The anaerobic gram-positive cocci
most commonly encountered in infection are
*Peptostreptococcus magnus, P. asaccharolyti-
cus, P. prevotii, P. micros,* and *P. anaerobius.*

As with other anaerobic organisms, disruption of a mucosal surface or introduction of anaerobic cocci into a normally sterile site may
lead to infection with the anaerobic cocci (usually as part of a mixed flora). Virulence factors
have not been studied as extensively in the
case of anaerobic cocci as with clostridia and
anaerobic gram-negative rods, but such factors
as lipopolysaccharides, hyaluronidase, collagenase, and capsules have been described. Again,
with the anaerobic cocci as with all anaerobes,
specimen collection and transport are critical
for meaningful bacteriologic data.

**37.1.a. Morphology and general character-
istics.** Gram-positive anaerobic cocci produce
minute to small, convex colonies that are gray
to white and opaque (Plate 37.1). The edges
are entire, and the colony surface may appear
stippled or pock marked. Colony size is usually
<0.5-2 mm in diameter. There may be a halo
of discoloration surrounding the colonies (*P.
micros*). *Peptococcus niger,* an organism that is
rarely encountered, produces black-pigmented
colonies. *Veillonella* (gram-negative) produces
small, convex, translucent to transparent colonies with an entire edge. These colonies may
show red fluorescence under long-wave UV
light, but, unlike the pigmented *Bacteroides,*
fluorescence does not depend on blood in the
medium and is lost rapidly after exposure of
colonies to air. Growth of anaerobic cocci in
broth is typically slow and results in balls,
clumps or aggregates of growth rather than diffuse turbidity. Microscopically, the anaerobic
cocci are not as distinctive as the gram-negative
anaerobic rods, but there are some notable features. *P. anaerobius* (Plate 37.2) and *P. pro-
ductus* are large coccobacilli often found in
chains. *P. magnus* cells are >0.6 μm in diameter and are found singly or in masses; they
look like staphylococcal cells (Plate 37.3).
Other peptostreptococci may also be mistaken

FIGURE 37.1
Flow chart for anaerobic cocci. (From Sutter, V.L., Citron, D.M., Edelstein, M.A.C., and Finegold, S.M. 1985. Wadsworth anaerobic bacteriology manual, ed. 4. Star Publishing Co., Belmont, Calif.)

for staphylococci on the basis of microscopic appearance. Indeed, such an appearance on direct Gram stain, with no staphylococci recovered on aerobic culture after 18-24 h, should suggest the possibility of *Peptostreptococcus*. *P. micros* cells are <0.6 μm in diameter and usually form short chains (Plate 37.4). The anaerobic streptococci (*S. intermedius, S. constellatus,* and *S. morbillorum*) vary in size and may be seen either in chains or pairs. Some anaerobic cocci can be shown to possess a capsule by staining with ruthenium red and examining under electron microscopy. *Veillonella* are tiny (<0.5 μm in diameter) **gram-negative cocci** that occur in masses or as diplococci. Negative staining of *Veillonella* cells reveals a convoluted surface. Unusually large cocci, especially when found in groups or packets, may suggest *Megasphaera* or *P. tetradius*. *Megasphaera* commonly stains gram-positive but is really gram-negative on the basis of cell-wall composition.

37.1.b. Differentiation of anaerobic cocci. Differentiation between genera of anaerobic cocci is based on Gram stain reaction and cell wall characteristics, metabolic endproducts, and whether or not a fermentable carbohydrate is required (Table 37.1). Figure 37.1 is a flow

chart illustrating the major means for differentiating between major groups and certain species of anaerobic cocci. Differentiation between various gram-positive anaerobic cocci is based on indole production, butyric and isocaproic acid production, production of lactic acid as the only major endproduct, fermentation of various carbohydrates, and cell size (Table 37.2). The anaerobic gram-negative cocci are differentiated on the basis of nitrate reduction, catalase production, glucose fermentation and fatty acid endproducts (Table 37.3).

37.2. Anaerobic Gram-Positive Cocci

37.2.a. Structure and extracellular products. This group includes one species of *Peptococcus, P. niger,* that is rarely encountered in clinical infection, three anaerobic species in the genus *Streptococcus* (*S. intermedius, S. constellatus,* and *S. morbillorum*), and the genus *Peptostreptococcus,* seven species of which may be encountered in infection (Table 37.2). Some strains of *Peptostreptococcus* and of anaerobic *Streptococcus* are encapsulated (the capsule is demonstrable by electron microscopy after ruthenium red staining). Hyaluronidase is produced by some oral strains of *Pep-*

TABLE 37.2
Characteristics of Anaerobic Gram-Positive Cocci

	Indole production	Butyric acid production	Isocaproic acid production	Lactic acid only major endproduct	Glucose	Cellobiose	Lactose	Maltose	Sucrose	Urease	Cell size ≥0.6 μm	Fatty acids from peptone yeast glucose broth
					Fermentation of							
Peptostreptococcus asaccharolyticus	+	+	−	−	−	−	−	−	−	−		B (A l p)
P. prevotii	−	+	−	−	−w	−	−	W−	W−	−+		B (A L p)
P. tetradius	−	+	−	−	+	−	−	+	+	+		B L (a p)
P. anaerobius	−	V	+	−	W−	−	−	W−	W−	−		A IC (ib b iv)
P. productus	−	−	−	+	+	+	+	+	+	−		A l s
P. micros	−	−	−	+	−	−	−	−	−	−		A (s)
P. magnus	−	−	−	−	+	−	−	−	−	−	+	A
Streptococcus sp.	−	−	−	+	+	V	V	+	+	−		L (a)

Modified from Sutter, V.L., Citron, D.M., Edelstein, M.A.C., and Finegold, S.M. 1985. Wadsworth anaerobic bacteriology manual, ed. 4. Star Publishing Co., Belmont, Calif.

Reactions: − = negative reaction; + = positive reaction for majority of strains; includes weak as well as strong acid production from carbohydrates in saccharolytic organisms; −+ = most strains negative; reaction helpful if negative; W− = most strains weakly positive, some negative; −w = most strains negative, some weakly positive; V = variable reaction.

PRAS carbohydrates: + = pH <5.5; W = pH 5.5-5.7; − = pH >5.7.

Fatty acids: A = acetic; P = propionic; IB = isobutyric; B = butyric; IV = isovaleric; V = valeric; IC = isocaproic; C = caproic; C′ = caprylic; L = lactic; S = succinic; PA = phenylacetic. NOTE: (1) Capital letters indicate major metabolic products. (2) Small letters indicate minor products. (3) Parentheses indicate a variable reaction. (4) Isoacids are primarily from carbohydrate-free media (such as PY) in the case of saccharolytic organisms.

tostreptococcus. Both the capsule and the hyaluronidase are felt to be virulence factors. The morphology of the anaerobic gram-positive cocci has been described under 37.1.a.

37.2.b. Identification methods. A discussion of preliminary grouping and identification procedures for the anaerobic gram-positive cocci appears in Chapter 34. Tables 37.1 and 37.2 and Figure 37.1 present data on differentiation within the group of anaerobic gram-positive cocci. Definitive identification of the anaerobic cocci depends on gas chromatographic analysis of endproducts, but the use of a number of simple tests permits species identification of many of these organisms. *P. anaerobius* is unique among anaerobic gram-positive cocci in degrading tyrosine crystals in a tyrosine medium; it is also the only species inhibited by sodium polyanetholsulfonate (SPS disk test [Plate 37.5]; see Chapter 34). Cellular fatty acid content is distinct in certain species of *Peptostreptococcus*. The species of *Peptostreptococcus* are serologically distinct from each other and are distinct from members of the genera *Peptococcus* and *Streptococcus*; unfortunately, there are no commercial serologic products available that would facilitate identification. As noted above, organisms resembling staphylococci on direct Gram stain of a clinical specimen may be anaerobic cocci; if there are no staphylococci recovered aerobically after 18-24 h incubation, this strongly suggests the possibility of anaerobic cocci.

37.2.c. Susceptibility to antimicrobial agents. The drug of choice for anaerobic gram-positive coccal infections has generally been considered to be penicillin G. However, some strains require as much as 8 μg/ml for inhibition and rare strains may require as much as 32 μg/ml. The latter strains would best be treated with another, more active agent. Chloramphenicol, the carboxypenicillins and ureidopenicillins, and cefoxitin are active against all strains, although some strains require 16 μg/ml of cefoxitin for inhibition. Metronidazole is active against all but rare strains of obligately an-

aerobic gram-positive cocci. Clindamycin is not active at achievable serum levels against about 10% of strains of cocci formerly classified in the genus *Peptococcus*. Cephalothin is quite active against all anaerobic gram-positive cocci. Occasional strains are resistant to cefamandole and ceftazidime; other cephalosporins are active against all strains, as is imipenem. Erythromycin is inactive at achievable levels against 20%-30% of strains formerly classified in the genus *Peptococcus*. Tetracycline has poor activity against anaerobic gram-positive cocci; doxycycline is somewhat better but should not be used unless susceptibility of a given strain from an infection has been documented.

37.2.d. Noncultural methods of identification. Little work has been done in this area with the anaerobic gram-positive cocci. The distinct serologic differences referred to earlier suggest that it should be possible to develop good fluorescent antibody or other reagents for direct identification, but this has not been done to date.

37.3. Anaerobic Gram-Negative Cocci

37.3.a. Structure and extracellular products. Distinctive morphologic features have been discussed under 37.1.a. *Veillonella* (Plate 37.6) cells have, on electron microscopic examination, a solid membrane between the outer membrane and the plasma membrane. The lipopolysaccharides (LPS) of *Veillonella* are potent endotoxins and contain 2-keto-3-deoxyoctonate (KDO) and heptose as well as a number of other sugars and amino sugars. Some strains of *Veillonella* have been shown to produce collagenase.

37.3.b. Identification methods. Fatty acid endproducts are the key means for differentiation among the three genera of anaerobic gram-negative cocci (Table 37.1), but, as noted in Table 37.3, nitrate reduction, catalase production and glucose fermentation are also useful in characterizing strains.

37.3.c. Susceptibility to antimicrobial agents. *Veillonella* is seldom a significant

TABLE 37.3
Characteristics of Anaerobic Gram-Negative Cocci

	NITRATE REDUCTION	CATALASE	GLUCOSE	FATTY ACIDS FROM PEPTONE YEAST GLUCOSE BROTH
Veillonella sp.	+	V	−	A p
Acidaminococcus fermentans	−	−	−	A B
Megasphaera elsdenii	−	−	+	a ib b iv v C

Modified from Sutter, V.L., Citron, D.M., Edelstein, M.A.C., and Finegold, S.M. 1985. Wadsworth anaerobic bacteriology manual, ed. 4. Star Publishing Co., Belmont, Calif.

Reactions: − = negative reaction; + = positive reaction for majority of strains; includes weak as well as strong acid production from carbohydrates in saccharolytic organisms; V = variable reaction.

PRAS carbohydrates: + = pH <5.5; W = pH 5.5-5.7; − = pH >5.7.

Fatty acids: A = acetic; P = propionic; IB = isobutyric; B = butyric; IV = isovaleric; V = valeric; IC = isocaproic; C = caproic; C′ = caprylic; L = lactic; S = succinic; PA = phenylacetic. NOTE: (1) Capital letters indicate major metabolic products. (2) Small letters indicate minor products. (3) Parentheses indicate a variable reaction. (4) Isoacids are primarily from carbohydrate-free media (such as PY) in the case of saccharolytic organisms.

pathogen, and *Acidaminococcus* and *Megasphaera* are rarely encountered in infection, so that specific therapy directed against the anaerobic gram-negative cocci is seldom indicated. Penicillin G is quite active against these organisms, but other penicillins, including the carboxypenicillins and ureidopenicillins are not always active against all strains. Metronidazole, chloramphenicol, clindamycin, and cefoxitin are all very active against the gram-negative coccal anaerobes, as are cephalothin, the newer cephalosporins, and imipenem.

BIBLIOGRAPHY

Babcock, J.B. 1979. Tyrosine degradation in presumptive identification of *Peptostreptococcus anaerobius*. J. Clin. Microbiol. 9:358.

Bourgault, A.-M., Rosenblatt, J.E., and Fitzgerald, R.H. 1980. *Peptococcus magnus*: a significant human pathogen. Ann. Intern. Med. 93:244.

Ezaki, T., Yamamoto, N., Ninomiya, K., et al. 1983. Transfer of *Peptococcus indolicus*, *Peptococcus asaccharolyticus*, *Peptococcus prevotii*, and *Peptococcus magnus* to the genus *Peptostreptococcus* and proposal of *Peptostreptococcus tetradius* sp. nov. Int. J. Sys. Bacteriol. 33:683.

Finegold, S.M. 1977. Anaerobic bacteria in human disease. Academic Press, Inc., New York.

Moss, C.W., Lambert, M.A., and Lombard, G.L. 1977. Cellular fatty acids of *Peptococcus variabilis* and *Peptostreptococcus anaerobius*. J. Clin. Microbiol. 5:665.

Pien, F.D., Thompson, R.L., and Martin, W.J. 1972. Clinical and bacteriologic studies of anaerobic gram-positive cocci. Mayo Clin. Proc. 47:251.

Rolfe, R.D., and Finegold, S.M. 1981. Comparative in vitro activity of new beta-lactam antibiotics against anaerobic bacteria. Antimicrob. Agents Chemother. 20:600.

Sutter, V.L., Citron, D.M., Edelstein, M.A.C., and Finegold, S.M. 1985. Wadsworth anaerobic bacteriology manual, ed. 4. Star Publishing Co., Belmont, Calif.

Sutter, V.L., and Finegold, S.M. 1976. Susceptibility of anaerobic bacteria to 23 antimicrobial agents. Antimicrob. Agents Chemother. 10:736.

Thomas, C.G.A., and Hare, R. 1954. The classification of anaerobic cocci and their isolation in normal human beings and pathological processes. J. Clin. Pathol. 7:300.

Wong, M., Catena, A., and Hadley, W.K. 1980. Antigenic relationships and rapid identification of *Peptostreptococcus* species. J. Clin. Microbiol. 11:515.

38 *Chlamydia, Mycoplasma,* and *Rickettsia*

38.1. Introduction

Organisms of the genera *Chlamydia, Mycoplasma,* and *Rickettsia* are prokaryotes that differ from most other bacteria in their very small size, their unusual cell wall structure, or, in the case of *Rickettsia* and *Chlamydia,* their obligate intracellular parasitism. *Chlamydia* and *Mycoplasma* genera each include species that cause pneumonia and species that cause venereal disease. The fastidious nature of both of these organisms is at least one reason for the parallel development of similar disease syndromes; the organisms must adhere to and multiply within a protective environment, and the mucous membranes of the respiratory tract and the genitourinary tract provide favorable conditions at the first site at which the pathogen impinges on a hospitable host. Isolation of pathogenic chlamydiae and mycoplasma is possible for hospital clinical laboratories but rickettsiae are extremely difficult to cultivate and too hazardous to work with for routine isolation attempts. These three genera will be treated separately in this chapter.

38.2. Chlamydiae

38.2.a. General properties. There are only two species of *Chlamydia,* obligate intracellular parasites within the family Chlamydiaceae. *Chlamydia psittaci* is the agent of pneumonia and systemic disease associated with contact

TABLE 38.1
Differences Among Three Groups of *Chlamydia*

	C. TRACHOMATIS (NON-LGV STRAINS)	C. TRACHOMATIS (LGV STRAINS)	C. PSITTACI
Sensitive to sulfonamides	+	+	–
Grow in cytoplasmic vesicles	+	+	–
Iodine-staining inclusions	+	+	–
Grow in mucosal surface cells	+	–	+
Grow in lymphoid cells	–	+	+
Intracerebral injection lethal to mice	+	–	+

with birds; the disease is variously known as **psittacosis** or **ornithosis**. Although many species variants occur, they have not been separated further. *Chlamydia trachomatis* is associated with four primary syndromes: **endemic trachoma** (repetitive conjunctival infection ultimately leading to blindness), **sexually transmitted chlamydial disease** (including nongonococcal urethritis and cervicitis), **inclusion conjunctivitis** (caused by the sexually transmitted strains and not leading to blindness), and **lymphogranuloma venereum (LGV)**. The organism may, in some cases, infect the entire genital tract and may cause pneumonia in infants. Table 38.1 outlines some biological differences among these groups of organisms.

Although the chlamydiae possess a cell wall similar to that of gram-negative bacteria, their cell wall is distinctive in lacking a peptidoglycan layer. They do produce an endotoxin-like lipopolysaccharide antigen. Unlike any other bacteria, chlamydiae undergo an unusual developmental cycle (Figure 38.1). The infectious particles, rigid-enveloped structures approximately 0.3 μm in diameter called **elementary bodies,** attach to the surface of a susceptible host cell. They induce endocytosis and are enclosed within a cytoplasmic vesicle, a **phagosome.** The organisms are able to prevent lysosomal fusion. After the initial stage, elementary bodies reorganize to a more metabolically active form, the **reticulate body.** Reticulate bodies multiply by binary fission until approxi-

mately 18-24 h after infection, at which point many of the reticulate bodies reorganize again into infectious elementary bodies. Newly formed reticulate and elementary bodies are still enclosed within the phagosomic intracellular vesicle, which is visible microscopically as an **inclusion** after it has been highlighted with a special stain. The inclusions of *C. trachomatis* can be stained with iodine, since they consist primarily of glycogen and exist in a rather compact form, in contrast to the diffuse, Giemsa-staining inclusions of *C. psittaci*. At 48-72 h after initial attachment, the cell ruptures to release a large number of infectious elementary bodies. The diseases caused by each of the species and the laboratory diagnosis of those diseases differ in several important ways. Each entity, *C. trachomatis* (LGV-associated), *C. trachomatis* (non-LGV), and *C. psittaci*, will be discussed separately.

38.2.b. Psittacosis: general features and laboratory diagnostic methods. *C. psittaci* is an endemic pathogen of birds of all species. Psittacine birds (such as parrots and parakeets) are the major reservoir for human disease, but outbreaks have occurred among turkey processing workers and pigeon aficionados. The birds may show diarrheal illness or may be asymptomatic. Humans acquire the disease by inhalation of aerosols. The organisms are deposited in the alveoli, from which some are ingested by alveolar macrophages and carried to regional lymph nodes. From there, they are disseminated sys-

FIGURE 38.1
Life cycle of *Chlamydia*. *EB*, Elementary body. *RB*, Reticulate body. (From Boyd, R.F. 1984. General microbiology. The C.V. Mosby Co., St. Louis.)

temically, growing within cells of the reticuloendothelial system. Findings include pneumonia, severe headache, changes in mentation, and hepatosplenomegaly.

Diagnosis of psittacosis is almost always by serologic means. Because of hazards associated with working with the agent, only laboratories with type III biohazard containment facilities (Chapter 2) can safely culture *C. psittaci*. State health departments take an active role in consulting with clinicians about possible cases. Complement fixation (Chapter 12) has been most commonly used to detect psittacosis infection. A more recent test, microindirect immunofluorescence, seems to be more sensitive but is difficult to perform. For this test, various strains of *C. psittaci* are grown in hens' egg yolk sac cultures. The cultures, rich with elementary bodies, are diluted and vigorously dispersed in buffer. The tester uses a small pipette or pen and places a dot of each antigen in a geometric array on the surface of a glass slide. Several identical arrays, each containing a dot of every antigen, are prepared on a single

slide. These slides are fixed and frozen until use. At the time of the test, serial dilutions of patients' serum are placed over the antigen arrays. After incubation and washing steps, fluorescein-conjugated antihuman immunoglobulin (either IgG or IgM) is overlayed on the slide. The slide is finally read for fluorescence of particular antigen dots with an ultraviolet microscope (Chapter 7). Either a fourfold rise in titer between acute and convalescent serum samples or a single IgM titer of 1:32 in a patient with clinically suspicious illness is diagnostic.

38.2.c. Lymphogranuloma venereum: general features and laboratory diagnostic methods. Lymphogranuloma venereum (LGV) is a sexually transmitted disease that is unusual in Europe and North America but not uncommon in Africa, Asia, and South America. The disease is characterized by a primary genital lesion of short duration at the site of initial infection. This lesion is often small and may be unrecognized, especially by female patients. The second stage, that of acute lymphadenitis, often involves the inguinal lymph nodes, causing them to enlarge, forming buboes. During this stage, infection may spread systemically to cause fever or locally to cause granulomatous proctitis. In a small number of cases (more women than men) the disease progresses to the third stage, that of a chronic inflammatory response that contributes to the development of genital hyperplasia, rectal fistulae, rectal stricture, draining sinuses, and other manifestations. Occasionally, chronic ulcerative or infiltrative lesions of the penis and scrotum may develop.

Diagnosis of LGV is usually made serologically, although a skin test called the **Frei test** was used extensively until recently. For the Frei test, LGV antigen grown in yolk sac culture was injected into one forearm of the patient and yolk sac control material was injected into the other arm. Development of a delayed type hypersensitivity reaction at the site of LGV antigen at 48 h was diagnostic. This test was not sensitive during early disease (before 6-8 weeks) and was not specific, as any chlamydial disease would induce a positive Frei test. Since chlamydial disease has become more widespread, the utility of the Frei test is questionable.

The microimmunofluorescence test, as described above for psittacosis, is the most sensitive serologic test for LGV. Very few laboratories perform the test, however; complement fixation is more commonly employed for diagnosis. Titers of 1:16 are considered to be significant. Material aspirated from buboes can be cultured for chlamydiae, as outlined below. Specimen collection procedures are discussed in Chapter 19.

38.2.d. *Chlamydia trachomatis* as a cause of non-LGV disease: general features and laboratory identification. Chlamydial infections have surpassed gonococcal infections as the most prevalent sexually transmitted disease in the United States. In addition to causing a spectrum of disease similar to that of gonococci, including urethritis, cervicitis, bartho-linitis, proctitis, salpingitis, inclusion conjunctivitis (ophthalmia neonatorum), perihepatitis (Fitz-Hugh-Curtis syndrome), epididymitis, and endocarditis, chlamydiae are a significant cause of pneumonia in neonates. Chlamydiae have been found as one cause of the urethral syndrome in women, characterized by symptoms of a urinary tract infection with pyuria but few or no conventional bacteria. Both chlamydiae and gonococci are major causes of pelvic inflammatory disease (PID), contributing significantly to the rising rate of infertility and ectopic pregnancies in young women. After only one episode of PID, as many as 10% of women may become infertile due to tubal occlusion. The risk increases dramatically with each additional episode of PID. Chlamydial salpingitis leading to infertility may be asymptomatic. Chlamydial infection can be transmitted to an infant from an infected mother during delivery. Approximately 0.5% of live births are complicated by neonatal chlamydial inclusion conjunctivitis or pneumonia.

Many genital chlamydial infections in people of either sex are asymptomatic. It is estimated that as many as 22% of women and 7% of men in some populations are asymptomatic carriers. The highest risk group is patients with gonococcal infection; 20%-35% of men with gonorrhea and 50% of women with gonorrhea are likely to harbor *C. trachomatis* concomitantly. Furthermore, in the United States, 60% of cases of nongonococcal urethritis (NGU) are caused by chlamydiae. The incidence of this disease is even higher in Scandinavian countries. With the recently developed diagnostic tests outlined below, we expect that a much clearer epidemiologic picture and ultimately better control of this wide-spread disease are attainable goals for the near future.

Although the microimmunofluorescent test is useful for diagnosis of chlamydial infection, it is difficult to perform and not generally available. High background levels of antibody in populations with increased prevalence of sexually transmitted diseases make serologic testing for *C. trachomatis* infection very difficult, even with microimmunofluorescence. Other serologic tests are not sensitive enough. Fortunately, a fluorescein-conjugated monoclonal antibody test system (Micro-Trak, Syva Co.) that is both reasonably sensitive and specific for the direct detection of chlamydia antigen is available. The system has been widely evaluated with favorable results. Most evaluations have screened patients with symptomatic disease; the sensitivity of this test for the detection of asymptomatic carriers has not been established. Material containing cells from male or female urethral discharge, scrapings from genital sites and infected conjunctivae, or tissue biopsies are suitable specimens for either culture or direct antigen detection. Collection procedures are detailed in the appropriate chapters in Part II, particularly Chapter 19. Material must contain epithelial (not just pus) cells, since the elementary bodies in infected tissue are primarily intracellular in such cells. The single most important determinant of success in detecting chlamydiae is the quality of the specimen.

All necessary supplies are included with the commercial kit. Slides with material to be examined for direct detection of antigen are prepared and fixed with acetone. The conjugate is added to the slide and incubated at room temperature for 15 min. After distilled water rinse, the slides are covered with coverslips and examined using a fluorescent microscope. Elementary bodies show up as apple-green fluorescing tiny spheres or short coccal forms (Plate 38.1). This method has been shown to be almost comparable to conventional culture techniques (outlined below), with some false positive and false negative results, and requires only 30 min in all to perform. As with any immunofluorescent procedure, experience is necessary to be able to distinguish artifacts from true positive results. It is suggested that at least between five and ten definite fluorescing elementary bodies should be seen in order for the specimen to be called positive.

In addition to direct visual observation, *Chlamydia* antigens can be detected by a recently introduced enzyme-linked immunosorbent assay, Chlamydiazyme (Abbott Laboratories). Patient specimen material to be tested for the presence of *Chlamydia* antigens is placed in the wells of a microdilution plate in which the reaction takes place; results are read on the Quantum II reader (Abbott). This system has shown specificity and sensitivity equal to that of the direct immunofluorescent assay in the hands of some investigators. Advantages are that expertise in fluorescence microscopy is unnecessary and that large numbers of specimens may be processed with relatively little hands-on time. Disadvantages are the initial cost of the equipment and the necessity for batching specimens to make the test cost effective. Because of the cumbersome methods necessary for culturing chlamydiae (described below), however, either the new direct fluorescent antibody stain or the ELISA diagnostic system offer an attractive alternative to conventional culture. Both methods are easily adaptable to the workflow of routine clinical laboratories that otherwise might offer no diagnostic tests for *Chlamydia*.

Direct examination of Giemsa-stained scrapings from conjunctiva and cervical and urethral cells may also be performed. Only in severe inclusion conjunctivitis of the newborn is this method sensitive enough for routine use and here, again, experience is extremely important, as is examination of the slide for many minutes. Examination of the stained smear is usually performed by cytologists or pathologists rather than microbiologists.

The current standard for diagnosis of chlamydial diseases is cell culture. McCoy cells (a line of mouse fibroblasts), grown on coverslips in the bottom of 1-dram vials, are commercially available (M. A. Bioproducts). Only laboratories proficient in tissue culture methods should try to maintain their own cell lines (Chapter 42). The chlamydial isolation procedure, outlined in Procedure 38.1, consists of (1) adding the specimen to the cell layer which is then treated with a cytostatic agent (cycloheximide) to prevent cell division and enhance infectivity; (2) centrifuging the specimen onto the cells to force contact and adherence; and (3) incubating.

Iodine has been used traditionally to detect the inclusions of *C. trachomatis* in cell culture, prepared as a wet mount. Lugol's iodine (Chapter 46) applied for 3-5 min to absolute methanol-fixed monolayers is adequate for this purpose. The iodine may remain on the cells until the culture is examined. If this stain is used, however, the cell culture must be incubated for 72 h before staining to achieve good sensitivity. Iodine-stained monolayers may be decolorized with methanol and restained with Giemsa to produce a permanent record. For those laboratories that do not use monoclonal staining reagents, a second passage of inclusion-negative cell culture supernatants to a fresh cell culture will result in a higher yield of positive cultures. The sensitivity of the fluorescent stain seems to obviate the need for blind passage.

PROCEDURE 38.1. CELL CULTURE METHOD FOR ISOLATION OF CHLAMYDIAE

1. Swab or tissue is collected in sucrose transport medium containing antibiotics as outlined in Chapter 19.
2. After vigorously vortexing the medium to remove most material from the swab, remove swab from transport tube and add a couple of sterile glass beads to homogenize the specimen if it is thick, as in tracheobronchial aspirates. Tissue should be ground or minced and diluted in transport medium. Vortex vigorously with the beads.
3. Aspirate the cell culture medium above the monolayer with a sterile pipette and add 0.5 ml of the specimen solution and 0.5 ml of maintenance medium (Chapter 45).
4. Centrifuge the vial for at least 1 h at 4,000 × g or greater at ambient temperature in a temperature controlled centrifuge to infect the cell monolayer. Do not allow the temperature to increase past 40° C.
5. Incubate for 2 h at 37° C. If the specimen is likely to be toxic, such as in the case of a rectal swab or sputum, the incubation step should be deleted.
6. Remove the supernatant medium and add 2 ml fresh maintenance medium containing 1 μg/ml cycloheximide.
7. Stopper the vials tightly and incubate at 37° C in air (or in 5% CO_2 if vials are capped loosely) for 48 h.
8. Air dry the coverslips and fix in cold acetone. Stain as for direct detection of antigen using the fluorescein-conjugated monoclonal antibody designed for detection of tissue-culture infected cells (Syva Co.).
9. Visualization of fluorescent inclusions and tiny elementary bodies is diagnostic.

38.3. Mycoplasmas

38.3.a. General properties. Members of the class *Mollicutes*, these organisms are found throughout the animal and plant kingdom as free-living saprophytes and parasites. Because the first recognized mycoplasma was isolated from a case of pleuropneumonia in a cow, the organism was designated **pleuropneumonia-like organism** or **PPLO.** That term is still used today, particularly for certain mycoplasma media. The smallest organisms able to survive extracellularly, they are highly pleomorphic because they lack a cell wall, which also renders them completely resistant to beta lactam and other cell wall active drugs. Although some species are normal human respiratory tract flora, *M. pneumoniae* is a major cause of respiratory disease (primary atypical pneumonia, sometimes called "walking pneumonia"), and *M. hominis* and *Ureaplasma urealyticum* are important pathogens of the human genital tract. None of the other species, shown in Table 38.2, are definitely pathogenic for humans. These organisms colonize the mucosa of the respiratory and genital tracts of humans, growing extracellularly. By an unknown mechanism, infection with mycoplasma causes injury to mucosal cells. The tissue damage leads to impairment of ciliary function. Although *M. pneumoniae* rarely causes invasive disease, *M. hominis* has been recovered from the blood of febrile postpartum patients.

38.3.b. *Mycoplasma pneumoniae:* general features and laboratory identification. It is estimated that *M. pneumoniae* may cause as many as 50% of all community-acquired pneumonias during noninfluenza periods. The disease is primarily one of children and young adults, spreading from person to person via respiratory tract secretions. The most common syndrome produced is tracheobronchitis, but pneumonia, pharyngitis, rhinitis, ear infection (including bullous myringitis), meningitis, myocarditis, and pericarditis also occur.

Although culture methods are available, very few laboratories offer them. Similarly, there has been little progress in the direct detection of mycoplasma or their antigens in clinical specimens. The advent of monoclonal antibodies may alleviate this diagnostic need. Accurate, rapid diagnosis is highly desirable, since penicillin and other beta lactam agents

TABLE 38.2

Mycoplasmas Recovered from Humans

GENUS AND SPECIES	HEMADSORPTION	H_2O_2 PRODUCED	GLUCOSE FERMENTED	ARGININE HYDROLYZED	UREA HYDROLYZED
Mycoplasma					
pneumoniae	+	+	+	−	−
salivarium	−	−	−	+	−
orale	−	−	−	+	−
buccale	−	−	−	+	−
faucium	−	−	−	+	−
lipophilum	−	−	−	+	−
primatum	−	−	−	+	−
fermentans	−	−	+	+	−
hominis	−	−	−	+	−
genitalium	+	+	+	−	−
Ureaplasma					
urealyticum	+/−		−	−	+
Acholeplasma					
laidlawii	−		+	−	−

are ineffective treatment; erythromycin and tetracycline are the antibiotics of choice. Diagnosis is usually made serologically. Nonspecific production of **cold agglutinins** occurs in approximately half of patients with atypical pneumonia. The most widely used serologic test today is complement fixation (Chapter 12). A fourfold rise in titer between the acute serum and the convalescent serum drawn 2-4 weeks later is diagnostic. Titers in single serum specimens greater than or equal to 1:128 suggest recent infection. New immunologic tests for detection of *M. pneumoniae* antibodies, such as indirect immunofluorescence and ELISA, have recently

PROCEDURE 38.2. ISOLATION OF *M. PNEUMONIAE*

1. Place 0.1-0.2 ml of liquid specimen or dip and twirl a specimen received on a swab in a vial of SP-4 culture medium (Chapter 45). After expressing as much fluid as possible from the swab by "wringing" it at the mouth of the vial, remove the swab to prevent contamination.
2. Seal the vial tightly and incubate in air at 37° C for up to 3 weeks.
3. Inspect the vial daily. During the first 5 days a change in pH, indicated by a color shift from orange to yellow or violet, or increased turbidity is a sign that the culture is contaminated and should be discarded.
4. If either a slight acid pH shift (yellow color) with no increase in turbidity or no change occurs after 7 days' incubation, subculture several drops of the broth culture to Edward-Hayflick agar (Chapter 45). Continue to incubate the original broth.
5. If broth that exhibited no changes at 7 days shows a slight acid pH shift at any time, subculture to agar as above. Broths that show no change at 3 weeks are blindly subcultured again, to agar.
6. Incubate the agar plates in a very moist atmosphere with 5% CO_2 at 37° C for 7 days.
7. Observe the agar surface under 40 × magnification after 5 days for colonies, which appear as spherical, grainy, yellowish forms, embedded in the agar, with a thin outer layer ("fried egg").
8. Definitive identification of *M. pneumoniae* is accomplished by overlaying Edward-Hayflick agar plates showing suspicious colonies with 5% sheep or guinea pig erythrocytes in 1% agar made in physiologic saline (0.85% NaCl) instead of water. The 1% agar is melted and cooled to 50° C, the blood cells are added, and a thin layer is poured over the original agar surface.
9. Reincubate the plate for 24 h and observe for beta hemolysis around colonies of *M. pneumoniae* caused by production of hydrogen peroxide (Plate 38.2). Additional incubation at room temperature overnight will enhance the hemolysis. No other species of mycoplasma produce this reaction.

Modified from Clyde, Kenny, and Schachter. 1984. Cumitech 19. American Society for Microbiology, Washington, D.C.

38.1

38.2

PLATE 38.1.   Appearance of fluorescein-conjugated monoclonal antibody–stained elementary bodies in direct smear of urethral cell scraping from patient with chlamydial urethritis.
PLATE 38.2.   *Mycoplasma pneumoniae* colonies with sheep red blood cell overlay.

38.3

PLATE 38.3.   Colonies of *Ureaplasma urealyticum* after 48 h incubation, overlaid with urea-manganese chloride reagent.

39.1

39.2

PLATE 39.1.   Colonies of violet-pigmented *Chromobacterium violaceum* on blood agar.
PLATE 39.2.   Colonies of *Dermatophilus congolensis* on 5% sheep blood agar. (Organisms courtesy Dr. Morris Gordon.)

39.3

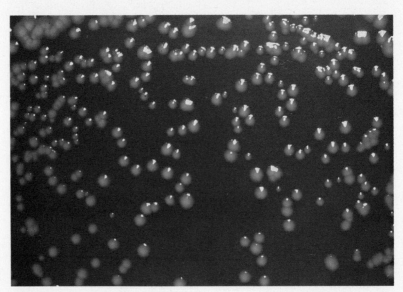

39.4

PLATE 39.3. Culture of vaginal discharge after 48 h incubation. Colonies of *Gardnerella vaginalis* growing in large numbers on CNA agar that also supports the growth of some normal flora.
PLATE 39.4. Colonies of *Legionella pneumophila* on BCYE agar. (Organism courtesy Dr. Clifford Mintz.)

39.5

39.6

PLATE 39.5. Giménez stain of *Legionella pneumophila* from a colony grown on BCYE.
PLATE 39.6. Fluorescent-antibody stained *Legionella pneumophila* from a positive control slide.

39.7

PLATE 39.7. *Streptobacillus moniliformis* smear made from a standard colony. Stained with Giemsa and visualized under oil immersion magnification (1,000 ×).

been developed and show much promise. There have been no published trials of the commercially available reagents at this time, but they should be as sensitive and specific as other ELISA and IFA methods described for detection of other antibodies (Chapter 12).

Collection and transport of respiratory tract specimens, including nasopharyngeal and throat swabs and washings, tracheal aspirates, sputa, and lung biopsy specimens, are detailed in Chapters 16 and 21. A procedure for isolation of *M. pneumoniae* (Procedure 38.2) is modified from Clyde, Kenny, and Schachter.[1]

Other methods are available for identifying mycoplasma colonies isolated by the above procedure, including hemadsorption, immunofluorescent stain of colonies, and inhibition by specific antisera impregnated onto filter paper disks.

38.3.c. Genital mycoplasmas: general properties and laboratory identification. Of the seven species of mycoplasma found in the human genital tract (Table 38.2), only *U. urealyticum* and *M. hominis* are unequivocally known to be pathogens. Under what circumstances they are pathogenic is still unclear, as a large number of adults are asymptomatically colonized with both species. Ureaplasmas are a cause of nongonococcal urethritis in males, but they also colonize sexually active males without urethritis. Further studies are needed to elucidate the role of this organism in disease in males. In females, ureaplasmas do not seem to cause disease, but they may possibly contribute to low birth weight of newborns born to colonized mothers. *M. hominis* does not seem to cause disease commonly in males, but it is a cause of postpartum fevers in women. Additionally, strains of the organism can be isolated significantly more often from patients with pelvic inflammatory disease than from controls.

Specimens are collected on swabs, as described in Chapter 19. Transport media such as modified Stuart's, 2-SP (used for chlamydiae),

or trypticase soy broth (BBL Microbiology Systems) with 0.5% albumin and 400 U/ml penicillin will preserve viability for up to 24 h at refrigerator temperatures. Specimens that must be held longer should be frozen at $-70°$ C in a medium containing protein. Culture media may also be used for transport. Culture methods described here (Procedures 38.3 and 38.4) are modified from Mårdh[2] and from Clyde, Kenny, and Schachter.[1]

PROCEDURE 38.3.
ISOLATION OF *U. UREALYTICUM*

1. Inoculate one *Ureaplasma* agar plate and one *Ureaplasma* broth (Chapter 45) each with 0.1 ml specimen from transport medium.
2. Incubate broth in tightly sealed test tubes for 5 days. Observe twice daily for a color change in the broth to red with no increase in turbidity. If color change occurs, transfer one loopful to a *Ureaplasma* agar plate and streak for isolated colonies.
3. Agar plates are incubated in a candle jar or, optimally, in an anaerobic jar at 37° C. Colonies will appear on agar within 48 h. Plates are inspected in the same way as described for *M. pneumoniae* (Procedure 38.2). *Ureaplasma* colonies will appear as small, granular, yellowish spheres that simulate the "white" of the "fried egg."
4. To definitively identify colonies on *Ureaplasma* agar after 48 h incubation, pour a solution of 1% urea and 0.8% $MnCl_2$ in distilled water over the agar surface. *U. urealyticum* will stain dark brown due to production of urease (Plate 38.3).

PROCEDURE 38.4.
ISOLATION OF *M. HOMINIS*

1. Inoculate one *M. hominis* agar plate and two *M. hominis* broth tubes (Chapter 45), one broth containing phenol red indicator and one without the possibly inhibitory phenol red, each with 0.1 ml specimen from transport media.
2. Incubate broths in tightly sealed test tubes for 5 days. If the phenol red-containing broth changes color to red or violet, both broths are subcultured to *M. hominis* agar. After 48 h incubation, transfer 0.1 ml or a loopful of broth from tubes that exhibited no change or only a slight increase in turbidity to *M. hominis* agar and streak for isolated colonies.
3. *M. hominis* agar plates are incubated in the same manner as *Ureaplasma* cultures. Plates should be observed daily for up to 5 days for colonies.

Although serologic tests such as indirect hemagglutination and metabolism inhibition for genital mycoplasmas are available, they are rarely used. It is possible that ELISA tests of sufficient specificity for diagnosis may be available in the future.

38.4. *Rickettsia* and *Coxiella*

38.4.a. General properties. The Rickettsiaceae are a group of organisms that infect wild animals, with humans acting as accidental hosts in most cases. Most of these organisms are passed between animals by an insect vector. All rickettsiae multiply only intracellularly. *Coxiella burnetii*, which is similar to but distinct from the rickettsiae, can survive extracel-

TABLE 38.3
Vectors of Selected Diseases Caused by *Rickettsia* and *Coxiella*

AGENT	DISEASE	VECTOR
Rickettsia akari	Rickettsialpox	Mites
R. conorii	Boutonneuse fever	Ticks
R. prowazekii	Epidemic typhus Brill-Zinsser disease	Lice
R. rickettsii	Rocky Mountain spotted fever	Ticks
R. tsutsugamushi	Scrub typhus	Mites
R. typhi	Murine (endemic) typhus	Fleas
Rochalimaea quintana	Trench fever	Lice
Coxiella burnetii	Q fever	Ticks, aerosols

lularly. The rickettsiae cannot even survive outside of their animal hosts or insect vectors. The diseases caused in humans are usually characterized by fever, headache, and rash. With the exception of Q fever, caused by *C. burnetii*, the rickettsiae multiply in the endothelial cells of blood vessels, causing cell injury and death. Damage to cells results in vascular changes and the influx of inflammatory cells that serve to magnify the host's immune response and increase overall morbidity.

All rickettsiae are pleomorphic gram-negative coccobacilli. The organisms multiply by binary fission in the cytoplasm of host cells, which are finally lysed during release of mature rickettsiae. The rickettsiae, but not *C. burnetii*, infect humans following the bite of an infected arthropod vector. The agents, their vectors, and diseases are shown in Table 38.3. *Coxiella burnetii* is more hardy than the others, resisting desiccation and sunlight. They infect humans by the aerosol route. In contrast to rickettsiae, *Coxiella* is passively phagocytized by host cells and multiplies within vacuoles. The other agents, after being deposited directly into the bloodstream through the bite of a louse, Ixodid tick, flea, or mite, induce

TABLE 38.4
Reactions of *Proteus* Strains in Weil-Felix Test

DISEASE	OX-19	OX-2	OX-K
Brill-Zinsser	V	V	−
Epidemic typhus	+	V	−
Murine typhus	+	V	−
Rickettsialpox	−	−	−
Rocky Mountain spotted fever	+	+	−
Scrub typhus	−	−	V
Q fever	−	−	−

+ = >90% positive agglutination; − = >90% negative agglutination; V = variable results.

host cells to engulf them, after which they quickly escape the vacuole to become free in the cytoplasm. *Coxiella* is inhaled into the alveoli, picked up by macrophages, and carried to lymph nodes, from which it disseminates into the bloodstream. Granulomatous hepatitis and endocarditis are common sequelae.

Early diagnosis is usually made on clinical grounds based on the symptoms of fever, rash, and exposure to ticks. The characteristic spread of the rash from the extremities to the trunk help to distinguish Rocky Mountain spotted fever (RMSF) from meningococcemia.

38.4.b. Laboratory identification. Biopsy specimens of skin tissue from the rash of RMSF can be stained directly with a specific immunofluorescent reagent. This test, available at certain state health laboratories and the Centers for Disease Control, can provide a diagnosis as early as 3-4 days after symptoms have appeared. The Giménez stain (Chapter 46) is also used for examination of clinical material.

Although the rickettsiae can be cultured in embryonated eggs and in tissue culture, the risk of laboratory-acquired infection is extremely high, limiting culture techniques to a few specialized laboratories. Diagnosis of rickettsial disease is primarily accomplished serologically. The least specific but most widely used test in the United States is the **Weil-Felix**

reaction, the fortuitous agglutination of certain strains of *Proteus vulgaris* by serum from patients with rickettsial disease. Table 38.4 outlines the positive reactions associated with each disease. Commercial suppliers produce kits that contain all necessary antigens and human antirickettsial control antisera for performance of the Weil-Felix test. This test is only presumptive, however, and a more specific serologic test such as complement fixation or direct immunofluorescence must be used for confirmation of disease. These tests are performed primarily by reference laboratories and kits are obtainable from CDC for performing tests for IgG antibody. The microimmunofluorescent dot test, as described for diagnosis of psittacosis, has also shown excellent sensitivity for detecting antibodies to rickettsiae. By overlaying the antigen dots on the slide with fluorescein-conjugated antihuman IgM after the patient's serum has been allowed to form complexes, early diagnosis of RMSF can be achieved (within 7-10 days after onset of symptoms). Both immunofluorescent and a recently developed latex agglutination test methods have shown good sensitivity for diagnosis of RMSF within the first week. Neither Q fever nor rickettsialpox induces Weil-Felix antibody in infected patients. Especially in those cases, specific immunofluorescent tests are valuable.

Coxiella burnetii undergoes an antigenic **phase variation** during infection. The organisms exist in phase II during initial infection, and humans produce antibody to phase II early in disease. If infection progresses to chronic disease, such as endocarditis or hepatitis, antibodies to phase I are present and can be measured by complement fixation or immunofluorescence.

Except for latex agglutination, immunofluorescence, and direct fluorescent antibody testing for diagnosing RMSF, none of the serologic tests is useful for diagnosing disease in time to influence therapy, since antibodies to rickettsiae other than *R. rickettsii* often cannot be detected until at least 2 weeks after the patient has become ill. With newer immunologic reagents being developed, we can hope that more easily performed, sensitive, and specific tests for all rickettsial diseases will soon be available.

REFERENCES

1. Clyde, W.A. Jr., Kenny, G.E., and Schachter, J. 1984. Cumitech 19: laboratory diagnosis of chlamydial and mycoplasmal infections. Drew, W.L., coordinating editor. American Society for Microbiology, Washington, D.C.
2. Mårdh, P.-A. 1984. Laboratory diagnosis of sexually transmitted diseases. In Holmes, K.K., Mårdh, P.-A., Sparling, P.F., and Wiesner, P.J., editors. Sexually transmitted diseases. McGraw-Hill Book Co., New York.

BIBLIOGRAPHY

Baca, O.G., and Paretsky, D. 1983. Q fever and *Coxiella burnetii:* a model for host-parasite interactions. Microbiol. Rev. 47:127.

Couch, R.C. 1984. Mycoplasma diseases. In Holmes, K.K., Mårdh, P.-A., Sparling, P.F., and Wiesner, P.J., editors. Sexually transmitted diseases. McGraw-Hill Book Co., New York.

Gutman, L.T. 1980. Chlamydia. In Joklik, W.K., Willett, H.P., and Amos, D.B., editors. Zinsser microbiology, ed. 17. Appleton-Century-Crofts, New York.

Hechemy, K.E. 1980. Rocky Mountain spotted fever: the clinical and immunoserologic picture. Clin. Immunol. Newsletter 1(10):1.

Moulder, J.W. 1984. Looking at chlamydiae without looking at their hosts. Am. Soc. Microbiol. News 50:353.

Peter, J.B., and Lovett, M.A. 1982. Genital infection from *Chlamydia trachomatis.* Diagn. Med. 5:17.

Philip, R.N., Casper, E.A., Ormsbee, R.A., et al. 1976. Microimmunofluorescence test for the serological study of Rocky Mountain spotted fever and typhus. J. Clin. Microbiol. 3:51.

Saah, A.J., and Hornick, R.B. 1985. *Coxiella burnetii* (Q fever). In Mandell, G.L., Douglas, R.G., Jr., and Bennett, J.E., editors. Principles and practice of infectious diseases, ed. 2. John Wiley & Sons, New York. (Note: several other chapters by the same authors contain valuable information.)

Schachter, J. 1984. Biology of *Chlamydia trachomatis.* In Holmes, K.K., Mårdh, P.-A., Sparling, P.F., and Wiesner, P.J., editors. Sexually transmitted diseases. McGraw-Hill Book Co., New York.

Weissfeld, A.S. 1983. Genital mycoplasma. Clin. Microbiol. Newsletter 5:65.

Woodward, W.E., and Hornick, R.B. 1985. *Rickettsia rickettsii* (Rocky Mountain spotted fever). In Mandell, G.L., Douglas, R.G., Jr., and Bennett, J.E., editors. Principles and practice of infectious diseases, ed. 2. John Wiley & Sons, New York.

39

Unclassified or Unusual Cultivatable Etiologic Agents of Infectious Disease

The microorganisms discussed in this chapter were not placed in any of the previous chapters, either because they are unusual enough to fail to fit into existing classifications, or because they are isolated rarely or only in association with a defined syndrome. Several of the organisms discussed here require very special isolation techniques for their cultivation, necessitating a high index of suspicion on the part of the clinician. Only by communicating with the laboratory the need for special procedures can the physician ensure that certain of the organisms listed below will be isolated. In other cases, isolates of these organisms might be dismissed as contaminants if technologists have not been warned to expect something unusual.

39.1. Genus *Bartonella*

39.1.a. Epidemiology and pathogenesis of *Bartonella* infection. *Bartonella bacilliformis*, the only species in the genus *Bartonella*, is closely related to *Chlamydia* (Chapter 38), differing in the site of infection in the vertebrate host and in the requirement of intracellular multiplication. Although *Chlamydia* parasitize the epithelial cells of the respiratory and genital mucous membranes, *Bartonella* grow within and on the surface of erythrocytes and occasionally in vascular endothelium. In contrast to *Chlamydia*, *Bartonella* can be cultivated in vitro on nonliving media.

564

The disease bartonellosis is confined to the Andes region of Peru, Ecuador, and Colombia, where the arthropod vector, the sand fly, *Phlebotomus*, and susceptible humans both exist. Humans acquire the disease from the bite of the fly and humans serve as a reservoir for the organism in the region. Two forms of the disease are common, a febrile, systemic disease characterized by anemia, called **Oroya fever,** and a chronic, cutaneous disease characterized by tumorlike lesions of the skin and mucous membranes, called **verruga peruana.** Verruga peruana usually follows an episode of Oroya fever. The bacteria on the surface of and within erythrocytes seem to contribute to the anemia. Patients with partial immunity develop verruga peruana. It is not known exactly how the organisms damage the red blood cells.

39.1.b. Laboratory diagnosis of bartonellosis. The organisms can be isolated from blood and from material aspirated from lymph nodes or cutaneous lesions. Organisms grow best at room temperature and do not require increased CO_2 in the atmosphere. Brain heart infusion agar, modified to contain 0.4% agar, with the addition of 5% human, rabbit, or horse blood, should support growth of *B. bacilliformis*. The organisms stain gram-negative and are visualized best with the carbol-fuchsin counterstain (Chapter 46). They are curved or coccoid, with mixtures of rods and granules, which tend to grow in aggregates. In vitro, cells produce a polar tuft of flagella. Biochemically, *B. bacilliformis* is quite inert.

According to Ristic and Kreier,[9] the organisms may also be visualized in blood films from infected patients. They stain red-violet with Giemsa stain (Chapter 46), appearing as cocci or bacilli, with occasional curved or ringlike forms. The cells may show polar enlargements (appearing only at one end).

39.1.c. Therapy of bartonellosis. The disease seems to respond rapidly to therapy with penicillin, chloramphenicol, tetracycline, or streptomycin. Because patients with Oroya fever appear to be at increased risk for contracting *Salmonella* infection, chloramphenicol may be the drug of choice.

39.2. Genus *Calymmatobacterium*

39.2.a. Epidemiology and pathogenesis of *Calymmatobacterium* infection. *Calymmatobacterium granulomatis* is the etiologic agent of **granuloma inguinale,** or **donovanosis** (Chapter 19), a venereally transmitted disease characterized by subcutaneous nodules that enlarge and evolve to form beefy, erythematous, granulomatous, painless lesions that bleed easily. The lesions, which usually occur on the genitalia, have been mistaken for neoplasms. Patients often have inguinal lymphadenopathy. The organism has been isolated only from human lesions and the disease is confined primarily to the tropics, although it has been reported in the United States. Infectivity of this bacillus must be low, since sexual partners of infected patients often do not themselves become infected.

39.2.b. Laboratory diagnosis of granuloma inguinale. The organism can be visualized in scrapings of lesions stained with Wright's or Giemsa stain. Subsurface infected cells must be present; surface epithelium is not an adequate specimen. Groups of organisms are seen within mononuclear endothelial cells; this pathognomonic entity is known as a **Donovan body,** named after the physician who first visualized the organism in such a lesion. The organism stains as a blue rod with prominent polar granules giving rise to a "safety pin" appearance, surrounded by a large, pink capsule. The capsular polysaccharide shares several crossreactive antigens with *Klebsiella* species, fueling speculation that *Calymmatobacterium* is closely related to *Klebsiella*.

Cultivation in vitro is very difficult, but it can be done using media containing some of the growth factors found in egg yolk (Procedure 39.1). A medium described by Dienst has been

PROCEDURE 39.1. CULTIVATION OF *CALYMMATOBACTERIUM GRANULOMATIS*

1. Prepare medium as follows:

Peptone (Difco Laboratories)	10 g
Tryptone (Difco Laboratories)	3 g
Glucose	3 g
Commercial sea salts (any chemical supplier)	2 g
Agar (Bacto agar, Difco Laboratories)	1.2 g
Distilled water	1,000 ml

Dissolve all ingredients by heating gently. Adjust pH to 7.3. Autoclave at 121° C for 15 min and cool to 45° C. Soak fresh eggs in 70% alcohol for 10 min before aseptically removing egg yolks. Dilute egg yolks with equal volume of sterile saline (0.85% NaCl) and mix with equal parts of the basal medium. Dispense the medium in sterile 16 × 125 mm tubes, 20 ml per tube. (Commercially available egg yolk may be suitable as a substitute for fresh egg yolks.)

2. A physician aspirates lymph node material or obtains material from the lesion with a sterile scalpel. The lesion is cleansed by carefully swabbing the surface of the lesion with a sterile gauze pad soaked in sterile saline to remove surface contamination. A small slice near the edge of the lesion will allow removal of subsurface material. The best material is obtained from under the surface of the lesion near the edge.

3. Inoculate the medium well below the surface with the scraping or aspirated material. Incubate for at least 72 h at 37° C. Incubating the tubes in a candle jar may help to retain the low oxygen concentration of the medium. Gram stain the broth, using a carbol-fuchsin counterstain. *C. granulomatis* is gram-negative.

Modified from Dienst and Brownell. 1984. In Krieg and Holt, editors. Bergey's manual of systematic bacteriology, ed. 9. Williams & Wilkins, Baltimore.

used to culture *Calymmatobacterium* from aspirated bubo material, as described by Dienst and Brownell.[1]

39.2.c. Therapy of granuloma inguinale. Although gentamicin and chloramphenicol are effective, tetracycline or ampicillin are usually the drugs of first choice. Trimethoprim-sulfamethoxazole has also been shown to be an effective treatment for granuloma inguinale. Erythromycin may also be used.

39.3. Genus *Capnocytophaga*

39.3.a. Epidemiology and pathogenesis of *Capnocytophaga* infection. The *Capnocytophaga* are **capnophilic** (carbon dioxide-loving) gram-negative bacilli, found as normal oral flora in humans. These organisms are often found in significantly larger numbers within the gingival pockets of patients with periodontal disease. The organisms produce proteases that are able to cleave secretory immunoglobulins, which are postulated to have a protective effect in preventing oral disease. An additional possible virulence factor is production by *Capnocytophaga* of a heat stable factor that alters polymorphonuclear neutrophil chemotactic activity. Interestingly, young patients with severe periodontitis also often display a neutrophil dysfunction that may spontaneously revert with the effective treatment of their periodontitis. The role of the extracellular products of *Capnocytophaga* in virulence of the organism has not yet been fully elucidated.

In addition to periodontal disease, *Capnocytophaga* is associated with systemic disease, usually in leukemic and/or granulocytopenic patients. However, there are several reports of osteomyelitis, septic arthritis, endocarditis, and soft tissue infections in normal hosts from which *Capnocytophaga* has been isolated. The portal of entry is thought to be the oral cavity. Many of the patients with predisposing immunosuppression had bleeding gums or oral mucosal erosion before they developed sepsis.

39.3.b. Laboratory identification of *Capnocytophaga*. The organism grows well on trypticase soy agar with 5% sheep blood, the standard blood agar plate used by most microbiology laboratories for routine cultures, as well as on chocolate or trypticase soy agar without blood. After 48-72 h incubation at 37° C in 5% CO_2 or anaerobically (Chapter 8), colonies are 1-5 mm in diameter, opaque, shiny, and nonhemolytic, with a pale beige or yellowish color. The color may be more apparent if growth is scraped from the surface with a loop and examined against a white background. The organism will not grow in air. Occasionally, gliding motility of the organism may be observed as outgrowths from the colonies or as a haze on the surface of the agar (Figure 39.1). The gliding motility is best observed on media containing 3% agar. The organism fails to grow on MacConkey agar.

Gram stain reveals gram-negative, fusiform shaped bacilli with one rounded end and one tapered end and occasional filamentous forms (Figure 39.2). The organisms may appear as aggregates. They are oxidase and catalase negative. A negative spot indole test (Chapter 9) is also helpful. There are three named species of *Capnocytophaga*, *C. ochracea*, *C. sputigena*, and *C. gingivalis*, and one unnamed group, that can be distinguished with difficulty biochemically (Table 39.1). Commercially available anaerobic identification systems, such as the RapID ANA (Innovative Diagnostics, Inc.), Minitek System (BBL Microbiology Systems), and API AnIdent (Analytab Products), and the multiparameter API ZYM enzymatic identification system can be used to differentiate *Capnocytophaga* species. For most situations in clinical microbiology laboratories, however, a presumptive identification to genus is as beneficial to clinicians as is definitive identification. All species share the traits of acid production from glucose and sucrose, negative urease, lysine and ornithine decarboxylases, as well as the characteristics listed above. The organism differs from morphologically similar organisms, such as *Actinobacillus actinomycetemcomitans* (Chapter 29), *Haemophilus aphrophilus* (Chapter 29), *Eikenella corrodens* (Chapter 28), *Gardnerella vaginalis* (below), and CDC Group HB-5 (an unclassified fastidious gram-negative coccobacillus that has been isolated from genitourinary tract specimens and occasionally from blood). Table 39.2 outlines some of the major differential characteristics among these fastidious gram-negative organisms.

39.3.c. Treatment of *Capnocytophaga* infections. Sepsis caused by this organism is severe, especially in immunocompromised patients, and must be approached aggressively. Bactericidal activity has been shown for penicillin, carbenicillin, clindamycin, and erythromycin. All strains are resistant to aminoglycosides.

FIGURE 39.1
Colonies of *Capnocytophaga* growing on 5% sheep blood agar. Note haze of growth extending from colonies, evidence of gliding motility of the bacteria.

FIGURE 39.2
Gram stain of *Capnocytophaga*.

TABLE 39.1
Key Differential Characteristics Among Species of *Capnocytophaga**

TEST	*C. OCHRACEA*	*C. SPUTIGENA*	*C. GINGIVALIS*	GROUP IV
Fructose	100	46	0	0
Lactose	82	31	0	100
Maltose	93	100	0	100
Mannitol	79	0	0	0
Raffinose	75	0	0	0
Rhamnose	71	92	79	0
Trehalose	93	0	7	80
NO_2 to nitrogen	82	92	100	0

Modified from Forlenza, S.W. 1985. *Capnocytophaga:* an opportunistic pathogen. Clin. Microbiol. Newsletter 7:17.
*Carbohydrate fermentations were performed in buffered single substrate medium. Results are given as a percentage of positive reactions observed from testing 60 strains.

TABLE 39.2
Key Differential Characteristics of Morphologically Similar Species of Fastidious Gram-Negative Bacilli

	OXI-DASE	CAT-ALASE	CELL SHAPE		INDOLE	NITRATE TO NITRITE	PRODUCE ACID		
			COCCOID	FUSIFORM			GLU-COSE	MAL-TOSE	LAC-TOSE
Actinobacillus	−	+	+	−	−	+	+	+	−
Capnocytophaga	−	+	−	+	−	+/−	+	+	+/−
Cardiobacterium	+	−	−	−	+ (weak)	−	+	+	−
Eikenella	+	−	−	−	−	+	−	−	−
Gardnerella	−	−	−	−	−	−	+	+	+/−
H. aphrophilus	−/+ (weak)	−/+ (weak)	+/−	−	−	+	+	+	+
HB-5	+ (weak)	−	+/−	−	+ (weak)	+	+	−	−

+ = positive (>90%); − = negative (>90%); +/− = variable.

39.4. Genus *Cardiobacterium*

39.4.a. Epidemiology and pathogenesis of *Cardiobacterium* infection.
Cardiobacterium hominis, the only species in the genus, is normal flora in the human mouth, and perhaps on other mucous membranes. It is noninvasive and has not been associated with any type of infection other than bacteremia or endocarditis. The incidence of *Cardiobacterium*-related bacteremia, however, is increasing. This may be due to the increased number of susceptible hosts, or, more likely, to increased awareness among microbiologists as well as better blood culturing techniques. Only 34 cases of *C. hominis* infection had been reported until 1983. Most patients had prior cardiac valvular disease. No specific virulence factors have been delineated for this organism.

39.4.b. Laboratory identification of *Cardiobacterium hominis.*
As an etiologic agent of disease, this organism has been isolated only from blood. It grows well in standard blood culture media (Chapter 14) and can be subcultured to 5% sheep blood agar, chocolate agar,

and trypticase soy agar without blood. The organism does not grow on MacConkey agar. Incubation of blood agar subcultures at 37° C in 5% CO_2 or in air with increased humidity (a candle jar probably provides the best atmosphere) for 48 h yields colonies that are 1-2 mm in diameter, slightly alpha hemolytic, smooth, round, glistening, and opaque. The organism will grow equally well at 30° and 37° C. Colonies grown on trypticase soy agar without blood should be observed microscopically under low power (100 ×) after 24 h incubation for typical rough appearance with an internal serpentine pattern of bacilli, some of which stream from the edge of the colony toward adjacent colonies. This appearance is in contrast to the prominent star-like pattern seen in colonies of *Actinobacillus actinomycetemcomitans* (Chapter 29), with which *Cardiobacterium* may be confused. *Cardiobacterium* is a pleomorphic gram-negative bacillus that tends to form rosettelike arrangements.

The organism is oxidase positive. *C. hominis* is able to utilize carbohydrates in media with sufficient nutritional factors. The addition of 10% horse serum to standard fermentation media will allow sufficient growth of the organism. A key biochemical parameter of *C. hominis* is the production of indole. The conventional indole test (Chapter 27), even after 48 h incubation, may not demonstrate the weak production of indole characteristic of this species. The spot indole test (Chapter 9), performed on a colony grown on blood agar for 72 h, may be positive. Alternatively, the more sensitive indole reagent described in Chapter 28, that of Ehrlich, combined with xylene extraction, may be required for demonstration of this property. *C. hominis* is urease negative, catalase negative, and nitrate negative, as outlined in Table 39.2.

39.4.c. Treatment of infection due to Cardiobacterium hominis.

The organism is susceptible in vitro to penicillin, ampicillin, cephalothin, chloramphenicol, aminoglycosides, and tetracycline. Penicillin is probably the drug of choice, although the organism's identity must be certain, as *A. actinomycetemcomitans* and *H. aphrophilus*, with which *C. hominis* may be confused, are often resistant to penicillin.

39.5. Genus Chromobacterium

39.5.a. Epidemiology and pathogenesis of Chromobacterium infection.

Chromobacterium violaceum, instantly recognizable by its purple pigment, is the etiologic agent of a particularly devastating and virulent bacteremia, usually acquired in the southeastern United States, particularly in Florida. The organism has been recovered from soil and water in tropical countries. Patients usually acquire the organism from puncture wounds or wounds that come into contact with soil or contaminated water. One patient, however, presumably acquired the infection by swallowing large amounts of water during a near-drowning accident. Since at least three of twelve patients were known to have chronic granulomatous disease and the status of several other patients is unknown, Macher, Casale, and Fauci[5] have suggested that an underlying neutrophil dysfunction places patients at increased risk for developing fulminant *C. violaceum* infections.

The organism is extremely virulent; there is an overall mortality rate of 57% in patients with infection acquired in the United States. The infection often presents as a febrile illness, and skin lesions are common. Liver abscess and pulmonary involvement are also prominent features. Virulence factors have not been studied much, but extracellular proteases are produced by species of *C. violaceum*.

39.5.b. Laboratory identification of Chromobacterium violaceum.

The organisms are usually recognized by their violet pigment (Plate 39.1), produced on media containing tryptophan, such as 5% sheep blood agar. Although the organisms grow best at 25° C, they will grow at 37° C. *C. violaceum* is facultatively anaerobic. Cultures may smell of ammonium cyanide, since the organisms produce HCN. *C. violaceum* is resistant to penicillin and to the vibriostatic agent 0/129 (Chapter 30). Although it is usually oxidase positive, the purple color may mask the reaction. It is catalase, Voges-Proskauer, and esculin negative. The rarely encountered pigment-negative strains may be confused with *Vibrio* species or *Aeromonas* species (Chapter 30). Resistance to 0/129 will distinguish *Chromobacterium* from vibrios, which are susceptible, and lack of indole production will differentiate *Chromobacterium* from *Aeromonas* and *Plesiomonas,* both of which are indole positive. Unlike many of the other unusual gram-negative bacilli, *C. violaceum* grows well on MacConkey agar.

The organisms are always motile, as demonstrated by wet preparation. On Gram stain, they are medium to long bacilli with rounded ends; the bacilli are occasionally slightly curved. *Chromobacterium* possesses the unusual flagellar arrangement of both a single polar flagellum and lateral flagella. The other species of *Chromobacterium, C. fluviatile,* has not been associated with human infection. A former additional nonpathogenic species, *C. lividum,* has now been transferred to the genus *Janthinobacterium.*

39.5.c. Treatment of infections due to *Chromobacterium violaceum.*

Most isolates are susceptible in vitro to chloramphenicol, aminoglycosides, tetracycline, and trimethoprim-sulfamethoxazole. Resistance to ampicillin, cephalothin, carbenicillin, and penicillins has been reported. Those patients that recovered from septicemia in the series reported by Macher et al.[5] were treated with gentamicin, with or without chloramphenicol.

39.6. Genus *Dermatophilus*

39.6.a. Epidemiology and pathogenesis of *Dermatophilus* infection.

Within the same family as the *Actinomyces* species, and therefore classified as a bacterium, *Dermatophilus con-* *golensis* is the etiologic agent of dermatophilosis (also called strawberry foot rot, lumpy wool, mycotic dermatitis, and streptotrichosis), a disease of the skin that is characterized by acute or chronic development of an exudative, scabbing dermatitis. The disease occurs worldwide in domestic animals, including cattle, sheep, goats, horses, other mammals, and humans. Manifestations of the disease are more severe in tropical regions. The organism has been isolated from both patients and wild animals in New York. As with the fungi, pathogenesis is probably related to the large size of the organism and its ability to resist cell-mediated killing. Extracellular enzymes may contribute to pathogenesis.

39.6.b. Laboratory identification of *Dermatophilus.*

Biopsy material and touch preparations of the underside of scabs should be stained by Giemsa or methenamine silver. Typical organisms displaying septate hyphallike forms, tapering and dividing transversely, with production of packets of coccoid spores as a final morphotype, are visible, particularly around hair follicles. The organism is gram-positive, but fine structure is not visible with the Gram stain.

As described by Gordon,[3] biopsy specimens and tissue scrapings from skin lesions, as well as exudate aspirated from unopened pustules should be streaked to blood agar, which is incubated in air at 37° C. Brain heart infusion agar with 5% sheep blood, recommended for primary inoculation of all specimens for isolation of fungi, will also support growth of *D. congolensis.* Colonies develop to a diameter of approximately 5 mm after 2-4 days growth. Colonies are grayish and usually become orange after several days, heaped, rough, glabrous, and adherent to the agar; pitting may be observed with early growth (Plate 39.2). In heavy areas, the colonies are beta hemolytic and in later stages they may become mucoid. The organisms will also grow in brain heart infusion-peptone broth, but they do not grow on Sabouraud's dextrose agar. Direct wet prepa-

FIGURE 39.3
Methylene blue–stained organisms of *Dermatophilus congolensis* from colony on blood agar plate.
(Courtesy Dr. Morris Gordon.)

ration from colonies will show branching filaments from 0.5-5 μm in width; branches are at right angles. The filaments divide longitudinally and transversely, finally becoming aggregates of motile coccoid-shaped spores (Figure 39.3). If only coccoid forms are seen on wet preparation from a colony, a younger subculture should be examined for filaments. Because the Gram stain tends to obscure details, a plain methylene blue stain (such as Loeffler's methylene blue, Chapter 46) should be used. Although cellular morphology is characteristic, biochemical reactions may help confirm the identification. The organisms are catalase and urease positive. *D. congolensis* produces extracellular enzymes, such as protease and gelatinase. All strains are indole, nitrate, and Voges-Proskauer negative.

39.6.c. Treatment of infections caused by *Dermatophilus congolensis*. The organism is susceptible in vitro to penicillin, streptomycin, chloramphenicol, tetracycline, erythromycin, and sulfonamides. It is resistant to the antidermatophyte griseofulvin. The drugs of choice appear to be a pencillin in combination with an aminoglycoside.

39.7. Genus *Gardnerella*

39.7.a. Epidemiology and pathogenesis of *Gardnerella* infection. This pleomorphic gram-variable bacillus, *Gardnerella vaginalis*, is found in the genital and urinary tract of humans, where it may play a role in **bacterial vaginosis,** a possibly sexually transmitted disease of women characterized by copious, malodorous discharge. Although male partners of women with bacterial vaginosis can be found to harbor the organism in the genital tract, it does not seem to cause symptoms in males. In addition to women with the characteristic discharge, approximately two-thirds of asymptomatic normal controls also harbor the organism, although the number of colony forming units is often lower in asymptomatic females.

Bacterial vaginosis, formerly called "nonspecific vaginitis," is one of the most common complaints of postpubescent women visiting their gynecologists. The vaginal discharge associated with *Gardnerella* is usually homogeneous, unaccompanied by pain or itching. Unlike the purulent discharge of gonococcal urethritis, *Trichomonas* vaginitis, and most yeast infections, there is a paucity of neutrophils in the discharge of patients infected with *G. vaginalis*. For this reason, the term vaginosis, rather than "vaginitis," was coined. Recent studies by Spiegel and others[11] have implicated anaerobic bacteria in the etiology of bacterial vaginosis. The contribution of *G. vaginalis* to this syndrome is thus not known. The organism does display some virulence for humans in addition to its role in vaginosis; a number of reports of postpartum sepsis, both in mothers and neonates, have been published. The difficulty in cultivating the organism from blood has probably led to a lack of recognition for its role in postpartum bacteremia and fever.

39.7.b. Laboratory identification of *Gardnerella vaginalis*. Specimens most likely to be sent to the microbiology laboratory for cultivation of *G. vaginalis* include cervical, urethral, and vaginal swabs from patients with discharge, as well as urethral cultures from male sexual partners. Women suffering from postpartum fevers, and neonates showing signs of sepsis, may be infected with *G. vaginalis*, which can be isolated from blood. The sodium polyanetholsulfonate (SPS) currently used as an anticoagulant in most commercial blood culture media (Chapter 14) has been found to inhibit growth of *Gardnerella*, however, and these media are not suitable for culture. Good results have been achieved by direct plating of blood onto agar. Although there have been no studies, it seems likely that the lysis-centrifugation blood culture method (Chapter 14) would allow growth of *G. vaginalis* plated onto chocolate or other supportive agar, such as Columbia agar with colistin and nalidixic acid (Chapter 8).

Most specimens of genital origin are contaminated with other flora. The fastidious nature of *G. vaginalis*, therefore, requires the use of a semiselective medium. The best selective and differential medium for detection of *G. vaginalis*, particularly from normal controls in which the number of organisms is small, was described by Totten and others,[12] called **HBT (human blood tween)** agar (Chapter 45). This medium consists of a basal layer made of colistin-nalidixic acid-Columbia agar base (BBL Microbiology Products) with 1% Proteose Peptone No. 3 (Difco Laboratories), 0.0075% Tween 80 (Difco), and 2 mg/liter amphotericin B (see Chapter 13 for suppliers). This basal agar is cooled to 50° C and poured into 90 mm diameter Petri plates, approximately 18 ml per plate. The basal layer is allowed to solidify and an overlayer, consisting of the basal layer formulation with the addition of 5% human blood, preserved with citrate, phosphate, and dextrose and added to the cooled agar at 50° C, is poured over each basal layer, approximately 5 ml per plate. HBT medium is also available commercially. Material from genital discharge is inoculated within 4-6 h of collection onto this medium and the plates are incubated in 5%-10% CO_2 or in a candle jar for 48 h. The organism has been shown to survive poorly in commonly used transport media. Colonies of *G. vaginalis* on HBT agar are convex, opaque, and gray surrounded by a diffuse zone of beta hemolysis. On sheep blood agar these organisms are not hemolytic and are barely visible. They grow well on CNA agar, without yielding any hemolysis (Plate 39.3). The ability of the organism to hemolyze human erythrocytes forms the basis for the differential nature of the HBT agar. *G. vaginalis* will not grow on MacConkey agar.

Gram stain of colonies reveals small, pleomorphic coccobacilli, some with pointed ends, that appear to stain gram-variable to gram-negative (Figure 39.4.). As described by Greenwood,[4] the cell wall of *G. vaginalis* is unusual,

FIGURE 39.4
Gram stain of *Gardnerella vaginalis* from growth on CNA agar.

resembling gram-negative cell walls more than gram-positive, but possessing a laminated structure and possibly a glycocalyx, which may participate in enhancing adherence of the organisms to genital epithelium. *G. vaginalis* is oxidase and catalase negative. It will utilize certain carbohydrates, but its fastidious growth requirements and resemblance to other coryneform organisms isolated from genital tract specimens have contributed to some difficulty in routine clinical laboratories in performing the tests necessary for its identification. Many laboratories report a presumptive identification of *G. vaginalis* for gram-variable, pleomorphic coccobacilli recovered from vaginal cultures, showing diffuse beta hemolysis on HBT and negative catalase and oxidase tests, which is acceptable for most circumstances. Yong and Thompson[13] report a rapid (1 h) biochemical identification based on fermentation of starch and raffinose and hydrolysis of hippurate. Recently, Reimer and Reller[8] have described two

simple tests that served to correctly identify *G. vaginalis* (Procedure 39.2).

Presumptive diagnosis of bacterial vaginosis can be made without performing cultures, as described in Chapter 19. Aside from the distinctive clinical picture, a direct wet mount of vaginal discharge material will usually show "clue cells," squamous epithelial cells covered with tiny bacilli, especially around the periphery, giving the cell a stippled appearance. Discharge material will have a characteristic fishy odor, particularly after addition of 10% KOH (the sniff test), and the pH of the material will be greater than 4.5.

39.7.c. Treatment of *Gardnerella vaginalis* vaginosis. Although in vitro susceptibility of *G. vaginalis* to metronidazole is variable, metronidazole has consistently yielded the best cure of bacterial vaginosis. Since metronidazole is effective primarily against anaerobic bacteria, the ability of metronidazole to affect this syndrome speaks against a primary causative role

PROCEDURE 39.2. SCREENING TESTS FOR *GARDNERELLA VAGINALIS*

1. Prepare *Brucella* blood agar plates containing *Brucella* agar base (Difco Laboratories), 5% defibrinated sheep blood, 5 μg/ml hemin (Eastman Chemical Co.), and 10 μg/ml vitamin K_1 (ICN Pharmaceuticals). These plates may be purchased commercially, but the components must be the same as those listed here for proper performance of the test.

2. Prepare chocolate agar plates containing GC agar base (BBL Microbiology Systems), 1% IsoVitaleX (BBL), and 10 mg/ml hemoglobin (Difco). These plates may also be available commercially, but the components must be those listed here for proper performance of the test.

3. Prepare sodium polyanetholsulfonate (SPS) disks (5%) by pipetting a 5% solution of SPS (Becton-Dickinson Vacutainer Systems) in water to each of a number of 6 mm diameter blank filter paper disks (BBL), 20 μl per disk. Allow the disks to dry and then store them with a desiccator in the refrigerator. Five percent SPS disks may also be purchased commercially.

4. Grow the test organism overnight on a *Brucella* blood agar plate in 5% CO_2 at 37° C. Using a cotton swab, emulsify enough growth from the agar surface into 2 ml of sterile saline to equal a McFarland 0.5 turbidity standard.

5. Using another cotton swab, streak one *Brucella* blood agar plate and one chocolate agar plate for confluent growth, much as for a disk diffusion susceptibility test.

6. Place an SPS disk in the center of the inoculated *Brucella* blood agar plate.

7. Place a streak of *Streptococcus sanguis I* (ATCC 35557; American Type Culture Collection) down the center of the chocolate agar plate.

8. Incubate both plates for 24-48 h at 37° C in 5% CO_2.

9. Only *G. vaginalis* will show both a zone of >12 mm inhibition around the SPS disk and a very small zone of inhibition of growth close to the line of streptococcal growth.

10. Other genera may be positive in one or the other of these tests, but not in both.

Modified from Reimer and Reller. 1985. J. Clin. Microbiol. 21:146.

for *Gardnerella*. All strains have been susceptible in vitro to ampicillin, carbenicillin, oxacillin, penicillin, and vancomycin. Susceptibility to the latter three agents is usually a characteristic of gram-positive organisms, another enigmatic finding for *Gardnerella*.

39.8. Genus *Legionella*

39.8.a. Epidemiology and pathogenesis of *Legionella* infection. Species of *Legionella*, the only genus in the newly described family Legionellaceae, are distributed worldwide in surface water, soil, mud, lakes, and streams. The organisms are not known to have an animal reservoir. The causative agents of Legionnaires' disease, a febrile and pneumonic illness, *Legionella* were discovered in 1976 after an epidemic of pneumonia among Pennsylvania state American Legion members attending a convention in Philadelphia focused worldwide attention on this new entity. Workers at the Centers for Disease Control, Atlanta, isolated the agent, a fastidious gram-negative bacillus that was unlike previously described organisms. Although the agent was first discovered in 1976, there is evidence of *Legionella* infection as far back as 1947. Most of the studies to date have centered around *Legionella pneumophila*, the type species of the genus and the most prevalent etiologic agent of Legionnaire's disease. Many other species of *Legionella* have now been characterized, isolated from sporadic cases of pneumonia and from other outbreaks, as well as from environmental sources. Extrapulmonary disease is rare with *Legionella* infection. Most of the reported cases of non-*L. pneumophila* pneumonia have been nosocomial in nature. Much of the discussion that follows is related to information gathered about *L. pneumophila*. To what extent the characteristics of *L. pneumophila* are shared by the other species has not yet been fully determined.

Legionella live in natural waters and can be found in air conditioning cooling tower water, air conditioning condensate, and reservoir waters, often in association with blue-green algae. The organisms can also multiply in relatively hot water, and can be found in shower heads, whirlpool baths, and institutional potable water systems. They are able to grow at temperatures from 25°-43° C on artificial media, and at even higher temperatures in nature. Patients usually acquire the organism by breathing in aerosols; no person-to-person transmission occurs. Eradication of *Legionella* from institutional water systems requires increased heat (hot water tanks must be heated to >70° C for 72 h) or increased chlorination (to 2 parts per million of

free chlorine). Surgical patients, those who are immunosuppressed (particularly those on corticosteroids), and persons who smoke are at increased risk for acquiring Legionnaires' disease.

The disease occurs sporadically, at low levels endemically, or as epidemics among susceptible hosts. It is not a rare infection (it is estimated that 25,000-50,000 cases occur annually in the United States); there is usually a seasonal peak during late summer. The disease involves multiple organ systems, but it is manifested primarily as severe, consolidated pneumonia. Bacteremia is probably not uncommon, especially in the immunosuppressed patient. Another manifestation of disease caused by *Legionella pneumophila* is Pontiac fever, a multisystem disease with respiratory symptoms but without pneumonia. Pontiac fever is a mild self-limited disease with no mortality, in contrast to Legionnaires' disease which has a significant mortality. The clinical manifestations exhibited by infection with a particular species primarily are due to differences in the immune response of the host and perhaps to inoculum size; the same *Legionella* species gives rise to different expressions of disease in different individuals. Schlanger et al.[10] have reported a patient with sinusitis and no presenting pneumonia caused by *L. pneumophila*. The cellular immunodeficiency of this patient no doubt contributed to his acquisition of the infection.

Pathogenesis of *Legionella* infection has been studied quite extensively. Although the organisms produce several extracellular enzymes, including a phosphatase, a lipase, and nucleases, these have not been shown to contribute significantly to virulence. An extracellular toxin, however, may contribute to intracellular survival of the organisms by impairing the ability of phagocytic cells to utilize oxygen, and thus carry out oxidative bactericidal activities. The primary virulence mechanism of *Legionella* is its ability to survive within phagocytic host cells. Cell-mediated immune responses are necessary for the host to overcome disease. Serologic evidence exists for the presence of asymptomatic disease, since many healthy people surveyed possess antibodies to *Legionella* species and in a hospital outbreak (VA Wadsworth Medical Center) there was a significant incidence of asymptomatic seroconversion.

39.8.b. Laboratory diagnosis of Legionnaires' disease by culture. An excellent manual that covers all aspects of laboratory diagnosis of Legionnaires' disease is that of Edelstein (listed in the bibliography of this chapter), from which some of the material presented here has been taken. The monograph prepared by the CDC, *"Legionnaires'": the disease, the bacterium and methodology* (also listed in the bibliography), is another important sourcebook. Animal inoculation is probably not necessary for clinical purposes. Specific serotyping is not within the capability of routine microbiology laboratories, but the general isolation and direct detection of *Legionella* can be done effectively by all laboratories that possess a class II biological safety cabinet (Chapter 2).

Specimens from which *Legionella* can be isolated include respiratory tract secretions of all types, including sputum, pleural fluid, other sterile body fluids such as blood, and lung, transbronchial, or other biopsy material. Sputum specimens are preferable to bronchial washings, which are likely to contain small amounts of inhibitory local anesthetics and are diluted by saline. Sputum from patients with Legionnaires' disease is usually nonpurulent and may appear bloody or watery. Therefore the grading system used for screening sputum for routine cultures is not applicable. Patients with Legionnaires' disease usually have detectable numbers of organisms in their respiratory secretions, even for quite some time after antibiotic therapy has been initiated. If the disease is present, the initial specimen is often likely to be positive. However, additional specimens should be processed if suspicion of the

disease persists. Pleural fluid has not yielded many positive cultures in studies performed in several laboratories, but it may contain organisms. Specimens should be transported without holding media, buffers, or saline, which may be inhibitory to growth of *Legionella*. The organisms are actually very hardy and are best preserved by maintaining specimens in a small, tightly closed container to prevent desiccation and transporting them to the laboratory within 30 min of collection. If longer delay is anticipated, specimens should be refrigerated. If specimens cannot be assured of remaining moist, a small amount (1 ml) of sterile, nonbacteriostatic distilled water may be added.

Material should be inoculated to culture plates and applied to slides for direct fluorescent antibody testing (as described below) as soon as it is received in the laboratory. Technologists should work in a biological safety cabinet. As described in Chapter 16, sputum can be best picked from upper respiratory secretions with a wooden applicator stick, to which the mucus and pus cells will adhere. Edelstein recommends diluting sputum specimens that may contain contaminating bacteria 1:10 in trypticase soy broth, vortexing the suspension with sterile glass beads, and inoculating plates with several drops of the diluted specimen. Lesser dilutions are recommended for aspirates. Sputum and respiratory secretions for direct fluorescent antibody tests are applied to slides without dilution. As described in Chapter 21, tissues are homogenized before smears and cultures are performed and clear sterile body fluids are centrifuged for 30 min at 4,000 × g. The sediment is then vortexed and used for culture and smear preparation. Blood for culture of *Legionella* should probably be processed with the lysis-centrifugation tube system (DuPont Isolator, described in Chapter 14) and plated directly to buffered charcoal yeast extract agar (BCYE), as described below. A biphasic culture medium containing BCYE agar and yeast extract broth, designed for isolation of *Legionella* from blood, is available from Remel Laboratories.

Specimens should be inoculated to two agar plates for recovery of *Legionella*, at least one of which is buffered charcoal yeast extract agar (BCYE) without inhibitory agents. This medium, developed at the CDC, contains charcoal to detoxify the medium, remove carbon dioxide, and modify the surface tension to allow the organisms to proliferate more easily. BCYE is also prepared with ACES buffer to stabilize pH, cysteine (required for growth of the organism), yeast extract, alpha-ketoglutarate, and an iron compound (growth supplements). A second medium, BCYE base with polymyxin B, anisomycin (to inhibit fungi), and cefamandole, is recommended for specimens such as sputum that are likely to be contaminated with other flora. Although these media can be prepared in the laboratory, they are complex and cumbersome to make (Chapter 45). Fortunately, they are commercially avail-

able from Remel Laboratories. Mueller-Hinton agar with 1% hemoglobin and 1% IsoVitaleX, first developed for susceptibility testing of *Haemophilus influenzae*, also will support the growth of most legionellae. Several other media, including a selective agar containing vancomycin and a differential agar containing bromthymol blue and bromcresol purple, are also available from Remel. Specimens obtained from sterile body sites may be plated to two media without selective agents, and perhaps also inoculated into the special blood culture broth without SPS. Of course, specimens should always be plated to standard media for recovery of pathogens other than *Legionella* that may be responsible for the disease.

Plates should be incubated in air or in a candle jar at 35°-37° C in a humid atmosphere. Only growth of *L. gormanii* is stimulated by increased CO_2, so air incubation is preferable to 5%-10% CO_2, which may inhibit some legionellae. Within 3-4 days, colonies should be visi-

FIGURE 39.5
Gram stain of *Legionella pneumophila* from a colony grown on BCYE after 72 h incubation.

ble. Plates should be held for a maximum of 2 weeks before discarding. Blood cultures in biphasic media should be held for 1 month. At 5 days, colonies are 3-4 mm in diameter, gray-white to blue-green, glistening, convex, circular, and may exhibit a cut-glass sort of internal granular speckling (Plate 39.4). A Giménez stain (Chapter 46) reveals small, coccobacillary organisms with occasional filamentous forms (Plate 39.5). A Gram stain yields thin, gram-negative bacilli (Figure 39.5). All *Legionella* species are weakly catalase positive (strongly catalase positive organisms may not be legionellae). Oxidase test results are variable. Another rapid differential screening test is the production of fluorescent pigment, visible under long-wave fluorescent light (long-wave light is generated at 365 nm, a Wood's light generates light of wavelength near 250 nm). *L. pneumophila*, *L. micdadei*, *L. jordanis*, *L. wadsworthii*, *L. oakridgensis*, and *L. longbeachae* fluoresce pale yellow-green; whereas *L. gormanii*, *L. dumoffii*, *L. bozemanii*, and *L. morrisii* fluoresce blue-white. All *Legionella* species described so far are able to liquefy gelatin

---

CURRENTLY RECOGNIZED SPECIES OF *LEGIONELLA*

L. anisa	*L. maceachernii**
*L. bozemanii**	*L. micdadei**
L. cherrii	*L. oakridgensis*
L. dumoffii·	*L. parisiensis*
L. erythra	*L. pneumophila**
*L. feeleii**	*L. rubrilucens*
*L. gormanii**	*L. sainthelensi*
*L. hackeliae**	*L. santicrucis*
L. jamestowniensis	*L. spiritensis*
L. jordanis	*L. steigerwaltii*
*L. longbeachae**	*L. wadsworthii**

*Isolated from patient specimens.

(Chapter 27). The box below lists some of the currently recognized species of legionellae. Over 90% of all cases of Legionnaires' disease are associated with *L. pneumophila*. Definitive identification requires the facilities of a specialized reference laboratory. Although specific antisera, developed primarily for direct fluorescent antibody tests (described below), can be used for species identification, there does appear to be some cross reactivity. Emulsions of organisms from isolated colonies are made in 10% neutral formalin, diluted 1:100 (to produce a very thin suspension) and placed on slides for fluorescent antibody staining, as described below. Clinical laboratories can probably perform sufficient service to clinicians by indicating the presence or probable presence of *Legionella* species in a specimen. A monoclonal antibody conjugated to fluorescein is available for genus identification of isolated colonies (Genetic Systems). If further identification is necessary, the isolate should be forwarded to an appropriate reference laboratory. There seem to be a large number of serogically separate subtypes and species that are just being recognized with the new found ability to cultivate the organisms in vitro. Rapid expansion of our knowledge about this ubiquitous family of bacteria is expected to take place over the next several years.

39.8.c. Direct detection of *Legionella* in infected clinical material. The most rapid means of diagnosing Legionnaires' disease is to directly detect the presence of the bacilli in clinical specimens. Although *Pseudomonas* species and other contaminating material may cause cross-reactive and nonspecific fluorescence, **direct fluorescent antibody (DFA)** tests should be performed on specimens received in the laboratory for *Legionella* detection. Antisera conjugated with fluorescein are available from several commercial suppliers, including BioDx, Biological Products Division of Centers for Disease Control, Litton Bionetics, and Zeus Technologies. Specimens are first tested with pools of antisera containing antibodies to several species or serotypes of *L. pneumophila*. Those that exhibit positive results are then reexamined with specific conjugated antisera. Methods are basically the same as those described for direct fluorescent antibody detection of *Bordetella pertussis* (Chapter 16). Manufacturers' directions should be followed explicitly and material from commercial systems should never be divided and used separately. Laboratories should decide which serotypes to routinely test for based on the prevalence of isolates in their geographic area. Culture of specimens must always be done as well, as it will detect those organisms that are not included within the usual battery of serotypes and because culture is more sensitive than DFA. Briefly, material from the specimen is applied directly to two marked circles on an alcohol-cleaned microscope slide. Tissue is applied to the slide by touch preparation with adequate pressure to express bacteria from spaces. The slide is allowed to air dry, is heat-fixed, and then fixed by overlaying the slide with 10% buffered (pH 7.0) formalin for 10 min. The formalin is rinsed from the slides with sterile distilled water and the slide is allowed to air dry. If it cannot be stained immediately (delay is not acceptable for clinical specimens from living patients), the slide may be frozen at $-20°$ C in the dark for several weeks. One of the two specimen areas is tested against pooled antisera, and the other is tested against specific antiserum in the event of a positive result. The sensitivity of the DFA test is low, since 10^4 to 10^5 bacteria per milliliter of specimen are required for detection. Slides should be examined for quite a long time, especially by technologists who rarely perform the test. The organisms appear as brightly fluorescent rods, with a velvety texture (Plate 39.6). Examination for as long as 15-20 min is recommended before a slide can be confidently declared negative.

Two recently developed immunologic tests for Legionnaires' disease have shown great promise. Detection of antigen in urine by

means of an RIA (Chapter 11) or ELISA (Chapter 10) test has yielded very specific and sensitive results. ELISA methods are also being used to detect circulating antigens in serum with good results. Neither of these tests is commercially available yet. The CDC has reported excellent preliminary results with a nucleic acid probe that specifically detects genetic material of *L. pneumophila*, either in clinical specimens or from isolated colonies. A radiolabeled RNA probe that recognizes all species of *Legionella* (Gen-Probe) is under study for utilization as a diagnostic reagent. The continued development of nucleic acid probe technology (Chapter 10) should aid microbiologists in the difficult task of isolating and identifying the myriad species of *Legionella* that have been found to be the etiologic agents of human disease.

39.8.d. Serologic and immunologic diagnosis of Legionnaires' disease. Most cases of legionellosis have been diagnosed retrospectively by detection of a fourfold rise in anti-*Legionella* antibody with an indirect fluorescent antibody test (Chapter 12). Serum specimens no closer than 2 weeks apart should be tested. Confirmation of disease is accomplished by a fourfold rise in titer to >128, or, for unusual cases, a single serum with a titer of >256 and a characteristic clinical picture. As many as 12% of healthy persons will yield titers as high as 1:256, and unfortunately, individuals with Legionnaires' disease may not exhibit serologic titers until as long as 8 weeks after the primary illness or may never have significant titer rises. Commercially prepared antigen-impregnated slides are available from Zeus Technologies, Litton Bionetics, and BioDx.

39.8.e. Treatment of Legionnaires' disease. Erythromycin is the drug of choice for treatment of disease caused by *Legionella*. Penicillins, cephalosporins of all generations, and aminoglycosides are not effective and should not be used. High dose trimethoprim-sulfamethoxazole and tetracyclines have been effective in some cases. The concomitant administration of rifampin along with erythromycin may prove beneficial, especially in severe cases. For patients who cannot take erythromycin, doxycycline (plus rifampin for moderately and severely ill patients) is recommended. Clinical response usually follows the introduction of effective therapy within 48 h.

39.9. Genus *Prototheca*

39.9.a. Epidemiology and pathogenesis of *Prototheca* infection. *Prototheca* are algae without chlorophyll that morphologically resemble green algae. The organisms are worldwide in distribution, found in water and soil. They enter the body through breaks in the skin, usually associated with minor trauma. The primary syndrome is a chronic, nodular skin lesion, although the organism can cause joint infection, wound infection, and rare disseminated disease in humans. The presence of the organism, which is resistant to killing by phagocytes, results in a granulomatous response. Spontaneous recovery does not occur.

39.9.b. Laboratory identification of *Prototheca*. There are two species of *Prototheca* associated with human disease, *P. wickerhamii* and *P. zopfii*. The organisms grow very well on Sabouraud's dextrose agar, and presumably on any other agar that will support the growth of yeast, such as brain heart infusion agar and Sabouraud's dextrose with heart infusion. Colonies are opaque, white to tan, smooth, heaped, moist, and resemble those of yeast. Examination under wet mount (Chapter 7), however, reveals the characteristic structure of *Prototheca* (Figure 39.6). Cells are spherical, varying in size from tiny (1.5 μm diameter) to large (three times the size of a red blood cell). Within the cells (called sporangia), endospores can be seen developing.

For most laboratories, identification of *Prototheca* to genus by observation of typical cel-

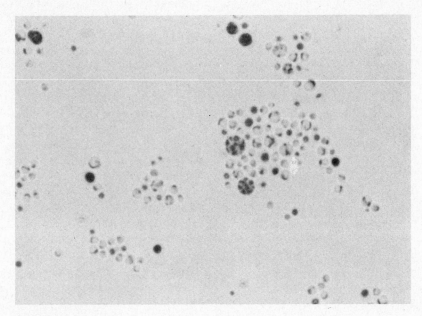

FIGURE 39.6
Prototheca organisms seen in wet mount stained with lactophenol cotton blue.

lular morphology is sufficient. If definitive identification is required, Padhye, Baker and D'Amato[6] have shown that the API 20C system (Analytab Products, Inc.), a multiwell identification system for yeasts, will accurately determine the assimilation pattern and other biochemical parameters of *Prototheca* species within 4 days.

39.9.c. Treatment of *Prototheca* infections. The infections caused by this organism must be treated or surgically excised. Most patients respond to amphotericin B, although ketoconazole has been used successfully in at least one patient. *Prototheca* species are resistant to flucytosine.

39.10. Genus *Streptobacillus*

39.10.a. Epidemiology and pathogenesis of *Streptobacillus* infection. *Streptobacillus moniliformis*, the only species within the genus, is one of the etiologic agents of **rat-bite fever.** Humans acquire the infection via the bite of an infected rat (including laboratory rats), or less commonly via contaminated milk, food, or water. When the organism is acquired by ingestion, the disease is called **Haverhill fever.** The organism is normal oral flora of wild and laboratory rats, although it is also associated with respiratory disease and fatal systemic disease in laboratory animals. Virulence factors have not been defined. The organism is known to spontaneously develop L forms (without cell walls), which may allow persistence of the organism in some sites.

Patients develop acute onset of chills, fever, headache, and severe joint pains. Within the first 2 days, patients exhibit a maculopapular, petechial, or morbilliform rash on the palms, soles of the feet, and the extremities. Complications include endocarditis, septic arthritis, and pneumonia.

39.10.b. Laboratory identification of *Streptobacillus*. Organisms may be cultured from blood, material aspirated from infected joints or lymph nodes, or aspirated from the pus within lesions. The organism requires the presence of blood, ascitic fluid, or serum for growth. Growth will occur on blood agar, incubated in a very moist environment with 5%-10% CO_2, after 48 h incubation at 37° C. Colonies are not hemolytic. Addition of 10%-30% ascitic fluid (available commercially from some media suppliers, such as Difco Laboratories) or 20% horse serum should allow recovery of the organism. The organism grows as "fluff balls" or "breadcrumbs" near the bottom of the tube of broth or on the surface of the sedimented red blood cell layer in blood culture media. Colonies grown on brain heart infusion agar supplemented with 20% horse serum are small, smooth, glistening, colorless or grayish, with irregular edges. Colonies may also exhibit a "fried egg" appearance, with a dark center and a flattened, lacy edge. These colonies have undergone the spontaneous transformation to the L form. Stains of L form colonies will yield coccobacillary or bipolar staining coccoid forms; usually a special stain, such as the Dienes stain (performed by pathologists) is required. Gram-stained organisms from standard colonies will show extreme pleomorphism, with long filamentous forms, chains, and swollen cells. The carbol fuchsin counterstain or Giemsa may be necessary for visualization (Plate 39.7). With the same stains, organisms may be visualized directly in clinical material for rapid diagnosis.

S. moniliformis does not produce indole, is catalase, oxidase, and nitrate negative, in contrast to organisms with which *Streptobacillus* may be confused, including *Actinobacillus*, *Haemophilus aphrophilus*, and *Cardiobacterium*. In addition, the clinical history of a rat bite is usually elicited. The other agent of rat-bite fever, *Spirillum minus* (Chapter 40), cannot be grown in vitro. Serological diagnosis is also useful, as patients develop agglutinating titers to the causative organism. The specialized serologic tests are performed only at national reference laboratories, since the disease is extremely rare in the United States.

39.10.c. Treatment of *Streptobacillus moniliformis* infections. The organism is susceptible to penicillin and streptomycin. Therapy with a combined regimen of a penicillin and an aminoglycoside is probably most effective. The organism is only weakly susceptible to tetracycline in vitro. *S. moniliformis* is resistant to sulfonamides.

39.11. Thermophilic Bacteria

A recent report by Rabkin, Galaid, Hollis, and others from the CDC[7] implicates a new group of bacteria as etiologic agents of human disease. Isolated from specimens such as cerebrospinal fluid, blood, and heart valves, these organisms are able to grow at increased temperatures. Called **thermophilic bacteria,** most isolates grew better at 42°-50° C than they did at 37° C, the temperature at which they were first isolated. All species were grown on tryptone-glucose-yeast extract agar. None were able to grow at room temperature. No strains were fermentative, and only a few strains were able to utilize glucose and/or maltose oxidatively in O-F media (Chapter 28). No organisms grew on MacConkey agar and none grew on TSIA or KIA agar slants. All strains were oxidase positive, none were indole positive. There are probably several species among this group, but further studies are needed to delineate them. It is certain that at least several isolates were etiologic agents of disease in humans who had no predisposing conditions. They were all susceptible to penicillin and cephalosporins, and most were susceptible to aminoglycosides. Since the isolates grew poorly at normal incubator temperatures, they might be dismissed by microbiologists unless there is an index of suspicion. Other thermophilic microorganisms, such as certain actinomycetes and *Cytophaga* species, found in environmental sources, have been implicated as etiologic agents of human allergic pneumonitis, although they do not grow within the human body. The unusual thermophilic bacteria described here are another newly recognized group among the ubiquitous microorganisms able to infect humans.

39.12. Unnamed Bacteria

A number of unnamed bacterial groups, morphologically similar but not yet definitively characterized, have been implicated as etiologic agents of human disease. Because the Centers for Disease Control is the national reference laboratory, most clinically significant isolates that cannot be identified by other laboratories in the United States are ultimately sent to CDC. Such organisms, designated by letters that reflect their characteristics (EF stands for eugonic fermenter, which means good-growing fermenter; DF stands for dysgonic fermenter, which means poor-growing fermenter; EO stands for eugonic oxidizer) or other letters (Ve-1, IVc-2, HB, etc.) so that they can be categorized by microbiologists, may be isolated from clinical specimens. Although the individual groups are not discussed in this text, they may be listed in some tables and charts because they resemble organisms being discussed. Limited discussion of some species is found in Chapter 28. Identification tables published by the CDC and in the *Manual of Clinical Microbiology,* fourth edition, published by the American Society for Microbiology, should be consulted for further details concerning these organisms.

REFERENCES

1. Dienst, R.B., and Brownell, G.H. 1984. Genus *Calymmatobacterium Aragao and Vianna 1913.* In Krieg, N.R., and Holt, J.G., editors. Bergey's manual of systematic bacteriology, ed. 9. Williams & Wilkins, Baltimore.
2. Forlenza, S.W. 1985. *Capnocytophaga:* an opportunistic pathogen. Clin. Microbiol. Newsletter 7:17.
3. Gordon, M.A. 1985. Aerobic pathogenic Actinomycetaceae. In Lennette, E.H., Balows, A., Hausler, W.J. Jr., and Shadomy, H.J., editors. Manual of clinical microbiology, ed. 4, American Society for Microbiology, Washington, D.C.
4. Greenwood, J.R. 1983. Current taxonomic status of *Gardnerella vaginalis.* Scand. J. Infect. Dis. Suppl. 40:11.

5. Macher, A.M., Casale, T.B., and Fauci, A.S. 1982. Chronic granulomatous disease of childhood and *Chromobacterium violaceum* infections in the southeastern United States. Ann. Intern. Med. 97:51.

6. Padhye, A.A., Baker, J.G., and D'Amato, R.F. 1979. Rapid identification of *Prototheca* species by the API 20C system. J. Clin. Microbiol. 10:579.

7. Rabkin, C.S., Galaid, E.I., Hollis, D.G., et al. 1985. Thermophilic bacteria: a new cause of human disease. J. Clin. Microbiol. 21:553.

8. Reimer, L.G., and Reller, L.B. 1985. Use of a sodium polyanetholesulfonate disk for the identification of *Gardnerella vaginalis*. J. Clin. Microbiol. 21:146.

9. Ristic, M., and Kreier, J.P. 1984. Bartonellaceae Gieszczykiewicz 1939. In Krieg, N.R., and Holt, J.G., editors. Bergey's manual of systematic bacteriology, ed. 9. Williams & Wilkins, Baltimore.

10. Schlanger, G., Lutwick, L.I., Kurzman, M., et al. 1984. Sinusitis caused by *Legionella pneumophila* in a patient with the acquired immune deficiency syndrome. Am. J. Med. 77:957.

11. Spiegel, C.A., Amsel, R., Eschenbach, D., Schoenknecht, R., and Holmes, K.K. 1980. Anaerobic bacteria in nonspecific vaginitis. N. Engl. J. Med. 303:601.

12. Totten, P.A., Amsel, R., Hale, J., Piot, P., and Holmes, K.K. 1982. Selective differential human blood bilayer media for isolation of *Gardnerella (Haemophilus) vaginalis*. J. Clin. Microbiol. 15:141.

13. Yong, D.C.T., and Thompson, J.S. 1982. Rapid microbiochemical method for identification of *Gardnerella (Haemophilus) vaginalis*. J. Clin. Microbiol. 16:30.

BIBLIOGRAPHY

Bennett, J.E. 1985. Miscellaneous fungi. In Mandell, G.L., Douglas, R.G. Jr., and Bennett, J.E., editors. Principles and practice of infectious diseases, ed. 2. John Wiley & Sons, New York.

Branson, D. 1984. *Legionella*. Microbiology Newsletter, Remel Laboratories, 2:33.

Csango, P.-A., Holmes, K.K., Jerve, F., Mårdh, P.A., and Piot, P., editors. 1983. First international conference on vaginosis. Scand. J. Infect. Dis. Suppl. 40.

Edelstein, P.H. 1985. Legionnaires' disease laboratory manual. Legionnaires' disease laboratory. Wadsworth V.A. Medical Center, Los Angeles.

Edelstein, P.H., Meyer, R.D., and Finegold, S.M. 1980. Laboratory diagnosis of Legionnaires' disease. Am. Rev. Respir. Dis. 121:317.

Forlenza, S.W. 1985. *Capnocytophaga:* an opportunistic pathogen. Clin. Microbiol. Newsletter 7:17.

Fung, J.C., and Baron, E.J. 1985. *Gardnerella vaginalis* vaginitis. In Sun, T., editor. Sexually related infectious disease: laboratory and clinical aspects. Field and Rich Associates, New York.

Fung, J.C., Berman, M., and Fiorentino, T. 1983. *Capnocytophaga:* a review of the literature. Am. J. Med. Technol. 49:589.

Goldberg, J. 1959. Studies on granuloma inguinale. IV. Growth requirements of *Donovania granulomatis* and its relationship to the natural habitat of the organism. Br. J. Vener. Dis. 35:266.

Greenwood, J.R., and Pickett, M.J. 1984. Genus *Gardnerella Greenwood and Pickett 1980*. In Krieg, N.R., and Holt, J.G., editors. Bergey's manual of systematic bacteriology, ed. 9. Williams & Wilkins, Baltimore.

Gutman, L. 1980. *Pasteurella, Actinobacillus, Streptobacillus, Calymmatobacterium*. In Joklik, W.K., Willett, H.P., and Amos, D.B., editors. Zinsser microbiology, ed. 17. Appleton-Century-Crofts, New York.

Jones, G.L., and Hébert, G.A. 1979. "Legionnaires':" the disease, the bacterium, and methodology. United States Department of Health, Education, and Welfare, Atlanta. H.E.W. Publ.: C.D.C. 79-8375.

Jones, G.L., and Hébert, G.A. 1980. *Legionella* update. United States Department of Health, Education, and Welfare, Atlanta. H.E.W. Publ.: C.D.C. 80-8387.

Meyer, R.D. 1983. *Legionella* infections: a review of five years of research. Rev. Infect. Dis. 5:258.

Lee, T.S., and Wright, B.D. 1981. Fulminating chromobacterial septicaemia presenting as respiratory distress syndrome. Thorax 36:557.

Morse, S.A. 1980. Sexually transmitted diseases. In Lennette, E.H., Balows, A., Hausler, W.J. Jr., and Truant, J.P., editors. Manual of clinical microbiology, ed. 3. American Society for Microbiology, Washington, D.C.

Sneath, P.H.A. 1984. Genus *Chromobacterium Bergonzini 1881*. In Krieg, N.R., and Holt, J.G., editors. Bergey's manual of systematic bacteriology, ed. 9. Williams & Wilkins, Baltimore.

Starr, A.J., Cribbett, L.S., Poklepovic, J., et al. 1981. *Chromobacterium violaceum* presenting as a surgical emergency. South. Med. J. 74:1137.

Wormser, G.P., and Bottone, E.J. 1983. *Cardiobacterium hominis:* review of microbiologic and clinical features. Rev. Infect. Dis. 5:680.

40

New, Controversial, or Noncultivatable Etiologic Agents of Disease

In addition to those diseases caused by agents that cannot be grown in culture using existing methods, there are a number of diseases that appear to be caused by an infectious agent, although such an agent has not been identified. Reasons for which an infectious agent might be considered to be associated with a disease include an epidemiologic pattern suggestive of dissemination by an agent or a clinical presentation that is similar to that produced by known etiologic agents. Once the suggestion of infectious etiology is advanced, tools of science can be used to investigate the problem. Within the last several years, a number of diseases, either newly recognized or described long ago, have been definitely traced to an etiologic agent for the first time. For example, diligent effort by scientists in many laboratories in the United States, particularly the Centers for Disease Control in Atlanta, over an intense 6-month period in 1976 discovered *Legionella* species as the cause of pneumonia that had suddenly struck a group of American Legion state conventioneers with great morbidity. Since the etiologic agent was isolated, it has been linked by serologic and other studies with epidemics of pneumonia that occurred years before. A new entity, *Legionella* (Chapter 39), could thus be held responsible for infections that had previously been undiagnosed or misdiagnosed. The diseases mentioned in this chapter are ei-

585

ther well-described syndromes for which no etiologic agent has been found, although the diseases appear to be of an infectious nature, diseases with which a newly described agent is associated, or well-described syndromes for which an etiologic agent has been discovered but not yet isolated. None of the agents mentioned in this chapter are routinely sought by clinical microbiology laboratories at this time.

40.1. Diseases Associated with an Etiologic Agent

Lyme disease is an example of a newly recognized infectious disease for which the agent has been identified and isolated (Chapter 31). The geographic and seasonal incidence of Lyme disease, a complex of a cutaneous manifestation (erythema chronicum migrans), large joint arthritis, and other symptoms, suggested an infectious etiology. Scientists determined that the symptoms were most compatible with an arthropod-borne spirochetal disease, and set out to find such a spirochete. Within a short time, they successfully visualized the agent in ticks, subsequently identified it in special stains made from lesion material, and eventually developed an artificial medium that could support the growth of the spirochete.

Several diseases are in various stages of investigation that will lead to isolation and characterization of an etiologic agent, but the agent has not yet been cultivated. These diseases will be mentioned here.

There are, of course, a number of infectious diseases for which the agent is well known but cannot be cultivated easily, if at all, such as syphilis, leprosy, granuloma inguinale, hepatitis, warts (papillomavirus), and the slow virus diseases of progressive multifocal leukoencephalopathy (JC virus) and subacute sclerosing panencephalitis (measleslike paramyxovirus). Recently, a new mycobacterium has been isolated from the gastrointestinal tracts of patients with Crohn's disease (Chapter 41) although it is not established as a cause. Only with great difficulty can this agent be cultivated in the laboratory.

40.1.a. _Spirillum minus_–caused rat-bite fever. _Spirillum minus_ (formerly called _S. minor_, an incorrect Latin usage), an agent of rat-bite fever, has never been grown in culture. The organism has been visualized in Giemsa- or Wright-stained blood films and can be seen under darkfield microscopy. _Spirillum minus_ is a thick, spiral, gram-negative organism with two or three windings and polytrichous polar flagella. Infection can be transmitted by the bite or scratch of an infected animal. The bite wound heals spontaneously, but 1-4 weeks later reulcerates to form a granulomatous lesion at the same time that the patient develops constitutional symptoms of fever, headache, and a generalized, blotchy purplish maculopapular rash. Although it is rare that the organism can be seen in blood, it may be visualized in darkfield preparations made from the lesion. Diagnosis is definitively made by injection of lesion material or blood into experimental white mice or guinea pigs, which then develop the disease. Differentiation between rat-bite fever caused by _Spirillum minus_ and that caused by _Streptobacillus moniliformis_ (Chapter 39) is usually accomplished based on clinical presentations of the two infections. The incubation period for _Spirillum minus_ is much longer than that of streptobacillary rat-bite fever, which has occurred within 12 h of the initial bite.

40.1.b. Cat-scratch disease. Cat-scratch disease was first recognized by Robert Debre in Paris during the 1930s. The disease is not uncommon, with over 750 reported cases and probably more than 100 cases occurring annually in the United States. Patients are usually children (80%), and the primary sites of lesions are the hands, arms and legs, and face and neck. Most cases are acquired following the scratch, bite, or lick of a cat or kitten, usually newly arrived to the household. Patients exhibit regional tender lymphadenopathy, anorexia, fatigue, fever, and headache, usually beginning 2 weeks after the cat scratch or contact. They may display a rash, generalized lymphadenopathy, seizures, and other systemic findings. The disease is usually self-limited; complications such as a suppurative lymph node or encephalitis have been reported. Until 1983, clinical diagnosis required that a patient fulfill three of the following four criteria: (1) history of animal contact plus a site of primary inoculation, (2) negative laboratory studies for other causes of lymphadenopathy, (3) characteristic histopathology of the lesion or lymph node, and (4) a positive skin test. The skin test antigen is prepared from heat-treated pus taken from another patient's lesion. Injection of 0.1 ml of this material intradermally elicits a wheal or papule within 72 h, although the reaction can be the result of previous infection. Approximately 5% of patients will have false negative skin test results, and 5% will have false positive results.

In 1983, Wear, Margileth, Hadfield, and others[8] reported visualization of organisms in the lesions of cat-scratch disease. The organisms are gram negative, 0.3-0.5 μm in diameter, and 0.5-1.0 μm in length. They are best visualized with the Warthin-Starry silver stain, such as that of Luna[5] (Procedure 40.1), usually used for spirochetes (Chapter 31) but which also stains *Legionella* in tissue. The bacilli are not acid fast and do not stain with the Gomori methenamine silver stain. They appear to be intracellular pathogens; the delayed-type hypersensitivity response to skin test antigen would appear consistent with an intracellular pathogen. Electron micrographs further support their findings.[3] At the time of this writing, transmission to an experimental animal has not been published, although such studies are being actively pursued. Evidence that the gram-negative organism does cause the disease, however, is based on the fact that patients produce antibodies which, when coupled with immunoperoxidase or fluorescein, can be

seen to bind to the organisms in lymph node material taken from newly diagnosed patients. No specific reactions have occurred between these sera and preparations of any other infectious agents, and bacteria in lesion tissue sections do not react with immune sera made against any other morphologically similar bacteria. Gerber and co-workers have cultivated an organism from a lymph node from a patient with cat-scratch disease. They consider the bacterium to be gram-positive, a conclusion that has generated controversy.[2] A definitive etiologic agent has not been conclusively proved.

Treatment with antibiotics is not recommended, and one episode of disease probably imparts lifelong immunity. Once the etiologic agent has been unequivocally grown in culture, specific serologic reagents for diagnosis can be prepared and the need for lymph node biopsy will disappear. An excellent general discussion of this disease is found in the article by Hadfield, Schlagel, and Margileth.[4]

40.1.c. Gastritis and gastric ulcer. Reports from the Australian workers Marshall and Warren[6] implicate a spiral-shaped bacterium in the etiology of some cases of gastritis and perhaps peptic ulcer in humans. Warthin-Starry silver stain (Procedure 40.1) of gastroscopic biopsy of stomach tissue from 58 of 100 patients revealed an S-shaped bacterium, resembling *Campylobacter* species, but possessing four polar sheathed flagella. The organism grew on chocolate or blood agar after 3 days of incubation at 37° C, under the same microaerophilic conditions as for *Campylobacter* species (Chapter 30). Colonies were 1 mm in diameter and nonpigmented. The isolates were oxidase, catalase, and H_2S positive and negative for nitrate, glucose fermentation, indole, and urease. The bacterium has been cultivated in vitro from material obtained by gastroscopic biopsy of 11 patients, but its role in the etiology of gastritis remains controversial. The name *Campylobacter pyloridis* has been proposed for this organism.[6]

PROCEDURE 40.1. WARTHIN-STARRY STAIN

1. Make solutions as follows:
   a. Acidulated water
      Add enough 1% aqueous citric acid to bring 1,000 ml of triple distilled water to pH 4.0.
   b. 1% silver nitrate solution

Silver nitrate, crystalline	1 g
Acidulated water	100 ml

   c. 2% silver nitrate solution

Silver nitrate, crystalline	2 g
Acidulated water	100 ml

   d. 5% gelatin solution

Sheet gelatin, high grade	10 g
Acidulated water	200 ml

   e. 0.15% hydroquinone solution

Hydroquinone crystals, photographic quality	0.15 g
Acidulated water	100 ml

   All chemicals should be available from a standard chemical supply company, such as Sigma Chemical Co. or E. Merck Darmstadt.
2. Fix tissue sections in buffered neutral formalin. Avoid chromate fixatives. This fixative is standard for most pathology laboratories. The tissue is embedded in paraffin; sections are cut at a thickness of 6 μm.
3. Warm the 2% silver nitrate, the 5% gelatin, and the 0.15% hydroquinone in 50 ml beakers in a water bath heated to 54° C.
4. Deparaffinize the patient's tissue slide and a known positive control slide through a series of xylene changes with increasing concentrations of water, until the slide is finally placed into triple distilled water for final hydration. These procedures are standard histologic methods. Place the slides into a Coplin jar containing the 1% silver nitrate solution, preheated in a 43° C water bath. Allow the silver to impregnate the slides for 30 min at 43° C in the water bath.
5. While the slides are being impregnated, prepare the developer as follows:

Silver nitrate solution (2%)	1.5 ml
Gelatin solution (5%)	3.75 ml
Hydroquinone solution (0.15%)	2 ml

   Prepare this developer, immediately before it is used, in a small beaker or flask.

Modified from Luna, L.G. 1968. Warthin-Starry method for spirochetes and Donovan bodies. In Manual of histologic staining methods of the Armed Forces Institute of Pathology. McGraw-Hill Book Co., New York.

PROCEDURE 40.1. WARTHIN-STARRY STAIN—cont'd

6 Remove the slides from the impregnator, lay them flat across a slide holder, and immediately flood them with the warm developer solution. Allow the sections to develop until they are light brown or yellow. Check the known control periodically, which should show black spirochetes or bacteria against a yellow or light brown background. When handling the slides, use paraffin-coated or plastic forceps.
7. Wash quickly and thoroughly in hot tap water, approximately 50° C. Rinse in distilled water.
8. Dehydrate in 95% alcohol, then absolute alcohol, and clear in xylene by placing the slides in two jars of each solution for 5 min each jar.
9. Mount with Permount or Histoclad (available from American Scientific Products). Observe for characteristic black organisms against a light brown or yellow background.

40.1.d. Hepatitis associated with hepatitis B virus and delta agent. The viruses of hepatitis A and B have been identified and characterized, but only hepatitis A virus has been grown in culture. The infectious particle of hepatitis B virus, the Dane particle, is present in the blood and hepatocytes of patients and can be visualized by electron microscopy. Several different antigenic constituents are released during infection. Diagnosis is based on detection of either antibodies to the constituents or the antigens themselves. Newer methods for detecting the surface antigen (HBsAg), an early protein antigen (HBeAg), and antibodies to HBsAg, HBeAg, and hepatitis core antigen (HBc) include radioimmunoassay (Chapter 11) and ELISA (Chapter 10). Microbiology laboratories usually do not perform these tests.

Coinfection of patients with hepatitis B virus and a newly recognized cytopathic virus, the **delta agent,** may be responsible for some proportion of the most severe cases of hepatitis. The delta agent may be a defective virus, requiring coinfection with hepatitis B in the delta-infected cell for damage to occur. Persons at risk of acquiring delta agent hepatitis are those with chronic asymptomatic hepatitis B infection.

40.1.e. Rhinosporidiosis. Rhinosporidiosis is a chronic, celluloproliferative infection of the mucous membranes of the face and other areas, usually in the nose and less often in the conjunctiva, thought to be caused by a fungus that produces a spherulelike body similar to that of *Coccidioides immitis*. The disease is much more common in men than in women. The lesions ultimately develop into pedunculated polyps. Most prevalent in India, the infection has been described in the United States. A similar disease occurs in horses, cattle, and other animals. The agent, seen macroscopically in the polyp as tiny white dots, seems to consist of large, thick-walled cysts or sporangia containing many endospores. The endospores, each about the size of a red blood cell, are released through a pore in the wall of the sporangium once it has matured to its full size of 200-300 μm. The agent of rhinosporidiosis, called *Rhi-*

nosporidium seeberi, has never been cultivated in vitro nor been shown to cause infection in experimental animals injected with lesion material from humans. The cyst can be stained with mucicarmine; histologic studies are the only diagnostic tool available at this time.

40.1.f. Lobomycosis. Lobomycosis is another presumed fungal infection from which an etiologic agent has not been cultured. Found in adult males, primarily living in the Amazon River basin, and in bottle-nose dolphins off the coast of Florida, the disease is characterized by chronic, progressive, subcutaneous nodules, usually on the face or extremities. The lesions can become verrucous or ulcerative. The organism, *Loboa loboi,* can be seen in scrapings and histological sections from the lesions as a large, thick-walled, spheroidal or oval yeast. The yeasts possess multiple buds and often appear in short chains. The buds are the same size as the mother cells, unlike the multiple buds of *Paracoccidioides brasiliensis.* The yeasts can be visualized with 10% KOH and stain with methenamine silver or PAS. Diagnosis is made histologically.

40.1.g. Kuru and Creutzfeldt-Jakob disease. Kuru, a progressively fatal dementing disease of head-hunting tribes of New Guinea, was first thought to be of sex-linked genetic origin, since female adults were involved more often than males, and children were universally affected. When it was realized that the histologic lesions in the brains of patients with kuru resembled those found in sheep with a naturally occurring neurologic disease with similar symptoms, scrapie, the search began in earnest for an etiologic agent. Scrapie was known to be transmissible. In 1965, kurulike disease was transmitted to monkeys after intracerebral injection of material from the brains of humans who died from kuru. Brains of humans, monkeys, and sheep suffering from the disease show a characteristic spongiform degeneration of tissue (abnormal spaces in the tissue), with vacuoles in the neurons and extensive glial cell proliferation with almost no inflammatory changes. A similar histologic and clinical picture was characteristic of another rare human disease, Creutzfeldt-Jakob disease (CJD). This disease, found in humans throughout the world, consists of a very slowly progressive first stage of intellectual deterioration and behavioral abnormalities, followed by a shorter, rapidly progressive terminal stage characterized by myoclonic contractions of various muscle groups. Patients suffer from ataxia, dementia, and delirium which progresses to stupor, coma, and death. There is no treatment for any of these diseases. Another histologic feature of the brain of patients and laboratory animals with CJD, shared by patients with Alzheimer's disease (another progressive dementing disease of humans), is the presence of characteristically staining areas called amyloid plaques. The nature of these plaques in CJD has only recently been described as consisting of aggregates of the putative agent of the disease.

Only within the last 2 years has a candidate agent been purified by workers, including Prusiner.[7] First isolated from brains of scrapie-infected sheep, the agent was found to consist primarily of a single protein of approximately 27,000 molecular weight, designated PrP 27-30. PrP 27-30 was found to be the primary structural component of the agent itself, called a **prion** (proteinaceous infectious agent) by Prusiner. Antibodies to PrP 27-30 reacted with the "amyloid" plaques found in brains of patients with CJD and with the same structures found in the brains of scrapie-infected experimental animals. Prusiner proposed that the amyloid plaques found in patients with CJD are composed of crystalline arrays of prions, and that prions are the etiologic agent of CJD, scrapie, and perhaps kuru. Since brains of patients with Alzheimer's disease also demonstrate similar-appearing amyloid plaques, a prionlike illness may account for this disease as well.

It is not yet known whether the scrapie prion and the CJD prion are identical, although the scrapie prion protein has now been sequenced and found to share no homology with any other known proteins. The prions are extremely resistant to denaturation by proteases, nucleases, heat, ultraviolet light, and/or chemicals. Phenolic compounds and dilute chlorine bleach, active against most other infectious agents, have no effect on prions. Dilute (1 N) NaOH has been shown by Brown et al.[1] to effectively render the prion noninfectious. It is not known how or even whether they reproduce. The pathogenesis of disease is still largely unknown; however, cases of CJD have been diagnosed in several individuals who ate the brains of wild or domestic animals. Ingestion of brains, even well cooked, cannot be recommended at this time, since cooking practices would be entirely unable to reduce infectivity of an agent such as a prion. Direct inoculation of infectious material has been known to transmit disease, as has transplantation of corneas and administration of growth hormone from infected humans. Organs and tissues from any patients with degenerative neurologic diseases should not be used for transplantation.

Laboratory workers who must handle tissue from the brains of patients with CJD should take extra precautions. Double gloves, masks, and gowns should be worn, and all manipulations should take place within a biological laminar flow safety cabinet (Chapter 2). A solution of 1 N NaOH should be used to soak all instruments and even the hands of technologists can be soaked briefly in this alkali if accidental exposure occurs.

40.1.h. Whipple's disease. Whipple's disease, found primarily in middle-aged men, is characterized by the presence of macrophages in almost every organ system. Patients develop diarrhea, weight loss, arthralgia, often a long history of joint pain, and a distended and tender abdomen. Neurologic and sensory changes often occur. Patients may respond well to antibacterial agents, including trimethoprim-sulfamethoxazole, tetracycline, and penicillin.

Within the macrophages and numbers of other cells of involved tissue can be seen bacterial forms. These bacteria are 0.25 μm in diameter and as long as 2.5 μm. Their cell wall stains gram variably, but there appears to be a trilaminar structure to the plasma membrane on electron microscopy, which is more characteristic of gram-negative organisms. An outer trilaminar cell membrane superficially resembles that found on the surface of *Gardnerella vaginalis*. The organisms are antigenically similar to certain streptococci. Electron microscopy is the most definitive diagnostic tool, since the organism has not been cultivated in vitro or passed to laboratory animals, although the bacteria can be seen with certain stains.

40.2. Diseases for Which No Etiologic Agent Has Been Demonstrated

40.2.a. Kawasaki disease. Kawasaki disease occurs in children, usually less than 8 years old, primarily in Japan, but many cases have been reported in the United States. The symptoms include fever which lasts at least 5 days, congestion of the conjunctivae, dry, red lips and red, fissured or "strawberry" tongue, reddening of the palms of hands and soles of feet with ultimate desquamation, a rash over the trunk and face, and cervical lymphadenopathy. The disease has also been called **mucocutaneous lymph node syndrome.** Patients are usually ill for 1 month with the convalescent phase lasting 6-10 weeks. The most important sequela of the disease is cardiopathy, which occurs in 20% of patients. Diagnosis of Kawasaki disease can be made in patients in whom other etiologies are excluded and who meet five of the six criteria, providing also that antibiotic treatment does not ameliorate the fever. The rash and subsequent desquamation resemble that caused by staphylococci, particularly toxic shock syndrome staphylococci, but efforts to isolate an organism from patients with Kawasaki disease have been unsuccessful.

40.2.b. Non-A, non-B hepatitis. Although non-A, non-B hepatitis (NANB) is presumed to have a viral etiology, no agent or agents have been definitively associated with this syndrome. Approximately 90% of cases of hepatitis following blood transfusion cannot be linked to an etiologic agent and thus are designated NANB hepatitis. In addition, one fourth to one half of all patients with hepatitis who have not had a transfusion meet the criteria for NANB hepatitis. Transmission has occurred through water and food, and the disease has been experimentally transmitted to chimpanzees. Therefore, epidemiologically, clinically, and experimentally, the disease(s) resembles viral hepatitis A and B. Acute infection often leads to chronic hepatitis. Because the etiologic agent or agents are unknown, there are no diagnostic tests available. Diagnosis is currently made on clinical grounds in the absence of evidence for any other cause of hepatitis. It is probably only a matter of time until an etiologic agent or several agents are associated with this common syndrome.

40.2.c. Other diseases. Two childhood exanthems, **roseola** and **erythema infectiosum (fifth disease)**, are thought to have a viral etiology, although no agent has been implicated. Both illnesses are mild and self-limited and appear to be somewhat contagious. The rash of roseola occurs within 48 h after the febrile period, which usually lasts 3-5 days. The rash of fifth disease begins on the cheeks, causing them to resemble slapped cheeks. The rash then moves to the extremities, where it may disappear and recur several times. Headache and fever may be associated with the rash in one fourth of patients. No infectious agent has been clearly associated with either of these infectious syndromes.

It seems reasonable to mention multiple sclerosis in this section. Epidemiologic studies point to an infectious agent, and the pattern of pathologic findings in the neural tissue resembles that found in a progressive multifocal leukoencephalopathy, a slow virus infection. No definite virus particles have been seen in electron microscopic studies of brain tissue from patients with multiple sclerosis, but these patients do exhibit high levels of serum antibodies against a number of known viruses. The pathogenesis of this relatively common demyelinating disease is unknown, but an infectious etiology has not been ruled out.

REFERENCES

1. Brown, P., Rohwer, R.G., and Gajdusek, D.C. 1984. Sodium hydroxide decontamination of Creutzfeldt-Jakob disease virus. N. Engl. J. Med. 310:727.
2. Gerber, M.A., MacAlister, T.J., Ballow, M., et al. 1985. The aetiological agent of cat scratch disease. Lancet 1:1236.
3. Hadfield, T.L., Malaty, R.H., Van Dellen, A., et al. 1985. Electron microscopy of the bacillus causing cat-scratch disease. J. Infect. Dis. 152:643.
4. Hadfield, T.L., Schlagel, C., and Margileth, A. 1985. Stalking the cause of cat-scratch disease. Diagn. Med. 8:23.
5. Luna, L.G. 1968. Warthin-Starry method for spirochetes and Donovan bodies. In Manual of histologic staining methods of the Armed Forces Institute of Pathology. McGraw-Hill Book Co., New York.
6. Marshall, B.J., and Warren, J.R. 1984. Unidentified curved bacilli in the stomach of patients with gastritis and peptic ulceration. Lancet 1:1311.
7. Prusiner, S.B. 1982. Novel proteinaceous infectious particles cause scrapie. Science 216:136.
8. Wear, D.J., Margileth, A.M., Hadfield, T.L., et al. 1983. Cat scratch disease: a bacterial infection. Science 221:1403.

BIBLIOGRAPHY

Bockman, J.M., Kingsbury, D.T., McKinley, M.P., et al. 1985. Creutzfeldt-Jakob disease prion proteins in human brains. N. Engl. J. Med. 312:73.
Dobbins, W.O. III. 1985. Whipple's disease. In Mandell, G.L., Douglas, R.G. Jr., and Bennett, J.E., editors. Principles and practice of infectious diseases, ed. 2. John Wiley & Sons, New York.

Gajdusek, D.C., Gibbs, C.J., Asher, D.M., et al. 1977. Precautions in medical care of, and in handling materials from, patients with transmissible virus dementia (Creutzfeldt-Jakob disease). N. Engl. J. Med. 297:1253.

Gutman, L.T. 1980. *Spirillum* and *Campylobacter*. In Joklik, W.K., Willett, H.P., and Amos, D.B., editors. Zinsser microbiology, ed. 17. Appleton-Century Crofts, New York.

Lohr, J.A. 1985. Kawasaki disease (mucocutaneous lymph node syndrome). In Mandell, G.L., Douglas, R.G. Jr., and Bennett, J.E., editors. Principles and practice of infectious diseases, ed. 2. John Wiley & Sons, New York.

McKinley, M.P., Bolton, D.C., and Prusiner, S.B. 1983. A protease-resistant protein is a structural component of the scrapie prion. Cell 35:57.

Mitchell, T.G. 1980. Subcutaneous mycoses. In Joklik, W.K., Willett, H.P., and Amos, D.B., editors. Zinsser microbiology, ed. 17. Appleton-Century-Crofts, New York.

Murray, H.W., 1985. *Spirillum minor* (rat-bite fever). In Mandell, G.L., Douglas, R.G. Jr., and Bennett, J.E., editors. Principles and practice of infectious diseases, ed. 2. John Wiley & Sons, New York.

Taylor, A.F., Stephenson, T.G., Giese, H.A., and Petterson, G.R., 1984. Rat-bite fever in a college student. Calif. Morbid., no. 13. Department of Health Services, Sacramento, Calif.

41 Mycobacteria

□We are indebted to George Kubica of the CDC for allowing us to present many of the biochemical testing methods used in the Mycobacteriology Section of the CDC, as presented in their training manuals.

594

Mycobacteria have caused disease in humans since recorded history began; lesions clearly caused by mycobacteria have been identified in Egyptian mummies. Related to the corynebacteria and to *Nocardia* species, the mycobacteria contain several species pathogenic to humans, as well as those pathogenic to animals and fish. Many species are soil and water saprophytes, and one species, *Mycobacterium smegmatis*, is normal flora of human skin and mucous membranes. The primary human pathogen, *M. tuberculosis*, is found only in humans, however, who provide its reservoir. Tuberculosis still remains one of the most important infectious diseases in the world socioeconomically, particularly in parts of Asia and India.

41.1. Epidemiology and Pathogenesis of Mycobacterial Infections

41.1.a. *Mycobacterium tuberculosis*. Tuberculosis accounts for a large number of deaths and great morbidity worldwide. The disease is most common in parts of the world where overcrowding and lack of native resistance exist. For example, a large epidemic among North American Eskimos began in the 1950s, when that population first became exposed to the organism. Infection is spread from person to person by inhalation of airborne **droplet nuclei,** small drops of respiratory secretions containing infectious mycobacteria expelled from patients with disease during coughing, sneezing, or talking. These droplets are small enough that they remain aloft in the air for some time. If they are within the size range of 5-10 μm, they are small enough to avoid being trapped by nasal turbinates or mucociliary membranes and may reach and impinge on the alveolar walls and be taken up by alveolar macrophages. The pathogenesis of tuberculosis was discussed in Chapter 16.

Tuberculosis was spread by ingestion of milk from infected cows before pasteurization became commonplace. Almost all tuberculosis acquired in the United States today is by aerosol inhalation. With the exceptions of leprosy and *M. avium-intracellulare* infection in certain populations (discussed in Chapter 23), no other mycobacterial diseases are presumed contagious. Patients with cavitary disease are the primary reservoir for dissemination of *M. tuberculosis*. Although the disease incidence among Americans is falling, increasing numbers of cases are being discovered among Latin American and Southeast Asian immigrants and refugees. These patients, often infected with antibiotic-resistant strains of *M. tuberculosis*, pose new problems for public health officials and represent new foci for spread of the disease in certain locations, notably larger cities. Elderly patients, alcoholics, and non-Caucasians are more likely to develop disease.

It has been shown that inhalation of a single viable organism can lead to infection, although close contact is usually necessary for acquisition of infection. Of persons who become infected, 15%-20% go on to develop disease. Disease usually occurs some years after the initial infection, when the patient's immune system breaks down for some reason other than the presence of tuberculosis bacilli within the lung. In a small percentage of infected hosts, the disease becomes systemic, affecting such organs as the kidneys, spleen, bone marrow, central nervous system, and intestinal tract. In most patients, however, the disease is restricted to the lungs, with granuloma formation, caseous necrosis, and ultimately cavitary disease (Chapter 16). Diagnosis is made by isolating and identifying the etiologic agent, *M. tuberculosis*.

41.1.b. Other cultivatable mycobacteria. *M. bovis*, the agent of bovine tuberculosis, is an uncommon cause of disease in the United States today, although it used to be one of the primary agents of human intestinal tuberculosis, acquired through ingestion of contaminated milk. An attenuated strain of *M. bovis*, **bacille Calmette-Guérin (BCG),** has been used extensively in many parts of the world to immunize susceptible individuals against tuberculosis. BCG has recently been used as part of a controversial protocol to boost the nonspecific cellular immune response of certain immunologically deficient patients, particularly those with malignancies. Because mycobacteria are the classic examples of intracellular pathogens, and the body's response to BCG hinges on cell mediated immunoreactivity, immunized individuals are expected to react more aggressively against all antigens that elicit cell mediated immunity. Rarely, the unfortunate individual's immune system will be so compromised that it cannot handle the BCG, and systemic BCG infection may develop.

Respiratory infection in immunocompetent hosts is usually caused by *M. tuberculosis*, but *M. kansasii* and *M. avium-intracellulare* complex also cause tuberculosis-like disease. Other mycobacteria cause pulmonary disease, as well. Person-to-person spread is believed not to occur for any nontuberculous mycobacterial species other than *M. avium-intracellulare*. *M. avium-intracellulare* is the most common mycobacterial species isolated in many large hospital laboratories in the United States today due to its high prevalence in patients suffering from acquired immune deficiency syndrome (AIDS; see Chapter 23). In homosexual patients with AIDS the mode of acquisition of *M. avium-intracellulare* is believed to be through the gastrointestinal tract, often by sexual transmission

via infected semen. The first symptom of mycobacterial disease in many of these patients is protracted diarrhea. Acid fast stains of feces or intestinal biopsy specimens reveal huge numbers of acid fast bacilli. The infection usually disseminates in AIDS patients, with organisms being recovered from multiple sites including blood, sputum, feces, semen, lymph nodes, and internal organs.

Isolation of *M. tuberculosis* or *M. bovis* is always indicative of disease, whereas isolation of other mycobacteria may or may not be clinically significant. *M. gordonae*, for example, one of the more common mycobacteria isolated from clinical specimens, is a normal inhabitant of tap water and rarely causes disease in humans. Table 41.1 lists the **mycobacteria other than tuberculosis (MOTT)** that have been implicated as etiologic agents of human disease. There are other species that may be isolated from human clinical specimens, such as *M. gastri*, *M. terrae* complex, *M. triviale*, *M. gordonae*, *M. flavescens*, *M. phlei*, *M. vaccae*, and *M. smegmatis*, as mentioned in the sections that follow, but they are believed to be of no clinical significance at this time. However, on rare occasions *M. gordonae* may be involved in prosthetic valve endocarditis and meningitis.

41.1.c. Crohn's disease–associated *Mycobacterium*. Isolation of a new species of *Mycobacterium* from the bowel mucosa of patients with Crohn's disease has been reported by Chiodini and co-workers.[3] This news is particularly interesting, since the etiology of Crohn's disease, a chronic inflammatory bowel disease, has not been previously considered to be infectious. The organism is extremely fastidious, seems to require a growth factor, **mycobactin,** produced by other species of mycobacteria, such as *M. phlei*, a saprophytic strain, and may take as long as 18 months for primary isolation. Three strains of the new mycobacteria were isolated from terminal ileum biopsies taken from 14 patients with Crohn's disease. Cultural characteristics of these newly described strains

TABLE 41.1
Mycobacteria Other Than *M. tuberculosis* That Cause Human Disease

SPECIES	NATURAL HABITAT	TYPE OF INFECTION
M. africanum	Animals, soil	Pulmonary
M. asiaticum	Animals	Pulmonary
M. avium-intracellulare	Seawater, soil, animals	Pulmonary, systemic, gastrointestinal, lymphadenitis
M. chelonei subsp. *abscessus*	Seawater, soil, animals	Cutaneous, surgical wound, pulmonary, systemic
M. chelonei subsp. *chelonei*	Seawater, soil, animals	Porcine heart valves, surgical wound
M. fallax	Water, soil	Pulmonary
M. fortuitum	Water, soil, animals	Pulmonary, surgical wound, cutaneous, systemic, bone and joint, etc.
M. haemophilum	Unknown	Cutaneous and subcutaneous lesions
M. kansasii	Water, animals	Pulmonary, systemic, skin, joint, lymph nodes, etc.
M. leprae	Armadillos	Cutaneous, systemic, pulmonary, peripheral nervous system
M. malmoense	Unknown	Pulmonary
M. marinum	Aquariums, water, fish	Cutaneous ("swimming pool granuloma"), joints
M. scrofulaceum	Soil, water, fomites	Lymphadenitis (usually cervical), pulmonary, disseminated
M. shimoidei	Unknown	Pulmonary
M. simiae	Primates, water	Pulmonary
M. szulgai	Unknown	Pulmonary, lymphadenitis, cutaneous, subcutaneous, bursitis
M. ulcerans	Unknown	Cutaneous
M. xenopi	Soil, water	Pulmonary, epididymitis

are further discussed below. Whether these mycobacteria actually contribute to development of Crohn's disease or are simply colonizing an environmental niche in the bowel of these patients remains to be elucidated.

41.1.d. *Mycobacterium leprae*. Possibly second to *M. tuberculosis* in worldwide importance is *M. leprae*, the agent of leprosy (also called **Hansen's disease**). The organism has not yet been cultivated in vitro. Leprosy is a chronic disease of the skin, mucous membranes, and nerve tissue, with a strong immunologic component to the pathology. Understanding of the pathogenesis and epidemiology of the disease is hampered by our inability to grow the organism in culture. In tropical countries, where the disease is most prevalent, the disease may be acquired from infected humans; however, infectivity is very low. Prolonged close contact and host immunologic status play a role in infectivity. Recently, several reports

have detailed the development of leprosy among high school boys in the southwestern United States. These boys acquired the disease over widespread areas of their upper bodies after wrestling with wild armadillos. The armadillo appears to be a natural reservoir for the leprosy bacillus.

However leprosy is acquired, it passes through many stages in the host, characterized by various clinical and histopathologic features. Although there are many intermediate stages, the primary stages include a silent phase, during which leprosy bacilli multiply in the skin within macrophages, and an indeterminate phase, in which the bacilli multiply in peripheral nerves and begin to cause sensory impairment. More severe disease states that may follow are called **tuberculoid,** in which granulomas and hyperactive tissue are evident in the skin, and **lepromatous,** in which the patient's immune response is virtually absent and the bacilli multiply rapidly, often within many organs of the body and the reticuloendothelial system. A patient may spontaneously recover at any stage, and there are several borderline stages defined by subtle differences in the host response to infection. Berlin and Martin[2] have summarized current knowledge about leprosy.

Diagnosis is usually made through histopathologic examination of material taken from a skin lesion or from the earlobe of a suspected patient. Acid fast bacilli are evident by the Ziehl-Neelsen or other stain, often in great numbers. Other sites from which positive smears may be seen include lymph nodes, bone marrow, and human milk. The stages of leprosy can be additionally pinpointed by a patient's response to **lepromin,** a crude suspension of material taken from excised nodules of patients with Hansen's disease. Treatment consists of dapsone or DDS (4,4′-diaminodiphenylsulfone), often given in combination with rifampin. Excellent results have also been seen with clofazimine, which requires several months to build up active concentrations within the patient's tissues.

41.2. Morphologic Characteristics of Mycobacteria

The mycobacteria possess cell walls that contain mycolic acids, long-chain multiply crosslinked fatty acids. Corynebacteria and *Nocardia* also have similar fatty acids in their cell walls; the number of carbon atoms in the mycolic acid chain differentiates the three genera. Mycobacterial mycolic acids are quite long; their crosslinks probably serve to complex basic dyes, contributing to the characteristic of **acid fastness** that distinguishes the genus *Mycobacterium*. Acid fast organisms stain with carbol fuchsin but are very resistant to decolorization, even with strong decolorizers, such as **acid-alcohol (3% concentrated HCl in 95% ethanol).** Organisms with shorter mycolic acid chains, such as *Nocardia*, are only partially acid fast (Chapter 33). The fatty acids and lipids in the mycobacterial cell wall probably account for

the organism's unusual resistance to the effects of drying and harsh decontaminating agents, both acid and alkaline, as well as for acid fastness.

On Gram stain, mycobacteria usually appear as slender gram-positive bacilli. They may be mistaken for aerobic actinomycetes or corynebacteria, especially when isolated from clinical material from patients in whom mycobacterial disease was not suspected. The organisms are nonmotile. With a classical acid fast stain (Chapter 7), the mycobacteria appear as red, slender, delicate bacilli, from 1-4 μm long. They often have a beaded or banded appearance. Microscopic morphology cannot reliably distinguish among different mycobacterial species, but certain general guidelines about microscopic appearance follow. *M. tuberculosis* appears to have tapered ends and may exhibit **cording** (intertwining of bacilli in serpentine coils, particularly when grown in liquid media containing Tween-80), whereas *M. avium-intracellulare* often appears as short, almost coccobacillary forms. Cells of *M. kansasii* may appear as longer, banded and beaded bacilli, resembling a "barber pole"; *M. kansasii* may also display cording. Cells of MOTT are usually thicker and more beaded than cells of *M. tuberculosis*.

Preliminary identification of mycobacteria is based on their colonial morphologic characteristics, including **pigmentation** before and after exposure to light (Plate 41.1), and **rate of growth**. Excluding the *M. tuberculosis* complex, which includes *M. tuberculosis*, *M. bovis*, *M. africanum*, and *M. ulcerans*, the mycobacteria are loosely assigned to groups based on these two gross morphologic characteristics. **Photochromogens** are defined as organisms which produce yellow or orange pigment after exposure to light but remain buff-colored in the dark. Colonies of **scotochromogens** are pigmented even in the absence of exposure to light. Another group of MOTT are slow-growing, nonpigmented strains, called **nonphotochromogens**. The rapid growing mycobacteria

Acid fast bacilli

Subculture/growth rate

<7 days
Pigment

Scotochromogen	Photochromogen	Nonphotochromogen
M. scrofulaceum	M. fortuitum	M. kansasii (rare)
M. flavescens	M. chelonei	M. marinum
	M. fallax (30° C)	
	Other	

>7 days
Pigment

Nonphotochromogen	Photochromogen	Scotochromogen
M. tuberculosis	M. kansasii	M. avium complex
M. bovis	M. marinum	M. xenopi
M. simiae	M. asiaticum	M. terrae
M. africanum	M. simiae	M. malmoense
M. ulcerans		M. scrofulaceum
M. xenopi		M. szulgai
M. avium complex		M. gordonae
M. shimoidei		M. flavescens
M. gastri		
M. terrae		
M. triviale		
M. malmoense		
M. haemophilum		

FIGURE 41.1
Flow chart for identification of mycobacteria.

are those which produce a visible colony on subculture of a minimal inoculum in less than 7 days; organisms exhibiting this characteristic are called **rapid growers**. These groupings are still useful for preliminary species differentiation, as illustrated by the key in Figure 41.1. Certain species do not fit easily into one single group, and may exhibit characteristics of two groups; for this reason the semidichotomous key is partially redundant. Once isolated, the mycobacteria are identified by a series of biochemical and enzymatic reactions that are unlike those used for most other etiologic infectious agents. Performance of these tests will be discussed in this chapter.

41.3. Collection and Transport of Specimens

Special collection methods are required for certain specimens for isolation of mycobacteria. Although collection techniques are discussed in Chapter 6, those procedures that are unique to mycobacteriology will be mentioned here. A high index of suspicion on the part of the clinician is usually necessary for detection of acid fast bacilli, since most mycobacteria grow slowly and would not be expected to appear on standard media within the incubation times used for routine bacterial cultures. Occasionally an unsuspected rapidly growing *Mycobacterium* species will be isolated from clinical material, such as a surgical wound aspirate, on routine culture. Unless an acid fast stain is performed, such an isolate will be an identification problem. Chapter 33 contains a flow chart for identification of filamentous, aerobic, nonspore-forming gram-positive bacilli, which include mycobacteria.

41.3.a. Respiratory secretions. The most common clinical specimens received for isolation of acid fast bacilli are pulmonary secretions. Spontaneously coughed or induced sputum, bronchial aspirations and lavages, and gastric contents (expected to contain swallowed sputum) are all acceptable. Patients who are able to produce sputum should be given clearcut instructions as to the collection of such a specimen. The best specimen is obtained from patients when supervision, or better yet, assistance, is available from health care professionals during collection. Purulent material from the first productive deep cough of the morning should be expelled into a sterile container without contaminating saliva or nasal secretions. The patient should rinse his or her mouth out vigorously with water, **not mouthwash**, before producing sputum. Approximately 5-10 ml of sputum should be collected for each specimen. The sputum is transported immediately to the laboratory in a sterile container, such as a screw-top plastic urine cup or in a special container designed for the purpose, such as the Falcon sputum collection kit (Falcon Plastics, Becton-Dickinson Co.). If the specimen must be held, it should be refrigerated. Mycobacteria will survive in refrigerated sputa for at least several days. Pooled sputum samples collected over several hours and deposited in the same container are not satisfactory, as they are more likely to be contaminated. For optimal recovery of mycobacteria, three to five separate specimens, collected over a period of several days, are recommended. Early morning samples containing the collected secretions accumulated during the night will yield the most isolates.

Patients who are unable to produce sputum may be induced to cough up deep respiratory secretions by allowing them to breathe nebulized (aerosolized), warm 10% sodium chloride, or 10% glycerin and 15% sodium chloride solutions for approximately 10 min. Although these specimens appear watery and resemble saliva, they may produce positive cultures. Such specimens should be labeled **induced sputum** so that they are not mistaken for saliva. Although sputum specimens for routine bacteriologic studies are routinely monitored for acceptability (Chapter 16), specimens received for acid fast bacilli are usually always accepted and cultured without prescreening.

41.3.b. Gastric aspirates. Patients unable to produce sputum, uncooperative patients (including small children), or those too ill to ex-

pectorate usually swallow sputum during the night, which pools in the stomach. Because of the relative acid resistance of mycobacteria and the slow rate of host metabolism during sleep, such swallowed sputum will retain viable acid fast bacilli. Gastric contents can then be collected for culture. Specimens are collected first thing in the morning or after the patient has fasted for at least 8 h. A disposable plastic gastric tube is inserted through the nose or mouth and gently threaded down the esophagus into the stomach. The patient is instructed to sip small amounts of water to help the tube down. When the tube reaches the stomach, the gastric contents are aspirated into a 50 ml syringe and immediately placed into a sterile container. Then 20-30 ml of sterile distilled water (for parenteral administration, obtained from the pharmacy) is injected into the stomach through the tube or swallowed by the patient. This fluid, the **gastric lavage,** is then aspirated into the syringe and added to the original specimen. The specimen is hand carried **immediately** to the laboratory, where it is processed rapidly or neutralized with pellets of NaOH until pH 7.0 is reached. Pellets are added a few at a time, mixed to dissolve, and the pH is measured using hydrion paper. This procedure, as for all procedures that require manipulation of specimens, must be carried out within a laminar flow safety cabinet (Chapter 2). Some laboratories advocate the use of masks for technologists during handling of respiratory secretions that may contain tubercle bacilli.

41.3.c. Other specimens received for mycobacterial culture. Tuberculous meningitis is uncommon, but still occurs in both immunocompetent and immunosuppressed patients. Most critical for isolation of acid fast bacilli from cerebrospinal fluid is that the quantity of specimen be sufficient. There may be very few organisms in the spinal fluid, which makes their detection difficult. At least 10 ml of cerebrospinal fluid is recommended for recovery of mycobacteria.

The discovery of circulating mycobacteria in the blood of patients with AIDS has led to increased requests for such cultures. Best recovery can be achieved by collecting the blood in a lysis-centrifugation system (DuPont Isolator, Chapter 14). If the blood is allowed to remain in the lysing solution for approximately 1 h, lysis of phagocytic cells may occur, allowing release and enhanced recovery of intracellular mycobacteria. In patients with AIDS, quantitation of such organisms can be used to monitor therapy and determine prognosis. For this purpose the 1.5 ml Pediatric Isolator tubes can be used, since the entire contents are plated and colony forming units can be determined per milliliter of initial specimen. Other traditional methods have been described for isolation of mycobacteria from blood, including biphasic blood culture media, but the lysis-centrifugation system is the most practical so far. Automated radiometric detection of mycobacteria in blood is another alternative for such cultures. Use of this system is discussed below.

Urine from patients with renal disease may contain mycobacteria, usually *M. tuberculosis*. The first morning voided urine collected 3 days in a row will usually yield the organism, if present. For recovery of mycobacteria, the entire volume of urine should be collected, if possible. Pooled 24 h urine collections are not recommended. Specimens should be refrigerated if they are not processed immediately. Urine collected by suprapubic aspiration (Chapter 18) is presumed to be free of other microorganisms and should be centrifuged (as for sterile body fluids, as discussed below) and cultured without decontamination.

Sterile body fluids of all types, tissue, and other such specimens are also suitable for recovery of mycobacteria. The least desirable specimen is a swab. Small tissue biopsies or aspirated material are recommended for isolation of mycobacteria from skin lesions. Feces, although often received in earlier years for diagnosis of gastrointestinal tuberculosis, has not been a common specimen for routine clinical laboratories until the recent epidemic of AIDS. Feces are commonly the first specimen to become positive for *M. avium-intracellulare* in patients with AIDS and laboratories are again receiving fecal samples. We recommend performing a direct acid fast stain on a thin smear of stool and processing the culture only if acid fast bacilli are seen on smear. We have found that emulsifying a swab of fecal material in 5 ml of Dubos albumin broth (available commercially), incubating the broth overnight, and then processing the entire broth as if it were a sputum or other contaminated specimen, yields reasonable results without undue loss of cultures due to overgrowth by contaminating bacteria. Specimens such as tissues and feces that cannot be immediately processed should be frozen at $-20°$ C until they can be handled. Viability of mycobacteria in frozen liquid samples is not as well preserved.

41.4. Primary Laboratory Services

41.4.a. Levels of laboratory service. Not all laboratories have a biological safety cabinet in which to safely handle mycobacterial specimens. For those laboratories that lack such facilities, only a limited number of procedures can be performed. Other laboratories may isolate mycobacteria so infrequently that it is not cost effective for them to maintain the necessary products required for further studies. Additionally, laboratories that isolate mycobacteria infrequently cannot be expected to gain proficiency in handling these organisms. To assist laboratories in making decisions about the level of service they can reasonably and reliably provide, Wayne and associates[12] have suggested four levels of proficiency for laboratories:

1. Collection and transport of specimens; preparation and examination of smears for acid fast bacilli
2. Detection, isolation, and identification of *M. tuberculosis*

3. Determination of drug susceptibility of mycobacteria

4. Identification of mycobacteria other than *M. tuberculosis*

One thousand specimens annually has been suggested as the minimum number of specimens that a laboratory claiming level 4 proficiency should receive. Laboratories could then refer all studies beyond those they are capable and willing to perform to a reference laboratory. With cost containment becoming ever more critical for hospitals, such a policy makes good sense (depending on the charges, if any by the reference laboratory).

41.4.b. Direct Examination of Clinical Material

Smears made directly from specimens may be examined for acid fast bacilli. Sputum may be examined directly as a stat procedure for confirmation of the presence of mycobacteria in the respiratory secretions of patients newly suspected of having tuberculosis. This is an especially important procedure for hospitalized patients, as they must be placed in respiratory isolation, an expensive and time-consuming procedure, if they are actively disseminating mycobacteria. Microbiologists handling such specimens should take all necessary precautions, as outlined in Chapter 2. The sputum specimen is placed in a biologic safety cabinet, and a wooden applicator stick is used to select mucopurulent material for smear preparation. Material is spread over the surface of the slide in a thin layer. These slides should be heat-fixed within the hood or allowed to dry on a heating platform at 85° C for 15 min before staining. Even heat-fixed and stained smears may harbor a few infectious mycobacteria. All smears should be handled as if they were contaminated.

For those laboratories without biological safety cabinets, handling of specimens beyond preparation of acid fast stains should not be attempted. A contaminated specimen, such as

---

PROCEDURE 41.1. PREPARATION OF ACID FAST SMEARS FROM INFECTIOUS MATERIAL

1. Mix the sputum or stool with an equal part of 5% sodium hypochlorite (undiluted household bleach, such as Clorox). Stir with a wooden stick to ensure even mixing. Then shake the tightly closed container for 2-3 min.

2. Allow the mixture to remain at room temperature for at least 10 min, or until the mixture is homogeneous when swirled, and then centrifuge in a 15 ml disposable conical centrifuge tube for 10 min at 3,000 rpm.

3. Decant the supernatant and transfer a portion of the now sterile creamy white sediment to a slide with a cotton-tipped applicator.

4. Air dry the smear and stain for acid fast bacilli. No fixation is necessary.

---

stool or sputum, can be rendered noninfectious for staining purposes (see Procedure 41.1).

Cerebrospinal fluid must be concentrated to increase the chance of detection of small numbers of organisms. The specimen should be centrifuged for at least 30 min at $2,000 \times g$ to concentrate the bacteria. The supernatant is decanted (and held for testing for cryptococcal antigen and other procedures that do not require cells, such as protein and glucose concentrations, discussed in Chapter 15), and the sediment is vortexed thoroughly. The well-mixed sediment is then applied to a slide in heaped drops. A heaped drop is allowed to air dry, and a second application of sediment is placed on the same spot and allowed to dry. A minimum of three layers, applied to the same 1 cm di-

PROCEDURE 41.2. KINYOUN'S COLD ACID FAST STAIN

1. Heat-fix slides by flaming, or allow to dry on an 85° C slide-warming tray for at least 15 min. Stain a known positive and negative control slide with each staining procedure.
2. Flood slides with Kinyoun's carbol fuchsin and allow to stain for 5 min at room temperature.
3. Rinse with distilled water to prevent tap water contaminants from being introduced.
4. Decolorize with acid-alcohol for 3 min and rinse again with distilled water.
5. Redecolorize with acid-alcohol for 1-2 min or until no more red color runs from the smear.
6. Rinse with distilled water and drain standing water from slide surface by tipping slide.
7. Flood slide with methylene blue counterstain and allow to stain for 4 min.
8. Rinse with distilled water and allow to air dry.
9. Examine under high dry (400 ×) magnification, and confirm acid fast structures under oil immersion (1,000 ×).

Modified from Kinyoun. 1915. Am. J. Public Health 5:867.

ameter circle, should facilitate detection of small numbers of bacilli. This dried slide is heat fixed before staining. As with all smears, even after staining, some mycobacteria may be viable on the slide, which should be handled as if it were contaminated.

Other material, including ground or homogenized tissue, touch preparations of cut surfaces of tissue, centrifuged sediments of body fluid material, and abscess contents, are deposited on slides directly, allowed to air dry, and stained. Tissue that cannot be processed immediately may be frozen until cultures and smears can be prepared.

The stains used for detection of acid fast bacilli are of two types: **carbol fuchsin** and **fluorochromic.** The carbol fuchsin stains used are the classic **Ziehl-Neelsen,** which requires heating the slide to fix the carbol fuchsin within the lipid cell walls of mycobacteria, and the cold **Kinyoun's,** which increases the concentration of basic fuchsin and phenol, avoiding the need for heat. The procedure for the Ziehl-Neelsen stain was given in Chapter 7, and the components of the stain solutions are listed in Chapter 46. Kinyoun's stain (Procedure 41.2) is shown below. Any specimen that is not going to be subjected to decontamination and concentration procedures is suitable for direct acid fast stain.

For those laboratories that possess an ultraviolet microscope, a fluorochromic staining procedure (Chapter 7) is recommended for initial screening of smears. Fluorescent stains are much more sensitive than the conventional carbol fuchsin stains because the fluorescent bacilli stand out brightly against the background; the smear can be initially examined at lower magnifications than that required for examination under oil immersion, and thus more fields can be visualized in the same amount of time. In addition, a positive fluorescent smear may be restained with Ziehl-Neelsen directly over the previous stain without destaining, as long as the immersion oil has been completely removed with xylene. Such restaining is unnecessary, however, because rhodamine is as specific for acid fast bacilli as are the traditional stains. Screening of specimens with rhodamine or rhodamine-auramine will result in a higher yield of positive smears and will substantially reduce the amount of time needed for examining smears. One drawback associated with the fluorochrome stains is that most strains of *M. fortuitum* and *M. chelonei* do not stain well with these reagents. It is recommended that Ziehl-Neelsen stained smears be examined for approximately 3 min before being reported as negative; a similar fluorochrome smear can be examined as thoroughly in less time. It is important to wipe the immersion oil from the objective lens after examining a positive smear, since stained bacilli can float off the slide into the oil and may possibly contribute to a false positive reading for the next smear examined.

Smears should be examined thoroughly; the technologist should scan each area before reporting a smear as "negative." When acid fast bacilli are seen, they are reported as "acid fast bacilli seen." Enumeration of numbers of organisms should be reported following the convention of the American Lung Association, assuming examination of the smear under 1,000 × magnification, as shown in Table 41.2.[1] The clinical relevance of very rare numbers of acid

TABLE 41.2
Reporting Numbers of Acid Fast Bacilli Observed in Stained Smears

NUMBER AFB OBSERVED	REPORT*
None	Negative for AFB (−)
1-2/300 fields†	Actual number seen (+); request another specimen
1-9/100 fields	Average number/100 fields (1+)
1-9/10 fields	Average number/10 fields (2+)
1-9/field	Average number/field (3+)
>9/field	>9/field (4+)

Modified from American Thoracic Society. 1981. Diagnostic standards and classification of tuberculosis and other mycobacterial diseases. Am. Rev. Respir. Dis. 123:343.
*Note that it should be stated in the report whether the smear was direct or concentrated.
†Oil immersion field (1,000 ×).

fast bacilli is difficult to assess. The technologist should report the number of acid fast organisms seen on the smear with the notation that such numbers are of doubtful diagnostic value. Detection of larger numbers of acid fast bacilli seen on initial smear (five or six per high-power field, 400 ×) is indicative of infection.

41.5. Specimen Handling in the Laboratory: Digestion, Decontamination, and Concentration Procedures

41.5.a. Specimens that can be inoculated to media without decontamination. Specimens received from sites that do not contain normal flora are suitable for direct inoculation to media. Body fluids that are in danger of clotting should be collected in sterile citrated tubes (Vacutainer citrate tubes, Becton-Dickinson Co.) or in sterile tubes containing some other anticoagulant such as 1 mg/ml ethylenediaminetetraacetic acid (EDTA) or 0.1 mg/ml heparin. Body fluids, including cerebrospinal fluid, received in amounts greater than 1 ml should be centrifuged before staining or inoculating. A force of at least 2,000 × g, usually achieved by centrifuges spinning at 3,000 rpm, for at least 30 min is required to concentrate mycobacteria. These organisms, because of the high lipid content of their cell walls, are more buoyant in liquid (have less density) than other bacteria, and thus require more vigorous concentration techniques. Laboratories that do not have centrifuges that generate enough force should consider spinning specimens for a longer period, perhaps for 1 h. Supernatants are decanted and held for other studies, as necessary.

Even after vigorous centrifugation, many mycobacteria may not sediment. The specific gravity and lipid content of the liquid specimen are determinants of the buoyant density of mycobacteria suspended in it. For this reason, although mycobacteria have been shown to be retained in the sediment of sputum, they are often carried along with other particulate matter. Certain specimens, such as cerebrospinal fluid and urine, may not share the same components, and thus do not aid the sedimentation of mycobacteria. Until new methods are developed for handling such specimens, centrifugation at high speeds is required. Another method recommended for concentrating the bacilli in cerebrospinal fluid is to pass the fluid through a 0.45 μm pore size membrane filter, which will collect all acid fast bacilli. This filter may then be aseptically cut into pieces which can be placed on the surface of media and into broth cultures. If spinal fluid is treated in this way, examination of a smear is not possible.

Tissue specimens should be ground or homogenized. Large tissue specimens should be minced with sterile scissors or scalpel blades before grinding in a glass tissue grinder (Figure 41.2) or mortar and pestle. The addition of a small amount of Dubos albumin broth will assist emulsification. This procedure will inevitably create aerosols; therefore technologists must be very careful to work well within the biohazard cabinet and manipulate the material gently.

We have found that a homogenizing instrument (Stomacher Lab-Blender 80, Tekmar Co.) that uses rapid pounding of tissue placed in a small amount of broth in a sterile plastic bag does an excellent job of preparing tissue specimens (except lung, which should be minced or ground) for culture. A piece of tissue (minimum size, 1 cm³) is placed into one of the sterile plastic bags that are recommended by the manufacturer along with a minimum of 2 ml of sterile Dubos albumin broth, and the Stomacher is allowed to run for at least 30 seconds. The liquid in the bag containing the bacteria that have been expressed from the tissue is then used for culture and smears. If the material is very dilute, the liquid can be concentrated by centrifugation. The method does not create aerosols, since the bag is sealed during homogenization. Bone cannot be ground with this instrument, as the bone chips can pene-

trate the plastic bag. Tissue from contaminated sites, such as tonsils or autopsy material, should be decontaminated and concentrated after it has been homogenized. The liquid is handled as if it were sputum.

As mentioned above and in Chapter 14, blood for mycobacterial culture should be drawn into DuPont Isolator tubes. A second method of culturing blood (and other material) for acid fast bacteria utilizes radiometric detection of the products of carbon metabolism (Bactec, Johnston Laboratories), as outlined in Chapter 11. Use of the Bactec instrument for mycobacterial culturing is discussed below.

41.5.b. Specimens that require decontamination and concentration before inoculation to media. Sputum and other respiratory secretions contain normal flora, and therefore are decontaminated to inhibit overgrowth of slowly growing mycobacteria by faster growing bacteria or fungi. Other specimens from nonsterile body sites are also decontaminated. Culture of feces from patients suspected of harboring *M. tuberculosis* is rarely attempted by hospital laboratories. If such a request is received, methods detailed in the CDC laboratory manual by Vestal[10] should be followed. Feces from pa-

FIGURE 41.2
Glass tissue grinder suitable for homogenizing tissue for inoculation to media for isolation of mycobacteria.

PROCEDURE 41.3. ACETYLCYSTEINE-ALKALI METHOD FOR DIGESTION AND DECONTAMINATION OF SPECIMENS FOR MYCOBACTERIAL CULTURE

1. Prepare 0.676 (1/15) M phosphate buffer as follows:
   Solution A

Sodium monohydrogen phosphate (anhydrous)	9.47 g
Distilled water	1,000 ml

   Solution B

Potassium dihydrophosphate	9.08 g
Distilled water	1,000 ml

   Add 625 ml of solution B to 375 ml of solution A and adjust pH to 6.8. Dispense in small volumes, such as 250 ml screw cap bottles, and autoclave for 15 min at 121° C. Store at room temperature.

2. For each day's cultures, add up the total volume of specimens to be treated and prepare an equal volume of the digestant-decontamination mixture, N-acetylcysteine sodium hydroxide (NALC-NaOH) as follows:

1 N (4%) NaOH	50 ml
0.1 M (2.94%) trisodium citrate · $3H_2O$	50 ml
N-acetyl-L-cysteine powder	0.5 g

   All reagents are available from Sigma Chemical Co. and several other manufacturers (Appendix). The amount of digestant can be varied depending on the volume of material to be digested, by doubling or halving the components. It is useful to use sterile distilled water for preparation of solutions to minimize chances of inadvertently adding acid fast tap water contaminants to the specimens. This solution should be used within 24 h.

3. Work within a biological safety cabinet and wear gloves. Transfer a maximum of 10 ml of sputum, urine, or other fluid to be processed to a sterile, disposable plastic 50 ml conical centrifuge tube with a leakproof and aerosol-free plastic screw cap. Tubes with easily visible volume indicator marks are best.

4. Add an equal volume of freshly prepared digestant to the tube, being very careful when pouring digestant not to touch the lip of the specimen container, which might inadvertently transfer positive material to a negative specimen. Tighten the cap completely.

5. Vortex the specimen for approximately a slow count of 15, or for a maximum of 30 seconds, being certain to create a vortex in the liquid and not to merely agitate the material. Check for homogeneity by inverting the tube. If clumps remain, vortex the specimen intermittently while the rest of the specimens are being digested. An extra pinch of N-acetylcysteine crystals may be necessary to liquefy really mucoid sputa.

6. Start a 15 min timer as the first specimen is finished being vortexed. Continue digesting the other specimens, noting the amount of time that the entire run takes. The digestant should remain on the specimens for no longer than 15

PROCEDURE 41.3. ACETYLCYSTEINE-ALKALI METHOD FOR DIGESTION AND DECONTAMINATION OF SPECIMENS FOR MYCOBACTERIAL CULTURE—cont'd

min. After this 15 min period at room temperature, buffer is added to stop the decontamination process. Buffer should be added to the specimens so as to be sure that they are each allowed a 15 min period of digestion.

7. After 15 min of digestion, add enough phosphate buffer to reach within 1 cm of the top, screw the cap tightly closed, and invert the tube to mix the solutions and stop the digestion process. Addition of this solution also reduces the specific gravity of the specimen, aiding sedimentation of the bacilli during centrifugation.

8. Centrifuge all tubes at greater than $1,800 \times g$, or at least 3,000 rpm, for 15 min.

9. Carefully pour off the supernatant into a splash-proof container (Figure 41.3) containing 5% phenol, Amphyl, or other germicide (Appendix). The lip of the tube may be wiped with an Amphyl- or phenol-soaked gauze to absorb drips. Be careful not to touch the lip of any tube to another container. It is very helpful to carefully watch the sediment as the supernatant is being decanted, since sometimes a very mucoid sediment can be loose and may pour right out with the supernatant. The technologist who sees the sediment beginning to slip can then stop decanting and use a sterile capillary pipette to remove the supernatant without losing the sediment.

10. Inoculate the sediment to culture media and to slides for staining and examination.

FIGURE 41.3
Supernatant from acid fast specimen concentrates is carefully decanted into a splash-proof container that can be autoclaved and reused.

tients with AIDS, suspected of containing large numbers of *M. avium-intracellulare*, are handled as stated above, culturing only specimens that were positive on direct smear. A swab of material from smear-positive specimens is placed into 5 ml of Dubos albumin broth and twirled to evenly disperse the contents. After overnight incubation, this 5 ml broth can be decontaminated and concentrated as if it were sputum.

Urine specimens (except for those collected so as to avoid contamination with normal flora, such as suprapubic aspirates or specimens collected surgically) are also subjected to digestion and decontamination. Although the method is not ideal, the entire voided urine is placed into sterile, 50 ml plastic centrifuge tubes and centrifuged at 2,000 × g for 30 min. The sediments are combined and resuspended in 2-5 ml sterile distilled water. This sample is then decontaminated and concentrated as if it were sputum. An alternative method described by Vestal[10] is to add an equal volume of 4% H_2SO_4 to the combined sediment after centrifugation. This suspension is vortexed and allowed to stand for 15 min at room temperature. The tube is then filled to within 1 cm of the top with sterile distilled water to dilute the sulfuric acid and prevent it from destroying the mycobacteria. This suspension is centrifuged as above, the supernatant is decanted, and the sediment is diluted with 0.2% albumin before smears and cultures are prepared.

Gastric aspirate material may be contaminated and require some manipulation. If processed immediately, the gastric aspirate can be digested with the addition of a pinch of *N*-acetylcysteine per 25 ml of aspirate material. This suspension is vortexed and centrifuged for 30 min at 1,800 × g, or 3,000 rpm. After the supernatant is discarded, the sediment is processed as if it were sputum.

Three decontamination methods are currently acceptable; all of them destroy contaminating bacteria without undue loss of viability of the mycobacteria in the specimen. Although sodium hydroxide acts as both an emulsifier and a decontaminant, breaking down mucus as it inhibits growth of contaminants, a mucus liquefier such as acetylcysteine may be used with sodium hydroxide to shorten the decontamination time and preserve more viable mycobacteria. Sputum samples digested with acetylcysteine and decontaminated with sodium hydroxide (Procedure 41.3) or digested with trisodium phosphate and decontaminated with benzalkonium chloride (Procedure 41.4) yield similar numbers of positive results, as discussed by Krasnow.[5] The chapter on mycobacteria by Sommers and Good in the American Society for Microbiology *Manual of Clinical Microbiology* contains an excellent discussion of techniques for handling mycobacterial cultures.[7]

Occasional specimens will be so contaminated with bacteria, particularly *Pseudomonas* and *Klebsiella* species, that mycobacterial cultures will be overgrown despite standard decontamination. If sediment material is left over, it may be redigested with a stronger alkali solution. Usually, another specimen from that patient must be requested. In these cases, 3% or 4% NaOH digestant may be substituted for the standard 2% NaOH in the NALC-NaOH digestant. The timing is quite critical for this reagent, as for the NALC-NaOH procedure. Longer digestion times should not be used, but increased NaOH concentrations may be necessary. Oxalic acid (6%) has been used to decontaminate specimens contaminated with *Pseudomonas aeruginosa*. It is acceptable to add certain antibiotics (penicillin or nalidixic acid, for example) to the sediment if most mycobacteria are resistant to these agents.

The sediment material from any concentration procedure is inoculated to culture media and spread on slides. The addition of 0.5-1 ml of 0.2% bovine albumin (Bovine albumin fraction V, Sigma) adjusted to pH 6.8 (with 4%

PROCEDURE 41.4. BENZALKONIUM CHLORIDE (ZEPHIRAN)–TRISODIUM PHOSPHATE METHOD FOR DIGESTION AND DECONTAMINATION OF SPECIMENS FOR MYCOBACTERIAL CULTURE

1. Prepare Zephiran–trisodium phosphate digestant as follows:

   Trisodium phosphate ($Na_3PO_4 \cdot 2H_2O$)   500 g

   Hot, sterile distilled water   2,000 ml

   To this solution, add 3.25 ml of Zephiran concentrate (17% benzalkonium chloride, Winthrop Laboratories). Mix. Store at room temperature.
2. Mix equal parts of the specimen and digestant, exactly as detailed in Procedure 41.3. Instead of vortexing, however, the tubes must be shaken for exactly 30 min on a shaking apparatus (a paint mixer works well).
3. Allow the mixtures to stand without agitation for an additional 30 min.
4. Centrifuge as in Procedure 41.3 for 30 min.
5. Decant supernatant as in Procedure 41.3.
6. Resuspend the supernatant in 20 ml of neutralizing buffer (obtained from Difco Laboratories). Although the $\frac{1}{15}$ M phosphate buffer described in Procedure 41.3 may be used, the commercial buffer contains components to specifically neutralize the Zephiran.
7. Recentrifuge the tubes as above for 20 min.
8. Decant supernatant fluids as above, and retain the sediments for smears and cultures.

FIGURE 41.4
The sediment from concentrated specimens is spread across a glass slide for staining. To prevent the material from being washed off, it may be allowed to extend to the edges of the slide.

NaOH) will dilute the sediment slightly, increasing the volume of material for cultures, and will assist the material to remain adherent to the slide during staining. To avoid material from very thick or viscous sediments from washing off the slide during staining, the sediment may be spread across the center of each slide so that the surface tension overlaps the top and bottom edge of the slide (Figure 41.4). Only one specimen should be placed on a slide. Approximately 3 drops of the sediment should be inoculated to each of the media used for culture. Gentle aspiration of the sediment up and down several times into a sterile Pasteur pipette or a sterile disposable plastic transfer pipette will mix the sediment adequately. All manipulations, of course, are performed within the safety cabinet. The same pipette full of material can be used to inoculate culture media and prepare the slide, using the pipette tip to spread the smear. The albumin-sediment suspension may be refrigerated for several days without substantial loss of viability of mycobacteria, since the solution is well buffered. It is useful to retain part of the sediment, at least until smears are read, so that material will be available for direct susceptibility testing if the smears are positive. Additionally, cultures that become contaminated within a few days can be redecontaminated and recultured.

The isolation rates of a tap water saprophyte can help a laboratory to judge the efficacy of its digestion, decontamination, and concentration procedures. *M. gordonae* serves as a good marker organism since it is ubiquitous. In areas where *M. gordonae* is present in the tap water, microbiologists should be expected to isolate this organism from approximately 5% of all clinical specimens. Laboratories with a substantially lower isolation rate for *M. gordonae* should reexamine their decontamination technique since it may be too harsh.

41.6. Culture Media and Methods

41.6.a. Conventional cultures. Concentrated decontaminated material, concentrated material from sterile body sites, or unconcentrated specimens from sterile body sites should be inoculated to at least two, and preferably three, different media. All specimens should be inoculated to one egg-based medium, such as Löwenstein-Jensen, Wallenstein's, or Petragnani (all available from commercial sources of prepared media, Appendix) and one clear agar medium, such as Middlebrook 7H11. The addition of 2% glycerol to Middlebrook 7H11 agar will enhance the growth of *M. avium-intracellulare* and other MOTT.

Wallenstein and Petragnani agars both contain added glycerol to support the growth of MOTT, but they also contain increased amounts of malachite green, which inhibits growth of contaminants and mycobacteria somewhat. For specimens that may be contaminated, one of the more selective media should

also be inoculated. Components of several selective media are shown in Table 41.3. Principles of selective media are discussed in Chapter 8. Culture media prepared in medicine bottles with screw caps are recommended, since the agar slants provide more surface area for growth, allowing isolated colonies to be picked for subculture. For laboratories with limited incubator space, however, tubed media may be used.

We recommend the use of Löwenstein-Jensen, Middlebrook 7H11, and Mycobactosel (selective Löwenstein-Jensen, available from BBL Microbiology Systems) or the Gruft modification of Löwenstein-Jensen for initial isolation. Several drops of the sediment from sterile fluid specimens (cerebrospinal fluid, joint fluid, pleural fluid, etc.) are additionally inoculated to 5 ml of Dubos albumin or Middlebrook 7H9 broth for enrichment. Alternatively, the fluid may be inoculated directly, 1 ml of fluid into 5 ml of broth. The broths are incubated along with the agar media and examined once every week by acid fast stain. If smears are negative, the broths are subcultured to Löwenstein-Jensen agar after 4, 6, and 8 weeks before being discarded. Material from Isolator tubes after lysis centrifugation is inoculated to Middlebrook 7H11 agar plates, following the manufacturer's recommendations. Egg-based media should be purchased, unless the laboratory has the personnel and facilities to prepare such media. Middlebrook agar powder base and premeasured, presterilized vials of the **oleic acid, albumin, dextrose, catalase, sodium chloride enrichment (OADC)** for preparation of plates are available from several commercial media manufacturers, or prepared tubed media may be purchased.

Cultures are incubated at 35° C in the dark. A second set of cultures of material from skin lesions suspected of harboring *M. marinum* are incubated at room temperature (or at 30° C if such an incubator is available). All tubes should be incubated with loose caps in an atmosphere

TABLE 41.3

Selective Mycobacterial Isolation Media

MEDIUM	COMPONENTS	INHIBITORY AGENTS
Gruft modification of Löwenstein-Jensen	Fresh whole eggs, defined salts, glycerol, potato flour, ribonucleic acid (5 mg/100 ml)	Malachite green, 0.025 g/100 ml Penicillin, 50 U/ml Nalidixic acid, 35 μg/ml
Mycobactosel* Löwenstein-Jensen	Fresh whole eggs, defined salts, glycerol, potato flour	Malachite green, 0.025 g/100 ml Cycloheximide, 400 μg/ml Lincomycin, 2 μg/ml Nalidixic acid, 35 μg/ml
Middlebrook 7H10	Defined salts, vitamins, cofactors, oleic acid, albumin, catalase, glycerol, dextrose	Malachite green, 0.0025 g/100 ml Cycloheximide, 360 μg/ml Lincomycin, 2 μg/ml Nalidixic acid, 20 μg/ml
Selective 7H11 (Mitchison's medium)	Defined salts, vitamins, cofactors, oleic acid, albumin, catalase, glycerol, dextrose, casein hydrolysate	Carbenicillin, 50 μg/ml Amphotericin B, 10 μg/ml Polymyxin B, 200 U/ml Trimethoprim lactate, 20 μg/ml
Wallenstein	Egg yolk, glycerol	Malachite green, 2 g/100 ml

Modified from Sommers, H.M., and Good, R.C. 1985. In Lennette, E.H., Balows, A., Hausler, W.J. Jr., and Shadomy, H.J., editors. Manual of clinical microbiology, ed. 4. American Society for Microbiology, Washington, D.C.
*BBL Microbiology Systems.

of 5%-10% CO_2, at least for the first 2 weeks. If possible, tubes should be laid horizontally on a slant, to allow the liquid inoculum to spread evenly over the agar surface. After 2 weeks the caps are tightened to prevent evaporation and desiccation of the media. Plates may be taped closed on either side with a small length of cellophane tape (to prevent accidental opening) and enclosed within polyethylene bags, which are taped closed after excluding all air to prevent the media from drying during the extended incubation. Alternatively, plates may be poured to double thickness to prevent the media from drying.

Cultures are examined twice weekly for growth. Contaminated cultures are discarded and reported as "contaminated, unable to detect presence of mycobacteria," and repeat specimens are requested. If sediment is still available, it may be recultured after enhanced decontamination or by inoculating the sediment to a more selective medium, as mentioned above. After 8 weeks of incubation, neg-

ative cultures (those showing no growth) from smear-negative specimens are reported, and the cultures are discarded. On occasion, mycobacteria may require as long as 12 weeks for initial isolation. Accordingly, cultures from specimens that showed acid fast bacilli on the original smears must be held for an additional 4 weeks (for a total of 12 weeks of incubation) before being reported as negative.

41.6.b. Susceptibility testing. In addition to routine cultures, sediments from those respiratory specimens that yielded positive smears may also be inoculated directly to susceptibility testing media, as discussed in Chapter 13. Isolates of mycobacteria may be tested for susceptibility to primary drugs used for their treatment, as outlined in Chapter 13. In areas where resistant mycobacteria are commonly seen, susceptibility testing of all isolates is recommended. Laboratories that see very few positive cultures should consider sending isolates to a reference laboratory for testing. Those isolates that must be saved for the future possibility of additional studies (such as susceptibilities if the patient does not respond well to treatment) can be frozen in sterile 10% skim milk in distilled water at $-70°$ C. They can then be defrosted and subcultured for future studies. Methods have also been developed for testing rapid growers (see Swenson et al.[9]).

One important consideration to take into account when testing isolates of *M. avium-intracellulare* is that colony morphology relates to virulence in this species. The more transparent, glossy colonies are more virulent than the opaque, dull, white or yellow colonies often seen on isolation media. Growth in vitro selects for the opaque, less virulent morphotype. Isolated colonies of the transparent type should be chosen for in vitro susceptibility testing of these organisms; testing a sweep of growth from the surface of an agar slant may not yield results that correlate with the in vivo situation.

41.6.c. Radiometric cultures. An exciting, relatively recent development for the rapid detection of mycobacteria in clinical specimens is the use of radiometric monitoring (outlined in Chapter 11). Inoculation of a portion of the digested and decontaminated specimen (using NALC-NaOH methods) or the uncontaminated sterile body fluid into special 7H12 broth media developed for use with the Bactec instrument (Johnston Laboratories) can result in much more rapid detection of the presence of mycobacteria than can usually be achieved by conventional culture. Detection times for the Bactec average approximately 10 days, as opposed to 17 days for conventional culture methods. Briefly, the organisms multiply in the broth and metabolize ^{14}C-containing metabolites, producing radioactively labeled $^{14}CO_2$ in the atmosphere that collects above the broth in the bottle. The Bactec instrument withdraws this CO_2-containing atmosphere and measures the amount of radioactivity present. Those bottles that yield a radioactive index, called a "growth index," greater than 10 are considered to be positive. The broth culture can be further

tested for identification of tuberculosis complex organisms by an additional procedure.

Although the exact procedure for culturing specimens using the Bactec should be obtained from the manufacturer, a brief outline of the use of this instrument is presented here. After the specimen has been digested and decontaminated, using 4% NaOH and NALC, the sediment is resuspended in sterile distilled water to a total volume of approximately 2 ml. A small quantity of this suspension (0.1-0.2 ml) is injected into each of two Bactec bottles, one containing Middlebrook 7H12 broth and one containing 7H12 with added antimicrobial agents. The rest of the sediment is used for inoculation to conventional media and smear preparation. Cultures are incubated as above, and Bactec bottles are incubated in air at 37° C. The bottles are tested for $^{14}CO_2$ production three times weekly for 6 weeks. Bottles that register a growth index greater than 10 are subcultured to media and smeared for acid fast stain. Broth from bottles registering a growth index greater than 50 are split into two samples, each of which is injected into a fresh bottle of medium. A 5 µg quantity of para-nitro-alpha-acetylamino-beta-hydroxypropiophenone (NAP) is added to one of the bottles, and they are both reincubated. These two bottles are then tested on the Bactec daily for 4 days. An increase in the growth index in the unaltered control bottle without a corresponding increase of the growth index in the bottle containing NAP indicates the presence of *M. tuberculosis* or *M. bovis*, both of which are susceptible to NAP. NAP does not inhibit growth of MOTT. An additional medium containing TCH (thiophene-2-carboxylate hydrazide), to which only *M. bovis* is susceptible, can be used to separate *M. tuberculosis* and *M. bovis*. Definitive identification of mycobacteria other than the tuberculosis complex requires biochemical testing of isolated colonies, of course.

The Bactec system has also been adapted for performance of mycobacterial susceptibility testing. Sediments from acid fast, smear-positive specimens are inoculated into Bactec bottles containing special Middlebrook 7H12 with antimicrobial agents and a control broth without antimicrobial agents. The bottles are incubated for a maximum of 2 weeks, and the growth index readings from the antibiotic-containing bottles are compared to those of the control. Once the growth index in the control bottle reaches 20, the test can be reported. A change in the growth index in the antibiotic media that is equal to or greater than that in the control medium indicates resistance, and a greater change in the control indicates susceptibility. Results of trials of this method compared with the conventional direct susceptibility testing method indicate that the Bactec agreed very well with conventional results, especially when large numbers of organisms were present in the sediment. The radiometric mycobacterial culturing and susceptibility testing systems are continuously improving. At this time, conventional media should be inoculated in addition to Bactec media for detection and isolation of mycobacteria.

41.7. Initial Identification Tests: Pigment Production and Growth Rate

The preliminary identification of mycobacterial isolates depends on their colony morphology, pigment production, and growth rates, as outlined in Figure 41.1. Some guidelines for initial handling of colonies that appear after several days of incubation are outlined here. These procedures are modified from material published by George Kubica and the Bacteriology Training Section of the Centers for Disease Control. Quality control organisms should be tested along with unknowns, as listed in Table 41.4. The commonly used quality control organisms can be maintained in broth at room temperature and transferred monthly. In this way, they will always be available for inoculation to test media along with suspensions of the unknown mycobacteria being tested.

The first test that must always be performed on colonies growing on mycobacterial media is an acid fast stain to confirm that the colonies are indeed mycobacteria. At this point, inoculate several colonies of the organism to 5 ml of Middlebrook 7H9 broth (available from several commercial suppliers) and incubate the broth at 35° C for 5-7 days with daily agitation (with the cap tightened shut) to enhance growth. If there is sufficient growth on the original Löwenstein-Jensen medium, the Löwenstein-Jensen slant can be used for performance of the niacin test, as outlined below. The broth subculture can be used for inoculation of all test media, including biochemical tests as well as pigmentation and growth rate determinations (Procedure 41.5). It is up to the microbiologist to determine whether all tests are inoculated initially at the same time or whether the results of growth rate and pigment production are determined before additional tests are set up. Some observations about colony morphology and permissive incubation temperatures of mycobacteria that may be found in clinical specimens are listed in Table 41.5.

The dilution of the organism used to assess growth rate is critical. Even slow-growing mycobacteria will appear to produce colonies in less than 7 days if the inoculum is too heavy. One organism particularly likely to exhibit false positive rapid growth is *M. flavescens*. This species therefore serves as an excellent quality control organism for this procedure.

41.8. Performance of Specific Identification Tests and Quality Control

Once an unknown acid fast bacillus is placed into a category based on growth rate and pigment production, a series of other tests is used to identify species. Not all tests are necessary for the identification of most species. The performance of each of the important tests is described below, as well as the primary organ-

Text continued on p. 618.

TABLE 41.4
Controls and Media Used and Duration of Tests

NO.	BIOCHEMICAL TEST	CONTROL ORGANISMS		RESULT		MEDIUM USED AND AMOUNT	DURATION OF TEST	REMARKS
		POSITIVE	NEGATIVE	POSITIVE	NEGATIVE			
1	Niacin	M. tuberculosis	M. avium	Yellow	No change of color	0.5 ml DH$_2$O	30 min	Room temperature
2	Nitrate	M. tuberculosis M. szulgai (weak)	M. avium	Pink or red	No change of color	0.3 ml 7H9	2 h	37° C bath
3	Urease	M. tuberculosis	M. avium	Pink or red	No change of color	0.5 ml DH$_2$O	2 h	37° C bath
4	68° C Catalase	M. avium	M. tuberculosis	Bubbles	No bubbles	0.5 ml phosphate buffer [pH 7]	30 min	68° C bath
5	S.Q. Catalase	M. kansasii	M. avium	>45 mm	≤40 mm	Commercial medium	14 days	37° C incubator [with CO$_2$]
6	Tween 80	M. kansasii	M. tuberculosis	Pink or red	No change of color	1 ml DH$_2$O	5 days	37° C incubator [without CO$_2$]
7	Tellurite	M. avium	M. tuberculosis	Smooth fine black precipitate (smokelike action)	Gray clumps (no smokelike action)	Middlebrook 7H9 broth	10 days	37° C incubator [with CO$_2$]
8	Arylsulfatase	M. fortuitum	Medium	Pink or red	No change of color	Wayne's aryl-sulfatase medium	3 days	37° C incubator [without CO$_2$]
9	5% NaCl	M. fortuitum	M. tuberculosis	Substantial growth	Little or no growth	Commercial slant	28 days	37° C incubator [with CO$_2$]
10	TCH	M. bovis	M. tuberculosis	No growth	Growth	TCH flat and L-J	8 weeks	37° C incubator [with CO$_2$]

From Berlin, O.G.W., and Martin, W.J. 1980. Clin. Microbiol. Newsletter 2:4, 1980.

PROCEDURE 41.5. DETERMINATION OF PIGMENT PRODUCTION
AND GROWTH RATE

1. After the broth culture has incubated for 5-7 days, adjust the turbidity to that of a McFarland 0.5 standard by adding additional broth to more turbid suspensions. If the broth is less turbid than a McFarland 0.5, use a correspondingly lower dilution for the inoculum.
2. Dilute the broth (McFarland 0.5 turbidity) 10^{-4} by adding 0.1 ml broth suspension to 9.9 ml sterile distilled water (making a 1:100 dilution) and then repeating the same procedure for a final dilution of 1:10,000.
3. Inoculate 0.1 ml of the broth to each of three tubes of Löwenstein-Jensen agar. Completely wrap two of the tubes in aluminum foil so as to block all light. If the isolate was obtained from a skin lesion, or the initial colony was yellow pigmented (possible *M. szulgai*), six tubes should be inoculated. The second set of tubes, two of them also wrapped with aluminum foil, is incubated at 30° C, or at room temperature if a 30° C incubator is not available.
4. Examine the cultures after 5 and 7 days for the appearance of grossly visible colonies. Examine again at intervals of 3 days.
   Interpretation: Rapid growers produce visible colonies in less than 7 days; slow growers require more than 7 days.
5. As soon as growth is visible in the unwrapped culture, one of the aluminum foil–wrapped tubes is unwrapped and exposed to a bright light, such as a desk lamp, for 2 h. The cap must be loose during exposure, since pigment production is an oxygen-dependent reaction. The tube is rewrapped and returned to the incubator, and the cap is left loose.
6. The three tubes are examined 24 and 48 h after light exposure. For tubes incubating at 30° C, pigment may require 72 h for development.
7. Results are interpreted as shown in Plate 41.1.

TABLE 41.5
Distinctive Properties of Cultivable Mycobacteria Encountered in Clinical Specimens[a]

COMPLEX[b]	SPECIES	CLINICAL SIGNIFI-CANCE[c]	GROWTH RATE[d] AT				COLONY TYPE		NIACIN	SUSCEPTIBILITY TO T2H[g] (5 µG/ML)	NITRATE REDUCTION
			45° C	37° C	31° C	24° C	USUAL COLONY MORPHOLOGY[e]	PIGMENTATION[f]			
	M. ulcerans	1	–	–	S	–	R	N	–	–	–
TB	M. tuberculosis	1	–	S	S	–	R	N	+	–	+
	M. bovis	1	–	S		–	Rt	N	–	+	–
	M. marinum	2		∓	M	M	S/SR	P	∓	–	–
	M. kansasii	2		S	S	S	SR/S	P	–	–	+
	M. simiae	3-2	–	S			S	P	+	–	–
	M. asiaticum		–	S		S	S	P	–	–	–
M. scrofula-ceum	M. scrofula-ceum	3-2		S	S	S	S	S	–	–	–
	M. szulgai	1		S	S	S	S or R	S/P	–	–	+
	M. gordonae	4		S		S	S	S	–	–	–
	M. flavescens	4		M		M	S	S[j]	–	–	+
	M. xenopi	3	S	S			Sf	S	–	–	–
M. avium	M. avium	2	–/+	S		±	St/R	N	–	–	–
	M. intracel-lulare	2	–/+	S		±	St/R	N	–	–	–
	M. gastri	4		S		S	S/SR/R	N	–	–	–
	M. mal-moense	1		S	S	S	S	N	–	–	–
	M. haemo-philum	1	–	–	S[k]	S	R	N	–	–	–
	M. nonchro-mogenicum	4		S		S	SR	N	–	–	+
M. terrae	M. terrae	4		S		S	SR	N	–	–	+
	M. triviale	4		M		S	R	N	–	–	+
M. fortuitum	M. fortuitum	4-3	–	R		R	Sf/Rf	N	–	–	+
	M. chelonei	4-3	–	R		R	S/R	N	V	–	–
	M. phlei	4	R	R	R	R	R	S			+
	M. smegmatis	4	R	R	R	R	R/S	N			+
	M. vaccae	4		R		R	S	S			+

From Sommers, H.M., and Good, R.C. 1985. *Mycobacterium.* In Lennette, E.H., Balows, A., Hausler, W.J. Jr., and Shadomy
[a]Plus and minus signs indicate the presence or absence, respectively, of the feature; blank spaces indicate either that the infor
[b]For most clinical laboratories, designation to the complex is usually sufficient.
[c]Potential clinical significance: 1, present only as pathogens; 2, present usually as pathogens; 3, present commonly as nonpatho
[d]S, Slow; M, moderate; R, rapid.
[e]R, Rough, S, smooth; SR, intermediate in roughness; t, thin or transparent; f, filamentous extensions.
[f]P, Photochromogenic; S, scotochromogenic; N, nonphotochromogenic. Note: *M. szulgai* is scotochromogenic at 37° C an
[g]TCH, Thiophene-2-carboxylic acid hydrazide.
[h]Tween hydrolysis may be + at 10 days.
[i]Arylsulfatase, 14 days, is +.
[j]Young cultures may be nonchromogenic or possess only pale pigment which may intensify with age.
[k]Requires hemin as a growth factor.
[l]*M. chelonei* subsp. *chelonei* is –, *M. chelonei* subsp. *abscessus* is +.

SEMIQUANTI-TATIVE CATALASE (>45 MM)	68° C CATA-LASE	TWEEN HYDROLYSIS, 5 DAYS	TELLURITE REDUCTION	TOLERANCE TO 5% NaCl	IRON UPTAKE	ARYLSUL-FATASE, 3 DAYS	MacCONKEY AGAR	UREASE	PYRAZIN-AMIDASE, 4 DAYS
−	+	−		−		−		−	−
−	−	−ʰ	∓	−	−	−	−	+	+
−	−	−	∓	−	−	−	−	+	−
−	−	+	∓	−	−	∓ⁱ	−	+	+
+	+	+	∓	−	−	−	−	+	−
+	+	−	+	−	−	−		+	+
+	+	+	−	−	−	−		−	−
+	+	−	∓	−	−	V	−	+	±
+	+	∓ʰ	±	−	−	V	−	+	+
+	+	+	−	−	−	V	−	−	∓
+	+	+	∓	+	−	−	−	+	+
−	+	−	∓	−	−	+	−	−	V
−	±	−	+	−	−	−	∓	−	+
−	±	−	+	−	−	−	∓	−	+
−	−	+	∓	−	−	−	−	+	−
−	±	+	+	−	−	−	−	V	+
−	−	−	−	−	−	−	−	−	+
+	+	+	−	−	−	−	V	−	V
+	+	+	−	−	−	−	V	−	V
+	+	+	−	+	−	∓	−	−	V
+	+	V	+	+	+	+	+	+	+
+	V	V	+	Vˡ	−	+	+	+	+
+	+	+	+	+	+	−	−		
+	+	+	+	+	+	−	−		
+	+	+	+	V	+	−	−		

J., editors. Manual of clinical microbiology, ed. 4. American Society for Microbiology, Washington, D.C.
ation is not currently available or that the property is unimportant. V, Variable; ±, usually present; ±, usually absent.

ns; 4, present usually as nonpathogens.

otochromogenic at 25° C.

isms for which the test is used. At the same time that the unknown organism is inoculated to test media, the quality control organisms (Table 41.4) are also inoculated to test media for performance of the same tests.

41.8.a. Niacin test. The most important organism to identify quickly is *M. tuberculosis*, since it is the only one that can be easily spread from human to human, and thus its detection is a matter of public health importance. Niacin serves as a precursor in the biosynthetic pathways of coenzyme production in all mycobacteria. *M. tuberculosis*, *M. simiae*, occasional *M. chelonei*, *M. marinum*, and BCG lack an enzyme that further converts niacin to another metabolite. Niacin therefore accumulates in the medium in which these organisms are growing. A positive niacin test is preliminary evidence that an organism that exhibits a buff-colored, slow-growing, rough colony may be *M. tuberculosis*. This test is not sufficient, however, for confirmation of the identification. If sufficient growth is present on the initial Löwenstein-Jensen slant (the egg-base medium enhances accumulation of free niacin), a niacin test can be performed immediately. If growth on the initial culture was scanty, the subculture used for growth rate determination can be used. If this culture yields only rare colonies, the colonies should be spread around with a sterile cotton swab (after the growth rate has been determined) to distribute the inoculum over the entire slant, which is then reincubated until light growth over the surface of the medium is visible. For reliable results, the niacin test should be performed only from cultures on Löwenstein-Jensen that are at least 3 weeks old and show at least 50 colonies.

PROCEDURE 41.6. NIACIN TEST WITH COMMERCIALLY AVAILABLE PAPER STRIPS (AVAILABLE FROM DIFCO LABORATORIES)

1. Add 1 ml sterile distilled water to the surface of the egg-based medium on which the colonies to be tested are growing.
2. Lay the tube horizontal, so that the fluid is in contact with the entire surface. With the pipette used to add the water, scratch or lightly poke through the surface of the agar; this allows niacin in the medium to dissolve in the water.
3. Allow the tube to sit for 15 min at room temperature. It can incubate longer to achieve a stronger reaction.
4. Remove 0.6 ml of the distilled water (which appears cloudy at this point) to a clean, 12 × 75 mm screw cap or snap top test tube. Insert a niacin test strip with the arrow down, following manufacturer's instructions.
5. Cap the tube tightly and incubate at room temperature, occasionally shaking the tube to mix the fluid with the reagent on the bottom of the strip.
6. After 20 min, observe the color of the liquid against a white background (Plate 41.2). Yellow liquid indicates a positive test. The color of the strip should not be considered when evaluating results. If the liquid is clear, the test is negative.
7. Discard the strip into alkaline disinfectant (10% NaOH) to neutralize the cyanogen bromide.
8. Negative tests may be repeated after an additional 3-5 weeks of incubation of the test medium.

Classic tests for niacin involve cyanogen bromide, which is hazardous to use and presents disposal problems. For this reason, a method that utilizes reagent-impregnated paper strips should be used. The results are comparable and the procedure is simple (Procedure 41.6). Control organisms are inoculated at the same time as the test organisms, as listed in Table 41.4.

41.8.b. Nitrate test. The test for reduction of nitrate, carried out by the enzyme nitroreductase, distinguishes between several species of mycobacteria within all morphologic groups (Table 41.6). Rapid growers may be tested after 2 weeks of incubation, but most organisms require 4 weeks of incubation of the subculture for demonstration of a positive nitrate test. Commercially available nitrate strips yield acceptable results only with strongly nitrate positive organisms, such as *M. tuberculosis*. This test (Procedure 41.7) may be tried first because of its ease of performance. The *M. tuberculosis* positive control must be strongly positive in

TABLE 41.6
Nitrate Reduction Test

GROUP	POSITIVE	NEGATIVE
Slow-growing nonphoto-chromogens	*M. tuberculosis*	*M. bovis* *M. simiae*
Slow-growing scotochromogens	*M. szulgai* (weak) *M. flavescens*	*M. scrofulaceum* *M. gordonae*
Rapid-growing nonphoto-chromogens	*M. fortuitum*	*M. chelonei*
Photochromogens	*M. kansasii*	*M. marinum* *M. asiaticum* *M. simiae*

PROCEDURE 41.7. NITRATE TEST WITH COMMERCIALLY AVAILABLE PAPER STRIPS (AVAILABLE FROM DIFCO LABORATORIES)

1. Add 1 ml sterile saline to a sterile 13 × 100 ml screw cap test tube.
2. Emulsify two very large clumps of growth from a 4-week-old culture in the saline. The solution should be very turbid (milky).
3. Using sterile forceps, carefully insert a nitrite test strip according to the package insert instructions. The strip should only touch the fluid at the bottom of the tube, not the sides. These strips should be stored refrigerated in the dark. Discolored strips have deteriorated and should not be used.
4. Cap the tube tightly and incubate upright for 2 h at 37° C. Incubation in a water bath will insure maintenance of adequate temperature.
5. After the first hour, shake the tube gently without tilting.
6. After the 2 h incubation, tilt the tube six times, wetting the entire strip.
7. Place the tube in a slanted position for 10 min with the liquid covering the strip.
8. Observe the top portion of the strip for any blue color change, indicating a positive reaction. A negative reaction (lack of nitroreductase) yields no color change.

PROCEDURE 41.8. NITRATE TEST USING CHEMICAL REAGENTS

1. Prepare the dry crystalline reagent as follows:

Sulfanilic acid (Sigma Chemical Co.)	1 part
N-(1-naphthyl) ethylenediamine dihydrochloride	1 part
(Eastman Chemical Co.)	
1-Tartaric acid (Sigma)	10 parts

   These crystals can be measured out with any small scoop or tiny spoon, since the proportions are by volume, not weight. The mixture should be ground in a mortar and pestle to insure adequate mixing, because the crystals are of different textures. The reagent can be stored in a dark glass bottle at room temperature for at least 6 months.
2. Add 0.2 ml sterile distilled water to a 16 × 125 mm screw cap tube. Emulsify two very large clumps of growth from a 4 week culture on Löwenstein-Jensen agar in the water. The suspension should be milky.
3. Add 2 ml nitrate substrate broth (Difco Laboratories or Remel Laboratories) to the suspension and cap tightly.
4. Shake gently and incubate upright for 2 h in a 37° C waterbath.
5. Remove from water bath and add a small amount of the crystalline reagent. A wooden stick or a small spatula can be used to add crystals; the amount is not critical.
6. Examine immediately for a pink to red color, indicating the presence of nitrite, demonstrating the ability of the organism to reduce nitrate to nitrite.
7. If no color results, the organisms may have reduced nitrate beyond nitrite (as in the conventional nitrate test, Chapter 9). Add a small amount of powdered zinc to the negative tube. If a red color develops, that indicates that unreduced nitrate was present in the tube and the organism was nitroreductase negative. Compare results to those obtained using the quality control organisms, including the weakly positive control.

the strip test or the test results will be unreliable. If the paper strip test is negative or if the control test result is not strongly positive, the chemical procedure (Procedure 41.8) must be carried out, using strong and weakly positive controls. Steps and reagents used for performing the classic chemical nitrate procedure are outlined in detail in the CDC manual by Vestal.[10]

41.8.c. Catalase test. Acid fast bacilli produce the enzyme **catalase**, which is detected by the breakdown of hydrogen peroxide and the subsequent active ebullition of gas (oxygen) bubbles. Detection of catalase activity, which should be tested routinely, has proved useful in several ways: (1) tubercle bacilli that become resistant to INH lose or show reduced catalase activity, (2) the catalase activity of human or bovine strains may be selectively inhibited by heat, and (3) *M. gastri* and isolates of clinically insignificant *M. kansasii* also lose their catalase activity at pH 7 and at 68° C.

Catalase is measured in two ways: (1) by the relative activity of the enzyme, as determined

PROCEDURE 41.9. SEMIQUANTITATIVE (S.Q.) CATALASE TEST

1. Prepare 10% Tween 80 solution as follows:

Tween 80 (Difco Laboratories)	10 ml
Distilled water	90 ml

   Mix together and autoclave for 10 min at 121° C. Swirl solution after autoclaving to disperse Tween. Store in refrigerator. This reagent is also available from Remel Laboratories and can be stored for at least 6 months.
2. Inoculate the surface of a 5 ml Löwenstein-Jensen agar butt tube (available commercially) with 0.1 ml of the broth subculture originally made for preparing the inoculum for the growth rate and pigment tests (described above). Inoculate tubes with the quality control organisms at the same time.
3. Incubate tubes with caps loose for 2 weeks at 35° C.
4. Prepare hydrogen peroxide reagent fresh for each use:

30% hydrogen peroxide (Superoxol, Merck Chemical Co.)	1 part
10% Tween 80	1 part

   Make 1 ml of the hydrogen peroxide reagent for each test to be performed.
5. Place the tubes upright in a rack which is standing in a tray lined with paper towels soaked with disinfectant. The tray must be autoclavable and waterproof. The column of bubbles produced by this test often tends to overflow; the tray will catch the overflow. If the microbiologist is quick enough, he or she can tighten the cap on a vigorously bubbling tube before it flows out the top.
6. Add 1 ml hydrogen peroxide reagent to each tube and to a control tube that was not inoculated with bacteria.
7. Allow tubes to stand and column of bubbles to develop for 5 min before measuring the height of the column of bubbles above the surface of the medium. Alternatively, a line can be drawn on the side of each tube at a height of 45 mm above the agar surface before the reagent is added. Cultures whose bubbles rise above the line are considered positive; those with bubble column heights less than 45 mm are considered negative (Plate 41.3).
8. If the height of the column of bubbles is between 31 and 45 mm, the test should be considered equivocal and repeated.

by the height of a column of bubbles of oxygen formed by the action of untreated enzyme produced by the organism (**semiquantitative [S.Q.] catalase test,** Procedure 41.9), and (2) by the ability of the catalase enzyme to remain active after heating, a measure of the heat stability of the enzyme (**heat stable catalase test,** Procedure 41.10).

41.8.d. Hydrolysis of Tween 80. The commonly nonpathogenic slow-growing scotochromogens and nonphotochromogens produce a lipase that is able to hydrolyze Tween 80 (the detergent polyoxyethylene sorbitan monooleate) into oleic acid and polyoxyethylated sorbitol, whereas pathogenic species do not. Intact Tween 80 binds the phenol red indicator, caus-

PROCEDURE 41.10. HEAT STABLE (68° C, pH 7.0) CATALASE TEST

1. Prepare 1/15 M phosphate buffer, pH 7.0 as follows:
   Solution A

Na_2HPO_4 (anhydrous)	9.47 g
Distilled water	1,000 ml

   Solution B

KH_2PO_4	9.07 g
Distilled water	1,000 ml

   Mix 61.1 ml of solution A with 38.9 ml of solution B and check that the pH is 7.0. Adjust if necessary. Since the suspension will only be tested for a short time, the buffer need not be sterile. Store the two solutions in the refrigerator.
2. Suspend several large clumps of growth from an actively growing agar slant in 0.5 ml of the phosphate buffer in a 16 × 125 mm screw cap test tube. Prepare control organisms in the same way.
3. Incubate all tubes for exactly 20 min in a 68° C heat block or water bath. The temperature must be strictly monitored during the entire incubation.
4. Cool the suspensions to room temperature.
5. Add 0.5 ml of the Tween–hydrogen peroxide solution (same as above) and observe for formation of bubbles. Negative tubes should be held for 20 min before reporting as negative. Observe very carefully, since even a few tiny bubbles are indicative of a positive result. The tubes must not be agitated in any way, since Tween will bubble if shaken.

PROCEDURE 41.11. TWEEN 80 HYDROLYSIS TEST

1. Prepare Tween 80 hydrolysis substrate from concentrate according to manufacturer's instructions.
2. Inoculate the substrate with one large clump of actively growing mycobacteria from an agar slant. Inoculate control substrate tubes at the same time.
3. Incubate at 35° C.
4. Examine after 1, 5, and 10 days for a change in the substrate from orange to pink. Compare the color to an uninoculated substrate control. Tubes should not be shaken during reading.

TABLE 41.7
Tween 80 Hydrolysis Test

GROUP	POSITIVE	NEGATIVE
Photochromogens	M. kansasii M. marinum M. asiaticum	M. simiae
Nonphotochromogens	M. gastri M. terrae complex M. malmoense	M. bovis M. avium complex M. xenopi M. simiae M. haemophilum
Scotochromogens	M. szulgai (slow) M. gordonae M. flavescens	M. scrofulaceum M. xenopi

41.1

PLATE 41.1.   Initial grouping of mycobacteria based on pigment production before and after exposure to light. In one test system, subcultures of each isolate are grown on two agar slants. One tube is wrapped in aluminum foil to prevent exposure of the organism to light, and the other tube is allowed light exposure. After sufficient growth is present, the wrapped tube is unwrapped, and the tubes are examined together. **Photochromogens** are unpigmented when grown in the dark (tube A) and develop pigment after light exposure (tube B). **Scotochromogens** are pigmented in the dark (tube C); the color does not intensify after exposure to light (tube D). **Nonphotochromogens** are nonpigmented when grown in the dark (tube E) and remain so even after light exposure (tube F).

41.2

41.3

41.4

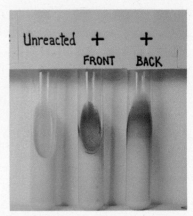

41.5

PLATE 41.2.   Niacin test performed with filter paper strips. The positive test *(right)* displays a yellow color and the negative result remains milky white or clear.

PLATE 41.3.   Semiquantitative catalase test. The tube on the left contains a column of bubbles that has risen past the line indicating 45 mm height (a positive test). The tube on the right is the negative control.

PLATE 41.4.   A positive arylsulfatase test is shown on the left; the tube containing the negative control is on the right.

PLATE 41.5.   Iron uptake test for mycobacteria.

41.6

41.7

PLATE 41.6. *Mycobacterium tuberculosis* colonies on Lowenstein-Jensen agar after 8 weeks of incubation.
PLATE 41.7. *Mycobacterium kansasii* colonies exposed to light.

41.8

41.9

PLATE 41.8. Scotochromogen *Mycobacterium* with yellow colonies.
PLATE 41.9. *Mycobacterium avium* complex. Smooth colonies on L-J medium.

41.10

PLATE 41.10. *Mycobacterium phlei* (rapid grower). Rough colonies.

41.11

PLATE 41.11. Smooth, multilobate colonies of *Mycobacterium fortuitum* on L-J medium.

PROCEDURE 41.12. ARYLSULFATASE TEST

1. Prepare enzyme substrate stock solution as follows:

Phenolphthalein disulfate, tripotassium salt (Sigma Chemical Co.)	2.6 g
Distilled water	50 ml

   a. Mix thoroughly to make a 0.08 M solution. Sterilize through a 0.2 μm pore size membrane filter. Store refrigerated.

   b. Prepare two flasks of 180 ml each of basal Middlebrook 7H9 or Dubos-Tween-albumin broth (from commercial dry powder). Autoclave for 15 min at 121° C and cool to room temperature. Aseptically add one 20 ml vial of Middlebrook albumin-dextrose-catalase (ADC) enrichment to each flask.

   c. For the 3 day test, aseptically add 2.5 ml of the enzyme substrate stock to one flask, for a final concentration of 0.001 M phenolphthalein substrate.

   d. For the 14 day test, add 7.5 ml of the substrate stock, to the other flask, for a concentration of 0.003 M substrate.

   e. These two reagents should be dispensed in 2 ml amounts into 16 × 125 mm screw cap test tubes. Store at room temperature. The substrates are also available commercially (ready-made) from Remel Laboratories.

2. Prepare the alkaline indicator solution (6 N sodium carbonate) as follows:

Na_2CO_3, anhydrous	10.6 g
Distilled water	100 ml

   Mix together

3. Inoculate tubes of the 3 day substrate and the 14 day substrate with 0.1 ml of the broth culture originally set up for determination of growth rates and pigment production. Alternatively, a heavy inoculum of material from an agar slant is acceptable.

4. After 3 days' incubation at 35° C, 6 drops of the sodium carbonate is added to the 3 day 0.001 M substrate.

5. After 14 days' incubation, 6 drops of the sodium carbonate solution is added to the 14 day 0.003 M substrate.

6. Observe for an immediate color change to pink or red after addition of carbonate, indicating a positive result for arylsulfatase (Plate 41.4).

ing it to assume the structure it would normally assume only at a more acid pH. When Tween 80 is hydrolyzed, it no longer binds the indicator, allowing it to assume its normal configuration at pH 7.0, which is visible to us as pink or red. This pink color, which is the sign of a positive reaction, does not result from a pH shift, but results from a breakdown of the Tween 80.

Tween 80 hydrolysis (Procedure 41.11) is useful for separating species of photochromogens, nonphotochromogens, and scotochromogens, as shown in Table 41.7. Because laboratory-prepared media have a very short shelf life, the CDC recommends the use of a commercial Tween 80 hydrolysis substrate (Difco Laboratories or Remel Laboratories) which is stable for up to 1 year.

41.8.e. Arylsulfatase test (Procedure 41-12). The enzyme arylsulfatase, which splits free phenolphthalein from the tripotassium salt of phenolphthalein disulfate, is present in most mycobacteria. Varying the test conditions helps to differentiate different forms of the enzyme. The 3 day test is particularly useful for identifying the potentially pathogenic rapid growers, *M. fortuitum*, *M. triviale*, and *M. chelonei*. Slow growing *M. marinum* and *M. szulgai* are positive in the 14 day test.

41.8.f. Growth inhibition by thiophene-2-carboxylic acid hydrazide (TCH). Only *M. bovis* is unable to grow in the presence of 5 μg/ml TCH. Because small amounts of niacin may be produced by some strains of *M. bovis*, it is recommended that all isolates resembling *M. tuberculosis* be tested against this compound. Performance of this test is outlined in Procedure 41.13.

41.8.g. Other tests. Tests other than those mentioned here are often performed to make more subtle distinctions between species. They include the ability to grow using only sodium citrate or mannitol as a sole source of carbon, used to distinguish between certain rapid growers. *M. fortuitum* and most other rapid growers are able to convert ferric ammonium citrate to iron oxide. The **iron uptake test** is useful for separating *M. chelonei*, which is unable to convert iron in this way (Plate 41.5). **Ability to grow on MacConkey agar** without crystal violet can help to identify *M. fortuitum*, which is not inhibited by the medium. Pyrazinamide can be deaminated by *M. tuberculosis* and the *M. avium* complex, as well as by *M. marinum*, whereas *M. bovis* and *M. kansasii* do not possess the enzyme **pyrazinamidase**. The inability of *M. chelonei* to grow in 5% NaCl is yet another test for differentiating this organism from *M. fortuitum*. Most rapid growers and some *M. flavescens* strains will grow on medium containing such high salt concentrations. **Reduction of potassium tellurite** to a

---

PROCEDURE 41.13. TCH SUSCEPTIBILITY

1. Prepare the TCH agar as follows:
   Prepare Middlebrook 7H10 agar according to manufacturer's instructions, adding the enrichment when the agar has cooled to 55° C. At this time, also add sufficient filter-sterilized TCH (Aldrich Chemical Co.) to make a final concentration of 5 μg/ml. Chapter 13 discusses methods for making such solutions. Mix the agar thoroughly. Also prepare drug-free control agar. Pour the molten agar into quadrants of Felsen Petri dishes, 5 ml per quadrant. Allow the plates to set.
2. Make dilutions of the 7-day-old broth culture that was originally inoculated for preparation of the growth control, 1:1,000 and 1:10,000, in sterile water or saline, as described in Procedure 41.5.
3. Inoculate 0.1 ml of each dilution to one drug-containing and one control agar medium. Incubate for 3 weeks in 10% CO_2 at 35° C.
4. Organisms are resistant to TCH if growth in the TCH-containing medium is equal to or exceeds 1% of the growth on the control agar. Results are interpreted much as are those of susceptibility tests, described in Chapter 13.

black precipitate within 3 days by rapid growers and *M. avium* complex distinguishes these organisms. The tellurite reduction test is also important for differentiating *M. malmoense* (very unusual isolate) from the saprophytes *M. gastri* and *M. terrae*. The **urease test** for hydrolysis of urea by mycobacteria can provide valuable information. As it is currently performed, however, results vary among laboratories, and no reliable method can be recommended.

It is not cost-effective for routine clinical microbiology laboratories to be able to perform all of the procedures necessary for definitive identification of mycobacteria, since excellent reference laboratories are available in every state. With a minimal number of basic procedures, however, the great bulk of all strains isolated can be presumptively identified and those that require further testing can be identified as such and forwarded to regional laboratories.

41.8.h. New approaches to mycobacterial identification. New approaches are being explored for identification of the mycobacteria because, as can be appreciated from the number of tests necessary, the difficulty in performing them, and the time needed for the organisms to grow, the state of the art is somewhat archaic. Thin-layer chromatography and gas liquid chromatography have seemed logical choices for test systems, because cell wall lipids lend themselves to such procedures. Workers such as Tisdall, De Young, Roberts, and Anhalt and Brennan, Heifers, and Ullom have used chromatographic methods for identification of clinical isolates of mycobacteria. Citations from these authors are listed in the bibliography. The patterns produced by the mycobacterial nucleic acids after restriction endonuclease treatment and gel electrophoresis have also proved useful for separating the bacilli into species. These tests are not yet within the realm of routine microbiology laboratories, although a number of larger laboratories are beginning to use such methods on a routine basis.

Many of the MOTT mycobacterial groups have been characterized by serotyping schemes and phage typing. In particular, the *M. avium* complex has been studied and defined serologically and by phage grouping. Once serovars are established, more sensitive techniques, such as ELISA, may prove useful for rapid identification of clinically relevant strains. At this time, there are no commercial products to aid microbiologists in the slow task of identifying mycobacterial species.

41.9. Brief Discussion of Individual Organisms

41.9.a. *Mycobacterium tuberculosis.* Colonies of human tubercle bacilli generally appear on egg media after 2-3 weeks at 35° C; no growth occurs at 25° or 45° C. Growth first appears as small (1-3 mm), dry, friable colonies that are rough, warty, granular, and buff colored. After several weeks these increase in size (up to 5-8 mm); typical colonies have a flat irregular margin and a "cauliflower" center (Plate 41.6). Because of their luxuriant growth, these mycobacteria are termed **eugonic.** Colonies are easily detached from the medium's surface but are difficult to emulsify. After some experience with mycobacteria has been gained, one can recognize typical colonies of human-type tubercle bacilli without great difficulty. However, final confirmation by biochemical tests must be carried out in all cases.

Virulent strains tend to orient themselves in tight, **serpentine cords,** best observed in smears from the condensation water or by direct observation of colonies on a cord medium. Catalase is produced in moderate amounts but not after heating at 68° C for 20 min in pH 7 phosphate buffer; human strains resistant to isoniazid (INH) are frequently catalase negative and yield smooth colonies on egg media. Nitrate reduction is positive. The niacin test (Procedure 41.5) is useful in that most **niacin-positive** strains encountered in the diagnostic laboratory prove to be *M. tuberculosis.* Susceptibility to antituberculous drugs is characteristically high.

41.9.b. *Mycobacterium bovis*. Bovine tubercle bacilli are rarely isolated in the United States but remain significant pathogens in other parts of the world. They require a longer incubation period—generally 3-6 weeks—and appear as tiny (less than 1 mm), translucent, smooth, pyramidal colonies when grown at 35° C. They adhere to the surface of the medium but are emulsified easily. On the basis of these characteristics, their growth is termed **dysgonic.** On 7H10 the colonies are rough and resemble those of *M. tuberculosis*.

M. bovis grows only at 35° C. It forms serpentine cords in smears from colonies on egg media; the niacin reaction and nitrate reduction tests are negative. *M. bovis* is also susceptible to thiophene-2-carboxylic acid hydrazide (TCH) (unless it is isoniazid resistant), a useful test to differentiate it from other mycobacteria. The susceptibility of *M. bovis* to the primary antituberculous drugs is similar to that of *M. tuberculosis*.

41.9.c. *Mycobacterium ulcerans*. *M. ulcerans* is associated with skin lesions and is considered the causative agent of Buruli ulceration, a necrotizing ulcer found in African natives. The organism requires several weeks' incubation at 32° C. Unlike *M. marinum*, this organism is **nonphotochromogenic.** It is resistant to isoniazid, ethambutol, PAS, and ethionamide, but it is susceptible to rifampin, streptomycin, viomycin, kanamycin, and cycloserine.

41.9.d. *Mycobacterium africanum*. Rarely isolated in the United States, *M. africanum* resembles *M. tuberculosis*. It is very inactive biochemically, showing only positive urease and variably positive ability to grow in the presence of TCH. This species has been isolated from pulmonary cultures of humans as well as from monkeys.

41.9.e. Photochromogens. Four well-defined photochromogenic mycobacteria display pigment after exposure to light: *M. kansasii*, *M. marinum*, *M. simiae*, and *M. asiaticum*. All species in this category are potential pathogens.

M. kansasii organisms are responsible for pulmonary disease in humans, often appearing in white, emphysematous men older than 45 years. The disease with its complications is indistinguishable from that caused by *M. tuberculosis*, but it follows a more chronic and indolent course. Other types of disease, including disseminated infection, may occur. The disease is not communicable, in distinct contrast with that caused by the tubercle bacillus.

Optimal growth of *M. kansasii* occurs after 2-3 weeks at 35° C (slower at 25° C); growth does not occur at 45° C. Colonies are generally smooth, although there is a tendency to develop roughness. They are cream colored when grown in the dark and become a bright **lemon yellow** if exposed to light (Plate 41.7).

If cultures are grown continuously under light (2-3 weeks), bright orange crystals of beta-carotene form on the surface of colonies, especially where growth is heavy. Nonphotochromogenic and scotochromogenic variants of *M. kansasii* occur very rarely.

Clinically significant strains of *M. kansasii* are strongly catalase positive, even after heating at 68° C at pH 7 (especially when using the semiquantitative test of Wayne, Procedure 41.8). Low-catalase strains of *M. kansasii* have been described; these were not associated with human pathogenicity. Most strains do not produce niacin, although aberrant strains have been noted; nitrates are reduced; mature colonies show loose cords.

Stained preparations of *M. kansasii* show characteristically **long, banded, and beaded cells** that are strongly acid fast. There is variable susceptibility to INH and streptomycin, moderate susceptibility to rifampin, and resistance to para-aminosalicylic acid (PAS), but *M. kansasii* infections typically respond to conventional antituberculous therapy; however, triple therapy, including rifampin, is desirable.

Primarily associated with granulomatous lesions of the skin, particularly of the extremities, *M. marinum* infection usually follows exposure of the abraded skin to contaminated water. Known best for causing "swimming pool granuloma," this organism also has been implicated in infections related to home aquariums, bay water, and industrial exposures involving water. It grows best at **25°-32° C,** with sparse to no growth at 35° C (corresponding to the reduced skin temperature of the extremities), and is never isolated from sputum. It may be distinguished from *M. kansasii* by its source, its more rapid growth at 25° C, negative nitrate reduction, and weaker catalase production. The drugs most active against *M. marinum* are amikacin and kanamycin. Tetracyclines are inhibitory, chiefly at concentrations slightly below the expected blood levels.

First isolated from monkeys, *M. simiae* has subsequently been recovered from humans with pulmonary disease. Pigmentation may be erratic. It has a positive niacin reaction, a high thermostable catalase activity, and a negative nitrate test; hydrolyzes Tween 80 slowly (more than 10 days); and is resistant to all first-line antituberculous drugs. It is sensitive to cycloserine and ethionamide.

M. asiaticum grows at 37° C and yields smooth colonies; photochromogenicity may vary with different growth conditions. This species is rarely encountered in the United States. It has been isolated from cases of pulmonary disease in humans and from monkeys. More isolates are needed in order to better define the characteristics of *M. asiaticum.*

41.9.f. Scotochromogens. The **scotochromogens** are **pigmented in the dark** (Greek *scotos*, dark), usually a deep yellow to orange, which darkens to an orange or dark red when the cultures are exposed to continuous light for 2 weeks (Plate 41.8). This pigmentation in the dark occurs on nearly all types of media at all stages of growth—characteristics that clearly aid in their identification.

The scotochromogens include the potential pathogens *M. scrofulaceum, M. szulgai,* and *M. xenopi;* the so-called tap water scotochromogen, isolated from laboratory water stills, faucets, soil, and natural waters (now classified as *M. gordonae*); and *M. flavescens.*

Since the tap water scotochromogen is rarely associated with human disease, it is important to differentiate it from the potentially pathogenic mycobacteria. The former may contaminate equipment used in specimen collection, as in gastric lavage.

M. scrofulaceum is a slow-growing organism, producing smooth, domed to spreading, **yellow** colonies in both light and darkness. When exposed to continuous light, the colonies may increase in pigment to an **orange** or **brick red;** the aluminum foil shield should remain in place (Procedure 41.5) until visible growth occurs in the unshielded tube; then colonies in the shielded tube should be exposed to continuous light. Initial growth may be inhibited by too much light. The hydrolysis of Tween 80 (and urease activity) separates *M. scrofulaceum* from the tap water organisms in that the latter hydrolyze it within 5 days, whereas *M. scrofulaceum* remains negative up to 3 weeks. *M. scrofulaceum* is a cause of cervical adenitis and bone and other infections, particularly in children. It is often resistant to INH and PAS.

M. szulgai has been associated with pulmonary disease, cervical adenitis, cutaneous infection, tenosynovitis, and olecranon bursitis. It gives a positive nitrate reduction test. It is relatively susceptible to ethionamide, rifampin, ethambutol, and higher levels of INH.

M. xenopi has been isolated from the sputum of patients with pulmonary disease. The optimal temparature for its growth is 42° C, and it fails to grow at 22°-25° C. Four to five weeks' incubation is required to produce tiny dome-shaped colonies of a characteristic yellow color; branching **filamentous extensions** are seen around colonies on 7H10 agar, resembling a miniature bird's nest. Tween 80 hydrolysis and tellurite reduction tests are negative. Therapy with standard antituberculous drugs is generally successful.

Growth of *M. gordonae* appears late on L-J and 7H10 media, usually after 2 weeks and frequently after 3-6 weeks, as scattered small yellow-orange colonies in both light and darkness. Hydrolysis of Tween 80 characteristically occurs. *M. flavescens*, another nonpathogenic organism, also produces a yellow-pigmented colony in both light and darkness but is considerably more rapid in growth (usually within 1 week) and reduces nitrate as well as hydrolyzing Tween 80.

41.9.g. Nonphotochromogens. This group of mycobacteria is made up of a heterogeneous variety of both pathogenic and nonpathogenic organisms that do not usually develop pigment on exposure to light. The *M. avium* complex, including *M. avium-intracellulare*, and possibly some strains of *M. scrofulaceum*, grow slowly at 35° C (10-21 days) and 25° C and usually produce thin, translucent, radially lobed to smooth, cream colored colonies (Plate 41.9). Isolates often undergo rapid phase variation to a domed, opaque, yellow colony. This colony is commonly the predominant morphotype initially isolated from patients with AIDS. It has been shown that the rough or opaque colony type is less virulent and that its cell wall is more permeable to antibacterial agents.

Another variant of *M. avium* complex bacilli resembles *M. scrofulaceum* in certain biochemical characteristics; the colonies also become darker yellow with age (unlike other *M. avium* strains). Although biochemical results vary, the majority of isolates of the *M. avium* complex are niacin negative (with rare exceptions), do not reduce nitrate, and produce only a small amount of catalase. Tween 80 is not hydrolyzed in 10 days, but most of these organisms **reduce tellurite** within 3 days, a useful test to differentiate these potential pathogens from clinically insignificant nonphotochromogens.

The *M. avium* complex causes serious tuberculosislike disease that is most difficult to treat. However, these organisms may also occur in clinical specimens as nonpathogens. The organisms are resistant to most antituberculosis drugs. Newer agents such as ansamycin and clofazimine may be partially active against these organisms. Combinations of drugs including ethambutol, rifampin, and amikacin have also had limited success, at least for treatment (but not cure) of the disseminated infection commonly seen in patients with AIDS (Chapter 23). Standard practice has been to use five drugs in combination therapy (if five drugs with in vitro activity can be found).

Mycobacterium gastri ("J" bacillus) has been described as occurring primarily as single colony isolates from gastric washings. However, it has not been associated with disease in humans. It is closely related to the low catalase-producing strains of *M. kansasii*, from which it may be readily differentiated by the photochromogenic ability of the latter. *M. gastri* may be differentiated from other nonphotochromogens by its ability to hydrolyze Tween 80 rapidly, loss of catalase activity at 68° C, and nonreduction of nitrate.

M. malmoense was first described in 1977 in Sweden, where it was found associated with pulmonary disease. Subsequently, it has been found in human pulmonary disease in Australia and Wales. The organism is nonphotochromogenic and grows slowly (2-3 weeks at 37° C and up to 6 weeks at 22° C). Colonies are colorless, smooth, glistening, grayish white, opaque, domed, and circular, 0.5-1.5 mm in diameter. The organism does not produce niacin, is nitrate negative, hydrolyzes Tween 80 and pyrazinamide, and produces heat-labile catalase. It is resistant to isoniazid, streptomycin, PAS, and rifampin and is susceptible to ethambutol, cycloserine, kanamycin, and ethionamide.

M. haemophilum is a recently described organism isolated from skin lesions.[8] It requires hemin for growth and may be isolated on chocolate agar, 7H10 agar containing hemolyzed but not whole sheep red blood cells, or L-J medium containing 1% ferric ammonium citrate. Incubation should be at 32° C for a minimum of 2-4 weeks. The organism does not grow at 37° C. It should not be expected in specimens of sputum or gastric lavage. It is highly resistant to INH, streptomycin, and ethambutol but is susceptible to PAS.

M. terrae complex organisms have been called "radish" bacilli. A number of these mycobacteria have been isolated from soil and vegetables as well as from humans, where their pathogenicity remains questionable. The slow-growing (35° C) colonies may be circular or irregular in shape and smooth or granular in texture. They actively hydrolyze Tween 80, reduce nitrate, and are strong catalase producers, but they do not reduce tellurite in 3 days. *M. terrae* is resistant to INH.

M. triviale ("V" bacilli) occurs on egg media as rough colonies that may be confused with *M. tuberculosis* or rough variants of *M. kansasii*. These bacilli have been recovered from patients with previous tuberculous infections but are considered to be unrelated to human infections. There is one report of human infection with this organism. They are nonphotochromogenic, moderate to strong nitrate reducers, and maintain a high catalase activity at 68° C. They hydrolyze Tween 80 rapidly and do not reduce tellurite.

M. shimoidei was first isolated from a patient in Japan in 1975. It has since been isolated from other patients with pulmonary disease. The organism hydrolyzes Tween 80 and produces heat-stable catalase. Colonies are rough, and growth occurs from 37°-45° C.

41.9.h. Rapid growers. These mycobacteria are characterized by their ability to **grow in 3-5 days** on a variety of culture media, incubated either at 25° or 35° C. Two members, *M. fortuitum* and *M. chelonei*, are associated with human pulmonary infection, although *M. fortuitum* is also a common soil organism and may frequently be recovered from sputum without necessarily being implicated in a pathologic process.

M. smegmatis, *M. phlei* (Plate 41.10) and *M. vaccae* are considered **saprophytes** and are nonpathogenic. *M. smegmatis* and *M. phlei* produce pigmented colonies and show filamentous extensions from colonies growing on cornmealglycerol agar. The ability of *M. phlei* ("hay bacillus") to produce large amounts of CO_2 has been utilized to stimulate primary growth of *M. tuberculosis* on 7H10 agar plates incubated in CO_2-impermeable (Mylar) bags. *M. phlei* also produces the growth factor **mycobactin,** required by some species of *M. avium* complex and the putative Crohn's disease–associated *Mycobacterium.*

M. fortuitum has been incriminated in progressive pulmonary disease, usually with a severe underlying complication, and has resulted in death. This potential pathogen also grows rapidly (2-4 days), is generally nonchromogenic, and may be readily separated from the rapidly growing saprophytes by its **positive 3-day arylsulfatase reaction** and by growing on MacConkey agar within 5 days, producing a change in the indicator. Both rough and smooth colonies are produced, with increased dye absorption (greening) on L-J medium (Plate 41.11). The niacin test is negative.

M. fortuitum is usually resistant to PAS, streptomycin, and INH but is susceptible to amikacin and cefoxitin and often the tetracyclines.

M. chelonei (formerly *M. borstelense*) comprises two distinct subspecies: *M. chelonei* subsp. *chelonei*, which fails to grow on 5% NaCl medium, and *M. chelonei* ss. *abscessus*, which grows on the NaCl medium. *M. fortuitum* and *M. chelonei* are distinguished from each other by the combined use of five tests. *M. fortuitum* is typically nitrate reductase positive, beta-glucosidase positive, penicillinase negative, and trehalose negative and produces acid from fructose. *M. chelonei* has the opposite reactions.

M. chelonei subsp. *abscessus* has been isolated from pulmonary, postsurgical wound, and other infections. There have been several cases of disseminated disease attributed to this species since 1978. *M. chelonei* subsp. *chelonei* is less common, and it has not been isolated from sputum. Infection occurs at the site of an injury that penetrates the skin. The paper by Wallace et al.[11] beautifully describes the current status of rapidly growing mycobacteria as causes of human disease.

M. fallax resembles *M. tuberculosis*, with cord formation on solid media. The organisms grow rapidly only at 30° C and slowly at 37° C. Several strains have been isolated from humans with pulmonary disease; other strains are found in soil and water. The species is nitrate reductase positive and negative for thermostable catalase, arylsulfatase, and urease.

41.9.i. Unclassified *Mycobacterium* associated with Crohn's disease. After long incubation (18 months), colonies are brilliant white and mucoid. With the exception of a weak niacin result, positive 14 day arylsulfatase, and positive thermostable catalase, the isolates are biochemically inactive. Since the organism has been isolated from only 3 of 14 bowel sections from patients with Crohn's disease, definitive characterization is not possible at this time. It is not known whether these organisms contribute to the pathologic condition seen in patients with Crohn's disease.

41.10. Nonculture Methods for Diagnosis

Because the mycobacteria are difficult to isolate, and because there are no serological methods for detecting mycobacterial disease, much attention has been focused on developing ways to diagnose disease without requiring isolation and identification of the organism. The Bactec system is the first step in that direction, but growth of the organism is still a requirement. Recently, an ELISA system (explained in Chapter 12) was developed for detection of antimycobacterial antibody in cerebrospinal

fluid of patients with tuberculous meningitis.[4] This type of rapid diagnostic test should prove very useful. Some studies utilizing GLC analyses of body fluids and serum samples from patients with mycobacterial disease have shown promise, by detecting unusual lipid profiles in patients with disease. No commercial product is yet available for rapid diagnosis of mycobacterial disease.

REFERENCES

1. American Thoracic Society. 1981. Diagnostic standards and classification of tuberculosis and other mycobacterial diseases. American Lung Association Publication. Am. Rev. Respir. Dis. 123:343.
2. Berlin, O.G.W., and Martin, W.J. 1981. Leprosy or Hansen's disease. Clin. Microbiol. Newsletter 3:135.
3. Chiodini, R.J., Van Kruiningen, H.J., Merkal, R.S., et al. 1984. Characteristics of an unclassified *Mycobacterium* species isolated from patients with Crohn's disease. J. Clin. Microbiol. 20:966.
4. Hernandez, R., Munoz, O., and Guiscafre, H. 1984. Sensitive enzyme immunoassay for early diagnosis of tuberculous meningitis. J. Clin. Microbiol. 20:533.
5. Krasnow, I. 1978. Primary isolation of mycobacteria. Lab. Med. 9:26.
6. Kubica, G.P., Gross, W.M., Hawkins, J.E., et al. 1975. Laboratory services for mycobacterial diseases. Am. Rev. Respir. Dis. 112:773.
7. Sommers, H.M., and Good, R.C. 1985. *Mycobacterium*. In Lennette, E.H., Balows, A., Hausler, W.J. Jr., and Shadomy, H.J., editors. Manual of clinical microbiology, ed. 4. American Society for Microbiology, Washington, D.C.
8. Sompolinsky, D., Lagziel, A., Naveh, D., and Yankilevitz, T. 1978. *Mycobacterium haemophilum* sp. nov.: a new pathogen of humans. Int. J. Syst. Bacteriol. 28:67.
9. Swenson, J.M., Thornsberry, C., and Silcox, V. 1982. Rapidly growing mycobacteria: testing of susceptibility to 34 antimicrobial agents by broth microdilution. Antimicrob. Agents Chemother. 22:186.
10. Vestal, A.L. 1975. Procedures for the isolation and identification of mycobacteria. DHEW (CDC 75-8230). Centers for Disease Control, Atlanta.
11. Wallace, R.J. Jr., Swenson, J.M., Silcox, V.A., et al. 1983. Spectrum of disease due to rapidly growing mycobacteria. Rev. Infect. Dis. 5:657.
12. Wayne, L.G., David, H., Hawkins, J.E., et al. 1976. Referral without guilt or how far should a good lab go? ATS News 2:8.

BIBLIOGRAPHY

Bacteriology Training Section. 1983. Identification test techniques for mycobacteria. Centers for Disease Control, Atlanta.

Brennan, P.J., Heifers, M., and Ullom, B.P. 1982. Thin-layer chromatography of lipid antigens as a means of identifying nontuberculous mycobacteria. J. Clin. Microbiol. 15:447.

Good, R.C., and Snidery, D.E. Jr. 1982. Isolation of non-tuberculous mycobacteria in the United States, 1980. J. Infect. Dis. 146:829.

Inderlied, C.B., Baron, E.J., and Gagné, C. 1984. Disseminated mycobacterial disease in a patient with acquired immune deficiency syndrome. ASCP Check Sample No. MB 84-9 (MB-140). American Society of Clinical Pathologists, Chicago.

Kubica, G.P. 1984. Culture examination and identification. Centers for Disease Control, Atlanta.

Levy-Frebault, V., Rafidinarivo, E., Prome, J.-C., et al. 1983. *Mycobacterium fallax* sp. nov. Int. J. Syst. Bacteriol. 33:336.

Righter, J., Hart, G.D., and Howes, M. 1983. *Mycobacterium chelonei:* report of a case of septicemia and review of the literature. Diagn. Microbiol. Infect. Dis. 1:323.

Ryan, C.G., and Dwyer, B.W. 1983. New characteristics of *Mycobacterium haemophilum*. J. Clin. Microbiol. 18:976.

Sommers, H.M. 1978. The identification of mycobacteria. Lab. Med. 9:34.

Tisdall, P.A., DeYoung, D.R., Roberts, G.D., and Anhalt, J.P. 1982. Identification of clinical isolates of mycobacteria with gas-liquid chromatography: a 10-month follow up study. J. Clin. Microbiol. 16:400.

Wayne, L.G., Good, R.C., Krichevsky, M.I., et al. 1981. First report of the cooperative, open-ended study of slowly growing mycobacteria by the International Working Group on Mycobacterial Taxonomy. Int. J. Syst. Bacteriol. 31:1.

Yanagihara, D.L., Barr, V.L., Knisely, C.V., et al. 1985. Enzyme-linked immunosorbent assay of glycolipid antigens for identification of mycobacteria. J. Clin. Microbiol. 21:569.

42 Laboratory Methods in Basic Virology

W. Lawrence Drew, M.D., Ph.D.

42.1. General Principles

42.1.a. Viral structure. With the electron microscope, viruses can be seen to consist of capsid, or protein coat, and a core of nucleic acid. Some viruses, such as members of the herpes family, may also have a lipid-containing envelope. Figure 42.1 shows numerous herpes simplex viruses in various stages of development. Each viral particle has a dark central core and an outer coat of one or more layers, creating a halo effect.

42.1.b. Virus classification. All true viruses have a nucleic acid which is either DNA or RNA. Nucleic acid composition is the basis for a simple system of classifying viruses of clinical importance. The DNA viruses comprise six groups which cause human disease (Table 42.1); the RNA viruses may be divided into 11 such groups (Table 42.2).

42.1.c. Viral replication (Figure 42.2). Unlike bacteria, viruses can reproduce only within cells, where they utilize cellular "machinery" for synthesis of daughter viruses. A typical cycle of viral replication involves the following steps:

1. Attachment of the virus to the cell.
2. Penetration of the cell by the virus.
3. Uncoating of the viral coat, exposing nucleic acid. In this eclipse phase, intact virus is not detectable within the cell by electron microscopy.

4. Viral nucleic acid functions as a template for the production of "messenger" RNA, which codes for the synthesis of viral proteins (structural and enzymatic) using cellular polysomes. In the case of retroviruses, RNA is the template for the production of complementary DNA, via the enzyme reverse transcriptase. This intermediary DNA is then the template for production of messenger RNA, and virus synthesis proceeds as described above.
5. Synthesis of "daughter" viral nucleic acid using the "parent" viral nucleic acid as template.
6. Assembly of intact viral particles within the cell.
7. Release of viral particles from the cell. In this process of extrusion, cell lipid or membrane may envelop the virus and form its outer coat.

42.1.d. Viral infection. Within the intact animal, viral infection may be pictured as follows:

1. Invasion of susceptible superficial cells by a specific virus. For example, enteroviruses may initially attack cells lining the gastrointestinal tract.
2. Viral replication within these cells may lead to local spread and may yield sufficient virus progeny to cause viremia.
3. This primary viremia may lead to parasitism of reticuloendothelial cells.
4. Following replication within reticuloendothelial cells, a secondary viremia may occur with parasitism of distal visceral cells, e.g., neural cells by poliomyelitis virus.

Symptoms may develop at the time of initial invasion of superficial living cells, as with rhinoviruses and the common cold, or may not appear until after secondary viremia and invasion of visceral target organs, as with poliomyelitis. In the case of "slow" virus infections such as progressive multifocal leukoencephalo-

FIGURE 42.1
Electron micrograph of herpes simplex virus.

TABLE 42.1
Viruses of Human Importance: DNA

FAMILY	VIRAL MEMBERS
Pox	Variola, vaccinia, molluscum contagiosum
Herpes-virus	Herpes simplex, varicella-zoster, cyto-megalovirus, Epstein-Barr virus
Adenovirus	Types 1 to 8 most implicated in causing human disease
Papovavirus	Human papilloma (wart), progressive multifocal leukoencephalopathy agents (JC, SV40), BK
Hepatitis B	Hepatitis B
Parvovirus	Norwalk agent

TABLE 42.2
Viruses of Human Importance: RNA

FAMILY	VIRAL MEMBERS
Orthomyxovirus	Influenza A, B, C
Paramyxovirus	Parainfluenza, mumps, measles, respiratory syncytial virus
Togavirus	Encephalitis (western equine, eastern equine, St. Louis, etc.), yellow fever, dengue, rubella
Bunyavirus	California encephalitis, Rift Valley fever
Coronavirus	Coronavirus
Reovirus	Types 1 to 3, rotavirus, Colorado tick fever
Picornavirus	Enterovirus Polio, Coxsackie A, Coxsackie B, Echovirus, enterovirus 68-71, 72 (hepatitis A) Rhinovirus Calicivirus, Norwalk virus
Arenavirus	Lymphocytic choriomeningitis, Lassa, Tacaribe (hemorrhagic fever agents)
Rhabdovirus	Rabies
Marburg, Ebola	
Retrovirus	Human T cell leukemia, probable AIDS agent (HTLV III/LAV)

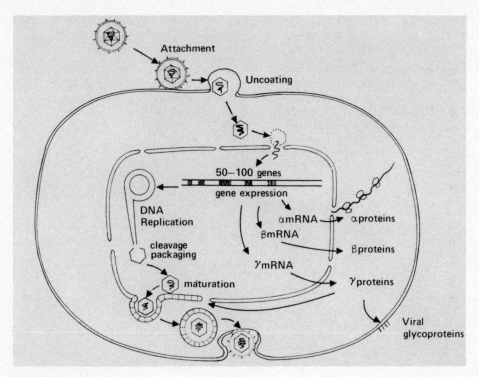

FIGURE 42.2
Schematic of virus replication.

pathy (PML), symptoms may not develop for many years.

42.2. Etiology of Viral Syndromes

Certain specific syndromes may be caused by several different viruses. This is especially true of respiratory diseases, such as bronchiolitis, which may be caused by either respiratory syncytial or parainfluenza virus (Tables 42.3 and 42.4). Similarly, the spectrum of disease potential for any one virus type is quite broad. For example, influenza virus may cause illness ranging from upper respiratory tract infection (URI) to pneumonia. Table 42.5 illustrates similar considerations in several nonrespiratory diseases.

Despite the broad range of viruses respon-

sible for human illness, Table 42.6 indicates that relatively few are recovered with any frequency in a clinical virology laboratory. This simplifies the problem of recognition for the technologist, since in most instances these commonly isolated viruses develop distinctive cytopathic effect (CPE; described below) in tissue culture. If the CPE does not permit ready identification, a few simple immunologic tests suffice for recognition of the commonly isolated viruses. It is apparent from Table 42.6 that if one can learn to isolate and identify the eight virus groups listed, 96% of all isolates can be reported correctly. Despite the impressive results cited above, however, more rapid methods of viral diagnosis are highly desirable, especially for slow-growing viruses.

TABLE 42.3
Most Common Etiologic Agents of Viral Respiratory Diseases in Infants and Children

Upper respiratory tract infection	Rhinovirus, coronavirus, parainfluenza, adenovirus, respiratory syncytial virus, influenza
Pharyngitis	Adenovirus, coxsackie A, herpes simplex, EB virus, rhinovirus, parainfluenza, influenza
Croup	Parainfluenza, respiratory syncytial virus
Bronchitis	Parainfluenza, respiratory syncytial virus
Bronchiolitis	Respiratory syncytial virus, parainfluenza
Pneumonia	Respiratory syncytial virus, adenovirus, influenza, parainfluenza

TABLE 42.4
Most Common Etiologic Agents of Viral Respiratory Disease in Adults

Upper respiratory tract infection	Rhinovirus, coronavirus, adenovirus, influenza, parainfluenza
Pneumonia	Influenza, adenovirus
Pleurodynia	Coxsackie B

TABLE 42.5
Etiologic Agents of Common Viral Syndromes

SYNDROME	AGENTS
Myocarditis	Coxsackie B
Pleurodynia	Coxsackie B
Herpangina	Coxsackie A
Febrile illness ± rash	Echo, coxsackie
Infectious mononucleosis	EB virus, cytomegalovirus
Aseptic meningitis	Echo, coxsackie A & B,
Encephalitis	Herpes simplex, togavirus, rabies, enteroviruses

TABLE 42.6
Frequency of Occurrence and Average Detection Time for Commonly Isolated Viruses at Mount Zion Hospital and Medical Center

VIRUS	ISOLATES		AVERAGE DETECTION TIME (DAYS)
	NO.	%	
Herpes simplex virus	416	42	2.7
Influenza A	66	7	3.8
Enteroviruses (echo, coxsackie A, B)	79	8	4.2
Cytomegalovirus (CMV)	213	21	5.8
Respiratory syncytial virus (RSV)	35	3	6.1
Varicella-zoster	41	4	6.1
Adenovirus	80	8	6.4
Parainfluenza 1, 3	29	3	6.4
Other	41	4	
TOTALS	1,000	100	4.1

42.3. Overview of Rapid Viral Diagnostic Methods

42.3.a. Cytology. The most readily available rapid technique is cytologic examination for the presence of characteristic viral inclusions. These intracellular structures may represent aggregates of virus within an infected cell or may be abnormal accumulations of cellular materials consequent to the viral-induced metabolic disruption. Papanicolaou (Pap) smears may show these inclusions in single cells or in large syncytial (large aggregates of cells containing more than one nucleus) groups, as in a patient with herpes simplex infection of the cervix (Figure 42.3). Cytology is most commonly used to detect infections with herpes simplex virus or cytomegalorivus, but is definitely less sensitive than culture. Rabies infection may also be detected by use of the Seller stain for the detection of Negri bodies (rabies inclusions in brain tissue).

42.3.b. Detection of viral antigen. Direct examination of virus-infected tissues or exudates may be performed with specific fluorescein-labeled viral antibody as described below in 42.5.a. This test can be completed within 1 h and is a sensitive method for detecting the presence of viral antigen. However, the performance of the test and the preparation of high-titered, labeled antisera both require considerable technological expertise. Fluorescent antibody identification has been used regularly for the diagnosis of infections with herpes simplex, varicella-zoster, and rabies viruses. We have found that varicella-zoster virus (VZV), which grows slowly or not at all in tissue culture, can be readily detected in smears from skin lesions by a fluorescent antibody method.[5] Good commercial conjugates are available for the direct detection of herpes simplex, varicella-zoster, respiratory syncytial, and influenza viruses in clinical specimens. Many of these antigens also

FIGURE 42.3
Herpes simplex virus cytology.

may be detected by indirect fluorescent antibody techniques. Immunofluorescent antibody may also be used to rapidly detect the presence of a virus such as CMV in tissue culture. By centrifuging urine onto tissue culture monolayers and staining at 24-36 h after inoculation, this virus may be detected without waiting many days for cytopathogenic effect (CPE) to develop.[7] Radioimmunoassay has been used to detect hepatitis B and herpes simplex antigens. More recently other immunologic techniques such as ELISA (enzyme-linked immunosorbent assay) have been applied to the detection of these and other viral antigens. Immunoperoxidase assays to detect HSV in clinical specimens directly or after 1-2 days in tissue culture have usually proven less sensitive than the standard tissue culture isolation procedures.[10]

Nucleic acid hybridization techniques for the detection of viral nucleic acids in clinical specimens have been described recently. CMV has been successfully identified in urine by dot blot hybridization (Chapter 10), but this method is less sensitive (although more rapid) than tissue culture.[3] The converse has been reported in blood samples where dot blot hybridization was positive in samples negative by culture, although the specificity of this procedure needs to be confirmed.[11] RNA viruses, specifically rotaviruses, have also been detected by a dot hybridization assay of fecal samples.[6]

42.3.c. Electron microscopy (EM). EM is particularly useful for detecting viruses that grow poorly or not at all in tissue culture. At present, EM is being used to examine feces for rotavirus and other candidate viruses as causes of gastroenteritis. The procedure is surprisingly simple for an experienced electron microscopist (as described below in 42.5.b) and can be completed within 15 min of receipt of the specimen. Although it would be inappropriate to purchase an electron microscope solely for a diagnostic virology laboratory, an existing electron microscope in an institution could be used.

42.3.d. Viral serology. Certain viruses, e.g., hepatitis A and B, rubella, measles, and coronaviruses, are difficult to isolate in tissue culture, and infections caused by them are best diagnosed serologically as discussed in 42.7 and Chapter 12. Arboviruses, which cause some types of encephalitis, require suckling mice for isolation; serologic techniques are also the most practical means for diagnosing infections with these viruses (in this chapter, the term "arbovirus" is used in preference to the more correct toga- or bunyavirus because of its familiarity). Serologic studies, especially complement fixation, are much less useful in infants, who may not mount an antibody response detectable by this method.

In practice, we encourage the submission of an acute-phase serum specimen in all patients suspected of having a viral illness. A convalescent serum specimen is requested only if a virus etiology has not been established by culture or other methods.

42.4. Laboratory Methods in Diagnostic Virology

42.4.a. Laboratory equipment. Necessary equipment includes the following items:

1. A 35° C aerobic incubator equipped to hold at least two roller drum racks and with sufficient shelf space to store a week's supply of cell cultures.
2. Two or three roller drums with motor-driven bases to rotate the drums.
3. An inverted microscope with 4 and 10 × objectives to examine the cell culture flasks and tubes.
4. An ultracold freezing unit ($-70°$ C) to store reagents, antigens, and other materials.
5. A laminar flow hood (Chapter 2) in which to carry out cell culture procedures.
6. A conventional horizontal head centrifuge.

7. Refrigerator (4° C) with −20° C freezer
for reagent and media storage.
8. Fluorescent microscope.

Other equipment includes vortex mixers, a 56° C water bath, a vibrating platform, electric pipetters, and a sonic oscillator (helpful but not essential). Many of these items can be shared with other sections of the laboratory.

The remaining equipment is minor and includes such items as disposable pipettes, assorted glassware, hemacytometer, plastic cell culture flasks and membrane filtration units, along with the usual furnishings for storage of laboratory requisitions and other records.

42.4.b. Selection of specimens for viral culture. Selection of appropriate specimens is complicated since several different viruses may cause the same clinical disease (Table 42.7). For example, several different types of specimens may be submitted from patients with central nervous system (CNS) disease: cerebrospinal fluid (CSF) (enterovirus, mumps virus, and perhaps herpes simplex virus [HSV type 2]); throat (enterovirus); stool or rectal swab (enterovirus). In addition, blood should be collected as an acute-phase specimen in case subsequent serological tests are necessary (mumps virus, HSV, arbovirus). Many considerations, however, allow the clinician to select the most appropriate specimens. For example, during the summer, when enteroviral meningitis is prevalent, throat and stool specimens should certainly be submitted, in addition to CSF. On the other hand, the development of encephalitis in children after the acquisition of several mosquito bites in wooded areas endemic for California encephalitis virus would suggest that a blood specimen for antibody testing would be optimal. Further examples include CNS disease following parotitis (urine and CSF specimens for mumps virus) or a focal encephalitis with a temporal lobe localization preceded by headaches and disorientation (brain biopsy for

HSV). In respiratory syndromes it is generally only necessary to submit a throat or nasopharyngeal specimen; stool and urine isolates would be irrelevant. Table 42.8 summarizes the procedures for obtaining and transporting specimens for viral studies. Other considerations are as follows.

Throat, nasopharyngeal swab, aspirate. For recovering viruses, nasopharyngeal aspirates are superior to swabs, but the latter are considerably more convenient. Throat swabs are probably adequate for recovering entero- and adenoviruses and HSV, whereas nasopharyngeal specimens are definitely superior for recovering respiratory syncytial virus and probably better for parainfluenza viruses. Nasal specimens are optimal for recovering rhinoviruses.

Rectal swabs and stool specimens. Most cases of viral gastroenteritis are now known to be due to viruses which cannot be cultivated in cell cultures. Fecal specimens from such cases may be examined for nonculturable agents, e.g., rotavirus, by electron microscopy or by antigen detection (see below). Stool cultures are useful in patients suspected of having enterovirus disease, e.g., aseptic meningitis, myopericarditis, and hand, foot, and mouth disease. Enteroviruses in the feces of such patients support the possibility but do not definitely prove that these agents are causing the illness. Available evidence indicates that stool specimens are more productive than rectal swabs. Generally, infectivity of viruses which are surrounded by a lipid membrane (e.g., HSV, cytomegalovirus [CMV]) is destroyed by gastric acidity, and therefore they will not be excreted in active form in the feces.

Urine. CMV, mumps, and adenovirus are the viruses most frequently recovered from urine by the laboratory. In cases of CNS disease due to mumps, the virus can be isolated from urine when specimens from other sites are negative. The recovery of CMV from urine is increased twofold to threefold by processing

TABLE 42.7
Appropriate Specimens for Viral Isolation*

SYNDROMES AND PROBABLE VIRAL AGENTS	THROAT/ NASOPHARYNX	STOOL	CSF	URINE	OTHER
Respiratory syndrome	+ + + +				
Adenoviruses					
Enteroviruses					
Influenza virus					
Parainfluenza virus					
Respiratory syncytial virus (RSV)					
Rhinoviruses					+ + + nasal
Dermatologic and mucous membrane disease	+				+ + + +
Vesicular					
Enterovirus (hand, foot, mouth syndrome)	+ +	+ + +			+ + + (Vesicle fluid or scraping)
Herpes simplex†					
Varicella-zoster†	+ +				
Exanthematous	+ +				
Enterovirus		+ + +			
Measles‡					
Rubella‡					
Meningoencephalitis	+ +		+ + +		
Arboviruses					
Enteroviruses		+ + + +			
Herpes simplex					(Brain biopsy)
Lymphocytic choriomeningitis§					
Mumps virus					
Gastrointestinal		+ +			
Adenoviruses‡					
Parvovirus‡					
Rotavirus‖					
Congenital and Perinatal	+ +	+	+ +		+ +
Cytomegalovirus				+ + +	(Blood)
Enteroviruses					
Herpes simplex virus					(Vesicle fluid)
Eye syndrome					+ + + +
Adenoviruses	+ +				(Conjunctival swab or scraping)
Herpes simplex virus					
Vaccinia virus					
Varicella-zoster virus					
(Chlamydiae¶)					
CMV infection	+ +			+ + + +	+
Cytomegalovirus (CMV)					(Blood)
Myocarditis, pericarditis, and pleurodynia	+ +	+ + + +			+
Coxsackie B					(Pericardial fluid)

*Specimens indicated beside the disease categories should be obtained in all instances; others should be obtained if the specific virus is suspected.

†Direct fluorescent antibody studies are available for herpes simplex virus and varicella-zoster.

‡Best diagnosed by EM since the adenoviruses responsible for gastroenteritis are not culturable by standard techniques.

§Best diagnosed serologically.

‖Best diagnosed by antigen detection or EM.

¶Chlamydiae were once considered viruses because they are obligate intracellular parasites. They are included here because they can be isolated in cell culture. (See Chapter 38.)

TABLE 42.8
Summary of Procedures for Obtaining and Transporting Specimens for Viral Studies

General
  Do not freeze specimens. Obtain specimens as early in the patient's illness as possible. Inoculate tissue cultures at patient's bedside if possible.
Throat
  Swab inflamed area. Use Culturette swab (Marion Scientific Corp.) as for bacteriologic culture.
Nasopharynx
  Obtain a nasopharyngeal swab or a nasal wash specimen using a bulb syringe or a suction apparatus and 3-7 ml buffered saline.
Stool
  Obtain as for bacteriologic culture. If a specimen cannot be passed, a rectal swab of feces may be obtained with a Culturette.
Cerebrospinal fluid (CSF)
  Obtain 1 ml as for bacteriologic culture.
Urine
  Obtain a clean-voided specimen (10-20 ml) as for bacteriologic culture and transport in sterile screw-capped tube.
Skin or mucosal lesion
  Use Culturette swab to obtain vesicle fluid and scrape cells from base of lesion.
Biopsy material
  Use aseptic technique and submit in a sterile container (e.g., urine container).
Blood for culture
  Submit at least 3 ml of heparinized blood (green-top Vacutainer tube, Becton-Dickinson Co.). Some laboratories prefer citrated blood because of evidence suggesting that heparin has antiviral properties.
Blood for serologic studies
  Submit at least 5 ml of clotted whole blood (red-top Vacutainer tube). In certain viral syndromes (e.g., lower respiratory) an acute-phase specimen should be submitted. If a virus is not isolated, a convalescent specimen should be obtained at least 7 days after the acute specimen. Certain viral illnesses (e.g., rubella, rubeola, hepatitis, and arbovirus encephalitis) are diagnosed most readily by serologic studies.
Transportation
  Transport specimens as rapidly as possible, using a messenger service. Specimens should be stored and transported at refrigerator temperature (4° C). **Do not freeze.** If transportation of swabs will be delayed, place them in a tube of buffered bacteriologic broth medium rather than in the Culturette.

several specimens. Urine specimens submitted for culture of CMV can be inoculated directly into cell cultures. Alternatively, they may be centrifuged, and either the supernatant urine or the sediment, resuspended in a small volume, can be used as inoculum. Recent studies indicate that centrifuging the urine onto the tissue culture monolayer is the best of all these procedures.[7]

Generally, examination of the urine sediment for cytomegalic inclusion-bearing cells is not a sensitive method for diagnosing CMV infections. Viral isolation is at least four times more sensitive in both infants and adults than is examination of urine sediment.

Dermal lesions. Fluid and cells from vesicles are superior to specimens from ulcers or crusts for both culture and direct stains.

CSF, other "sterile" fluids, e.g., pleural, peritoneal, pericardial, joint. These fluids should be inoculated as quickly as possible into tissue culture.

Eye. A nasopharyngeal swab may be used to obtain secretions from the palpebral conjunctiva. Eye scrapings should be obtained by an ophthalmologist or other trained person.

Blood. CMV viremia may be present in symptomatic infection and has been correlated with lethal pneumonia in bone marrow transplant recipients. Leukocytes, in which this and other viruses reside, may be collected more efficiently by a Ficoll-Hypaque-Macrodex sedimentation technique than by the conventional buffy coat method. Anticoagulated blood or a clot can be used for isolation of arboviruses, and serum is suitable for recovering enteroviruses.

Tissue. Tissue explants and cells grown in cell cultures after dispersal of the cells from tissue fragments have provided higher rates of viral isolation than homogenized specimens. Presumably, viral inhibitors may be released into the homogenate, resulting in lower recovery rates in the disrupted cells. Lung (CMV, influenza virus, adenovirus,) and brain (HSV) are the most productive tissue sources for viral isolates. As with urine sediment, the cytological detection of CMV inclusions in tissue is at least three to six times less sensitive than viral isolation.

∙ ∙ ∙

Proper timing of specimen collection is essential for adequate recovery of viruses. Specimens should be collected early in the acute phase of infection. Studies with respiratory viruses indicate that the mean duration of viral shedding may be 3-7 days. Also, HSV and varicella-zoster virus (VZV) may not be recovered from lesions beyond 5 days after onset. Isolation of an enterovirus from the CSF may only be possible within 2 to 3 days after onset of the CNS manifestations.

42.4.c. Transport of specimens to the laboratory. The shorter the interval between collection of a specimen and its delivery to the laboratory, the greater the potential for isolating an agent. When feasible, inoculate all specimens other than blood, feces, and tissue into culture tubes at the patient's bedside. These are then transported to the laboratory promptly. Any material may be used for swabs; however, calcium alginate may inactivate HSV. In general, the following statements hold, but there may be a few exceptions:

1. Never leave a specimen at room or incubator temperature.
2. When it is impossible to deliver a specimen immediately, it should be refrigerated and packed in shaved ice for delivery to the laboratory within 12 h of collection.

Several types of media have been used for the transport of viral specimens. Most of these have been selected for this purpose based either on tradition or on data obtained by testing the survival of laboratory strains of virus. A re-

cent double-blind prospective study to compare the recovery of viruses from the upper respiratory tracts or dermal lesions of children, using three types of transport media, showed no statistically significant differences between modified Stuart's (Chapter 45), modified Hanks', or Leibovitz-Emory media.[9] It is generally believed that protein (serum, albumin, gelatin) incorporated into a transport medium enhances the survival of viruses in transit; however, two studies have indicated that HSV survives as well in Stuart's or Hanks' protein-free medium.[13] The Culturette (Modified Stuart's Bacterial Transport Medium, Marion Laboratories) appears to be satisfactory for short-term (i.e., up to 4 h) transport.

Improper storage can significantly reduce viral culture yields. After a freeze-thaw cycle, significant losses in infectivity titer occur with lipid-envelope viruses (HSV, CMV), but not with agents such as adenoviruses and enteroviruses, which have a coat of protein only. For example, a laboratory strain of HSV held for 1-3 days at $-20°$ C and then thawed had reductions in infectious titer of 10^2 or more. In contrast, when stored for 1-3 days at $4°$ C in Hanks' or broth medium there was no loss of infectivity in two-thirds of the specimens.[13] In another study only 3 of 45 (7%) strains of CMV failed to produce cytopathic effects after storage for 7 days at $4°$ C.[12] Storage at room temperature was unsatisfactory. Alternatively, once a specimen is received in the laboratory, cryoprotectants such as sorbitol may be added, but even then viral suspensions must be frozen and thawed under rigid conditions ($-70°$ C when freezing, $25°$ C/min when thawing) to achieve maximum recovery of the virus. Thus, **for short term (<5 days) transit or storage of specimens for viral culture, specimens should be held at $4°$ C rather than frozen.**

Specific requirements for shipping specimens have been published by the U.S. Public Health Service (Fed. Reg., vol. 45, no. 141, 21

FIGURE 42.4
Label for etiologic agents.

July 1980) and by the Department of Transportation and Interstate Quarantine regulations (49 CFR, Section 173.386.388, and 42 CFR, Section 72.25, Etiologic Agents). These regulations can be obtained from the Biohazards Control Officer, Centers for Disease Control, Atlanta, Georgia. In essence, regulations require that the specimen be wrapped in sufficient absorbent material to absorb the entire contents of the specimen in case of leakage or breakage. The wrapped specimen must be enclosed in a durable watertight container, which is then enclosed in an outer shipping container. The watertight container must be secured with shock-absorbent material or tape so that it does not become loose as the dry ice sublimates (see Chapter 2).

The label Etiologic Agents/Biomedical Material must appear on the outside of the shipping container (Figure 42.4).

42.4.d. Media and cells used for viral isolation. Several kinds of cell culture systems are routinely used for isolation of viruses (also see Chapter 8). Cell cultures may be primary, low passage, or established cell lines. Primary cells, e.g., monkey or human embryonic kidney, are most receptive to viruses after only one or two passages, whereas diploid fibroblast cells may remain virus sensitive through 20-50 passages. Continuous cell lines such as Hep-2 are virus sensitive even after hundreds of passages.

1. *Primary Monkey Kidney (PMK)* is an excellent system for recovery of myxoviruses and many enteroviruses, and also may support growth of adenoviruses, respiratory syncytial viruses, and measles viruses. These cells are occasionally contaminated by simian viruses (most commonly SV5 and SV40), a problem minimized by the addition of antisera to these agents in the cell culture media.

2. *Human fetal diploid (HFD)*, e.g., foreskin fibroblasts (**Figure 42.5**). These fibroblastic cells have the dual advantages of being relatively inexpensive and susceptible to a broad spectrum of viruses. They are useful in the isolation of varicella-zoster virus (VZV), herpes simplex virus (HSV), adenovirus, picornavirus, and respiratory syncytial virus (RSV), and are the only cells in which cytomegalovirus (CMV) is recovered.

FIGURE 42.5
Foreskin fibroblast monolayer.

3. *Hep-2 continuous cell line.* These epithelial cells, derived from a human cancer, are an excellent cell system for recovering adenovirus, HSV, and especially RSV.

The availability of commercial cell cultures and media greatly facilitates the work involved in virus isolation. If purchased commercially, upon arrival in the laboratory, tubes are examined microscopically. If an adequate monolayer of cells is present, the growth medium is replaced by 2-3 ml of fresh maintenance medium prior to storage at 35° C. If the monolayer is incomplete, the growth medium is replaced by 2-3 ml of fresh growth medium. HFD and Hep-2 cultures can be prepared in a clinical laboratory rather than purchased commercially.

The majority of clinically significant viruses can be recovered in the cell systems described above. Specimens submitted for the isolation of viruses requiring other types of cell cultures (e.g., coxsackie A, togaviruses) are forwarded to reference laboratories. Some laboratories prefer additional cell cultures such as RD (rhabdomyosarcoma) or BGM (continuous monkey kidney) for recovering coxsackie A and B viruses, respectively.

Two kinds of media, growth and maintenance, are used for cell culture. These media are prepared with Eagle's minimum essential medium (MEM) in Earle's balanced salt solution (EBSS). Suppliers are listed in the Appendix, and formulas are given in Chapter 45. Growth medium is a serum-rich nutrient medium designed to support rapid cell growth. We use this medium for initiating growth of Hep-2 cells in tubes or for feeding tubes or purchased tissue culture cells that have incomplete cell monolayers. Maintenance medium, on the other hand, is used to keep cells in a steady state of metabolism and is, therefore, less rich in growth factors such as serum.

42.4.e. Specimen processing. Because specimens submitted for virus isolation are

TABLE 42.9
Laboratory Processing of Viral Specimens

SOURCE	SPECIMEN	PROCESSING*	TISSUE CULTURE
Blood	Heparinized blood	Obtain buffy coat by centrifuging at 2,500 rpm for 10-15 min. Inoculate directly.	PMK, HFD, Hep-2
Cerebrospinal fluid (CSF)	1 ml CSF	Inoculate directly.	PMK, HFD, Hep-2
Feces (preferred to rectal swab)	Pea-sized aliquot of feces	Place in 2 ml of viral antibiotic mixture (Chapter 45). Shake with mixer and hold at RT† for 60 min. Centrifuge at 2,500 rpm for 15 min and use supernatant fluid for inoculum.	PMK, HFD, Hep-2
Genital, skin	Culturette or swab in HFD tube	Insert swab in HFD tube for 30 min at RT. Use fluid from that tube to inoculate additional tubes.	PMK, Hep-2
Miscellaneous	Culturette, fluids	Swab: insert into PMK tube for 30 min at RT; use fluid from that tube to inoculate additional tubes. Fluid: inoculate directly.	PMK, HFD, Hep-2
Respiratory tract	Culturette, nasopharyngeal or throat swab or washings	Insert swab directly into PMK tube for 30 min at RT. Use fluid from that tube to inoculate additional tubes. If infant specimen, inoculate Hep-2 first.	PMK, HFD, Hep-2
Tissue	Tissue in sterile container	Mince with sterile scalpel and scissors. Prepare 20% suspension in viral antibiotic mixture (Chapter 45) and grind with sterile sand. Centrifuge at 2,500 rpm for 15 min and use supernatant fluid for inoculum.	PMK, HFD
Urine	Fresh refrigerated urine or frozen with equal volume of sterile 70% sorbitol in distilled water	Inoculate directly‡ into HFD. Also, treat 5-10 ml urine with 0.3 ml viral antibiotic mixture (Chapter 45) for 60 min at RT. Centrifuge at 2,500 rpm for 15 min. Discard all but 1 ml of the supernate, resuspend the sediment in the remaining fluid, and use for inoculum.	HFD, PMK (if mumps or adenovirus suspected)

*All inocula into tissue culture tubes are 0.25 ml volumes.
†RT = room temperature.
‡Treatment of urine with antibiotics is not necessary for direct inoculation of HFD tube.

similar to those submitted for routine bacterial isolation, they can be inoculated in a bacteriology laboratory by the same technologist who handles all the other microbiology cultures. This system assures that viral cultures are set up promptly and that they are processed during evening shifts and on weekends.

Virus specimens are inoculated according to the guidelines presented in Table 42.9. In all cases the volume of fluid inoculated into a single tissue culture tube is 0.25 ml.

If not inoculated directly at the patient's bedside, body fluids or swabs taken from sterile or minimally contaminated areas such as the nasopharynx or throat may be inserted directly into a tissue culture tube in the laboratory. The type of tissue culture used for this inoculation is selected according to the type of specimen, as outlined in Table 42.9.

After 30 min the swab is removed from the culture tube, and 0.25 ml aliquots of the tissue culture fluid from the tube are used as the inocula for additional necessary cultures. Swabs of specimens such as feces that are heavily contaminated with bacteria must first be treated with antibiotic-antifungal mixtures to reduce the chances of tissue culture contamination.

Inoculated cell cultures are transferred daily from the processing area to the virus laboratory where they are incubated at 35° C in roller drums and examined daily for cytopathogenic effect (CPE) for a period of 10-14 days. CPE may be quantitated as follows:

± = < 25% of monolayer exhibits CPE
1+ = 25% of monolayer exhibits CPE
2+ = 50% of monolayer exhibits CPE
3+ = 75% of monolayer exhibits CPE
4+ = 100% of monolayer exhibits CPE

Human fetal diploid (HFD) cultures are kept at least 21 days to allow for the isolation of cytomegalovirus (CMV). The longer incubation of these culture cells necessitates weekly media changes (Procedure 42.1). Because toxic specimens such as stool, urine and tissues can

---

PROCEDURE 42.1. CHANGING MEDIA

When changing inoculated tissue culture media, it is important to avoid cross-contamination between specimens. Different pipettes should be used to remove and to add media. Pipettes should also be changed between specimens. It might be helpful to set up a vacuum flask assembly to which the pipettes may be attached when removing media.

When changing uninoculated tissue culture media, one pipette may be used to remove the media and another to add it. Contamination of media with cells of different types should be avoided by using separate containers of media for changing one particular cell type.

---

cause degeneration of monolayers, media must be changed the day following their inoculation.

Tubes of primary monkey kidney (PMK) inoculated with respiratory specimens are hemadsorbed routinely at 5 and 10 days after inoculation (or earlier if myxovirus-like CPE is detected) with a 0.4% suspension of guinea pig erythrocytes to aid detection of myxoviruses as described in Procedure 42.2. Hemadsorption may be performed at 3 days postinoculation during periods of influenza virus prevalence to accelerate detection of this virus.

Our laboratory does not make a practice of "blind passing" negative specimens. However, cell cultures that show nonspecific or ambiguous CPE are passed into appropriate cell systems by scraping the monolayer off the sides of the culture tube with a 1 ml pipette and inoculating 0.25 ml of the resulting suspension into new cell cultures. If CMV or varicella-zoster virus (VZV) is suspected in a specimen, such

PROCEDURE 42.2. HEMADSORPTION OF PRIMARY MONKEY KIDNEY (PMK) MONOLAYERS TO DETECT MYXOVIRUSES

Perform on cultures of respiratory specimens (or urine in the case of suspected mumps) at 3 days postinoculation during influenza season and at 5 and 10 days postinoculation or when CPE first appears during the rest of the year. Note: RSV is not detected by this method.

1. **Preparation of 0.4% suspension of guinea pig erythrocytes (RBCs)**
   a. Wash fresh guinea pig erythrocytes three times in dextrose-gelatin-veronal (DGV) buffer (purchased commercially). Centrifuge cells at 1,500 rpm for 5 min after the first two washes, and at 2,000 rpm for 10 min after the last wash.
   b. Prepare a 10% suspension of the washed erythrocytes in DGV (3.6 ml DGV and 0.4 ml packed RBCs). Store at 4° C; cells will last approximately 1 week.
   c. On the day of testing, prepare a 0.4% suspension of the RBCs by diluting the 10% suspension with PMK maintenance medium (Chapter 45) (0.4 ml of 10% suspension plus 9.6 ml medium).

2. **Hemadsorption procedure**
   a. To each inoculated PMK culture to be tested, to two uninoculated negative controls, and to two positive controls (influenza A, parainfluenza 2), add 0.2 ml of the 0.4% RBC suspension. Be careful not to cross-contaminate tubes; positive controls should be tested last.
   b. Place tubes horizontally in the rack so that the erythrocyte suspension covers the monolayer. Refrigerate at 4° C for 30 min.
   c. Invert tubes quickly to dislodge RBCs lying on the cell sheet. Examine each tube microscopically for RBCs that adhere to the monolayer (Figure 42.6). Culture fluids should be inspected for hemagglutination.

Viruses which both hemadsorb and hemagglutinate guinea pig erythrocytes are usually either influenza A or B. Mumps virus and the parainfluenza viruses (PIV) generally produce only hemadsorption. Certain simian viruses, most notably SV5, contaminate monkey kidney tissue cultures and also hemadsorb at 4° C. Examine all tubes as soon as possible after removal from the refrigerator, because the neuraminidase of myxoviruses is active at room temperature, and hemadsorbing viruses will begin to elute if left for extended periods at this temperature.

passages should be made by trypsinizing the monolayer. Absence of CPE in the subpassages indicates that the initial changes were not caused by a virus.

42.4.f. Isolation and identification of viruses. Although there are many ways to detect the presence of viruses in cell culture, only two are commonly used in the clinical laboratory: (1) the observation of CPE and (2) hemadsorption/hemagglutination of guinea pig erythrocytes. Often determining the type, rapidity, and selectivity of CPE in cell cultures is

FIGURE 42.6
Parainfluenza virus
hemadsorption.

TABLE 42.10
Cultivation and Identification of Commonly Isolated Viruses

VIRUS	PMK	HEP-2	HFD	CPE DESCRIPTION	RATE OF GROWTH (DAYS)	IDENTIFICATION AND COMMENTS
Adenovirus	+ +*	+ +	+ +	Rounding and aggregation of infected cells in grapelike clusters	2-10	Confirm by FA.† Serotype by cell culture neutralization.
Cytomegalovirus (CMV)	−	−	+ +	Discrete small foci of rounded cells.	5-21	Distinct CPE sufficient to identify. Cell associated virus; requires trypsin for passage. Confirm by FA.
Enterovirus	+ + + +	±	+ +	Characteristic refractile angular or tear-shaped CPE; progresses to involve entire monolayer.	2-8	Identify by cell culture neutralization test with intersecting pools of hyperimmune sera. Stable at pH 3.

*Relative sensitivity of cell cultures for recovering the virus: − = none recovered; ± = rare strains recovered; + = few strains recovered; + + + + = ≥ 80% of strains recovered.
†FA = fluorescent antibody; HAD = hemadsorption; HI = hemagglutination inhibition.

TABLE 42.10

Cultivation and Identification of Commonly Isolated Viruses—cont'd

VIRUS	PMK	HEP-2	HFD	CPE DESCRIPTION	RATE OF GROWTH (DAYS)	IDENTIFICATION AND COMMENTS
Herpes simplex (HSV)	± (type 2)	+ + + +	+ + + +	Rounded, swollen refractile cells. Occasional syncytia, especially with type 2. Rapidly involves entire monolayer.	1-3 (may take up to 7)	Ether, chloroform labile. Distinct CPE. Confirmation may be performed by FA.
Influenza	+ + + +	−	±	Destructive degeneration with swollen, vacuolated cells.	2-10	Detect by hemadsorption or hemagglutination with guinea pig RBCs. Identify by FA, HAD, or HI.†
Mumps	+ + +	±	±	CPE usually absent. Occasionally syncytia are seen.	5-10	Detect by hemadsorption with guinea pig RBCs. Confirm by FA or HAD.
Parainfluenza (PIV)	+ + +	−	−	CPE is often minimal or absent. PIV 3 produces fibroblast-like appearance at edges of cell sheet.	4-10	Detect by hemadsorption with guinea pig RBCs. Identify by FA or HAD.
Respiratory syncytial virus (RSV)	+	+ + +	+	Syncytia in Hep-2, PMK. In HFD degeneration of cell sheet in definite foci.	3-10	Distinct CPE in Hep-2 is sufficient for presumptive identification. Confirm by FA.
Rhinovirus	±	−	+ + +	Characteristic refractile rounding of cells. In PMK, CPE is identical to that produced by enteroviruses.	4-10	Labile at pH 3.
Varicella-zoster	−	−	+ +	Discrete foci of rounded, swollen, refractile cells. Slowly involves entire monolayer.		Confirm by FA.

enough to enable preliminary or final identification of an isolate.

Examples of viruses that are frequently identifiable on initial isolation include herpes simplex virus (HSV) when it produces typical rapid CPE in HFD and Hep-2 cells, and cytomegalovirus, a slow-growing virus that produces clusters of refractile cells only in human fibroblasts. Table 42.10 lists the viruses most commonly isolated in the clinical laboratory and the cell cultures in which they can be cultivated.

FIGURE 42.7
Herpes simplex virus cytopathic effect. **A**, normal cell monolayer. **B**, Infected cells.

In this section the recognition and identification of these viruses are described. The reader is referred to standard textbooks[1, 2] for additional information about these viruses and other less commonly isolated viruses.

Herpes simplex virus (HSV). Herpes simplex virus is the most frequently isolated virus in the clinical laboratory. It grows well in a variety of cell cultures including HFD and epithelial cell lines such as Hep-2. CPE appears an average of 1-3 days after culture inoculation. Typically, the CPE begins in focal areas and may progress to involve the entire monolayer within 24 h. Infected cells become enlarged "giant cells" and may clump together to form cellular clusters called syncytia (Figure 42.7). Type 2 HSV is especially prone to develop syncytia, and in addition may produce CPE in PMK, a property not shared by type 1 HSV.

The necessity for confirming an isolate as HSV is controversial but may be achieved with specific fluorescent antisera as described in Procedure 42.3. Fluorescein-conjugated antisera may also be used to identify HSV isolates as type 1 or 2, but the distinction is not always clear-cut.

Varicella-zoster virus (VZV). Varicella-zoster virus is a member of the herpesvirus group. Occasionally VZV is confused with HSV because both are apt to be recovered from skin lesions and both can produce CPE in human fibroblasts. Usually the CPE produced by VZV is focal, spreads slowly, and appears several days later than that of HSV. The CPE is characterized by foci of enlarged refractile cells appearing 5-7 days after inoculation. To confirm the presence of VZV in culture, we employ fluorescent antisera (Procedure 42.3).

Cytomegalovirus (CMV). Cytomegalovirus, another member of the herpesvirus family, is a frequent clinical isolate. As mentioned earlier, CMV is characterized by the slow development of discrete foci of rounded cells in cell culture (Figure 42.8) and its inability to produce CPE in any cells other than human diploid fibroblasts (HFD). CMV is by far the most common virus recovered from urine; rarely an adenovirus, enterovirus, mumps or herpes simplex virus also may be recovered from urine.

HFD cultures inoculated with specimens of suspected CMV should be held for at least 21 days to enable the CPE of the virus to develop, although 92% of our isolates from infants have been detectable in 10 days and 98% in 14 days of incubation. Direct inoculation of urine into cell culture often enables CPE to develop in less than 10 days. As mentioned earlier, centrifugation of the urine onto the monolayer and staining with monoclonal antibody may enable CMV to be detected after just 24 h in tissue culture.[7] Because it may be confused with certain strains of adenovirus, immunofluorescent confirmation (FA, Procedure 42.3) should be performed using available antibodies.

Adenoviruses. Adenoviruses, of which there are more than 30 serotypes, cause a variety of clinical syndromes ranging from pneumonia to acute pharyngitis to conjunctivitis. The virus may be recovered from conjunctiva, stool, body fluids, and urine.

Growth in cell culture tends to be slow, with CPE appearing in an average of 6 days after inoculation. Adenoviruses may be recovered in a variety of cell systems, including PMK and HFD, although human embryonic kidney (HEK) is probably the best culture system. The CPE is characterized by marked rounding and clumping, producing the appearance of grapelike clusters. Continuous cell lines such as HeLa and Hep-2 are also sensitive to adenovirus growth and are possible substitutes. CPE in Hep-2 has the appearance of rounded, tightly clumped, **very granular** cell aggregates.

Since adenoviruses possess a common group antigen, isolates are confirmed easily by fluorescent antibody methods. Precise typing, however, requires a cell culture neutralization method (Procedure 42.4).

Because adenovirus types 1-7 are more frequently associated with illness than are other serotypes, a neutralization test with antisera to these specific types can be performed on isolates from respiratory and fecal specimens. If typing of an isolate is not possible with these antisera, the virus is forwarded to a reference laboratory for further identification. Adenoviruses recovered from specimens such as urine and conjunctiva are not usually typed since these sites are not normally colonized with any adenoviruses. If an adenovirus is responsible for respiratory illness, it should be recoverable from respiratory secretions and not from feces alone.

Picornaviruses. The picornaviruses include two major groups of viruses: (1) rhinoviruses, agents of the common cold, and (2) enteroviruses, which include polioviruses, coxsackieviruses types A and B, echoviruses, and miscellaneous other enteroviruses and hepatitis A virus. Both rhinoviruses and enteroviruses tend to be seasonal isolates with peak isolations occurring from late summer to early winter. Epidemics caused by a single type of enterovirus are not uncommon.

ENTEROVIRUSES. Presently a large number of enteroviruses are known: poliovirus 1-3, coxsackie A 1-24, coxsackie B 1-6, echovirus 1-34, enterovirus 68-71, and enterovirus 72 (hepatitis A). Despite this large number, only a relative few tend to be recovered in the clinical laboratory. Of the nonpolio enteroviruses typed in our laboratory, 75% were one of the following: coxsackie A9, A16, B2-5, and echo 9, 11, and 30. Polioviruses are recovered frequently from recently immunized infants and children.

Most enteroviruses can be isolated in cell culture, although some types of coxsackie A require inoculation of suckling mice. PMK is an excellent cell culture system for recovering these viruses, but they grow in other systems (such as rhabdomyoma [RD], African green

PROCEDURE 42.3. IDENTIFICATION OF ISOLATES BY FLUORESCENT ANTIBODY (FA) METHOD

This method of virus identification is currently used in our laboratory in preference to the hemadsorption inhibition (HadI) and hemagglutination inhibition (HI) methods. FA is also used for identification of measles, VZV, CMV, and adenovirus, as well as for typing of HSV isolates.

Each virus isolate to be identified should have developed 2-3 + CPE (or demonstrate pronounced hemadsorption) without appreciable loss of cells from the glass. Pool three tubes of uninoculated homologous cell cultures with one tube of infected cells to (1) assure adequate cell numbers for making the required numbers of smears, and (2) provide contrast between fluorescent infected cells and nonfluorescent uninfected cells.

Each test must include known positive controls for each fluorescent antiserum to be used, controls to detect heterologous staining, and negative controls of uninfected homologous cells. Positive control slides and controls for heterologous staining are prepared by pooling the cells from four tubes of infected cells. Negative control slides are prepared by pooling the cells from four tubes of uninfected cell cultures. Control smears may be prepared in advance, fixed, and stored at $-70°$ C until needed.

1. **Determination of the working dilution of fluorescent conjugates**
   a. Prepare serial doubling dilutions of the conjugate in phosphate buffered saline (PBS).
   b. Test each conjugate dilution for its ability to stain homologous and heterologous virus-infected cell culture smears as well as normal uninfected cell culture smears.
   c. The working dilution of the antiserum should be the highest dilution producing 3-4 + fluorescence on the homologous virus smears, no fluorescence in negative smears, and $\leq 1+$ fluorescence on heterologous virus smears.

2. **Preparation of slides**
   a. Discard media from all tubes. Wash monolayers with 2 ml PBS, pH 7.5 (Chapter 45).
   b. To washed monolayers, add 1 ml prewarmed 0.25% trypsin (Chapter 45). Bathe cell sheets by rotating tubes 10-15 seconds.
   c. Pour off trypsin, and incubate tubes at 35° C for 10 min in a slanted position so that the residual trypsin covers the monolayers. After incubation, examine microscopically to assure that the cells are detached from the glass (occasionally PMK cells require an additional 4-5 min).
   d. Pool the resulting cell suspensions in 3 ml PBS containing 2% fetal bovine serum (FBS). Disperse cells by vigorous pipetting or shaking on vortex mixer.

PROCEDURE 42.3. IDENTIFICATION OF ISOLATES BY FLUORESCENT ANTIBODY (FA) METHOD—cont'd

  e. Centrifuge pooled cells at 2,000 rpm for 10 min and carefully remove supernatant.
  f. Resuspend the cell pellet in 0.05 ml PBS with 2% FBS. Examine microscopically to assure that cells are not overdiluted or underdiluted and that they are adequately dispersed.
  g. Using a Pasteur pipette, place 2 small (5 mm) drops of the cell suspension on cleaned and labeled slides. Prepare enough smears to test with antisera to all viruses under consideration. Remaining cells can be suspended in a few milliliters of growth medium and stored at −70° C.
  h. Allow slides to air dry and fix for 10 min in acetone. Store at −70° C.
3. **Fluorescent antibody staining procedure**
    Fluorescent antisera should be titrated in advance (see above, step 1). This staining procedure is used for both direct smears (see 42.5.a.) and slides prepared as described above.
  a. Circle areas to be stained with permanent ink marker.
  b. Prior to each run, dilute conjugate to predetermined working dilution with PBS. Allow 0.05 ml diluted conjugate per smear.
  c. Apply diluted conjugates to appropriate areas without touching pipette to slide. Cover circles completely.
  d. Place slides in a moist chamber and cover the chamber to minimize evaporation. Incubate slides at 35° C for 20 min. Be careful not to tilt slides, since conjugates will run together.
  e. After staining, tip slides to drain conjugate from smear, place slides in a slide carrier, and rinse with running PBS, pH 7.2-7.5 (Chapter 45). Soak in two changes of PBS for a total of 20 min.
  f. Rinse slides in distilled water to remove PBS salt crystals.
  g. Allow slides to air dry, taking care to protect them from bright light. Mount with 25% buffered glycerol in PBS and cover with no. 1 coverslips.
  h. Examine with fluorescent microscope using Schott UG2 exciter filter or equivalent.
4. **Interpretation of smears**
  a. Uninfected cell culture smears (negative controls) should exhibit no fluorescence.
  b. Positive controls should exhibit 3-4＋ fluorescence with homologous antisera. Cross-reactions with heterologous antigens must be minimal, i.e., no greater than 1＋. This should not present a problem if initial titration of the conjugate was performed properly.
  c. Specific staining of an isolate with acceptable control reactions constitutes positive identification.

FIGURE 42.8
Cytomegalovirus cytopathic effect.

monkey kidney [BGMK], and HFD) with varying degrees of success. Tear-shaped or angular refractile CPE is characteristic for the group and is usually detectable 3-5 days after inoculation.

Unfortunately, enteroviruses have no group antigen, and except for hepatitis A, identification is based on **neutralization tests** with intersecting pools of specific antisera. During enterovirus epidemics, it is often useful to attempt identification of an isolate by first testing with antisera to the prevailing virus(es) in an effort to avoid the use of all antisera pools. In addition, enteroviral isolates from small children who have a history of recent oral poliomyelitis immunization can be tested with trivalent poliomyelitis antisera to rule out these agents prior to neutralization attempts with serum pools. A clue to the presence of vaccine strains of polioviruses is the very rapid development of CPE, often in 1 or 2 days. The Lim-Benyesh-Melnick intersecting pools (A-H) of hy

perimmune serum are available through the Research Resources Branch of the National Institute of Allergy and Infectious Diseases (NIAID), Department of Health and Human Services, Bethesda, MD 20014. These eight pools identify poliovirus 1-3, coxsackie A7, 9, 16; coxsackie B1, 2, 4-6; and echovirus 1-7, 9, 13-21, 24-27, 29-33. In addition to the pools, our laboratory employs specific antisera to identify coxsackie A24, coxsackie B3, and echo 8 viruses. These antisera are not included in any of the pools. Instructions for rehydration of the serum pools and performance of the neutralization test are provided by NIAID on receipt of the antisera, and therefore are not included here. A presumptive identification of the isolate usually is possible and can be confirmed using specific antisera.

If an enterovirus cannot be identified by the serum pools and the individual antisera mentioned above, the isolate may represent a new virus type or antigenic variant, a mixture

PROCEDURE 42.4. ADENOVIRUS NEUTRALIZATION TEST

This test is used in the typing of adenovirus isolates.

1. **Principle**

    Serotyping of a virus isolate is based on the ability of specific immune sera to neutralize 100 $TCID_{50}$ (median tissue culture infective dose) of virus and to inhibit its growth (i.e., CPE production) in cell culture.

2. **Type-specific antisera**

    We keep antisera to adenovirus types 1-7 on hand. If typing of an isolate cannot be accomplished with these, the virus can be forwarded to a reference laboratory for further identification.

    a. Inactivate sera at 56° C for 30 min and dilute to a working dilution (determined by the supplier) with maintenance medium.

    b. The working dilution should contain a minimum of 20 standard antibody units. If this titration has not been done by the commercial suppliers, it can be performed in the laboratory using 100 $TCID_{50}$ per 0.1 ml of the reference adenovirus type and an equal volume of serial doubling dilutions of the antisera. The highest serum dilution that neutralizes 100 $TCID_{50}$ of the reference virus is 1 standard antibody unit; 20 U are used in the test.

3. **Neutralization test procedure**

    a. Harvest culture fluids when culture shows 3-4+ CPE. Viral titers in the fluid can be boosted by sonication or alternate cycles of freezing and thawing. The infectivity titer of the fluid may be determined by the Reed-Muench method (consult any standard virology text such as those listed in the Bibliography). A convenient alternative to titrating the virus by the Reed-Muench method is to select arbitrarily the dilution that is most apt to approximate 100 $TCID_{50}$. For adenovirus, a 1:10 dilution of a culture showing 3-4+ CPE is usually adequate; for enteroviruses, a 10^{-2} or 10^{-3} dilution should be used. This alternative is used in our laboratory. To check on this estimate of virus titer, make serial log dilutions of the virus in maintenance medium; 0.1 ml of each dilution (10^{0}-10^{-4}) is inoculated into single tissue culture tubes of Hep-2 or HFD cells, and the virus titer can be calculated approximately from the dilutions which exhibit CPE.

    b. Neutralization test:

    (1) Mix 0.2 ml of diluted virus (in this case 10^{-1}) with an equal volume of each antiserum at its working dilution, i.e., the dilution containing 20 antibody units.

    (2) Allow the serum-virus mixture to incubate for 1 h at room temperature.

    (3) Use 0.2 ml of each serum-virus mixture to inoculate duplicate tubes of appropriate cell cultures.

    (4) Incubate all inoculated tubes (titration and neutralization assays) at 35° C and examine daily for 7 days.

    c. Interpretation: Inhibition of CPE by specific antisera, when control tubes (in this case, the 10^{-1} dilution) show 2-3+ CPE, constitutes identification of the serotype. Complete inhibition is not always possible, but there should be at least a 2+ difference in CPE between the positive control and the inhibited serotype.

PROCEDURE 42.5. ACID LABILITY TEST TO DIFFERENTIATE RHINOVIRUS FROM ENTEROVIRUS

1. **Principle**
   Rhinoviruses are labile at pH 3, while enteroviruses are not.
2. **Preparation of media**
   a. Eagle's minimum essential medium (MEM) prepared without sodium bicarbonate (Chapter 45) is approximately pH 3; test with pH meter and adjust with 2N HCl if necessary.
   b. The same medium prepared with sodium bicarbonate should be pH 7; check with pH meter and adjust if necessary.
3. **Performance of test**
   a. Make a 1:10 dilution of the virus to be tested in each of the above media (0.2 ml virus and 1.8 ml medium) and incubate for 3 h at room temperature.
   b. Use stock rhinovirus and enterovirus as controls.
   c. Make serial $\log_{10}$ dilutions in Hanks' BSS (Chapter 45) of each mixture (10^{-1}-10^{-5}).
   d. Inoculate 0.1 ml of each dilution in each medium, in duplicate, into tubes of HFD, incubate at 35° C and observe for a period of 7-10 days for CPE.
   e. A 2 log decrease of infectivity due to pH 3 treatment and no decrease at pH 7 indicates that the isolate is a rhinovirus. The isolate is an enterovirus if no reduction of infectivity by pH 3 treatment occurs.

---

of viruses, or a very high titer of virus which is able to overcome the antibody used in the test. Occasionally enteroviruses form aggregates that are incompletely neutralized by antisera. In these cases, there will be an apparent neutralization for several days; then the virus will "break through" the antisera and produce CPE.

Hepatitis A is not recovered in tissue culture and is diagnosed by serologic methods (see Section 42.7.b.).

RHINOVIRUSES. These viruses are a major cause of the common cold or URI (upper respiratory infection). They differ from enteroviruses in that they are labile at pH 3 and grow better in HFD cells than in cells of monkey origin.

Rhinoviruses are rarely recovered in the clinical laboratory, in part because patients with mild illness usually are not cultured. In addition, they grow best at 33° C rather than at the 35° C of most laboratory incubators. To detect the occasional rhinovirus, all viruses producing picornavirus-like CPE in respiratory specimens are tested for acid lability (Procedure 42.5) unless a picornavirus is isolated from a stool or CSF specimen.

Myxoviruses. Myxoviruses are generally separated into two groups: (1) orthomyxoviruses, including influenza A, B, and C, and (2) paramyxoviruses, including parainfluenza types 1-4, respiratory syncytial virus, and mumps virus. They are identified by hemadsorption inhibition (Procedure 42.6).

PROCEDURE 42.6. HEMADSORPTION INHIBITION TEST (HadI) TO IDENTIFY MYXOVIRUS ISOLATES

Viruses to be considered are influenza A and B, PIV 1, 2, and 3, mumps, and SV5. Treat immune sera to these seven virus agents with receptor-destroying enzyme (RDE) of *Vibrio cholerae* to remove nonspecific inhibitors of hemadsorption (see step 2 below).

1. **Principle**

   Inhibition of hemadsorption by specific antisera.

2. **Receptor-destroying enzyme (RDE) treatment of immune sera**

   a. Mix 0.3 ml of each antiserum to be used with an equal volume of RDE and incubate in a 37° C water bath overnight. The RDE should have a titer of 128 U. (For RDE titration procedure, see standard texts.)

   b. Inactivate treated sera in a 56° C water bath for 30 min.

   c. Dilute serum 1:10 by adding 2.4 ml phosphate-buffered saline (PBS).

   d. To remove nonspecific agglutinins, add 0.1 ml 50% guinea pig RBCs for each ml of the 1:10 dilution. Refrigerate with occasional agitation at 4° C for 1 h.

   e. Centrifuge at 2,000 rpm for 10 min. Remove supernatant and use in HadI test. Freeze excess treated sera at −20° C.

3. **Test procedure**

   a. Scrape cells and fluid together with a 1 ml pipette and pass 0.1 ml into each of 10 tubes of PMK. After 72 h incubation, hemadsorb one PMK tube to determine whether the virus titer is adequate to perform the inhibition test. Hemadsorption by 50% or greater of the cell sheet generally is adequate.

   b. Wash remaining infected monolayers twice with Hanks' balanced salt solution (BSS) plus antibiotics (Chapter 45).

   c. Add 0.6 ml Hanks' BSS plus 0.2 ml of each RDE-treated antiserum to labeled tubes. The two remaining tubes include one positive control and one to be saved for further studies if necessary.

   d. After incubation for 30 min at room temperature, add 0.2 ml of a 0.4% guinea pig erythrocyte suspension to each tube and reincubate cultures at 4° C for 30 min. Place tubes in rack, cell sheet down.

   e. Examine tubes as in hemadsorption procedure (Procedure 42.2). Inhibition of hemadsorption by a specific antiserum is sufficient evidence to identify the isolate. This inhibition may not be complete, but must show at least a 2+ difference from the control.

Note: Occasional influenza A isolates cannot be identified by this method. In such cases, perform a hemagglutination inhibition (HI) test. Strain identification of influenza A isolates is beyond the scope of the hospital laboratory and should be performed by a reference facility.

Influenza viruses. These viruses are notable for their epidemic potential, particularly influenza A which affects all age groups and tends to cause pandemics every 10 years and lesser outbreaks almost yearly. Influenza B virus may be recovered sporadically or in association with true outbreaks, while influenza C is rarely if ever isolated. The ability of influenza virus to cause epidemics is related to its antigenic variations, a feature especially notable with type A. The first isolates of an outbreak are apt to be of great interest to the medical community and should be sent to a reference laboratory for strain identification.

Influenza viruses are readily recovered in PMK cell cultures although occasional strains of type A virus may grow only in embryonated hen's eggs. CPE production varies among different types of influenza A viruses, but may be observed in 2-4 days with certain strains. Influenza virus CPE consists of destructive degeneration of the cell sheet; infected cells become granular and swollen and eventually detach from the glass.

Parainfluenza viruses (PIVs). PIVs are important agents of acute respiratory illness among infants and small children. Infection with parainfluenza type 1 is seasonal in nature, with peak isolations occurring in fall and early winter, often during epidemics of croup. Type 3 infections occur sporadically throughout the year as well as in seasonal outbreaks.

PIVs, like influenza virus, grow well in PMK but often do not produce CPE. As a result, PMK cells inoculated with respiratory specimens are routinely hemadsorbed at 5 and 10 days postinoculation (or earlier if CPE is present) with a suspension of guinea pig erythrocytes (Procedure 42.2). If virus is present, these erythrocytes will hemadsorb to the infected monolayer due to the presence of a viral hemagglutinin elaborated at the cell surface (Figure 42.6). This adherence can be minimal in cases where large amounts of virus have been liberated into the culture fluid, and the erythrocytes are agglutinated before they can adsorb to the monolayer. Consequently, it is important that both fluids and the monolayer surface be examined in the performance of this test.

Monolayers exhibiting hemadsorption during an influenza outbreak are tested with fluorescent antibody to confirm the presence of influenza A. If this test is negative, the isolate should be passed and tested further with fluorescent antisera to other hemadsorbing viruses, or identified by the hemadsorption inhibition or hemagglutination inhibition tests.

Respiratory syncytial virus. RSV is a major cause of pneumonia and bronchiolitis in infants and small children. RSV is very labile, and best isolation results are obtained when respiratory specimens are inoculated directly into tubes of Hep-2 cells. CPE may take up to 14 days to first appear, but direct inoculation can reduce isolation time to an average of 4-5 days. This virus does not hemadsorb and tends to show little or no CPE in PMK and HFD. The slow production of refractile giant cell syncytia in Hep-2 is highly suggestive of RSV in a patient with respiratory disease, and confirmation is optional. Troublesome isolates can be confirmed by fluorescent antibody methods.

Mumps virus. This virus is recovered infrequently in the clinical laboratory, probably because the disease is recognized easily by physicians and preventive vaccination is widespread. It is, however, an important agent of aseptic meningitis in children, and it is occasionally associated with orchitis in adult males. Specimens submitted for isolation of this virus include respiratory swabs, urine and CSF. PMK tubes inoculated with such specimens should be hemadsorbed with guinea pig erythrocytes (by the same procedure [Procedure 42.2] described for influenza and parainfluenza viruses) since CPE in culture is not regularly caused by mumps virus. When present, CPE consists of a destructive degeneration of the monolayer with occasional syncytia. Isolates are confirmed with fluorescent antisera.

42.4.g. Additional tissue culture techniques (Procedures 42.7 to 42.10).

42.4.h. Interpretation of viral culture results. The interpretation of virological data must be based on knowledge of the normal viral flora in the site sampled, the clinical findings, and the epidemiological behavior of viruses. In some situations, serological studies may be necessary to support or refute the possible association of a virus isolate with a disease.

Viruses in tissue and body fluids. In general, the detection of any virus in host tissues, CSF, blood, or vesicular fluid can be considered highly significant. Recovery of viruses other than CMV in urine may be diagnostic of significant infection, e.g., adenovirus type 2, associated with acute hemorrhagic cystitis, and mumps. However, recovery of CMV from urine can be difficult to interpret. The CMV isolate may merely reflect active, asymptomatic virus replication or may indicate a significant infection in the patient. Viruria in the first 3 weeks of life establishes a diagnosis of congenital CMV infection, whereas the onset of viral excretion after 4 weeks of life reflects intrapartum or postpartum infection. Diagnosis of acquired CMV infections in older patients usually results from a combination of findings, including positive cultures from any site, illness known to be compatible with CMV, reasonable exclusion of other potential etiological agents, and support by specific serological or histological data or both.

Virus isolation from other sites. Upper respiratory tract (or specimens obtained by traversing the upper airways), vaginal, and fecal cultures vary greatly in terms of their significance. At one extreme, isolates such as measles, mumps, influenza, parainfluenza, and respiratory syncytial virus are very significant

since asymptomatic carriage and prolonged shedding of these viruses is unusual. Conversely, other viruses can be shed without symptoms and for periods ranging from several weeks (enteroviruses) to many months (adenoviruses, HSV, CMV). Examples include HSV and CMV in the oropharynx and vagina, adenoviruses in the oropharynx and intestinal tract, and enteroviruses in the intestinal tract. VSV, HSV, CMV, adenoviruses, and Epstein-Barr virus (EBV) may remain latent for long periods and then become reactivated in response to a variety of stressful stimuli, including other infectious agents. In this setting, their detection may have no significance (VZV is an exception) or may merely represent a secondary problem complicating the primary infection (e.g., HSV "cold sores" in patients with bacterial sepsis).

Adenovirus isolates are common in infants and young children. Based on the epidemiology and observed serological responses, it has been found that, in febrile and respiratory syndromes, simultaneous isolation of these agents from both the throat and feces has greater probability of association with that illness; isolation from the throat, but not the feces, has a lesser probability of association, and isolation from the feces alone has the least diagnostic significance. In these latter situations, interpretation of the significance of the culture results can be aided by adenovirus serological studies.

Enteroviruses are also most commonly found in infants and children, particularly during the late summer and early autumn seasons. A knowledge of the relative frequency of virus shedding among various age groups in a particular locale is extremely helpful in assessing significance of results of throat or stool cultures; for example, the peak prevalence of enteroviruses in the stools of toddlers during the late summer may range from greater than 20% in subtropical climates to 5% in temperate zones.

PROCEDURE 42.7. CULTIVATION AND SUBPASSAGE OF Hep-2 CELLS

Cell passage

1. Remove maintenance medium from stock flask and rinse cell sheet once with 10-20 ml PBS, pH 7.5 (Chapter 45).
2. Add 1-2 ml 0.24% trypsin (Chapter 45) to flask and incubate at 35° C for 5-10 min.
3. When cells detach from the plastic, add 10 ml of growth medium (Chapter 45) and disperse cells by pipetting vigorously. Examine the suspension microscopically to ensure adequate cell dispersal.
4. Seed new 250 ml plastic culture flasks with 2-3 ml of this suspension, and then add an additional 20 ml of growth medium per flask.
5. Inoculate cell culture tubes with 0.05 ml of the suspension from step 4, and then add 1 ml of the growth medium to each tube.
6. Close tubes and flasks tightly and incubate horizontally in a stationary position at 35° C for 72 h. Once cells are sufficiently sheeted, replace growth medium in culture tubes with 3 ml maintenance medium (Chapter 45). Replace growth medium in flasks with 20 ml of maintenance medium.

PROCEDURE 42.8. PRESERVATION AND STORAGE OF Hep-2 CELLS BY FREEZING

1. Repeat steps 1-3 in Procedure 42.7.
2. Transfer the cell suspension to a test tube and centrifuge at 1,500 rpm for 5 min. Decant supernatant.
3. Resuspend pellet thoroughly in 2 ml of growth medium (Chapter 45) containing 10% DMSO (dimethyl sulfoxide) or 50% glycerol. Dispense 1 ml aliquots of this suspension into sterile glass ampules. Seal ampules by flaming and freeze to −70° C slowly.
4. For reconstitution of the frozen cells, the ampule should be thawed rapidly in a 35° C water bath and the contents used to seed a new flask. Add 10 ml of growth medium and incubate the flask at 35° C until a confluent monolayer has formed. Replace growth medium with 20 ml of maintenance medium (Chapter 45) and reincubate.

PROCEDURE 42.9. PASSAGE OF CMV AND VZV ISOLATES

Most viruses can be passed by subculturing the culture medium. CMV and VZV are cell-associated viruses and must be passed by trypsinizing infected monolayers.

1. Discard media from infected cell sheet and wash the monolayer two times with PBS, pH 7.5 (Chapter 45).
2. To washed monolayer, add 2 ml 0.25% trypsin (Chapter 45). Bathe cell sheet by rotating tube for 10-15 seconds. Pour off trypsin.
3. Allow monolayer to incubate in residual trypsin for 5-10 min at 35° C. (Occasionally a subpassage will rapidly deteriorate because of the presence of excess trypsin in the inoculum. Care must be exercised to assure that most of the trypsin is removed prior to the incubation step.)
4. After cells detach from the glass, add 1 ml growth medium (Chapter 45) to the cell-trypsin suspension and pipette vigorously to disperse cell aggregates.
5. Inoculate fresh monolayers with 0.2 ml of the suspension from step 4.

PROCEDURE 42.10. PRESERVATION AND STORAGE OF VIRUSES BY FREEZING

1. **CMV and VZV**

    CMV- and VZV-infected monolayers having 2-3+ CPE are trypsinized as described in Procedure 42.9. Instead of adding growth medium to the trypsin-cell suspension, resuspend cells in 1-2 ml of growth medium containing 10% DMSO for VZV and 35% sorbitol for CMV. Disperse monolayer by vigorous pipetting and store at −70° C in flame-sealed glass ampules.

2. **Other viruses**

    There are two acceptable methods of preparing infected monolayers for storage. DMSO or sorbitol are not necessary for the preservation of viruses other than VZV and CMV.

    a. Scrape monolayers exhibiting 3-4+ CPE (or hemadsorption) into their own culture media, pipette vigorously to disperse cell aggregates, and aliquot 1 ml amounts into glass ampules which are then flame-sealed and stored at −70° C. For short-term storage, tightly sealed screw-cap vials or test tubes may be used.

    b. Trypsinize infected monolayers (Procedure 42.9). Resuspend cells in 2-3 ml of fresh growth medium (Chapter 45), aliquot 1 ml amounts into glass ampules or test tubes, seal, and freeze at −70° C.

Even in the latter areas, carriage rates may approach 30% in infants during periods of enterovirus activity. Shedding of enteroviruses in the throat is relatively transient (usually 1-2 weeks), whereas fecal shedding may last 4-16 weeks. Thus, with a clinically compatible illness, isolation of an enterovirus from the throat supports a stronger temporal relationship to the disease than an isolate from the feces alone. When echovirus or coxsackievirus is recovered from the stool only, it may be helpful to study the patient's serum for an antibody rise against that particular viral isolate.

HSV is unusual in a fecal culture; in such cases, it usually represents either severe disseminated infection or infection of the anus or perianal areas. If this virus is obtained from an anal or rectal culture of a sexually active patient with signs of nervous system disease, e.g., aseptic meningitis or lumbosacral myeloradiculitis, it may indicate the etiology. Detection of HSV in the upper respiratory tract may have no meaning other than nonspecific stress reactivation unless typical vesicles or ulcers are also seen. Because of the stress-related phenomenon, isolation of HSV in the throat or mucocutaneous lesions of patients with encephalitis cannot be interpreted as causative of the CNS disease. Currently, the definitive way to establish a diagnosis of herpes simplex encephalitis is by direct demonstration of the virus in a brain biopsy. In newborn infants, however, isolation of the virus from any site should raise the possibility that a potentially severe infection exists.

Isolation of adenoviruses, HSV, VZV, and some enteroviruses from the cornea and conjunctiva in cases of inflammatory disease at these sites usually establishes the etiology of the infection.

Significance of negative virological results. There are numerous occasions when the laboratory is asked to perform studies with the intent of ruling out specific viral agents. The ability to exclude the presence of a virus depends greatly on the sensitivity of the detection systems being used. The most important prerequisites include (1) proper communication with the laboratory **before** initiating studies, (2) procurement of the appropriate specimens in the **early** phase of acute illness, (3) careful attention to the procedures of collection, transportation, and processing of specimens, and (4) avoidance of fungal or bacterial contamination of processed cultures. When all these criteria are fulfilled, it is usually possible to interpret negative data with a high degee of confidence.

42.5. Visual Methods for Detection of Viruses in Clinical Specimens

42.5.a. Fluorescent antibody techniques. Much of the original work on immunofluorescent (IF) applications in the diagnostic laboratory utilized indirect methods which were considered to be economical and widely applicable; however, more recent studies have shown that direct methods are feasible. Commercially prepared direct conjugates are available for many of the common viruses (sources include Flow Laboratories, Whittaker M.A. Bioproducts, and Northeast Biomedical Laboratories), and others may be prepared by animal immunization with cell culture harvests (Table 42.11). Whenever possible, it is desirable to produce antibody with tissue culture harvests prepared from cells of the homologous animal species. The recent development of in vitro production of monoclonal antibodies (Chapter 10) should greatly enhance the specificity and sensitivity of IF as well as other immunodiagnostic methods in the future. In fact, IF is probably superior to culture for the diagnosis of RSV and VZV infections since culture of these two viruses takes several days and may be falsely negative.[5]

A suggested approach to direct IF diagnosis is given in Procedure 42.11.

TABLE 42.11
Detection of Viral Antigens by Fluorescent Antibody

SYNDROME	POSSIBLE VIRAL AGENTS DETECTABLE BY IF	USUAL TISSUE OR CELL SOURCE
Colorado tick fever	Colorado tick fever virus	Erythrocytes
Congenital infections	Rubella virus, cytomegalovirus, herpes simplex virus	Nasopharyngeal, throat, lesion scrapings, tissue
Conjunctivitis, keratitis	Herpes simplex, adenovirus	Conjunctival cells, corneal scrapings
Disseminated disease	Herpes simplex virus, cytomegalovirus, varicella zoster, virus	Tissue, lesion scrapings
Encephalitis	Herpes simplex virus	Brain biopsy
	Mumps virus	Throat, urine sediment
	Rabies virus	Brain biopsy, corneal scrapings, neck skin biopsy
Infectious mononucleosis	Epstein-Barr virus	Lymphocytes, lymphoid tissue
Macular or maculopapular exanthems	Measles, rubella, adenoviruses	Nasopharyngeal, throat, urine sediment
Mucocutaneous vesicles and ulcers	Herpes simplex, varicella-zoster viruses	Lesion or vesicle scrapings, mucosal cells
Respiratory tract infection	Influenza A, B; parainfluenza 1, 2, 3; adenovirus; respiratory syncytial virus	Nasopharyngeal, throat, lung biopsy

42.5.b. Electron microscopy. Several reviews of the procedures and utility of electron microscopy (EM) in diagnostic virology have been published.[1, 2, 4, 8] EM techniques are most applicable for the investigation of viral infections in which the titer of virus in specimens is at least 10^6-10^7 particles per milliliter. EM is most commonly utilized for feces examination since rotaviruses as well as adenoviruses, coronaviruses, and caliciviruses may be seen and identified as the cause of the illness (Figure 42.9). The Norwalk agent virus, an important cause of gastroenteritis, is not easily visible by standard EM in feces, and usually requires enhancement by immune EM to permit detection. Immune EM allows visualization of virus particles that may be present in numbers too small for easy direct detection. The addition of specific antiserum to the test suspension causes the virus particles to form antibody-bound aggregates, which are more easily detected by EM than are single virus particles. Other spec-

imens, such as vesicle fluid, biopsy tissue, solid wart tissue, urine, or serum, can be negatively stained with minimum preparation to yield positive results. If concentrations of viruses are lower in these specimens or others, techniques to enhance visualization are necessary. Enhancement techniques may include pseudoreplication, agar gel diffusion, ultracentrifugation, or immune EM.

Diseases in which EM can play a role in rapid identification of viruses include gastroenteritis, herpes simplex infections, varicella-zoster (especially in the immunocompromised patient), congenital CMV infection, hepatitis B, molluscum contagiosum, and warts.

In most instances, viruses seen by EM can be detected by alternative methods. For example, HSV and VZV viral antigens can be detected by IF techniques, and rotavirus in stool specimens can be detected by latex agglutination, ELISA, or counterimmunoelectroosmo-

PROCEDURE 42.11. RAPID DIAGNOSIS OF VIRAL INFECTION BY DIRECT FLUORESCENT ANTIBODY STAINING

1. Specimens

Four types of specimens can be used for IF diagnosis: frozen sections, impression smears, lesion scrapings, and resuspended cells in centrifuged sediment.

Frozen sections should be cut to 3-4 μm in thickness, and lesion scrapings are best obtained with a scalpel blade and then smeared in spots on the slide. Swabs of lesions may be **rolled** onto the slide; rubbing should be avoided since this can distort cell morphology.

Cell suspensions can usually be readily recovered from urine or other body fluids (e.g., amniotic fluid by centrifugation). In addition, if appropriate vigor has been applied in the collection of swabs from the respiratory tract, conjunctiva, vagina, or skin lesions, the specimens in viral transport media can be utilized. These samples are blended thoroughly on a Vortex mixer, and the swabs are removed. The samples are then centrifuged at 1,200 to 1,500 × g for 30 min, and the supernatant is used for cell culture inoculation. The remaining sediment is suspended in just enough PBS (without phenol red) to yield a slightly turbid suspension, which is spotted on the wells of slides with a Pasteur pipette. The amount of PBS required for resuspension usually varies from 0.1-1 ml. All slides are labeled appropriately, allowed to air dry completely, and then fixed in acetone at −20° C for 10 min. If slides must be transported from one laboratory to another, they may be sent air-dried at ambient temperature, or acetone fixed at 4° C. Formalin fixed tissues are **not** suitable for IF studies.

2. Slides

Clean, plain, 1 mm thick glass slides can be used for frozen sections or impression smears. For examination of resuspended cells, preprinted slides are preferred to slides prepared by spraying with Fluoroglide.

3. Conjugates

Fluorescein isothiocyanate–conjugated antisera are reconstituted with phosphate-buffered saline (PBS), pH 7.4 to 8.0, aliquoted, and stored at −60° C until the time of use. These samples are then titrated at 1:5, 1:10, 1:20, and 1:40 dilutions in PBS to determine optimal working dilutions in infected cell cultures. (Optimal dilution is defined as that which gives 3+ to 4+ specific fluorescence in cells infected with homologous virus and no fluorescence in cells infected with heterologous virus or in uninfected cells.) This optimal dilution is then tested for cross-reactivity with heterologous viruses, as well as for nonspecific fluorescence in impression smears or frozen sections of normal, noninfected human tissues, such as brain and lung. In clinical use, appropriate controls include preimmune conjugates derived from the homologous animal source, conjugated antisera to heterologous viruses, and, when tissue sections or impression smears are used, normal, noninfected tissue controls. The conjugates are used on clinical specimens at a twofold lower dilution than for typing of tissue culture isolates. Slides submitted for VZV

PROCEDURE 42.11. RAPID DIAGNOSIS OF VIRAL INFECTION BY DIRECT FLUORESCENT ANTIBODY STAINING—cont'd

or HSV fluorescent antibody examination should be stained with both conjugates. The HSV conjugate used in our laboratory is bivalent, i.e., contains antibody to both types 1 and 2 HSV, and is obtained commercially. The working dilution is determined as described in Procedure 42.3.

Positive and negative controls for each conjugate are necessary. For example, HSV and VZV positive controls should be stained with the heterologous conjugate to ascertain the extent (if any) of cross-reactions.

4. Staining

The procedure used is the same as that outlined for identification of cell culture isolates (Procedure 42.3). Appropriately diluted conjugate is overlaid on each specimen, and the slides are incubated at 35° C for 30-60 min in a humidified chamber. The slides are then washed with gentle agitation for two 5 min periods in PBS. Coverslips (no. 1) are mounted with buffered glycerol (pH 8.0), and specimens are examined for fluorescence. A halogen-source microscope equipped with epifluorescence is ideal for this purpose, with observation at 600 × magnification. If oil immersion is used, low-fluorescence oil is necessary.

5. Interpretation

Strict criteria for interpreting fluorescence patterns must be applied. For example, nuclear and cytoplasmic staining are typical for influenza virus, adenoviruses, and the herpesviruses (Figure 42.10); cytoplasmic staining only is seen with respiratory syncytial (Figure 42.11), parainfluenza, and mumps viruses; staining within multinucleated giant cells is typical of measles viruses. If the pattern of fluorescence is appropriate, and proper controls have been employed, the specificity of the test is high. In fact, for some agents such as VZV, direct IF is often considerably more sensitive than culture. Smears that have insufficient (<6) epithelial cells, or that have primarily pus or tissue fragments, are considered unsatisfactory and should be reported as such. (Note: The technologist should be aware of nonspecific staining reactions. Leukocytes are notorious for nonspecific binding of fluorescein-conjugated antisera; only epithelial cells should be used to interpret direct smears. Tissues also may trap the conjugate and prevent it from being washed away.) False-positive results can be obtained if the above criteria are not strictly applied. Specimens which contain yeasts, mucus, or leukocytes can be especially misleading.

It is extremely important to attempt virus isolation on specimens submitted for fluorescent-antibody staining to verify results, to enhance the overall sensitivity of diagnosis, and to properly standardize the conjugates. When both cultures and IF examination are performed, false-negative IF tests will be observed. In some instances, these false-negative tests result from specimens with very low virus titer, requiring many days for detection in culture. False-negative fluorescent assay results have occurred with critical specimens such as brain biopsies for HSV encephalitis; **culture "backup" is therefore mandatory.**

FIGURE 42.9
Electron micrographs of viruses visualized in feces from patients with diarrhea. **A,** Adenovirus. **B,** Rotavirus.

FIGURE 42.10
Herpes simplex virus, fluorescent antibody stain.

FIGURE 42.11
Respiratory syncytial virus, fluorescent antibody stain.

phoresis. Nonetheless, EM can be quite useful in a diagnostic virology laboratory, especially for the examination of feces from patients with gastroenteritis.

EM can also be used to detect herpesvirus particles in a brain biopsy from a patient with encephalitis, and CMV particles may be seen in high concentration in the urine of congenitally infected infants but may require some form of enhancement for EM detection. Although hepatitis B viral particles can be seen in serum with EM, very sensitive and convenient methods for viral antigen detection such as RIA or ELISA are usually employed. Human papilloma virus (common warts), Orf virus, and molluscum contagiosum poxvirus can be viewed in homogenates of solid biopsy tissue, but examination of these specimens is rarely indicated. EM methods (Procedure 42.12) can also be used to hasten the identifi-

cation of a virus which has been recovered in tissue culture and to detect viral (and mycoplasma) contaminants in cell cultures.

42.6. Enzyme Immunoassays for Detection of Viral Antigens and Antibodies

42.6.a. Solid-phase immunoassays. Solid-phase immunoassays (SPIAs) for the detection of antigens or antibodies use, as an indicator, a radioactive label (for RIA) or the action of an enzyme label on a substrate (for ELISA). Several excellent reviews on these procedures and their application to viral diagnosis have been published. Chapters 10 and 12 describe the principles of such methods.

Most SPIAs for the detection of antigen have employed one of three methods: competitive, direct (double-antibody sandwich method), or indirect (double-antibody sandwich-antiglobulin method). In a competitive assay, la-

PROCEDURE 42.12. LABORATORY METHODS FOR ELECTRON MICROSCOPY

1. Specimen collection and preparation

Specimens should be collected as described below and transported at ambient temperature in sealed containers to prevent drying.

a. **Fluid specimens.** Depending on the type of clinical specimen, centrifugation may help to provide a better preparation. Feces can be prepared by making a 10%-20% suspension in distilled water and then clarifying with a bench centrifuge if necessary.

Vesicle fluid should be collected from unbroken lesions by using a tuberculin syringe containing a small amount of distilled water. A sheath should be placed over the needle and tape should be applied to the plunger and sheath before the syringe is transported to the laboratory inside an appropriate container.

Urine that is cloudy should be clarified by centrifugation at $2,500 \times g$ for 30 min. This supernatant fluid will usually yield virus more readily if as large a volume as possible, e.g., 10-20 ml, is centrifuged for 1 h at $15,000 \times g$ and then the resuspended pellet is stained. Techniques of enhancement (see below) have proven useful for urine specimens.

Serum contains many low-molecular-weight proteins which need to be washed out by diluting with an equal volume of distilled water. As with urine centrifugation for 1 h at $15,000 \times g$ is necessary, and the serum may even require recentrifugation to provide a clean specimen.

b. **Tissue specimens.** Biopsy or autopsy tissue is cut into small (1 mm) cubes and placed on a metal planchet for freezing and thawing (five cycles). An alternative method involves mechanical homogenization using a mortar and pestle or homogenizer. After this, a relatively smooth suspension can be achieved by mixing the homogenate in small amounts of distilled water by using a fine-bore Pasteur pipette. Best results are achieved by differential centrifugation and staining of the supernatant fluid with phosphotungstic acid.

c. **Other specimens.** Other, less commonly examined specimens may be submitted for EM examination. Conjunctival scrapings usually contain small amounts of tissue. CSF seldom yields a virus. Both of these specimens should be processed directly without centrifugation. Sputum specimens should be diluted in saline and then homogenized or treated with 20% N-acetyl-cysteine. Differential centrifugation or some form of enhancement is usually necessary to concentrate the specimen.

PROCEDURE 42.12. LABORATORY METHODS
FOR ELECTRON MICROSCOPY—cont'd

2. Staining

The most appropriate laboratory technique for the examination of clinical specimens is negative staining. The most commonly used stain is phosphotungstic acid as a 2%-4% solution adjusted to a pH of 6-8 with 1 N potassium hydroxide and stored as a working solution at 4° C. Formvar carbon-coated, 400-mesh copper grids provide the most versatile carriers for specimen viewing. Place a drop of the specimen on a drop of sterile distilled water on a waxed surface. Touch a grid held by fine forceps to the drop; hold it upright, and stain with a drop of phosphotungstic acid. Remove excess fluid with a torn strip of filter paper, and dry the specimen before examining by EM. The total process takes about 5 min.

3. Techniques to enhance virus visualization

Other techniques have been devised to enhance the sensitivity of EM for detecting viruses. These include pseudoreplication and agar gel diffusion for concentrating rotaviruses in feces and CMV in urine. Ultracentrifugation and immune EM (mentioned above) have also been employed for concentrating rubella virus, Norwalk agent, and hepatitis A virus.

---

beled antigen is mixed with the test sample containing antigen, and they compete for a limited amount of antibody attached to the solid phase. A negative control sample is included. Unbound antigen is washed away, and the difference in indicator activity between the specimen and control is measured. The less substrate detected, the more antigen was present in the specimen.

A direct SPIA for detection of antigen involves the addition of the clinical specimen to a capture antibody (CA) attached to a solid phase. Unbound antigen is washed away before the addition of a labeled detector antibody (DA). DA is measured spectrophotometrically or visually (ELISA) or in a radioactive counter (RIA). The more labeled substrate detected, the more antigen is present in the sample. An example of this procedure (ELISA) is seen in Figure 42.12.

The indirect test is similar to the direct assay employing a CA and a DA, but the DA is not labeled. Instead a third indicator antibody (IA), which is antispecies to the DA, is labeled, and the balance of the assay is then similar. This approach is the most popular because of the availability of IA conjugates from commercial sources. Although the indirect tests provide some amplification of the binding reaction, the additional antibody brings about more frequent nonspecific reactions.

SPIA techniques have been successfully applied to the detection of hepatitis B, rotavirus, hepatitis A antibody, adenovirus, HSV, respiratory syncytial virus, influenza A virus, CMV, and group A coxsackievirus. Commercial kits (Abbott, M.A. Bioproducts, Behring Diagnostics, Litton Bionetics) are available for the detection of rotaviruses as well as HBsAg, HBsAb, HBcAb, HAV, IgM, and IgG. Fluid specimens are most appropriate for detection of viral antigens by ELISA. Serum may be used directly in the test; urine and feces may need homogenization with saline and preliminary

FIGURE 42.12
Enzyme immunoassay (Rotazyme, Abbott Laboratories) for rotavirus.

clarification by centrifugation to be suitable for the test. Nasopharyngeal or sputum specimens should be collected in appropriate transport media and diluted 1:5 to a final concentration of 20% in N-acetyl-cysteine before use in the test.

Enzyme immunoassays provide the advantage of relatively stable and nonradioactive reagents, and the results can be either qualitative or quantitative. ELISAs are usually more sensitive than all other assays except RIA. The equipment necessary for ELISAs can be quite simple and objective. The major drawback of all SPIAs is that the quality of specimens such as respiratory, genital, or skin swabs cannot be assessed. This is in marked contrast to IF. Specific disadvantages of ELISAs include the variability of solid-phase carriers and the carcinogenicity of certain chromogenic substrates. RIAs require expensive equipment and also involve exposure to carcinogens. In addition, disposing of these hazardous materials poses considerable difficulty. Most SPIAs also require a day or overnight incubation with several washing procedures. For the optimal use of SPIAs in rapid viral diagnosis, several specimens should be examined for antigen in a given run. Thus these techniques are best suited for diseases such as viral gastroenteritis, viral hepatitis, or respiratory infections, in which many specimens are being submitted to the labora-

tory at a given time. Although a single specimen could be analyzed, quite often an alternative assay (IF, EM, etc.) might be more appropriate.

42.7. Viral Serology

Up to about a decade ago, serology was utilized as a primary procedure in diagnosing viral infections. More recently, this approach has been replaced in many cases by methods designed to detect the viral agents or their antigens as quickly as possible. However, several situations still exist in which serological diagnosis can be extremely helpful. These are outlined in Table 42.12. The specifics of the wide variety of serological testing procedures cannot be detailed in this chapter, but can be found in reference texts such as that edited by Lennette and Schmidt (Bibliography) and in Chapter 12.

Serologic tests in present use include complement fixation (CF), neutralization (Neut), hemagglutination inhibition (HI), passive hemagglutination (PHA), indirect fluorescent antibody (IFA), immune adherence hemagglutination (IAHA), immune electron microscopy (IEM), counterimmunoelectrophoresis (CIE), radioimmunoassay (RIA), enzyme-linked immunosorbent assay (ELISA), fluorescent-focus inhibition (FFI), anticomplement immunofluorescence (ACIF), and single radial hemolysis (SRH). Each of the above tests can be adapted

TABLE 42.12

Situations Where Serological Testing Can Be Helpful

SITUATION	VIRUSES UNDER CONSIDERATION	COMMON METHODS OF CHOICE*
CNS infections	Western equine encephalitis	HI, CF
	Eastern equine encephalitis	HI, CF
	California encephalitis virus	HI, CF, CIE
	St. Louis encephalitis virus	HI, CF
	Lymphocytic choriomeningitis virus	CF, IFA
	Measles	HI, CF
	Epstein-Barr virus	IFA
	Rabies	IFA, FFI, CF
Exanthems	Measles	HI, CF, Neut
	Rubella	HI, SRH, ELISA, RIA
Vesicular	Herpes simplex virus	CF, IFA
	Varicella-zoster virus	IFA, IAHA, RIA, ELISA
Hepatitis A	Hepatitis A virus	ELISA, RIA, RIA(IgM)
Hepatitis B	Hepatitis B virus	ELISA
Heterophile-negative infectious mononucleosis syndromes	Cytomegalovirus	IFA, ACIF, PHA, ELISA, CF
	Epstein-Barr virus	IFA, ELISA
Myocarditis-pericarditis	Group B coxsackievirus, types 1-5	Neut
	Influenza A, B	HI, CF
	Cytomegalovirus	IFA, ACIF, PHA, ELISA, CF
Respiratory	Influenza A, B	CF
	Respiratory syncytial virus	
	Parainfluenza 1-3	
	Adenovirus	
	(Also, *Mycoplasma pneumoniae, Chlamydia*)	
Serology needed to determine status (single serum)		
Rubella		HI, SRH, ELISA, RIA
Hepatitis B		RIA, PHA, ELISA
Varicella-zoster		IFA, IAHA, RIA, ELISA

*Abbreviations: Neut, neutralizing antibody; RIA, radioimmunoassay; HI, hemagglutination inhibition; CF, complement fixation; CIE, counterimmunoelectrophoresis; IFA, indirect immunofluorescence; FFI, fluorescent-focus inhibition; SRH, single radial hemolysis; PHA, passive hemagglutination; IAHA, immune adherence hemagglutination; ELISA, enzyme-linked immunosorbent assay; ACIF, anticomplement immunofluorescence.

to demonstrate antibody response or to identify a particular agent.

42.7.a. Tests available. Complement fixation (CF) is a highly satisfactory serologic test. Antibodies measured by this system generally develop slightly later in the course of an illness than those measured by other techniques; this lag provides a greater opportunity to demonstrate titer differences between acute and convalescent sera. Members of some virus groups, such as the adenoviruses, influenza A viruses, and influenza B viruses, possess common antigens demonstrable by complement fixation. Thus, antibody response to infection by any member of the particular group can be observed without resorting to a multiplicity of tests with individual antigens. Unfortunately other members of large virus groups such as enteroviruses do not possess a common antigen and must be tested individually.

The **neutralization test (Neut)** is essentially a protection test. When a virus is incubated with homologous type-specific antibody, the virus is rendered incapable of producing infection in an indicator host system. The test is technically more exacting than other serologic tests and is the principal method used for identifying virus isolates. A neutralizing antibody response is virus type specific and develops with the onset of symptoms. Titers peak rapidly to a plateau and persist for long intervals, and measurable titers may be maintained indefinitely.

The **hemagglutination inhibition test (HI)** can be performed with a variety of viruses that have the capacity to agglutinate selectively red blood cells of various animal species (chicken, guinea pig, human O group, and others). The hemagglutination capacity of a virus is inhibited by specific immune or convalescent serum. Hemagglutination-inhibiting antibody develops rapidly after the onset of symptoms, plateaus rapidly, declines slowly, and may last indefinitely at low levels.

In the **passive hemagglutination (PHA)** procedure, certain viruses can be chemically coupled to the surface of erythrocytes, which then serve as indicators of the presence of homologous antibody in serum by the hemagglutination reaction.

For the **indirect fluorescent antibody test (IFA)**, virus-infected cells are placed in prepared wells on microscope slides, then fixed in cold acetone and dried. Serum antibody is applied and, following incubation for antigen-antibody coupling, antihuman globulin-fluorescein conjugate is added to delineate, by fluorescence, the sites of antigen-antibody reaction. It is possible to identify specifically a virus in any adequately pre-

pared specimen containing virus-infected cells, but the current lack of high-titer, specific antisera limits the usefulness of this method.

42.7.b. Interpretation of viral serologic tests.

Acute-phase serum. When a virological workup is planned for an individual patient, it is generally useful to obtain at least 2-3 ml of acute-phase serum and store it in the freezer. This may become valuable, particularly if virus detection subsequently fails or the interpretation of an isolate is equivocal. In these instances a convalescent-phase serum may be requested 2-3 weeks after the first, and appropriate selection of antigens to be tested can be made.

Single sera. In some cases, a single serum may be studied and appropriately interpreted. Virus-specific immunoglobulin M (IgM) antibody usually rises during the first 2-3 weeks of infection and persists for several weeks to months, eventually becoming replaced by IgG antibody (Figure 42.13). Thus, an elevated titer of specific IgM antibody suggests a recent primary infection by the virus in question, and this may be further supported by demonstrating a fall in IgM antibody in follow-up sera. Detection of specific IgM has been used with success in the diagnosis of infections due to VZV, EBV, CMV, rubella, and coxsackieviruses and is currently the procedure of choice to establish a recent or acute infection due to hepatitis A or B (hepatitis A IgM and IgM antibody to hepatitis B core antigen, respectively). The methods to be employed in IgM-specific antibody determination vary considerably, including sucrose density gradient centrifugation, column chromatography, staphylococcal protein A absorption, and solid-phase immunoassays such as immunofluorescence (IF), enzyme-linked immunosorbent assay (ELISA), and radioimmunoassay (RIA). These methods vary in sensitivity, convenience, and

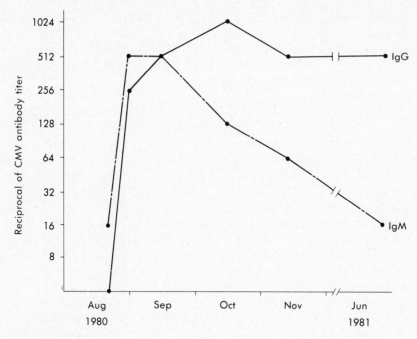

FIGURE 42.13
Time course of cytomegalovirus IgM antibody.

applicability. Several limitations of interpretation must be kept in mind. It is now recognized that IgM-specific antibody responses are not always restricted to primary infections; reactivation or reinfection may result in IgM responses, particularly in CMV, HSV, EBV, and VZV infections. In addition, patients may continue to produce IgM-specific antibody to rubella or CMV for many months after a primary infection. Heterotypic IgM responses can also occur, for example, antibody responses to CMV in EBV infections and vice versa. Other pitfalls include falsely low or negative IgM titers due to competition by IgG antibody for antigen-binding sites and false-positive reactions due to rheumatoid factor. Both these errors appear to be most common in solid-phase assays employing IF.

Both false-negative and false-positive IgM fluorescent antibody results have been frequently encountered in screening sera from newborns for specific antibody to CMV and rubella virus. In some, but not all cases, false-positive results can be attributed to rheumatoid factor of maternal origin. False-negative results might occur as a result of competition between high levels of maternal IgG and low levels of fetal IgM in cord sera.

Other uses of single sera include screening infant blood for certain antibodies of the IgG class, known popularly as the TORCH screen. Antibody to *Toxoplasma gondii (To)*, rubella *(r)*, CMV *(c)*, and HSV *(h)* is measured in an effort to determine possible congenital infection with these agents; however, the utility of these tests has been misunderstood (also discussed in Chapter 12). They are more useful in excluding a possible infection than in proving an etiology. If, for example, rubella antibody is absent, then the infant almost certainly does not have congenital rubella infection. To diagnose active rubella infection in such a baby, viral cultures and additional serologic studies are required. Other uses of single sera include CMV antibody screening to eliminate the transmission of CMV antibody–positive blood to seronegative babies or other immunocompromised patients and rubella antibody screening to identify women requiring vaccination.

If there is adequate knowledge of the specific levels of antibody titers achieved in individuals during acute infection and afterward, the height of a titer in a single serum sample may aid in a presumptive diagnosis of recent infection. For example, hemagglutination-inhibition antibody titer of 1:160 or greater to western equine encephalitis or St. Louis encephalitis virus or a complement fixation titer of 1:128 or greater to influenza B virus would be supportive of a recent experience with the agent. However, it is important to remember that such interpretive criteria cannot be applied to all infections, since titers to many viruses can persist at varying levels. Thus, titers in single sera must be interpreted cautiously in most cases.

False-positive serological results. The majority of serological interpretations are based upon conversion from seronegativity to positivity or a fourfold or greater rise in antibody titer between paired sera. However, such apparently significant antibody titer rises may not always be significant. An example of this is the occasional rise of antibody to CMV in patients with influenza A or *Mycoplasma pneumoniae* infections, suggesting stress reactivation of CMV by the latter agents. False-positive serologic responses may also result from cross-reactions to related antigens, e.g., an antibody rise to parainfluenza virus may actually result from infection with mumps virus. Also, anamnestic antibody responses may falsely suggest seroconversion or cause an apparent fourfold or greater rise in antibody titer.

False-negative serological results. Infants may not develop complement fixing and other antibody responses to respiratory syncytial virus, influenza virus, and other agents. They may also fail to develop IgM antibody responses despite congenital infection with CMV or rubella virus. Severely immunocompromised patients may fail to develop antibodies, although this is comparatively infrequent.

42.7.c. Combinations of several serologic tests for diagnosis of clinical syndromes. Selection of antigens for testing with paired sera in cases where a virus is suspected but not detected can sometimes be made on the basis of clinical syndrome, the known local epidemiology of particular viruses, and the age of the patient. This has led to the concept of serological **"batteries"** or "panels." Some examples of possible batteries are included in Table 42-12.

CNS syndromes. HSV, mumps, western equine encephalitis, eastern equine encephalitis, St. Louis encephalitis, and California encephalitis viruses and perhaps lymphocytic choriomeningitis virus and EBV may be included in a battery of tests for a CNS syndrome. Although herpes simplex antigen is included in the panel, a rise in antibody titer is not sufficient to diagnose HSV encephalitis. A large share of viral CNS illness, especially aseptic meningitis, is caused by the enterovirus group, but the multiplicity of serotypes and the cumbersome serological methods necessary for their diagnosis usually make it impractical to include them in a battery. When one or two enteroviruses have been shown to be epidemic in an area in one summer, it is possible to pick up some additional cases by carrying out neutralization tests on paired sera employing only the enterovirus or enteroviruses in question.

Respiratory syndromes. Depending upon the age of the patient, the antigen panel for

TABLE 42.13
Interpretation of Epstein-Barr Virus Serology

SITUATION	IgG-VCA	IgM-VCA	EA	EBNA
No past infection	−	−	−	−
Acute infection	+	+	+	−
Convalescent phase	+	+ or −	+ or −	+
Past infection	+	−	−	+
?Chronic or reactivation	+	−	+	+

testing respiratory syndromes might include influenza A and B, respiratory syncytial virus, parainfluenza 1, 2, and 3, and adenoviruses (and *M. pneumoniae* and *Chlamydia*). For example, respiratory syncytial virus and parainfluenza might be routinely tested for in infants and young children but not in adults.

Exanthems. To test for exanthems, an antigen battery would include measles and rubella. If the disease is vesicular, HSV and VZV should be included.

Myocarditis-pericarditis. Antigens from group B coxsackievirus types 1 through 5 and perhaps influenza A and B viruses (depending upon epidemiological circumstances) would make up the battery tested for myocarditis and pericarditis. Although there are numerous viruses that have been implicated in inflammatory diseases of the heart and its covering membranes, the group B coxsackieviruses types 1 through 5 have been considered to account for nearly 50% of the cases. Unfortunately, much of the clinical illness is expressed at a time when standard methods of virus detection are likely to fail, and serological diagnosis must be attempted.

42.7.d. Special considerations. The full interpretation of serological results may require testing for the presence of antibody to several different antigenic components of a single virus: two notable examples are EBV and hepatitis B virus. In those instances of EBV infections which cannot be diagnosed by the usual clinical criteria and heterophile antibody tests, specific IF antibody tests can be performed (Table 42.13). These include (1) IgG antibody to viral capsid antigen (VCA), which appears early in infection and usually persists for life; (2) antibody to early antigen (EA), which appears in most patients and persists only during the active phase of infection (weeks to months); and (3) antibody to EBV nuclear antigen (EBNA), detected by anti-complement IF, which appears 2-4 weeks after onset and usually persists for life. In the early phase of acute infection, IgM-specific VCA titers are usually elevated; however, reactivation of infection may also provoke a similar response. Presence of **both** VCA and EBNA antibody in an acute or convalescent-phase serum suggests a past infection. Recent EBV infection is suggested by any of the following: (1) IgM antibody to VCA, (2) presence of VCA antibody and absence of EBNA, (3) rising titer of EBNA, or (4) presence of elevated VCA and early antigen antibodies.

Acute hepatitis B virus infection is usually accompanied by the presence of surface antigen (HBsAg) in serum (Figure 42.14). Antibody to HBsAg (anti-HBs) appears weeks to months after the virus has been eliminated and is a marker of past infection with relative immunity to reinfection. IgM antibody to the core antigen (anti-Hbc IgM) appears early in infection and persists for variable periods thereafter. Anti-HBc IgM antibody is now considered to be the best serologic marker of acute hepatitis

FIGURE 42.14
Hepatitis B serology.

B, since in some patients with acute hepatitis B, HBsAg may decline to an undetectable titer. When this occurs, and the anti-HBs has not yet developed, the patient is said to be in the "core window." Another component of hepatitis B virus, known as e antigen, may also be sought in HBsAg-positive sera; its corresponding antibody may be sought as well. The presence of hepatitis B e antigen is correlated with infectivity, and its antibody is considered to be a marker for a lower risk of transmission.

REFERENCES

1. Almeida, J.D. 1980. Practical aspects of diagnostic electron microscopy. Yale J. Biol. Med. 53:5.
2. Chernesky, M.A. 1979. The role of electron microscopy in diagnostic virology. In Lennette, D., Specter, S., and Thompson, K., editors. Diagnosis of viral infections: The role of the clinical laboratory. University Park Press, Baltimore.
3. Chou, S., and Merigan, T.C. 1983. Rapid detection and quantitation of human cytomegalovirus in urine through DNA hybridization. N. Engl. J. Med. 308:921.
4. Doane, F.W., and Anderson, N. 1977. Electron and immune electron microscopic procedures for diagnosis of viral infections. In Kurstak, E., and Kurstak, C., editors. Comparative diagnosis of viral diseases, vol. 2. Academic Press, New York.
5. Drew, W.L., and Mintz, L. 1980. Rapid diagnosis of varicella-zoster virus infection by direct immunofluorescence. Am. J. Clin. Pathol. 73:699.
6. Flores, J., et al. 1983. A dot hybridization assay for detection of rotaviruses. Lancet 1:555.
7. Gleaves, C.A., Smith, T.F., Shuster, E.A., and Pearson, G.R. 1984. Rapid detection of cytomegalovirus in MRC-5 cells inoculated with urine specimens by using low-speed centrifugation and monoclonal antibody to an early antigen. J. Clin. Microbiol. 19:917.
8. Hsiung, G.D., Fong, C.K.Y., and August, M.J. 1979. The use of electron microscopy for diagnosis of virus infections: an overview. Prog. Med. Virol. 25:133.
9. Huntoon, C.J., House, R.F. Jr., and Smith, T.F. 1981. Recovery of viruses from three transport media incorporated into culturettes. Arch. Pathol. Lab. Med. 105:436.
10. Rubin, S.J., and Rogers, S. 1984. Comparison of Cultureset and primary rabbit kidney cell culture for the detection of herpes simplex virus. J. Clin. Microbiol. 19:920.
11. Spector, S.A., Rua, J.A., Spector, D.H., et al. 1984. Detection of human cytomegalovirus in clinical specimens by DNA-RNA hybridization. J. Infect. Dis. 150:121.
12. Stagno, S., Pass, R.F., Reynolds, D.W., et al. 1980. Comparative study of diagnostic procedures for congenital cytomegalovirus infection. Pediatrics 65:251.
13. Yeager, A.S., Morris, J.E., and Prober, C.G. 1979. Storage and transport of cultures for herpes simplex virus, type 2. Am. J. Clin. Pathol. 72:977.

BIBLIOGRAPHY

Drew, W.L., editor. 1976. Viral infections: a clinical approach. F.A. Davis Co., Philadelphia.

Hsiung, G.D., in collaboration with Fong, C.K.Y. 1982. Diagnostic virology (illustrated with light and electron micrographs). Yale University Press, New Haven, Conn.

Gardner, P.S., and McQuillin, J. 1974. Rapid virus diagnosis: application of immunofluorescence. Butterworth's, London.

Lennette, D.A., Specter, S., and Thompson, K.D., editors. 1979. Diagnosis of viral infections: the role of the clinical laboratory. University Park Press, Baltimore.

Lennette, E.H., and Schmidt, N.J., editors. 1979. Diagnostic procedures for viral, rickettsial, and chlamydial infections, ed. 5. American Public Health Association, Washington, D.C.

43 Laboratory Methods in Basic Mycology

Glenn D. Roberts, Ph.D.

Historically, the fungi have been regarded as relatively insignificant causes of infection and until recently clinical laboratories offered little more than interest in providing mycological services. During the past few years, however, the literature has shown a sharp increase in the number of case reports of fungal infections. The fungi are now well recognized causes of infection, and physician awareness of their importance is much more common. Some clinical microbiology laboratories have kept pace with the changing times, but unfortunately many still offer only minimal mycological services. The reasons for this are not easily defined, but the lack of emphasis in the area of mycology by medical technology educational programs has played a major role in the scant training in this area of microbiology. In addition, the myth that mycology is too hard to learn has probably been partly responsible for the lack of interest in mycology.

The emergence of continuing education programs presenting the practical aspects of clinical mycology and a number of recent textbooks in the same area, along with the increased number of journal publications, now make mycology available to all clinical microbiology laboratories where it should be included as an important component.

43.1. Importance of Fungi

There are more than 50,000 valid species of fungi, but only some 50-75 are generally recognized as being pathogenic for humans. These organisms normally live a saprophytic existence in nature, enriched by decaying nitrogenous matter, where they are capable of maintaining a separate existence, with a parasitic cycle in humans or animals. The mycoses are not communicable in the usual sense of person-to-person or animal-to-person transfer; humans become an accidental host by the inhalation of spores or by their introduction into tissue through trauma. With the exception of the dimorphic fungi, humans are relatively resistant to infections caused by these organisms. However, an alteration in the immune system of the host (Chapter 23) may lead to infection by fungi that are normally considered to be nonpathogenic. Such infections may occur in patients with debilitating diseases, diabetes, or impaired immunologic function resulting from corticosteroid or antimetabolite therapy. Other predisposing factors include long-term intravenous cannulation, gastrointestinal surgical procedures, and long-term antimicrobial chemotherapy. During recent years, there has been an increase in the number of infections caused by saprobic fungi in immunocompromised patients. This has resulted in an obligation for the laboratory to identify and report all organisms recovered from clinical specimens submitted for fungal culture.

43.2. Levels of Laboratory Service

To ensure adequate patient care, mycological services should be offered by all clinical microbiology laboratories. The extent to which these services are offered is dependent on the individual laboratory setting. The following are proposed levels of service:

I.   Performance of direct examination of clinical specimens for the presence of fungi and collection, culturing, and transport of appropriate clinical specimens to a reference laboratory.

II.   Performance of all functions of Level I laboratories as well as the identification of yeasts using commercially available systems, performance of the latex test for cryptococcal antigen, and performance of commercially available fungal immunodiffusion tests.

III. Performance of all functions of Level II laboratories as well as the identification of commonly encountered filamentous fungi.

IV.   Performance of all functions of laboratories at lower levels, the identification of all fungi, performance of all fungal serologic tests, and antifungal susceptibility tests.

Laboratories should choose the extent to which they are proficient and forward all additional procedures to a qualified reference laboratory. With the current emphasis on cost containment (Chapter 4), smaller clinical laboratories should carefully consider the extent to which they should provide mycological services.

43.3. Fungi Commonly Encountered in a Clinical Laboratory

Of the more than 50,000 valid species of fungi, less than 100 are likely to be encountered in clinical specimens. Laboratorians just beginning to work in clinical mycology might feel intimidated by this large number; however, it is commonplace for a laboratory to recover many of the same fungi on a day-to-day basis. During the period 1975 through 1983, 267,861 clinical specimens were submitted for fungal culture at the Mayo Clinic. Of these, 75,258 (28.1%) were positive for one or more fungi. Table 43.1 presents the fungi most commonly recovered from clinical specimens at the Mayo Clinic from 1975 through 1983. This listing is derived from the 94,358 fungi recovered from various

TABLE 43.1
Fungi Most Commonly Recovered from Clinical Specimens at the Mayo Clinic, 1975-1983

BLOOD	CEREBROSPINAL FLUID	GENITOURINARY TRACT	RESPIRATORY TRACT	SKIN
Candida albicans	Cryptococcus neoformans	Candida albicans	Yeast, not Cryptococcus	Trichophyton rubrum
Candida tropicalis	Candida albicans	Candida glabrata	Penicillium species	Trichophyton mentagrophytes
Candida parapsilosis	Candida parapsilosis	Candida tropicalis	Aspergillus species	Alternaria species
Cryptococcus neoformans	Candida tropicalis	Candida parapsilosis	Aspergillus fumigatus	Candida albicans
Histoplasma capsulatum	Coccidioides immitis	Penicillium species	Cladosporium species	Penicillium species
Candida lusitaniae	Histoplasma capsulatum	Candida krusei	Alternaria species	Scopulariopsis species
Candida krusei		Cryptococcus neoformans	Aspergillus niger	Epidermophyton floccosum
Saccharomyces species		Saccharomyces species	Geotrichum candidum	Candida parapsilosis
Candida pseudotropicalis		Histoplasma capsulatum	Fusarium species	Aspergillus species
Candida zeylanoides		Cladosporium species	Aspergillus versicolor	Acremonium species
Trichosporon beigelii		Aspergillus species	Aspergillus flavus	Aspergillus versicolor
Coccidioides immitis		Trichosporon beigelii	Acremonium species	Cladosporium species
Candida guilliermondii		Alternaria species	Scopulariopsis species	Fusarium species
			Beauveria species	Trichosporon beigelii
				Phialophora species

clinical sources, and organisms are listed in order of their frequency of occurrence. It is well known that there are differences in the geographical distribution of certain fungi; however, Table 43.1 should be of value to most laboratories in the interpretation of fungal culture results.

43.4. Collection, Transport, and Culturing of Clinical Specimens

The diagnosis of fungal infections is dependent entirely on the selection and collection of an appropriate clinical specimen for culture. Many fungal infections are similar clinically to mycobacterial infections and often the same specimen is cultured for both fungi and mycobacteria. Most infections have a primary focus in the lungs; respiratory secretions are almost always included among the specimens selected for culture. It should be emphasized that dissemination to distant body sites often occurs and fungi may be commonly recovered from nonrespiratory sites. The proper collection of specimens and their transport to the clinical laboratory are of major importance for the recovery of fungi. In many instances, specimens not only contain the etiologic agent but also contain contaminating bacteria or fungi that will rapidly overgrow some of the slower growing pathogenic fungi. Since overgrowth with contaminating organisms is common, it is important to transport the specimens to the clinical laboratory as soon as possible. Although collection methods are discussed in Chapter 6, a few specific comments concerning specimen collection and culturing will be included in this chapter.

43.4.a. Respiratory secretions. Respiratory secretions (sputum, induced sputum, bronchial washings and tracheal aspirations) are perhaps the most commonly submitted specimens for fungal culture. To ensure the optimal recovery of fungi and prevent overgrowth by contaminants, antibacterial antibiotics should be included in the battery of media to be used. Cycloheximide, an antifungal agent that prevents rapid overgrowth by contaminating organisms, should be included in at least one of the culture media used. As much specimen as possible (0.5 ml) should be used to inoculate each medium.

43.4.b. Cerebrospinal fluid. Cerebrospinal fluid (CSF) collected for culture should be filtered through a 0.45 μm pore size membrane filter attached to a sterile syringe. After filtration, the filter is removed and is placed onto the surface of an appropriate culture medium with the "organism" side down. Cultures should be examined daily and the filter moved to another location on an every-other-day basis. If less than 2 ml of specimen is submitted for culture, it should be centrifuged and 1-drop aliquots of the sediment should be placed onto several areas on the agar surface. Media used for the recovery of fungi from CSF should contain no antibacterial or antifungal agents. Once submitted to the laboratory, CSF specimens should be processed promptly. If prompt processing is not possible, samples should be kept at room temperature or placed in a 30° C incubator since most organisms will continue to replicate in this environment.

43.4.c. Blood. Disseminated fungal infections are more prevalent than previously recognized, and blood cultures provide an accurate method for determining their cause. Only a few fungal blood culture systems have been available over past years, and most are not used by clinical microbiology laboratories. In smaller laboratories, it may be adequate to use a biphasic brain-heart infusion agar-broth blood culture system.[59] However, larger laboratories are encouraged to use a lysis-centrifugation system, the DuPont Isolator tube, since it has been shown to be the optimal fungal blood cul-

ture system (Chapter 14). Using this system, red blood cells and white blood cells that may contain the microorganisms are lysed, and centrifugation serves to concentrate fungi and bacteria prior to culturing. The concentrate is inoculated onto the surface of appropriate culture media and most fungi are detected within the first 4 days of incubation. However, an occasional isolate of *Histoplasma capsulatum* may require approximately 10-14 days for recovery. The optimal temperature for fungal blood cultures is 30° C and the suggested incubation time is 30 days.

43.4.d. Hair, skin, and nail scrapings. These specimens are usually submitted for dermatophyte culture and are contaminated with bacteria and/or rapidly growing fungi. Samples collected from lesions may be obtained by scraping the skin or nails with a scalpel blade or microscope slide, and infected hairs are removed by plucking them with forceps. These specimens should be placed in a sterile Petri dish or paper envelope prior to culturing; they should not be refrigerated. Either Mycobiotic or Mycosel agar (Chapter 8), which contain chloramphenicol and cycloheximide, is satisfactory for the recovery of dermatophytes from hair, skin or nails. Cultures should be incubated for a minimum of 30 days at 30° C before being reported as negative.

42.3.e. Urine. Urine samples collected for fungal culture should be processed as soon as possible after collection. Twenty-four-hour urine samples are unacceptable for culture. After considering the arguments concerning the value of quantitating the growth of fungi recovered from urine cultures, I have concluded that quantitation should not be performed except as part of the routine urine culture procedure. All urine samples should be centrifuged and the sediment cultured using a loop to provide adequate isolation of colonies. Since urine is often contaminated with gram-negative bacteria, it is necessary to use media containing antibacterial agents to ensure the recovery of fungi.

43.4.f. Tissue, bone marrow, and sterile body fluids. All tissues should be processed prior to culturing by mincing or grinding or placement in a Stomacher (Tekmar; Chapter 21). Currently the optimal system is the use of the Stomacher, which expresses the cytoplasmic contents of cells by pressure exerted from the action of rapidly moving metal paddles against the tissue in a broth suspension. After processing, at least 1 ml of specimen should be spread onto the surface of appropriate culture media and incubation should be at 30° C for 30 days.

Bone marrow may be placed directly onto the surface of appropriate culture media and incubated in the manner previously mentioned. Sterile body fluids should be concentrated by centrifugation before culturing and at least 1 ml of specimen should be placed onto the surface of appropriate culture media. All specimens should be cultured as soon as they are received by the laboratory to ensure the recovery of fungi from these important sources. Chapter 21 discusses laboratory handling of these specimens.

43.5. Culture Media and Incubation Requirements

Any of a number of fungal culture media are satisfactory for use in the clinical microbiology laboratory. Most are adequate for the recovery of fungi and selection is usually left up to each individual laboratory director. Table 43.2 lists various fungal culture media and the indications for their use. Ideally, a battery of media should be used and the following recommendations should be met:

1. Media with and without blood enrichment should be used.
2. Media with and without cycloheximide should be used.
3. All media should contain antibacterial agents; if *Nocardia* is suspected, mycobacterial culture media should be used for this purpose.

Culture dishes or screw-capped culture tubes are satisfactory for the recovery of fungi. Culture dishes are optimal since they provide better aeration of cultures, a large surface area for better isolation of colonies and greater ease of handling by technologists making microscopic preparations for examination. Agar in culture dishes has a marked tendency to dehydrate during the extended incubation period required for fungi; however, this problem can be minimized by using culture dishes containing at least 40 ml of agar and placing them in an incubator which contains a pan of water to humidify the environment. Dishes should be opened and examined only within a certified biological safety cabinet (Chapter 2). Many laboratories discourage the use of culture dishes; however, the advantages of using them outweigh the disadvantages.

Culture tubes are more easily stored, require less space for incubation and are easily handled. In addition, they have a lower dehydration rate and laboratory workers feel that cultures are less hazardous to handle when in tubes. The disadvantages, which include relatively poor isolation of colonies, a reduced surface area for culturing and a tendency to promote anaerobiosis, discourage their routine use in a clinical microbiology laboratory.

Cultures should be incubated at room temperature or preferably at 30° C for 30 days before reporting as negative. A relative humidity of 40%-50% can be achieved by placing an open pan of water in the incubator. Cultures should be examined at least three times weekly during incubation.

As previously mentioned, most clinical specimens are contaminated with bacteria and rapidly growing fungi. The need for antibacterial and antifungal agents is obvious. The addition of 0.5 mg/ml of cycloheximide and 0.016 mg/ml of chloramphenicol to media has been traditionally advocated to inhibit the growth of contaminating saprobic molds and bacteria. Better results have been achieved using a combination of 5 µg/ml of gentamicin and 16 µg/ml of chloramphenicol as antibacterial agents.

Certain of the fungi seem to have a requirement for blood, and a concentration of 5%-10% sheep blood is recommended for inclusion into at least one of the culture media used. Cycloheximide may be added to any of the media which contain or lack antibacterial antibiotics. However, if cycloheximide is included as a part of the battery of culture media used, a medium lacking this ingredient should also be included.

Certain of the pathogenic fungi are partially or completely inhibited by this compound; included are *Cryptococcus neoformans*, *Candida krusei* and other species of *Candida*, *Trichosporon beigelii*, *Pseudallescheria boydii*, and species of *Aspergillus*.

The use of antibiotics in fungal culture media is necessary for the optimal recovery of organisms; however, the use of decontamination and concentration methods advocated for the recovery of mycobacteria is not appropriate for fungal cultures.[57]

TABLE 43.2
Fungal Culture Media: Indications for Use

MEDIA	INDICATIONS FOR USE
Primary recovery media	
Brain-heart infusion agar	Primary recovery of saprobic and pathogenic fungi
Brain-heart infusion agar with antibiotics	Primary recovery of pathogenic fungi exclusive of dermatophytes
Brain-heart infusion biphasic blood culture bottles	Recovery of fungi from blood
Dermatophyte test medium	Primary recovery of dermatophytes, recommended as screening medium only
Inhibitory mold agar	Primary recovery of pathogenic fungi exclusive of dermatophytes
Mycosel or mycobiotic agar	Primary recovery of dermatophytes
SABHI agar	Primary recovery of saprobic and pathogenic fungi
Yeast-extract phosphate agar	Primary recovery of pathogenic fungi exclusive of dermatophytes
Differential test media	
Ascospore agar	Detection of ascospores in ascosporogenous yeasts such as *Saccharomyces* sp.
Cornmeal agar with Tween 80 and trypan blue	Identification of *Candida albicans* by chlamydospore production; identification of *Candida* by microscopic morphology
Cottonseed conversion agar	Conversion of dimorphic fungus *Blastomyces dermatitidis* from mold to yeast form
Czapek's agar	Recovery and differential identification of *Aspergillus* sp.
Niger seed agar	Identification of *Cryptococcus neoformans*
Nitrate reduction medium	Detection of nitrate reduction in confirmation of *Cryptococcus* sp.
Potato dextrose agar	Demonstration of pigment production by *Trichophyton rubrum*; preparation of microslide cultures
Rice medium	Identification of *Microsporum audouinii*
Trichophyton agars 1-7	Identification of members of *Trichophyton* genus
Urea agar	Detection of *Cryptococcus* sp.; differentiate *Trichophyton mentagrophytes* from *Trichophyton rubrum*; detection of *Trichosporon* sp.
Yeast fermentation broth	Identification of yeasts by determining fermentation
Yeast nitrogen base agar	Identification of yeasts by determining carbohydrate assimilation

From Koneman, E.W., and Roberts, G.D. 1985. Practical laboratory mycology, ed. 3. The Williams and Wilkins Co., Baltimore.

43.6. Direct Microscopic Examination of Clinical Specimens

Direct microscopic examination of clinical specimens has been used for many years; however, its usefulness should be reemphasized.[55] Since the charge of the clinical microbiology laboratory is to provide a rapid and accurate diagnosis, the mycology laboratory can provide this service in many instances by direct examination of the clinical specimen submitted for culture. Microbiologists are encouraged to become familiar with the diagnostic features of fungi commonly encountered in clinical specimens. This very important procedure can often provide the first microbiologic proof of etiology in patients with fungal infection.

Tables 43.3 and 43.4 present the methods available for the direct microscopic detection of fungi in clinical specimens and a summary of

Text continued on p. 690.

TABLE 43.3

Characteristics of Methods Available for the Direct Microscopic Detection of Fungi in Clinical Specimens

METHOD	USE	TIME REQUIRED	ADVANTAGES	DISADVANTAGES
Acid fast stain	Detection of mycobacteria and *Nocardia*	12 min	Detects *Nocardia** and *B. dermatitidis*.	Tissue homogenates are difficult to observe due to background staining.
Calcofluor white	Detection of fungi	1 min	Can be mixed with KOH; detects fungi rapidly due to bright fluorescence.	Requires use of a fluorescence microscope; background fluorescence prominent, but fungi exhibit more intense fluorescence. Vaginal secretions are difficult to interpret.
Gram stain	Detection of bacteria	3 min	Is commonly performed on most clinical specimens submitted for bacteriology and will detect most fungi, if present.	Sone fungi stain well; however, others, e.g., *Cryptococcus* sp., stain weakly in some instances. Some isolates of *Nocardia* fail to stain or stain weakly.
India ink	Detection of *C. neoformans* in CSF	1 min	When positive in CSF, is diagnostic of meningitis.	Positive in less than 50% of cases of meningitis; not reliable.
Potassium hydroxide (KOH)	Clearing of specimen to make fungi more readily visible	5 min; if clearing is not complete, an additional 5-10 min is necessary	Rapid detection of fungal elements.	Experience required since background artifacts are often confusing. Clearing of some specimens may require an extended time.

From Roberts, G.D., Goodman, N.L., Land, G.A., Larsh, H.W., and McGinnis, M.R. 1985. Detection and recovery of fungi in clinical specimens. In Lennette, E.H., Balows, A., Hausler, W.J. Jr., and Shadomy, H.J., editors. Manual of clinical microbiology, ed. 4. American Society for Microbiology, Washington, D.C.
*Acid-fast bacterium.   *Continued.*

TABLE 43.3

Characteristics of Methods Available for the Direct Microscopic Detection
of Fungi in Clinical Specimens—cont'd

METHOD	USE	TIME REQUIRED	ADVANTAGES	DISADVANTAGES
Methenamine silver stain	Detection of fungi in histologic section	1 h	Best stain to detect fungal elements.	Requires a specialized staining method that is not usually readily available to microbiology laboratories.
Papanicolaou stain	Examination of secretions for presence of malignant cells	30 min	Cytotechnologist can detect fungal elements.	
Periodic acid–Schiff (PAS) stain	Detection of fungi	20 min; 5 min additional if counterstain is employed	Stains fungal elements well; hyphae of molds and yeasts can be readily distinguished.	*Nocardia* sp. do not stain well; *B. dermatitidis* appears pleomorphic.
Wright stain	Examination of bone marrow or peripheral blood smears	7 min	Detects *H. capsulatum*.	Detection is limited to *H. capsulatum*.

TABLE 43.4

Summary of Characteristic Features of Fungi Seen in Direct Examination
of Clinical Specimens

MORPHOLOGIC FORM FOUND IN SPECIMENS	ORGANISM(S)	SIZE RANGE (DIAMETER, μm)	CHARACTERISTIC FEATURES
Yeastlike	*Histoplasma capsulatum*	2-5	Small; oval to round budding cells; often found clustered within histiocytes; difficult to detect when present in small numbers.
	Sporothrix schenckii	2-6	Small; oval to round to cigar-shaped; single or multiple buds present; uncommonly seen in clinical specimens.
	Cryptococcus neoformans	2-15	Cells exhibit great variation in size; usually spherical but may be football shaped; buds single or multiple and "pinched off"; capsule may or may not be evident; occasionally pseudohyphal forms with or without a capsule may be seen in exudates or CSF.

From Roberts, G.D., Goodman, N.L., Land, G.A., Larsh, H.W., and McGinnis, M.R. 1985. Detection and recovery of fungi in clinical specimens. In Lennette, E.H., Balows, A., Hausler, W.J. Jr., and Shadomy, H.J., editors. Manual of clinical microbiology, ed. 4. American Society for Microbiology, Washington, D.C.

TABLE 43.4

Summary of Characteristic Features of Fungi Seen in Direct Examination
of Clinical Specimens—cont'd

MORPHOLOGIC FORM FOUND IN SPECIMENS	ORGANISM(S)	SIZE RANGE (DIAMETER, μm)	CHARACTERISTIC FEATURES
	Blastomyces dermatitidis	8-15	Cells are usually large, double refractile when present; buds usually single; however, several may remain attached to parent cells; buds connected by a broad base.
	Paracoccidioides brasiliensis	5-60	Cells are usually large and are surrounded by smaller buds around the periphery ("mariner's wheel appearance"); smaller cells may be present (2-5 μm) and resemble H. capsulatum; buds have "pinched off" appearance.
Spherules	Coccidioides immitis	10-200	Spherules vary in size; some may contain endospores, others may be empty. Adjacent spherules may resemble B. dermatitidis; endospores may resemble H. capsulatum but show no evidence of budding. Spherules may produce multiple germ tubes if a direct preparation is kept in a moist chamber for ≥24 h.
	Rhinosporidium seeberi	6-300	Large, thick-walled sporangia containing sporangiospores are present; mature sporangia are larger than spherules of C. immitis; hyphae may be found in cavitary lesions.
Yeast and pseudohyphae or hyphae	Candida sp.	3-4 (yeast) 5-10 (pseudohyphae)	Cells usually exhibit single budding; pseudohyphae, when present, are constricted at the ends and remain attached like links of sausage; hyphae, when present, are septate.
	Malassezia furfur	3-8 (yeast) 2.5-4 (hyphae)	Short curved hyphal elements are usually present along with round yeast cells that retain their spherical shape in compacted clusters.
Nonseptate hyphae	Zygomycetes; Mucor, Rhizopus, and other genera	10-30	Hyphae are large, ribbonlike, often fractured or twisted; occasional septa may be present. Smaller hyphae are confused with those of Aspergillus sp., particularly A. flavus.
Hyaline septate hyphae	Dermatophytes Skin and nails	3-15	Hyaline, septate hyphae are commonly seen. Chains of arthroconidia may be present.

Continued.

TABLE 43.4
Summary of Characteristic Features of Fungi Seen in Direct Examination
of Clinical Specimens—cont'd

MORPHOLOGIC FORM FOUND IN SPECIMENS	ORGANISM(S)	SIZE RANGE (DIAMETER, μm)	CHARACTERISTIC FEATURES
Hyaline septate hyphae—cont'd	Hair	3-15	Arthroconidia on periphery of hair shaft producing a sheath are indicative of ectothrix infection. Arthroconidia formed by fragmentation of hyphae within the hair shaft are indicative of endothrix infection.
		3-15	Long hyphal filaments or channels within the hair shaft are indicative of favus hair infection.
	Aspergillus sp.	3-12	Hyphae are septate and exhibit dichotomous, 45-degree angle branching; larger hyphae, often disturbed, may resemble those of Zygomycetes.
	Geotrichum sp.	4-12	Hyphae and rectangular arthroconidia are present and are sometimes rounded. Irregular forms may be present.
	Trichosporon sp.	2-4 by 8	Hyphae and rectangular arthroconidia are present and are sometimes rounded. Occasionally blastoconidia may be present.
	Pseudallescheria boydii (cases other than mycetoma)		Hyphae are septate and are impossible to distinguish from those of other hyaline molds, e.g., *Aspergillus* sp.
Dematiaceous septate hyphae	*Cladosporium* sp. *Curvularia* sp. *Drechslera* sp. *Exophiala* sp. *Phialophora* sp. *Wangiella dermatitidis*	2-6	Dematiaceous polymorphous hyphae are seen; budding cells with single septa and chains of swollen rounded cells are often present. Occasionally aggregates may be present in infection caused by *Phialophora* and *Exophiala* sp.
	Exophiala werneckii	1.5-5	Usually large numbers of frequently branched hyphae are present along with budding cells.
Sclerotic bodies	*Cladosporium carrionii* *Fonsecaea compacta* *Fonsecaea pedrosoi* *Phialophora verrucosa* *Rhinocladiella aquaspersa*	5-20	Brown, round to pleomorphic, thick-walled cells with transverse septations. Commonly, cells contain two fission planes that form a tetrad of cells. Occasionally, branched septate hyphae may be found along with sclerotic bodies.

TABLE 43.4

Summary of Characteristic Features of Fungi Seen in Direct Examination
of Clinical Specimens—cont'd

MORPHOLOGIC FORM FOUND IN SPECIMENS	ORGANISM(S)	SIZE RANGE (DIAMETER, μm)	CHARACTERISTIC FEATURES
Granules	Acremonium A. falciforme A. kiliense A. recifei	200-300	White, soft granules without a cementlike matrix.
	Curvularia C. geniculata C. lunata	500-1,000	Black, hard grains with a cementlike matrix at periphery.
	Aspergillus A. nidulans	65-160	White, soft granules without a cementlike matrix.
	Exophiala E. jeanselmei	200-300	Black, soft granules, vacuolated, without a cementlike matrix, made of dark hyphae and swollen cells.
	Fusarium		White, soft granules without a cementlike matrix
	F. moniliforme	200-500	
	F. solani	300-600	
	Leptosphaeria		
	L. senegalensis	400-600	Black, hard granules with cementlike matrix present.
	L. tompkinsii	500-1,000	Periphery composed of polygonal swollen cells and center of a hyphal network.
	Madurella		
	M. grisea	350-500	Black, soft granules without a cementlike matrix, periphery composed of polygonal swollen cells and center of a hyphal network.
	M. mycetomatis	200-900	Black to brown, hard granules of two types: (1) Rust brown, compact, and filled with cementlike matrix (2) Deep brown, filled with numerous vesicles, 6-14 μm in diameter, cementlike matrix in periphery, and central area of light-colored hyphae.
	Neotestudina		White, soft granules with cementlike matrix present at periphery.
	N. rosatti	300-600	
	Pseudallescheria		White, soft granules composed of hyphae and swollen cells at periphery in a cementlike matrix.
	P. boydii	200-300	
	Pyrenochaeta		Black, soft granules composed of polygonal swollen cells at periphery, center is network of hyphae, no cementlike matrix present.
	P. romeri	300-600	

the characteristic microscopic features of each method. More information regarding specific procedures is given in Chapter 7. Figures 43.1 to 43.10 and Plates 43.1 to 43.12 present photomicrographs of some of the fungi commonly seen in clinical specimens.

Traditionally, the potassium hydroxide preparation has been the recommended method for the direct microscopic examination of specimens.[52] However, it is currently felt that the calcofluor white stain[23] (Chapter 7) is preferred. Slides prepared by this method may be observed using fluorescent microscopy or brightfield microscopy as used for the potassium hydroxide preparation; the former is optimal since fungal cells will fluoresce.

FIGURE 43.1
Potassium hydroxide preparation of skin, phase contrast, dermatophyte, showing septate hyphae intertwined among epithelial cells (500 ×).

FIGURE 43.2
Potassium hydroxide preparation of skin, phase contrast, *Malassezia furfur*, showing spherical yeast cells and short hyphal fragments (500 ×).

FIGURE 43.3
Gram stain of urine, *Candida albicans*, showing
blastoconidia and pseudohyphae.

FIGURE 43.4
Papanicolaou stain of sputum, *Aspergillus fumigatus*,
showing dichotomously branching septate hyphae.

FIGURE 43.5
Potassium hydroxide preparation of sputum, phase
contrast, *Rhizopus* species, showing fragmented portions
of nonseptate hyphae of varying size.

FIGURE 43.6
Calcofluor white stain of sputum, *Histoplasma
capsulatum*, showing intracellular yeast cells 2–5 μm in
diameter.

FIGURE 43.7
Periodic acid-Schiff stain of exudate, *Sporothrix schenckii*, showing cigar- to oval-shaped yeast cells.

FIGURE 43.8
Potassium hydroxide preparation of pleural fluid, phase contrast, *Cryptococcus neoformans*, showing encapsulated, spherical yeast cells of varying sizes.

FIGURE 43.9
Potassium hydroxide preparation of exudate, phase contrast, *Blastomyces dermatitidis*, showing large budding yeast cells with a distinct broad base between the cells.

FIGURE 43.10
Potassium hydroxide preparation of sputum, bright field, *Coccidioides immitis*, showing two spherules, filled with endospores, lying adjacent to each other that resemble *B. dermatitidis*.

43.7. Characteristics of Fungi (Informal Glossary)

The fungi, a term which includes both yeasts and molds, differ significantly from the bacteria. The fungi are eukaryotic and contain a definite nucleus with a surrounding nuclear membrane; their cell wall is primarily composed of glucose and mannose polymers (chitin); their cell membrane contains sterols, and the organisms are resistant to antibacterial antibiotics. They show marked susceptibility to polyene antifungal agents and all reproduce asexually; however, some reproduce sexually as well.

The fungi seen in the clinical laboratory can easily be separated into two groups based on the macroscopic appearance of the colonies formed. The **yeasts** produce moist, creamy, opaque or pasty colonies on culture media while the **molds** (filamentous fungi) produce fluffy, cottony, woolly or powdery colonies. Certain of the slow-growing pathogenic fungi are dimorphic and produce a mold form at 25°-30° C and a yeast or spherule form at 35°-37° C under certain circumstances.

The identification of the yeasts requires not only recognition of certain microscopic features, but also the use of biochemical tests to provide a definitive species identification. The definitive identification of the molds requires recognition of the characteristic microscopic features of the organism. The following paragraphs will describe the basic microscopic morphologic features of fungi and representative photomicrographs will be used to illustrate them.

The yeasts are unicellular organisms that reproduce by budding; their microscopic morphologic features usually appear similar for different genera and are not particularly helpful in their separation. The basic structural units of the molds are tubelike projections known as hyphae (Figures 43.11 to 43.13). As the **hyphae** grow, they become intertwined to form a loose network called the **mycelium** which penetrates

FIGURE 43.11
Hyaline hyphae showing septations (430 ×).

FIGURE 43.12
Dematiaceous hyphae showing pigmentation and septations (430 ×).

FIGURE 43.13
Hyaline hyphae lacking septations (aseptate).

FIGURE 43.14
Antler hyphae showing swollen hyphal tips resembling antlers, with lateral and terminal branching (favic chandeliers) (500 ×).

FIGURE 43.15
Racquet hyphae showing a swollen area resembling a tennis racquet.

the substrate from which it obtains the necessary nutrients for growth. The nutrient absorbing and water exchanging portion of the fungi is called the **vegetative mycelium.** The portion projecting above the substrate surface is known as the **aerial mycelium;** aerial mycelia often give rise to fruiting bodies from which the asexual spores are borne. Recognition of certain types of vegetative hyphae is helpful in placing the organism into a certain group. For example, dermatophytes often produce several types of hyphae including **antler hyphae** (Figure 43.14) that are curved, freely branching, and antlerlike in appearance. **Racquet hyphae** are often found that are enlarged, club-shaped hyphae with the smaller end attached to the large end of an adjacent club-shaped hyphal strand (Figure 43.15). In addition, certain of the dermatophytes produce **spiral hyphae** that are coiled or corkscrewlike turns seen within the hyphal strand (Figure 43.16). These structures are not characteristic for any certain group of organisms; however, they are frequently found in the dermatophytes.

The features by which most fungi are identified are related to the mode of sporulation and the morphology and arrangement of the spores produced. Fungi may reproduce sexually, asexually or by both means. **Sexual reproduction** is associated with the production of specialized structures that result in nuclear fusion and the production of specialized spores. Some species of fungi produce sexual spores in a large saclike structure called an **ascocarp** (Figure 43.17). This, in turn, contains smaller sacs called **asci,** each of which contains four or eight **ascospores.** This type of sexual reproduction is sometimes seen in the fungi recovered in the clinical microbiology laboratory. Most of the fungi of clinical importance reproduce asexually. There is a consensus that perhaps all fungi possess a sexual form; however, this form has not been observed on artificial culture media for most of the clinically important species. **Asexual sporulation** is the type of sporulation seen in most fungi encountered in a clinical laboratory. The type of spores, their morphology and arrangement are important criteria for establishing the definitive identification of an organism.

FIGURE 43.16
Spiral hyphae exhibiting corkscrew-like turns (430 ×).

FIGURE 43.17
Ascocarp showing dark appearing ascospores (430 ×).

The simplest type of sporulation is the development of the spore directly from the vegetative hyphae. Three types of spores are recognized. **Arthroconidia** are formed directly from the hyphae by fragmentation through the points of septation. When mature, they appear as square, rectangular or barrel-shaped, thick-walled cells (Figure 43.18). These result from the simple fragmentation of the hyphae into spores which are easily dislodged and disseminated into the environment. **Chlamydospores** are round, thick-walled resistant spores formed directly from the differentiation of the hyphae in which there is a concentration of protoplasm and nutrient material (Figure 43.19). These spores appear to be resistant resting spores produced by the rounding up and enlargement of the terminal cells of the hyphae. **Blastoconidia**, most often found in the yeasts, are cells produced by budding with the daughter cells

being pinched off from portions of the mother cell through a constricted area (Figure 43.20). In some species of yeasts, most commonly *Candida*, blastoconidia may elongate and remain attached and form structures called **pseudohyphae** (Figure 43.21).

A variety of other types of spores occur with many species of fungi. **Conidia** are asexual spores produced singly or in groups by specialized vegetative hyphal strands called **conidiophores.** In some instances, the conidia are freed from their point of attachment by pinching off, or abstriction. Some conidiophores terminate in a swollen structure called a **vesicle.** From the surface of the vesicle are formed secondary small flask-shaped **phialides** which in turn give rise to long chains of **conidia.** This type of fruiting structure is characteristic of the aspergilli (Figure 43.22). A single slender, tubular conidiophore (phialide) that supports a

FIGURE 43.18
Arthroconidia formation produced by the breaking down of a hyphal strand into individual rectangular units (430 ×).

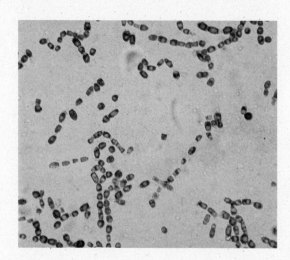

FIGURE 43.19
Chlamydospores composed of thick-walled spherical cells (430 ×).

FIGURE 43.20
Blastoconidia (budding cells) characteristic of the yeasts (430 ×).

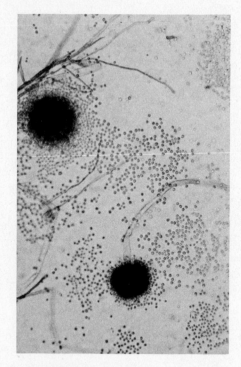

FIGURE 43.21
Pseudohyphae consisting of elongated cells with constrictions where attached (430 ×).

FIGURE 43.22
Conidia (asexual spores) produced on specialized structures (conidiophores) of *Aspergillus* (430 ×).

cluster of conidia, held together as a gelatinous mass, is characteristic of certain fungi, including the genus *Acremonium* (Figure 43.23). In other instances, conidiophores branch into a structure known as a penicillus where each branch terminates in secondary branches (**me-**

FIGURE 43.23
Simple tubular phialide with a cluster of conidia at its tip, characteristic of *Acremonium* (430 ×).

tulae) and phialides from which chains of conidia are borne (Figure 43.24). Species of *Penicillium* and *Paecilomyces* are representative of this type of sporulation. In other instances, fungi may produce conidia of two sizes: **microconidia** are small, unicellular, round, elliptical or pyriform in shape (Figure 43.25); **macroconidia** are large, usually multiseptate, and club- or spindle-shaped (Figure 43.26). Microconidia may be borne directly on the side of the hyphal strand or at the end of a long or short conidiophore. Macroconidia are usually borne on a short to long conidiophore and may be smooth-walled or rough-walled. Microconidia and macroconidia are seen in many fungal species and are not specific, except as they are used to differentiate the different genera of dermatophytes.

One group of fungi, the **zygomycetes,** produce structures different from the ones previously described. The hyphae are **nonseptate** and asexual spores are produced in a large sac-like structure called a **sporangium** which is borne on the tip of a supporting structure (**sporangiophore**) (Figure 43.27).

FIGURE 43.24
Complex method of sporulation where conidia are borne on phialides produced on secondary branches (metulae), characteristic of *Penicillium* (430 ×).

FIGURE 43.25
Numerous small, spherical microconidia contrasted with a large, elongated macroconidium (430 ×).

FIGURE 43.26
Large, rough-walled macroconidium of *Microsporum canis* (430 ×).

FIGURE 43.27
Large, saclike sporangium that contains sporangiospores, characteristic of the zygomycetes (250 ×).

Sporulation takes place by progressive cleavage during maturation within the sporangium; the spores are produced and released by the rupture of the sporangial wall. This type of sporulation is characteristic of the zygomycetes.

43.8. Classification of Fungi

The botanical taxonomic scheme for grouping the fungi has very little value in a clinical microbiology laboratory. Table 43.5 is a simplified taxonomic scheme illustrating the major groups to which the clinically important fungi belong. Using this classification scheme, the fungi can be included within four major divisions: **Zygomycota, Ascomycota, Basidiomycota,** and **Deuteromycota.**[13] The division Zygomycota includes organisms which have aseptate hyphae and reproduce asexually by spores produced inside of sporangia and reproduce sexually by

the production of zygospores. *Mucor, Rhizopus,* and *Absidia* are the most common members of this group. The Ascomycota includes organisms which have septate hyphae, produce conidia, or reproduce sexually by means of ascospores produced within an ascus. Common members of this group include *Pseudallescheria boydii* and species of *Aspergillus.* The Basidiomycota includes a group of organisms which have septate hyphae and reproduce asexually by conidia or sexually by means of basidiospores. *Filobasidiella (Cryptococcus)* is the major genus within this division that is encountered in a clinical laboratory. The major group to which most of the clinically important fungi belong is the Deuteromycota. This group of organisms has septate hyphae and reproduces asexually with the production of conidia. Whether they reproduce sexually is not known. As previously mentioned, the botanical taxo-

TABLE 43.5
Phylogenetic Position of Medically Significant Fungi

CLASS	ORDER	FAMILY	GENUS/SPECIES
Phylum Zygomycota			
Zygomycetes	Entomophthorales	Entomophthoraceae	*Basidiobolus*
	Mucorales	Mucoraceae	*Absidia*
			Cunninghamella
			Mucor
			Rhizopus
			Syncephalastrum
Phylum Ascomycota			
Hemiascomycetes	Endomycetales	Endomycetaceae	*Endomyces (Geotrichum* sp.)*
		Saccharomycetaceae	*Kluyveromyces (Candida pseudotropicalis)**
Loculoascomycetes	Myriangiales	Saccardinulaceae	*Piedraia hortae*
	Microascales	Microascaceae	*Pseudallescheria boydii*
Plectomycetes	Eurotiales	Eurotiaceae	*Emericella (Aspergillus nidulans)**
			*Sortorya (Aspergillus fumigatus)**

Modified from Chandler, F.W., Kaplan, W., and Ajello, L., 1980. Histopathology of mycotic disease. Year Book Medical Publishers, Chicago.
*Genus/species designations for the sexual, imperfect forms are shown in parentheses.

TABLE 43.5
Phylogenetic Position of Medically Significant Fungi—cont'd

CLASS	ORDER	FAMILY	GENUS/SPECIES
		Gymnoascaceae	*Ajellomyces (Histoplasma capsulatum, Blastomyces dermatitidis)**
			*Arthroderma (Trichophyton sp.)**
			*Nannizzia (Microsporum sp.)**
Phylum Basidiomycota			
Teliomycetes	Ustilaginales	Filobasidiaceae	*Filobasidiella (Cryptococcus neoformans)**
Form Phylum Deuteromycota			
Blastomycetes		Cryptococcaceae	*Candida*
Hyphomycetes	Moniliales	Moniliaceae	*Acremonium*
			Aspergillus
			Blastomyces
			Chrysosporium
			Coccidioides
			Epidermophyton
			Geotrichum
			Gliocladium
			Histoplasma
			Microsporum
			Paecilomyces
			Paracoccidioides
			Penicillium
			Sepedonium
			Scopulariopsis
			Sporothrix
			Trichoderma
			Trichophyton
		Dematiaceae	*Alternaria*
			Aureobasidium
			Cladosporium
			Curvularia
			Drechslera
			Exophiala
			Fonsecaea
			Helminthosporium
			Madurella
			Nigrospora
			Phialophora
			Rhinocladiella
			Stemphylium
			Ulocladium
			Wangiella
		Tuberculariaceae	*Epicoccum*
			Fusarium
Coelomycetes	Sphaeropsidales		*Phoma*

TABLE 43.6
Clinical Classification of Pathogenic Fungi

CUTANEOUS	SUBCUTANEOUS	OPPORTUNISTIC	SYSTEMIC
Superficial mycoses	Chromoblastomycosis	Aspergillosis	Aspergillosis
Tinea	Sporotrichosis	Candidosis	Blastomycosis
Piedra	Mycetoma (eumycotic)	Cryptococcosis	Candidosis
Candidosis	Phaeohyphomycosis	Geotrichosis	Coccidioidomycosis
Dermatophytosis		Zygomycosis	Histoplasmosis
			Cryptococcosis
			Geotrichosis
			Paracoccidioido-mycosis
			Zygomycosis

nomic scheme has little role in the clinical laboratory. Clinicians find more value in categorizing the fungi into three or four categories: (1) the **superficial** or **cutaneous mycoses;** (2) **subcutaneous mycoses;** (3) the **systemic mycoses;** and (4) the **opportunistic mycoses.**

The superficial or cutaneous mycoses are fungal infections that involve the hair, skin, or nails without invasion of the tissue. The group of fungi in this category that are most commonly recovered are the dermatophytes; also included are agents of infections such as tinea versicolor, tinea nigra, and piedra which involve the outermost keratin layer of the skin.

Subcutaneous mycoses are infections confined to the subcutaneous tissue without dissemination to distant sites. Examples include sporotrichosis, chromoblastomycosis, and mycetoma.

The systemic mycoses are caused primarily by fungi belonging to the genera *Blastomyces*, *Coccidioides*, *Histoplasma*, and *Paracoccidioides*. Infections caused by these organisms involve the lungs primarily, but also may become widely disseminated and involve any organ of the body.

The group of fungi included in the opportunistic mycoses includes an ever-expanding list of organisms. These infections are commonly found in patients who are immunocompromised, usually by an underlying disease process or by immunosuppressive agents. Fungi previously thought to be nonpathogenic can cause infection in the compromised host; commonly encountered infections include aspergillosis, zygomycosis, candidosis, and cryptococcosis.

This type of classification allows the clinician to logically categorize organisms into groups having clinical relevance. Table 43.6 presents an example of the clinical classification of fungi that will be useful to the clinician. This type of classification also plays little role in the identification of fungi in the clinical microbiology laboratory.

43.9. Clinical Laboratory Working Schema

To assist persons working in clinical microbiology laboratories with the identification of clinically important fungi, Koneman and Roberts[35] have suggested the use of a practical working schema which is designed to (1) assist in the recognition of fungi most commonly encountered in clinical specimens; (2) assist with the recognition of fungi recovered on culture media that belong to the strictly pathogenic fungi; and (3) provide a pathway that is easy to follow and that allows a positive identification of an organism to be made on the basis of a few colonial and microscopic features of the organism. Table 43.7 presents these features; however, it must be recognized that the table includes only

TABLE 43.7
Commonly Encountered Fungi of Clinical Laboratory Importance: A Practical Working Schema

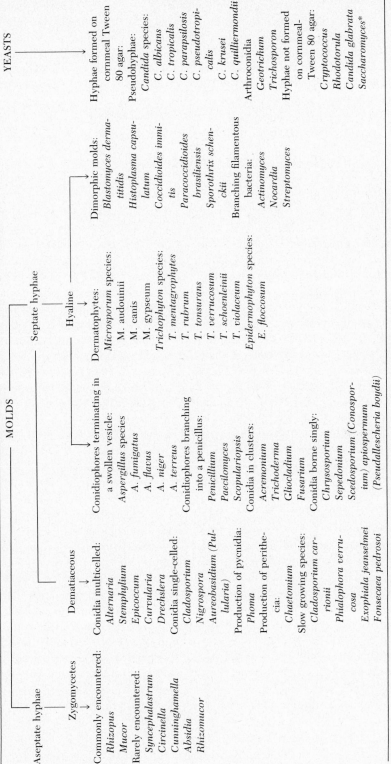

MOLDS

Aseptate hyphae → Zygomycetes

Commonly encountered:
Rhizopus
Mucor
Rarely encountered:
Syncephalastrum
Circinella
Cunninghamella
Absidia
Rhizomucor

Septate hyphae → Dematiaceous

Conidia multicelled:
Alternaria
Stemphylium
Epicoccum
Curvularia
Drechslera
Conidia single-celled:
Cladosporium
Nigrospora
Aureobasidium (Pullularia)
Production of pycnidia:
Phoma
Production of perithecia:
Chaetomium
Slow growing species:
Cladosporium carrionii
Phialophora verrucosa
Exophiala jeanselmei
Fonsecaea pedrosoi

Septate hyphae → Hyaline

Conidiophores terminating in a swollen vesicle:
Aspergillus species
A. fumigatus
A. flavus
A. niger
A. terreus
Conidiophores branching into a penicillus:
Penicillium
Paecilomyces
Scopulariopsis
Conidia in clusters:
Acremonium
Trichoderma
Gliocladium
Fusarium
Conidia borne singly:
Chrysosporium
Sepedonium
Scedosporium (Conosporium) apiospermum (Pseudallescheria boydii)

Dermatophytes:
Microsporum species:
M. audouinii
M. canis
M. gypseum
Trichophyton species:
T. mentagrophytes
T. rubrum
T. tonsurans
T. verrucosum
T. schoenleinii
T. violaceum
Epidermophyton species:
E. floccosum

Dimorphic molds:
Blastomyces dermatitidis
Histoplasma capsulatum
Coccidioides immitis
Paracoccidioides brasiliensis
Sporothrix schenckii
Branching filamentous bacteria:
Actinomyces
Nocardia
Streptomyces

YEASTS

Hyphae formed on cornmeal Tween 80 agar:
Pseudohyphae:
Candida species:
C. albicans
C. tropicalis
C. parapsilosis
C. pseudotropicalis
C. krusei
C. quilliermondii
Arthroconidia
Geotrichum
Trichosporon
Hyphae not formed on cornmeal Tween 80 agar:
Cryptococcus
Rhodotorula
Candida glabrata
Saccharomyces*

From Koneman, E.W., and Roberts, C.D. 1985. Practical laboratory mycology, ed. 3. The Williams and Wilkins Co., Baltimore.
*Rudimentary hyphae may be present.

those organisms commonly seen in the clinical laboratory. With practice, most laboratorians should be able to recognize the fungi commonly encountered on a day-to-day basis. The identification of others will require the use of various texts containing photomicrographs which are useful for their identification.

The use of this schema requires that one first examine the culture for the presence or absence of septae. If the hyphae appear to be predominately nonseptate, zygomycetes should be considered. If the hyphae are septate, they must be examined further for the presence or absence of pigment. If a dark pigment is present in the conidia or the hyphae, the organism is considered to be dematiaceous and the conidia are then examined for their morphological features and their arrangement on the hyphae. If the hyphae are nonpigmented, they are considered to be hyaline. They are then examined for the type and the arrangement of the conidia produced. The molds are identified by recognition of their characteristic microscopic features.

The yeasts may be presumptively identified by the presence or absence of hyphae, pseudohyphae, blastoconidia, and arthroconidia on cornmeal agar. The identification of yeasts will be discussed later within the chapter.

43.10. Extent of Identification of Fungi Recovered from Clinical Specimens

The question of when and how far to go with identification of fungi recovered from clinical specimens presents an interesting situation. The current emphasis on cost containment (Chapter 4) and the ever-increasing number of opportunistic fungi causing infection in compromised patients cause one to consider whether or not all fungi recovered from clinical specimens should be thoroughly identified and reported. Murray et al.[45] in 1975 were concerned with the time and expense associated with the identification of yeasts from respiratory tract specimens. Since these are the specimens most commonly submitted for fungal culture, they questioned whether it was important to provide an identification for every organism recovered. After evaluating the clinical usefulness of information provided by the identification of yeast recovered from respiratory tract specimens, they suggested that (1) the routine identification of yeasts recovered in culture from respiratory secretions is not warranted, but that all yeasts should be screened for the presence of *Cryptococcus neoformans;* (2) that all respiratory secretions submitted for fungal culture, regardless of the presence or absence of oropharyngeal contamination, should be cultured since such pathogens as *Histoplasma capsulatum, Blastomyces dermatitidis, Coccidioides immitis* and *Sporothrix schenckii* may be recovered; and (3) that the routine identification of yeast in respiratory secretions is of little or no value to the clinician and probably represents "normal flora" with the exception of *C. neoformans.*

When and how far to proceed with an identification of the molds is a much more difficult question to answer. A consensus of a number of clinical mycologists is that all commonly encountered molds should be identified and reported regardless of the clinical source. Those organisms which fail to sporulate after a reasonable time should be reported as being present but the identification need not be attempted if the dimorphic fungi have been ruled out or if the clinician feels that the organism is not clinically significant. Ideally, all laboratories should identify all fungi recovered from clinical specimens; however, the limits of practicality and economic considerations play a definite role in making a decision as to how far to go with their identification. Each individual laboratory director, in consultation with the clinicians being served, will have to make this decision after considering the patient population, laboratory practice, and economic impact.

43.11. Laboratory Safety Considerations

Although there are risks associated with the handling of fungi recovered from clinical specimens, a commonsense approach concerning their handling will protect the laboratory from contamination and workers from infection.

It is necessary that all mold cultures and clinical specimens be handled in a class II biological safety cabinet (Chapter 2), **with no exceptions.** Some laboratory directors feel that it is necessary to handle mold cultures within an enclosed biological safety cabinet equipped with gloves; however, this is not necessary if a laminar flow biological safety cabinet is used. It is permissible, however, to handle yeast cultures on the bench top; they must be treated as infectious agents. The use of a Bacti-incinerator or a gas flame is suitable for the decontamination of a loop used for transfer of yeast cultures. Cultures of organisms suspected of being pathogens should be sealed with tape to prevent laboratory contamination and should be autoclaved as soon as a definitive identification of the organism is made.

Few problems concerning laboratory contamination or infection of laboratory personnel will be associated with the handling of fungi if common safety precautions and careful handling of cultures are observed.

43.12. General Considerations for the Identification of Molds

The identification of molds is made using a combination of (1) the growth rate, (2) colonial morphologic features, and (3) microscopic morphologic features. In most instances the latter provides the most definitive means for identification. The determination of the growth rate of a culture is one of the most helpful observations made when examining a mold culture. However, this information may be of limited value since the growth rate of certain fungi is variable, depending upon the amount of inoculum present in a clinical specimen. In general, the growth rate for the dimorphic fungi, including *Blastomyces dermatitidis*, *Coccidioides immitis*, *Histoplasma capsulatum*, and *Paracoccidioides brasiliensis*, is slow; 1-4 weeks are usually required before colonies become visible. In some instances, however, cultures of *B. dermatitidis* and *C. immitis* may be detected within 3-5 days. This is a somewhat unusual circumstance and is encountered only when large numbers of the organism are present on the culture medium. In contrast, colonies of the zygomycetes may appear within 24 h while the other hyaline and dematiaceous fungi often exhibit growth within 1-5 days. The growth rate of an organism is an important observation but it must be used in combination with other features before the definitive identification of an organism can be made.

The colonial morphologic features are also of limited value in identifying the molds, due to natural variation among isolates and variation of colonies on different culture media. Although it may be possible to recognize certain species recovered repeatedly in the laboratory based on their colonial morphologic features, this is an unreliable criterion and should be used only to supplement the information obtained by microscopic examination of the culture. When examining the colonial morphological features, the type of culture media used and the incubation conditions must be considered. For example, *H. capsulatum*, which appears as a white to tan mold on brain heart infusion agar, may appear yeastlike in appearance when grown on the same medium containing blood enrichment. It is recommended that the colonial morphologic features be used to supplement the information obtained from the growth rate and microscopic morphologic features.

In general, the microscopic morphologic features of the molds are stable and exhibit minimal variation. The definitive identification is based on the characteristic shape, method of

PROCEDURE 43.1. WET MOUNT

1. With a wire bent at a 90-degree angle, cut out a small portion of an isolated colony. The portion should be removed from a point intermediate between the center and periphery. The portion removed should contain a small amount of the supporting agar.
2. Place the portion of the culture onto a slide to which has been added a drop of lactophenol cotton (Chapter 46) or aniline blue (Figure 43.28).
3. Place a coverslip into position and apply gentle pressure with a pencil eraser or other suitable object to disperse the growth and agar. Examine microscopically.

FIGURE 43.28
Wet mount, showing dispersion of growth under coverslip using pressure.

production, and arrangement of spores; however, the size of the hyphae also provides helpful information. The large ribbonlike hyphae of the zygomycetes are easily recognized, while small hyphae, 1-2 μm in size, may suggest the presence of one of the dimorphic fungi.

The fungi may be prepared for microscopic observation using several techniques. The procedure traditionally used by most laboratories is the wet mount examination (Procedure 43.1). The wet mount can be prepared easily and quickly and often is sufficient to make the identification for many of the fungi commonly encountered in the clinical laboratory.

The major disadvantage of the wet mount is that the characteristic arrangement of spores is disrupted when pressure is applied to the coverslip. This method is suitable in many instances since characteristic spores are often seen but, when their arrangement cannot be determined, it is not adequate to make a definitive identification.

The easiest, most economical and most suitable method for the microscopic identification of fungi is the Scotch (cellophane) tape preparation (Procedure 43.2). This method is recommended for routine use in clinical microbiology laboratories of all sizes.

The transparent tape preparation allows one to observe the organism microscopically approximately the way it grows in culture. The spores are usually intact, and the microscopic identification of an organism can be made with ease. If the tape is not pressed firmly enough to the colonies' surface, the sample may not be adequate for an identification. In instances where spores are not observed, a wet mount should be made as a backup step. There have been situations where the macroconidia of *Histoplasma capsulatum* were seen in wet mount

PROCEDURE 43.2. SCOTCH OR CELLOPHANE TAPE PREPARATION

1. Touch the adhesive side of a small length of transparent tape to the surface of the colony.
2. Adhere the length of tape to the surface of a microscope slide to which has been added a drop of lactophenol cotton or aniline blue (Figure 43.29).
3. Observe microscopically for the characteristic shape and arrangement of the spores.

FIGURE 43.29
Scotch tape preparation, showing placement of tape onto slide containing lactophenol cotton blue.

preparations when the Scotch tape preparation revealed only hyphal fragments. On the contrary, there have been instances where cultures have sporulated heavily and revealed only the presence of conidia when the Scotch tape preparation is observed. In this type of situation, a second Scotch tape preparation should be made from the periphery of the colony where sporulation is not as heavy.

Some laboratories prefer to use the microslide culture (Procedure 43.3) for making the microscopic identification of an organism. This method might appear to be the most suitable since it allows one to microscopically observe the fungus growing directly underneath the coverslip. Microscopic features should be easily discerned, structures should be intact, and a large number of representative areas of growth are available for observation.

Although this method is ideal for making a definitive identification of an organism, it is the least practical of all the methods described. It should be reserved for those instances where an identification cannot be made on the basis of a Scotch tape preparation or wet mount. **Caution:** do not make slide cultures of slowly growing organisms suspected of being di-

morphic pathogens such as *H. capsulatum*, *B. dermatitidis*, *C. immitis*, *P. brasiliensis*, or *S. schenckii*. Microslide cultures should be observed only after a coverslip has been removed from the agar plug and not while it is in position on top of the agar plug. This method of observation is highly dangerous in the case of the above species and should not be used in the clinical laboratory.

43.13. Superficial and Cutaneous Mycoses

The superficial fungal infections are produced by fungi of very low virulence. They exhibit little tissue invasion and evoke minimal host response, the infections they produce are asymptomatic, and aesthetically displeasing lesions are usually produced. Lesions usually exhibit hyperpigmentation, hypopigmentation, or nodular mass production on the hair shaft distal to the skin. Most are uncommonly seen except for tinea versicolor.

43.13.a. Tinea versicolor (pityriasis versicolor). Tinea versicolor is a skin infection characterized by superficial brownish scaly areas on light-skinned persons and lighter areas on dark-skinned persons. The lesions occur on the smooth surfaces of the body, namely, the

PROCEDURE 43.3. MICROSLIDE CULTURE

1. Cut a small block of a suitable agar medium that has been previously poured into a Petri dish to a depth of approximately 2 mm. The block may be cut using a sterile scalpel blade or with a sterile test tube that has no lip (which produces a round block).
2. Place a sterile microscope slide onto the surface of a Petri dish containing sterile 2% agar. Alternatively, place a round piece of filter paper or paper towel into a sterile Petri dish, add 2 applicator sticks and position the microscope slide on top.
3. Add the agar block to the surface of the sterile microscope slide.
4. With a right angle wire, inoculate the 4 quadrants of the agar plug with the organisms (Figure 43.30).
5. Apply a sterile coverslip onto the surface of the agar plug.
6. If the filter paper applicator stick method is used, add a small amount of sterile water to the bottom of the Petri dish. Replace the lid of the culture and allow it to incubate at 30° C.
7. After a suitable incubation period, remove the coverslip (working inside of a biological safety cabinet) and place it on a microscope slide containing a drop of lactophenol cotton or aniline blue. It is often helpful to place the coverslip near the opening of a Bacti-incinerator to allow rapid drying of the organism on the coverslip to occur prior to adding it to the stain.
8. Observe microscopically for the characteristic shape and arrangement of spores.
9. The remaining agar block may be used later (if the microslide culture is unsatisfactory for the microscopic identification) if it is allowed to incubate further. The agar plug is then removed and a drop of lactophenol cotton or aniline blue is placed on the area of growth and a coverslip is positioned into place. Many laboratorians like to make two cultures on the same slide so that if characteristic microscopic features are not observed on examination of the first culture, the second will be available after an additional incubation period.

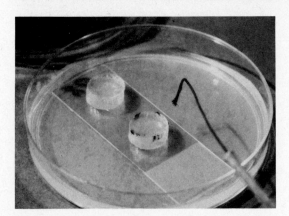

FIGURE 43.30
Microslide culture, showing inoculation of agar plug.

trunk, arms, shoulders, and face. It has a worldwide distribution. It is caused by *Malassezia furfur*, an organism not usually cultured in the clinical laboratory. Recovery of the organism is not required to establish a diagnosis and it is seldom attempted; if one wishes to culture the organism, an agar medium overlaid with a fatty acid (olive oil) is used. Most often, the diagnosis of *Malassezia furfur* is made by the direct microscopic examination of skin scales. Here the organism will easily be recognized as oval or bottle shaped cells that exhibit monopolar budding in the presence of a cell wall with a septum at the site of the bud scar (Plate 43.2). In addition, small hyphal fragments are observed. *Malassezia pachydermatis*, another species, may be recovered from skin lesions of patients; however, it requires no lipid additives.

It should be mentioned that *Malassezia furfur* is currently being seen as the cause of disseminated infection in infants and young children and even adults given lipid replacement therapy.[51] The organism is readily cultured from blood or skin lesions without the use of a fatty acid additive. The morphologic form seen in the direct microscopic examination of specimens from these patients is the yeast form without the presence of pseudohyphae.

43.13.b. Tinea nigra. Tinea nigra is an infection which is manifested by blackish-brown macular patches on the palm of the hand or sole of the foot. Lesions have been compared to silver nitrate staining of the skin. The etiologic agent is *Exophiala werneckii*, a dematiaceous fungus. Initial colonies of *E. werneckii* may be black, shiny, and yeastlike in appearance. With age, colonies become filamentous with velvety-gray aerial hyphae. Microscopically, the yeastlike growth consists of olive-colored budding cells which are one- or two-celled. Older colonies exhibit one- or two-cell conidia that are produced by annelides, which bear successive rings (annelations).

43.13.c. Piedra. Black piedra is a fungal infection of the hair of the scalp and rarely of axillary and pubic hair. The etiologic agent is a dematiaceous fungus called *Piedraia hortae*. The disease occurs primarily in tropical areas of the world; cases have been reported in Africa, Asia, and in Latin America. Portions of hair are examined (in wet mounts using potassium hydroxide which is gently heated) for the presence of nodules which are composed of cemented mycelium. When mature nodules are crushed, oval asci, containing 2-8 aseptate ascospores, 19-55 μm long by 4-8 μm in diameter, are seen (Figure 43.31 and Plate 43.3). The asci are spindle shaped and have a filament at each pole. The organism is easily cultured on any fungal culture medium lacking cycloheximide.

White piedra is an uncommon fungal infection found in both tropical and temperate regions of the world. It is characterized by the development of soft, yellow or pale brown ag-

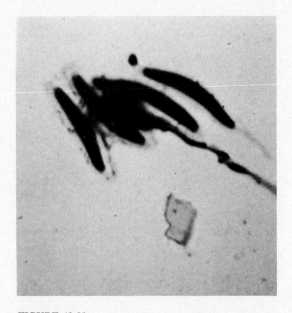

FIGURE 43.31
Piedra, showing curved, fusiform ascospores of *Piedraia hortae* (430 ×).

gregations around hair shafts in the axillary, facial, genital and scalp regions of the body. The etiologic agent is *Trichosporon beigelii*. It frequently invades the cortex of the hair and causes damage. White nodules are removed and observed using the potassium hydroxide preparation after applying light pressure to the coverslip so that crushing of the nodule occurs (Plate 43.4). Hyaline hyphae, 2 to 4 μm in width, and arthroconidia are found in the preparation of the cementlike material binding the hyphae together. The organism may be identified in culture by blastoconidia and arthroconidia formation. *Trichosporon beigelii* may be distinguished from the other species in the genus by its inability to ferment carbohydrates and ability to aerobically utilize certain substrates. *Trichosporon beigelii* may produce systemic infection in immunocompromised hosts, particularly patients with leukemia.

43.14. Cutaneous Infections (Dermatomycoses)

Dermatomycoses are fungal infections that involve the superficial areas of the body including the hair, skin and nails. The genera *Trichophyton*, *Microsporum*, and *Epidermophyton* are the only fungi associated with the dermatomycoses. Such cutaneous mycoses are perhaps the most common fungal infections of humans and are usually referred to as "tinea" (Latin for 'worm' or 'ringworm'). The gross appearance of the lesion is that of an outer ring of an active, progressing infection with central healing within the ring. These infections may be characterized by another Latin noun to designate the area of the body involved. For example, **tinea corporis** (body), **tinea cruris** (groin), **tinea capitis** (scalp and hair), **tinea barbae** (beard), and **tinea unguium** (nail) are used to designate the type of infection observed. The group of fungi commonly called dermatophytes break down and utilize keratin as a source of nitrogen but are usually incapable of penetrating the subcutaneous tissue. The genus *Trichophyton* is capable of invading the hair, skin and nails, whereas the genus *Microsporum* involves only the hair and skin; the genus *Epidermophyton* involves the skin and nails.

43.14.a. Common species. Common species of dermatophytes recovered from clinical specimens, in order of frequency, include *Trichophyton rubrum*, *T. mentagrophytes*, *Epidermophyton floccosum*, *T. tonsurans*, *Microsporum canis*, *T. verrucosum*, *T. violaceum*, and *T. schoenleinii*.[4]

Since the dermatophytes generally present a similar microscopic appearance within infected hair, skin or nails, the final identification can be made only by culture. A summary of the colonial and microscopic morphologic features of these fungi is presented in Table 43.8. Figure 43.32 presents an identification schema which will be of use to the clinical microbiologist for the identification of commonly encountered dermatophytes.

Descriptions of the common species of fungi causing dermatomycoses in the United States follow; other geographically limited species which are uncommonly encountered are described in the references cited.

Figure 43.32 begins with the microscopic features of the dermatophytes as they might be observed in an initial examination of the culture. In many instances the primary recovery medium fails to function well as a sporulation medium. It is commonly necessary to subculture the initial growth onto **cornmeal agar** or **potato dextrose agar** so that sporulation will occur.

The genus *Trichophyton* is recognized by the presence of microconidia borne either laterally along the side of the hyphae or in clusters. Microconidia are usually numerous, except for some of the slower growing species such as *T. violaceum*, *T. schoenleinii* and *T. verrucosum*, which rarely exhibit sporulation. Macroconidia are uncommonly produced by

TABLE 43.8

Characteristics of More Commonly Isolated Dermatophytes

DERMATOPHYTE	COLONIAL MORPHOLOGY	GROWTH RATE	MICROSCOPIC IDENTIFICATION
Microsporum audouinii	Downy white to salmon pink colony; reverse tan to salmon pink	2 weeks	Sterile hyphae: terminal chlamydospores, favic chandeliers, and pectinate bodies; macroconidia rarely seen—bizarre shaped if seen; microconidia rare or absent.
Microsporum canis	Colony usually membranous with feathery periphery; center of colony white to buff over orange-yellow; lemon yellow or yellow-orange apron and reverse	1 week	Thick-walled, spindle-shaped, multiseptate, rough-walled macroconidia, some with a curved tip; microconidia rarely seen
Microsporum gypseum	Cinnamon-colored, powdery colony; reverse light tan	1 week	Thick-walled rough, elliptical multiseptate macroconidia; microconidia few or absent.
Epidermophyton floccosum	Center of colony tends to be folded and is khaki green; periphery is yellow; reverse yellowish brown with observable folds	1 week	Macroconidia large, smooth-walled, multiseptate, clavate, and borne singly or in clusters of two or three; microconidia not formed by this species
Trichophyton mentagrophytes	Different colonial types; white to pinkish, granular and fluffy varieties; occasional light yellow periphery in younger cultures; reverse buff to reddish brown	7-10 days	Many round to globose microconidia most commonly borne in grapelike clusters or laterally along the hyphae; spiral hyphae in 30% of isolates; macroconidia are thin-walled, smooth, club-shaped, and multiseptate; numerous or rare depending upon strain
Trichophyton rubrum	Colonial types vary from white downy to pink granular; rugal folds are common; reverse yellow when colony is young; however, wine red color commonly develops with age	2 weeks	Microconidia usually teardrop, most commonly borne along sides of the hyphae; macroconidia usually absent, but when present are smooth, thin-walled, and pencil-shaped
Trichophyton tonsurans	White, tan to yellow or rust, suedelike to powdery; wrinkled with heaped or sunken center; reverse yellow to tan to rust red	7-14 days	Microconidia are teardrop or club-shaped with flat bottoms; vary in size but usually larger than other dermatophytes; macroconidia rare and balloon forms found when present
Trichophyton schoenleinii	Irregularly heaped, smooth white to cream colony with radiating grooves; reverse white	2-3 weeks	Hyphae usually sterile; many antler-type hyphae seen (favic chandeliers)
Trichophyton violaceum	Port wine to deep violet colony, may be heaped or flat with waxy-glabrous surface; pigment may be lost on subculture	2-3 weeks	Branched, tortuous hyphae that are sterile; chlamydospores commonly aligned in chains
Trichophyton verrucosum	Glabrous to velvety white colonies; rare strains produce yellow-brown color; rugal folds with tendency to sink into agar surface	2-3 weeks	Microconidia rare; large and tear-drop when seen. Macroconidia extremely rare, but form characteristic "rat-tail" types when seen; many chlamydospores seen in chains, particularly when colony is incubated at 37° C

From Koneman, E.W., and Roberts, G.D. 1985. Practical laboratory mycology, ed. 3. The Williams and Wilkins Co., Baltimore.

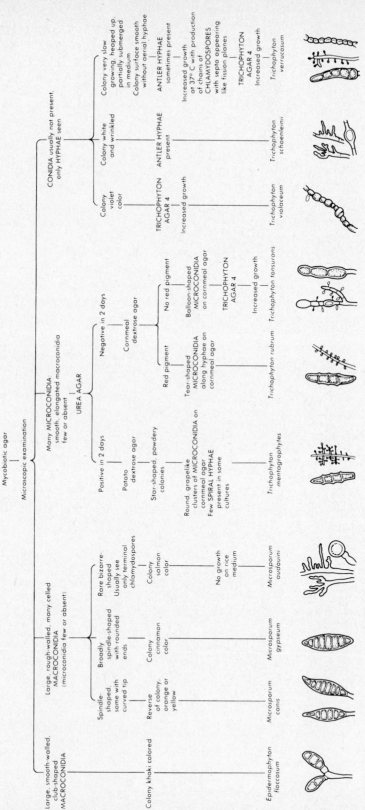

*Schema used for dermatophytes commonly recovered by Mayo Clinic Mycology Laboratory.

FIGURE 43.32
Dermatophyte identification schema. (From Koneman, E.W., and Roberts, G.D. 1985. Practical laboratory mycology, ed. 3. The Williams & Wilkins Co., Baltimore.)

most species of *Trichophyton*. When present, they are smooth-walled, elongated, pencil- to cigar-shaped, and are borne from short delicate conidiophores.

The genus *Epidermophyton* is characterized by the presence of large, club-shaped, multi-segmented, smooth-walled macroconidia that are commonly produced either singly or in clusters of two to three from the tips of short conidiophores; microconidia are not produced. This organism is easily identified.

The genus *Microsporum* is characterized by the production of large, rough-walled, multi-segmented macroconidia that are produced singly from short conidiophores or are produced directly from the hyphae. Macroconidia may be numerous and are usually spindle shaped to elongated. Microconidia are uncommonly produced except for the occasional isolate where their production may predominate.

43.14.b. Genus *Trichophyton*. Species of this genus are widely distributed and are the most important and common causes of infections of the feet and nails; they may be responsible for tinea corporis (Plate 43.13), tinea capitis, and tinea barbae. They are most commonly seen in adult infections, which vary considerably in their clinical manifestations. Most cosmopolitan species are **anthropophilic,** or 'man-loving'; few are **zoophilic,** primarily infecting animals.

Generally, hairs infected with members of the genus *Trichophyton* do not fluoresce under a Wood's lamp (Plate 43.1); the demonstration of fungal elements inside, surrounding and penetrating the hair shaft, or within a skin scraping is necessary to make a diagnosis of the dermatophyte infection. The recovery and identification of the causative organism are necessary for confirmation.

Microscopically, the genus *Trichophyton* is characterized by smooth, club-shaped, thin-walled macroconidia with 8-10 septa ranging in size from 4 by 8 μm to 8 by 15 μm. The ma-

croconidia are borne singly at the terminal ends of hyphae or on short conidiophores; the microconidia predominate and are usually spherical, pyriform (teardrop shaped), or clavate (club shaped), and 2-4 μm in size. Only the common species of *Trichophyton* is described in this chapter.

Trichophyton rubrum and *T. mentagrophytes* are the most common species recovered in the clinical laboratory. *T. rubrum* is a slow growing organism that produces a flat or heaped-up colony that is generally white to reddish with a cottony or velvety surface. The characteristic cherry-red color is best observed on the reverse side of the colony; however, this is only produced after 3 or 4 weeks of incubation. Occasional strains may lack the deep red pigmentation on first isolation. Colonies may be of two types, fluffy and granular. Microconidia are uncommon in most of the fluffy strains but are more common in the granular strains and occur as small, teardrop-shaped conidia often borne laterally along the sides of the hyphae (Figure 43.33). Macroconidia are uncom-

FIGURE 43.33
Trichophyton rubrum, showing an elongated macroconidium and numerous pyriform microconidia borne singly on hyphae (750 ×).

PROCEDURE 43.4. HAIR PERFORATION TEST[5]

1. Place a filter paper disk into the bottom of a sterile Petri dish.
2. Cover surface of paper disk with sterile distilled water.
3. Add a small portion of sterilized prepubertal hair into the water.
4. Inoculate a portion of the colony to be studied directly onto the hair.
5. Incubate at 25° C for 10-14 days.
6. Observe hairs at regular intervals by placing them into a drop of water on a microscope slide. Position a coverslip and examine microscopically for the presence of conical perforations of the hair shaft (Figure 43.34; Plate 43.14).

monly seen, although they are sometimes found in the granular strains, where they appear as thin-walled, smooth-walled, multicelled, pencil-shaped conidia with 3 to 8 septa. *T. rubrum* has no specific nutritional requirements. It does not perforate hair in vitro (Procedure 43.4) or produce urease.

T. mentagrophytes produces two distinct colonial forms: the downy variety recovered from cases of tinea pedis and the granular variety recovered from lesions acquired by contact with animals.

T. mentagrophytes produces rapidly growing colonies which appear as white, cottony or downy colonies to cream-colored or yellow colonies that are coarsely granular to powdery. Granular colonies may show evidence of red pigmentation. The reverse side of the colony is usually rose-brown, occasionally orange to deep red and may be confused with *T. rubrum*. The white downy colonies produce only a few spherical microconidia; the granular colonies sporulate freely with numerous small, spherical microconidia produced in grapelike clusters and thin-walled, smooth-walled, cigar-shaped macroconidia measuring 6 by 20 μm to

FIGURE 43.34
Hair perforation by *Trichophyton mentagrophytes;* wedge-shaped areas illustrate hair perforation (100 ×).

8 by 50 μm in size, with 2-5 septa (Figure 43.35). Macroconidia characteristically exhibit a definite narrow attachment to their base. Spiral hyphae may be found in one-third of the isolates recovered.

T. mentagrophytes produces urease within 2-3 days after inoculation onto Christensen's urea agar (Chapter 9). In addition, *T. mentagrophytes* perforates hair, in contrast to *T. rubrum* which does not. This latter criterion may be used when there is difficulty in distinguishing between the two species.

T. tonsurans, along with *Microsporum audouinii*, is responsible for an epidemic form of tinea capitis occurring most commonly in children, but occasionally in adults. It has displaced *M. audouinii* as a primary cause of tinea capitis in most of the United States. The fungus causes a low-grade superficial lesion of varying severity and produces circular, scaly patches of alopecia (loss of hair). The stubs of hair remain in the epidermis of the scalp after the brittle hairs have broken off and may give the typical "black dot" ringworm appearance. Since the infected hairs do not fluoresce under a Wood's lamp, a careful search for the embedded stub should be carried out by the physician using a bright light.

The direct microscopic examination of infected hairs in a potassium hydroxide preparation (Chapter 7) reveals the hair shaft to be filled with masses of large (4-7 μm) arthroconidia in chains, characteristic of an **endothrix** type of invasion. Cultures of *T. tonsurans* develop slowly and are typically buff to brown, wrinkled and suedelike in appearance (Plate 43.15). The colony surface shows radial folds, often developing a craterlike depression in the center with deep fissures. The reverse side of the colony is yellowish to reddish brown. Microscopically, numerous microconidia with flat bases borne on the sides of hyphae are observed. With age, the microconidia tend to become pleomorphic and are swollen to elongated and are referred to as "balloon forms" (Figure 43.36). Chlamydospores are abundant

FIGURE 43.35
Trichophyton mentagrophytes, showing numerous microconidia in grapelike clusters. Also shown are several thin-walled macroconidia (500 ×).

FIGURE 43.36
Trichophyton tonsurans, showing numerous microconidia borne singly or in clusters. A single macroconidium (rare) is also present (600 ×).

in old cultures; swollen and fragmented hyphal cells resembling arthroconidia may be seen. *T. tonsurans* grows poorly on media lacking vitamins; however, growth is greatly enhanced by the presence of thiamine.

T. verrucosum causes a variety of lesions in cattle and in humans; it is most often seen in farmers who acquire their infection from cattle. The lesions are found chiefly on the beard, neck, wrist and back of the hands; they are deep, pustular, and inflammatory. With pressure, short stubs of hair may be recovered from the purulent lesion. Direct examination of the outside of the hair shaft reveals sheaths of isolated chains of large (5-10 μm) spores (**ectothrix**) and hyphae within the hair (**endothrix**). Masses of these conidia may also be seen in exudate from the lesions.

T. verrucosum grows very slowly (14-30 days) and growth is enhanced at 35°-37° C. Growth is also enhanced on media enriched with thiamine and inositol. *T. verrucosum* may be suspected when colonies appear to embed themselves into the agar surface. Kane and Smitka[29] described a new medium for the early detection and identification of *T. verrucosum*. The ingredients for this medium are 4% casein and 0.5% yeast extract. The organism is recognized by its early hydrolysis of casein and very slow growth rate. Chains of chlamydospores are formed regularly at 37° C. The early detection of hydrolysis, formation of characteristic chains of chlamydospores (Figure 43.37), and the restrictive slow growth rate of *T. verrucosum* differentiates it from *T. schoenleinii*, another slowly growing organism. Colonies are small, heaped and folded, occasionally flat and disk shaped. At first they are glabrous and waxy, with a short aerial mycelium. Colonies range from gray and waxlike to a bright ochre. The reverse of the colony is most often nonpigmented but may be yellow.

Chlamydospores in chains and antler hyphae may be the only forms observed microscopically. Chlamydospores are produced abundantly at 35°-37° C. Microconidia may be produced by some cultures if the medium is enriched with yeast extract or a vitamin. Conidia, when present, are borne laterally from the hyphae and are large and clavate. Macroconidia are rarely formed, vary considerably in size and shape and are referred to as "rat tail."

Trichophyton schoenleinii causes a severe type of infection called "favus" (Plate 43.16). It is characterized by the formation of yellowish cup-shaped crusts or scutulae, resulting in considerable scarring of the scalp and sometimes permanent alopecia. A distinctive invasion of the infected hair, the favic type, is demonstrated by the presence of large inverted cones of hyphae and arthroconidia at the base of the hair follicle and branching hyphae throughout the length of the hair shaft. Longitudinal tunnels or empty spaces appear in the hair shaft where the hyphae have disintegrated. In potassium hydroxide preparations, these tunnels are readily filled with fluid; air bubbles may also be

FIGURE 43.37
Trichophyton verrucosum, showing multicelled, smooth thin-walled macroconidia, which are rarely seen (500 ×).

seen in these tunnels. *T. schoenleinii* is a slowly growing organism (30 days or longer) and produces a white to light gray colony that has a waxy surface. Colonies have an irregular border which consists mostly of submerged hyphae and which tends to crack the agar. The surface of the colony is usually nonpigmented or tan, furrowed and irregularly folded. The reverse side of the colony is usually tan or nonpigmented. Microscopically, conidia are not formed commonly. The hyphae tend to become knobby and club-shaped at the terminal ends, with the production of many short lateral and terminal branches (antler hyphae) (Figure 43.38). Chlamydospores are generally numerous. All strains of *T. schoenleinii* may be grown in a vitamin-free medium and grow equally well at room temperature or at 35°-37° C.

T. violaceum produces an infection of the scalp and body and is primarily seen in persons living in the Mediterranean region, the Middle and Far East, and Africa. Hair invasion is of the endothrix type; the typical "black dot" type of tinea capitis is observed clinically. Direct microscopic examination of the potassium hydroxide preparation of the nonfluorescing hairs shows dark thick hairs filled with masses of arthroconidia arranged in chains, similar to those seen in *T. tonsurans* infections.

Colonies of *T. violaceum* are very slow growing, beginning as cream-colored, glabrous, cone-shaped, and later becoming heaped up, verrucous (warty), and violet to purple in color and waxy in consistency. Colonies may often be described as being "port wine" in color. The reverse side of the colony is purple or nonpigmented. Older cultures may develop a velvety area of mycelium and sometimes lose their pigmentation. Microscopically, microconidia and macroconidia are generally not present; only sterile, distorted hyphae and chlamydospores are found. In some instances, however, swollen hyphae containing cytoplasmic granules may be seen (Figure 43.39). The growth of *T. violaceum* is enhanced on media containing thiamine.

FIGURE 43.38
Trichophyton schoenleinii, showing swollen hyphal tips with lateral and terminal branching (favic chandeliers). Microconidia and macroconidia are absent (500 ×).

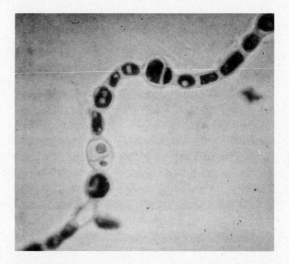

FIGURE 43.39
Trichophyton violaceum, showing chains of swollen cells containing cytoplasmic granules. Microconidia and macroconidia are usually absent (500 ×).

43.14.c. Genus *Microsporum*. The genus *Microsporum* is immediately recognized by the presence of large (8 × 8-15 μm × 35-150 μm) spindle-shaped, rough-walled macroconidia with thick (up to 4 μm) walls that contain 4-15 septa. The microconidia, when present, are small (3-7 μm) and club-shaped and are borne on the hyphae, either laterally or on short conidiophores. Species of *Microsporum* develop either slowly or rapidly and produce aerial hyphae that may be velvety, powdery, glabrous or cottony, varying in color from whitish, buff, to a cinnamon brown, with varying shades on the reverse side of the colony.

Microsporum audouinii was, in past years, the most important cause of epidemic tinea capitis among schoolchildren in the United States. This organism is anthropophilic and is spread directly by means of infected hairs on hats, caps, upholstery, combs or barber clippers. The majority of infections are chronic; some heal spontaneously, whereas others may persist for several years. Infected hair shafts fluoresce yellow-green using a Wood's lamp (Plate 43.1). Colonies of *M. audouinii* generally grow more slowly than other members of the genus *Microsporum* (10-21 days), and produce a velvety aerial mycelium that is colorless to light gray to tan. The reverse side often appears salmon-pink to reddish-brown. Colonies of *M. audouinii* do not usually sporulate in culture. The addition of yeast extract may stimulate growth and the production of macroconidia in some instances. Most commonly, atypical vegetative forms such as terminal chlamydospores (Figure 43.40) and antler and racquet hyphae are the only clues to the identification of this organism. It is common to identify *M. audouinii* by exclusion of all the other dermatophytes as a cause of infection.

Microsporum canis is primarily a pathogen of animals; it is the most common cause of ringworm infection in dogs and cats in the United States. Children and adults acquire the disease through contact with infected animals, particularly puppies and kittens, although human-to-human transfer has been reported. Hairs infected with *M. canis* fluoresce a bright yellow-green using a Wood's lamp, which is a useful tool for screening pets as possible sources of human infection. Direct examination of a potassium hydroxide preparation of infected hairs reveals small spores (2-3 μm) outside the hair, although culture procedures must be performed to provide specific identification.

Colonies of *M. canis* grow rapidly, are granular or fluffy with a feathery border, are white to buff, and characteristically have a lemon-yellow or yellow-orange fringe at the periphery. On aging, the colony becomes dense and cottony and a deeper brownish-yellow or orange and frequently shows an area of heavy growth in the center. The reverse side of the colony is bright yellow, becoming orange or reddish-brown with age. Rarely strains are recovered that show no reverse side pigment. Microscopically, *M. canis* shows an abundance of large

FIGURE 43.40
Microsporum audouinii, showing a distorted macroconidium. Macroconidia and microconidia are usually absent (1,800 ×).

43.1

43.2

PLATE 43.1.   Fluorescent hairs. Wood's lamp (mycotic infection).
PLATE 43.2.   *Malassezia furfur*, microscopic (400 ×). (Courtesy Upjohn Co.)

43.3

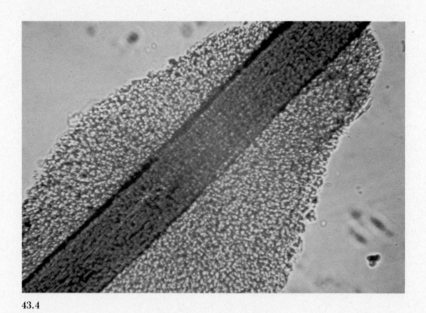

43.4

PLATE 43.3. *Piedraia hortae.* Hair (400 ×). (Courtesy Upjohn Co.)
PLATE 43.4. *Trichosporon beigelii.* Hair (40 ×). (Courtesy Upjohn Co.)

43.5

43.6

PLATE 43.5. *Sporothrix schenkii* in mouse testis.
PLATE 43.6. Sclerotic bodies of chromoblastomycosis in tissue (400 ×). (Courtesy Upjohn Co.)

43.7

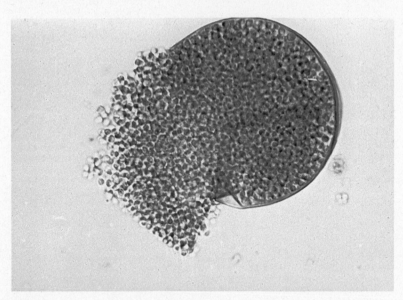

43.8

PLATE 43.7. *Candida albicans.* Acridine orange stain. (Courtesy Upjohn Co.)
PLATE 43.8. *Coccidioides immitis.* Ruptured spherule with endospores.

43.9

43.10

PLATE 43.9. *Histoplasma capsulatum* in mononuclear cells of liver (1,000 ×). (Courtesy Upjohn Co.)

PLATE 43.10. *H. capsulatum* in neutrophil on peripheral blood smear (1,000 ×).

43.11

43.12

PLATE 43.11.   *Blastomyces dermatitidis* in tissue. Gridley stain (1,000 ×).
PLATE 43.12.   Zygomycosis. Note large, nonseptate branched hyphae.

43.13

43.14

PLATE 43.13. *Trichophyton verrucosum*, ringworm of skin. (Courtesy Upjohn Co.)
PLATE 43.14. *Trichophyton mentagrophytes*. In vitro hair perforation test.

43.15

43.16

PLATE 43.15.   *Trichophyton tonsurans* colony.
PLATE 43.16.   Scalp infection. *Trichophyton schoenleinii*. (Courtesy Upjohn Co.)

43.17

43.18

PLATE 43.17. *S. schenkii* colony. (Courtesy Upjohn Co.)
PLATE 43.18. *Phialophora* infection of foot. (Courtesy Upjohn Co.)

43.19

43.20

PLATE 43.19. Lesions of paracoccidioidomycosis about lips. Note purulent exudate at right edge of mouth. (Courtesy Upjohn Co.)

PLATE 43.20. *Paracoccidioides brasiliensis*. Numerous small buds.

43.21

43.22

PLATE 43.21. *Aspergillus fumigatus* conidiophore and conidia (400 ×).
PLATE 43.22. *Rhizopus* colony.

43.23

43.24

PLATE 43.23. *Mucor*. Spores inside sporangia.
PLATE 43.24. *C. albicans*. Germ tubes.

43.25

43.26

PLATE 43.25.   *C. albicans.* Blastospores and chlamydospores.
PLATE 43.26.   Disseminated coccidioidomycosis. Coccidioidal granuloma.

43.27

43.28

PLATE 43.27.   API Yeast-Ident system.
PLATE 43.28.   Uni-Yeast Tek (Flow Laboratories) system.

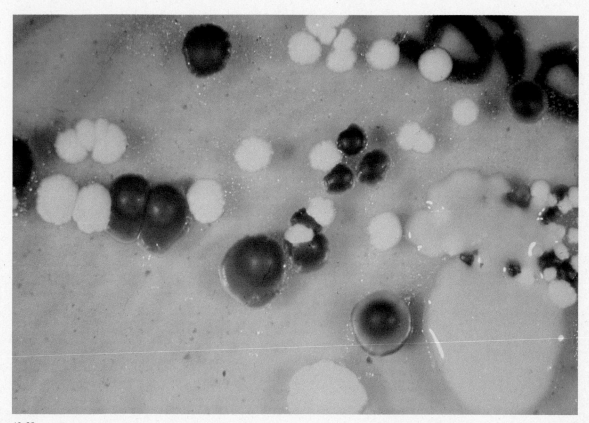

43.29

PLATE 43.29. Niger seed agar. *Cryptococcus neoformans* and *Candida albicans*.

(15 μm × 60-125 μm), spindle-shaped, multi-segmented (4-8) macroconidia with curved ends (Figure 43.41). These are thick-walled with warty (echinulate) projections on their surfaces. Microconidia are usually few in number; however, large numbers may occasionally be seen.

Microsporum gypseum, a free-living saprophyte of the soil (geophilic) that only rarely causes human or animal infection, may be seen occasionally in the clinical laboratory. Infected hairs generally do not fluoresce using a Wood's lamp. However, microscopic examination of the infected hairs shows them to be irregularly covered with clusters of spores (5-8 μm), some in chains. These arthroconidia of the ectothrix type are considerably larger than those of other *Microsporum* species.

Microsporum gypseum grows rapidly as a flat, irregularly fringed colony with a coarse powdery surface that appears to be buff or cinnamon color. The underside of the colony is conspicuously orange to brownish. Microscopi-

cally, macroconidia are seen in large numbers and are characteristically large, ellipsoidal, have rounded ends, and are multisegmented (3-9) with echinulated surfaces (Figure 43.42). Although they are spindle-shaped, these macroconidia are not as pointed at the distal ends as those of *M. canis.* The appearance of the colonial and microscopic morphologic features is sufficient to make the distinction between *M. gypseum* and *M. canis.*

43.14.d. Genus *Epidermophyton.* *Epidermophyton floccosum,* the only member of the genus *Epidermophyton,* is a common cause of tinea cruris and tinea pedis. In direct examination of skin scrapings using the potassium hydroxide preparation, the fungus is seen as fine branching hyphae. *E. floccosum* grows slowly and growth appears as an olive-green to khaki color, with the periphery surrounded by a dull orange-brown color. After several weeks, colonies develop a cottony white aerial mycelium that completely overgrows the colony and is sterile.

FIGURE 43.41
Microsporum canis, showing several spindle-shaped, thick-walled, multicelled macroconidia (500 ×).

FIGURE 43.42
Microsporum gypseum, showing ellipsoidal, multicelled macroconidia (750 ×).

FIGURE 43.43
Epidermophyton floccosum, showing numerous smooth, multiseptate, thin-walled macroconidia that appear club shaped (1,000 ×).

Microscopically, numerous smooth, thin-walled, club-shaped, multiseptate (2-4 μm) macroconidia are seen (Figure 43.43). They are rounded at the tip and are borne singly or in groups of two or three on a conidiophore. Microconidia are absent, spiral hyphae are rare, and chlamydospores are usually numerous.

This organism is very susceptible to cold temperatures and for this reason it is recommended that specimens submitted for dermatophyte culture not be refrigerated prior to culture.

43.15. Subcutaneous Mycoses

Subcutaneous mycoses are infections that involve the skin and subcutaneous tissue, generally without dissemination to other organs of the body. This classification is artificial; for example, sporotrichosis occasionally involves lungs, other viscera, meninges, or joints and may disseminate. The other agents causing subcutaneous infections may also produce disseminated infection occasionally. The etiologic agents are found in several unrelated fungal genera, all of which may exist as saprophytes in nature. Humans and animals serve as accidental hosts after traumatic inoculation of the fungal spores into cutaneous and subcutaneous tissues. Three subcutaneous mycoses are considered here: sporotrichosis, chromoblastomycosis, and mycetoma.

43.15.a. Sporotrichosis. Sporotrichosis is a chronic infection of worldwide distribution caused by the dimorphic fungus, *Sporothrix schenckii*, whose natural habitat is living or dead vegetation. Humans acquire the infection through trauma (thorns, splinters), usually to the hand, arm, or leg. The primary lesion begins as a small nonhealing ulcer, commonly of the index finger or the back of the hand. With time, the infection is characterized by the development of nodular lesions of the skin or subcutaneous tissues at the point of contact and later involves the lymphatic channels and lymph nodes draining the region. The subcutaneous nodules break down and ulcerate to form an infection that becomes chronic. Only rarely is the disease disseminated; pulmonary infection may be seen. The infection is an occupational hazard for farmers, nursery workers, gardeners, florists, and miners. It is commonly known as "rose gardener's" disease.

Exudate from unopened subcutaneous nodules or from open draining lesions is often submitted for culture and direct microscopic examination. Direct examination of this material is usually of little diagnostic value because it is difficult to demonstrate the characteristic yeast forms, even with special stains; reasons for this are unclear.

Colonies of *S. schenckii* grow rapidly (3-5 days) and are usually small, moist, and white to cream-colored in appearance. On further incubation, these become membranous, wrinkled, and coarsely matted, with the color becoming irregularly dark brown or black and the colony becoming leathery in consistency (Plate 43.17). It is common for the clinical microbiology lab-

FIGURE 43.44
Sporothrix schenckii, mycelial form, showing pyriform to ovoid microconidia borne in a flowerette at the tip of the conidiophore (750 ×).

FIGURE 43.45
Sporothrix schenckii, yeast form, showing cigar-shaped and oval budding cells (500 ×).

oratory to mistake a young culture of *Sporothrix schenckii* for that of a yeast until the microscopic features are observed.

Microscopically, hyphae are delicate (1-2 μm thick), septate, exhibit branching, and bear one-celled conidia, 2-5 μm in diameter. These are borne bouquetlike, in clusters from the tips of single conidiophores. Each conidium is attached to the conidiophore by an individual, delicate, threadlike structure (denticle) that may require examination under oil immersion to be visible. As the culture ages, single-celled, thick-walled, black pigmented conidia may also be borne along the sides of the hyphae, simulating the arrangement of microconidia produced by *T. rubrum*. The common designations for these types of sporulation are the "flowerette" and "sleeve" arrangements, respectively (Figure 43.44).

Because of similar morphologic features, saprophytic species of the genus *Sporothrix* may be confused with *S. schenckii*, and it is necessary to distinguish between them. During incubation of a culture at 37° C, the colony of *S. schenckii* transforms to a soft, cream-colored to white, yeastlike colony. Microscopically, singly or multiply budding, spherical, oval, or cigar-shaped yeast cells are observed without difficulty (Figure 43.45). Conversion from the mold form to the yeast form is easily accomplished, and usually occurs within 1-5 days after transfer of the culture to a medium containing blood enrichment; most isolates of *S. schenckii* are converted to the yeast form within 12-48 h at 37° C.

42.15.b. Chromoblastomycosis. Chromoblastomycosis is a chronic fungal infection acquired via traumatic inoculation of spores, primarily in the extremities. The infection is characterized by the development of a papule at the site of the traumatic insult that spreads to form warty or tumorlike lesions characterized as "cauliflower-like" (Plate 43.18). There may be secondary infection and ulceration. The lesions are usually confined to the feet and legs but may involve the head, face, neck, and other body surfaces. Histologic examination of lesion tissue reveals characteristic **sclerotic bodies**, copper-colored, septate cells that appear to be dividing (Plate 43.6). Brain abscess caused by the etiologic agents of chromoblastomycosis has been reported with some frequency.[9]

The disease is widely distributed, but most cases occur in tropical and subtropical areas of the world. Occasional cases are reported from temperate zones, including the United States. The infection is seen most often in areas where agricultural workers fail to wear protective clothing and suffer thorn or splinter puncture wounds through which the spores enter from the soil.

The group of fungi known to cause chromoblastomycosis are dematiaceous. All are slow growing and produce heaped up and slightly folded, darkly pigmented colonies with a grayish-velvety appearance. The reverse side of the colonies is jet black.

The taxonomy of the organisms which cause chromoblastomycosis is complex.[44] Their identification is based on distinct microscopic morphologic features. Three genera, *Cladosporium*, *Phialophora*, and *Fonsecaea*, are known to cause chromoblastomycosis.

The genus *Cladosporium* includes those species which produce long chains of conidia (blastoconidia) that have a dark septal scar present.

The genus *Phialophora* includes those species that produce short, flask-shaped to tubular phialides, usually with a well-developed collarette. Clusters of conidia are produced by the phialides through an apical pore.

The genus *Fonsecaea* includes those organisms which exhibit a mixed type of sporulation, that uniquely includes one-celled primary conidia that are produced on either side of conidiophores resembling a series of bent knees. Conidia are produced sympodially. The primary conidia give rise to secondary conidia that appear to occur in loose heads. This is known as the rhinocladiella type of sporulation and predominates, depending upon the strain isolated. A mixture of the rhinocladiella and cladosporium types may occur; moreover, phialides with collarettes may also be present. Two species, *Fonsecaea pedrosoi* and *Fonsecaea compacta*, are etiologic agents of chromoblastomycosis. Both are morphologically distinct: *F. pedrosoi* is differentiated from *F. compacta* by the production of loose heads, in contrast to the more compact heads produced by *F. compacta*.

FIGURE 43.46
Cladosporium species, showing *Cladosporium* type of sporulation with chains of elliptical conidia (430 ×).

The diagnostic features of the three genera are summarized as follows:

1. *Cladosporium* (*Cladosporium carrionii*)—cladosporium type of sporulation with long chains of elliptical conidia (2-3 μm × 4-5 μm) borne from erect, tall branching conidiophores (Figure 43.46).

2. *Phialophora* (*Phialophora verrucosa*)—tubelike or flask-shaped phialides, each with a distinct collarette. Conidia are produced endogenously and occur in clusters at the tip of the phialide (Figure 43.47).

3. *Fonsecaea* (*F. pedrosoi* and *F. compacta*)—conidial heads with sympodial arrangement of conidia, with primary conidia giving rise to secondary conidia (Figure 43.48). Cladosporium type of sporulation may occur and phialides with collarettes may also be present.

The laboratory diagnosis of chromoblastomycosis is made easily. Scrapings from crusted areas added to 10% potassium hydrox-

FIGURE 43.47
Phialophora verrucosa, showing flask-shaped phialide with a distinct collarette and conidia near its tip (750 ×).

FIGURE 43.48
Fonsecaea pedrosoi, showing conidial heads with sympodial arrangement of conidia (430 ×).

ide show the presence of the sclerotic bodies, which appear rounded, brown, and 4-10 μm in diameter and resemble "copper pennies" (Plate 43.6).

43.15.c. Mycetoma. Mycetoma is a chronic granulomatous infection that usually involves the lower extremities but may occur in any part of the body. The infection is characterized by swelling, purplish discoloration, and tumorlike deformities of the subcutaneous tissue and multiple sinus tracts that drain pus containing yellow, white, red, or black granules. The infection gradually progresses to involve the bone, muscle, or other contiguous tissue and ultimately requires amputation in most cases. Occasionally, there may be dissemination to other organs including the brain; however, this type of infection is relatively uncommon.

Mycetoma is common among persons who live in tropical and subtropical regions of the world, whose outdoor occupations and failure to wear protective clothing predispose them to trauma.

Two types of mycetoma are described, actinomycotic mycetoma which is caused by species of the aerobic actinomycetes including *Nocardia*, *Actinomadura*, and *Streptomyces* (Chapter 33); and eumycotic mycetoma caused by a heterogeneous group of species having true septate hyphae.[43] The most common etiologic agent of mycetoma in the United States is *Pseudallescheria boydii*, a member of the Ascomycota (because it produces ascospores). The organism is a common saprobe and is found in soil and sewage; humans acquire the infection by traumatic implantation of the organism into the skin and subcutaneous tissues.

Macroscopic examination of granules from lesions of mycetoma caused by *P. boydii* reveal them to be white to yellow, and 0.2-2 mm in diameter. Microscopically, the granules of *P. boydii* consist of loosely arranged, intertwined hyphae.

Pseudallescheria boydii is a hyaline organism that grows rapidly (5-10 days) on common laboratory media. Initial growth begins as a white fluffy colony that changes in several weeks to a brownish-gray (mousey) mycelium. The reverse of the colony is black. *P. boydii* has undergone several name changes in the past and is an example of an organism that reproduces both asexually and sexually. The asexual form is called *Scedosporium apiospermum* and microscopically produces elliptical (sperm-shaped), single-celled conidia borne singly from the tips of long or short conidiophores (annelophores) (Figure 43.49). Clusters of conidiophores with conidia produced at the ends sometimes occur and are referred to as "coremia."

Pseudallescheria boydii is the sexual form of the organism. The sexual form exhibits **cleistothecia,** which are saclike structures that contain asci and ascospores. When the latter are fully developed, the large (50-200 μm), thick-walled cleistothecia rupture and liberate the asci and ascospores (Figure 43.50). The ascospores are oval and delicately pointed at each end and resemble the conidia of the asexual form. Isolates of *P. boydii* may be induced to form cleistothecia by culturing on plain water agar.

P. boydii is also involved in causing a variety of infections elsewhere in the body. Included are infections of the nasal sinuses and septum, meningitis, arthritis, endocarditis, mycotic keratitis, external otomycosis, and brain abscess. Most of these more serious infections occur primarily in immunocompromised patients.

It should be mentioned that it is impossible to predict the specific etiologic agent of mycetoma. Culture media containing antibiotics should not be used alone for culturing clinical specimens, since species of the aerobic actinomycetes are susceptible to antibacterial antibiotics and may be inhibited by these agents incorporated into routine culture media. For further information on other fungi involved in mycetoma, one may refer to references listed at the end of this chapter.

FIGURE 43.49
Scedosporium apiospermum, showing asexually produced conidia borne singly on long or short conidiophores (annelophores) (430 ×).

FIGURE 43.50
Pseudallescheria boydii, showing cleistothecia and numerous ascospores (750 ×).

43.16. Systemic Mycoses

Systemic fungal infections may involve any of the internal organs of the body as well as lymph nodes, bone, subcutaneous tissue, and skin. Asymptomatic infection is common and may go unrecognized clinically and may be detected only by serologic testing; in some cases roentgenographic examination may reveal healed lesions. Symptomatic infections may present signs of only a mild or more severe but self-limited disease. with positive supportive evidence from cultural or immunologic findings. Disseminated or progressive infection may reveal severe symptoms, with spread of the initial disease to several organs as well as to the bone, skin, and subcutaneous tissues. Some cases of disseminated infection may exhibit little in the way of signs or symptoms of disease for long periods, only to exacerbate later.

Traditionally, the systemic mycoses have included blastomycosis, coccidioidomycosis, histoplasmosis and paracoccidioidomycosis. The fungi responsible for these infections, although unrelated generically and dissimilar morphologically, have one characteristic in common—that of **dimorphism**. The dimorphic fungi involved exist in nature as the saprobic form, sometimes called the mold form, which is quite distinct from the parasitic, or invasive form, sometimes called the tissue form. Distinct morphologic differences may be observed with the dimorphic fungi both in vivo and in vitro. Temperature (35°-37° C), certain nutritional factors, and stimulation of growth in tissue independent of temperature are among the factors necessary to initiate the transformation of the mold form to the parasitic form.

43.16.a. General features of dimorphic fungi. As a general rule, the dimorphic fungi are regarded as slowly growing organisms that require 7-21 days for visible growth to appear. However, exceptions to this rule occur with some frequency. Cultures of *Blastomyces der-*

matitidis and *Histoplasma capsulatum* are recovered in as short a time as 4-5 days when large numbers of organisms are present in the clinical specimen. In contrast, single colonies of *B. dermatitidis* and *H. capsulatum* sometimes require 21-30 days of incubation before they are detected. *Coccidioides immitis* is consistently recovered within 3-5 days of incubation, but when large numbers of colonies are present, colonies may be detected within 48 h. Single colonies may require 14-21 days before visible growth can be detected. Cultures of *Paracoccidioides brasiliensis* are commonly recovered within 5-25 days with a usual incubation period of 10-15 days. As one can see, the growth rate, if slow, might lead one to suspect the presence of a dimorphic fungus; however, a great deal of variation in the time for recovery exists.

Textbooks present descriptions for the dimorphic fungi that the reader assumes are typical for each particular organism. As is true in other areas of microbiology, a great deal of variation in the colonial morphologic features also occurs, commonly due to the type of medium used. One must be aware of this variation and must not rely heavily on colonial morphologic features for the identification of members of this group of fungi.

The color of the colony is sometimes helpful but varies widely; colonies of *B. dermatitidis* and *H. capsulatum* are described as being fluffy white with a change in color to tan or buff with age. Some isolates initially appear darkly pigmented with colors ranging from gray or dark brown to red. On media containing blood enrichment, these organisms appear heaped, wrinkled, glabrous and neutral in color, and yeastlike in appearance; often tufts of aerial hyphae project from the top of the colony. Some colonies may appear pink to red due to the adsorption of hemoglobin from the blood in the medium. *Coccidioides immitis* is described as being fluffy white with scattered areas of hyphae that are adherent to the agar surface so as to give an overall "cobweb" appearance to the colony. However, numerous morphologic forms including textures ranging from woolly to powdery and pigmentation ranging from pink-lavender or yellow to brown or buff have been reported. While the growth rate and colonial morphologic features may help one to recognize the presence of a dimorphic fungus, they should be used in combination with the microscopic morphologic features to make a tentative identification. The definitive identification of a dimorphic fungus has traditionally been made by observing both the mold and parasitic forms of the organism. Cultures of the mold form are easily recovered at 25°-30° C; however, the tissue form is usually not recovered from the clinical specimen. Previously the definitive identification was made by the in vitro conversion of a mold form to the corresponding yeast or spherule form by animal inoculation or by in vitro conversion on a blood enriched medium incubated at 35°-37° C. The conversion of dimorphic molds to the yeast form (except for *C. immitis*) can be accomplished with some difficulty as outlined in Procedure 43.5.

Since the conversion of the dimorphic molds to the corresponding yeast or spherule forms is technically cumbersome to perform and long delays are often experienced, the effort to convert the dimorphic fungi is not recommended and should be replaced by a relatively new procedure, **exoantigen testing** (Procedure 43.6). This technique is used in many laboratories to make a definitive identification of *B. dermatitidis*, *C. immitis*, *H. capsulatum* and *P. brasiliensis*. The exoantigen test relies on the principle that soluble antigens are produced and can be extracted from fungi; they are concentrated and subsequently reacted with serum known to contain antibodies directed against the specific antigenic components of the organism being tested. Reagents and materials for the exoantigen test are cur-

PROCEDURE 43.5. IN VITRO CONVERSION OF DIMORPHIC MOLDS

1. Transfer a large inoculum of the mold form of the culture onto the surface of a fresh, moist slant of brain heart infusion agar containing 5%-10% sheep blood. If *Blastomyces dermatitidis* is suspected, a tube of cottonseed conversion medium[71] should be inoculated.

2. Add a few drops of sterile distilled water to provide moisture if the surface of the culture medium appears to be dry.

3. Leave the cap of the screw-cap tube slightly loose to allow the culture to have adequate oxygen exchange.

4. Incubate cultures at 35°-37° C for several days; observe for the appearance of yeastlike portions of the colony. It may be necessary to make several subcultures of any growth that appears, since several transfers are often required to accomplish the conversion of many isolates. Cultures of *Blastomyces dermatitidis*, however, are usually easily converted and require 24-48 h on cottonseed agar medium. *Coccidioides immitis* may be converted in vitro to the spherule form using a chemically defined medium[67]; however, this method is of little use to the clinical laboratory and it should not be attempted.

PROCEDURE 43.6. EXOANTIGEN TEST[33,63,64]

1. A mature fungus culture on a Sabouraud's dextrose agar slant is covered with an aqueous solution of merthiolate (1:5,000 final concentration), which is allowed to remain in contact with the culture for 24 h at 25° C. It is necessary that the entire surface of the colony be covered so that effective killing of the organism is ensured.

2. Filter the aqueous solution through a 0.45 μm pore size membrane filter. This should be performed inside a biological safety cabinet.

3. Five milliliters of this solution is concentrated using a Minicon Macrosolute B-15 Concentrator (Amicon Corporation). The solution is concentrated 50 × when testing with *H. capsulatum* and *B. dermatitidis* antiserum and 5 × and 25 × for reaction with *C. immitis* antiserum.

4. The concentrated supernatant is used in the microdiffusion test. The supernatant is placed into wells punched into a plate of buffered, phenolized agar adjacent to the control antigen well and is tested against positive control antiserum obtained from commercial sources (Immunomycologics, Meridian Diagnostics, and Scott-Nolan Laboratories).

5. The immunodiffusion test is allowed to react for 24 h at 25° C and the plate is observed for the presence of precipitin bands of identity with the reference reagents. The sensitivity of the exoantigen test for the identification of *B. dermatitidis* may be increased by incubating the immunodiffusion plates at 37° C for 48 h; however, bands appear sharper at 25° C after 24 h. It is recommended that any culture suspected of being *B. dermatitidis* be incubated at both temperatures.

6. *C. immitis* may be identified for the presence of the CF, TP, or HL antigens while *H. capsulatum* and *B. dermatitidis* may be identified by the presence of H or M bands and the A band, respectively. Detailed instructions for the performance and interpretation of the tests are included with the manufacturers' package insert.

rently available commercially and provide all laboratories with the capability of identifying the dimorphic fungi with ease and rapidity.

The exoantigen test is now considered by most laboratories to be the most conclusive method for making a definitive identification of the dimorphic fungi.

The inclusion of only the dimorphic fungi in the group of systemic mycoses is a bit artificial, since other fungi, including *Cryptococcus neo-* *formans* and species of *Candida* and *Aspergillus*, also cause disseminated infection. They will not be discussed in this portion of the chapter since they are not dimorphic as previously defined and since they usually cause infection only in immunocompromised patients. They will be discussed in a subsequent section on the opportunistic mycoses.

43.16.b. Blastomycosis. Blastomycosis is a chronic suppurative and granulomatous infection caused by the dimorphic fungus *B. dermatitidis*. The disease is most commonly found on the continent of North America and extends southward from Canada to the Mississippi, Ohio and Missouri River valleys, Mexico and Central America. Some isolated cases have also been reported from Africa. The largest number of cases occur in the Mississippi, Ohio and Missouri River valley regions.

Blastomycosis begins as a respiratory infection and is probably acquired by inhalation of the conidia or hyphal fragments of the organism. The exact ecological niche for this organism in nature has not been determined; however, patients with a history of exposure to soil or wood have the highest incidence of infection. The infection may spread and involve the lungs, long bones, soft tissue, and skin. It is not transmitted from person to person and generally occurs as sporadic cases. Several outbreaks have been reported, however, and have been related to a common exposure. Blastomycosis is more common in men and seems to be associated with outdoor occupations.

The diagnosis of blastomycosis may easily be made when a clinical specimen is observed using the potassium hydroxide preparation. *B. dermatitidis* appears as a large, spherical, thick-walled cell 8-20 μm in diameter, usually with a single bud that is connected to the parent cell by a broad base.

B. dermatitidis usually requires 5 days to 4 weeks or longer for growth to be detected. On enriched culture media, the mold form develops initially as a glabrous or waxy appearing colony that may become off-white to white in color. With age, the aerial hyphae often turn gray to brown; however, on media enriched with blood, colonies appear to have a more waxy, yeastlike appearance. Tufts of hyphae often project upward from the colonies and are referred to as the "prickly state" of the organism.

Microscopically, hyphae of the mold form are septate and delicate and measure 1-2 μm in diameter. Commonly, ropelike strands of hyphae are seen; however, these are found with most of the dimorphic fungi. The characteristic microscopic morphologic features are single, pyriform conidia produced on long to short conidiophores that resemble lollipops (Figure 43.51). The production of conidia in some isolates is minimal or absent, particularly on a medium containing blood enrichment.

Colonies of the yeast form develop within 7 days and appear waxy and wrinkled, and cream to tan in color. Microscopically, large, thick-walled yeast cells with buds attached by a broad base are seen (Figure 43.52). During the conversion process, swollen hyphal forms and immature cells with rudimentary buds may be present.

As previously mentioned, the definitive identification of *B. dermatitidis* is based on the characteristic microscopic features of the mold form and the presence of a specific A band in the exoantigen test. In some instances, *P. boydii* and *T. rubrum* might be confused microscopically with *B. dermatitidis*. The relatively slow growth rate of *B. dermatitidis* and careful examination of the microscopic morphologic features will usually differentiate these fungi from *B. dermatitidis*.

43.16.c. Coccidioidomycosis. Coccidioidomycosis is a fungal infection that is primarily limited to the desert southwestern portion of the United States as well as semiarid regions of Mexico and Central and South America. Although the geographical distribution of the organism is well-defined, cases of coccidioidomycosis may be seen in any part of the world because of the ease of travel. The infection is acquired by inhalation of the infective arthroconidia of *Coccidioides immitis*. Approximately 60% of the cases are asymptomatic and self-limited respiratory tract infections. The infection, however, may become disseminated with extension to other organs, meninges, bone,

FIGURE 43.51

Blastomyces dermatitidis, mycelial form, showing oval conidia borne laterally on branching hyphae (1,000 ×).

skin, lymph nodes, and subcutaneous tissue. Fewer than 1% of persons who acquire coccidioidomycosis ever become seriously ill; dissemination does, however, occur most frequently in persons of dark-skinned races.

In direct microscopic examinations of sputum or other body fluids, *C. immitis* appears as a nonbudding, thick-walled spherule, 20-200 μm in diameter, containing either granular material or numerous small (2-5 μm in diameter) endospores (Figure 43.53). The endospores are freed by rupture of the cell wall of spherules; therefore empty and collapsed "ghost" spherules may be present. Small, immature spherules measuring 10-20 μm may be confused with *B. dermatitidis* when two are lying adjacent. In instances where the identification of *C. immitis* is questionable, a wet preparation of the clinical specimen may be made using sterile saline and the edges of the coverglass may be sealed with petrolatum and incubated overnight. When spherules are present, multiple hyphal strands will be produced from the endospores.

FIGURE 43.52

Blastomyces dermatitidis, yeast form, showing thick-walled, oval to round, single-budding yeastlike cells (500 ×).

FIGURE 43.53

Coccidioides immitis, tissue form, showing spherule containing numerous spherical endospores (1,000 ×).

Cultures of *C. immitis* represent a biohazard to laboratory workers and strict safety precautions must be followed when examining cultures. Mature colonies may appear within 3-5 days of incubation and may be present on most media, including those used for bacteriology. **Laboratory workers should be cautioned not to open cultures of fluffy white molds unless they are placed in a biological safety cabinet.** Colonies of *C. immitis* often appear as delicate, cobweblike growth after 3-21 days of incubation. Some portions of the colony will exhibit aerial hyphae whereas others will have the hyphae adherent to the agar surface. Most isolates appear fluffy white; however, colonies of varying colors have been observed. On blood agar, some colonies exhibit a greenish discoloration, whereas others appear yeastlike, smooth, wrinkled, and tan in color. Isolates of *C. immitis* have been reported to range in color from pink to yellow to purple and black.[28]

Microscopically, some cultures show small septate hyphae that often exhibit right-angle branches and racquet forms. With age, the hyphae form arthroconidia that are characteristically rectangular or barrel-shaped in appearance. The arthroconidia are larger than the hyphae from which they are produced and stain darkly with lactophenol cotton or aniline blue. The arthroconidia are separated from one another by clear or lighter staining nonviable cells and are referred to as **alternate arthroconidia** (Figure 43.54). Arthroconidia have been reported to range in size from 1.5-7.5 μm in width and 1.5-30 μm in length, whereas most are 3-4.5 μm in width and 3.1 μm in length. Variation has been reported in the shape of arthroconidia and ranges from rounded to square to curved; however, most are barrel shaped. Even if alternate arthroconidia are observed microscopically, the definitive identification should be made using only the exoantigen test.

If a culture is suspected of being *C. immitis*, it should be sealed with tape to prevent chances of laboratory acquired infection. Since *C. immitis* is the most infectious of all the fungi, extreme caution should be used when handling cultures of this organism. The following safety precautions should be observed:

1. If culture dishes are used, they should be handled only in a biological safety cabinet. Cultures should be sealed with tape if the specimen is suspected of containing *C. immitis*.

2. The use of cotton plug test tubes is discouraged and screw-cap tubes should be used if this mode of culture is preferred. If *C. immitis* is suspected, the culture should be overlayed with sterile water or saline before using an inoculating wire to remove a portion for microscopic examination. All handling of cultures of *C. immitis* in screw-capped tubes should be performed inside a biological safety cabinet.

3. All microscopic preparations for examination should be prepared in a biological safety cabinet.

FIGURE 43.54
Coccidioides immitis, mycelial form, showing numerous, thick-walled, rectangular or barrel-shaped alternate arthroconidia (500 ×).

4. Cultures should be autoclaved as soon as the final identification of *C. immitis* is made.

Some members of the Gymnoascasceae are found in the environment and may microscopically resemble *C. immitis*. Some species pro-

duce alternate arthroconidia that tend to be more rectangular and it is necessary to consider them when making an identification. *Geotrichum candidum* and species of *Trichosporon* produce hyphae that disassociate into arthroconidia (Figures 43.55 and 43.56). The colonial

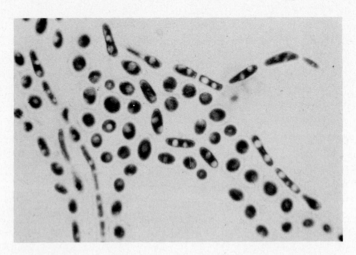

FIGURE 43.55
Trichosporon species, showing arthroconidia and an occasional blastoconidium.

FIGURE 43.56
Geotrichum candidum, showing numerous arthroconidia. Note that arthroconidia do not alternate with a clear cell as in the case of *C. immitis* (430 ×).

morphologic features of older cultures may resemble *C. immitis*. Microscopically, the arthroconidia do not appear to be alternate and are even staining. Confusion rarely occurs between members of the Gymnoascasceae and *C. immitis*. It is also important to remember that there are occasional strains of *C. immitis* that fail to sporulate and may be identified only by the exoantigen test.

43.16.d. Histoplasmosis. Histoplasmosis is a chronic, granulomatous infection that is primary in the lung and eventually invades the reticuloendothelial system. Approximately 95% of cases are asymptomatic and self-limited. Chronic pulmonary infections occur and dissemination to the lymphatic tissue, liver, spleen, kidneys, meninges, and heart has been reported. Ulcerative lesions of the upper respiratory tract may occur. Histoplasmosis is another infection that is prevalent in the Ohio, Mississippi River, and Missouri River valleys where conditions are optimal for growth of the organism in soil enriched with bird manure or bat guano.

Outbreaks of histoplasmosis have been associated with activities which disperse the microconidia or hyphal fragments into the air. Infection is acquired via inhalation of these infective units from the environment. The severity of the disease is generally related directly to the inoculum size. Numerous cases of histoplasmosis have been reported in persons cleaning a chicken house or barn that has been undisturbed for long periods or from working in or cleaning those areas which have served as roosting places for starlings and similar birds.

It is estimated that 500,000 persons are infected annually by *H. capsulatum*, the etiologic agent of histoplasmosis. It is perhaps one of the most common fungal infections seen in the midwestern and southern parts of the United States.

The direct microscopic examination of respiratory tract specimens and other similar specimens is usually unsatisfactory for the detection of *H. capsulatum*. The organism, however, may be detected by an astute laboratorian when examining Wright- or Giemsa-stained specimens of bone marrow or peripheral blood. *H. capsulatum* is found intracellularly within mononuclear cells as small round to oval yeast cells 2-5 μm in diameter.

H. capsulatum is easily cultured from clinical specimens; however, it may be overgrown by bacteria or rapidly growing molds. A procedure useful for the recovery of *H. capsulatum*, *B. dermatitidis* and *C. immitis* from contaminated specimens utilizes a yeast extract phosphate medium[59] and a drop of concentrated ammonium hydroxide (NH_4OH) placed on one side of the inoculated plate of medium. In the past, it has been recommended that specimens not be kept at room temperature prior to culture since *H. capsulatum* would not survive. It has been shown that *H. capsulatum* will survive transit in the mail for as long as 16 days.[24] It is, however, recommended that specimens be cultured as soon as possible to ensure the optimal recovery of *H. capsulatum* and other dimorphic fungi.

H. capsulatum is considered to be a slow growing mold at 25°-30° C and usually requires 2-4 weeks or more for colonies to appear. It is not uncommon to recover the organism in 7 days or less if large numbers of cells are present in the clinical specimen. Isolates of *H. capsulatum* have been reported to be recovered from blood cultures in a mean time of 8 days.[8] Textbooks describe the colonial morphology of *H. capsulatum* as being a white fluffy mold that turns brown to buff with age. Some isolates ranging from gray to red have also been reported. The organism commonly produces wrinkled, moist, heaped, yeastlike colonies which are soft and cream, tan or pink in color. Tufts of hyphae often project upwards from the colonies as described with *B. dermatitidis*.

Microscopically, the hyphae of *H. capsula-*

FIGURE 43.57
Histoplasma capsulatum, mycelial form, showing
characteristic tuberculate macroconidia (1,000 ×).

FIGURE 43.58
Histoplasma capsulatum, yeast form, showing
intracellular, oval yeast cells, deeply stained (2,000 ×).

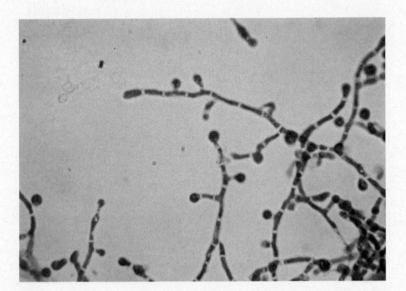

FIGURE 43.59
Paracoccidioides brasiliensis, mycelial form, showing septate hyphae and pyriform conidia singly borne
(430 ×).

tum are small (1-2 μm in diameter) and are often intertwined to form ropelike strands. Commonly, large (8-14 μm in diameter) spherical or pyriform, smooth-walled macroconidia are seen in young cultures. With age, the macroconidia become roughened or tuberculate and provide enough evidence to make a tentative identification (Figure 43.57). The macroconidia are produced either on short or long lateral branches of the hyphae. Some isolates produce round to pyriform smooth microconidia (2-4 μm in diameter) in addition to the characteristic tuberculate macroconidia. Some isolates of *H. capsulatum* fail to sporulate despite numerous attempts to induce sporulation.

Conversion of the mold form to the yeast form is usually difficult and requires several successive transfers at 3- to 5-day intervals. Yeast colonies appear bacteria-like, mucoid, and membranous and are white to tan. Microscopically, a mixture of swollen hyphae and small budding yeast cells 2-5 μm in size are observed (Figure 43.58). These are similar to the intracellular yeast cells seen in mononu-

clear cells in infected tissue. The yeast form of *H. capsulatum* cannot be recognized unless the corresponding mold form is present on another culture or unless the yeast form is converted directly to the mold form by incubation at 25°-30° C after yeast cells have been observed. The observation of both the mold and yeast form of *H. capsulatum* is satisfactory for the definitive identification. However, the exoantigen test is recommended as the most definitive means of providing an identification of this organism.

Sepedonium, a saprobic organism found growing on mushrooms, is always mentioned as being confused with *H. capsulatum*, since it produces similar tuberculate macroconidia. This organism is almost never recovered from clinical specimens, does not have a yeast form and fails to produce the characteristic H or M bands seen in the exoantigen test with *H. capsulatum*.

43.16.e. Paracoccidioidomycosis. Paracoccidioidomycosis is a chronic granulomatous infection that begins as a primary pulmonary infection. It is often asymptomatic and then disseminates to produce ulcerative lesions of the mucous membranes. Ulcerative lesions are commonly present in the nasal and oral mucosa, gingivae, and less commonly in the conjunctivae. Lesions occur most commonly on the face in association with oral mucous membrane infection (Plate 43.19). The lesions are characteristically ulcerative, with a serpiginous active border and a crusted surface. Lymph node involvement in the cervical area is common. Pulmonary infection is seen most often, and progressive chronic pulmonary infection is found in approximately 50% of cases. Dissemination to other anatomical sites, including the lymphatic system, spleen, intestines, liver, brain, meninges, and adrenals, occurs in some patients.

The infection is most commonly found in South America with the highest prevalence in Brazil, Venezuela and Colombia. It also has

FIGURE 43.60
Paracoccidioides brasiliensis, yeast form, showing multiple budding (400 ×).

TABLE 43.9
Summary of the Characteristic Features of Fungi Known To Be the Most Common Causes of Fungal Infection of Man

INFECTION	ETIOLOGIC AGENT	GROWTH RATE (DAYS)	CULTURAL CHARACTERISTICS AT 30° C	
			BLOOD-ENRICHED MEDIUM	MEDIUM LACKING BLOOD ENRICHMENT
Blastomycosis	*Blastomyces dermatitidis*	5-30	Colonies are cream to tan, soft, moist, wrinkled, waxy, flat to heaped, and yeastlike. "Tufts" of hyphae often project upward from colonies	Colonies are white to cream to tan, some with drops of exudate present, fluffy to glabrous, and adherent to the agar surface
Cryptococcosis	*Cryptococcus neoformans*	3-10	Colonies are usually dome-shaped, dry, cream to tan, and smaller than those on media lacking blood enrichment	Colonies are dry to mucoid and shiny, dome-shaped, smooth and cream to tan in color; however, some isolates appear golden to orange on certain media, i.e., inhibitory mold agar
Histoplasmosis	*Histoplasma capsulatum*	5-45	Colonies are heaped, moist, wrinkled, yeastlike, soft, and cream, tan or pink in color. "Tufts" of hyphae often project upward from colonies	Colonies are white, cream, tan or gray, fluffy to glabrous. Some colonies appear yeast-like and adherent to the agar surface. Many variations in colonial morphology occur
Paracoccidioidomycosis	*Paracoccidioides brasiliensis*	21-28	Colonies are heaped, wrinkled, moist, and yeast-like; with age, colonies may become covered with short aerial mycelium and may turn brown	

From Thomson, R.B., and Roberts, G.D. 1982. A practical approach to the diagnosis of fungal infections of the respira-

MICROSCOPIC MORPHOLOGIC FEATURES		SCREENING TESTS	MICROSCOPIC MORPHOLOGIC FEATURES OF TISSUE FORM	CONFIRMATORY TESTS FOR IDENTIFICATION
BLOOD-CONTAINING MEDIUM	NON-BLOOD-CONTAINING MEDIUM			
Hyphae 1-2 μm in diameter are present; some are aggregated in ropelike clusters. Sporulation is rare	Hyphae 1-2 μm in diameter are present; single pyriform conidia are produced on short to long conidiophores. Some cultures produce few conidia	Not available	8-15 μm, broad-based budding cells with double contoured walls are seen. Cytoplasmic granulation is often obvious	1. Broad-based budding cells may be seen after in vitro conversion on cottonseed agar 2. Exoantigen test positive with A or B bands. Seventy percent exhibit A bands
Cells are usually spherical, vary in size, and may be encapsulated. Cells may have more than one "pinched off" bud present on parent cell		1. Urease production 2. Phenol oxidase production 3. Nitrate reductase production	2-15 μm, single or multiply budding spherical cells that vary in size are seen. Evidence of encapsulation may be present	1. Carbohydrate utilization 2. Pigment on niger seed agar
Hyphae 1-2 μm in diameter are present; some are aggregated in ropelike clusters. Sporulation is rare	Young cultures usually have a predominance of smooth-walled macroconidia that become tuberculate with age. Macroconidia may be pyriform or spherical. Some isolates produce small pyriform microconidia in the presence or absence of macroconidia	Not available	2-5 μm, small, oval to spherical budding cells often seen inside of mononuclear cells	Exoantigen test positive with H, M, or H and M bands
Hyphae 1-2 μm in diameter are present; some isolates produce conidia similar to those of *B. dermatitidis*. Chlamydospores may be numerous and multiple budding yeast cells 10-25 μm in diameter may be present		Not available	10-25 μm, multiply budding cells (buds 1-2 μm) resembling a "mariner's wheel" may be present. Buds are attached to the parent cell by a narrow neck	Exoantigen test positive for bands 1, 2, 3

tory tract. Clin. Lab. Med. 2:321.   *Continued.*

TABLE 43.9
Summary of the Characteristic Features of Fungi Known To Be the Most Common Causes of Fungal Infection of Man—cont'd

INFECTION	ETIOLOGIC AGENT	GROWTH RATE (DAYS)	CULTURAL CHARACTERISTICS AT 30° C	
			BLOOD-ENRICHED MEDIUM	MEDIUM LACKING BLOOD ENRICHMENT
Candidosis	*Candida albicans* and other *Candida* species	2-4	Colonies vary in their morphology but are usually white to tan, shiny to dull, flat to heaped, smooth to wrinkled, and moist to dry. Some colonies produce pseudohyphal fringes at the periphery. Colonies growing on blood enriched media are somewhat smaller and drier than on non-blood-containing media	
Zygomycosis	*Rhizopus* species, *Mucor* species, and other *Zygomycetes*	1-3	Colonies are extremely fast growing, woolly, and gray to brown to gray-black in color	
Aspergillosis	*Aspergillus fumigatus* *Aspergillus flavus* *Aspergillus niger* *Aspergillus* species	3-5	Colonies of *A. fumigatus* are usually blue-green to gray-green while those of *A. flavus* and *A. niger* are yellow-green and black, respectively. Other species of *Aspergillus* exhibit a wide range of colors. Blood enriched media usually have little effect on the colonial morphologic features	
Coccidioidomycosis	*Coccidioides immitis*	2-21	Colonies may be white and fluffy to greenish on blood enriched media. Some isolates are yeast-like, heaped, wrinkled, and membranous	Colonies usually are fluffy white but may be pigmented gray, orange, brown, or yellow. Mycelium is adherent to the agar surface in some portions of the colony

been seen in many other areas, including Mexico, Central America, and Africa. Occasional imported cases have been seen in the United States and Europe.

The exact mechanism by which paracoccidioidomycosis is acquired is unclear; however, it is speculated that its origin is pulmonary and it is acquired by the inhalation of the organism from the environment. Since mucosal lesions are an integral part of the disease process, it is also speculated that the infection may be acquired through trauma to the oropharynx caused by vegetation that is commonly chewed by residents of the endemic areas. The exact ecological niche of the organism in nature is undetermined.

MICROSCOPIC MORPHOLOGIC FEATURES		SCREENING TESTS	MICROSCOPIC MORPHOLOGIC FEATURES OF TISSUE FORM	CONFIRMATORY TESTS FOR IDENTIFICATION
BLOOD-CONTAINING MEDIUM	NON-BLOOD-CONTAINING MEDIUM			
Most species produce either blastoconidia, pseudohyphae, or true hyphae. Chlamydospores are produced by *C. albicans* and certain isolates of *C. tropicalis*		Germ tube production by *C. albicans*	Blastoconidia 2-5 μm in diameter and pseudohyphae are present	1. Germ tube production for *C. albicans* 2. Carbohydrate utilization
1. *Rhizopus* species—rhizoids are produced at the base of a sporangiophore 2. *Mucor* species—no rhizoids are produced		Not available	Large ribbon-like (10-30 μm), twisted; often distorted pieces of aseptate hyphae may be present. Septae may occasionally be seen	Identification is based on characteristic morphologic features
1. *A. fumigatus*—uniserate heads with phialides covering the upper one half to two thirds of the vesicle 2. *A. flavus*—uniserate or biserate or both with phialides covering the entire surface of a spherical vesicle 3. *A. niger*—biserate with phialides covering the entire surface of a spherical vesicle. Conidia are black		Not available	Septate hyphae 5-10 μm in diameter that exhibit dichotomous branching	Identification is based on microscopic morphologic features and colonial morphology. *A. fumigatus* can tolerate elevated temperatures at ≥15° C
Chains of alternate, barrel-shaped arthroconidia are characteristic; some arthroconidia may be elongated. Hyphae are small and often arranged in ropelike strands and racquet forms are seen in young cultures		Not available	Round spherules 30-60 μm in diameter containing 2-5 μm endospores are characteristic	Exoantigen test positive for III, F, or TP bands

Specimens submitted for direct microscopic examinations are important for the diagnosis of paracoccidioidomycosis. Large, round or oval, multiply budding yeast cells (8-40 μm in diameter) are usually recognized in sputum, mucosal biopsy and other exudates. Characteristic multiply budding yeast forms resemble a "mariner's wheel." The yeast cells surrounding the periphery of the parent cell range from 8-15 μm in diameter.

Colonies of *P. brasiliensis* grow very slowly (21-28 days) and are heaped, wrinkled, moist, and yeastlike. With age, colonies may become covered with a short aerial mycelium and turn tan to brown in color. The surface of colonies is often heaped with crater formations.

Microscopically, the mold form is similar to that seen with *B. dermatitidis*. Small hyphae (1-2 μm in diameter) are seen along with numerous chlamydospores. Small, delicate (3-4 μm) globose or pyriform conidia may be seen arising from the sides of the hyphae or on very short conidiophores (Figure 43.59). Most often, cultures reveal only fine septate hyphae and numerous chlamydospores.

After conversion on a blood enriched medium, the colonial morphology of the yeast form is characterized by smooth, soft-wrinkled, yeastlike colonies that are cream to tan in color. Microscopically, the colonies are composed of yeast cells 10-40 μm in diameter which are surrounded by narrow-necked yeast cells around the periphery as previously described (Figure 43.60; Plate 43.20).

If in vitro conversion to the yeast form is unsuccessful, the exoantigen test[63] (Procedure 43.6) should be used to make the definitive identification of *P. brasiliensis*.

Table 43.9 presents a summary of the colonial and microscopic morphologic features of the dimorphic fungi.

43.17. Opportunistic Mycoses

The opportunistic mycoses are a group of fungal infections that occur almost exclusively in immunocompromised patients. The type of patient who acquires an opportunistic fungal infection is one who is compromised by some underlying disease process such as lymphoma, leukemia, diabetes mellitus, or an underlying defect of the immune system. Patients are often on treatment with corticosteroids, cytotoxic drugs or other immunosuppressive agents. A host of fungi previously thought to be nonpathogenic are known to be the etiologic agents of the opportunistic fungal infections. Since most of the organisms known to cause infection in this group of patients are commonly encountered in the clinical laboratory as saprobes, it is impossible for the laboratory to determine the clinical significance of an isolate recovered from the specimens of immunocompromised patients. It is necessary for the laboratory to completely identify and report the presence of all fungi recovered from immunocompromised patients.

While there is an ongoing list of opportunistic mycoses, a certain few are seen with the greatest frequency and include aspergillosis, zygomycosis, candidosis (candidiasis), and cryptococcosis. The etiologic agents of each will be discussed; however, the fungi associated with the less common opportunistic mycoses will be presented in Section 43.22, Saprobic Fungi.

43.17.a. Aspergillosis. Several species of aspergilli are among the most frequently encountered organisms in the clinical laboratory; some are pathogenic whereas others are infrequently associated with infection or do not cause infection at all. The aspergilli are widespread in the environment where they colonize grain, leaves, soil, and living plants. Conidia of the aspergilli are easily dispersed into the environment and humans become infected by inhaling them. These organisms are capable not only of causing disseminated infection, as is seen in immunocompromised patients, but also of causing a whole host of other types of infections including invasive lung infection, pulmonary mycetoma, allergic bronchopulmonary aspergillosis, external otomycosis, mycotic keratitis, onychomycosis, sinusitis, endocarditis and central nervous system infection. Most often, immunocompromised patients acquire a primary pulmonary infection which rapidly disseminates and causes infection in virtually every organ.

It is difficult to assess the significance of members of the genus *Aspergillus* in a clinical specimen. They are found frequently in cultures of respiratory secretions, skin scrapings and other specimens. Table 43.10 presents the Mayo Clinic experience with the recovery of species of *Aspergillus* from clinical specimens. It has been reported that *Aspergillus* is signifi-

TABLE 43.10

Recovery of *Aspergillus* from Clinical Specimens, Mayo Clinic, 1975-1984

ORGANISM	TYPE OF CLINICAL SPECIMEN				
	RESPIRATORY SECRETIONS	GASTRO-INTESTINAL	GENITO-URINARY	SKIN, SUBCUTANEOUS TISSUE	BLOOD, BONE, CNS, ETC.
Aspergillus clavatus	97/93*	1/1	—	1/1	—
A. flavus	1298/740	10/10	11/11	177/131	2/2
A. fumigatus	3247/2656	11/9	14/14	175/137	8/8
A. glaucus	307/503	1/1	—	8/8	1/1
A. nidulans	52/48	—	—	5/3	—
A. niger	1484/1376	18/18	17/17	151/124	11/11
A. terreus	164/146	—	—	23/21	3/3
A. versicolor	1237/1202	6/6	24/22	226/224	16/16
Other species of *Aspergillus*	3463/3418	14/18	32/32	319/314	16/16

*Numerator = number of cultures; *denominator* = number of patients.

cant in only 10% of cases[66]; however, this depends upon the hospital setting and type of patient population seen.

Since aspergilli are recovered frequently, it is imperative that the organism be demonstrated by the direct microscopic examination of fresh clinical specimens and that the organism be recovered repeatedly from a patient with an appropriate clinical picture to ensure that the organism is clinically significant.

Aspergillus fumigatus is most commonly recovered from immunocompromised patients; moreover, it is the species most often seen in the clinical laboratory. In addition, *Aspergillus flavus* is commonly recovered from immunocompromised patients and represents a frequent isolate in the clinical microbiology laboratory. The recovery of *A. fumigatus* or *A. flavus* from surveillance nasal cultures is strongly correlated with subsequent invasive aspergillosis.[3] The absence of a positive nasal culture does not preclude infection, however. *Aspergillus niger* is seen commonly in the clinical laboratory, but its association with clinical disease is somewhat limited. *Aspergillus ter-*

reus, a previously uncommon isolate, is recognized currently as a significant cause of infection in immunocompromised patients, but its frequency of recovery is much lower than the previously mentioned species.

Specimens submitted for direct microscopic examination may contain septate hyphae that show evidence of dichotomous branching. In addition, some hyphae may show the presence of rounded, thick-walled cells.

It should be mentioned that most species of *Aspergillus* are susceptible to cycloheximide and should not be cultured onto media containing this ingredient.

Aspergillus fumigatus is a rapidly growing mold (2-6 days) which produces a fluffy to granular, white to blue-green colony. Mature sporulating colonies most often exhibit the blue-green powdery appearance. Microscopically, *Aspergillus fumigatus* is characterized by the presence of septate hyphae and short or long conidiophores having a characteristic cell at their base. The tip of the conidiophore expands into a large, dome-shaped vesicle which has bottle-shaped phialides occurring in a single

FIGURE 43.61
Aspergillus fumigatus, showing chains of conidia, arising from a single row of phialides on the upper portion of the vesicle (500 ×).

row and around the upper half or two-thirds of its surface. Long chains of small (2-3 μm in diameter), spherical, rough-walled, green conidia form a columnar mass on the vesicle (Figure 43.61; Plate 43.21). Cultures of *Aspergillus fumigatus* are thermotolerant and are able to withstand temperatures up to 45° C.

Aspergillus flavus, somewhat more rapidly growing (1-5 days), produces a yellow-green colony. Microscopically, vesicles are globose and phialides are produced directly from the vesicle surface (uniserate) or from a primary row of branches (metulae; biserate). The phialides give rise to short chains of yellow-orange elliptical or spherical conidia that become roughened on the surface with age (Figure 43.62).

Aspergillus niger, sometimes referred to as being dematiaceous, produces mature colonies within 2-6 days. Growth begins initially as a yellow colony that soon develops a black, dotted surface as conidia are produced. With age, the colony becomes jet black and powdery while the reverse remains buff or cream color.

Microscopically, *A. niger* exhibits septate hyphae, long conidiophores that support spherical vesicles which give rise to large metulae

and smaller phialides from which long chains of brown, rough-walled conidia are produced (Figure 43.63). The entire surface of the vesicle is involved in sporulation.

Only the previously mentioned species of aspergilli are discussed; however, the reader is referred to the chapter by Swatek et al.[68] for further information regarding other species.

43.17.b. Zygomycosis. Zygomycosis is a somewhat less common infection when compared to aspergillosis; however, it is a significant cause of morbidity and mortality in immunocompromised patients. The organisms involved have a worldwide distribution and are commonly found on decaying vegetable matter or in soil. The infection is generally acquired by inhalation of spores followed by subsequent development of infection. Immunocompromised patients, particularly those having uncontrolled diabetes and patients receiving prolonged corticosteroid, antibiotic, or cytotoxic therapy, are particularly at risk. The organisms involved in causing zygomycosis have a marked propensity for vascular invasion and rapidly produce thrombosis and necrosis of tissue. One of the most common forms observed is the rhinocerebral form where the nasal mucosa,

FIGURE 43.62
Aspergillus flavus, showing spherical vesicles that give rise to metulae and phialides that produce chains of conidia (430 ×).

FIGURE 43.63
Aspergillus niger, showing large spherical vesicle that gives rise to metulae, phialides, and chains of dark brown conidia (750 ×).

palate, sinuses, orbit, face, and brain are involved; each shows massive necrosis with vascular invasion and infarction. Other types of infection involve the lungs and gastrointestinal tract; some patients develop disseminated infection. Organs including the liver, spleen, pancreas and kidney may be involved. The zygomycetes have also been reported to be the etiologic agent of infection in the skin of burn patients and in subcutaneous tissue of patients undergoing surgery.

The rapid diagnosis of zygomycosis may be made by examination of tissue specimens or exudate from infected lesions using the potassium hydroxide preparation. Branching, predominantly nonseptate hyphae will be observed. It is highly important that the laboratory notify the clinician of these findings since zygomycetes grow very rapidly and vascular invasion occurs at about the same rate.

The colonial morphologic features of the zygomycetes allow one to immediately suspect organisms belonging to this group. Colonies characteristically produce a fluffy, white to gray or brown hyphal growth that diffusely covers the surface of the agar within 24-96 h (Plate 43.22). The hyphae appear to be coarse and fill the entire culture dish or tube rapidly with loose grayish hyphae dotted with brown or black sporangia. It is impossible to distinguish between the different genera and species of zygomycetes based on their colonial morphologic features since most are identical in appearance.

Microscopically, the zygomycetes characteristically produce large ribbonlike hyphae that are irregular in diameter and nonseptate; however, occasional septa may exist in older cultures. The specific identification of these organisms is confirmed by observing the characteristic saclike fruiting structures (**sporangia**) which produce internally spherical, yellow or brown spores (**sporangiospores**) (Plate 43.23). Each sporangium is formed at the tip of a supporting structure (**sporangiophore**). During maturation, the sporangium becomes fractured and sporangiospores are released into the environment. Sporangiophores are usually connected to each other by nonseptate hyphae called **stolons,** which attach at contact points where rootlike structures (**rhizoids**) anchor the organism to the agar surface. The identification of the three most common zygomycetes, *Mucor*, *Rhizopus*, and *Absidia*, is based on the presence or absence of rhizoids and the position of the rhizoids in relation to the sporangiophores. *Mucor* is characterized by sporangiophores that are singularly produced or branched and have at their tip a round sporangium filled with sporangiospores. *Mucor* does not have rhizoids or stolons and this distinguishes it from the other genera of zygomycetes (Figure 43.64).

Rhizopus has unbranched sporangiophores with rhizoids which appear at the point where the stolon arises (Figure 43.65).

Absidia, an uncommon isolate in the clinical laboratory, is characterized by the presence of rhizoids which originate between sporangiophores (Figure 43.66). The sporangia are pyriform and have a swollen portion of the sporangiophore at the junction of the sporangium. Usually a septum is formed in the sporangiophore just below the sporangium.

The other genera of zygomycetes which may be encountered in the clinical laboratory include *Saksenaea*, *Cunninghamella*, *Conidiobolus* and *Basidiobolus*. For additional information on these and other species, the reader is referred to the chapter by Greer and Rogers.[21]

43.17.c. Candidosis (candidiasis). Candidosis is the most frequently encountered opportunistic fungal infection. It is caused by a number of species of *Candida* with *Candida albicans* being the most frequent etiologic agent, followed by *Candida tropicalis* and *Candida (Torulopsis) glabrata*. A number of other spe-

FIGURE 43.64
Mucor species, showing numerous sporangia in the absence of rhizoids (430 ×).

FIGURE 43.65
Rhizopus species, showing sporangium on long sporangiophore arising from nonseptate hyphae. Note presence of characteristic rhizoids at the base of the sporangiophore (250 ×).

FIGURE 43.66
Absidia species, showing sporangia on long sporangiophores arising from nonseptate hyphae. Note that rhizoids are produced between sporangiophores and not at their bases (250 ×).

cies have been involved in infection in immunocompromised patients; however, their incidence is not nearly as high, as previously mentioned. *Candida albicans* and others are a part of the normal endogenous microbial flora and infections are believed to be endogenous in origin. The organisms may be recovered from the oropharynx, gastrointestinal tract, genitourinary tract, and skin. *Candida* species are responsible for a number of different types of infections in normal and immunocompromised patients. Included are intertriginous candidosis where skin folds are involved, paronychia, onychomycosis, perlèche, vulvovaginitis, thrush, pulmonary infection, eye infection, endocarditis, meningitis, fungemia and disseminated infection. The latter two types of infections are most commonly seen in immunocompromised patients while the others mentioned may occur in normal hosts.

The clinical significance of *Candida* recovered from specimens is difficult to evaluate, since it is considered to be part of the normal flora of humans.[61] A study at Mayo Clinic eval-

uated the clinical significance of yeasts recovered from respiratory secretions, except for *Cryptococcus neoformans*, and concluded that they are part of the normal flora and that their routine identification is unnecessary.[45] The repeated recovery of different species of yeasts from multiple specimens from the same patient usually indicates colonization. The simultaneous recovery of the same species of yeast from several body sites including urine is a good indicator of disseminated infection and the subsequent development of fungemia.

The direct microscopic examination of clinical specimens containing *Candida* will reveal budding yeast cells (blastoconidia) 2-4 μm in diameter or pseudohyphae showing regular points of constriction, resembling lengths of sausages; or true septate hyphae. The blastoconidia, hyphae, and pseudohyphae are strongly gram-positive. It is advisable to report the approximate number of such forms since the presence of large numbers in a fresh clinical specimen may be of diagnostic significance.

The colonial and microscopic morphological features of the species of *Candida* are of little value in making a definitive identification. *Candida albicans*, however, may be identified by the production of germ tubes (Plate 43.24) or presence of chlamydospores (Plate 43.25). Other species of *Candida* must be identified by the utilization of and sometimes fermentation of specific carbohydrate substrates. Specific detailed procedures for the identification of yeast, including *Candida* species, will be presented later in this section.

43.17.d. Cryptococcosis. Cryptococcosis, specifically caused by *Cryptococcus neoformans*, is a subacute or chronic fungal infection which has several manifestations. In the immunocompromised patient, it is not uncommon to see disseminated disease with or without meningitis; meningitis occurs in approximately two-thirds of patients with disseminated infection. Occasionally, patients with disseminated infection will exhibit painless skin lesions which may ulcerate (Plate 43.26). Other uncommon manifestations of cryptococcosis include endocarditis, hepatitis, renal infection and pleural effusion. It is of interest to note that a recent review of patient records from 1975 through 1984 at the Mayo Clinic revealed over 100 cases of colonization of the respiratory tract with *C. neoformans* without subsequent development of infection. Follow-up on these patients was as long as 6 years; none in this group was considered to be immunocompromised. This makes the clinical significance of *C. neoformans* somewhat difficult to assess; however, its presence in clinical specimens from immunocompromised patients should be considered to be significant. In many instances the clinical symptoms are suppressed by corticosteroid therapy and culture or serologic evidence provides the earliest proof of infection. There is a strong association of cryptococcal infection with such debilitating diseases as leukemia and lymphoma and the immunosuppressive therapy that may be required for these and other underlying diseases. The presence of *C. neoformans* in clinical specimens in some instances precedes the symptoms of an underlying disease. The infection is probably more frequent than is commonly recognized; it is estimated that there may be 300 new cases each year in the United States.[26]

Four serotypes of *C. neoformans* have been described (A, B, C, and D) with somewhat different geographic distribution.[37] The organism has been proved to be a basidiomycete by the discovery of its sexual form. The name of the sexual form is *Filobasidiella*, with two species. *F. neoformans* and *F. bacillisporus;* the latter includes serotypes B and C.[38] The term *Cryptococcus* will continue to be used since it is well established by tradition. Despite the discovery of two species of *Cryptococcus*, there is no difference in disease produced or in the response to chemotherapy between the two species.

Cryptococcus neoformans exists as a saprobe in nature. It is most often found associated with the excreta of pigeons. The hypothesis that pigeon habitats serve as reservoirs for human infection is substantiated by numerous reports; the pigeon manure apparently serves as an enrichment for *C. neoformans* because of its chemical makeup. It is believed that *C. neoformans* is widely distributed in nature, becomes aerosolized, and is inhaled prior to infection.

Traditionally, the India ink preparation has been the most widely used method for the rapid detection of *C. neoformans* in clinical specimens. An evaluation of 39 consecutive patients with cryptococcal meningitis seen at Mayo Clinic showed that only 40% gave positive India ink preparations of the cerebrospinal fluid. The purpose of the India ink preparation is to delineate the large capsule of *C. neoformans*, since the ink particles cannot penetrate the capsular polysaccharide material. **Because**

FIGURE 43.67
Cryptococcus neoformans, showing colonies that appear shiny and mucoid due to the presence of a polysaccharide capsule.

of the low positivity rate of the India ink preparation, it is not recommended as a routine tool in the clinical microbiology laboratory. It should be replaced with the cryptococcal latex test for antigen that will be described in a subsequent section.

The microscopic examination of other clinical specimens, including respiratory secretions, can be of value in making a diagnosis of cryptococcosis. *C. neoformans* appears as a spherical, single or multiple budding, thick-walled, yeastlike organism 2-15 μm in diameter, usually surrounded by a wide, refractile polysaccharide capsule. Perhaps the most important characteristic of *C. neoformans* is the extreme variation in the size of the yeast cells; this is unrelated to the amount of polysaccharide capsule present. It is important to remember that not all isolates of *C. neoformans* exhibit a capsule.

Cryptococcus neoformans is easily cultured on routine fungal culture media without cycloheximide. The organism is inhibited by the presence of cycloheximide at 25°-30° C. For the optimal recovery of *C. neoformans* from cerebrospinal fluid, it is recommended that a 0.45 μm pore size membrane filter be used

with a sterile syringe. The filter is placed on the surface of the culture medium and is removed at daily intervals so that growth under the filter can be visualized. An alternative to the membrane filter technique is the use of centrifugation. Contrary to a prior report[70] the centrifugation of cerebrospinal fluid has no effect on the viability of the organism.

Colonies of *C. neoformans* usually appear on culture media within 1-5 days and begin as a smooth white to tan colony which may become mucoid and cream to brown in color. It is important to recognize the colonial morphology on different culture media since variation does occur; e.g., on inhibitory mold agar, *C. neoformans* appears as a golden yellow, nonmucoid colony. Textbooks typically characterize the colonial morphology as being *Klebsiella*-like because of the large amount of polysaccharide capsule material present (Figure 43.67). In reality, most isolates of *C. neoformans* do not have large capsules and may not have the typical mucoid appearance.

The microscopic examination of colonies of *C. neoformans* may be of help in providing a tentative identification of *C. neoformans* since the cells will be spherical and exhibit a wide variation in their size. A presumptive identification of *C. neoformans* may be based on urease production, rapid phenol oxidase production, and failure to utilize an inorganic nitrate substrate. The final identification of *C. neoformans* is based on typical carbohydrate utilization patterns and pigment production on niger seed agar. Specific tests useful for the identification of *C. neoformans* and other species of cryptococci will be presented in a subsequent section.

43.18. General Considerations for the Identification of Yeasts

During the past few years, a significant increase in the number of fungal infections caused by yeasts has been reported in the literature. Numerous species of *Candida* and other yeasts have been implicated. These infections are primarily seen in immunocompromised patients, and some of the yeasts have proved to be resistant to antifungal therapy.[6,19,22,42] It is now recognized that these infections are associated with patients having surgery and patients on long-term intravenous therapy without adequate catheter care. Microbiologists should be aware that any of the genera and species of yeast can be potential pathogens in this group of patients.

Just how far the laboratory should go with a complete identification of all yeast species is of question. It is recommended that:

1. All yeasts recovered from sterile body fluids, including cerebrospinal fluid, blood, urine, paracentesis and other fluids, should be identified to the species level.
2. Yeasts from all seriously ill or immunocompromised patients or in whom a mycotic infection is suspected should be identified to the species level.
3. Yeasts from respiratory secretions should not be identified on a routine basis; however, they should be screened for the presence of *Cryptococcus neoformans*.
4. Yeasts recovered in large amounts from any clinical source should be identified to the species level.
5. Yeasts recovered from several successive specimens, except respiratory secretions, should be identified to the species level. Each laboratory director will have to decide how much time, effort, and expense is to be spent on the identification of yeasts in the laboratory.

During the past few years, a definite change has occurred in the methods used for the identification of yeasts. The development of commercially available systems has provided laboratories of all sizes with the capability of accurate and standardized methods. These systems have extensive computer-based data bases which include information based on thousands of isolates of yeasts. Variations in the reactions of carbohydrates and other substrates utilized are considered in the identification of yeasts provided by these systems. The use of commercially available systems is recommended for all laboratories; however, they should be used in conjunction with some rapid screening tests which will provide the presumptive identification of *C. neoformans* and a definitive identification of *C. albicans*. In addition, some laboratories might prefer the use of conventional systems; therefore, the information presented within this section will discuss rapid screening methods for the presumptive identification of yeasts, commercially available systems, and a conventional schema that will provide for the identification of commonly encountered species of yeast seen in the clinical laboratory.

43.19. Rapid Screening Tests for the Identification of Yeast

43.19.a. Rapid urease test (Procedure 43.7). The rapid urease test is a most useful

PROCEDURE 43.7.
RAPID UREASE TEST [56]

1. Reconstitute a vial of dehydrated Difco urea broth with 3 ml of sterile distilled water on the day of use.
2. Dispense 3-4 drops into each well of a microdilution plate. Determine the exact number of wells to be used for the day and use only the number necessary.
3. Transfer a heavy inoculum of a yeast colony (not including pink yeasts) to a well containing the urea broth. Colonies tested should be no older than 7 days and should be free of contamination with bacteria. In some instances, it might be necessary to make a subculture to obtain enough growth to provide the inoculum for the test.
4. Include positive and negative controls using *C. neoformans* and *C. albicans*, respectively.
5. Seal the microdilution wells with plastic tape and incubate 4 h at 37° C.
6. Observe for the production of a pink to purple color which is indicative of urease production.

PROCEDURE 43.8. RAPID SELECTIVE
UREASE TEST [73]

1. Sweep a cotton-tipped applicator impregnated with the dehydrated urea substrate over the surface of two or three colonies so that the tip is well covered with the organism.
2. Place the applicator containing the yeast into a tube containing 3 drops of 1% benzalkonium chloride (pH 4.86 ± 0.01) and whirl firmly against the bottom of the tube to place the organisms into contact with the cotton fibers.
3. Add a cotton plug to the tube and incubate at 45° C for up to 30 min.
4. Examine after 10, 15, 20, and 30 min for the presence of a color change from yellow to purple. A red or purple color indicates urease production by *C. neoformans*.

tool for screening for urease-producing yeasts recovered from respiratory secretions and other clinical specimens.[56] Alternatives to this method include the heavy inoculum of the tip of a slant of Christensen's urea agar and subsequent incubation at 35°-37° C. In many instances, a positive reaction will occur within several hours; however, 1-2 days of incubation may be required. It is of interest to note that strains of *Rhodotorula, Candida,* and *Trichos-*

poron occasionally hydrolyze urea. Therefore the microscopic morphologic features will be of help in interpreting the usefulness of the urease test for the detection of *Cryptococcus.* Another alternative method is the rapid selective urease test (Procedure 43.8) developed by Zimmer and Roberts.[73] An evaluation of this method showed that the urease activity of 99.6% of 286 isolates of *C. neoformans* was detected within 15 min. This test appears to be useful in detecting *C. neoformans* from specimens cultured onto Sabouraud's dextrose agar. It has not been evaluated using isolates tested from other media.

All of the above mentioned tests are useful for helping to provide a tentative identification of *C. neoformans*; however, they must be sup-

PROCEDURE 43.9. NITRATE REDUCTION TEST[27]

1. Sweep the tip of an applicator impregnated with the nitrate reduction test reagents across two or three colonies of yeast.
2. Swirl the applicator containing the yeast against the bottom of an empty test tube to get the yeast cells in contact with the cotton fibers.
3. Incubate the tube and swab at 45° C for 10 min.
4. Remove the swab and add 2 drops each of N-naphthylethylenediamine and sulfanilic acid reagents to the tube and replace the applicator. A change in color to red indicates a positive test. Positive and negative controls using C. neoformans and C. albicans should be compared to all test organisms.

PROCEDURE 43.10. LEVODOPA–FERRIC CITRATE TEST

1. Remove the number of frozen levodopa–ferric citrate disks necessary for testing. Place in a Petri dish and moisten disks with 2 or 3 drops of distilled water prior to testing. Disks may be obtained commercially from Remel Laboratories.
2. Smear a liberal amount of the test organism onto the surface of each moistened disk.
3. Incubate disks at 37° C and examine at 30 min intervals for up to 6 h. Other reactions produced by C. neoformans should occur in less than 3 h.
4. Positive and negative controls using C. neoformans and C. albidus should be included with each test performed.

plemented with new additional tests before a preliminary identification can be reported. These include the rapid nitrate reduction test and the levodopa test for the detection of phenol oxidase production.

43.19.b. Rapid nitrate reductase test (Procedure 43.9). A characteristic feature of *Cryptococcus neoformans* is that it does not utilize an inorganic nitrate substrate. A rapid method described by Hopkins and Land[27] is recommended for the detection of nitrate reductase by species of cryptococci; however, it is not useful for the pink yeasts, including *Rhodotorula*.

43.19.c. Levodopa–ferric citrate test (Procedure 43.10). *Cryptococcus neoformans* is the only member of the genus *Cryptococcus*

known to produce the enzyme phenol oxidase. Phenol oxidase will react with dihydroxyphenylalanine in the presence of ferric citrate to form the dark pigmented compound, melanin.[31]

If an organism suspected of being *C. neoformans* produces urease, fails to reduce nitrate, and produces phenol oxidase, a presumptive identification of *C. neoformans* may be reported; all this can be accomplished within 3-4 h.

A commercially available product, C/N-Screen (Flow Laboratories) is useful for the presumptive identification of *C. neoformans*. Levodopa is used as a substrate for the detection of phenol oxidase production. The major disadvantage of this product is that it requires 48-72 h before positive reactions are visible.[14]

PROCEDURE 43.11. GERM-TUBE TEST

1. Suspend a very small inoculum of yeast cells obtained from an isolated colony in 0.5 ml of sheep serum (or normal human serum).
2. Incubate the tubes at 35°-37° C for no longer than 3 h.
3. After incubation, remove a drop of the suspension and place on a microscope slide. Examine under low power magnification for the presence of germ tubes. A germ tube is defined as an appendage which is one half the width and 3-4 times the length of the yeast cell from which it arises (Figure 43.68). In most instances, there is no point of constriction at the origin of the germ tube from the cell.

Although it is ideal to use all three screening tests to make a presumptive identification of *Cryptococcus neoformans*, it is not always possible to perform all three since the inoculum size available may be limited. In instances where inoculum is limited, the laboratorian must use the tests which he or she feels can be performed and then make a subculture so that additional tests can be performed at a subsequent time. The Mycology Laboratory at Mayo Clinic has found that it is often just as fast to inoculate the organism onto the surface of a plate of niger seed agar; results may be obtained during the same day of incubation. This will be discussed further within this section.

43.19.d. Germ-tube test (species of *Candida*) (Procedure 43.11). The germ-tube test is the most economical method used in the clinical laboratory for the identification of yeasts.[2] Approximately 75% of the yeasts recovered from clinical specimens are *C. albicans* and the germ-tube test usually provides a definitive identification of this organism within 3 h.

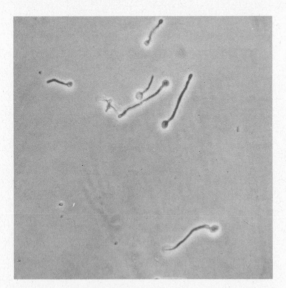

FIGURE 43.68
Candida albicans, germ-tube test, showing yeast cells with germ tubes present (430 ×).

Germ tubes appear as hyphallike extensions of yeast cells, produced usually without a constriction at the point of origin from the cell. In the past, it has been emphasized that *Candida stellatoidea* also produces germ tubes and the distinction between *C. albicans* should be made. The latest edition of the text entitled *The Yeasts: A Taxonomic Study* by Kreger-Van Rij[36] indicates that *C. stellatoidea* is no longer a species and has been combined with *C. albicans*. The germ-tube test is specific for the identification of *C. albicans*.

Another method of identification of *C. albicans* is based on the presence of chlamydospores on cornmeal agar containing 1% Tween 80 and trypan blue incubated at room temperature for 24-48 h. In addition, the appearance of spiderlike colonies on eosin methylene blue agar is characteristic of *C. albicans* and may be used to make a final identification by persons having experience with this method.

43.20. Commercially Available Yeast Identification Systems

As previously mentioned, commercially available yeast identification systems have provided laboratories of all sizes with standardized identification methods. The methods for the most part are rapid, and results are available within 72 h. The major advantage is that the systems provide an identification based on a data base of thousands of yeast biotypes which considers a number of variations and substrate utilization patterns. The identification systems range in price from $3.50 to $4.50. Another advantage is that manufacturers of these products provide computer consultation services to help the laboratorian with the identification of isolates which give an atypical result.

43.20.a. API-20C yeast system. The API-20C yeast identification system has perhaps the most extensive computer-based data set of all commercial systems available. The system consists of a strip that contains 20 microcupules, 19 of which contain dehydrated carbohydrate substrates for determining carbohydrate utilization profiles of yeasts (Figure 43.69). Reactions are compared to growth in the first cupule, which lacks a carbohydrate substrate. Reactions are read and results are converted to a seven-digit biotype profile number and the yeast identification is made from a profile register (Analytab Products). Chapter 9 discusses the principle of such systems. Most of the yeasts are identified within 48 h using this system; however, species of *Cryptococcus* and *Trichosporon* may require up to 72 h. It should be mentioned that the API-20C yeast identification system, as well as all the other commercially available products, require that the mi-

FIGURE 43.69
API-20C yeast identification system.

croscopic morphologic features of yeast grown on cornmeal agar containing 1% Tween 80 and trypan blue be used in conjunction with the carbohydrate utilization patterns. This is particularly helpful when more than one possibility for an identification is provided and the microscopic morphologic features can be used to distinguish between the possibilities given by the profile register. Several evaluations of the API-20C yeast identification system have been made and results have all been favorable.[12,40,58]

43.20.b. API Yeast-Ident system. The API Yeast-Ident system is a newly introduced product which utilizes both miniaturized conventional and chromogenic tests for the identification of yeasts and yeastlike organisms.[50] It consists of a series of 20 cupules containing dehydrated substrates or nutrient media (Plate 43.27). Inoculated strips are incubated for 4 h at 30° C and reactions are monitored by various indicator systems after the addition of a specific reagent, cinnamaldehyde, to certain substrates. Reactions are based on the degradation of carbohydrate substrates or the enzymatic hydrolysis of other substrates. The advantage of the system is that it will provide an identification within 4 h. Since this is a new product, the data base is not nearly as extensive as that of the API-20C system; however, in time the system should have an adequate data base for comparison of reactions. This system was not designed to replace the API-20C system, but rather to supplement it and to provide laboratories the option of using either system.

43.20.c. Uni-Yeast Tek system. The Uni-Yeast Tek yeast identification system (Flow Laboratories) consists of a sealed, multicompartment plate containing media to determine carbohydrate utilization, nitrate utilization, urease production and cornmeal agar morphology (Plate 43.28). In addition, media for performing the germ-tube test and the phenol oxidase test may be obtained from the manufacturer and used in conjunction with this sys-

tem. Evaluation of this product has shown that it is satisfactory for the identification of commonly encountered yeasts.[10,16] The major disadvantage of this system is that it requires up to 7 days for the complete identification of some yeasts. It, too, has a profile index provided by the manufacturer which is generated with computer-based data.

The use of commercially available yeast identification systems is recommended for all laboratories. In general, the systems are easy to use, easy to interpret, and relatively inexpensive when compared to testing using conventional methods. In most instances, they are faster than conventional systems and certainly require less media preparation prior to testing.

Several other systems, including the AutoBac I instrument,[46] the AutoMicrobic System,[25,47] and the Abbott Quantum II system[17] have been shown to be satisfactory for the rapid identification of yeasts. For laboratories that have this instrumentation available, these systems should be satisfactory.

43.21. Conventional Yeast Identification Methods

Some laboratories still prefer to use conventional methods for the identification of yeasts. Regardless of the type of identification system used, the germ-tube test is a beginning step in screening a large number of isolates. As previously mentioned, approximately 75% of yeast recovered in the clinical laboratory can be identified using the germ-tube test. Figure 43.70 presents a practical approach to the laboratory identification of yeast using the germ-tube test as a beginning step.

43.21.a. Cornmeal agar morphology (Procedure 43.12). The second major step using this practical identification schema is to use cornmeal agar morphology as a means to determine if the yeast produces blastoconidia, arthroconidia, pseudohyphae, true hyphae or chlamydospores. In the past, cornmeal agar

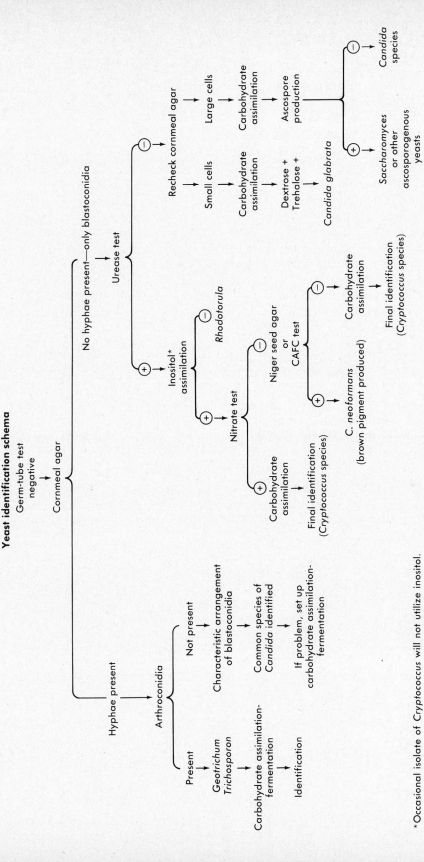

FIGURE 43.70

Schema for the practical laboratory identification of yeasts. (From Koneman, E.W., and Roberts, G.D. 1985. Practical laboratory mycology, ed. 3. The Williams and Wilkins Co., Baltimore.

PROCEDURE 43.12. CORNMEAL AGAR MORPHOLOGY

1. Obtain an isolated colony from the primary culture medium.
2. Inoculate a plate of cornmeal agar containing 1% Tween 80 and trypan blue by making three parallel cuts about ½ inch apart at a 45-degree angle to the culture medium. A sterile coverslip may be added to 1 area.
3. Incubate the cornmeal agar plate at 30° C for 48 h.
4. After 48 h, remove and examine the areas where the cuts into the agar were made for the presence of blastoconidia, arthroconidia, pseudohyphae, hyphae or chlamydospores.[20] Table 43.11 presents the microscopic morphologic features of the commonly encountered yeasts on cornmeal Tween 80 agar.

PROCEDURE 43.13. CARBOHYDRATE ASSIMILATION TESTS

1. Prepare a suspension of the yeast in saline or distilled water to a density equivalent to a McFarland no. 4 standard.
2. Cover the surface of a yeast nitrogen base agar plate containing bromcresol purple with the suspension of the yeast cells.
3. Remove the excess inoculum and allow the surface of the agar medium to dry.
4. With a sterile forceps, place selected carbohydrate disks (Difco Laboratories and BBL Laboratories) onto the surface of the agar. These should be spaced approximately 30 mm apart from each other.
5. Incubate the carbohydrate utilization plate at 30° C for 24-48 h.
6. Remove the plate and observe for the presence of a color change around the carbohydrate containing disks or the presence of growth surrounding them.

PROCEDURE 43.14. PHENOL OXIDASE DETECTION USING NIGER SEED AGAR

1. Place a heavy inoculum onto the surface of a plate of niger seed agar medium.
2. Incubate at 35°-37° C for at least 7 days.
3. Observe daily for the presence of a dark brown or black pigment which is indicative of phenol oxidase specifically produced by *C. neoformans* (Plate 43.29). It is important to note that many isolates of *C. neoformans* will produce phenol oxidase on this medium within 2-24 h.

morphology was used successfully for the detection of characteristic chlamydospores produced by *Candida albicans*. This method is currently satisfactory for the definitive identification of *C. albicans* when the germ-tube test is negative. In other instances, microscopic morphologic features on cornmeal agar differentiate the genera *Cryptococcus*, *Saccharomyces*, *Candida*, *Geotrichum*, and *Trichosporon*. Previously, it was believed that the morphologic features of the common species of *Candida* were distinct enough to provide a presumptive identification. This can be accomplished for *C. albicans*, *C. (Torulopsis) glabrata*, *C. krusei*, *C. parapsilosis*, *C. tropicalis*, and *C. pseudotropicalis* if one keeps in mind that there are numerous other species, uncommonly recovered in the clinical laboratory, that might resemble microscopically any of the previously mentioned species. In general, this method performs well since the previously mentioned genera and species are more commonly seen in clinical laboratories. For the uncommonly encountered isolates, cornmeal agar morphology will have less value. It is, however, recommended for use with most commercially available yeast identification systems and plays a major role in the differentiation between genera which yield similar biochemical profiles.

43.21.b. Carbohydrate assimilation (utilization). Carbohydrate utilization tests are the most commonly used conventional methods for the definitive identification of yeast recovered in a clinical laboratory. A number of different methods have been advocated for use in determining carbohydrate utilization patterns by clinically important yeast[1,41,42,53] and all work equally as well. Procedure 43.13 outlines the method found most useful by the Mayo Clinic Mycology Laboratory.

Once the carbohydrate utilization profile is obtained, reactions may be compared to those listed in tables in most mycology laboratory manuals.[35] In most instances, carbohydrate utilization tests provide the definitive identification of an organism and additional tests are unnecessary. Carbohydrate fermentation tests are preferred by some laboratories and are simply performed using purple broth containing different carbohydrate substrates. In general, carbohydrate fermentation tests are unnecessary and are not recommended for routine use.

43.21.c. Phenol oxidase detection using niger seed agar (Procedure 43.14). As has been previously mentioned, the levodopa–ferric citrate test is a useful screening test for the presumptive identification of *C. neoformans*. It is felt that a simplified *Guizotia abyssinica* medium (niger seed medium) is the definitive method to detect phenol oxidase production.[48] Most isolates of *C. neoformans* readily produce phenol oxidase; however, some isolates have been described that are deficient in their ability to produce this enzyme. In addition, there have been instances where cultures of *C. neoformans* have been shown to contain both phenol oxidase–producing and phenol oxidase–deficient colonies within the same culture. It is necessary to use all the criteria, including the nitrate reductase test, urease production, carbohydrate utilization, and the phenol oxidase test, before making a final identification of *C. neoformans*.

43.22. Saprobic Fungi Commonly Encountered in the Clinical Laboratory

As shown in Table 43.11, there are a number of fungi seen in the clinical microbiology laboratory that have not been discussed thus far. They are considered by many to be laboratory contaminants, but in reality they must be regarded as potential pathogens since infections with a number of these organisms have been reported. It is necessary for the laboratory to identify and report all organisms that are present in clinical specimens so that the clinician can determine their significance to the patient. In many instances, the presence of saprobic fungi is unimportant; however, that is not always the case. The following section will present the molds most commonly recovered from clinical specimens and a brief description of their colonial and morphologic features. In addition, Tables 43.12 and 43.13 present the common molds and yeasts implicated in causing human infection, the time required for their identification, most likely site for their recovery, and the clinical implications of each.

Text continued on p. 763.

TABLE 43.11
Characteristic Microscopic Features of Commonly Encountered Yeasts on Cornmeal Tween-80 Agar

ORGANISM	ARTHROCONIDIA	BLASTOCONIDIA	PSEUDOHYPHAE OR HYPHAE
Candida albicans	—	Spherical clusters at regular intervals on pseudohyphae	Chlamydospores present on pseudohyphae
C. glabrata	—	Small, spherical and tightly compacted	—
C. krusei	—	Elongated; clusters occur at septae of pseudohyphae	Branched pseudohyphae
C. parapsilosis	—	Present but not characteristic	Sagebrush appearance; large (giant) hyphae present
C. pseudotropicalis	—	Elongated, lie parallel to pseudohyphae	Pseudohyphae present but not characteristic
C. tropicalis	—	Produced randomly along hyphae or pseudohyphae	Pseudohyphae present but not characteristic
Cryptococcus	—	Round to oval, vary in size, separated by a capsule	—
Saccharomyces	—	Large and spherical	Rudimentary hyphae sometimes present
Trichosporon	Numerous; resemble *Geotrichum*	May be present but difficult to find	Septate hyphae present

TABLE 43.12
Common Filamentous Fungi Implicated in Human Mycotic Infections

ETIOLOGIC AGENT	TIME REQUIRED FOR IDENTIFICATION	PROBABLE RECOVERY SITES	CLINICAL IMPLICATION
Alternaria species	2-6 days	Skin, nails, conjunctiva, and respiratory secretions	Skin and nail infections, conjunctivitis, hypersensitivity pneumonitis
Aspergillus flavus	1-4 days	Skin, respiratory secretions, gastric washings, nasal sinuses	Skin infections, allergic bronchopulmonary infection, sinusitis, myocarditis, disseminated infection, renal infection, subcutaneous mycetoma
Aspergillus fumigatus	2-6 days	Respiratory secretions, skin, ear, cornea, gastric washings, nasal sinuses	Allergic bronchopulmonary infection, fungus ball, invasive pulmonary infection, skin and nail infections, external otomycosis, mycotic keratitis, sinusitis, myocarditis, renal infection
Aspergillus niger	1-4 days	Respiratory secretions, gastric washings, ear, skin	Fungus ball, pulmonary infection, external otomycosis, mycotic keratitis
Blastomyces dermatitidis	6-21 days (recovery time) (additional 3-14 days required for confirmatory identification)	Respiratory secretions, skin, oropharyngeal ulcer, bone, prostate	Pulmonary infection, skin infection, oropharyngeal ulceration, osteomyelitis, prostatitis, arthritis, CNS infection
Cephalosporium species	2-6 days	Skin, nails, respiratory secretions, cornea, vagina, gastric washings	Skin and nail infections, mycotic keratitis
Cladosporium species	6-10 days	Respiratory secretions, skin, nails, nose, cornea	Skin and nail infections, mycotic keratitis. Chromoblastomycosis, brain abscess, and tinea nigra palmaris caused by *Cladosporium carrioni, C. bantianum,* and *C. werneckii,* respectively
Coccidioides immitis	3-21 days	Respiratory secretions, skin, bone, cerebrospinal fluid, synovial fluid, urine, gastric washings	Pulmonary infection, skin infection, osteomyelitis, meningitis, arthritis, disseminated infection
Drechslera species	2-6 days	Respiratory secretions, skin, peritonitis (following dialysis)	Pulmonary infection (rare)
Epidermophyton floccosum	7-10 days	Skin, nails	Tinea cruris, tinea pedis, tinea corporis, onychomycosis

From Koneman, E.W. and Roberts, G.D. 1984. Mycotic disease. In Henry, J.B., editor. Clinical diagnosis and management by laboratory methods. W.B. Saunders Co., Philadelphia.   *Continued.*

TABLE 43.12
Common Filamentous Fungi Implicated in Human Mycotic Infections—cont'd

ETIOLOGIC AGENT	TIME REQUIRED FOR IDENTIFICATION	PROBABLE RECOVERY SITES	CLINICAL IMPLICATION
Fusarium species	2-6 days	Skin, respiratory secretions, cornea	Mycotic keratitis, skin infection (in burn patients)
Geotrichum species	2-6 days	Respiratory secretions, urine, skin, stool, vagina, conjunctiva, gastric washings, throat	Bronchitis, skin infection, colitis, conjunctivitis, thrush
Histoplasma capsulatum	10-45 days (recovery time) (additional 7-21 days required for confirmatory identification)	Respiratory secretions, bone marrow, blood, urine, adrenals, skin, cerebrospinal fluid, eye, pleural fluid, liver, spleen, oropharyngeal lesions, vagina, gastric washings, larynx	Pulmonary infection, oropharyngeal lesions, CNS infection, skin infection (rare), uveitis, peritonitis
Microsporum audouinii	10-14 days (recovery time) (additional 14-21 days required for confirmatory identification)	Hair	Tinea capitis
Microsporum canis	5-7 days	Hair, skin	Tinea corporis, tinea capitis, tinea barbae, tinea manuum
Microsporum gypseum	3-6 days	Hair, skin	Tinea capitis, tinea corporis
Mucor species	1-5 days	Respiratory secretions, skin, nose, brain, stool, orbit, cornea, vitreous humor, gastric washings, wounds, ear	Rhinocerebral infection, pulmonary infection, gastrointestinal infection, mycotic keratitis, intraocular infection, external otomycosis, orbital cellulitis
Penicillium species	2-6 days	Respiratory secretions, gastric washings, skin, urine, ear, cornea	Pulmonary infection, skin infection, external otomycosis, mycotic keratitis, endocarditis
Pseudallescheria (Petriellidium) boydii	2-6 days	Respiratory secretions, gastric washings, skin, cornea	Pulmonary fungus ball, mycetoma, mycotic keratitis
Phialophora species	6-21 days	Respiratory secretions, gastric washings, skin, cornea, conjunctiva	Some species produce chromoblastomycosis or mycetoma; mycotic keratitis, conjunctivitis, intraocular infection
Rhizopus species	1-5 days	Respiratory secretions, skin, nose, brain, stool, orbit, cornea, vitreous humor, gastric washings, wounds, ear	Rhinocerebral infection, pulmonary infection, mycotic keratitis, intraocular infection, orbital cellulitis, external otomycosis

TABLE 43.12

Common Filamentous Fungi Implicated in Human Mycotic Infections—cont'd

ETIOLOGIC AGENT	TIME REQUIRED FOR IDENTIFICATION	PROBABLE RECOVERY SITES	CLINICAL IMPLICATION
Scopulariopsis species	2-6 days	Respiratory secretions, gastric washings, nails, skin, vitreous humor, ear	Pulmonary infection, nail infection, skin infection, intraocular infection, external otomycosis
Sporothrix schenckii	3-12 days (recovery time) (additional 2-10 days required for confirmatory identification)	Respiratory secretions, skin, subcutaneous tissue, maxillary sinuses, synovial fluid, bone marrow, bone, cerebrospinal fluid, ear, conjunctiva	Pulmonary infection, lymphocutaneous infection, sinusitis, arthritis, osteomyelitis, meningitis, external otomycosis, conjunctivitis, disseminated infection
Trichophyton mentagrophytes	7-10 days	Hair, skin, nails	Tinea barbae, tinea capitis, tinea corporis, tinea cruris, tinea pedis, onychomycosis
Trichophyton rubrum	10-14 days	Hair, skin, nails	Tinea pedis, onychomycosis, tinea corporis, tinea cruris
Trichophyton tonsurans	10-14 days	Hair, skin, nails	Tinea capitis, tinea corporis, onychomycosis, tinea pedis
Trichophyton verrucosum	10-18 days	Hair, skin, nails	Tinea capitis, tinea corporis, tinea barbae
Trichophyton violaceum	14-18 days	Hair, skin, nails	Tinea capitis, tinea corporis, onychomycosis

TABLE 43.13

Common Yeastlike Organisms Implicated in Human Infection*

ETIOLOGIC AGENT	PROBABLE RECOVERY SITES	CLINICAL IMPLICATION
Candida albicans	Respiratory secretions, vagina, urine, skin, oropharynx, gastric washings, blood, stool, transtracheal aspiration, cornea, nails, cerebrospinal fluid, bone, peritoneal fluid	Pulmonary infection, vaginitis, urinary tract infection, dermatitis, fungemia, mycotic keratitis, onychomycosis, meningitis, osteomyelitis, peritonitis, myocarditis, endocarditis, endophthalmitis, disseminated infection, thrush, arthritis
Candida glabrata	Respiratory secretions, urine, vagina, gastric washings, blood, skin, oropharynx, transtracheal aspiration, stool, bone marrow, skin (rare)	Pulmonary infection, urinary tract infection, vaginitis, fungemia, disseminated infection, endocarditis

*Arranged in order of occurrence in the clinical laboratory.
From Koneman, E.W., and Roberts, G.D. 1984. Mycotic disease. In Henry, J.B., editor. Clinical diagnosis and management by laboratory methods. W.B. Saunders Co., Philadelphia.   *Continued.*

TABLE 43.13
Common Yeastlike Organisms Implicated in Human Infection—cont'd

ETIOLOGIC AGENT	PROBABLE RECOVERY SITES	CLINICAL IMPLICATION
Candida tropicalis	Respiratory secretions, urine, gastric washings, vagina, blood, skin, oropharynx, transtracheal aspiration, stool, pleural fluid, peritoneal fluid, cornea	Pulmonary infection, vaginitis, thrush, endophthalmitis, endocarditis, arthritis, peritonitis, mycotic keratitis, fungemia
Candida parapsilosis	Respiratory secretions, urine, gastric washings, blood, vagina, oropharynx, skin, transtracheal aspiration, stool, pleural fluid, ear, nails	Endophthalmitis, endocarditis, vaginitis, mycotic keratitis, external otomycosis, paronychia, fungemia
Saccharomyces species	Respiratory secretions, urine, gastric washings, vagina, skin, oropharynx, transtracheal aspiration, stool	Pulmonary infection (rare), endocarditis
Candida krusei	Respiratory secretions, urine, gastric washings, vagina, skin, oropharynx, blood, transtracheal aspiration, stool, cornea	Endocarditis, vaginitis, urinary tract infection, mycotic keratitis
Candida guilliermondii	Respiratory secretions, gastric washings, vagina, skin, nails, oropharynx, blood, cornea, bone, urine	Endocarditis, fungemia, dermatitis, onychomycosis, mycotic keratitis, osteomyelitis, urinary tract infection
Rhodotorula species	Respiratory secretions, urine, gastric washings, blood, vagina, skin, oropharynx, stool, cerebrospinal fluid, cornea	Fungemia, endocarditis, mycotic keratitis
Trichosporon species	Respiratory secretions, skin, oropharynx, stool	Pulmonary infection, brain abscess, disseminated infection, piedra
Cryptococcus neoformans	Respiratory secretions, cerebrospinal fluid, bone, blood, bone marrow, urine, skin, pleural fluid, gastric washings, transtracheal aspiration, cornea, orbit, vitreous humor	Pulmonary infection, meningitis, osteomyelitis, fungemia, disseminated infection, endocarditis, skin infection, mycotic keratitis, orbital cellulitis, endophthalmic infection
Candida pseudotropicalis	Respiratory secretions, vagina, urine, gastric washings, oropharynx	Vaginitis, urinary tract infection
Cryptococcus albidus subsp. *albidus*	Respiratory secretions, skin, gastric washings, urine, cornea	Meningitis, pulmonary infection
Cryptococcus luteolus	Respiratory secretions, skin, nose	Not commonly implicated in human infection
Cryptococcus laurentii	Respiratory secretions, cerebrospinal fluid, skin, oropharynx, stool	Not commonly implicated in human infection
Cryptococcus albidus subsp. *diffluens*	Respiratory secretions, urine, cerebrospinal fluid, gastric washings, skin	Not commonly implicated in human infection
Cryptococcus terreus	Respiratory secretions, skin, nose	Not commonly implicated in human infection

43.23. Dematiaceous (Darkly Pigmented) Molds

43.23.a. *Alternaria* species. Colonies of *Alternaria* are rapidly growing and appear to be fluffy and gray to gray-brown or dark to gray-green in color. Microscopically, hyphae are septate and golden-brown pigmented, and conidiophores are simple but sometimes branched. Conidiophores bear a chain of large brown conidia resembling a drumstick which contain both horizontal and longitudinal septae (Figure 43.71). It is difficult to observe chains

FIGURE 43.71
Alternaria species, showing muriform, dematiaceous conidia with horizontal and longitudinal septae.

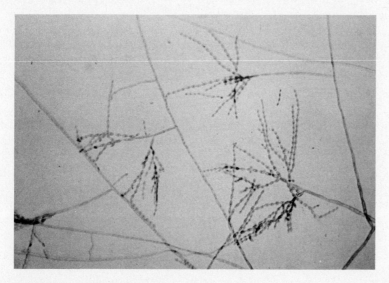

FIGURE 43.72
Cladosporium species, showing branching chains of dematiaceous blastoconidia that are easily dislodged during the preparation of a microscopic mount (430 ×).

FIGURE 43.73
Drechslera species, showing dematiaceous multicelled conidia produced sympodially (430 ×).

of conidia since they are easily dislodged as the culture mount is prepared.

43.23.b. *Cladosporium.* Colonies of *Cladosporium* most commonly appear as velvety or suedelike, heaped and folded. Microscopically, hyphae are septate and brown in color. Conidiophores are long and branched and give rise to chains of darkly pigmented conidia. Conidia are usually single celled and exhibit prominent attachment scars (disjunctors) that may resemble "shield" cells (Figure 43.72). This organism also fails to reveal chains of conidia on wet mounts due to the ease of dislodging of conidia.

43.23.c. *Drechslera.* *Drechslera* is a dematiaceous organism that has been described erroneously as *Helminthosporium* by many textbooks. Colonies of *Drechslera* are fluffy to velvety and gray to brown or black in color. Microscopically, the hyphae are septate and darkly pigmented and conidiophores are twisted where the large multiseptate elongate conidia are attached. A zigzag appearance is produced by the production of conidia on alternate sides of the conidiophore where growth continued until a conidium was formed on the alternate side (Figure 43.73).

43.24. Hyaline Molds

43.24.a. *Acremonium.* Colonies of *Acremonium* are rapidly growing and often appear yeastlike when initial growth is observed. Mature colonies become white to gray to rose or reddish orange in color. Microscopically, small septate hyphae that produce single unbranched tubelike phialides are observed. Phialides give rise to clusters of elliptical, single-celled conidia contained in a cluster at the tip of the phialide (Figure 43.74).

43.24.b. *Fusarium.* Colonies of *Fusarium* are fluffy to cottony and may appear in colors of pink, purple, yellow, green and other shades. Microscopically, the hyphae are small and septate and give rise to phialides which produce either single-celled microconidia usually borne in gelatinous heads similar to those seen in *Acremonium* or large macroconidia which are sickle or boat shaped and contain numerous septae (Figure 43.75). It is common to find numerous chlamydospores produced by some cultures of *Fusarium*.

43.24.c. *Penicillium.* Colonies of *Penicillium* may be shades of green, blue-green, pink, white or other colors. The surface of the colo-

FIGURE 43.74
Acremonium species, showing single unbranched phialides that give rise to clusters of elliptical conidia at their tips (500 ×).

FIGURE 43.75
Fusarium species, showing characteristic multicelled, sickle-shaped macroconidia (500 ×).

FIGURE 43.76
Penicillium species, showing typical brushlike conidiophores (penicillus) (430 ×).

FIGURE 43.77
Scopulariopsis species, showing a large penicillus with echinulate conidia having a flat base (430 ×).

nies may be velvety to powdery due to the presence of conidia. Microscopically, hyphae are hyaline and septate and produce brushlike conidiophores. Conidiophores exhibit branching metulae from which phialides producing chains of conidia arise (Figure 43.76).

43.24.d. *Scopulariopsis*. Colonies of *Scopulariopsis* initially appear white but later become light brown and powdery in appearance. Colonies often resemble those of *M. gypseum*. Microscopically, *Scopulariopsis* resembles a large *Penicillium* at first glance. The hyaline and septate conidiophores are branched and produce a penicillium-like structure. Conidia are produced from annellides. Annellides may be produced singly directly from the hyphae. Conidia are large, have a flat base, and are rough-walled (Figure 43.77).

A number of other saprobic fungi may be encountered in the clinical laboratory but are seen less commonly than those previously mentioned. The chapters by McGinnis[44] and Swatek et al.[68] provide more detailed information on their identification. In many instances, it will be necessary to use reference texts to make an identification.

43.25. Fungal Serologic Tests

A confirmed diagnosis of mycotic infection is based on the recovery and identification of a specific etiologic agent from a clinical specimen. However, the presence and identification of characteristic etiologic agents in clinical specimens observed microscopically also allow for the definitive diagnosis. There are instances, however, when either cultural proof or pathologic proof of infection cannot be obtained and other laboratory information must be utilized. Fungal serologic tests often provide this supplemental information for the diagnosis of mycotic infections, and in some instances provide the only means of diagnosis.[54]

Most clinical microbiology laboratories do not offer fungal serologic testing since the methods require precise technical expertise,

difficult reagent preparation, and costly reagents. In the past few years, commercial sources for reagents have become available and now fungal serologic tests can be offered by laboratories if they wish. Most often, these tests are performed by reference laboratories.

The usefulness of fungal serologic tests is hampered by false-negative results when blood is drawn at an inappropriate time or if blood is drawn from immunocompromised patients before antibodies are produced to the infection. Antigens used in fungal serologic testing are not purified and contain many cross-reacting components in common with other fungi. Antigens of *H. capsulatum*, *B. dermatitidis*, and *C. immitis* often cross-react and provide for difficulty in interpretation of results. It is recommended that a battery of antigens be used for testing to simplify the interpretation of these cross-reactions. As with other tests, false-negative and false-positive results can occur, but in most instances fungal serologic tests provide helpful and reliable results, particularly when used in combination with cultural and histopathologic proof of the etiologic agent.

The most simple and useful fungal serologic test available to the clinical laboratory is the cryptococcal latex test for antigen. Determination of the presence of cryptococcal polysaccharide by this method has proved to be extremely reliable and sensitive.[72] All laboratories are encouraged to provide this test on a routine basis because of its simplicity, sensitivity, and reliability. As previously mentioned, when compared with the India ink preparation, positive results are obtained in approximately 90% of the cases of cryptococcal meningitis when cerebrospinal fluid from the first lumbar puncture is tested. All false-positive reactions have been eliminated using an enzymatic method[65] that makes the test highly specific. The decision of whether to offer additional tests other than the cryptococcal latex test for antigen depends on the individual situation for each laboratory. Table 43.14 presents a summary of the

TABLE 43.14
Commonly Available Fungal Serologic Tests

INFECTION	ANTIGEN(S)	TEST(S)	INTERPRETATION
Aspergillosis	*Aspergillus fumigatus* *Aspergillus niger* *Aspergillus flavus*	Immunodiffusion	One or more precipitin bands suggestive of active infection. Precipitin bands shown to correlate with complement-fixation titers—the greater the number of bands, the higher the titer. When cultural proof is present in the presence of a positive test, it is diagnostic of active infection. Precipitins can be found in 95% of the fungus ball cases and 50% of the allergic bronchopulmonary cases. Sometimes positive in invasive infection, depending on the immunologic status of the patient.
Blastomycosis	*Blastomyces dermatitidis*		
	Yeast form	Complement-fixation	Titers of 1:8 to 1:16 are highly suggestive of active infection; titers of 1:32 or greater are indicative. Cross-reactions occur in patients having coccidioidomycosis or histoplasmosis; however, titers are usually lower. A decreasing titer is indicative of regression. Most patients (75%) having blastomycosis have negative tests.
	Yeast culture filtrate	Immunodiffusion	Preliminary results show that it is more sensitive than complement-fixation—80% detection rate.
Candidosis	*Candida albicans*	Immunodiffusion, counterimmuno-electrophoresis	Test difficult to interpret because precipitins are found in 20%-30% of the normal population, and reports in the literature are conflicting. Clinical correlation must exist for the test to be useful.
Coccidioidomycosis	Coccidioidin	Complement-fixation	Titers of 1:2 to 1:4 have been seen in active infection. Low titers should be followed by repeat testing at 2-3 week intervals. Titers of greater than 1:16 are usually indicative of active infection. Cross-reactions occur in patients having histoplasmosis, and false-negative results occur in patients with solitary pulmonary lesions. Titer parallels severity of infection.

From Koneman, E.W., and Roberts, G.D. 1984. Mycotic disease. In Henry, J.B., editor. Clinical diagnosis and management by laboratory methods. W.B. Saunders Co., Philadelphia.

TABLE 43.14
Commonly Available Fungal Serologic Tests—cont'd

INFECTION	ANTIGEN(S)	TEST(S)	INTERPRETATION
	Coccidioidin	Immunodiffusion	Results correlate with complement-fixation test and can be used as a screening test—should be confirmed by performing complement-fixation test.
	Coccidioidin	Latex agglutination	Precipitins occur during first 3 weeks of infection and are diagnostic, but not prognostic. Useful as a screening test for precipitins in early infection. False-positive tests frequent when diluted serum or cerebrospinal fluid specimens are used.
Cryptococcosis	No antigen—latex particles coated with hyperimmune anti-cryptococcal globulin	Latex agglutination for cryptococcal antigen	Presence of cryptococcal polysaccharide in body fluids is indicative of cryptococcosis. Rheumatoid factor presents false-positive reactions and RA test must be performed as a control. Decrease in antigen titer indicates regression. Positive tests (in CSF) have been seen in 95% of cryptococcal meningitis cases and 30% of nonmeningitis cases. Serum is less frequently positive than CSF. Disseminated infections usually present positive results in serum. Test may be performed using serum, CSF, and urine. Test more sensitive than India ink preparation.
Histoplasmosis	Histoplasmin and yeast form of *Histoplasma capsulatum*	Complement-fixation	Titers of 1:8 to 1:16 are highly suspicious of infection; however titers of 1:32 or greater are usually indicative of active infection. Cross-reactions occur in patients having aspergillosis, blastomycosis, and coccidioidomycosis, but titers are usually lower. Several follow-up serum samples should be tested—drawn at 2- to 3-week intervals. Rising titers indicate progressive infection and decreasing titers indicate regression. Some disseminated infections are nonreactive to the complement-fixation test. Recent skin tests in persons who have had prior exposure to *H. capsulatum* will cause an elevation in the complement-fixation titer. This occurs in 17%-20% of persons tested. The yeast antigen gives positive reactions in 75%-80% of cases, and the histoplasmin gives positive reactions in 10%-15% of cases. In 10% of cases both are positive simultaneously.

Continued.

TABLE 43.14
Commonly Available Fungal Serologic Tests—cont'd

INFECTION	ANTIGEN(S)	TEST(S)	INTERPRETATION
Histoplasmosis—cont'd	Histoplasmin	Immunodiffusion	H and M bands appearing simultaneously are indicative of active infection. M band may appear alone and can indicate early infection or chronic infection. Also the M band may appear after a recent skin test. The H band appears later than the M band and disappears earlier, and its disappearance may indicate regression of the infection.
	Histoplasmin	Latex agglutination	Test is unreliable. Many false-positive and false-negative tests may be observed. Any positive test should be confirmed by the complement-fixation test.
Sporotrichosis	Yeast of *Sporothrix schenckii*	Agglutination	Titers of 1:80 or greater usually indicative of active infection. Some cutaneous infections present negative tests; however, extracutaneous infections present positive tests.

common fungal serologic tests available and information regarding their interpretation. More detailed methods can be found in the text by Palmer et al.[49] and the chapter written by Kaufman and Reiss.[32] Perhaps these new methods will be available in a few years.

43.26. Antifungal Susceptibility Testing

Antifungal susceptibility tests are performed to provide information that will allow the physician to select the appropriate antifungal agent useful for treating a specific infection. Unfortunately, antifungal susceptibility testing has not progressed as far as tests used for determining susceptibility of bacteria to antimicrobial agents. There is no standard method used by all laboratories and there is disagreement concerning specific conditions of incubation and other variables necessary for performing the test.

Despite the problems associated with antifungal susceptibility testing, many physicians believe that these tests are important for the selection of an appropriate antifungal agent and as a method to detect the development of resistance of certain organisms during chemotherapy. The method described by Shadomy et al.[60] is perhaps the most commonly used procedure in the United States. Table 43.15 provides information on the susceptibility of the various fungi to amphotericin B, 5-fluorocytosine, miconazole and ketoconazole, the common antifungal agents available at the present time.

TABLE 43.15
In Vitro Antifungal Activities of Four Antifungal Agents Against Pathogenic Fungi*

ORGANISM	AMPHOTERICIN B		FLUCYTOSINE (5-FC)		MICONAZOLE		KETOCONAZOLE
	MIC (μg/ml)	MFC (μg/ml)	MIC (μg/ml)	MFC (μg/ml)	MIC (μg/ml)	MFC (μg/ml)	MIC (μg/ml)
Pathogenic yeasts							
Cryptococcus neoformans	0.05-0.78†	0.1-12.5	0.10-100‡	0.39->100	0.05-3.13	0.05-25	0.1-32
Candida albicans	0.2-0.78§	0.39-0.78	0.05-12.5‡	0.10->100	0.1-2.0§	0.1-10	<0.1-80
Candida spp. not *C. albicans*	0.2-1.56§	0.39-6.25	0.10-50‡	0.20->100	<0.1-2.0	0.1->10	<0.1-64
Candida glabrata	0.1-0.4	0.2-0.78	0.05-1.56	0.4->100	0.5-10	2-10	1-64
Trichosporon sp.	0.78-3.13	1.56-3.13	25-100	>100	0.2-25	0.2->100	
Geotrichum sp.	0.4-1.56	0.78-3.13	1.56-12.5	25->100	0.1-2	0.5->10	
Filamentous fungi							
Pseudallescheria boydii	1.56->100‡	>100	Resistant		0.05‖	0.05	0.1-4‡
Aspergillus sp. including *A. fumigatus*	0.05-8	6.25->100	0.2-1.56‡	>100	0.4->100	0.8->100	0.1-100¶
Blastomyces dermatitidis	0.05-0.2	0.1-0.4	Resistant		≤0.25	ND	0.1-2
Cladosporium trichoides	3.13->100	3.13->100	3.13-12.5‡	12.5->100	0.5->64	ND	0.1-64
Coccidioides immitis	0.1-0.78	0.78-1.56	Resistant		0.25-1.0	ND	0.1-0.8
Histoplasma capsulatum	0.05-1.0	0.05-0.2	Resistant		≤0.25	ND	0.1-0.5
Phialophora sp. and other dematiaceous fungi	0.05->128	6.25->128	Variable susceptibility	Resistant	0.05-32	ND	0.1-64
Sporothrix schenckii	1.56-12.5	3.13->100	Resistant	Resistant	1-2	ND	0.1-16
Zygomycetes	0.78-1.56	1.56->100	Variable susceptibility				
Dermatophytic fungi							
Epidermophyton floccosum					0.5-10	2-10	0.1-8
Microsporum sp.					0.5-10	0.5->10	0.1-64
Trichophyton sp.					0.5-10	0.5-10	<0.05-128
Control organisms							
S. cerevisiae ATCC 36375	0.1	0.2	0.05	0.10	0.20	0.39	0.20
C. pseudotropicalis ATCC 28838			0.05	0.10	0.10	0.20	0.05

From Shadomy, S., Espinel-Ingroff, A., and Cartwright, R.Y. 1985. Susceptibility testing with antifungal drugs. In Lennette, E.H., Balows, A., Hausler, W.J. Jr., and Shadomy, H.J., editors. Manual of clinical microbiology, ed. 4. American Society for Microbiology, Washington, D.C.

*Based upon both data obtained at the Medical College of Virginia, Virginia Commonwealth University, Richmond, and a review of the literature. In vitro data for nystatin is not included because of the narrow clinical spectrum of this agent; however, most isolates of *Candida* species should be clinically susceptible (MIC [minimum inhibitory concentration] of ≤10 μg/ml) to nystatin. MFC, Minimal fungicidal concentration; ND, not determined.

†Expected ranges of MICs and MFCs.

‡Resistance not uncommon.

§Resistance reported but rare.

‖Only limited data available.

¶In vitro susceptibility of *Aspergillus* sp. to ketoconazole is highly species dependent.

REFERENCES

1. Adams, E.D. Jr., and Cooper, B.H. 1984. Evaluation of modified Wickerham medium for identification of medically important yeasts. Am. J. Med. Technol. 40:377.

2. Ahearn, D.G. 1973. Identification and ecology of yeasts of medical importance. In Prier, J.E., and Friedman, H., editors. Opportunistic pathogens. University Park Press, Baltimore.

3. Aisner, J., Murillo, J., Schimpff, S.C., and Steere, A.C. 1979. Invasive aspergillosis in acute leukemia: correlation with nose cultures and antibiotic use. Ann. Intern. Med. 90:4.

4. Ajello, L. 1968. A taxonomic review of the dermatophytes and related species. Sabouraudia 6:147.

5. Ajello, L., and Georg, L.K. 1957. In vitro hair cultures for differentiating between atypical isolates of *Trichophyton mentagrophytes* and *Trichophyton rubrum.* Mycopathologia 8:3.

6. Baker, J.G., Nadler, H.L., Forgacs, P., and Kurtz, S.R. 1984. *Candida lusitaniae:* a new opportunistic pathogen of the urinary tract. Diag. Microbiol. Infect. Dis. 2:145.

7. Bille, J., Edson, R.S., and Roberts, G.D. 1984. Clinical evaluation of the lysis-centrifugation blood culture system for detection of fungemia and comparison with a conventional biphasic broth blood culture system. J. Clin. Microbiol. 19:126.

8. Bille, J., Stockman, L., Roberts, G.D., Horstmeier, C.D., and Ilstrup, D.M. 1983. Evaluation of a lysis-centrifugation system for recovery of yeasts and filamentous fungi from blood. J. Clin. Microbiol. 18:469.

9. Binford, C.H., Thompson, R.K., Gorham, M.E., and Emmons, C.W. 1952. Mycotic brain abscess due to *Cladosporium trichoides*, a new species. Am. J. Clin. Pathol. 22:535.

10. Bowman, P.I., and Ahearn, D.G. 1975. Evaluation of the Uni-Yeast-Tek kit for the identification of medically important yeasts, J. Clin. Microbiol. 2:354.

11. Brock, E.G., Reiss, E., Pine, L., and Kaufman, L. 1984. Effect of periodate-oxidation on the detection of antibodies against the M-antigen of histoplasmosis by enzyme immunoassay (EIA) inhibition. Curr. Microbiol. 10:177.

12. Buesching, W.J., Kurek, K., and Roberts, G.D. 1979. Evaluation of the modified API 20C system for identification of clinically important yeasts. J. Clin. Microbiol. 9:565.

13. Chandler, F.W., Kaplan, W., and Ajello, L. 1980. Color atlas and text of the histopathology of mycotic diseases. Year Book Medical Publishers, Chicago.

14. Cooper, B.H. 1980. Clinical laboratory evaluation of a screening medium (CN screen) for *Cryptococcus neoformans*. J. Clin. Microbiol. 11:672.

15. Cooper, B.H. 1980. Taxonomy classification and nomenclature of fungi. In Lennette, E.H., Balows, A., Hausler, W.J. Jr., and Truant, J.P., editors. Manual of clinical microbiology, ed. 3. American Society for Microbiology, Washington, D.C.

16. Cooper, B.H., Johnson, J.B., and Thaxton, E.S. 1978. Clinical evaluation of the Uni-Yeast-Tek system for rapid presumptive identification of medically important yeasts. J. Clin. Microbiol. 7:349.

17. Cooper, B.H., Prowant, S., Brunson, D., and Alexander, B.A. 1984. Collaborative evaluation of the Abbott automated yeast identification system. J. Clin. Microbiol. 11:853.

18. deRepentigny, L., Marr, L.D., Keller, J.W., Carter, A.W., Kuykendall, R.S., Kaufman, L., and Reiss, R. 1985. Comparison of enzyme immunoassay and gas-liquid chromatography for the rapid diagnosis of invasive candidiasis in cancer patients. J. Clin. Microbiol. 21:972.

19. Dick, J.D., Merz, W.G., and Saral, R. 1980. Incidence of polyene-resistant yeasts recovered from clinical specimens. Antimicrob. Agents Chemother. 18:158.

20. Dolan, C.T. 1971. A practical approach to identification of yeast-like organisms. Am. J. Clin. Pathol. 55:580.

21. Greer, D.L., and Rogers, A.L. 1985. Agents of zygomycosis (phycomycosis). In Lennette, E.H., Balows, A., Hausler, W.J. Jr., and Shadomy, H.J., editors. Manual of clinical microbiology, ed. 4. American Society for Microbiology, Washington, D.C.

22. Guinet, R.J., Chanas, J., Goullier, A., Bonnefoy, G., and Ambroise-Thomas, P. 1983. Fatal septicemia due to amphotericin B-resistant *Candida lusitaniae*. J. Clin. Microbiol. 18:443.

23. Hageage, G.J., and Harrington, B.J. 1984. Use of calcofluor white in clinical mycology. Lab. Med. 15:109.

24. Harari, A.R., Hempel, H.O., Kimberlin, C.L., and Goodman, N.L. 1982. Effects of time lapse between sputum collection and culturing on isolation of clinically significant fungi. J. Clin. Microbiol. 15:425.

25. Hasyn, J.J., and Buckley, H.R. 1982. Evaluation of the Automicrobic System for the identification of yeasts. J. Clin. Microbiol. 16:901.

26. Hoeprich, P.D. 1977. Cryptococcosis. In Hoeprich, P.D., editor. Infectious diseases. Harper & Row, Hagerstown, Md.

27. Hopkins, J.M., and Land, G.A. 1977. Rapid method for determining nitrate utilization by yeasts. J. Clin. Microbiol. 5:497.

28. Huppert, M., Sun, S.H., and Bailey, J.W. 1967. Natural variability in *Coccidioides immitis*. In Ajello, L., editor. Coccidioidomycosis. University of Arizona Press, Tucson.

29. Kane, J., and Smitka, C. 1978. Early detection and identification of *Trichophyton verrucosum*. J. Clin. Microbiol. 8:740.

30. Kaufman, L. 1984. Antigen detection: its role in the diagnosis of mycotic disease and the identification of fungi. In Sanna, A., and Morace, G., editors. New horizons in microbiology. Elsevier Science Publishing Co., Amsterdam.

31. Kaufman, C.S., and Merz, W.G. 1982. Two rapid pigmentation tests for identification of *Cryptococcus neoformans*. J. Clin. Microbiol. 15:339.

32. Kaufman, L., and Reiss, E. 1985. Serodiagnosis of fungal diseases. In Lennette, E.H., Balows, A., Hausler, W.J. Jr., and Shadomy, H.J., editors. Manual of clinical microbiology, ed. 4. American Society for Microbiology, Washington, D.C.

33. Kaufman, L., and Standard, P. 1978. Improved version of the exoantigen test for identification of *Coccidioides immitis* and *Histoplasma capsulatum* cultures. J. Clin. Microbiol. 8:42.

34. Koneman, E.W., and Roberts, G.D. 1984. Mycotic disease. In Henry, J.B., editor. Clinical diagnosis and management by laboratory methods. W.B. Saunders Co., Philadelphia.

35. Koneman, E.W., and Roberts, G.D. 1985. Practical laboratory mycology, ed. 3. The Williams & Wilkins Co., Baltimore.

36. Kreger-Van Rij, N.J.N. 1984. The yeasts: a taxonomic study. Elsevier Science Publishing Co., New York.

37. Kwon-Chung, K.J., Bennett, J.E., and Theodore, T.S. 1978. *Cryptococcus neoformans* sp. nov.: serotype B-C of *Cryptococcus neoformans*. Int. J. Sys. Bacteriol. 28:616.

38. Kwon-Chung, K.S. 1976. A new species of *Filobasidiella*, the sexual state of *Cryptococcus neoformans* B and C serotypes. Mycologia 68:942.

39. Land, G.A., Fleming, W.H. III, Beadles, T.A., and Foxworth, J.H. 1979. Rapid identification of medically important yeasts. Lab. Med. 10:533.

40. Land, G.A., Harrison, B.A., Hulme, K.L., Cooper, B.H., and Byrd, J.C. 1979. Evaluation of the new API 20C strip for yeast identification against a conventional method. J. Clin. Microbiol. 10:357.

41. Land, G.A., Stotler, R., Land, K.J., and Staneck, J.L. 1984. Updating and evaluation of the Vitek AMS yeast identification system. J. Clin. Microbiol. 4:649.

42. Libertin, C.R., Wilson, W.R., and Roberts, G.D. 1985. *Candida lusitaniae*—an opportunistic pathogen. Diag. Microbiol. Infect. Dis. 3:69.

43. Mahgonb, E.S., and Murray, I.G. 1973. Mycetoma. William Heineman Medical Books, London.

44. McGinnis, M.R. 1985. Dematiaceous fungi. In Lennette, E.H., Balows, A., Hausler, W.J. Jr., and Shadomy, H.J., editors. Manual of clinical microbiology,

ed. 4. American Society for Microbiology, Washington, D.C.

45. Murray, P.R., Van Scoy, R.E., and Roberts, G.D. 1977. Should yeasts in respiratory secretions be identified? Mayo Clin. Proc. 52:42.

46. Ngui Yen, J.H., and Smith, J.A. 1978. Use of Autobac 1 for rapid assimilation testing of *Candida* and *Torulopsis* species. J. Clin. Microbiol. 7:118.

47. Oblack, D.L., Rhodes, J.C., and Martin, W.J. 1981. Clinical evaluation of the AutoMicrobic system yeast biochemical card for rapid identification of medically important yeasts. J. Clin. Microbiol. 13:351.

48. Paliwal, D.K., and Randhawa, H.S. 1978. Evaluation of a simplified *Guizotia abyssinica* seed medium for differentiation of *Cryptococcus neoformans*. J. Clin. Microbiol. 7:346.

49. Palmer, D.F., Kaufman, L., Kaplan, W., and Cavallano, J.J. 1977. Serodiagnosis of mycotic diseases. Charles C Thomas, Publisher, Springfield, Ill.

50. Pincus, D.H., Leun, I.L., Baecher, C., Taylor, S.J., and McKinley, G.A. 1985. Development of a same day yeast identification system. Abstracts of the Annual Meeting of the American Society for Microbiology, no. 344.

51. Redline, R.W., and Dahms, B.B. 1981. *Malassezia* vasculitis in an infant on long-term intralipid therapy. N. Engl. J. Med. 305:1395.

52. Roberts, G.D. 1975. Detection of fungi in clinical specimens by phase-contrast microscopy. J. Clin. Microbiol. 2:261.

53. Roberts, G.D. 1976. Laboratory diagnosis of fungal infections. Hum. Pathol. 7:161.

54. Roberts, G.D. 1979. Serodiagnosis of mycotic infections. Ill. Med. J. 156:406.

55. Roberts, G.D., Goodman, N.L., Land, G.A., Larsh, H.W., and McGinnis, M.R. 1985. Detection and recovery of fungi in clinical specimens. In Lennette, E.H., Balows, A., Hausler, W.J. Jr., and Shadomy, H.J., editors. Manual of clinical microbiology, ed. 4. American Society for Microbiology, Washington, D.C.

56. Roberts, G.D., Horstmeier, C.D., Land, G.A., and Foxworth, J.H. 1978. Rapid urea broth test for yeasts. J. Clin. Microbiol. 7:584.

57. Roberts, G.D., Karlson, A.G., and DeYoung, D.R. 1976. Recovery of pathogenic fungi from clinical specimens submitted for mycobacterial culture. J. Clin. Microbiol. 3:47.

58. Roberts, G.D., Wang, H.S., and Hollick, G.E. 1976. Evaluation of the API 20C microtube system for the identification of clinically important yeasts. J. Clin. Microbiol. 3:302.

59. Roberts, G.D., and Washington, J.A. II. 1975. Detection of fungi in blood cultures. J. Clin. Microbiol. 1:309.

60. Shadomy, S., Espinel-Ingroff, A., and Cartwright, R.Y. 1985. Susceptibility testing with antifungal drugs. In Lennette, E.H., Balows, A., Hausler, W.J. Jr., and Shadomy, H.J., editors. Manual of clinical microbiology, ed. 4. American Society for Microbiology, Washington, D.C.

61. Silva-Hutner, M., and Cooper, B.H. 1985. Yeasts of medical importance. In Lennette, E.H., Balows, A., Hausler, W.J. Jr., and Shadomy, H.J., editors. Manual of clinical microbiology, ed. 4. American Society for Microbiology, Washington, D.C.

62. Smith, C.D., and Goodman, N.L. 1975. Improved culture method for the isolation of *Histoplasma capsulatum* and *Blastomyces dermatitidis* from contaminated specimens. Am. J. Clin. Pathol. 68:276.

63. Standard, P.G., and Kaufman, L. 1980. A rapid and specific method for the immunological identification of mycelial form cultures of *Paracoccidioides brasiliensis*. Curr. Microbiol. 4:297.

64. Standard, P.G., and Kaufman, L. 1982. Safety considerations in handling exoantigen extracts from pathogenic fungi. J. Clin. Microbiol. 15:663.

65. Stockman, L., and Roberts, G.D. 1983. Corrected version. Specificity of the latex test for cryptococcal antigen: a rapid, simple method for eliminating interference factors. J. Clin. Microbiol. 17:945.

66. Strimlan, C.V., Dines, D.E., Rodgers-Sullivan, R.F., Roberts, G.D., and Sheehan, W.C. 1980. Respiratory tract *Aspergillus*—clinical significance. Minn. Med. 63:25.

67. Sun, S.H., Huppert, M., and Vukovich, K.R. 1976. Rapid in vitro conversion and identification of *Coccidioides immitis*. J. Clin. Microbiol. 3:186.

68. Swatek, F., Halde, C., Rinaldi, M.J., and Shadomy, H.J. 1985. *Aspergillus* and other opportunistic saprophytic hyaline hyphomycetes. In Lennette, E.H., Balows, A., Hausler, W.J. Jr., and Shadomy, H.J., editors. Manual of clinical microbiology, ed. 4. American Society for Microbiology, Washington, D.C.

69. Thomson, R.B., and Roberts, G.D. 1982. A practical approach to the diagnosis of fungal infections of the respiratory tract. Clin. Lab. Med. 2:321.

70. Utz, J.P. 1967. Recognition and current management of the systemic mycoses. Med. Clin. North Am. 51:519.

71. Weeks, R.J. 1964. A rapid simplified medium for converting the mycelial phase of *Blastomyces dermatitidis* to the yeast phase. Mycopathologia 22:153.

72. Wu, T.C., and Koo, S.Y. 1983. Comparison of three commercial cryptococcal latex kits for detection of cryptococcal antigen. J. Clin. Microbiol. 18:1127.

73. Zimmer, B.L., and Roberts, G.D. 1979. Rapid selective urease test for presumptive identification of *Cryptococcus neoformans*. J. Clin. Microbiol. 10:380.

BIBLIOGRAPHY

Beneke, E.S., and Roger, A.L. 1980. Medicine mycology manual, ed. 4. Burgess Publishing Co., Minneapolis.

Emmons, C.W., Binford, C.H., Utz, J.P., and Kwon-Chung, K.J. 1977. Medical mycology, ed. 3. Lea & Febiger, Philadelphia.

Koneman, E.W., and Roberts, G.D. 1985. Practical laboratory mycology, ed. 3. The Williams & Wilkins Co., Baltimore.

Larone, D.H. 1976. Medically important fungi: a guide to identification. Harper & Row, Hagerstown, Md.

Lennette, E.H., Balows, A., Hausler, W.J. Jr., and Shadomy, H.J. 1985. Manual of clinical microbiology, ed. 4. American Society for Microbiology, Washington, D.C.

McGinnis, M.R. 1980. Laboratory handbook of medical mycology. Academic Press, New York.

Rippon, J.W. 1982. Medical mycology—the pathogenic fungi and pathogenic actinomycetes. W.B. Saunders Co., Philadelphia.

44

Laboratory Methods for Diagnosis of Parasitic Infections

Lynne Shore Garcia, M.S., CLS(NCA) MT(ASCP)

DIAGNOSTIC TECHNIQUES

44.1. Introduction

The field of parasitology is often associated with tropical areas; however, many parasitic organisms that infect humans are worldwide in distribution and occur with some frequency in the temperate zones. Many organisms endemic elsewhere are seen in the United States in persons who have lived or traveled in those areas. The influx of a number of refugee populations into the United States has also served as both a source of infected patients and possible transmission of certain parasites. Another factor to be considered is the increase in numbers of compromised patients, particularly those who are immunodeficient or immunosuppressed. Those persons are very much at risk for certain parasitic problems. Consequently, clinicians and laboratory personnel should be aware of the possibility that these organisms may be present and should be trained in the ordering and the performance of appropriate procedures for their recovery and identification. The clinician must be able to recognize and interpret the relevance of the laboratory data, and the laboratorian must be able to review the pros and cons of each procedure, selecting those that will provide the most accurate diagnostic test results.

Although common names are frequently used to describe parasitic organisms, these

776

names may represent different parasites in different parts of the world. To eliminate these problems, a binomial system of nomenclature is used in which the scientific name consists of the genus and species. On the basis of life histories and morphology, systems of classification have been developed to indicate the relationship among the various parasite species.

Parasites of humans are classified into five major subdivisions. These include the Protozoa (Amebas, Flagellates, Ciliates, Sporozoans, Coccidia), the Platyhelminthes or flatworms (Cestodes, Trematodes), the Acanthocephala or thorny-headed worms, the Nematoda or roundworms, and the Arthropoda (insects, spiders, mites, ticks, etc.). The main groups presented here include Protozoa, Nematoda, Platyhelminthes, and Arthropoda. This information is presented in Table 44.1. This classification scheme is designed to provide some order and meaning to a widely divergent group of organisms. No attempt has been made to include every possible organism, but only those that are considered to be clinically relevant in the context of human parasitology. It is hoped this table will provide some insight into the parasite groupings, thus leading to a better understanding of organism morphology, parasitic infections, and the appropriate clinical diagnostic approach.

The identification of parasitic organisms is dependent on morphologic criteria; these criteria are in turn dependent on correct specimen collection and adequate fixation. Improperly submitted specimens may result in failure to find the organisms or in their misidentification. Tables 44.2 and 44.3 contain information on the body sites and possible parasites recovered and the most commonly used specimen collection approaches.

The information presented in this chapter should provide the reader with appropriate laboratory techniques and examples of morphologic criteria to permit the correct identification of the more common human parasites.

Several excellent resource texts are also available.*

44.2. Fecal Specimens

44.2.a. Collection. The ability to detect and identify intestinal parasites (particularly protozoa) is directly related to the quality of the specimen submitted to the laboratory. Certain guidelines (below) are recommended to ensure proper collection and accurate examination of specimens.

Collection of fecal specimens for intestinal parasites should always be performed **prior to** radiologic studies involving barium sulfate. Because of the excess crystalline material in the stool specimen, the intestinal protozoa may be impossible to detect for at least 1 week after the use of barium. Certain medications may also prevent the detection of intestinal protozoa; these include mineral oil, bismuth, nonabsorbable antidiarrheal preparations, antimalarials, and some antibiotics (e.g., tetracyclines). The organisms may be difficult to detect for several weeks after the medication is discontinued.

Fecal specimens should be collected in clean, widemouthed containers; most laboratories use a waxed, cardboard half-pint container with a tight-fitting lid. The specimen should not be contaminated with water that may contain free-living organisms. Contamination with urine should also be avoided to prevent destruction of motile organisms in the specimen. All specimens should be identified with the patient's name, physician's name, hospital number if applicable, and the time and date collected. Every fecal specimen represents a potential source of infectious material (e.g., bacteria, viruses, and parasites) and should be handled accordingly.

The number of specimens required to demonstrate intestinal parasites will vary depending on the quality of the specimen submitted, the accuracy of the examination performed,

*References 3, 6, 9, 13, 24, 29, 35.

TABLE 44.1
Classification of Human Parasites

I. Protozoa
  1. Amebas—intestinal
     Entamoeba histolytica
     Entamoeba hartmanni
     Entamoeba coli
     Entamoeba polecki
     Entamoeba gingivalis
     Endolimax nana
     Iodamoeba bütschlii
  2. Flagellates—intestinal
     Giardia lamblia
     Chilomastix mesnili
     Dientamoeba fragilis
     Trichomonas hominis
     Trichomonas tenax
     Enteromonas hominis
     Retortamonas intestinalis
  3. Ciliates—intestinal
     Balantidium coli
  4. Coccidia, *Blastocystis hominis*—intestinal
     Cryptosporidium sp.
     Isospora belli
     Sarcocystis hominis
     Sarcocystis suihominis
     Sarcocystis "lindemanni"
     Blastocystis hominis
  5. Amebas, flagellates—from other body sites
     Amebas
       Naegleria fowleri
       Acanthamoeba culbertsoni
     Flagellates
       Trichomonas vaginalis
  6. Coccidia, sporozoa—from other body sites
     Coccidia
       Toxoplasma gondii
     Sporozoa
       Pneumocystis carinii
  7. Sporozoa, flagellates—from blood and tissues
     Sporozoa (malaria and *Babesia*)
       Plasmodium vivax
       Plasmodium ovale
       Plasmodium malariae
       Plasmodium falciparum
       Babesia sp.
     Flagellates (leishmaniae, trypanosomes)
       Leishmania tropica complex
       Leishmania mexicana complex
       Leishmania braziliensis complex
       Leishmania donovani
       Trypanosoma gambiense
       Trypanosoma rhodesiense
       Trypanosoma cruzi
       Trypanosoma rangeli

II. Nematodes
  1. Intestinal
     Ascaris lumbricoides
     Enterobius vermicularis
     Ancylostoma duodenale
     Necator americanus
     Strongyloides stercoralis
     Trichuris trichiura
  2. Tissue
     Trichinella spiralis
     Visceral larva migrans (*Toxocara canis* or *T. cati*)
     Cutaneous larva migrans (*Ancylostoma braziliense* or *A. caninum*)
     Angiostrongylus cantonensis
     Angiostrongylus costaricensis
     Gnathostoma spinigerum
     Anisakis sp. (larvae from saltwater fish)
     Phocanema sp. (larvae from saltwater fish)
  3. Filarial worms—blood
     Wuchereria bancrofti
     Brugia malayi
     Loa loa
     Onchocerca volvulus
     Mansonella ozzardi
     Mansonella streptocerca
     Mansonella perstans
     Dirofilaria immitis (usually lung lesion/dog heartworm)
     Dirofilaria sp.

III. Cestodes
  1. Intestinal
     Diphyllobothrium latum
     Dipylidium caninum
     Hymenolepis nana
     Hymenolepis diminuta
     Taenia solium
     Taenia saginata
  2. Larval forms—tissue
     Taenia solium
     Echinococcus granulosus
     Echinococcus multilocularis
     Multiceps multiceps
     Diphyllobothrium sp.

IV. Trematodes
  1. Intestinal
     Fasciolopsis buski
     Echinostoma ilocanum
     Heterophyes heterophyes
     Metagonimus yokogawai
  2. Liver/lung
     Opisthorchis sinensis
     Opisthorchis viverrini
     Fasciola hepatica
     Paragonimus westermani

TABLE 44.1
Classification of Human Parasites—cont'd

3. Blood
   Schistosoma mansoni
   Schistosoma haematobium
   Schistosoma japonicum
   Schistosoma intercalatum
   Schistosoma mekongi
V. Arthropoda
  1. Arachnida
    Scorpions
    Spiders (black widow, brown recluse)
    Ticks *(Dermacentor, Ixodes, Argas, Ornithodoros)*
    Mites *(Sarcoptes)*
  2. Crustacea
    Copepods *(Cyclops)*
    Crayfish, lobsters, crabs

3. Pentastomida
   Tongue worms
4. Diplopoda
   Millipedes
5. Chilopoda
   Centipedes
6. Insecta
   Anoplura: sucking lice *(Pediculus, Phthirus)*
   Dictyoptera: cockroaches
   Hemiptera: true bugs *(Triatoma)*
   Coleoptera: beetles
   Hymenoptera: bees, wasps, etc.
   Lepidoptera: butterflies, moths, etc.
   Diptera: flies, mosquitos, gnats, midges *(Phlebotomus, Aedes, Anopheles, Glossina, Simulium)*
   Siphonaptera: fleas *(Pulex, Xenopsylla)*

TABLE 44.2
Body Sites and Possible Parasites Recovered*

SITE	PARASITES	SITE	PARASITES
Blood			*Isospora belli*
Red cells	*Plasmodium* sp.		*Ascaris lumbricoides*
	Babesia sp.		*Enterobius vermicularis*
White cells	*Leishmania donovani*		Hookworm
	Toxoplasma gondii		*Strongyloides stercoralis*
Whole blood/plasma	*Trypanosoma* sp.		*Trichuris trichiura*
	Microfilariae		*Hymenolepis nana*
Bone marrow	*Leishmania donovani*		*Taenia saginata*
Central nervous system	*Taenia solium* (cysticercosis)		*Taenia solium*
	Echinococcus sp.		*Diphyllobothrium latum*
	Naegleria fowleri		*Opisthorchis sinensis (Clonorchis)*
	Acanthamoeba/Hartmanella sp.		*Paragonimus westermani*
	Toxoplasma gondii		*Schistosoma* sp.
	Trypanosoma sp.	Liver, spleen	*Echinococcus* sp.
Cutaneous ulcers	*Leishmania* sp.		*Entamoeba histolytica*
Intestinal tract	*Entamoeba histolytica*		*Leishmania donovani*
	Entamoeba coli	Lung	*Pneumocystis carinii*
	Entamoeba hartmanni		*Paragonimus westermani*
	Endolimax nana	Muscle	*Taenia solium* (cysticerci)
	Iodamoeba bütschlii		*Trichinella spiralis*
	Giardia lamblia		*Onchocerca volvulus*
	Chilomastix mesnili	Skin	*Leishmania* sp.
	Dientamoeba fragilis		Microfilariae
	Trichomonas hominis	Urogenital system	*Trichomonas vaginalis*
	Cryptosporidium sp.		*Schistosoma* sp.
	Blastocystis hominis		

*This table does not include every possible parasite that could be found in a particular body site. However, the most likely organisms have been listed.

TABLE 44.3
Body Sites and Specimen Collection

SITE	SPECIMEN OPTIONS	COLLECTION METHOD
Blood	Smears of whole blood	Thick and thin films (first choice)
	Anticoagulated blood	Anticoagulated blood (second choice)
		EDTA (first choice)
		Heparin (second choice)
Bone marrow	Aspirate	Sterile
Central nervous system	Spinal fluid	Sterile
Cutaneous ulcers	Aspirates from below surface	Sterile plus air-dried smears
	Biopsy	Sterile; nonsterile to histology
Intestinal tract	Fresh stool	½ pint waxed container
	Preserved stool	5% or 10% formalin, MIF, SAF, Schaudinn's PVA
	Sigmoidoscopy material	Fresh, PVA, or Schaudinn's smears
	Duodenal contents	Entero-Test or aspirates
	Anal impression smear	Cellophane tape (pinworm examination)
	Adult worm/worm segments	Saline, 70% alcohol
Liver, spleen	Aspirates	Sterile, collected in 4 separate aliquots (liver)
	Biopsy	Sterile, nonsterile to histology
Lung	Sputum	True sputum (not saliva); no preservative (10% formalin if time delay)
	Lavage (centrifuged sediment)	No preservative
		Air-dried smears
	Transbronchial aspirate	Same as above
	Tracheobronchial aspirate	Same as above
	Brush biopsy	Same as above
	Open lung biopsy	
Muscle	Biopsy	Fresh-squash preparation, nonsterile to histology
Skin	Scrapings	Aseptic, smear or vial
	Skin snip	No preservative
	Biopsy	Nonsterile to histology
Urogenital system	Vaginal discharge	Saline swab, Culturette (no charcoal), culture medium
	Urethral discharge	Same as above
	Prostatic secretions	Same as above
	Urine	Single unpreserved specimen (24 h unpreserved specimen)

and the severity of the infection. For a routine examination for parasites **prior to treatment, a minimum of three fecal specimens** is recommended—two specimens collected from normal movements and one specimen collected after a cathartic, such as magnesium sulfate or Fleet Phospho-Soda. A cathartic with an oil base should not be used, and all laxatives are contraindicated if the patient has diarrhea or significant abdominal pain. Stool softeners are inadequate for producing a purged specimen. The examination of at least six specimens ensures detection of 90% of infections; six are usually recommended when amebiasis is suspected.

Many organisms do not appear in fecal specimens in consistent numbers on a daily basis; thus collection of specimens on **alternate days** tends to yield a higher percentage of positive findings. The series of three specimens should be collected within no more than 10 days and a series of six within no more than 14 days.

The number of specimens to be examined after therapy will vary depending on the diagnosis; however, a series of three specimens collected as previously outlined is usually recommended. A patient who has received treatment for a protozoan infection should be checked 3-4 weeks after therapy. Patients treated for helminth infections may be checked 1-2 weeks after therapy, and those treated for *Taenia* infections 5-6 weeks after therapy.

Since the age of the specimen directly influences the recovery of protozoan organisms, the **time the specimen was collected** should be recorded on the laboratory request form. Freshly passed specimens are mandatory for the detection of trophic amebas or flagellates. **Liquid specimens should be examined within 30 min of passage** (not 30 min from the time they reach the laboratory), or the specimen should be placed in polyvinyl alcohol fixative (PVA) or another suitable preservative (see following

section on preservation of specimens). **Semiformed or soft specimens should be examined within 1 h of passage;** if this is not possible, the stool material should be preserved. Although the time limits are not as critical for the examination of a formed specimen, it is recommended that the material be examined on the day of passage. If these time limits cannot be met, portions of the sample should be preserved. Stool specimens should not be held at room temperature but should be refrigerated at 3°-5° C and stored in closed containers to prevent desiccation. At this temperature eggs, larvae, and protozoan cysts remain viable for several days. Fecal specimens should never be incubated or frozen prior to examination. When the proper criteria for collection of fecal specimens are not met, the laboratory should request additional samples.

Collection kit for clinic use. A collection kit that can be used for outpatient laboratory services contains the following items:

1. One 5-7 dram screw-capped vial containing approximately 10 ml of PVA. Some laboratories also request that some fecal material be placed in a separate vial containing 10 ml of 10% formalin, whereas others may also request a vial containing a portion of the unpreserved sample. Some workers recommended using a vial of Schaudinn's fixative in place of PVA.[41]
2. One half-pint cardboard carton with a tight-fitting lid.
3. Four 6-inch applicator sticks.
4. Instruction sheet containing information on proper collection procedures.
5. Small paper bag in which all supplies can be returned to the laboratory after specimen collection.

A number of commercial collection systems are presently available, and one can select which vials are appropriate for a particular institution. Most manufacturers will package the kit according to individual specifications. (See

"PVA Fixative" section below for representative suppliers).

Since examination of three specimens is usually recommended, a kit can be prepared with three vials of preservatives, three cartons, and 10 or 12 applicator sticks. If the patient's clinical status permits, all preserved specimens in the requested series may be collected prior to delivery.

CAUTION: PVA solution contains a large amount of mercury; for safety reasons and protection of the patient, each vial containing PVA or any type of preservative should have a child-proof cap and should be marked **Poison.** In some areas of the country it may be helpful to label the vials in more than one language, depending on the population using the medical facility.

Collection kit delivered by mail service. Specimens may be submitted to a referral laboratory through the regular postal service; however, the following United States postal regulations must be followed: the final kit size may vary according to individual needs; there must be two separate containers—one screw-capped metal container, which is placed inside a screw-capped cardboard container. The inner mailing tube should contain one vial of PVA (individual laboratories may wish to include a vial of 10% formalin, one of Schaudinn's fixative, or an empty vial) and several applicator sticks. The instruction sheet may be placed around the inner tube, which is then placed in the cardboard mailing container. This kit would be adequate for a single specimen; if three examinations were requested, the patient should submit three separate mailing kits.

The PVA-preserved portion of the specimen may be used for the complete examination, although some laboratories may prefer to use the sample in 10% formalin for the concentration procedure. Other laboratories may prefer to use Schaudinn's fixative for collection. The unpreserved portion of the specimen (many laboratories do not request this sample unless an occult blood procedure is requested) may be examined to determine the specimen type (e.g., liquid, soft, or formed).

44.2.b. Preservation. Depending on specimen-to-laboratory transportation time, the laboratory work load, and the availability of trained personnel, it may often be impossible to examine the specimen within specified time limits. To maintain protozoan morphology and prevent further development of certain helminth eggs and larvae, the fecal specimen should be placed in an appropriate preservative for examination at a later time. A number of preservatives are available; four of these methods—PVA (Procedure 44.1), formalin (Procedure 44.2), Merthiolate (thimerosal)-iodine-formalin (MIF), and sodium acetate–formalin (SAF)—will be discussed. When selecting an appropriate fixative, it is important to realize the limitations of each. PVA and SAF are the only fixatives included here from which a permanent stained smear can be easily prepared. The stained smear is extremely important in providing a complete and accurate examination for intestinal protozoa. The other fixatives mentioned permit the examination of the specimen as a wet mount only, a technique much less accurate than the stained smear for the identification of protozoa.

Although there has been a great deal of interest in developing a preservative without the use of mercury compounds, studies indicate that substitute compounds may not provide the quality of preservation necessary for good protozoan morphology on the permanent stained smear. Copper sulfate is the compound that has been tried most frequently, but does not provide results equal to those seen with mercuric chloride. Work will probably continue in this area in order to provide a solution to the problem of mercury disposal, a problem many laboratories are trying to solve.

PVA fixative. PVA fixative solution is highly recommended as a means of preserving protozoan cysts and trophozoites for examination at a later time. The use of PVA also permits specimens to be shipped by regular mail service to a laboratory for subsequent examination. PVA, which is a combination of modified Schaudinn's fixative and a water-soluble resin, should be used in the ratio of 3 parts PVA to 1 part fecal material. Perhaps the greatest advantage in the use of PVA is that permanent stained slides can be prepared from PVA-preserved material. This is not the case with many other preservatives; some permit the specimen to be examined as a wet preparation only, a technique that may not be adequate for the correct identification of protozoan organisms. PVA can be prepared in the laboratory (Procedure 44.1) or purchased commercially.* This fixative remains stable for long periods (months to years) when kept in **sealed containers** at room temperature. However, when dispensed in small vials, PVA may become viscous and turn cloudy or white after 2 or 3 months; these vials should be discarded.

Commercial packaging and distribution of these vials have essentially eliminated the problem of moisture loss and shelf-life.

Procedure 44.1 for preparation of PVA fixative is modified from Brooke and Goldman.[5]

Protozoan cysts, helminth eggs, and larvae are well preserved for long periods in **10% formalin** (Procedure 44.2). It is recommended that hot formalin (60° C) be used for helminth eggs to prevent further development of the eggs to the infective stage. Formalin should be used in the ratio of at least 3 parts formalin to

---

*Elvanol, grades 71-24, 71-30, and 90-25, can be obtained from E. I. du Pont de Nemours and Co. (or their local representatives) in a minimum of 50-pound bags. One could check with a local chemical supply house to see if small quantities might be available. When ordering PVA powder, be sure to specify the pretested powder for use in PVA fixative. The PVA powder should be water soluble and of medium viscosity. Prepared liquid PVA (ready for use) can be obtained from Medical Chemical Corporation, Meridian Diagnostics, Marion Scientific Corporation, Remel, Trend Scientific, Medical Media Lab, and Bio Spec.

PROCEDURE 44.1. PVA FIXATIVE

1. **Formula**

PVA, Elvanol 71-24	10 g
95% ethyl alcohol	62.5 ml
Mercuric chloride, saturated aqueous	125 ml
Glacial acetic acid	10 ml
Glycerin	3 ml

2. **Preparation**
   a. Mix liquid ingredients in a 500 ml beaker.
   b. Add PVA powder (stirring not recommended).
   c. Cover beaker with a large Petri dish, heavy waxed paper, or foil and allow to soak overnight.
   d. Heat solution slowly to 75° C. When this temperature is reached, remove beaker and swirl mixture until a homogeneous, slightly milky solution is obtained (30 seconds).

PROCEDURE 44.2 FORMALIN PRESERVATION (10% FORMALIN)

1. **Formula**

Formaldehyde (USP)	100 ml
0.85% saline solution	900 ml

2. **Preparation.** Dilute 100 ml of formaldehyde with 900 ml of 0.85% saline solution (distilled water may be used instead of saline).

1 part fecal material; thorough mixing of the fresh specimen and fixative is necessary to ensure good preservation.

MIF solution. The Merthiolate (thimerosal)-iodine-formalin solution of Sapèro and Lawless[39] can be used as a stain preservative for most kinds and stages of intestinal parasites and may be helpful in field surveys. Helminth eggs, larvae, and certain protozoa can be identified without further staining in wet mounts, which can be prepared immediately after fixation or several weeks later. This type of wet preparation may not be adequate for the diagnosis of all intestinal protozoa. Although some workers prepare a permanent stained smear from MIF-preserved material, another fixative preparation may be preferred for the precise morphology necessary for protozoan identification on the permanent stained smear. There are certain disadvantages with the MIF method, which may include the instability of the iodine component of the fixative.

SAF fixative. SAF fixative contains formalin combined with sodium acetate, which acts as a buffer. This combination ensures good preservation and stability of morphology. It is a liquid fixative much like 10% aqueous formalin. When the sediment is used to prepare permanent stained smears, there may be some difficulty in getting material to adhere to the slide. Mayer's albumin has been recommended as an adhesive.[40] Although it has a long shelf life and is easy to prepare in the laboratory, this technique may be more difficult to use for less experienced laboratory personnel who are not familiar with fecal specimen differences in consistency related to adhesion to the slide.

44.2.c. Macroscopic examination. The consistency of the stool (formed, semiformed, soft, or liquid) may give an indication of the protozoan stages present. When the moisture content of the fecal material is decreased during **normal passage** through the intestinal tract, the trophozoite stages of the protozoa encyst to survive. **Trophozoites** (motile forms) of the in-

testinal protozoa are usually found in soft or liquid specimens and occasionally in a semiformed specimen; the **cyst stages** are normally found in formed or semiformed specimens, rarely in liquid stools.

Helminth eggs or larvae may be found in any type of specimen, although the chances of finding any parasitic organism in a liquid specimen will be reduced because of the dilution factor.

Occasionally adult helminths, such as *Ascaris lumbricoides* or *Enterobius vermicularis* (pinworm), may be seen in or on the surface of the stool. Tapeworm proglottids may also be seen on the surface, or they may actually crawl under the specimen and be found on the bottom of the container. Other adult helminths, such as *Trichuris trichiura* (whipworm), hookworms, or perhaps *Hymenolepis nana* (dwarf tapeworm), may be found in the stool, but usually this occurs only after medication.

The presence of blood in the specimen may indicate a number of things and should always be reported. Dark stools may indicate bleeding high in the gastrointestinal tract, whereas fresh (bright red) blood most often is the result of bleeding at a lower level. In certain parasitic infections blood and mucus may be present; a soft or liquid stool may be highly suggestive of an amebic infection. These areas of blood and mucus should be carefully examined for the presence of trophic amebas. Occult blood in the stool may or may not be related to a parasitic infection and can result from a number of different conditions. Ingestion of various compounds may give a distinctive color to the stool (iron, black; barium, light tan to white).

44.2.d. Microscopic examination. The identification of intestinal protozoa and helminth eggs is based on recognition of specific morphologic characteristics; these studies require a good binocular microscope, good light source, and the use of a calibrated ocular micrometer.

The microscope should have 5× and 10× oculars (widefield oculars are often recommended) and three objectives: low power (10×), high-dry (40×-44×), and oil immersion (97×-99×). The microscope should be kept covered when not in use, and all lenses should be carefully cleaned with lens paper. The light source should provide light of variable intensity in the blue-white range.

Calibration of microscope. Parasite identification depends on several parameters, one of which is size; any laboratory doing diagnostic work in parasitology should have a calibrated microscope available for precise measurements.

Measurements are made by means of a micrometer disk placed in the ocular of the microscope; the disk is usually calibrated as a line divided in 50 units. Since the divisions in the disk represent different measurements, depending on the objective magnification used, the ocular disk divisions must be compared with a known calibrated scale, usually a stage micrometer with a scale of 0.1 and 0.01 mm divisions. Specific directions may be found in the work of Garcia and Ash.[13]

NOTE: After each objective power has been calibrated on the microscope, **the oculars containing the disk or these objectives cannot be interchanged with corresponding objectives or oculars on another microscope.** Each microscope that will be used to measure organisms must be calibrated as a unit; **the original oculars and objectives that were used to calibrate the microscope must also be used when an organism is measured.**

In order to comply with quality control requirements, each calibrated microscope should be recalibrated once a year. The calibrations do change, and a slight error can be magnified, particularly using the oil-immersion objective, where measurements can be critical to accurate speciation.

44.2.e. Diagnostic procedures. A combination of techniques yields a greater number of positive specimens than does any one technique alone. Procedures recommended for a complete ova and parasite examination are discussed in the following section.

Direct smears. Normal mixing in the intestinal tract usually ensures even distribution of helminth eggs or larvae and protozoa. However, examination of the fecal material as a direct smear may or may not reveal organisms, depending on the parasite density. The direct smear is prepared by mixing a small amount of fecal material (approximately 2 mg) with a drop of physiologic saline; this mixture provides a uniform suspension under a 22 by 22 mm coverslip. Some workers prefer a 1½- by 3-inch glass slide for the wet preparations, rather than the standard 1- by 3-inch slide most often used for the permanent stained smear. A 2-mg sample of fecal material forms a low cone on the end of a wooden applicator stick. If more material is used for the direct mount, the suspension is usually too thick for an accurate examination; less than 2 mg results in the examination of too thin a suspension, thus decreasing the chances of finding any organisms. If present, blood and mucus should always be examined as a direct mount. The entire 22 by 22 mm coverslip should be systematically examined using the low-power objective (10×) and low light intensity; any suspect objects may then be examined under high-dry power (43×). The use of the oil immersion objective on mounts of this kind is not recommended unless the coverslip (no. 1 thickness coverslip is recommended when the oil immersion objective is used) is sealed to the slide with a cotton-tipped applicator stick dipped in equal parts of heated paraffin and petroleum jelly. Many workers believe the use of oil immersion on this type of preparation is impractical, especially since morphologic detail is most easily seen and the diagnosis confirmed with oil immersion examination of the permanent stained smear.

The **direct wet mount** is used primarily to detect motile trophozoite stages of the protozoa. These organisms are very pale and trans-

PROCEDURE 44.3. MODIFIED D'ANTONI'S IODINE

1. **Formula**

Distilled water	100 ml
Potassium iodide (KI)	1 g
Powdered iodine crystals	1.5 g

2. **Preparation.** The potassium iodide solution should be saturated with iodine, with some excess remaining in the bottle. Store in brown, glass-stoppered bottles in the dark. The solution is ready for use immediately and should be decanted into a brown-glass dropping bottle; when the solution lightens, it should be discarded and replaced with fresh stock. The stock solution remains good as long as an excess of iodine remains on the bottom of the bottle. The iodine solutions eventually lighten in color and lose their staining strength; fresh solutions should be prepared every 2-3 weeks.[27]

PROCEDURE 44.4. ACETATE BUFFER SOLUTION

Stock solution A consists of 0.2 M solution of acetic acid (11.55 ml in 1,000 ml of distilled water).

Stock solution B consists of 0.2 M solution of sodium acetate (16.4 g of $C_2H_3O_2Na$, or 27.2 g of $C_2H_3O_2Na \cdot 3H_2O$ in 1,000 ml of distilled water).

Proportions of A and B for specific pH are as follows: mix the indicated quantity of stock solutions A and B and dilute with distilled water to a total of 100 ml.

Desired pH	Stock Solution A (ml)	Stock Solution B (ml)
3.6	46.3	3.7
3.8	44.0	6.0
4.0	41.0	9.0
4.2	36.8	13.2
4.4	30.5	19.5
4.6	25.5	24.5

parent, two characteristics that require the use of low light intensity. Protozoan organisms in a saline preparation usually appear as refractile objects. If suspect objects are seen on high-dry power, one should allow at least 15 seconds to detect motility of slow-moving protozoa. Heat applied by placing a hot penny on the edge of a slide may enhance the motility of trophic protozoa.

Note: With few exceptions, protozoan organisms should not be identified on the basis of a wet mount alone. Permanent stained smears should be examined to confirm the specific identification of suspected organisms.

Helminth eggs or larvae and protozoan cysts may also be seen on the wet film, although these forms are more often detected after fecal concentration procedures.

After the wet preparation has been thoroughly checked for trophic amebas, a drop of iodine may be placed at the edge of the coverslip, or a new wet mount can be prepared with iodine alone. A weak iodine solution is recommended; too strong a solution may obscure the organisms. Several types of iodine solutions are available: Dobell and O'Connor's, Lugol's (Chapter 46), and D'Antoni's (Procedure 44.3). Gram's iodine used in bacteriologic work is not recommended for staining parasitic organisms.

NOTE: Many laboratories believe that the benefits gained in organism recovery and identification from receipt of preserved stool speci-

PROCEDURE 44.5. ZINC SULFATE FLOTATION PROCEDURE (MODIFIED)

Protozoan cysts may be more distorted using this method, and the technique is unsuitable for stool specimens containing large amounts of fatty material. The specific gravity of the zinc sulfate should be 1.18 and should be checked frequently with a hydrometer. If this technique is used to concentrate formalin-preserved material, the specific gravity should be increased to 1.20.

Zinc sulfate solution ($ZnSO_4$, specific gravity 1.18); consists of approximately 330 g of dry crystals in 670 ml of distilled water. A 33% solution usually approximates the correct specific gravity but may be adjusted to 1.18 by the addition of zinc sulfate or distilled water.

1. Prepare a fecal suspension of ¼-½ teaspoon of feces (more if the specimen is diarrheal) in 10-15 ml of tap water.
2. Filter this material through two layers of gauze into a small tube (Wassermann tube). Fill the tube with tap water to within 2-3 mm of the top, and centrifuge for 1 min at 2,300 rpm.
3. Decant the supernatant fluid, fill the tube with water, and resuspend the sediment by stirring with an applicator stick. Centrifuge for 1 min at 2,300 rpm.
4. Decant the water, add 2-3 ml zinc sulfate solution, resuspend the sediment, and fill the tube with zinc sulfate solution to within 0.5 cm of the top.
5. Centrifuge for 1-2 min at 2,500 rpm. Do not "brake" the centrifuge; allow the tubes to come to a stop without interference or vibration.
6. Without removing the tubes from the centrifuge, touch the surface film of the suspension with a wire loop (diameter 5-7 mm; loop should be parallel with the surface of the fluid). **Do not go below the surface of the film with the loop.** Add the material in the loop to a slide containing a drop of dilute iodine or saline.

NOTE: Material recovered from the zinc sulfate flotation procedure must be examined within several minutes; prolonged contact with the high specific gravity solution leads to organism distortion.

mens far outweigh the disadvantages of not receiving a fresh specimen that can be examined for motile organisms. This is particularly true with the intestinal protozoa.

Protozoan cysts correctly stained with iodine contain yellow-gold cytoplasm, brown glycogen material, and paler refractile nuclei. The chromatoidal bodies may not be as clearly visible as they were in the saline mount.

Several staining solutions are available that may be used to reveal nuclear detail in the tro-

phozoite stages. Nair's[31] buffered methylene blue stain is effective in showing nuclear detail when used at a low pH; a pH range of 3.6-4.8 allows more active penetration of the organism with the biologic dye. After 5-10 min, Nair's buffered methylene blue stain stains the cytoplasm a pale blue and the nuclei a darker blue. Methylene blue (0.06%) in an acetate buffer (Procedure 44.4) at pH 3.6 usually gives satisfactory results; the mount should be examined within 30 min.

Concentration procedures. Often a direct mount of fecal material fails to reveal the presence of parasitic organisms in the gastrointestinal tract. Fecal concentration procedures should be included for a complete examination for parasites; these procedures allow the detection of small numbers of organisms that may be missed using only the direct mount. Helminth eggs can usually be identified when recovered from a concentration procedure. Generally the identification of intestinal protozoa should be considered tentative and confirmed with the permanent stained smear. Those protozoa which might be routinely identified from a concentration procedure include cysts of *Giardia lamblia, Entamoeba histolytica, Entamoeba coli,* and *Iodamoeba bütschlii.* There are commercially available concentrating devices that may assist a laboratory in standardizing the methodology.*

A number of concentration procedures are available; they are either **flotation** or **sedimentation techniques** designed to separate the parasitic components from excess fecal debris through differences in specific gravity. A flotation procedure (Procedure 44.5) permits the separation of protozoan cysts and certain helminth eggs through the use of a liquid with a high specific gravity. The parasitic elements are recovered in the surface film, whereas the debris will be found in the bottom of the tube. This technique yields a cleaner preparation than does the sedimentation procedure; however, some helminth eggs (operculated eggs or very dense eggs, such as unfertilized *Ascaris* eggs) and some protozoa do not concentrate well with the flotation method. The specific gravity may be increased, although this may produce more distortion in the eggs and protozoa. Any laboratory that uses only a flotation procedure may fail to recover all the parasites

present; to ensure detection of all organisms in the sample, both the surface film and the sediment should be carefully examined.

NOTE: Directions for any flotation technique must be followed exactly to produce reliable results.

Sedimentation procedures (using gravity or centrifugation) allow the recovery of all protozoa, eggs, and larvae present; however, the sediment preparation contains more fecal debris. If a single technique is selected for routine use, the **sedimentation procedure** (Procedure 44.6) **is recommended** as the easiest to perform and least subject to technical error.

Permanent stained smears. The detection and correct identification of **intestinal protozoa** are frequently dependent on the examination of the permanent stained smear. These slides not only provide the microscopist with a permanent record of the protozoan organisms identified but also may be used for consultations with specialists when unusual morphologic characteristics are found. In view of the number of morphologic variations possible, organisms may be found that are very difficult to identify and do not fit the pattern for any one species.

The smaller protozoan organisms are often seen on the stained smear and missed with only the direct smear and concentration methods. Although an experienced microscopist can occasionally identify certain organisms on a wet preparation, most identifications should be considered tentative until confirmed by the permanent stained slide. For these reasons, **the permanent stain is recommended for every stool sample submitted for a routine examination for parasites.**

A number of staining techniques are available; individual selection of a particular method may depend on the degree of difficulty and amount of time necessary for staining. The older classical method is the long Heidenhain's iron-hematoxylin method; however, for routine

---

*Evergreen Scientific (FPC, fecal parasite concentrator), Trend Scientific (FeKal, CON-Trate System).

diagnostic work most laboratories select one of the shorter procedures, such as the **trichrome method** or one of several methods using iron-hematoxylin. Other procedures are available; however, those included here generally tend to give the best and most reliable results with both fresh and PVA-preserved specimens.

PREPARATION OF FRESH MATERIAL. When the specimen arrives, use an applicator stick or brush to smear a small amount of stool on two clean slides and immediately immerse them in Schaudinn's fixative. If the slides are prepared correctly, one should be able to read newsprint through the fecal smear. The smears should fix for a minimum of 30 min; fixation time may be decreased to 5 min if the Schaudinn's solution is heated to 60° C.

If a liquid specimen is received, mix 3 or 4 drops of PVA with 1 or 2 drops of fecal material on a slide, spread the mixture, and allow the slides to dry for several hours at 35° C or overnight at room temperature. The following fixative solutions may be used (Procedures 44.7 and 44.8).

PREPARATION OF PVA-PRESERVED MATERIAL. Stool specimens preserved in PVA should be allowed to fix at least 30 min. After fixation, the sample should be thoroughly mixed and a small amount of the material poured onto a paper towel to absorb excess PVA. This is an important step in the procedure; allow the PVA to soak into the paper towel for 2-3 min before preparing the slides. With an applicator stick apply some of the stool material from the paper towel to two slides and let them dry for several hours at 37° C or overnight at room temperature. The PVA-stool mixture should be spread to the edges of the glass slide; this causes the film to adhere to the slide during staining. It is also important to thoroughly dry the slides to prevent the material from washing off during staining.

TRICHROME STAIN. This stain was originally developed by Gomori[15] for tissue differentia-tion and was adapted by Wheatley[52] for intestinal protozoa (Procedure 44.9). It is an uncomplicated procedure that produces well-stained smears from both fresh and PVA-preserved material.

The trichrome stain can be used repeatedly, and stock solution may be added to the jar when the volume is decreased. Periodically, the staining strength can be restored by removing the lid and allowing the 70% alcohol carried over from the preceding jar to evaporate. Each lot number or batch of stain (either purchased commercially or prepared in the laboratory) should be checked to determine the optimum staining time, which is usually a few minutes longer for PVA-preserved material.

The 90% acidified alcohol is used as a destaining agent that will provide good differentiation; however, prolonged destaining (more than 3 seconds) may result in a poor stain. To prevent continued destaining, the slides should be quickly rinsed in 100% alcohol and then dehydrated through two additional changes of 100% alcohol.

INTERPRETATION OF STAINED SMEARS. Many problems in interpretation may arise when poorly stained smears are examined; these smears are usually the result of inadequate fixation or incorrect specimen collection and submission. An old specimen or inadequate fixation may result in organisms that fail to stain or that appear as pale pink or red objects with very little internal definition. This type of staining reaction may occur with *Entamoeba coli* cysts, which require a longer fixation time; mature cysts in general need additional fixation time and therefore may not be as well stained as immature cysts. Degenerate forms or those that have been understained or destained too much may stain pale green.

When the smear is well fixed and correctly stained, the background debris will be green, and the protozoa will have a blue-green to purple cytoplasm with red or purple-red nuclei

PROCEDURE 44.6. FORMALIN-ETHER SEDIMENTATION TECHNIQUE

1. Transfer ¼-½ teaspoon of fresh stool into 10 ml of 10% formalin in a 15 ml shell vial, unwaxed paper cup, or 16 by 125 mm tube (container may vary depending on individual preferences) and comminute thoroughly. Let stand 30 min for adequate fixation.
2. Filter this material (funnel or pointed paper cup with end cut off) through two layers of gauze into a 15 ml centrifuge tube.
3. Add physiologic saline to within ½ inch of the top and centrifuge for 2 min at 1,500 rpm (or 1 min at 2,000 to 2,500 rpm).
4. Decant, resuspend the sediment (should have 0.5-1 ml sediment) in saline to within ½ inch of the top, and centrifuge again for 2 min at 1,500 rpm (or 1 min at 2,000-2,500 rpm). This second wash may be eliminated if the supernatant fluid after the first wash is light tan or clear.
5. Decant and resuspend the sediment in 10% formalin (fill the tube only half full). If the amount of sediment left in the bottom of the tube is very small, do not add ether in step 6; merely add the formalin, then spin, decant, and examine the remaining sediment.
6. Add approximately 3 ml of ether (**do not use near open flames**), stopper, and shake vigorously for 30 seconds. Hold the tube so that the stopper is directed away from your face; remove stopper carefully to prevent spraying of material caused by pressure within the tube.
7. Centrifuge for 2-3 min at 1,500 rpm. Four layers should result: a small amount of sediment in the bottom of the tube, containing the parasites; a layer of formalin; a plug of fecal debris on top of the formalin layer; and a layer of ether at the top.
8. Free the plug of debris by ringing with an applicator stick, and decant all the fluid. After proper decanting, a drop or two of fluid remaining on the side of the tube will drain down to the sediment. Mix the fluid with the sediment and prepare a wet mount for examination.

The formalin-ether sedimentation procedure may be used on PVA-preserved material. Steps 1 and 2 differ as follows:

1. Fixation time with PVA should be at least 30 min. Mix contents of PVA bottle (stool-PVA mixture: 1 part stool to 2 or 3 parts PVA) with applicator sticks. Immediately after mixing, pour approximately 2-5 ml (amount will vary depending on the viscosity and density of the mixture) of the stool-PVA mixture into a 15 ml shell vial, 16 by 125 mm tube, or such, and add approximately 10 ml physiologic saline.
2. Filter this material (funnel or paper cup with pointed end cut off) through two layers of gauze into a 15 ml centrifuge tube.

Steps 3 through 8 will be the same for both fresh and PVA-preserved material.

PROCEDURE 44.6. FORMALIN-ETHER SEDIMENTATION TECHNIQUE—cont'd

NOTE: Tap water may be substituted for physiologic saline throughout this procedure; however, saline is recommended. Some workers prefer to use 10% formalin for all the rinses (steps 3 and 4).

NOTE: The introduction of ethyl acetate as a substitute for diethyl ether (ether) in the formalin-ether sedimentation concentration procedure provides a much safer chemical for the clinical laboratory. Tests comparing the use of these two compounds on formalin-preserved and PVA-preserved material indicate that the differences in organism recovery and identification are minimal and probably do not reflect clinically relevant differences.

When examining the sediment in the bottom of the tube:

1. Prepare a saline mount (1 drop of sediment and 1 drop of saline solution mixed together), and scan the whole 22 by 22 mm coverslip under low power for helminth eggs or larvae.

2. Iodine may then be added to aid in the detection of protozoan cysts and should be examined under high-dry power. If iodine is added prior to low-power scanning, be certain that the iodine is not too strong; otherwise, some of the helminth eggs will stain so darkly that they will be mistaken for debris.

3. Occasionally a precipitate is formed when iodine is added to the sediment obtained from a concentration procedure with PVA-preserved material. The precipitate is formed from the reaction between the iodine and excess mercuric chloride that has not been thoroughly rinsed from the PVA-preserved material. The sediment can be rinsed again to remove any remaining mercuric chloride, or the sediment can be examined as a saline mount without the addition of iodine.[13]

PROCEDURE 44.7. SATURATED MERCURIC CHLORIDE

Mercuric chloride ($HgCl_2$)   110 g
Distilled water   1,000 ml
Use a beaker as a water bath; boil (use a hood if available) until the $HgCl_2$ is dissolved; let stand until crystals form.

PROCEDURE 44.8. SCHAUDINN'S FIXATIVE (STOCK SOLUTION)

Saturated aqueous solution   600 ml
  of $HgCl_2$
95% ethyl alcohol   300 ml
Immediately before use add 5 ml of glacial acetic acid per 100 ml of stock solution.

PROCEDURE 44.9. TRICHROME STAIN

1. **Formula**

Chromotrope 2R	0.6 g
Light green SF	0.3 g
Phosphotungstic acid	0.7 g
Acetic acid (glacial)	1 ml
Distilled water	100 ml

2. **Preparation.** The stain is prepared by adding 1 ml of glacial acetic acid to the dry components. Allow the mixture to stand for 15-30 min to "ripen," then add 100 ml of distilled water. This preparation gives a highly uniform and reproducible stain; the stain should be purple. Store in Coplin jars.

3. **Procedure**

   a. Prepare fresh fecal smears or PVA smears as described.

   b. Place in 70% ethanol for 5 min.* (Step b may be eliminated for PVA smears.)

   c. Place in 70% ethanol plus D'Antoni's iodine (dark reddish brown) for 2-5 min.

   d. Place in two changes of 70% ethanol—one for 5 min* and one for 2-5 min.

   e. Place in trichrome stain solution for 10 min.

   f. Place in 90% ethanol, acidified (1% acetic acid) for up to 3 seconds (**do not leave the slides in this solution any longer**).

   g. Dip once in 100% ethanol.

   h. Place in two changes of 100% for 2-5 min each.*

   i. Place in two changes of xylene or toluene for 2-5 min each.*

   j. Mount in Permount or some other mounting medium; use a no. 1 thickness coverglass.

   *Slides can be held several hours or overnight.

and inclusions. The differences in colors between the background and organisms provide more contrast than in hematoxylin-stained smears.

Helminth eggs and larvae usually stain dark red or purple; they are usually distorted and difficult to identify. White blood cells, macrophages, tissue cells, yeast cells, and other artifacts still present diagnostic problems, since their color range on the stained smear approximates that of the parasitic organisms (Plates 44.1 to 44.3).

IRON-HEMATOXYLIN STAIN. Although the original method produces excellent results, most laboratories that use an iron-hematoxylin stain select one of the shorter methods. A number of procedures are available; both of those presented here can be used with either fresh or PVA-preserved material. Both background debris and the organisms stain gray-blue to black, with the cellular inclusions and nuclei appearing darker than the cytoplasm.

The method described by Spencer and Monroe[44] (Procedure 44.10) is a bit longer than

PROCEDURE 44.10. IRON HEMATOXYLIN STAIN

1. **Solution I.** Solution I is hematoxylin, 10 g in 1,000 ml of absolute ethanol. Keep the stain in a stoppered flask, and allow to ripen in sunlight for at least a week.
2. **Solution II**

Ferrous ammonium sulfate	10 g
Ferric ammonium sulfate	10 g
HCl, concentrated	10 ml
Distilled water	1,000 ml

3. **Working solution.** Mix equal parts of solutions I and II; this working solution will last for about 7 days.
4. **Procedure**
   a. Prepare fresh fecal smears or PVA-preserved smears as previously described.
   b. Place in 70% ethanol for 5 min.*
   c. Place in 70% ethanol plus D'Antoni's iodine (dark reddish brown) for 2-5 min.
   d. Place in 70% ethanol for 5 min.*
   e. Wash in running tap water for 10 min.
   f. Place in working solution of iron-hematoxylin staining solution for 4-5 min.
   g. Wash in running tap water for 10 min.
   h. Place in 70% ethanol for 5 min.*
   i. Place in 95% ethanol for 5 min.
   j. Place in two changes of 100% ethanol for 5 min each.*
   k. Place in two changes of xylene or toluene for 5 min each.*
   l. Mount in Permount or some other mounting medium; use a no. 1 thickness coverglass.

   *Slides can be held several hours or overnight.

the trichrome procedure. Although the slides do not require destaining, decolorizing in 0.5% hydrochloric acid after a longer initial staining time may provide better differentiation.

Another iron-hematoxylin method, described by Tompkins and Miller[50] (Procedure 44.11) includes the use of phosphotungstic acid as a destaining agent. This procedure also gives good, reproducible results.

General information. The most important step in preparing a well-stained fecal smear is adequate fixation of a specimen that has been submitted within specified time limits. To ensure best results, the acetic acid component of Schaudinn's fixative should be added just prior to use; fixation time (room temperature) may be extended overnight with no adverse effects on the smears.

After fixation it is very important to completely remove the mercuric chloride residue from the smears. The 70% alcohol-iodine mixture removes the mercury complex; the iodine solution should be changed often enough (at least once a week) to maintain a dark reddish-

PROCEDURE 44.11.
TOMPKINS AND MILLER
IRON-HEMATOXYLIN STAIN

1. Prepare fresh fecal smears or PVA-preserved smears as previously described.
2. Place in 70% ethanol plus D'Antoni's iodine (dark reddish brown) for 2-5 min.
3. Place in 50% ethanol for 3 min.
4. Wash in running tap water for 3 min.
5. Place in 4% ferric ammonium sulfate mordant for 5 min.
6. Wash in tap water for 1 min.
7. Place in 0.5% aqueous hematoxylin for 2 min.
8. Wash in tap water for 1 min.
9. Place in 2% aqueous phosphotungstic acid for 2-5 min.
10. Wash in running tap water for 10 min.
11. Place in 70% ethanol (plus a few drops of saturated aqueous lithium carbonate) for 3 min.
12. Place in 95% ethanol for 5 min.
13. Place in two changes of 100% ethanol for 5 min each.*
14. Place in xylene or toluene for 5 min.*
15. Mount in Permount or some other mounting medium; use a no. 1 thickness coverglass.

*Slides can be held several hours or overnight.

PROCEDURE 44.12.
HOT MODIFIED ACID FAST STAIN
FOR *CRYPTOSPORIDIUM*

1. Spin an aliquot of 10% formalinized stool for 2 min at $300 \times g$.
2. Remove upper layer of sediment with pipette and place a thin layer onto a microscope slide.
   NOTE: If the stool specimen contains a lot of mucus, 10 drops of 10% KOH can be added to the sediment (step 2), vortexed, rinsed with 10% formalin, and respun before smear preparation. Some laboratories use this approach routinely before smear preparation.
3. Heat fix the smear at 70° C for 10 min.
4. Place slide on staining rack and flood with carbol-fuchsin.*
5. Heat to steaming and allow to stain for 5 min. If the slide begins to dry, more stain is added without additional heating.
6. Rinse the smear with tap or distilled water.
7. Decolorize with 5% aqueous sulfuric acid for 30 seconds (thicker smears may require a longer time).
8. Rinse smear with tap or distilled water, drain, and flood smear with methylene blue counterstain* for 1 min.
9. Rinse with tap or distilled water, drain, and air dry.

*Reagents are prepared as for Ziehl-Neelsen stain (Chapter 46).

brown color. If the mercuric chloride is not completely removed, the stained smear may contain varying amounts of highly refractive granules, which may prevent finding or identifying any organisms present.

Good results in the final stages of dehydration (100% alcohol) and clearing (xylene) depend on the use of **fresh reagents.** It is recommended that solutions be changed at least weekly and more often if large numbers of slides (10-50 per day) are being stained. Stock containers and staining dishes should have well-fitting lids to prevent evaporation and absorption of moisture from the air. If the clearing agent turns cloudy on addition of the slides from 100% alcohol, there is water in the solution. When clouding occurs, immediately return the slides to 100% alcohol, replace all dehydrating and clearing agents with fresh stock, and continue with the dehydration process.

Modified acid fast stain for Cryptosporidium sp. Although a number of different procedures have been tried for the recovery and identification of *Cryptosporidium* sp. in humans, the best approach seems to be hot or cold modified acid fast stains (Procedure 44.12). The hot modified acid fast method presented here consistently provides excellent results (see Chapter 7, Plate 7.2).[14]

44.3. Additional Techniques for Gastrointestinal Tract Specimens

44.3.a. Sigmoidoscopy material. When repeated fecal examinations fail to reveal the presence of *Entamoeba histolytica,* material obtained during sigmoidoscopy may be valuable in the diagnosis of amebiasis. However, this procedure does not take the place of routine fecal examinations; a series of at least three (six is preferable) fecal specimens should be submitted for each patient having a sigmoidoscopy examination. Material from the mucosal surface should be obtained by **aspiration** or **scraping,** not with a cotton-tipped swab. If

swabs must be used, most of the cotton should be removed (leave just enough to safely cover the end) and should be tightly wound to prevent absorption of the material to be examined.

The specimen should be processed and examined immediately; the number of techniques used will depend on the amount of material obtained. If the specimen is sufficient for both wet preparations and permanent stained smears, proceed as follows. The direct mount should be examined immediately for the presence of moving trophozoites; it may take time for the organisms to become acclimated to this type of preparation, thus motility may not be obvious for several minutes. Care should be taken not to confuse protozoan organisms with macrophages or other tissue cells; any suspect cells should be confirmed with the use of the permanent stained slide. The smears for permanent staining should be prepared at the same time the direct mount is made by gently smearing some of the material onto several slides and immediately placing them into Schaudinn's fixative. The slides can then be stained by any of the techniques mentioned for routine fecal smears. If the material is bloody, contains a lot of mucus, or is a "wet" specimen, 1 or 2 drops of the sample can be mixed with 3 or 4 drops of PVA right on the slide. Allow the smears to dry (overnight if possible) prior to staining.

44.3.b. Duodenal contents. In some instances repeated fecal examinations may fail to confirm a diagnosis of *Giardia lamblia* and *Strongyloides stercoralis* infections. Since these two parasites are normally found in the duodenum, the physician may submit duodenal drainage fluid to the laboratory for examination. The specimen should be submitted without preservatives and should be received and examined within 1 h after being taken. The amount of fluid may vary. It should be centrifuged and the sediment examined as wet

PROCEDURE 44.13. HARADA-MORI FILTER PAPER STRIP CULTURE

1. To each 15 ml centrifuge tube add approximately 3-4 ml of distilled water.
2. In the center of each filter paper strip (3/8 inch by 5 inches) smear, in a relatively thin film, approximately 0.5-1 g of feces.
3. The identification of the specimen can be written in pencil on the piece of filter paper between the waterline and the fecal material.
4. Insert the strip in the tube so that the end of the filter paper strip, usually cut so that it is slightly tapered, is near the bottom of the tube. Caps are not required for the tubes.
5. Maintain the tube in a rack at 24°-28° C, and add water to original level as it is needed. Usually there is rapid evaporation over the first day or two, and then the culture becomes stabilized.
6. The capillary flow of water up the filter paper strip keeps the feces moist. Soluble elements in the feces will be carried out of the fecal mass and accumulate as a dark area at the top of the paper.
7. Tubes should be kept for approximately 10 days, but infective larvae may be found any time after the fifth day.
8. Using a glass pipette, one may withdraw a small amount of fluid from the bottom of the tube; larvae will generally be alive and very active. They may be heat killed within the tube or after removal to the slide; iodine may also be used to kill larvae.
9. Examination of the larvae for typical morphologic features reveals either hookworm, *Strongyloides*, or *Trichostrongylus*.

mounts for the detection of motile organisms. Several mounts should be prepared and examined; because of the dilution factor, the organisms may be difficult to recover with this technique.

Another convenient method of sampling duodenal contents, which eliminates the necessity for intubation, is the use of the Entero-Test. This device consists of a gelatin capsule containing a weighted, coiled length of nylon yarn. The end of the line protrudes through the top of the capsule and is taped to the side of the patient's face. The capsule is then swallowed, the gelatin dissolves, and the weighted string is carried by peristalsis into the duodenum. After approximately 4 h the string is recovered and the bile-stained mucus attached to the string is examined as a wet mount for the presence of organisms. This type of specimen should also be examined immediately after the string is recovered. When the mucus is examined from either duodenal drainage or the Entero-Test capsule, typical "falling leaf" motility of *G. lamblia* trophozoites is usually not visible. The flagella usually are visible as a rapid "flutter," with the organism remaining trapped in the mucus.

44.3.c. Estimation of worm burdens. Although these procedures are not routinely performed, circumstances may arise when it is

---

PROCEDURE 44.14. BAERMANN TECHNIQUE

1. Attach rubber tubing with pinch clamp to the bottom of a 6-inch funnel. Fill the funnel with water. Place wire gauze, with one or two layers of gauze padding, in the funnel.
2. Place a large amount of fecal material on the gauze so that it is covered with water. If the fecal matter is too firm, it should be broken up slightly.
3. Allow the apparatus to stand for at least 2 h. Draw off 10 ml of fluid by releasing the pinch clamp, spin down in a centrifuge, and examine the sediment for larvae.

---

helpful to know the degree of infection in a patient or perhaps to follow the effectiveness of therapy. In certain helminth infections that have little clinical significance, the patient may not be given treatment if the numbers of parasites are small. The parasite burden may be estimated by counting the number of eggs passed in the stool.

The dilution egg-count technique developed by Stoll and Hausheer[45] has been widely used to estimate the number of adult worms present in several helminth infections, specifically hookworm, *Ascaris*, and *Trichuris*. The value of this type of procedure is based on repeated egg counts to detect changes in the numbers present. The direct smear method of Beaver[1,2] has also proved to be helpful in estimating the parasite burden.

Generally *Trichuris trichiura* and hookworm are the only helminth infections in which the egg count will determine whether the patient will receive therapy; low egg counts usu-

ally correlate with a lack of clinical symptoms. Approximately 30,000 eggs of *T. trichiura* per gram indicate the presence of several hundred worms, a worm burden that usually causes definite symptoms. From 2,000 to 5,000 hookworm eggs per gram indicate a clinically significant infection.

NOTE: The presence of even one *Ascaris* is potentially dangerous; when irritated, the parasite tends to migrate while in the gastrointestinal tract, and this migratory habit may cause severe clinical symptoms in the patient.

44.3.d. Recovery of larval-stage nematodes. Nematode infections that give rise to larval stages, which hatch either in the soil or in tissues, may be diagnosed by using culture techniques designed to concentrate the larvae. These procedures are used in hookworm, *Strongyloides*, and *Trichostrongylus* infections. Some of these techniques, which permit the recovery of infective-stage larvae, may be helpful since the eggs of many species are identical and specific identifications are based on larval morphology.

Harada-Mori paper strip culture. As a means of detecting light infections and providing specific identifications, the Harada-Mori filter paper strip culture technique (Procedure 44.13) is very useful. The method was originally introduced by Harada and Mori[16] in 1955 and has been modified by several workers. Fecal specimens should not be refrigerated prior to culture; some of the nematodes are susceptible to cold and do not undergo further development. Since infective-stage larvae may be recovered from the culture system, gloves should be worn to handle the filter paper strip and other equipment.

Baermann technique. When the stools from a patient suspected of having strongyloidiasis are repeatedly negative, the Baermann technique (Procedure 44.14) may be helpful in recovering larvae. The apparatus is designed to allow the larvae to migrate from the fecal ma-

Soil or fecal material

Gauze

Wire screen

Water

Rubber tubing

Clamp

Beaker

N. Kitamura

FIGURE 44.1
Baermann apparatus.

terial through several layers of damp gauze into water, which is centrifuged, thus concentrating the larvae in the bottom of the tube (Figure 44.1). Specimens for this technique should be collected after a mild saline cathartic, not a stool softener.

44.3.e. Hatching procedure for schistosome eggs. When schistosome eggs are recovered from either urine or stool, they should be carefully examined to determine viability. The presence of living miracidia within the eggs indicates an active infection, which may require therapy. The viability of the miracidium larvae

can be determined in two ways: (1) the cilia on the flame cells (primitive excretory cells) may be seen on high-dry power and are usually actively moving, and (2) the larvae may be released from the eggs with the use of a hatching procedure (Procedure 44.15). The eggs usually hatch within several hours when placed in 10 volumes of dechlorinated or spring water. The eggs, which are recovered in the urine, are easily obtained from the sediment and can be examined under the microscope to determine viability.

44.3.f. Cellophane tape preparations. *Enterobius vermicularis* is a roundworm that is worldwide in distribution. It is very common in children and is known as the **pinworm** or the seatworm. The adult female migrates from the anus during the night and deposits her eggs on the perianal area. Since the eggs are deposited outside the gastrointestinal tract, examination of a stool specimen may produce negative results. Although some laboratories use the anal swab technique, pinworm infections are most frequently diagnosed by using the cellophane tape method (Procedure 44.16) for egg recovery. Another collection procedure is illustrated in Figure 44.2. Occasionally the adult female may be found on the surface of a formed stool or on the cellophane tape. Specimens should be taken in the morning **before bathing** or going to the bathroom. For small children, it is best to collect the specimen early in the morning, just before the child awakens.

A series of at least **four to six consecutive negative tapes** should be obtained before ruling out infection with pinworms. However, most laboratories rarely receive more than one or two tapes, and the clinician may decide to treat the patient on the basis of symptoms or recurrent symptoms after the initial diagnosis.

44.3.g. Identification of adult worms. Most adult worms or portions of worms that are submitted to the laboratory for identification are *Ascaris lumbricoides, Enterobius vermicularis,*

PROCEDURE 44.15. HATCHING PROCEDURE FOR SCHISTOSOMES

1. Thoroughly mix a stool specimen in saline and strain through two layers of gauze.
2. Allow the material to settle, pour off the supernatant fluid, and repeat the process.
3. Decant the saline, add spring water, and pour the solution into a 500 or 1,000 ml Erlenmeyer flask or side-arm flask. Add enough fluid so that the level rises into the neck of the flask.
4. Cover the flask with foil or black paper, leaving 1-2 ml of fluid in the neck of the flask exposed to light.
5. Leave the flask at room temperature in subdued light for 2-3 h.
6. Place a bright light at the side of the flask directly opposite and close to the surface of exposed water.
7. The miracidia will come to the illuminated portion of the fluid and can be identified with a hand lens.

PROCEDURE 44.16. EXAMINATION OF CELLOPHANE* TAPE PREPARATIONS

1. Place a strip of cellophane tape on a microscope slide, starting ½ inch from one end and, running toward the same end, continuing around this end across the slide; tear off the strip even with the other end. Place a strip of paper, ½ by 1 inch, between the slide and the tape at the end where the tape is torn flush.
2. To obtain the sample from the peri-anal area, peel back the tape by gripping the label, and with the tape looped adhesive side outward over a wooden tongue depressor held against the slide and extended about 1 inch beyond it, press the tape firmly against the right and left peri-anal folds.
3. Spread the tape back on the slide, adhesive side down.
4. Place name and date on the label. **Note:** Do not use Magic transparent tape, but regular clear cellophane tape.
5. Lift one side of the tape and apply 1 **small drop** of toluene or xylene; press the tape down onto the glass slide.
6. The tape is now cleared; examine under low power and low illumination. The eggs should be visible if present; they are described as football shaped with one slightly flattened side.

*Refers to cellulose (Scotch) tape.

or segments of tapeworms. The adult worms present no particular problems in identification (Section 44.15); however, identification of the *Taenia* species tapeworms is dependent on the gravid proglottids, which contain the fully developed uterine branches. Identification as to species is based on the number of lateral uterine branches that arise from the main uterine stem in the gravid proglottids. Often the uterine branches are not clearly visible; one technique that can be used is the injection of the branches with India ink (Procedure 44.17), allowing them to be easily seen and counted.

A. Use a piece of clear (not frosted) cellophane tape approximately 4 inches (10 cm) long.

B. Hold the tape between thumbs and fore-fingers with sticky side facing outward.

C. Before the patient has arisen from bed in the morning (preferably while the child is still asleep), press the sticky side of the tape against the skin across the anal opening with even, thorough pressure.

D. Gently place the sticky side of the tape down against the surface of a clear glass slide. Label the slide with the patient's name.

FIGURE 44.2
A method for collection of a cellulose (Scotch) tape preparation for pinworm diagnosis. This method dispenses with the tongue depressor (Procedure 44.16), requiring only tape and a glass microscope slide.

PROCEDURE 44.17. IDENTIFICATION OF ADULT WORMS

Using a 1 ml syringe and 25- to 26-gauge needle, India ink can be injected into the central stem or into the uterine pore, filling the uterine branches with ink. The proglottid can then be pressed between two slides and held up to the light, and the branches can be counted (see Figure 44.35). Euparol is another mounting medium that can be used for tapeworm proglottids.

NOTE: Caution should be used in handling proglottids of *Taenia* species, since the eggs of *T. solium* are infective for humans.

44.4. Urogenital Specimens (Trichomoniasis)

The identification of *Trichomonas vaginalis* is usually based on the examination of wet preparations of vaginal and urethral discharges and prostatic secretions. These specimens are diluted with a drop of saline and examined under low power with reduced illumination for the presence of actively motile organisms; urine sediment can be examined in the same way. As the jerky motility of the organisms begins to diminish, it may be possible to observe the undulating membrane, particularly under high-dry power (Figure 44.3). Stained smears are usually not necessary for the identification of this organism; often the number of false-positive and false-negative results reported on the basis of stained smears would strongly suggest the value of confirmation (i.e., observation of the motile organisms).

Some studies indicate that the most sensitive method of detecting *T. vaginalis* is culture. This technique may not be the most practical, and expense may limit its availability. Although commercial media are available, positive control strains should be used each time patient material is cultured.

44.5. Sputum (Paragonimiasis)

When sputum is submitted for examination, it should be "deep sputum" from the lower respiratory passages, not a specimen that is mainly saliva. The specimen should be collected early in the morning (before eating or brushing teeth) and immediately delivered to the laboratory. Sputum is usually examined as a saline or iodine wet mount under low and high-dry microscope power. If the quantity is sufficient, the formalin-ether sedimentation technique can be used. A very mucoid or thick sputum can be centrifuged after the addition of an equal volume of 3% sodium hydroxide. With any technique, the sediment should be carefully examined for the presence of brownish spots or "iron filings," which may be *Paragonimus* eggs.

FIGURE 44.3
Trichomonas vaginalis trophozoite. (Illustration by Nobuko Kitamura.)

NOTE: Care should be taken not to confuse *Entamoeba gingivalis*, which may be found in the mouth and might be seen in the sputum, with *E. histolytica* from a pulmonary abscess. *E. gingivalis* will contain ingested polymorphonuclear neutrophils (PMN); *E. histolytica* will not.

44.6. Aspirates

The diagnosis of certain parasitic infections may be based on procedures using aspirated material. These techniques include microscopic examination, animal inoculation, and culture.

Examination of aspirated material from lung or liver abscesses may reveal the presence of *E. histolytica* (Procedure 44.18); however, the demonstration of these parasites is often extremely difficult for several reasons. Hepatic abscess material taken from the peripheral area, rather than the necrotic center, may reveal organisms, although they may be trapped in the thick pus and not exhibit any motility. The Amoebiasis Research Unit, Durban, South Africa, has recommended using proteolytic enzymes to free the organisms from the aspirate material.

Aspiration of cyst material (usually liver or lung) for the diagnosis of hydatid disease is usually performed when open surgical techniques

PROCEDURE 44.18. EXAMINATION OF LIVER ASPIRATES FOR AMEBAS

1. A minimum of two separate portions of exudate should be removed. The first portion, usually yellowish white, seldom contains organisms. Later portions, which are reddish, are more likely to contain amebas. The best material to examine is the final portion from the wall of the abscess.
2. Ten units of the enzyme streptodornase are added to each 1 ml of thick pus; this mixture is incubated for 30 min at 37° C with repeated shaking.
3. Centrifuge the mixture at 1,000 rpm for 5 min. The sediment may be examined microscopically as wet mounts or used to inoculate culture media. Some of the aspirate can be mixed directly with PVA on a slide and examined as a permanent stained smear.

are used for cyst removal. The aspirated fluid is submitted to the laboratory and examined for the presence of hydatid sand (scolices) or hooklets; the absence of this material does not rule out the possibility of hydatid disease, since some cysts are sterile (Figure 44.4).

Material from lymph nodes, spleen, liver, bone marrow, or spinal fluid may be examined for the presence of trypanosomes or leishmanial forms. Part of the specimen should be examined as a wet preparation to demonstrate motile organisms. Impression smears can also be prepared and stained with Giemsa stain (see Section 44.12, Detection of Blood Parasites). This type of material can also be cultured (specific details are presented in Section 44.9, Culture Techniques).

Specimens obtained from cutaneous ulcers should be aspirated from below the ulcer bed rather than the surface; this type of sample will be more likely to contain the intracellular leishmanial organisms and will be free of bacterial contamination. A few drops of sterile saline may be introduced under the ulcer bed (through uninvolved tissue) by needle (25 gauge) and syringe (1 or 2 ml). The aspirated fluid should be examined as stained smears and should be inoculated into appropriate media (see Section 44.9, Culture Techniques).

44.7. Spinal Fluid

Cases of primary meningoencephalitis are infrequently seen, but the examination of spinal fluid may reveal the causative agent, *Naegleria fowleri* (Plate 44.4), if present. The spinal fluid may range from cloudy to purulent (with or without red blood cells). The cell count ranges from a few hundred to more than 20,000 white blood cells per milliliter, primarily neutrophils; the failure to find bacteria in this type of spinal fluid should alert one to the possibility of primary meningoencephalitis. Motile amebas may be found in unstained spinal fluid; however, one should be very careful not to confuse organisms with various blood and tissue cells that may also be motile.

The classification, transmission, virulence, and disease pathogenesis of the free-living amebic genera *Naegleria*, *Hartmannella*, and *Acanthamoeba* are receiving considerable attention at this time. The question of increasing infections has not been answered, although studies of thermally polluted or enriched waters indicate the presence of such amebas in these situations. Studies have also shown that these organisms have been recovered from asymptomatic human carriers (nasal passages, nasopharyngeal secretions) and have been implicated in chronic or subacute meningoencephalitis as well as acute primary amebic meningoencephalitis.

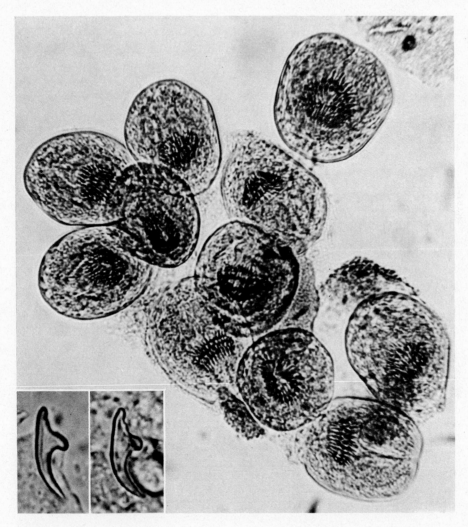

FIGURE 44.4
Echinococcus granulosus, hydatid sand. *Inset,* two individual hooklets (300 ×; inset 1,000 ×).

44.8. Biopsy Material

In some cases biopsy material may be used to confirm the diagnosis of certain parasitic infections. Most of these specimens are sent for routine tissue processing (fixation, embedding, sectioning, and staining). However, fresh material may be sent directly to the laboratory for examination; it is imperative that these specimens be received immediately to prevent deterioration of any organisms present.

Pneumocystis carinii is usually classified with the sporozoa and is recognized as an important cause of pulmonary infection in patients who are immunosuppressed as a result of therapy or patients with congenital or acquired immunologic disorders, including acquired immunodeficiency syndrome (AIDS). The organisms can be demonstrated in stained impression smears of lung material obtained by open, transbronchial, or brush biopsy. *Pneumocystis* can be seen in stained smears of tracheobronchial aspirates, although preparations of lung tissue are more likely to reveal the organisms.

Sputum specimens are generally considered unacceptable for the recovery of *Pneumocystis*.

Regardless of the technique used, multiple specimens may have to be examined to confirm the presence of *P. carinii* organisms. Although a number of different stains are available, the stain most often recommended is Gomori's silver methenamine (GMS), which clearly stains *Pneumocystis* organisms in dark brown or black (Figure 44.5). Both the long and shorter modifications of the silver stain (Chapter 16, Procedure 16.2) are relatively complex, and positive control slides should be included with each specimen to ensure accurate identification of the smears. Although the silver stain yields the most definitive results, toluidine blue O stains are much easier and faster to perform and yield reliable results in the hands of skilled technologists. One modified toluidine blue O method was given in Chapter 16, Procedure 16.3. A recent modification that has shown excellent clarity in our hands (E.J.B.) is that described in Procedure 44.19.

FIGURE 44.5
Pneumocystis carinii from tracheobronchial aspirate; stained with methenamine silver (1,600 ×). (From Markell, E.K., and Voge, M. 1981. Medical parasitology, ed. 5. W.B. Saunders Co., Philadelphia.)

PROCEDURE 44.19. MODIFIED TOLUIDINE BLUE O STAIN FOR *PNEUMOCYSTIS CARINII*

1. Work within a fume hood to prepare sulfation reagent as follows:
   a. Place a Coplin jar into a tub of cool tap water (not <10° C).
   b. Pour 45 ml glacial acetic acid into the Coplin jar.
   c. With a glass pipette, slowly add 15 ml concentrated sulfuric acid, being careful to avoid splashing. Mix gently with the pipette.
   d. Seal the Coplin jar with petroleum jelly or use a tightly capped screwcap.

   The solution can be stored at room temperature and must be prepared fresh each week.

2. Prepare toluidine blue O stain as follows:
   a. Toluidine blue O—actual dye (adjust amount for dye content of stain powder)   0.16 g
   b. Distilled water   60 ml
   c. Concentrated hydrochloric acid   2 ml
   d. Absolute ethanol   140 ml

   Dissolve the dye in the water. Working within a fume hood, slowly add the hydrochloric acid. Add the ethanol last. The solution is stable for 1 year at room temperature.

3. Prepare the specimen (usually bronchoalveolar lavage material) by centrifuging for 15 min at 1,500 × g. Spread the sediment thinly across several slides. If bronchial washing is received, choose mucoid flecks to stain. For particularly mucoid material, the sediment may be treated with Sputolysin and recentrifuged before making slides. Touch preparations of tissues are also suitable for staining. Allow the slides to air dry. Stain a known positive control with each patient specimen. Slides may be heat fixed gently before staining, although this is not necessary.

4. Place the slides in the sulfation reagent for 10 min. With a glass rod or pipette, mix the reagent thoroughly immediately after adding slides and again after 5 min.

5. Place the slides into a glass slide holder (or another Coplin jar) and rinse for 5 min by gently running cold tap water over the slides. Drain excess water by touching the slide edges to paper towels.

6. Place the slides in the toluidine blue O for 3 min. Drain excess stain onto paper towels.

7. Dip the slides into a Coplin jar filled with 95% ethanol for a few (approximately 10) seconds, until most of the blue dye has run off.

8. Further decolorize the slides in absolute ethanol for approximately 10 seconds.

9. Decolorize slides completely by passing them through two changes of xylene or Xyless (Columbia Diagnostics) for approximately 10 seconds.

10. Wipe the backs and sides of the slides to remove excess xylene and immediately coverslip the stained area with a large coverslip (20 × 50 mm) using Permount.

11. Slides can be examined immediately. *Pneumocystis* cysts appear as round, reddish blue structures, approximately 5 μm in diameter, often appearing punched-in or cup shaped, and usually are found in clusters.

Modified from Gosey, Howard, Witebsky, et al. 1985. J. Clin. Microbiol. 22:803.

Cryptosporidium sp. are coccidial protozoa found in the intestinal tract. Human cryptosporidiosis has been confirmed from gastrointestinal biopsies (and more recently from stool) from both patients whose immune responses were diminished (including AIDS patients) and those with normal immune systems. Cryptosporidia differ from other coccidia in that they are limited to the microvillus layer of gastrointestinal cells. Tissue diagnosis has been based on electron microscopy studies and Giemsa-stained smears from jejunal biopsy material and routine tissue processing (paraffin embedding and sectioning). This organism has definitely become more widely recognized as a potential pathogen in both immunosuppressed and immunocompetent hosts and other diagnostic procedures have been developed to facilitate organism recovery and identification, i.e., modified acid fast staining methods of stool (modified Kinyoun's stain, Procedure 44.12) (see Section 44.13.d). The organisms are also visible as refractile bodies in smears made directly or from concentrated feces.

Skin biopsy specimens for the diagnosis of cutaneous amebiasis or cutaneous leishmaniasis should be submitted for tissue processing. A portion of the tissue for the diagnosis of leishmaniasis can be teased apart with sterile needles and inoculated into appropriate culture media (see Section 44.9, Culture Techniques).

The diagnosis of onchocerciasis *(Oncho-cerca volvulus)* may be confirmed by the examination of "skin snips," very thin slices of skin, which are teased apart in saline to release the microfilariae.

Biopsy specimens taken from lymph nodes are submitted for routine tissue processing; impression smears can also be prepared and stained with Giemsa stain (see Section 44.12, Detection of Blood Parasites).

The diagnosis of trichinosis is usually based on clinical findings; however, confirmation may be obtained by the examination of a muscle biopsy (Plate 44.5). The encapsulated larvae can be seen in small pieces of fresh tissue, which are pressed between two slides and examined under low power of the microscope. At necropsy the larvae are most abundant in the diaphragm, masseter muscle, or tongue. Larvae can also be recovered from tissue that has undergone digestion in artificial digestive fluid at 37° C. Figure 44.6 shows the life cycle of this organism.

Tapeworm larvae may occasionally be recovered from a muscle specimen and should be carefully dissected from the capsules. They should then be pressed between two slides and examined under low power for the presence of a scolex with four suckers and a circle of hooks. If no hooks are present, it may be a species other than *Taenia solium*.

In some cases of schistosomiasis the eggs may not be recovered in the stool or urine;

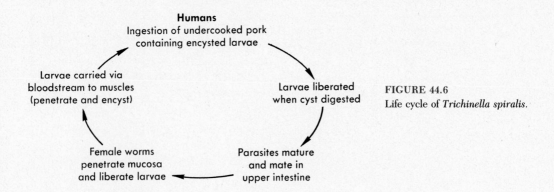

FIGURE 44.6
Life cycle of *Trichinella spiralis*.

however, examination of the rectal or bladder mucosa may reveal eggs of the appropriate species. The mucosal tissue should be compressed between two slides and examined under low power and decreased illumination. The eggs should be carefully examined to determine viability (Section 44.3.e). Small pieces of tissue may be digested with 4% sodium hydroxide for 2-3 h at 60° to 80° C. The eggs, which are recovered by sedimentation or centrifugation, can be examined under the microscope.

44.9. Culture Techniques

Most clinical laboratories do not provide culture techniques for the diagnosis of parasitic organisms; however, the lack of culture procedures should not prevent the correct identification of the majority of parasites. Isolation of intestinal amebas yields a higher number of positive results, provided fresh specimens are received by the laboratory within specified time limits. Most of the intestinal amebas do not culture as well as *Entamoeba histolytica*; however, once the organisms are established in culture, they must be speciated on the basis of morphology. Accurate identification of the organisms can be determined by the examination of permanent stained smears of culture sediment material, although the morphology may not appear typical from stained culture sediment.

Many different media have been developed for the culture of protozoan organisms (some of which are available commercially), and specific directions for their preparation are available in the literature. Types of media that have been widely used include: amebas—Balamuth's aqueous egg yolk infusion[27] and Boeck and Drbohlav's Locke-egg-serum medium[27]; *Trichomonas vaginalis*—Lash's casein hydrolysate serum medium[13] and Feinberg medium[12]; leishmaniae and trypanosomes—Novy-Mac-Neal-Nicolle medium,[13] diphasic blood agar medium (NIH method),[24] and Schneider's *Drosophila* medium.[18] Techniques for the culture

and isolation of other organisms (*Giardia lamblia, Plasmodium* species, and some of the helminths) are more difficult and are often reserved for research purposes.

44.10. Animal Inoculation

Most laboratories have neither the time nor facilities for animal care to provide animal inoculation procedures for the diagnosis of parasitic infections. Host specificity for many parasites also limits the kinds of laboratory animals available for these procedures. Occasionally animal studies may be requested; included here are several procedures that can be used.

The hamster is the animal of choice for inoculation procedures designed to recover leishmanial organisms. After intraperitoneal or intratesticular inoculation, the infection may develop very slowly over a period of several months; in some cases a generalized infection develops more quickly, and the animal may die in several days. Splenic and testicular aspirates should be examined for the presence of intracellular organisms; stained smears should be prepared and carefully examined with the oil immersion lens.

Mice are generally used for the isolation of *Toxoplasma gondii*, although most cases are diagnosed on clinical and serologic findings. Mice that are inoculated through the peritoneum develop a fulminating infection that leads to death within a few days. Organisms can be easily recovered from the ascitic fluid and should be examined as stained smears. Giemsa stain is recommended for both types of inoculation studies listed above (specific staining techniques are found in Section 44.12, Detection of Blood Parasites).

44.11. Serodiagnosis

Although serologic procedures for the diagnosis of parasitic diseases have been available for many years, they are generally not performed by most clinical laboratories. The procedures vary both in sensitivity and specificity and at times may be difficult to interpret. The Centers for Disease Control (CDC) offers several serologic procedures for diagnostic purposes, some of which are still in the experimental stages and not available elsewhere. For a discussion of specific procedures, see Chapter 12. The procedures mentioned here have been found to give fairly reproducible results at CDC.[20] Although commercial antigens and diagnostic kits are available, results from different reagents have been variable. Developmental work using monoclonal reagents is in progress, but commercially prepared kits or components are not yet available. Diagnostic tests for 18 parasitic infections are presented in Table 44.4.

TABLE 44.4
Immunodiagnostic Tests for Parasitic Diseases

PARASITIC DISEASES	COMPLEMENT FIXATION	AGGLUTINATION TESTS — BENTONITE FLOCCULATION	AGGLUTINATION TESTS — INDIRECT HEMAGGLUTINATION	AGGLUTINATION TESTS — LATEX	SPECIAL TESTS	INDIRECT IMMUNOFLUORESCENCE	IMMUNODIFFUSION	IMMUNOELECTROPHORESIS	COUNTERCURRENT IMMUNOELECTROPHORESIS	ENZYME-LINKED IMMUNOASSAY	RADIOIMMUNOASSAY	DETECTION OF CIRCULATING ANTIGEN
African trypanosomiasis	▲		▲			■	■			■		
Amebiasis	■	■	■	■	○AC	■	■	■	■	▲		○
Ancylostomiasis	○		▲			○	○					
Ascariasis	■	■				▲	▲	○		■	○	
Chagas	■		■	■	■A	■	○	▲		▲		○
Clonorchiasis	■					○	○	○				○
Cysticercosis	▲	▲	■	▲		▲	▲		○	○		
Echinococcosis	■	■	■	■		■	■	■	■	■	○	
Fascioliasis	■	○	■	▲		■	■	■	■	○		
Filariasis	▲	■	■	○		■		▲	▲	▲		▲
Giardiasis						▲	○					
Leishmaniasis	■		■	■	■A	■	○	○	○	▲	○	
Malaria	▲		■	▲		■	■	○	▲	■	○	▲
Paragonimiasis	■	○	○			▲	▲	○	○			○
Pneumocystosis	■			○		■	■					▲
Schistosomiasis	■	■	■	○	■BC	■	▲	■	▲	■	○	■
Strongyloidiasis			■			▲				○		
Toxocariasis	○	■				▲	■	○		■	○	○
Toxoplasmosis	■		■	■	■C	■	○			■	○	▲
Trichinellosis	■	■	■			■	■	▲	■			○

From Kagan, I.G.: personal communication.
○, reported in the literature; ■, evaluated test; ▲, experimental test; A, direct agglutination; B, circumoval precipitin test (COPT); C, FIAX automated fluoroimmunoassay.

The ELISA procedure is presently being evaluated for a number of parasitic infections. A significant contribution of the ELISA method will be detection of antigen in the body fluids of patients with parasitic diseases. With purified antigens the usefulness of techniques such as radioimmunoassay, ELISA, FIAX, and defined antigen substrate spheres (DASS) will be greatly expanded.

At the present time immunodiagnostic procedures are most widely used for amebiasis, toxoplasmosis, leishmaniasis, Chagas' disease, trichinosis, schistosomiasis, cysticercosis, and hydatid disease.

44.11.a. Amebiasis. The sensitivity of the procedures for amebiasis depends on the type of disease present; a very low degree of sensitivity is found with sera from asymptomatic carriers, increased sensitivity from patients with amebic dysentery, and the greatest sensitivity with sera from those patients with extraintestinal disease. The complement fixation (CF) procedure has generally been replaced by the indirect hemagglutination (IHA), countercurrent immunoelectrophoresis (CIE), and indirect fluorescent antibody (IFA) procedures; these three have approximately the same degree of sensitivity.

A new test that has been adapted to a routine diagnosis of amebiasis is the FIAX, a new fluorescence technique in which the fluorescence is measured in a fluorometer (Chapter 11).[19,49] Techniques have also been developed for detection of antigen in feces. The sensitivity is reported to be quite good, although the only organism detected would be E. histolytica.[34,42]

44.11.b. Toxoplasmosis. Approximately half of all adults in the United States have antibody to Toxoplasma. All infestations are acquired ultimately via cats, either directly with close contact or by ingestion of trophozoites or cysts in food (particularly raw meat) (Figure 44.7). The methylene blue dye test (MBD; Sabin-Feldman dye test) has been used for many years for the serologic diagnosis of toxoplasmosis. However, this procedure is being replaced by the IHA and IFA procedures, both of which are technically simple to perform and utilize a killed antigen rather than live organisms (used in the MBD test). Although all three procedures are approximately the same in terms of specificity and sensitivity, the IF procedure can be performed using specific conjugates of IgM, although interpretation of such results may be difficult and must be correlated with the patient's clinical status. Congenital infections are generally indicated when sera from newborns are positive with IgM conjugates.

However, IgM antibody methods have been subject to both false positive and false negative results because of rheumatoid factor, blocking antibody, and the induction of fetal IgM antibodies against maternal globulin.[43] Results from laboratories which employ test methods that do not try to eliminate the above sources of error may be subject to misinterpretation. The double sandwich ELISA IgM test has eliminated many of these problems.[38] In addition to this method, the ion exchange column chromatography methodology has successfully removed rheumatoid factor and blocking antibody from sera.

Because a different type of antigen is used for each test, the combination of the IFA and IHA procedures allows more accurate interpretation, particularly if the titers are borderline in terms of clinical significance.

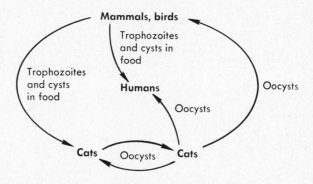

FIGURE 44.7
Life cycle of *Toxoplasma gondii.*

44.11.c. Pneumocystosis. The tests of choice for pneumocystosis are the CF and IFA tests. Antigens from either infected rat or human lung tissue are used in both tests and can detect disease in approximately 85% of infected patients. A direct fluorescent antibody test has been developed for the detection of organisms in mucus and sputum smears and tissue biopsies.[25]

During the past few years, additional work has been done in the development of diagnostic procedures designed to detect *Pneumocystis* antigenemia. These have included the CEP (also referred to as counterimmunoelectrophoresis, CIE) and the ELISA. Unfortunately these procedures are still not available commercially. None of these tests have been used successfully in routine clinical diagnosis because of a lack of specificity or sensitivity. Because a large portion of the general population is positive for antibody, the detection of specific antibody in selected patients may be of little value. Also, in addition to antigen being detected in a large number of patients with *Pneumocystis* pneumonia, it has also been detected in patients with no pneumonia and with pneumonia attributable to other causes. The development of culture techniques for this organism should lead to more specific antigen production.

44.11.d. Leishmaniasis. The serologic procedures (IHA, IFA, and CF) available for visceral leishmaniasis are quite helpful in making the diagnosis, and the IFA test is now being used routinely with excellent results being reported using amastigote antigen for cutaneous leishmaniasis. The IFA test is more specific than ELISA for the diagnosis of cutaneous leishmaniasis, but neither is as satisfactory as microscopic examinations. Both methods were acceptable for the diagnosis of visceral leishmaniasis when promastigote forms of *Leishmania donovani* were used as antigen.

44.11.e. Chagas' disease. Although both the IHA and CF procedures are used for the diagnosis of Chagas' disease, the CF is more sensitive. A direct agglutination technique introduced by Vattuone and Yanovsky[51] in 1971 is very sensitive when used with sera from patients with acute disease; the procedure also provides good specificity in terms of cross-reactivity with leishmaniasis. The ELISA technique has been used with a reported sensitivity of 98%, and eluates of blood samples collected on filter papers can be used. The CIE and CF techniques have shown a 92% agreement; however, the sensitivity of the CIE test was less than that of the CF test. Studies also indicate that serum from patients with a positive CF for Chagas' disease contains immunoglobins that bind to cryostat sections of heart muscle (animals, including the mouse). The antibody binds to the endothelial lining of the blood vessels, the vascular musculature around the arteries, and the interstitium of striated muscles; the fluorescence of the triad of tissues constitutes a positive test (essentially no false-positive tests with normal persons or patients with other cardiovascular diseases).

44.11.f. Trichinosis. A number of procedures are available for the diagnosis of trichinosis. The bentonite flocculation (BF) test has a high degree of specificity and is the standard procedure used at CDC; it is used to measure an increase or decrease in serum titers during the acute phase of the infection, yet it is not too sensitive and does not react with residual antibodies from past exposure to the parasite. It is important diagnostically when a series of serum samples from one patient show a rise in titers. When low titers are obtained, it is recommended that additional serologic tests (different types) may be valuable in confirming the diagnosis. The IFA procedure is the most sensitive[21,23,46] and can be used to detect antibodies in pigs infected with less than one larva per gram of diaphragm muscle tissue. The ELISA technique has also been found to be sensitive enough to detect low trichina infection in naturally infected pigs.[24]

44.11.g. Schistosomiasis. Several different tests (cholesterol-lecithin flocculation, BF, CF, and IFA) are used for the diagnosis of schistosomiasis; however, they all share problems of specificity and sensitivity. There has been increased use of the IFA procedure, which uses sections of adult worms for the antigen and which has proved to be the most sensitive technique (less cross-reactivity with trichina sera).

The circumoval precipitin test is used extensively in the Orient for the diagnosis of *Schistosoma japonicum* infection. There are also a number of studies using the ELISA technique; one study reports this test to be as sensitive as the IFA and CF tests with adult worms used as antigen but indicates that the ELISA was more specific.[28]

44.11.h. Cysticercosis. Extensive evaluation of the diagnostic tests for cysticercosis has been difficult to achieve because of the small number of sera available from proved human infections in the United States. Workers in South Africa reported the IHA procedure as providing 85% positive results with sera from proved cases of human infection.[36,37] Although the IHA was 100% reactive with sera from heavily infected animals, only 26% of those that were lightly infected were reactive. Biagi and associates[4] in Mexico reported the best results with the IHA. There are still difficulties with both specificity and sensitivity, and a higher positive titer with human sera may have to be selected as the standard to rule out false-positive reactions. The double-diffusion procedure, when evaluated by CDC, was found to be insensitive using both animal and human sera. Cross-reactions with sera from patients infected with *Echinococcus* species, *Taenia saginata*, and *Coenurus* species have been reported.

44.11.i. Echinococcosis. The IHA, IFA, and immunoelectrophoresis (IE) procedures are considered to be the tests of choice for the diagnosis of echinococcosis. The IHA and BF procedures are routinely used at CDC, the

IHA being the more sensitive test. High IHA titers usually indicate the presence of hydatid disease; however, low titers are difficult to interpret and have been found in sera from patients with collagen vascular diseases or hepatic cirrhosis. Hydatid cysts in the lung (sera, 33%-50% sensitivity) are less likely to be diagnosed by serologic means than those found in the liver (sera, 82%-86% sensitivity). The IE test has been evaluated in a number of countries; however, a double-diffusion band 5 (DD5) test has been reported to be more sensitive and more specific than the IE test.[8] CIE tests have also been reported to be very specific and sensitive, and the ELISA has also been evaluated.

44.12. Detection of Blood Parasites

44.12.a. Laboratory diagnosis of malaria. Malaria is one of the few acute parasitic infections that can be life threatening. For this reason any laboratory that offers this type of diagnostic service must be willing to provide technical expertise on a 24 h basis, 7 days per week.

The definitive diagnosis of malaria is based on the demonstration of the parasites in the blood. Two types of blood films are used. The **thick film** allows the examination of a larger amount of blood and is used as a screening procedure; the **thin film** allows speciation of the parasite.

Blood films are usually prepared when the patient is admitted; samples should be taken at intervals of 6-18 h for at least 3 successive days. Two hundred microscopic fields should be examined before a film is signed out as negative. If possible, the smears should be prepared from blood obtained from the finger or earlobe; the blood should flow freely. If patient contact is not possible and the quality of the submitted slides may be poor, a tube of fresh blood should be requested (EDTA anticoagulant is recommended) and smears prepared immediately after the blood is received.

PROCEDURE 44.20. GIEMSA STAIN

Giemsa stain is available commercially as a concentrated stock solution or as a powder for those who wish to make their own stain; there seems to be very little difference between the two preparations.

NOTE: Remember that automatic differential instruments used in hematology are not designed to recognize intracellular (red blood cell) parasites. Any suspected parasitic infection or presumptive diagnosis of fever of unknown origin (FUO) mandates a manual blood smear examination.

Reagents

1. Stock Giemsa stain:

Giemsa stain powder, certified	600 mg
Methanol, absolute and certified neutral, acetone free	50 ml
Glycerine, neutral, certified	50 ml

Grind well small portions of stain and glycerine in mortar and collect mixtures in a 500 or 1,000 ml flask until all measured material is mixed. Stopper flask with cotton plug, cover with heavy paper, place in 55°-60° C water bath for 2 h, making sure that the water reaches the level of the stain. Shake gently at ½ h intervals. Allow to cool; add alcohol.

Use a portion of the measured alcohol to wash out the mortar and add to the flask. Store in brown bottle. Allow to stand for 2-3 weeks. Filter before use.

2. 10% stock solution of Triton X-100:

Triton X-100	10 ml
Distilled water	100 ml

3. Stock buffers:
   a. Disodium phosphate buffer:

Na_2HPO_4 anhydrous	9.5 g
Distilled water	1,000 ml

   b. Sodium acid phosphate buffer:

$NaH_2PO_4 \cdot H_2O$	9.2 g
Distilled water	1,000 ml

4. Buffered water: pH range 7.0-7.2; check with pH meter before use.

Disodium phosphate buffer	61 ml
Sodium acid phosphate buffer	39 ml
Distilled water	900 ml

5. Triton–buffered water solutions:
   a. 0.01% Triton–buffered water:

Stock 10% aqueous Triton X-100	1 ml
Buffered water	1,000 ml

Use for thin blood films or combination of thin and thick blood films.

   b. 0.1% Triton–buffered water:

Stock 10% Triton X-100	10 ml
Buffered water	1,000 ml

Use for thick blood films.

PROCEDURE 44.21. STAINING THIN FILMS

1. Fix blood films in absolute methanol (acetone free) for 30 seconds.
2. Allow slides to air dry.
3. Immerse slides in a solution of 1 part Giemsa stock (commercial liquid stain or stock prepared from powder) to 10-50 parts of Triton-buffered water (pH 7.0-7.2). Stain 10-60 minutes (see note below). Fresh working stain should be prepared from stock solution each day.
4. Dip slides briefly in Triton X-100 buffered water.
5. Drain thoroughly in vertical position and allow to air dry.

   NOTE: A good general rule for stain dilution versus staining time is that if dilution is 1:20, stain for 20 min; if 1:30, stain for 30 min; and so forth. However, a series of stain dilutions and staining times should be tried to determine the best dilution/time for each batch of stock stain.

PROCEDURE 44.22. STAINING THICK FILMS

The procedure to be followed for thick films is the same as for thin films, except that the first two steps are omitted. If the slide has a thick film at one end and a thin film at the other, fix only the thin portion, and then stain both parts of the film simultaneously.

To prepare the thick film place 2 or 3 small drops of fresh blood on an alcohol-cleaned slide. With the corner of another slide, and using a circular motion, mix the drops and spread the blood over an area about 2 cm in diameter. Continue stirring for about 30 seconds to prevent formation of fibrin strands, which may obscure the parasites after staining. If the blood is too thick or any grease remains on the slide, the blood will flake off during staining. Allow the film to air dry (room temperature) in a dust-free area. Never apply heat to a thick film since heat will fix the blood, causing the red blood cells to remain intact during staining; the result is stain retention and subsequent inability to identify any parasites present.

The thin blood film is used primarily for specific parasite identification, although the number of organisms per field is much reduced compared with the thick film (see Plates 44.6 to 44.12). The thin film is prepared in exactly the same manner one used for the differential blood count. After the film has air dried (do not apply heat), it may be stained. The necessity for fixation before staining depends on the stain selected.

44.12.b. Staining blood films. For accurate identification of blood parasites, it is very important that a laboratory develop proficiency in the use of at least one good staining method. As a general rule, blood films should be stained as soon as possible, since prolonged storage results in stain retention.

The stains used are generally of two types. One has the fixative in combination with the staining solution, so that both fixation and staining occur at the same time. Wright stain (Chapter 46) is an example of this type of staining solution. Giemsa stain (Procedure 44.20) represents the other type of staining solution, in which the fixative and stain are separate; thus, the thin film must be fixed prior to staining (Procedures 44.21 and 44.22). There are also methods available for the identification of malarial parasites with the use of acridine orange (Chapter 46) and other DNA-binding dyes, the smears being examined using fluorescence microscopy.

When slides are removed from either type of staining solution, they should be dried in a vertical position. After being air dried, they may be examined under oil immersion by placing the oil directly on the uncovered blood film.

Specimens may be submitted from patients with *Plasmodium falciparum* infections who do not yet have gametocytes in the blood. Consequently, a low-level parasitemia with delicate ring forms might be missed without extensive oil immersion examination of the blood films (at least 200 oil immersion fields).

Results. Giemsa stain colors the components of blood as follows: erythrocytes, pale gray-blue; nuclei of white blood cells, purple and pale purple cytoplasm; eosinophilic granules, bright purple-red; neutrophilic granules, deep pink-purple.

There have been many studies using immunodiagnostic procedures for the diagnosis of malaria; However, these procedures are not routinely performed in most laboratories. Sulzer and Wilson[47] have reported the use of thick-smear antigens prepared from washed parasitized blood cells. This type of antigen is used in the IFA procedure, which has a 95% sensitivity and a false-positive rate of 1% at a titer of 1:16.[48] The IHA has also been used and evaluated by a number of workers.

In some areas of the world where *P. falciparum* is endemic, there is also a high incidence of hemoglobin S (HbS), thalassemia, and glucose-6-phosphate dehydrogenase (G-6-PD) deficiency carriers. The young heterozygous carrier of HbS gains some protection against *P. falciparum*. Apparently, G-6-PD deficiency and thalassemia are also associated with increased resistance.

Miller and co-workers[30] reported that Duffy-positive human erythrocytes are easily infected with *Plasmodium knowlesi*; however,

Duffy-negative human erythrocytes are resistant to infection. They suggest that the resistance of many west Africans and approximately 70% of American blacks to *Plasmodium vivax* may be related to the high incidence of Duffy-negative erythrocytes in these groups. In east Africa, where there is a higher incidence of Duffy-positive red cells, *P. vivax* is more common.

IDENTIFICATION OF ANIMAL PARASITES
44.13. Intestinal Protozoa

The protozoa are unicellular organisms, most of which are microscopic. They possess a number of specialized organelles, which are responsible for life functions and which allow further division of the group into classes.

The class Sarcodina contains the organisms that move by means of cytoplasmic protrusions called pseudopodia. Included in this group are free-living organisms, as well as nonpathogenic and pathogenic organisms found in the intestinal tract and other areas of the body.

The Mastigophora, or flagellates, contain specialized locomotor organelles called flagella: long, thin cytoplasmic extensions that may vary in number and position depending on the species. Different genera may live in the intestinal tract, the bloodstream, or various tissues. The blood- and tissue-dwelling flagellates are discussed in the section Detection of Blood Parasites.

The class Ciliata contains a number of species that move by means of cilia, short extensions of cytoplasm that cover the surface of the organism. This group contains only one organism that infects humans: *Balantidium coli* infects the intestinal tract and may produce severe symptoms.

Members of the class Sporozoa are found in the blood and other tissues and have a complex life cycle that involves both sexual and asexual generations. The four species of *Plasmodium*, the cause of malaria, are found in

44.1

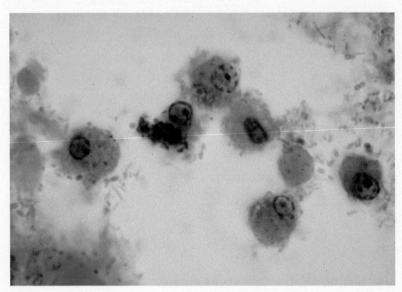

44.2

PLATE 44.1. Charcot-Leyden crystals.
PLATE 44.2. Polymorphonuclear leukocytes.

44.3

44.4

PLATE 44.3. *Blastocystis hominis* (larger objects) and yeast cells (smaller, more homogeneous objects).
PLATE 44.4. *Naegleria* in brain tissue. Hematoxylin and eosin stain.

44.5

PLATE 44.5. *Trichinella spiralis* larvae (encysted in muscle).

PLATE 44.6. *Plasmodium vivax* in thick smear. **1,** Ameboid trophozoites. **2,** Schizont, two divisions of chromatin. **3,** Mature schizont. **4,** Microgametocyte. **5,** Blood platelets. **6,** Nucleus of neutrophil. **7,** Eosinophil. **8,** Blood platelet associated with cellular remains of young erythrocytes. (From Wilcox.[53])

44.7

PLATE 44.7. *Plasmodium malariae.* **1,** Young ring form trophozoite of quartan malaria. **2-4,** Young trophozoite forms of parasite showing gradual increase of chromatin and cytoplasm. **5,** Developing ring form trophozoite showing pigment granule. **6,** Early band form trophozoite, elongated chromatin, some pigment apparent. **7-12,** Some forms that developing trophozoite of quartan may take. **13, 14,** Mature trophozoites, one a band form. **15-19,** Phases in development of schizont (presegmenting schizonts). **20,** Mature schizont. **21,** Immature microgametocyte. **22,** Immature macrogametocyte. **23,** Mature microgameotcyte. **24,** Mature macrogametocyte. (From Wilcox.[53])

PLATE 44.8. *Plasmodium malariae* in thick smear. **1,** Small trophozoites. **2,** Growing trophozoites. **3,** Mature trophozoites. **4-6,** Schizonts (presegmenting) with varying numbers of divisions of chromatin. **7,** Mature schizonts. **8,** Nucleus of leukocyte. **9,** Blood platelets. **10,** Cellular remains of young erythrocytes. (From Wilcox.[53])

44.9

PLATE 44.9. *Plasmodium falciparum.* 1, Very young ring form trophozoite. 2, Double infection of single cell with young trophozoites, one a marginal form, the other signet ring form. 3, 4, Young trophozoites showing double chromatin dots. 5-7, Developing trophozoite forms. 8, Three medium trophozoites in one cell. 9, Trophozoite showing pigment in cell containing Maurer's dots. 10, 11, Two trophozoites in each of two cells, showing variations of forms that parasites may assume. 12, Almost mature trophozoite showing haze of pigment throughout cytoplasm. Maurer's dots in cell. 13, Estivoautumnal "slender forms." 14, Mature trophozoite showing clumped pigment. 15, Parasite in process of initial chromatin division. 16-19, Various phases of development of schizont presegmenting (schizonts). 20, Mature schizont. 21-24, Successive forms in development of gametocyte, usually not found in peripheral circulation. 25, Immature macrogametocyte. 26, Mature macrogametocyte. 27, Immature microgametocyte. 28, Mature microgametocyte. (From Wilcox.[53])

PLATE 44.10. *Plasmodium falciparum* in thick film. **1,** Small trophozoites. **2,** Normal gametocytes. **3,** Slightly distorted gametocyte. **4,** "Rounded-up" gametocyte. **5,** Disintegrated gametocyte. **6,** Nucleus of leukocyte. **7,** Blood platelets. **8,** Cellular remains of young erythrocyte. (From Wilcox.[53])

PLATE 44.11. *Plasmodium ovale.* **1,** Young ring-shaped trophozoite. **2-5,** Older ring-shaped trophozoites. **6-8,** Older ameboid trophozoites. **9, 11, 12,** Doubly infected cells, trophozoites. **10,** Doubly infected cell, young gametocytes. **13,** First stage of the schizont. **14-19,** Schizonts, progressive stages. **20,** Mature gametocyte. (From Markell and Voge.[27])

44.12

44.13

PLATE 44.12.   *Entamoeba histolytica* trophozoite (contains ingested red blood cells).
PLATE 44.13.   *Entamoeba histolytica* trophozoite.

44.14

PLATE 44.14. *E. histolytica* cyst.

44.15

PLATE 44.15. *Entamoeba hartmanni* trophozoite. *Bottom, E. hartmanni* cyst.

44.16

PLATE 44.16. *Entamoeba coli* trophozoite.

44.17

PLATE 44.17. *Top, E. coli* cyst, iodine stain. *Bottom, E. coli* cyst, trichrome stain (poor preservation).

44.18

PLATE 44.18. *Top, Endolimax nana* trophozoite. *Bottom left, E. nana* cyst. *Bottom right, E. nana* cyst.

44.19

PLATE 44.19. *Top, Iodamoeba bütschlii* trophozoites. *Bottom left, I. bütschlii* cyst. *Bottom right, I. bütschlii* cyst.

this group and are discussed in the section Detection of Blood Parasites. Members of the genera *Isospora* and *Cryptosporidium* are found in the intestinal mucosa. Both *Isospora* and *Cryptosporidium* have been seen with increasing frequency in specimens from immunosuppressed patients, particularly those with AIDS.[7,32,33]

The majority of the intestinal protozoa live in the colon, with the exception of the flagellate *Giardia lamblia* and the coccidian parasites *Isospora belli* and *Cryptosporidium*, which are found in the small intestine. *I. belli* is the only protozoan that is an obligate tissue parasite in the intestinal tract and is passed in the stool as oocysts; the other members of the group, with the exception of *Cryptosporidium*, exist in the intestinal tract in the trophozoite or cyst stages. The important characteristics of the intestinal protozoa are found in Tables 44.5-44.10. The clinically important intestinal protozoa are generally considered to be *Entamoeba histolytica*, *Dientamoeba fragilis*, *G. lamblia*, *I. belli*, *Cryptosporidium*, and *Balantidium coli*. *E. histolytica* is the most important species and may invade other tissues of the body, resulting in severe symptoms and possible death. *D. fragilis* has been associated with diarrhea, nausea, vomiting, and other nonspecific abdominal complaints. *G. lamblia* is probably the most common protozoan organism found in persons in this country and is known to cause symptoms ranging from mild diarrhea, flatulence, and vague abdominal pains to acute, severe diarrhea to steatorrhea and a typical malabsorption syndrome. There have been a number of documented waterborne/foodborne outbreaks during the past several years, and the beaver has been implicated as an animal reservoir host for *G. lamblia*. It is speculated that other animals may be involved as well. With present improved culture techniques and the ability to harvest material for antigen, serologic tests for giardiasis have been developed for both antibody and antigen.

Another organism, *Blastocystis hominis* (Plate 44.3), is also now considered to be pathogenic for humans. It has been reclassified as a protozoan, and there are reports of *B. hominis* as an agent of human enteric disease.[54]

Sarcocystis sp. appears in Table 44.10 but will not be discussed in detail. According to the literature, extraintestinal human sarcocystosis is rare, with a much lower incidence than that seen with the intestinal infection.

The identification of intestinal protozoan parasites is difficult, at best, and the importance of the permanent stained slide should be reemphasized (Procedure 44.9). It is important to remember that many artifacts (vegetable material, debris, cells of human origin) may mimic protozoan organisms on a wet mount (Figure 44.8). The important diagnostic characteristics will be visible on the stained smear, and the final identification of protozoan parasites should be confirmed with the permanent stain.

44.13.a. Amebas. Occasionally when fresh stool material is examined as a direct wet mount, motile trophozoites may be observed. *E. histolytica* is described as having directional and progressive motility, whereas the other amebas tend to move more slowly and at random. The cytoplasm usually appears finely granular, less frequently coarsely granular, or vacuolated. Bacteria, yeast cells, or debris may be present in the cytoplasm. The presence of red blood cells in the cytoplasm is usually considered to be diagnostic for *E. histolytica* (Plates 44.12 to 44.14).

Nuclear morphology is one of the most important criteria used for identification; nuclei of the genus *Entamoeba* contain a relatively small karyosome and have chromatin material arranged on the nuclear membrane (Figures 44.9 to 44.11 and Plates 44.15 to 44.17). The nuclei of the other two genera, *Endolimax* and *Iodamoeba*, tend to have very large karyosomes with no peripheral chromatin on the nuclear

Text continued on p. 826.

TABLE 44.5
Morphologic Criteria Used To Identify Intestinal Amebic Trophozoites

	ENTAMOEBA HISTOLYTICA	ENTAMOEBA HARTMANNI	ENTAMOEBA COLI	ENDOLIMAX NANA	IODAMOEBA BÜTSCHLII
Size (diameter or length)*	12-60 µm; usual range, 15-20 µm; invasive forms may be > 20 µm	5-12 µm; usual range, 8-10 µm	15-50 µm; usual range, 20-25 µm	6-12 µm; usual range, 8-10 µm	8-20 µm; usual range, 12-15 µm
Motility	Progressive with hyaline, fingerlike pseudopods, motility may be rapid	Usually nonprogressive	Sluggish, nondirectional, with blunt pseudopods	Sluggish, usually nonprogressive	Sluggish, usually nonprogressive
Number of nuclei	One; difficult to see in unstained preparations, usually not seen	One; usually not seen in unstained preparations	One; often visible in unstained preparations	One; occasionally visible in unstained preparations	One; usually not visible in unstained preparations
Nucleus Peripheral chromatin (stained)	Fine granules, uniform in size, usually evenly distributed; may have beaded appearance	May appear as solid ring rather than beaded; nucleus may stain more darkly than E. histolytica, although morphology is similar	May be clumped and unevenly arranged on membrane; may also appear as solid, dark ring with no beads or clumps	No peripheral chromatin	No peripheral chromatin
Karyosome (stained)	Small, usually compact; centrally located but may also be eccentric	Usually small and compact; may be centrally located or eccentric	Large, not compact; may or may not be eccentric; may be diffuse and darkly stained	Large, irregularly shaped; may appear "blotlike"; many nuclear variations common	Large, may be surrounded by refractile granules that are difficult to see
Cytoplasm Appearance (stained)	Finely granular, "ground-glass" appearance; clear differentiation of ectoplasm and endoplasm; if present, vacuoles usually small	Finely granular	Granular with little differentiation into ectoplasm and endoplasm; usually vacuolated	Granular, vacuolated	Coarsely granular; may be highly vacuolated
Inclusions (stained)	Noninvasive organism may contain bacteria; presence of red blood cells diagnostic	May contain bacteria; no red blood cells	Bacteria, yeast, other debris	Bacteria	Bacteria, yeast, other debris

*These sizes refer to wet preparation measurements. Organisms on a permanent stained smear may be 1-1.5 µm smaller because of artificial shrinkage.

TABLE 44.6
Morphologic Criteria Used To Identify Intestinal Flagellate Trophozoites

	DIENTAMOEBA FRAGILIS	TRICHOMONAS HOMINIS	GIARDIA LAMBLIA	CHILOMASTIX MESNILI	ENTEROMONAS HOMINIS	RETORTAMONAS INTESTINALIS
Shape and size*	Shaped like amebas; 5-15 µm; usual range, 9-12 µm	Pear shaped; 8-20 µm; usual range, 11-12 µm	Pear shaped; 10-20 µm; usual range, 12-15 µm	Pear shaped; 6-24 µm; usual range, 10-15 µm	Oval; 4-10 µm; usual range, 8-9 µm	Pear shaped or oval; 4-9 µm; usual range, 6-7 µm
Motility	Usually nonprogressive; pseudopodia angular, serrated, or broad lobed and almost transparent	Jerky and rapid	"Falling leaf," organisms may be trapped in mucus; only flagella flutter seen.	Stiff, rotary	Jerky	Jerky
Number of nuclei	Percentage may vary, but approximately 40% of organisms have 1 nucleus and 60% 2 nuclei; not visible in unstained preparations; no peripheral chromatin, karyosome composed of cluster of 4-8 granules	One; not visible in unstained mounts	Two; not visible in unstained mounts	One; not visible in unstained mounts	One; not visible in unstained mounts	One; not visible in unstained mounts
Number of flagella (usually difficult to see)	No visible flagella	3-5 anterior, 1 posterior	4 lateral, 2 ventral, 2 caudal	3 anterior, 1 in cytostome	3 anterior, 1 posterior	1 anterior, 1 posterior
Other features	Cytoplasm finely granular and may be vacuolated with ingested bacteria, yeasts, and other debris	Axostyle (slender rod) protrudes beyond posterior end and may be visible; undulating membrane extends length of body	Sucking disk occupying ⅓ to ½ of ventral surface; pear-shaped front view, spoon-shaped side view	Prominent cytostome extending ⅓ to ½ length of body; spiral groove across ventral surface	One side of body flattened; posterior flagellum extends free posteriorly or laterally	Prominent cytostome extending approximately ½ length of body

*These sizes refer to wet preparation measurements. Organism on a permanent stained smear may be 1-1.5 µm smaller because of artificial shrinkage.

TABLE 44.7
Morphologic Criteria Used To Identify Intestinal Amebic Cysts

	ENTAMOEBA HISTOLYTICA	ENTAMOEBA HARTMANNI	ENTAMOEBA COLI	ENDOLIMAX NANA	IODAMOEBA BÜTSCHLII
Size*	10-20 μm; usual range, 12-15 μm	5-10 μm; usual range, 6-8 μm	10-35 μm; usual range, 15-25 μm	5-10 μm; usual range 6-8 μm	5-20 μm; usual range, 10-12 μm
Shape	Usually spherical	Usually spherical	Usually spherical, occasionally oval, triangular, or other shapes; may be distorted on stained slide if fixation poor	Spherical, ovoidal, or ellipsoidal	Ovoidal, ellipsoidal, or other shapes
Number of nuclei	Mature cyst 4; immature, 1 or 2 nuclei may be seen; nuclear characteristics difficult to see on wet preparation	Mature cyst 4; immature, 1 or 2 nuclei may be seen; 2 nucleated cysts very common	Mature cyst 8; occasionally 16 or more nuclei may be seen; immature cysts with 2 or more nuclei occasionally seen	Mature cyst, 4; immature cysts, 2 (very rarely seen and may resemble cysts of *Enteromonas hominis*)	Mature cyst, 1
Nucleus					
Peripheral chromatin (stained)	Peripheral chromatin present; fine, uniform granules, evenly distributed; nuclear characteristics may not be as clearly visible as in trophozoite	Fine granules evenly distributed on membrane; nuclear characteristics may be difficult to see	Coarsely granular and may be clumped and unevenly arranged on membrane; nuclear characteristics not as clearly defined as in trophozoite; may resemble *E. histoly-*	No peripheral chromatin	No peripheral chromatin

Karyosome (stained)	Small, compact, usually centrally located	Small, compact, usually centrally located	Large, may or may not be compact or eccentric; occasionally appears to be centrally located	Smaller than karysome seen in trophozoite, but generally larger than those of genus *Entamoeba*	Large, usually eccentric refractile granules may be on one side of karyosome ("basket nucleus")
Cytoplasm **Chromatoidal bodies (stained)**	May be present; bodies usually elongate with blunt, rounded, smooth edges	Often present; bodies elongate with blunt, rounded, smooth edges	May be present (less frequently than *E. histolytica*); splinter shaped with rough, pointed ends	No chromatoidal bodies present; occasionally small granules or inclusions seen; also, fine linear structures may be faintly visible on well-stained smears	No chromatoidal bodies present; occasionally small granules may be present
Glycogen (stained)	May be diffuse or absent in mature cyst; clumped chromatin mass may be present in early cysts (stains reddish brown in iodine)	May or may not be present, as in *E. histolytica*	May be diffuse or absent in mature cysts; clumped mass occasionally seen in immature cysts (stains reddish brown in iodine)	Usually diffuse if present (stains reddish-brown in iodine)	Large, compact, well-defined mass (stains reddish brown in iodine)

*These sizes refer to wet preparation measurements. Organisms on a permanent stained smear may be 1-1.5 µm smaller because of artificial shrinkage.

TABLE 44.8
Morphologic Criteria Used To Identify Intestinal Flagellate Cysts

	DIENTAMOEBA FRAGILIS	TRICHOMONAS HOMINIS	GIARDIA LAMBLIA	CHILOMASTIX MESNILI	ENTEROMONAS HOMINIS	RETORTAMONAS INTESTINALIS
Shape	No cyst	No cyst	Oval, ellipsoidal, or may appear round	Lemon shaped with anterior hyaline knob	Elongate or oval	Pear shaped or slightly lemon shaped
Size*			8-19 μm; usual range, 11-12 μm	6-10 μm; usual range, 8-9 μm	4-10 μm; usual range, 6-8 μm	4-9 μm; usual range 4-7 μm
Number of nuclei			Four; not distinct in unstained preparations; usually located at one end	One; not visible in unstained preparations	One to four; usually 2 lying at opposite ends of cyst; not visible in unstained mounts	One; not visible in unstained mounts
Other features			Longitudinal fibers in cyst may be visible in unstained preparations; deep-staining fibers usually lie across longitudinal fibers; there is often shrinkage, and cytoplasm pulls away from cyst wall; may also be "halo" effect around outside of cyst wall	Cytostome with supporting fibrils, usually visible in stained preparation; curved fibril along side of cytostome usually referred to as "shepherd's crook"	Resembles *E. nana* cyst; fibrils or flagella usually not seen	Resembles *Chilomastix* cyst; shadow outline of cytostome with supporting fibrils extending above nucleus

*These sizes refer to wet preparation measurements. Organisms on a permanent stained smear may be 1-1.5 μm smaller because of artificial shrinkage.

TABLE 44.9
Morphologic Criteria of *Balantidium coli*

	TROPHOZOITE	CYST
Shape and size*	Ovoid with tapering anterior end; 50-100 μm in length, 40-70 μm wide, usual range, 40-50 μm	Spherical or oval; 50-70 μm; usual range, 50-55 μm
Motility	Rotary or boring or both may be rapid	
Number of nuclei	1 large kidney-shaped macronucleus; 1 small round micronucleus, which is difficult to see even in stained smear; macronucleus may be visible in unstained preparation	1 large macronucleus visible in unstained preparation
Other features	Body covered with cilia, which tend to be longer near cytostome; cytoplasm may be vacuolated	Macronucleus and contractile vacuole visible in young cysts; in older cysts, internal structure appears granular

*These sizes refer to wet preparation measurements. Organisms on a permanent stained smear may be 1-1.5 μm smaller because of artificial shrinkage.

TABLE 44.10
Morphologic Criteria Used To Identify Intestinal Protozoa (Coccidia, *Blastocystis hominis*)

SPECIES	SHAPE/SIZE	OTHER FEATURES
Cryptosporidium sp.	Oocyst generally round, 4-6 μm, each mature oocyst containing 4 sporozoites	Oocyst, usual diagnostic stage in stool; various other stages in life cycle can be seen in biopsy specimens taken from gastrointestinal tract (brush border of epithelial cells) (intestinal tract)
Isospora belli	Ellipsoidal oocyst; range 20-30 μm in length, 10-19 μm in width; sporocysts rarely seen broken out of oocysts but measure 9-11 μm	Mature oocyst contains 2 sporocysts with 4 sporozoites each; usual diagnostic stage in feces is immature oocyst containing spherical mass of protoplasm (intestinal tract)
Sarcocystis hominis S. *suihominis* S. *bovihominis*	Oocyst thin-walled and contains 2 mature sporocysts, each containing 4 sporozoites; frequently thin oocyst wall ruptures; ovoidal sporocysts each measure 10-16 μm in length and 7.5-12 μm in width	Thin-walled oocyst or ovoid sporocysts occur in stool (intestinal tract)
S. "*lindemanni*"	Shapes and sizes of skeletal and cardiac muscle sarcocysts vary considerably	Sarcocysts contain from several hundred to several thousand trophozoites, each of which measures from 4-9 μm in width and 12-16 μm in length. The sarcocysts may also be divided into compartments by septa, not seen in *Toxoplasma* cysts (tissue/muscle)
Blastocystis hominis	Organisms are generally round, measure approximately 6-40 μm, and are usually characterized by a large, central body (looks like a large vacuole)	The more amebic form can be seen in diarrheal fluid, but will be difficult to identify

FIGURE 44.8

Various structures that may be seen in stool preparations. **1-8,** Various yeast cells. **9,** Macrophage with nucleus. **10, 11,** Deteriorated macrophage without nucleus. **12, 13,** Polymorphonuclear leukocytes. **14, 15,** Pollen grains. **16,** Charcot-Leyden crystals. (Adapted from Markell, E.K., and Voge, M. 1981. Medical parasitology, ed. 5. W.B. Saunders Co., Philadelphia. Illustration by Nobuko Kitamura.)

FIGURE 44.9

1, 2, Trophozoites of *Entamoeba histolytica*. **3, 4,** Early cysts of *E. histolytica*. **5-7,** Cysts of *E. histolytica*. **8, 9,** Trophozoites of *Entamoeba coli*. (1-18 from Garcia, L.S., and Ash, L.R. 1979. Diagnostic parasitology: clinical laboratory manual, ed. 2. The C.V. Mosby Co., St. Louis. Illustrations **4** and **11** by Nobuko Kitamura.)   *Continued.*

FIGURE 44.9, cont'd
10, 11, Early cysts of *E. coli.* **12-14,** Cysts of *E. coli.* **15, 16,** Trophozoites of *Entamoeba hartmanni.*
17, 18, Cysts of *E. hartmanni.*

10 μm

FIGURE 44.10
A-D, Trophozoites of *Entamoeba histolytica.* **E,** Early cysts of *E. histolytica.* **F-H,** Trophozoites of
Entamoeba coli. **I, J,** Cysts of *E. coli.*

A   B   C

D   E

10 μm

FIGURE 44.11
A-C, Trophozoites of *Entamoeba hartmanni.* **D, E,** Cysts of *E. hartmanni.*

membrane (Figures 44.12 to 44.14 and Plates 44.18 and 44.19).

The trophozoite stages may often be pleomorphic and asymmetrical, whereas the cysts are usually less variable in shape, with more rigid cyst walls. The number of nuclei in the cysts may vary, but their general morphology is similar to that found in the trophozoite stage. There are various inclusions in the cysts, such as chromatoidal bars or glycogen material, which may be helpful in identification.

44.13.b. Flagellates. Four common species of flagellates are found in the intestinal tract: *Giardia lamblia, Chilomastix mesnili, Trichomonas hominis,* and *Dientamoeba fragilis* (Plates 44.20 to 44.22). Several other smaller flagellates, such as *Enteromonas hominis* and *Retortamonas intestinalis* (Figure 44.15), are rarely seen, and none of the flagellates in the intestinal tract, with the exception of *G. lamblia* and *D. fragilis,* are considered pathogenic. *Trichomonas vaginalis* is pathogenic but occurs

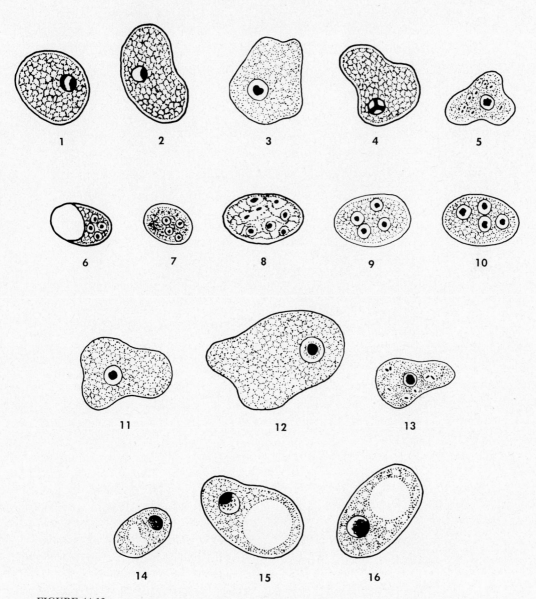

FIGURE 44.12
1-5, Trophozoites of *Endolimax nana*. **6-10,** Cysts of *E. nana*. **11-13,** Trophozoites of *Iodamoeba bütschlii*. **14-16,** Cysts of *I. bütschlii*. (From Garcia, L.S., and Ash, L.R. 1979. Diagnostic parasitology: clinical laboratory manual, ed. 2. The C.V. Mosby Co., St. Louis.)

A   B   C

D   E

├────────┤
10 μm

FIGURE 44.13
A-C, Trophozoites of *Endolimax nana*, **D**, **E**, Cysts of *E. nana*.

A   B   C

├────┤
10 μm

FIGURE 44.14
A, Trophozoites of *Iodamoeba bütschlii*. **B**, **C**, Cysts of *I. bütschlii*.

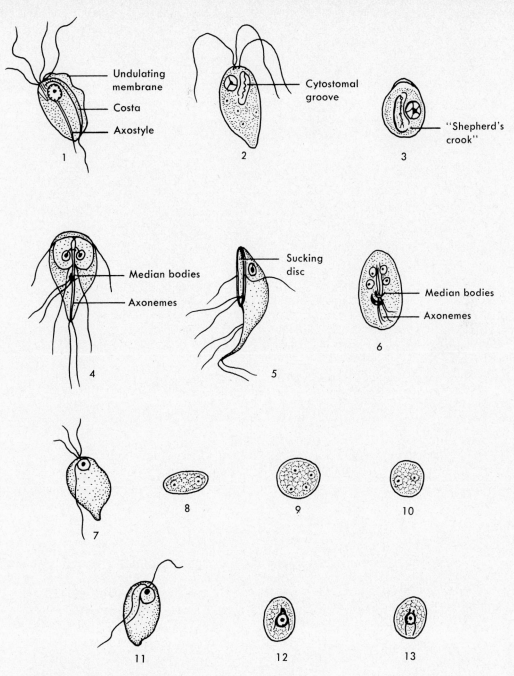

FIGURE 44.15

1, Trophozoite of *Trichomonas hominis.* **2,** Trophozoite of *Chilomastix mesnili.* **3,** Cyst of *C. mesnili.*
4, Trophozoite of *Giardia lamblia* (front view). **5,** Trophozoite of *G. lamblia* (side view). **6,** Cyst of *G. lamblia.* **7,** Trophozoite of *Enteromonas hominis.* **8-10,** Cysts of *E. hominis.* **11,** Trophozoite of *Retortamonas intestinalis.* **12, 13,** Cysts of *R. intestinalis.* (From Garcia, L.S., and Ash, L.R. 1979. Diagnostic parasitology: clinical laboratory manual, ed. 2. The C.V. Mosby Co., St. Louis. Illustration **5** by Nobuko Kitamura; illustrations **7** to **13** adapted from Markell, E.K., and Voge, M. 1981. Medical parasitology, ed. 5. W.B. Saunders Co., Philadelphia.)

10 μm

FIGURE 44.16
A-C, Trophozoites of *Giardia lamblia*. **D-F,** Cysts of *G. lamblia*.

in the urogenital tract. *Trichomonas tenax* is occasionally found in the mouth and may be associated with poor oral hygiene.

With the exception of *Dientamoeba*, the flagellates are easily recognized by their characteristic rapid motility, which has been described as a "falling leaf" motion for *Giardia* and a jerky motion for the other species. Most of the flagellates have a characteristic pear shape and possess different numbers and arrangements of flagella, depending on the spe-

cies. The sucking disk and axonemes of *Giardia*, the cytostome and spiral groove of *Chilomastix*, and the undulating membrane of *Trichomonas* are all distinctive criteria for identification (Figures 44.15 to 44.17).

Until recently *Dientamoeba* was grouped with the amebas; however, electron microscopy studies have confirmed its correct classification with the flagellates, specifically the trichomonads. *Dientamoeba* has no known cyst stage and is characterized by having one or two nuclei,

FIGURE 44.17
A-C, Trophozoites of *Chilomastix mesnili* (A, silver stain). D, E, Cysts of *C. mesnili.*

which have no peripheral chromatin and which have four to eight chromatin granules in a central mass. This organism is quite variable in size and shape and may contain large numbers of ingested bacteria and other debris. *Dientamoeba* is inconspicuous in the wet mount and is consistently overlooked without the use of the stained smear (Figures 44.18 and 44.19).

Organisms can be recovered in fecal specimens from asymptomatic persons, but reports in the literature describe a wide range of symp-

toms, which include intermittent diarrhea, abdominal pain, nausea, anorexia, malaise, fatigue, poor weight gain, and unexplained eosinophilia.

44.13.c. Ciliates. *Balantidium coli* is the largest protozoan and the only ciliate that infects humans (Plate 44.23). The living trophozoites have a rotatory, boring motion, which is usually rapid. The surface of the organism is covered by cilia, and the cytoplasm contains both a kidney-shaped macronucleus and a

FIGURE 44.18
Trophozoites of *Dientamoeba fragilis*. (From Garcia, L.S., and Ash, L.R. 1979. Diagnostic parasitology: clinical laboratory manual, ed. 2. The C.V. Mosby Co., St. Louis.

10 μm

FIGURE 44.19
A, B, Trophozoites of *Dientamoeba fragilis*.

FIGURE 44.20
1, Trophozoite of *Balantidium coli*. **2,** Cyst of *B. coli*. (From Garcia, L.S., and Ash, L.R. 1979. Diagnostic parasitology: clinical laboratory manual, ed. 2. The C.V. Mosby Co., St. Louis.)

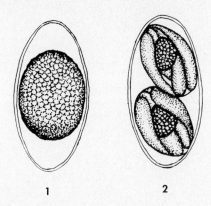

1   **2**

FIGURE 44.21
1, Immature oocyst of *Isospora belli.* **2,** Mature oocyst of
I. belli. (Illustration by Nobuko Kitamura.).

smaller, round micronucleus that is often difficult to see. The number of nuclei in the cyst
remains the same as that in the trophozoite. *B.
coli* infections are rarely seen in this country;
however, the organisms are quite easily recognized (Figure 44.20).

    44.13.d. Coccidia. *Isospora belli* is now
considered to be the only valid species of the
genus *Isospora* that infects humans, since *Isospora hominis* has been placed in the genus *Sarcocystis. I. belli* is released from the intestinal
wall as immature oocysts, so all stages from the
immature oocyst containing a mass of undiffer-
entiated protoplasm to those containing fully
developed sporocysts and sporozoites are found
in the stool (Figure 44.21). If passed in the immature condition, they mature within 4 or 5
days to form sporozoites. *I. belli* infections are
becoming increasingly important as a cause of
diarrhea in immunodeficient and immunosuppressed patients.[33] Many of the recently reported infections have occurred in patients
with AIDS. The diagnosis of *Isospora* infection
is usually accomplished by finding oocysts in
stool concentrates or rarely by direct wet
mount examination during routine ova and parasite examinations. Multiple stool exams are
recommended since the oocysts are not contin-

ually shed in the stool during infections.
Oocysts can be stained with rhodamine-auramine (Chapter 46), modified acid fast procedures, or Giemsa. The oocyst wall and sporocyst will fluoresce bright yellow when stained
with rhodamine-auramine. With the modified
acid fast stain (Procedure 44.12), the oocyst will
appear pink with bright red sporocysts.[33]
Giemsa (Procedure 44.20) stains both the oocyst
and sporocyst pale blue; however, trichrome
stain is not recommended because it stains the
oocyst poorly or not at all. Multiple biopsies of
the jejunal-duodenal brush border can also lead
to diagnosis, since in many patients apparently
only the asexual stages are seen.

    Cryptosporidium sp. is another coccidian
parasite that has been implicated in intestinal
disease, primarily in immunosuppressed patients and particularly those with AIDS.[14,32]
These organisms may not be host specific, are
probably transmitted by the fecal-oral route,
and may also infect persons with a competent
immune system. The developmental stages occur within a vacuole of host cell origin, which
is located at the microvillous surface of the host
epithelial cell (Figure 44.22). Although the infection is generally self-limiting in the immunocompetent person, the presence of autoinfective oocysts may explain why a small
inoculum can lead to an overwhelming infection in compromised patients and why they
may have persistent, life-threatening infections
in the absence of documentation of repeated
exposure to oocysts (Figure 44.22). Previously,
the majority of cases had been diagnosed by
light or electron microscopic examination of
small or large bowel biopsy material. However,
recent cases have been diagnosed from stool
specimens and suggest that the use of specific
stains and concentration techniques may be
more sensitive than intestinal biopsies in diagnosing *Cryptosporidium.* The oocysts range
from 4-6 μm and can be confused with yeast or
overlooked without special techniques, various
modified acid fast stains being one of the best

FIGURE 44.22
Proposed life cycle of *Cryptosporidium*. (*a*) Sporulated oocyst in feces.(*b*) Excystation in intestine. (*c*) Free sporozoite in intestine. (*d*) Type I meront (6 or 8 merozoites). (*e*) Recycling of Type I merozoite. (*f*) Type II meront (4 merozoites).(*g*) Microgametocyte, with approximately 16 microgametes. (*h*) Microgamete fertilizes macrogamete (*i*) to form zygote (*j*). Approximately 80% of the zygotes form thick-walled oocysts (*k*) which sporulate within the host cell. About 20% of the zygotes do not form an oocyst wall; their sporozoites are surrounded only by a unit membrane (*l*). Sporozoites within "autoinfective," thin walled oocysts (*l*) are released into the intestinal lumen (*m*) and reinitiate the endogenous cycle (at *c*). (Life cycle from William L. Current, Lilly Research Laboratories, Greenfield, Indiana.)

FIGURE 44.23
Cryptosporidium. **A,** Oocysts recovered from a Sheather's sugar flotation; organisms measure 4-6 μm. **B,** Scanning electron microscopy view of organisms at brush border of epithelial cells. (Courtesy Marietta Voge.)

approaches.[14] In wet preparations where iodine is added, yeast cells will stain with the iodine, but *Cryptosporidium* does not take up the stain. However, in light infections with few oocysts and many artifacts in the stool, this difference will be very difficult to visualize. The most widely used concentration method for obtaining the oocysts from stool is Sheather's sugar flotation (Figure 44.23),[13] although they may be visible in routine stool concentrates.

NOTE: The number of oocysts per stool specimen will vary considerably, both from patient to patient, but also during an infection in a single patient. Since therapy for this infection is less than optimal, even with the use of spiramycin, one should check multiple specimens before accepting the patient as being cured of the infection. With the development of very specific monoclonal reagents directed against components of the oocyst wall, the ability to screen large numbers of specimens quickly may be possible in the near future.

44.14 Blood Protozoa

44.14.a. Malaria. Malaria is caused by four species of the protozoan genus *Plasmodium*: *P. vivax*, *P. falciparum* (Plate 44.24), *P. malariae*, and *P. ovale* (Table 44.11). Humans become infected when the sporozoites are introduced into the blood from the salivary secretion of the infected mosquito when the mosquito vector takes a blood meal. These sporozoites then leave the blood and enter the parenchymal cells of the liver, where they undergo asexual multiplication. This development in the liver prior to red cell invasion is called the preerythrocytic cycle; if further liver development takes place after red cell invasion, it is called the exoerythrocytic cycle. The length of time for the preerythrocytic cycle and the number of asexual generations vary depending on the species; however, the schizonts eventually rupture, releasing thousands of merozoites into the bloodstream, where they invade the erythrocytes.

The early forms in the red cells are called **ring forms** or young trophozoites. As the parasites continue to grow and feed, they become actively ameboid within the red cell. They feed on hemoglobin, which is incompletely metabolized; the residue that is left is called malarial pigment and is a compound of hematin and of protein.

During the next phase of the cycle the chromatin (nuclear material) becomes fragmented throughout the organism, and the cytoplasm begins to divide, each portion being arranged with a fragment of nuclear material. These forms are called mature schizonts and are composed of individual merozoites. The infected red cell then ruptures, releasing the merozoites and also metabolic products into the bloodstream. If large numbers of red cells rupture simultaneously, a malarial paroxysm may result from the amount of toxic materials released into the bloodstream. In the early stages of infection or in a mixed infection with two species, rupture of the red cells is usually not synchronous; consequently, the fever may be continuous or daily rather than intermittent. After several days, a 48 or 72 h periodicity is usually established.

After several generations of erythrocytic schizogony, the production of gametocytes begins. These forms are derived from merozoites, which do not undergo schizogony but continue to grow and form the male and female gametocytes that circulate in the bloodstream. When the mature gametocytes are ingested by the appropriate mosquito vector, the sexual cycle is initiated within the mosquito with the eventual production of the sporozoites, the infective stage for humans (Figure 44.24).

The asexual and sexual forms just described circulate in the human bloodstream in three species of *Plasmodium*. However, in *P. falciparum* infections, as the parasite continues to grow the red cell membrane becomes sticky, and the cells tend to adhere to the endothelial lining of the capillaries of the internal organs;

TABLE 44.11
Microscopic Identification of Plasmodia of Humans in Giemsa-Stained Thin Blood Smears

	PLASMODIUM VIVAX	PLASMODIUM MALARIAE	PLASMODIUM FALCIPARUM	PLASMODIUM OVALE
Appearance of parasitized red blood cells: size and shape	1½ to 2 times larger than normal; oval to round	Normal shape; size may be normal or slightly smaller	Both normal	60% of cells larger than normal and oval; 20% have irregular, frayed edges (fimbriated)
Schüffner's dots (eosinophilic stippling)	Usually present in all infected cells except early ring forms	None	None; occasionally comalike red dots are present (Maurer's dots)	Present in all stages including early ring forms, dots may be larger and darker than in P. vivax
Color of cytoplasm	Decolorized, pale	Normal	Normal, bluish tinge at times	Decolorized, pale
Multiple infections	Occasional	Rare	Common	Occasional
All developmental stages present in peripheral blood	All stages present	Ring forms few, as ring stage brief; mostly growing and mature trophozoites and schizonts	Young ring forms and very rarely older stages in moribund patients; few gametocytes	All stages present
Appearance of parasite: young trophozoite (early ring form)	Ring is ⅓ diameter of cell; cytoplasmic circle around vacuole; heavy chromatin dot	Ring often smaller than in P. vivax, occupying ⅛ of cell; heavy chromatin dot; vacuole at times "filled in"; pigment forms early	Delicate, small ring with small chromatin dot (frequently 2); scanty cytoplasm around small vacuoles; sometimes at edge of red cell (appliqué form) or filamentous slender form; may have multiple rings per cell	Ring is larger and more ameboid than in P. vivax, otherwise similar to P. vivax
Growing trophozoite	Multishaped irregular ameboid parasite; streamers of cytoplasm close to large chromatin dot; vacuole retained until close to maturity; increasing amounts of	Nonameboid rounded or band-shaped solid forms; chromatin may be hidden by coarse dark brown pigment	Heavy ring forms fine pigment grains	Ring shape maintained until late in development

	or more small vacuoles retained until schizont stage; fills almost entire cell; fine brown pigment	cytoplasm compact, oval, band shaped, or nearly round, almost filling cell; chromatin may be hidden by peripheral coarse dark brown pigment	blood (except in severe infections); development of all phases following ring form occurs in capillaries of viscera	pear; pigment dark brown, less than in *P. malariae*
Schizont (presegmenter)	Progressive chromatin division; cytoplasmic bands containing clumps of brown pigment	Similar to *P. vivax* except smaller, darker, larger pigment granules peripheral or central	Not seen in peripheral blood (see above)	Smaller and more compact than *P. vivax*
Mature schizont	16 (12–24) merozoites, each with chromatin and cytoplasm, filling entire red cell, which can hardly be seen	8 (6–12) merozoites in rosettes or irregular clusters filling normal-sized cells, which can hardly be seen; central arrangement of brown-green pigment	Not seen in peripheral blood (rare exceptions)	¾ of cells occupied by 8 (8–12) merozoites in rosettes or irregular clusters
Macrogametocyte	Rounded or oval homogeneous cytoplasm; diffuse delicate light brown pigment throughout parasite; eccentric compact chromatin	Similar to *P. vivax*, but fewer in number, pigment darker and more coarse	Sex differentiation difficult; "crescent" or "sausage" shapes characteristic; may appear in "showers"; black pigment near chromatin dot, which is often central	Smaller than *P. vivax*
Microgametocyte	Large pink to purple chromatin mass surrounded by pale or colorless halo; evenly distributed pigment	Similar to *P. vivax*, but fewer in number, pigment darker and more coarse	See above	Smaller than *P. vivax*
Main criteria	Large, pale red cell; trophozoite irregular; pigment usually present; Schüffner's dots not always present; several phases of growth seen in one smear; gametocytes appear early	Red cell normal in size and color; trophozoites stain usually compact, intense, band forms not always seen; coarse pigment; no stippling of red cells; gametocytes appear late	Development following ring stage takes place in blood vessels in internal organs; delicate ring forms and crescent-shaped gametocytes are only forms normally seen in peripheral blood	Red cell enlarged, oval, with fimbriated edges; Schüffner's dots seen in all stages

FIGURE 44.24
Life cycle of *Plasmodium*. (Adapted from Wilcox, A. 1960. Manual for the microscopical diagnosis of malaria in man. U.S. Public Health Service, Washington, D.C. Illustration by Nobuko Kitamura.)

thus, only the ring forms and crescent-shaped gametocytes occur in the peripheral blood. Interference with normal blood flow in these vessels gives rise to additional problems, which are responsible for the different clinical manifestations of this type of malaria.

44.14.b. Babesiosis. *Babesia* are tick-borne (also can be transmitted via a blood transfusion) sporozoan parasites that have generally been considered parasites of animals (Texas cattle fever) rather than humans. However, there are now documented human cases, some infections occurring in splenectomized patients and others in patients with intact spleens.[3] *Babesia* organisms infect the red blood cells and appear as pleomorphic ringlike structures when

stained with any of the recommended stains used for blood films (Figure 44.25). They may be confused with the ring forms in *Plasmodium* infections; however, in a *Babesia* infection there are often many rings (four or five) per red cell and the individual rings are quite small compared with those found in malaria infections.[17]

44.14.c Hemoflagellates. Hemoflagellates are blood and tissue flagellates, two genera of which are medically important for humans: *Leishmania* and *Trypanosoma*. Some species may circulate in the bloodstream or at times may be present in lymph nodes or muscle. Other species tend to parasitize the reticuloendothelial cells of the hemopoietic organs. The

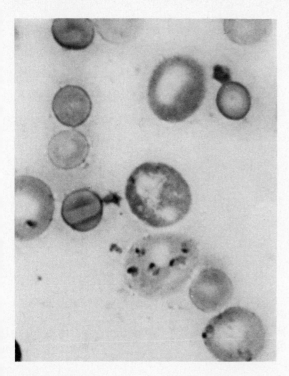

FIGURE 44.25
Babesia in red blood cells. (Photomicrograph by Zane Price. From Markell, E.K., and Voge, M. 1981. Medical parasitology, ed. 5. W.B. Saunders Co., Philadelphia.)

Amastigote

Promastigote

Epimastigote

Trypomastigote

N. Kitamura

FIGURE 44.26
Characteristic stages of species of *Leishmania* and *Trypanosoma* in human and insect hosts. (Illustration by Nobuko Kitamura.)

hemoflagellates of human beings have four morphologic types (Figure 44.26): amastigote (leishmanial form, or Leishman-Donovan body), promastigote (leptomonal form), epimastigote (crithidial form), and trypomastigote (trypanosomal form).

The amastigote form is an intracellular parasite in the cells of the reticuloendothelial system and is oval, measuring approximately 1½-5 μm, and contains a nucleus and kinetoplast. Species of the genus *Leishmania* usually exist as the amastigote form in humans and in the promastigote form in the insect host. The life cycle is essentially the same for all three species, and the clinical manifestations vary depending on the species involved. As the vector takes a blood meal, the promastigote form is introduced into a human, thus initiating the infection. Depending on the species, the parasites then move from the site of the bite to the organs of the reticuloendothelial system (liver, spleen, bone marrow) or to the macrophages of the skin (Figure 44.27).

Species based on clinical grounds are morphologically the same; however, there are differences in serologies and in growth requirements for culture. There is a great deal of biologic variation among the many strains that make up these groups. *Leishmania tropica* causes oriental sore or cutaneous leishmaniasis of the Old World; *Leishmania braziliensis* causes mucocutaneous leishmaniasis of the

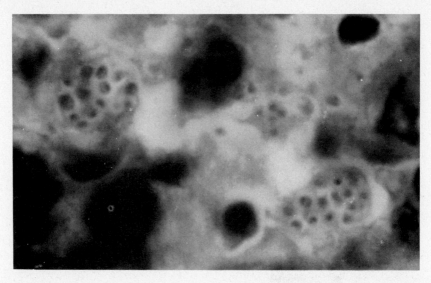

FIGURE 44.27
Leishmania donovani parasites in Küpffer cells of liver (2,000 ×).

FIGURE 44.28
Trypanosoma gambiense in blood film (1,600 ×).

New World; and *L. donovani* causes visceral leishmaniasis (Dumdum fever, or kala azar) (Plate 44.25). Additional species have been delineated based on the buoyant density of kinetoplast DNA, the isoenzyme patterns, and serologic testing.

In tissue impression smears or sections *Histoplasma capsulatum* must be differentiated from the Leishman-Donovan (L-D) bodies. *H. capsulatum* does not have a kinetoplast and stains with both periodic acid–Schiff (PAS) stain and Gomori methenamine silver stain, neither of which stains L-D bodies.

Diagnosis of leishmanial organisms is based on the demonstration of the L-D bodies or the recovery of the promastigote culture stages.

Three species of trypanosomes are pathogenic for humans: *Trypanosoma gambiense* (Figure 44.28) causes west African sleeping sickness; *Trypanosoma rhodesiense* causes east African sleeping sickness; and *Trypanosoma cruzi* causes South American trypanosomiasis, or Chagas' disease (Plate 44.26). The first two species are morphologically similar and pro-

FIGURE 44.29
A, *Trypanosoma cruzi* in blood film (1,600 ×). **B,** *Trypanosoma cruzi* parasites in cardiac muscle
(2,500 ×). (From Markell, E.K., and Voge, M.: Medical parasitology, ed. 5, Philadelphia, 1981, W.B.
Saunders Co.)

duce African sleeping sickness, an illness characterized by both acute and chronic stages. In the acute stage of the disease the organisms can usually be found in the peripheral blood or lymph node aspirates. As the disease progresses to the chronic stage the organisms can be found in the cerebrospinal fluid (CSF) (comatose stage: "sleeping sickness"). *T. rhodesiense* produces a more severe

infection, usually resulting in death within 1 year.

In the early stages of infection with *T. cruzi,* the trypomastigote forms appear in the blood but do not multiply (Figure 44.29, *A*). They then invade the endothelial or tissue cells and begin to divide, producing many L-D bodies, which are most often found in cardiac muscle (Figure 44.29, *B*). When these forms are liberated into the blood, they transform into the trypomastigote forms, which are then carried to other sites, where tissue invasion again occurs.

Diagnosis of the infection is based on demonstration of the parasites, most often on wet unstained or stained blood films. Both thick and thin films should be examined; these can be prepared from peripheral blood or buffy coat. The sediment recovered from CSF can also be examined for the presence of trypomastigotes. Specific techniques for culture, animal inoculation, handling of aspirate and biopsy material, and serologic procedures are presented in earlier sections of this chapter.

Another technique often used in endemic areas for the diagnosis of Chagas' disease is **xenodiagnosis**. Triatomids, the insect vector, are raised in the laboratory and are determined

to be free from infection with *T. cruzi*. These insects are allowed to feed on the blood of an individual suspected of having Chagas' disease, and after 2 weeks the intestinal contents are checked for the presence of the epimastigote forms. For additional information consult Maekelt.[26]

44.15. Intestinal Helminths

The intestinal helminths that infect humans belong to two phyla: the Nematoda, or roundworms, and the Platyhelminthes, or flatworms. The Platyhelminthes, most of which are hermaphroditic, have a flat, bilaterally symmetrical body. The two classes, Trematoda and Cestoda, contain organisms that are parasitic for human beings.

The trematodes (flukes) are leaf-shaped or elongate and slender organisms (blood flukes:

FIGURE 44.30
Life cycle of *Taenia saginata* and *Taenia solium*.

FIGURE 44.31
Life cycle of *Echinococcus granulosus* (hydatid disease).

Schistosoma species) that possess hooks or suckers for attachment. Members of this group, which parasitize humans, are found in the intestinal tract, liver, blood vessels, and lungs.

The cestodes (tapeworms) typically have a long, segmented, ribbonlike body, which has a special attachment portion, or scolex, at the anterior end. Adult forms inhabit the small intestine; however, humans may be host to either the adult or larval forms, depending on the species. The cestodes, as well as the trematodes, require (with few exceptions)

one or more intermediate hosts for the completion of the life cycle (Figures 44.30 and 44.31).

The phylum Nematoda, or roundworms, are elongate, cylindrical worms containing a well-developed digestive tract. The sexes are separate, the male usually being smaller than the female. Intermediate hosts are required for larval development in certain species; a large number of species parasitize the intestinal tract and certain tissues of humans (Figures 44.32 to 44.34).

FIGURE 44.32
Life cycle of *Strongyloides stercoralis*.

FIGURE 44.33
Life cycle of *Enterobius vermicularis* and *Trichuris trichiura* (direct type of cycle).

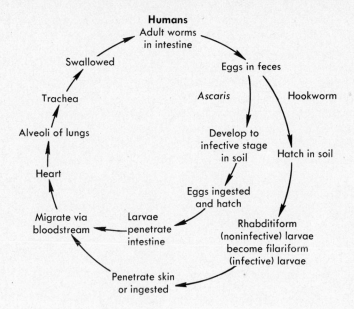

FIGURE 44.34

Life cycle of *Ascaris lumbricoides* and hookworms (indirect type of cycle).

KEY TO HELMINTH EGGS

a. Egg nonoperculated, spherical or subspherical, containing a six-hooked embryo   b
   Egg other than above   e
b. Eggs separate   c
   Eggs in packets of 12 or more   *Dipylidium caninum*
c. Outer surface of egg consists of a thick, radially striated capsule or embryophore   *Taenia* sp.
   Outer surface of egg consists of very thin shell, separated from inner embryophore by gelatinous matrix   d
d. Filamentous strands occupy space between embryophore and outer shell   *Hymenolepis nana*
   No filamentous strands between embryophore and outer shell   *Hymenolepsis diminuta*
e. Egg operculated   f
   Egg nonoperculated   j
f. Egg less than 35 μm long   *Clonorchis (Opisthorchis)* sp. or *Heterophyes heterophyes* or *Metagonimus yokogawai*
   Egg 38 μm or over   g
g. Egg 38-45 μm in length   *Dicrocoelium dendriticum*
   Egg over 60 μm in length   h
h. Egg with shoulders into which operculum fits   *Paragonimus westermani*
   Egg without opercular shoulders   i

i. Egg more than 85 μm long   *Fasciolopsis buski* or *Fasciola hepatica* or *Echinostoma* sp.
   Egg less than 75 μm long   *Diphyllobothrium latum*
j. Egg 75 μm or more in length, spined   k
   Egg less than 75 μm long, not spined   m
k. Spine terminal   *Schistosoma haematobium*
   Spine lateral   l
l. Lateral spine inconspicuous (perhaps absent)   *Schistosoma japonicum*
   Lateral spine prominent   *Schistosoma mansoni*
m. Egg with thick tuberculated capsule   *Ascaris lumbricoides*
   Egg without thick tuberculated capsule   n
n. Egg barrel shaped, with polar plugs   o
   Egg not barrel shaped, without polar plugs   p
o. Shell nonstriated   *Trichuris trichiura*
   Shell often striated   *Capillaria* sp.
p. Egg flattened on one side   *Enterobius vermicularis*
   Egg symmetrical   q
q. Egg with large blue-green globules at poles   *Heterodera marioni*
   Egg without polar globules   r
r. Egg bluntly rounded at ends, 56-76 μm long   Hookworm
   Egg pointed at one or both ends, 73-95 μm long   *Trichostrongylus* sp.

From Markell, E.K., and Voge, M. 1981. Medical parasitology, ed. 5. W.B. Saunders Co., Philadelphia.

Diagnosis of most intestinal helminth infections is based on the detection of the characteristic eggs (see Key) and larvae in the stool; occasionally adult worms or portions of worms may also be found. No permanent stains are required, and most diagnostic features can easily be seen on direct wet mounts or in mounts of the concentrated stool material.

44.15.a. Nematodes. The majority of nematodes are diagnosed by finding the characteristic eggs in the stool (Figure 44.35). The eggs of *Ancylostoma duodenale* and *Necator americanus* are essentially identical, so an infection with either species is reported as "Hookworm eggs present" (Plate 44.27). *Trichostrongylus* eggs may easily be mistaken for those of hookworms; however, the eggs of *Trichostrongylus* are somewhat larger, and one end tends to be more pointed.

Strongyloides stercoralis is passed in the feces as the noninfective rhabditiform larva (Plate 44.28). Although hookworm eggs are normally passed in the stool, these eggs may continue to develop and hatch if the stool is left at room temperature for several days. These larvae may be mistaken for those of *Strongyloides*. Figure 44.36 shows the morphologic differences between the rhabditiform larvae of

hookworm and *Strongyloides*. Recovery of *Strongyloides* larvae in duodenal contents is mentioned in Section 44.3.

The appropriate techniques for recovery of *Enterobius vermicularis* (pinworm) eggs are given in Section 44.3.f. (Plate 44.29). Eggs of the other nematodes are fairly easy to find and to differentiate from one another.

44.15.b. Cestodes. With the exception of *Diphyllobothrium latum*, tapeworm eggs are embryonated and contain a six-hooked oncosphere (Figure 44.37 and Table 44.12).

Taenia saginata and *Taenia solium* cannot be speciated on the basis of egg morphology; gravid proglottids or the scolices must be examined (Figure 44.38). *T. saginata* (beef tapeworm) proglottids have approximately 15-30 main lateral branches, and the scolex has no hooks; the proglottids of *T. solium* have 7-12 main lateral branches, and the scolex has a circle of hooks.

Hymenolepis nana has an unusual life cycle in that the ingestion of the egg can lead to the adult worm in humans (Figure 44.39). The eggs of *Hymenolepis nana* (more common) and *Hymenolepis diminuta* are very similar; however, *H. nana* eggs are smaller and have polar fila-

Text continued on p. 851.

A   B   C

FIGURE 44.35,
A, Immature hookworm egg. **B,** Embryonated hookworm egg. **C,** *Trichostrongylus orientalis,* immature egg.   *Continued.*

FIGURE 44.35, cont'd

D, *Strongyloides stercoralis,* rhabditiform larva (200 μm). **E,** *Enterobius vermicularis* egg. **F,** *Trichuris trichiura* egg. **G,** *Ascaris lumbricoides,* fertilized egg. **H,** *A. lumbricoides,* fertilized egg, decorticate. **I,** *A. lumbricoides,* unfertilized egg. **J,** *A. lumbricoides,* unfertilized egg, decorticate.

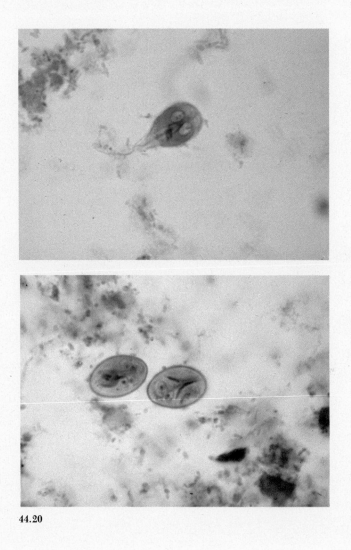

44.20

PLATE 44.20. *Top, Giardia lamblia* trophozoite. *Bottom left, G. lamblia* cyst.

44.21

PLATE 44.21. *Top, Chilomastix mesnili* trophozoite, silver stain. *Bottom left, C. mesnili* cyst.

44.22

PLATE 44.22. *Top, Dientamoeba fragilis*, two nuclei. *Bottom left, D. fragilis*, one nucleus.

44.23

PLATE 44.23. *Balantidium coli* trophozoite, iodine stain.

44.24

44.25

PLATE 44.24. *Plasmodium falciparum* early ring forms.
PLATE 44.25. *Leishmania donovani* amastigotes.

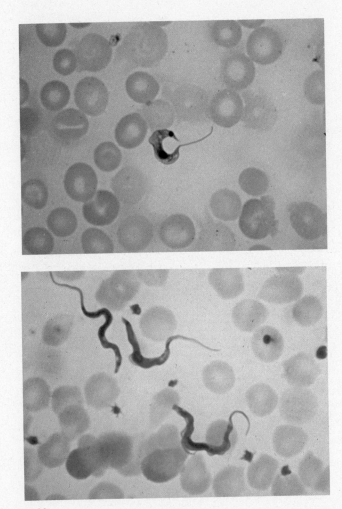

44.26

PLATE 44.26. *Top, Trypanosoma cruzi* trypomastigote. *Bottom, Trypanosoma brucei gambiense* trypomastigotes.

44.27

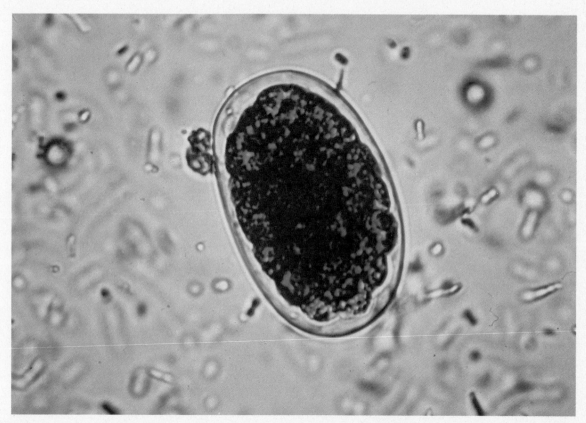

PLATE 44.27. Hookworm egg, iodine stain.

44.28

44.29

PLATE 44.28. *Strongyloides stercoralis* larva, iodine stain.
PLATE 44.29. *Enterobius vermicularis* eggs (cellophane [Scotch] tape preparation).

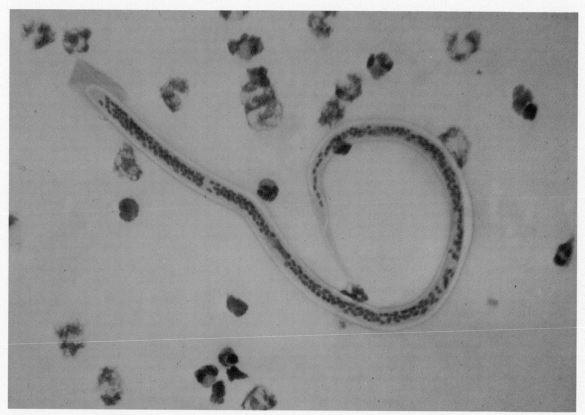

44.30

PLATE 44.30. *Wuchereria bancrofti* microfilaria.

FIGURE 44.36
Rhabditiform larvae. **A,** *Strongyloides.* **B,** Hookworm. **C,** *Trichostrongylus. bc,* Buccal cavity; *es,* esophagus; *gp,* genital primordia; *cb,* beadlike swelling of caudal tip. (Illustration by Nobuko Kitamura.)

50 μm

FIGURE 44.37
A, *Taenia* species egg. **B,** *Diphyllobothrium latum* egg. **C,** *Hymenolepis diminuta* egg. **D,** *Hymenolepis nana* egg. **E,** *Dipylidium caninum* egg packet.

TABLE 44.12
Differential Characteristics of Some Important Tapeworms of Humans

	TAENIA SAGINATA	*TAENIA SOLIUM*	*HYMENOLEPIS NANA*	*DIPHYLLOBOTHRIUM LATUM*
Length	4-8 m	3-5 m	2.5-4 cm	4-10 m
Scolex				
Shape	Quadrilateral	Globular	Usually not seen	Almondlike
Size	1 by 1.5 mm	1 by 1 mm		3 by 1 mm
Rostellum and hooklets	No	Yes		No
Suckers	4	4		2 (grooves)
Terminal proglottids (gravid)				
Size	19 by 7 mm, longer than wide	11 by 5 mm	Usually not seen	3 by 11 mm, wider than long
Primary lateral uterine branches	15-30 on each side	6-12 on each side		Rosette shaped
Color	Milky white	Milky white		Ivory
Appearance in feces	Usually appear singly	5 or 6 segments		Varies from a few inches to a few feet in length
Ova				
Shape	Spheroid	Spheroid	Broadly oval	Oval
Size	35 μm	35 μm	30 by 47 μm	45 by 70 μm
Color	Rusty brown	Rusty brown	Pale	Yellow-brown
Embryo with hooklets	Yes	Yes	Yes	No
Operculum	No	No	No	Yes (difficult to see)

KEY TO GRAVID PROGLOTTIDS OF THE MAJOR HUMAN TAPEWORMS

a. Uterus forms rosette in center of proglottid
   Diphyllobothrium latum
   Uterus otherwise disposed   b

b. Uterus with central stem running length of proglottid   c
   Uterus without central stem   d

c. Central stem with 7 to 13 main lateral branches
   Taenia solium
   Central stem with 15 to 20 main lateral
   branches   *T. saginata*

d. Proglottid wider than long   *Hymenolepis sp.*
   Proglottid longer than wide   *Dipylidium caninum*

From Markell, E.K., and Voge, M. 1981. Medical parasitology, ed. 5. W.B. Saunders Co., Philadelphia.

1   **2**   **3**   **4**

FIGURE 44.38
Gravid proglottids. **1,** *Taenia saginata.* **2,** *Taenia solium.* **3,** *Diphyllobothrium latum.* **4,** *Dipylidium caninum.* (From Garcia, L.S., and Ash, L.R. 1979. Diagnostic parasitology: clinical laboratory manual, ed. 2. W.B. Saunders Co., Philadelphia.)

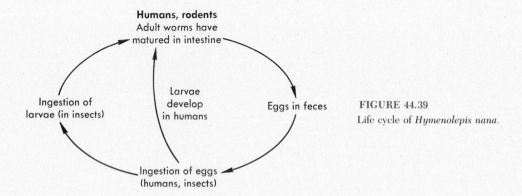

Humans, rodents
Adult worms have
matured in intestine

Ingestion of
larvae (in insects)

Larvae
develop
in humans

Eggs in feces

Ingestion of eggs
(humans, insects)

FIGURE 44.39
Life cycle of *Hymenolepis nana.*

ments, which are present in the space between the oncosphere and the egg shell (Figure 44.37).

Eggs of *Dipylidium caninum* are occasionally found in humans (particularly children) and are passed in the feces in packets of 5-15 eggs each (Figures 44.37 and 44.40). The proglottids may also be found; they may resemble cucum-ber seeds or, when dry, may look like rice grains (white).

The fish tapeworm, *Diphyllobothrium latum*, does not have embryonated eggs; these eggs have a somewhat thicker shell and are operculated, much like the trematode eggs (Figure 44.37). Humans acquire the parasite by eating undercooked or raw fish (Figure 44.41).

FIGURE 44.40
Dipylidium caninum egg packet. (Illustration by Nobuko Kitamura.)

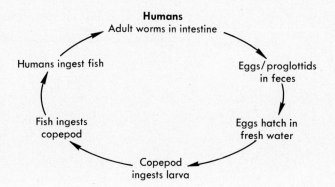

FIGURE 44.41
Life cycle of *Diphyllobothrium latum*.

44.15.c. Trematodes. Humans acquire most fluke infestations by ingesting the encysted metacercariae (Figure 44.42). Most of the trematodes have operculated eggs, which are best recovered by the sedimentation concentration technique rather than the flotation method. Many of these eggs are very similar, both in size and morphology, and often careful measurements must be taken to speciate the eggs (Figure 44.43). The eggs of *Clonorchis (Opisthorchis)*, *Heterophyes*, and *Metagonimus* are very similar and quite small; they are easily missed if the concentration sediment is examined with the 10× objective only. The eggs of *Fasciola hepatica* and *Fasciolopsis buski* are also very similar but much larger than those just mentioned.

Paragonimus westermani eggs are not only found in the stool but may be found in sputum (Figure 44.43). These eggs are very similar in size and shape to the egg of the fish tapeworm, *D. latum*. Schistosomiasis, a great source of morbidity in much of the developing world, is acquired during activities (such as bathing, swimming, doing laundry, planting rice, fishing, etc.) that involve contact with water infested with the intermediate snail host of the parasite. The free-swimming cercarial form attaches to a vertebrate host and penetrates through intact skin (Figure 44.44). In temperate zones such as in the areas near the Great Lakes, cercariae of other trematodes that normally infect birds or other animals can penetrate human skin and cause a strong local reaction (swimmer's itch), although they cannot go on to develop into adult worms in the unnatural human host. Probably the easiest trematode eggs to identify are those of the schistosomes: *S. mansoni* eggs are characterized by having a very prominent lateral spine, *S. haematobium* a terminal spine, and *S. japonicum* a small lateral spine that may be difficult to see. These eggs are nonoperculated. Schistosome eggs stain acid fast. Specific procedures for their recovery and identification are found in Section 44.3.e.

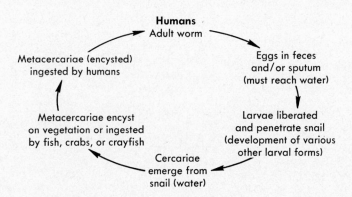

FIGURE 44.42
Life cycle of trematodes acquired by humans through ingestion of raw fish, crabs, or crayfish and vegetation.

50 μm

FIGURE 44.43
A, *Schistosoma mansoni* egg. **B,** *Schistosoma japonicum* egg. **C,** *Schistosoma haematobium* egg. **D,**
Paragonimus westermani egg. **E,** *Fasciola hepatica* egg. **F,** *Clonorchis (Opisthorchis) sinensis* egg.

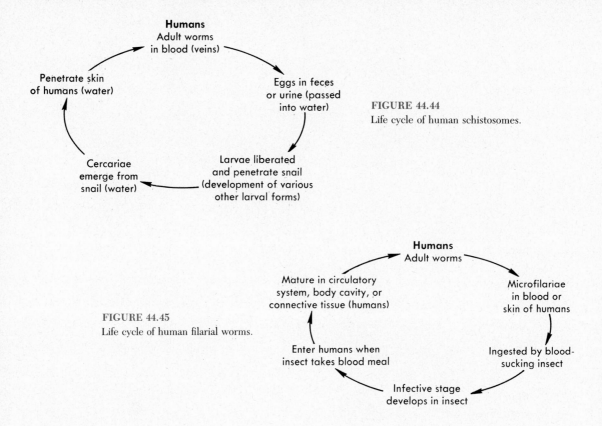

FIGURE 44.44
Life cycle of human schistosomes.

FIGURE 44.45
Life cycle of human filarial worms.

44.16. Blood Helminths

44.16.a. Filariae. The filarial worms are long, thin nematodes that inhabit parts of the lymphatic system and the subcutaneous and deep connective tissues. A life cycle has been included here to show the various stages present in the human host (Figure 44.45). Most species produce microfilariae, which can be found in the peripheral blood; two species, *Onchocerca volvulus* and *Dipetalonema strep-tocerca*, produce microfilariae found in the subcutaneous tissues and dermis.

Diagnosis of filarial infections is often based on clinical grounds, but demonstration of the parasite is the only accurate means of confirming the diagnosis (Figure 44.46). Fresh blood films may be prepared; actively moving micro-filariae can be observed in a preparation of this type. If the patient has a light infection, thick blood films can be prepared and stained. The Knott concentration procedure[22] and the membrane filtration technique[10,11] may also be helpful in recovering the organisms. Microfilariae of some strains tend to exhibit nocturnal periodicity; thus, the time the blood is drawn may be critical in demonstrating the parasite. The microfilariae of *O. volvulus* and *D. strep-tocerca* are found in "skin snips," very thin slices of skin, which are teased apart in normal saline to release the organisms. Differentiation of the species is dependent on (1) the presence or absence of the sheath and (2) the distribution of nuclei in the tail region of the microfilaria (Figure 44.47 and Plate 44.30).

FIGURE 44.46
Microfilaria of *Wuchereria bancrofti* in thick blood film. (From Markell, E.K., and Voge, M. 1981. Medical parasitology, ed. 5. W.B. Saunders Co., Philadelphia.

A   B   C   D   E   F   G

N. Kitamura

FIGURE 44.47

Anterior and posterior ends of microfilariae found in humans. **A,** *Wuchereria bancrofti.* **B,** *Brugia malayi.* **C,** *Loa loa.* **D,** *Onchocerca volvulus.* **E,** *Dipetalonema perstans.* **F,** *Dipetalonema streptocerca.* **G,** *Mansonella ozzardi.*

REFERENCES

1. Beaver, P.C. 1949. A nephelometric method of calibrating the photoelectric meter for making egg-counts by direct fecal smear. J. Parasitol. 35(Section 2):13.
2. Beaver, P.C. 1950. The standardization of fecal smears for estimating egg production and worm burden, J. Parasitol. 36:451.
3. Beaver, P.C., Jung, R.C., and Cupp, E.W. 1984. Clinical parasitology, ed. 9. Lea & Febiger, Philadelphia.
4. Biagi, F., Navarrete, F., Piña, A., Santiago, A.M., and Tapia, L. 1961. Estudio de tres reacciones serológicas en el diagnóstico de la cisticercosis. Rev. Med. Hosp. Gen. Mexico City 24:501.
5. Brooke, M.M., and Goldman, M. 1949. Polyvinyl alcohol-fixative as a preservative and adhesive for protozoa in dysenteric stools and other liquid material. J. Lab. Clin. Med. 34:1554.
6. Brooke, M.M., and Melvin, D. 1969. Morphology of diagnostic stages of intestinal parasites of man. DHEW Publ. No. (HSM)72-8116. U.S. Government Printing Office, Atlanta.
7. Cohen, J.D., Ruhlig L., Jayich, S.A., Tong, M.J., Lechago, J., and Snape, W.J. 1984. *Cryptosporidium* in acquired immunodeficiency syndrome. Dig. Dis. Sci. 29:773.
8. Coltorti, E.A., and Varela-Diaz, V.M. 1978. Detection of antibodies against *Echinococcus granulosus* arc 5 antigens by double diffusion test. Trans. R. Soc. Trop. Med. Hyg. 72:226.
9. Committee on Education, American Society of Parasitologists. 1977. Procedures suggested for use in examination of clinical specimens for parasitic infection. J. Parasitol. 63:959.
10. Dennis, D.T., and Kean, B.H. 1971. Isolation of microfilariae: report of a new method. J. Parasitol. 57:1146.
11. Desowitz, R.S., and Hitchcock, J.C. 1974. Hyperendemic bancroftian filariasis in the Kingdom of Tonga: the application of the membrane filter concentration technique to an age-stratified blood survey. Am. J. Trop. Med. Hyg. 23:877.
12. Feinberg, J.G., and Whittington, M.J. 1957. A culture medium for *Trichomonas vaginalis* Donne and species of *Candida*. J. Clin. Pathol. 10:327.
13. Garcia, L.S., and Ash, L.R. 1979. Diagnostic parasitology: clinical laboratory manual. ed. 2. The C.V. Mosby Co., St. Louis.
14. Garcia, L.S., Bruckner, D.A., Brewer, T.C., and Shimizu, R.Y. 1983. Techniques for the recovery and identification of *Cryptosporidium* oocysts from stool specimens. J. Clin. Micro. 18:185.

15. Gomori, G. 1950. A rapid one-step trichrome stain. Am. J. Clin. Pathol. 20:661.
16. Harada, Y., and Mori, O. 1955. A new method for culturing hookworm. Yonago Acta Med. 1:177.
17. Healy, G.R., and Ruebush, T.K. II. 1980. Morphology of *Babesia microti* in human blood smears. Am. J. Clin. Pathol. 73:107.
18. Hendricks, L., and Wright, N. 1979. Diagnosis of cutaneous leishmaniasis by in vitro cultivation of saline aspirates in Schneider's drosophila medium. Am. J. Trop. Med. Hyg. 28(6):962.
19. Kagan, I.G. 1979. Diagnostic epidemiologic and experimental parasitology: immunologic aspects. Am. J. Trop. Med. Hyg. 28:429.
20. Kagan, I.G. 1980. Serodiagnosis of parasitic diseases. In Lennette, E.H., Balows, A., Hausler, W.J., Jr., and Truant, J.P., editors: Manual of clinical microbiology, ed. 3. American Society for Microbiology, Washington, D.C.
21. Kagan, I.G., and Quist, K.D. 1970. An evaluation of five serologic tests for the diagnosis of trichinosis in lightly infected swine. *In* Singh, K.S., and Tandan, B.K., editors: H.D. Srivastava commemoration volume, Iznatnagar, U.P. India, India Veterinary Research Institute.
22. Knott, J.I. 1939. A method for making microfilarial surveys on day blood. Trans. R. Soc. Trop. Med. Hyg. 33:191.
23. Labzoffsky, N.A. Baratawidjaja, R.K., Kuitunen, E., Lewis F.N., Kavelman, D.A., and Morrissey, L.P. 1964. Immunofluorescence as an aid in the early diagnosis of trichinosis. Can Med. Assoc. J. 90:920.
24. Lennette, E.H., Balows, A., Hausler, W.J., Jr., and Shadomy H.J., editors. 1985. Manual of clinical microbiology, ed. 4. American Society for Microbiology, Washington, D.C.
25. Lim, S.K., Eveland, W.C., and Porter, R.J. 1974. Direct fluorescent-antibody for the diagnosis of *Pneumocystis carinii* pneumonia from sputa or tracheal aspirations from humans. Appl. Microbiol. 27:144.
26. Maekelt, G.A. 1964. A modified procedure of xenodiagnosis for Chagas' disease. Am. J. Trop. Med. Hyg. 13:11.
27. Markell, E.K., and Voge, M. 1981. Medical parasitology, ed. 5. W.B. Saunders Co., Philadelphia.
28. McLaren M., Draper, C.C., Roberts, J.M., Minter-Goedbloed, E., Ligthart, G.S., Teesdale, C.H., Amin, M.A., Omer, A.H.S., Bartlett, A., and Voller, A. 1978. Studies on the enzyme linked immunosorbent assay (ELISA) test for *Schistosoma mansoni* infections. Ann. Trop. Med. Parasitol. 72:243.
29. Melvin, D.M., and Brooke, M.M. 1974. Laboratory procedures for the diagnosis of intestinal parasites.

30. DHEW Pub. No. (CDC) 75-8282, Washington, D.C., U.S. Government Printing Office.
30. Miller, L.H., Mason, S.J., Dvorak, J.A., McGinniss, M.H., and Rothman, I.K. 1975. Erythrocyte receptors for (*Plasmodium knowlesi*) malaria: Duffy blood group determinants. Science 189:561.
31. Nair, C.P. 1953. Rapid staining of intestinal amoebae on wet mounts. Nature 172:1051.
32. Navin, T.R., and Juranek, D.D. 1984. Cryptosporidiosis: Clinical, epidemiologic and parasitologic review. Rev. Inf. Dis. 6:313.
33. Ng, E., Markell, E.K., Fleming, R.L., and Fried, M. 1984. Demonstration of *Isospora belli* by acid-fast stain in a patient with acquired immune deficiency syndrome. J. Clin. Micro. 20:384.
34. Palacios, B.O., de la Hoz, R., and Sosa, H. 1978. Determinación del antígeno amibiano en heces por el método elisa (enzyme linked immunosorbent assay) para la identificación de *Entamoeba histolytica*. Arch. Invest. Med. 1(Supp. 9):339.
35. Parasitology Subcommittee, Microbiology Section of Scientific Assembly, American Society for Medical Technology. 1978. Recommended procedures for the examination of clinical specimens submitted for the diagnosis of parasitic infections. Am. J. Med. Technol. 44:1101.
36. Proctor, E.M., and Elsdon-Dew, R. 1966. Serological tests in porcine cysticercosis. S. Afr. J. Sci. 62:264.
37. Proctor, E.M., Powell, S.J., and Elsdon-Dew, R. 1966. The serological diagnosis of cysticercosis. Ann. Trop. Med. Parasitol. 60:146.
38. Remington, J.S., Eimstad, W.M., and Fausto, G.A. 1983. Detection of immunoglobulin M antibodies with antigen-tagged latex particles in an immunosorbent assay. J. Clin. Microbiol. 17:939.
39. Sapero, J.J., and Lawless, D.K. 1953. The MIF stain-preservation technique for the identification of intestinal protozoa. Am. J. Trop. Med. Hyg. 2:613.
40. Scholten, T.H. 1972. An improved technique for the recovery of intestinal protozoa. J. Parasitol. 58:633.
41. Scholten, T.H., and Yang, J. 1974. Evaluation of unpreserved and preserved stools for the detection and identification of intestinal parasites. Am. J. Clin. Pathol. 62:563.
42. Serafin-Anaya, F.J., Castañeda-Castañeira, E., Diaz, S., Palacios, O., Gutierrez-Trujillo, G. 1978. Amebiasis intestinal en niños. II. Evaluación de diversas técnicas diagnósticas y distintos esquemas terapéuticos. Arch. Invest. Med. 1(Supp. 9):371.
43. Siegel, J.P., and Remington, J.S. 1983. Comparison of methods for quantitating antigen-specific immunoglobulin M antibody with a reverse enzyme-linked immunosorbent assay. J. Clin. Microbiol. 18:63.

44. Spencer, F.M., and Monroe, L.S. 1976. *The color atlas of intestinal parasites*, ed. 2. Charles C Thomas, Publisher, Springfield, Ill.
45. Stoll, N.R., and Hausheer, W.C. 1926. Concerning two options in dilution egg counting: small drop and displacement. Am. J. Hyg. 6:134.
46. Sulzer, A.J., and Chisholm, E.S. 1966. Comparison of the IFA and other tests for *Trichinella spiralis* antibodies. Public Health Rep. 81:729.
47. Sulzer, A.J., Wilson, M. 1967. The use of thick-smear antigen slides in the malaria indirect fluorescent antibody test. J. Parasitol. 53:1110.
48. Sulzer, A.J., Wilson, M., and Hall, E.C. 1969. Indirect fluorescent antibody tests for parasitic diseases. V. An evaluation of a thick-smear antigen in the IFA for malaria antibodies. Am. J. Trop. Med. Hyg. 18:199.
49. Taylor, R.G., and Perez, T.R. 1978. Serology of amebiasis using FIAX system. Arch. Invest. Med. 1:(Supp. 9):363.
50. Tompkins, V.N., and Miller, J.K. 1947. Staining intestinal protozoa with iron-hematoxylin-phosphotungstic acid. Am. J. Clin. Pathol. 17:755.
51. Vattuone, N.H. and Yanovsky, J.F. 1971. *Trypanosoma cruzi:* agglutination activity of enzyme-treated epimastigotes. Exp. Parasitol. 30:349.
52. Wheatley, W.B. 1951. A rapid staining procedure for intestinal amoebae and flagellates. Am. J. Clin. Pathol. 21:990.
53. Wilcox, A. 1960. Manual for the microscopical diagnosis of malaria in man. Public Health Service, Washington, D.C.
54. Zierdt, C.H. 1978. *Blastocystis hominis*, an intestinal protozoan parasite of man. Public Health Lab. 36:146.

45 Formulas and Preparation of Culture Media and Reagents

The basic principles governing the preparation of laboratory media were discussed in Chapter 8. The importance of testing each batch of media for proper performance was discussed in Chapter 3. Various specialized media formulations and uses have been mentioned throughout the text where appropriate; these media are cross-referenced in this chapter. The media formulas included in this chapter are those that can be used for more than one purpose or those that are so complicated that they cannot easily be placed within a chapter. Unless stated otherwise, storage of prepared media at 2°-8° C best preserves their usefulness. Tubed media should be stored tightly capped; tubed media that must be stored for long periods can be made airtight by dipping the tightly capped end into melted paraffin several times. Alternatively, several layers of Parafilm (American Can Co.) can be wrapped tightly around the cap end. Liquid media that have been stored for any length of time should be heated in a boiling water bath or in flowing steam (Arnold steam sterilizer, Chapter 8) for a few minutes to drive off dissolved gases and then cooled quickly to room temperature (in cold water, for example) before using. Agar tubes should be melted and allowed to resolidify to reconstitute sufficient moisture. Agar plates should be wrapped tightly in sealed plastic bags (polyethylene or other plastic) and stored upside down so that moisture does not collect on the agar surface. if agar plates of a particular medium will be used infrequently, tubes of the medium can be prepared (20 ml per tube) and stored, to be melted down and poured into Petri plates one at a time as needed. In the formulas given in this chapter and throughout the text, specific manufacturers of components have been mentioned if they were specified in the original reference, or if they are commonly available from that source. The substitution of similar ingredients should be confirmed by testing quality control strains of organisms before assuming that such media are equivalent. Instructions for proper preparation of all dry powder media are printed on the container or provided by the manufacturer in a supplemental publication, such as the *Difco Manual*, *Oxoid Manual*, and others. Almost every medium used for clinical microbiology, however, can be purchased prepared from at least one manufacturer. Specialty media can also be purchased, often at a slightly increased price. The most well-known large media suppliers are listed in the Appendix. Laboratories may often be able to find local suppliers for prepared media that are not cost effective for in-house preparation.

ACETATE AGAR

Acetate agar medium is prepared in the same manner as Simmons citrate agar except that 0.25% sodium acetate is used in place of citrate. It is used to determine whether an organism is able to utilize acetate as its sole carbon source. Growth on the slant and development of a **blue** color indicate a positive test. A negative test is no growth or color change.

This test is useful in differentiating *Escherichia coli* from shigellae in that the latter do not utilize acetate.

ALKALINE PEPTONE WATER FOR RECOVERY OF *VIBRIO CHOLERAE*

Peptone	10 g
NaCl	5 g
Distilled water	1,000 ml

Adjust to pH 9.0 with 1 N NaOH and autoclave for 15 min at 121° C.

AMIES TRANSPORT MEDIUM WITH CHARCOAL FOR MAINTENANCE OF FASTIDIOUS ORGANISMS IN ORIGINAL SPECIMENS

(Amies. 1967. Can. J. Public Health 58:296.)

1. Add 4 g of agar to 1 liter of distilled water, heat until dissolved, and while hot add:

Sodium chloride	3 g
Potassium chloride	0.2 g
Sodium thioglycollate	1 g
Disodium phosphate, anhydrous	1.15 g
(or disodium phosphate · 12 H_2O)	2.9 g
Monopotassium phosphate	0.2 g
Calcium chloride, 1% aqueous, freshly prepared	10 ml
Magnesium chloride · 6 H_2O, 1% aqueous	10 ml

(Final pH 7.3)

2. Stir until dissolved, and then add 10 g of pharmaceutical neutral charcoal. Dispense 5-6 ml per 13 by 100 mm screw-capped tube (or vial), with frequent stirring to keep the charcoal in suspension. Avoid cooling or gelling.
3. Sterilize at 121° C for 20 min. **Prior to solidification,** invert tubes to distribute the charcoal evenly. Store in refrigerator.
4. It should be emphasized that prolonged heating in open flasks should be avoided, since the reducing agent (sodium thioglycolate) is volatile.

ANAEROBIC INDICATORS USED TO VISUALLY DEMONSTRATE ANAEROBIC ATMOSPHERE WITHIN A JAR, CHAMBER, OR OTHER SYSTEM
Fildes and McIntosh Indicator

Prepare the following solutions:
1. 6% aqueous glucose (add a small crystal of thymol as a preservative).
2. Add 6 ml of 0.1 N sodium hydroxide to 94 ml of distilled water.
3. Add 3 ml of aqueous methylene blue (0.5%) to 100 ml of distilled water.

For use, mix 1 ml of each solution in a test tube, boil the mixture until colorless, then place in a loaded anaerobic jar before sealing. A blue color at the end of incubation indicates that anaerobiosis was not achieved.

Smith Modified Methylene Blue Indicator

(Smith. 1964. ASM meeting, Washington, D.C.)

Mix thoroughly 1 pound (450 g) of sodium bicarbonate (commercial grade is satisfactory) with 50 g of glucose and 20 mg of methylene blue. For use, add about 1 inch (2.5 cm) to a 16 × 100 mm test tube, half fill with tap water, invert to mix, and place within the anaerobic jar. The solution will slowly become colorless during incubation at 35° C; if more rapid decolorization is required, the solution may be heated to boiling and cooled rapidly immediately before placing in the jar. The indicator should be **colorless** at the end of incubation if anaerobiosis was maintained.

ANDRADE'S INDICATOR

(Modified from MacFaddin. 1980. Biochemical tests for identification of medical bacteria. Williams & Wilkins, Baltimore.)

Distilled water	100 ml
Acid fuchsin	0.5 g
1 N NaOH	16 ml

Dissolve the fuchsin in distilled water, and add the sodium hydroxide. If the fuchsin is not sufficiently decolorized after several hours, an additional 1 or 2 ml of sodium hydroxide is added. Continue to add NaOH (drop by drop) until the desired straw-yellow color is reached. Add Andrade's indicator to carbohydrate broth base used for phenol red carbohydrates (see Phenol red broth base, below) without the phenol red to a final concentration of 1% (10 ml indicator per liter broth base). Adjust the pH to 7.1-7.2 before adding carbohydrates. See *Carbohydrate media* for further information.

ASCOSPORE AGAR

Potassium acetate	10 g
Yeast extract	2.5 g
Dextrose	1 g
Agar	30 g
Distilled water	1,000 ml

Dissolve, tube, and autoclave at 121° C for 15 min. Ascospores are obtained in 2-6 days at room temperature (23°-25° C).

BACTEROIDES BILE ESCULIN AGAR (BBE AGAR)

Trypticase soy agar	40 g
Oxgall	20 g
Esculin	1 g
Ferric ammonium citrate	0.5 g
Hemin solution (5 mg/ml)	2 ml
Gentamicin solution (40 mg/ml)*	2.5 ml
Distilled water	1,000 ml

Adjust pH to 7.0, heat to dissolve, dispense in 100 ml bottles, autoclave at 121° C for 15 min, and cool to 50° C. Pour plates.

BEEF EXTRACT AGAR

Add 2.5% agar to beef extract broth, dissolve by boiling, adjust to pH 7.6, tube and autoclave at 121° C for 15 min, and slant before solidifying.

The medium is used for pure culture preparation of *Candida* species prior to carrying out fermentation tests.

BEEF EXTRACT BROTH

Beef extract	3 g
Peptone	10 g
Sodium chloride	5 g
Distilled water	1,000 ml

Dissolve ingredients by boiling, adjust to pH 7.2, tube in 10 ml amounts in 18 × 150 mm tubes, and autoclave at 121° C for 15 min. For use as a fermentation base broth, add 100 ml of a 0.04% aqueous solution of bromthymol blue before tubing and sterilizing.

---

*Garamycin injectable (Schering Corp.) may be used.

The medium is used for differentiation of *Candida* species by carbohydrate fermentation tests.

BILE

See Oxgall.

BILE ESCULIN AGAR

Beef extract	3 g
Peptone	5 g
Oxgall	40 g
Esculin	1 g
Ferric citrate	0.5 g
Agar	15 g
Distilled water	1,000 ml

1. Suspend 64 g of the dehydrated medium in water, heat to boiling to dissolve, and tube in screw-capped tubes.
2. Sterilize by autoclaving at 121° C for 15 min.
3. Cool to 55° C, add aseptically 50 ml of filter-sterilized horse serum (optional), and mix well.
4. Dispense in sterile tubes, and cool in a slanted position.

This medium is useful in the selective detection of group D streptococci. After inoculation, these organisms form brownish-black colonies surrounded by a black zone. *Listeria monocytogenes* also reacts positively, as do some other organisms. Other forms of agar and broth media also are available.

BIRDSEED AGAR

Guizottia abyssinica seeds (niger or thistle seeds)	70 g
Creatinine	0.78 g
Dextrose	10 g
Chloramphenicol (one 50 mg capsule)	0.05 g
Agar	20 g
Distilled water	1,000 ml
Diphenyl	100 mg
95% Ethyl alcohol	10 ml

1. Grind seed to powder in blender. Add 300 ml of water, and autoclave at 115° C for 10 min.
2. Filter through gauze, and bring volume to 1 liter.
3. Add other ingredients except diphenyl, and autoclave at 121° C for 15 min.
4. Cool to 50° C.
5. Add diphenyl to 10 ml of 95% ethanol, and add aseptically to medium.
6. Stir and pour into plates.

BISMUTH SULFITE AGAR

Beef extract	5 g
Peptone	10 g
Dextrose	5 g
Disodium phosphate	4 g
Ferrous sulfate	0.3 g
Bismuth sulfite indicator	8 g
Agar	20 g
Brilliant green	0.025 g
Distilled water	1,000 ml

Bismuth sulfite agar medium is highly recommended for the isolation of *Salmonella typhi*, as well as other salmonellae. It may be used for both streak and pour plates.

BLOOD AGAR PLATES FOR STREAKING

Blood agar base medium	500 ml
Sterile blood	20 ml

Sterilize the base medium (trypticase soy agar [BBL] or tryptic soy agar [Difco] are recommended*), cool to 48°-50° C, and add 5% sterile defibrinated sheep, horse, or rabbit blood, aseptically. Rotate to mix thoroughly, and pour into sterile Petri dishes in approximately 20 ml amounts. When agar is set, invert and incubate one or two plates per 100-200 ml batch overnight to test for sterility. Discard test plates. Blood agar plates may be refrigerated for 1 week without deterioration, but they should be packaged to minimize water loss, which could amount to 7% per week if unprotected.

---

*Brucella agar is an excellent base for blood agar for anaerobic bacteria. Columbia agar and Schaedler agar have also been recommended for this purpose.

The pouring should be done carefully to avoid air bubbles. If bubbles appear in the poured plate, pass a Bunsen flame over the agar before it sets. This causes the bubbles to break.

An alternative to pouring media from an Erlenmeyer flask is the use of a Kelly bottle with a release clamp on a piece of rubber tubing connected to a bell device at the other end. This assembly is mounted on a ring stand. Release of pressure on the clamp permits the heated medium to flow evenly into the plate. An advantage of this system is that bubbles (when present) rise to the top of the liquid medium in the bottle prior to its being poured into the plate.

BLOOD CYSTINE DEXTROSE AGAR

(Francis. 1928. J.A.M.A. 91:1155; Rhamy. 1933. Am. J. Clin. Pathol. 3:121.)

Beef heart infusion	500 g
Proteose peptone	10 g
Glucose	10 g
Sodium chloride	5 g
Cystine	1 g
Agar	15 g
Distilled water	1,000 ml

Blood cystine dextrose agar medium may be used satisfactorily for the cultivation of *Francisella tularensis*.

To prepare this medium dissolve 16.8 g of dehydrated product in 300 ml of distilled water. Adjust the medium to pH 7.3 and autoclave for 20 min at 15 pounds pressure. Cool to a temperature of 60°-70° C, add 18 ml of whole rabbit blood or dehydrated hemoglobin, mix well, and distribute into test tubes aseptically. Cool in a slanted position.

BORDET-GENGOU MEDIUM

Potatoes, infusion from	125 g
Sodium chloride	5.5 g
Agar	20 g
Distilled water	1,000 ml

Sterilize at 15 pounds for 15 min. Cool to 50° C and add 15%-20% sterile sheep, rabbit, or human blood aseptically.

The medium is recommended for cultivation of *Bordetella pertussis*.

BRAIN-HEART INFUSION BLOOD AGAR (BHIBA)

Brain-heart infusion agar (BBL, Difco, Gibco, Inolex)	26 g
Agar, powdered	2.5 g
Distilled water	500 ml
(Final pH approximately 7.4)	

Suspend the ingredients in the water, and dissolve by boiling. Autoclave for 15 min at 121° C. Cool to about 45° C, and add aseptically 30 ml of defibrinated animal blood. Mix well, and distribute aseptically in approximately 20 ml amounts in cotton-plugged and sterilized 25 × 150 mm Pyrex test tubes (without lips). Slant, allow to harden, and refrigerate. The medium may also be poured into plates, 40 ml/90 mm diameter Petri dish.

This medium is used for the isolation of fastidious fungi.

BRAIN-HEART INFUSION BROTH

Calf brain infusion	200 g
Beef heart infusion	250 g
Proteose peptone	10 g
Dextrose	2 g
Sodium chloride	5 g
Disodium phosphate	2.5 g
Distilled water	1,000 ml
(Reaction of medium pH 7.4)	

Brain-heart infusion broth is recommended for cultivating the pneumococcus for the liquid bile solubility test.

BRILLIANT GREEN AGAR

Yeast extract	3 g
Proteose peptone No. 3	10 g
Sodium chloride	5 g
Lactose	10 g
Sucrose	10 g

Phenol red	0.08 g
Brilliant green	0.0125 g
Agar	20 g
Distilled water	1,000 ml

(Final pH 6.9)

Brilliant green agar is a highly selective medium recommended for the isolation of salmonellae other than *Salmonella typhi*. It is not recommended for the isolation of shigellae.

BROMCRESOL PURPLE BROTH BASE FOR IDENTIFICATION OF STREPTOCOCCI

See Chapter 25.

BRUCELLA AGAR

Pancreatic digest of casein USP	10 g
Peptic digest of animal tissues USP	10 g
Yeast autolysate	2 g
Dextrose	1 g
Sodium chloride	5 g
Sodium bisulfite	0.1 g
Agar	15 g
Distilled water	1,000 ml

(Final pH 7.0 ± 0.02)

Heat with agitation until dissolved. Dispense and autoclave at 121° C for 15 min. Cool to 50° C and pour plates.

BRUCELLA SELECTIVE MEDIUM (FOR BRUCELLA)

Heart infusion agar	
Gelatin	1 g
Glucose	2.5 g
Distilled water	1,000 ml

Mix ingredients, autoclave for 15 min at 121° C, allow to cool to 50° C, and add 10 ml of sterile sheep blood and the following antibiotics:

1. Cycloheximide: 1 ml of a 100 mg/ml stock solution, final concentration = 100 μg/ml of agar.
2. Bacitracin (Upjohn Co.): 1 ml of a 25,000 U/ml stock solution; final concentration = 25 U/ml of agar.
3. Circulin (Upjohn Co): 1 ml of 25,000 U/ ml stock solution; final concentration = 25 U/ml of agar.
4. Polymyxin B (Burroughs Wellcome): 0.6 ml of a 10,000 U/ml stock solution; final concentration = 6 U/ml of agar.

BRUCELLA–VITAMIN K₁ BLOOD AGAR (BRBA)

1. Vitamin K_1 solution (see Chapter 44)
2. Preparation of base:

Brucella agar (BBL, Difco, Gibco)	43 g
Agar	2.5 g
Distilled water	1,000 ml

Sterilize by autoclaving at 121° C for 15 min, and cool to 50° C.

3. Add aseptically:

| Defibrinated or laked sheep blood | 50 ml |
| Vitamin K_1 solution | 1 ml |

Mix well and pour plates, using approximately 20 ml per plate. Store at room temperature. The medium is used for the isolation and subculture of anaerobes.

CAMPYLOBACTER MEDIA

The basic plate medium (Campy-BAP) consists of *Brucella* agar base and 5% sheep erythrocytes with the following amounts of antimicrobials per liter: vancomycin, 10 mg; trimethoprim, 5 mg; polymyxin B, 2,500 IU; amphotericin B, 2 mg; and cephalothin, 15 mg. The liquid medium (Campy-thio) is thioglycolate broth with 0.16% agar and the antimicrobials listed above.

CARBOHYDRATE BROTH

Prepare the following ingredients:
1. Heart infusion broth, 22.5 g, in 900 ml of distilled water.
2. Carbohydrate, 10 g, in 100 ml of distilled water.
3. Indicator, 1 ml (1.6 g of bromcresol purple in 100 ml of 95% ethanol).

Add 1, 2, and 3 together; dispense in 3 ml amounts in 13 × 100 mm screw-capped tubes. Autoclave for 10 min at 121° C.

A positive reaction is recorded when the indicator changes from purple to yellow.

CARBOHYDRATE MEDIA FOR FERMENTATION TESTS

When some carbohydrates are sterilized by heating in alkaline broth, they are more or less broken down into simple carbohydrates. It has been found definitely advantageous to sterilize sugar solutions by filtration through Seitz or membrane filters and to add these aseptically to the broth base in the required amounts. Although several carbohydrates can withstand autoclave temperature and pressure, one is advised to sterilize the following by **filtration**: xylose, lactose, sucrose, arabinose, trehalose, rhamnose, and salicin. These may be prepared as 5% or 10% solutions, depending on solubility, then sterilized by filtration and added aseptically to the base containing an indicator, to give 0.5%-1% final concentration.

Other less heat-susceptible carbohydrates may be added to the broth base containing indicator (e.g., bromcresol purple) before autoclaving at 116°-118° C (10-12 pounds pressure) for 15 min. Ten Broeck, in 1920, found that unheated serum contains an enzyme that hydrolyzes maltose to glucose. Serum to be added to maltose broth should therefore be heated for 1 h at 60° C to inactivate the enzyme. Incubate the carbohydrate broth to test sterility.

Cary and Blair Transport Medium for Feces

Disodium phosphate	1.1 g
Sodium chloride	5 g
Sodium thioglycolate	1.5 g
Agar	5 g
Distilled water	991 ml

Add the ingredients to a chemically clean flask rinsed with Sörensen's 0.067 M buffer (pH 8.1). Heat with frequent agitation until the solution just becomes clear. Cool to 50° C. Add 9 ml of freshly prepared aqueous 1% $CaCl_2$, and adjust the pH to 8.4.

Distribute 7 ml into previously rinsed and sterilized 9 ml screw-capped vials. Steam for 15 min, cool, and tighten caps.

CASEIN MEDIUM FOR SEPARATION OF NOCARDIA AND STREPTOMYCES

(Centers for Disease Control)

Prepare separately:

Skimmed milk (dehydrated or instant nonfat milk)	10 g
Distilled water	100 ml

Autoclave at 121° C for 20 min

Distilled water	100 ml
Agar	2 g

Autoclave as above.

Cool both solutions to approximately 45° C, mix, and pour into sterile Petri dishes.

Test for Hydrolysis

Streak or make point inoculations of each culture on casein plates, using half of a plate for each organism. Incubate at 25° C (or 35° C if it does not grow at room temperature). Observe for clearing of casein in 7 and 14 days. *Nocardia asteroides* does not hydrolyze casein. *N. brasiliensis* and *Streptomyces* species hydrolyze casein.

CETRIMIDE AGAR

(Lowbury and Collins. 1955. J. Clin. Pathol. 8:47.)

Peptone	20 g
Magnesium chloride	1.4 g
Potassium sulfate	10 g
Agar, dried	13.6 g
Cetrimide	0.3 g
Distilled water	1,000 ml
Glycerol	10 ml

(Final pH 7.2)

Suspend the powder in the water, add 10 ml of glycerol, heat with frequent agitation, and boil for 1 minute.

Dispense in 5 ml amounts in 15 × 125 mm

screw-capped tubes, autoclave at 118°-121° C for 15 min, and slant to give a generous slant.

This medium is used for the selective isolation or identification of *Pseudomonas aeruginosa*, whose growth is not inhibited by the cetrimide. Other members of the genus (except *P. fluorescens*) and related nonfermentative organisms are inhibited.

Cetrimide is cetyl trimethyl ammonium bromide (hexadecyltrimethylammonium bromide). This agent is called cetrimide per USP. It is available from Sigma and other suppliers. However, lots of cetrimide differ in their properties. For this reason, it is critical that cetrimide agar prepared from a new lot be tested with several quality control strains to ascertain that it is acceptable. Cetrimide agar is also available commercially.

(BUFFERED) CHARCOAL YEAST EXTRACT AGAR (BCYE)*

(Modified from Pasculle et al. 1980. J. Infect. Dis. 441:727.)

Yeast extract	10 g
Activated charcoal (Norit A or SG)	2 g
L-Cysteine HCl · H$_2$O	0.4 g
Ferric pyrophosphate, soluble	0.25 g
ACES buffer (Calbiochem, Behring, or Sigma)	10 g
Agar	17 g
α-Ketoglutarate, monopotassium salt (Sigma)	1 g
Purified water	980 ml

1. Dissolve the cysteine and ferric pyrophosphate separately in 10 ml of purified water. Place in a 37° C water bath for about 15 min to aid dissolution.
2. Add the ACES to 200 ml of purified water, and heat stir at lowest temperature for 30 min. Membrane filter sterilize, and store in a sterile container.

*Available in prepared plates from Remel Labs.

3. Add yeast extract, agar, and Norit to a flask containing 750 ml purified water.
4. Boil, add a stir bar, and sterilize by autoclaving for 15 min at 121° C.
5. Place the sterilized agar in a 50° to 52° C water bath for 1 h.
6. Place the melted agar on a heated stirrer, and rotate the stir bar slowly to avoid frothing.
7. Add filtered ACES slowly to stirring agar. **Note:** Preheat ACES in a 50° C water bath before adding.
8. Add the cysteine and then the ferric pyrophosphate to the stirred agar, using a syringe with an attached disk filter (e.g., Gelman Acrodisc 0.20 μm) in order to filter sterilize the small volume added.
9. Check the pH, and adjust it to 6.9 ± 0.05 using 1 N KOH. **Note:** 35-40 ml of KOH is required.
10. Pour into plates (15-20 ml per plate). **Note:** Swirl the bulk agar after pouring each plate to keep charcoal in suspension.
11. Incubate plates at room temperature for 24-48 h, and store packaged at 2°-8° C for a maximum of 8 weeks.

Selective Buffered Charcoal Yeast Extract Agar (Semiselective medium for Legionella pneumophila [BMPA-α])

(Edelstein. 1981. J. Clin. Microbiol. 14:298.)

Prepare buffered charcoal yeast extract agar base as described above. After the pH has been adjusted, add antimicrobial agents to the following final concentrations (using methods outlined in Chapter 13):

Anisomycin	80 μg/ml
Polymyxin B	80 U/ml
Cefamandole	4 μg/ml

This medium is also available in prepared plates from Remel Labs.

Differential Buffered Charcoal Yeast Extract Agar (DIFF/BCYE)

(Vickers et al. 1981. J. Clin. Microbiol. 13:380.)

Yeast extract	10 g
Activated charcoal (Norit A or SG)	1.5 g
L-Cysteine HCl	0.4 g
Ferric pyrophosphate (soluble)	0.25 g
ACES buffer	10 g
Agar	17 g
Bromcresol purple	0.01 g
Bromthymol blue	0.01 g
Polymyxin B (optional)	50,000 U
Vancomycin (optional)	0.001 g
Purified water	approx. 1,000 ml

1. Dissolve the cysteine and ferric pyrophosphate separately in 10 ml of purified water. Place in a 37° C water bath for about 15 min to aid dissolution.
2. Add the ACES to 200 ml of purified water, and heat stir at lowest temperature for 30 min. Membrane filter sterilize, and store in a sterile container.
3. Prepare separately 1% solutions (w/v) of bromcresol purple and bromthymol blue in 0.1 N KOH (1 g in 100 ml 0.1 N KOH). Membrane filter sterilize, and store at 2°-8° C.
4. Prepare a sterile solution of polymyxin B (50,000 U/ml) and vancomycin (1,000 μg/ml), and store in aliquots at −20° C.
5. Add yeast extract, agar, and Norit to a flask containing 750 ml of purified water.
6. Boil, add a stir bar, and sterilize by autoclaving for 15 min at 121° C.
7. Place the sterilized agar in a 50°-52° C water bath for 1 hr.
8. Place the melted agar on a heated stirrer, and rotate the stir bar slowly to avoid frothing.
9. Add filtered ACES slowly to stirring agar. **Note:** Preheat ACES in a 50° C water bath before adding.
10. Add the cysteine and then the ferric pyro-phosphate to the stirring agar using a syringe with an attached disk filter (e.g., Gelman Acrodisc 0.20 μm) to filter sterilize the small volume added.
11. Check the pH, and adjust it to 6.9 ± 0.05 using 1 N KOH. **Note:** 35-40 ml of KOH is required.
12. Add 1 ml each of the sterile 1% bromcresol purple and 1% bromthymol blue dye solutions to the adjusted agar.
13. Optional: Add the polymyxin B and vancomycin agents to the adjusted agar at final concentrations of 50,000 U and 1,000 μg, respectively, per liter of medium.
14. Pour into plates (15-20 ml per plate). **Note:** Swirl the bulk agar after pouring each plate to keep charcoal in suspension.
15. Incubate the plates at room temperature for 24-48 h, and store packaged at 2°-8° C for a maximum of 8 weeks.

CHLAMYDIA MEDIA

Growth Medium for McCoy Cell Cultures Used for Cultivation of Chlamydia trachomatis

RPMI 1640 (Flow Laboratories)	500 ml
Inactivated fetal bovine serum (Gibco)	50 ml
Glutamine (Sigma, 200 mmol/ml)	5 ml
Gentamicin (Schering Corp., 1,000 μg/ml)	1.4 ml

Add all ingredients together. Aseptically adjust pH to 7.4.

Maintenance Medium for McCoy Cell Cultures Used for Cultivation of C. trachomatis

RPMI 1640 (Flow Laboratories)	500 ml
Inactivated fetal bovine serum (Gibco)	25 ml
Glucose solution (filter sterilized, 1.1 g in 100 ml of distilled water)	25 ml
Glutamine (Sigma, 200 mmol/ml)	5 ml
Amphotericin B (E.R. Squibb & Sons, 250 μg/ml)	5.6 ml
Gentamicin (Schering Corp., 1,000 μg/ml)	5.6 ml

Add all ingredients together. Aseptically adjust pH to 7.4.

CHLAMYDOSPORE AGAR

Chlamydospore agar (BBL)	18.5 g
Distilled water	500 ml

Suspend the dehydrated product in a 1-liter Erlenmeyer flask, dissolve by heating, and tube in approximately 15 ml amounts in screw-capped, 20 × 150 mm test tubes. Autoclave at 121° C for 15 min with caps loosened. When cool, tighten caps and store at room temperature. When needed, melt a tube in a water bath, pour into a sterile Petri plate, and allow to solidify.

CHOCOLATE AGAR

Chocolate agar is agar to which blood or hemoglobin has been added and then heated until the medium becomes brown or chocolate colored. The recommended method of preparing this is as follows.

Suspend sufficient proteose No. 3 agar (Difco), Eugonagar (BBL), or GC agar base (BBL, Difco, Gibco) in distilled water to make a double strength base. Mix thoroughly, and heat to boiling for 1 minute with frequent agitation. Autoclave at 121° C for 15 min. At the same time, autoclave an equal volume of 2% hemoglobin (BBL, Difco, Gibco), which is made by the gradual addition of distilled water to the dehydrated hemoglobin, to obtain a **smooth suspension.** Cool both solutions to approximately 50° C, add the supplement (IsoVitaleX enrichment [BBL] or Supplement B or C [Difco] is recommended), combine with bacteriologic precautions, and then pour into sterile, disposable Petri plates. Best results are obtained when plates are **freshly prepared.** One or two plates per 100-200 ml batch should be incubated at 35° C overnight to determine sterility and later discarded.

Chocolate agar slants may be prepared individually by the method just described, slanting the medium after it has been tubed in 5-10 ml amounts in sterile screw-capped tubes. To prepare a large number of slants, use a flask containing 50-100 ml of agar, proceeding as before.

CHOCOLATE AGAR WITH ISOVITALEX AND VANCOMYCIN FOR RECOVERY OF *HAEMOPHILUS DUCREYI*

Chocolate agar is prepared as described above, using 1% IsoVitaleX enrichment. Before plates are poured, vancomycin (Upjohn Co.) is added for a final concentration of 3 μg/ml.

CHOPPED MEAT GLUCOSE (CMG)

Ground beef, fat free	500 g
Distilled water	1,000 ml
Sodium hydroxide, 1 N	25 ml

1. Mix ingredients, bring to boil, and simmer with frequent stirring for 20 min.
2. Cool to room temperature, skim off fat, and filter through three layers of gauze. Squeeze out gauze, retaining both meat particles and filtrate (filtered through coarse and fine paper).
3. Restore filtrate to 1 liter with distilled water, and add:

Trypticase	30 g
Yeast extract	5 g
Dipotassium phosphate	5 g
Resazurin solution (25 mg/100 ml water)	4 ml

4. Boil, cool, adjust to pH 7.8, and add 0.5% glucose and 0.5 g of cystine.
5. Dispense 6-7 ml amounts into tubes containing meat particles (step 2), 1 part meat to 4 or 5 parts broth, and autoclave at 121° C for 20 min.

This medium is recommended as a "backup" medium for the primary isolation of anaerobes and also for growing pure cultures for gas-liquid chromatographic analysis (available in prereduced tubes from Scott Laboratories). It may also be obtained as a dehydrated medium, cooked meat phytone [BBL, Gibco].

CHOPPED-MEAT MEDIUM

To 1 pound of finely ground beef heart and other muscle (fat free) add 500 ml of boiling sodium hydroxide (N/15-N/20) and boil for 20 min. Cool, strain off the fat, and filter through muslin. Adjust the fluid to pH 7.5, and add 1% peptone. Add approximately 2 inches (5 cm) of meat and a small ball of steel wool to each tube, and add enough broth to overlay the meat by about 1 inch (2.5 cm). Heat tubes for 30 min in boiling water, and sterilize by autoclaving at 121° C for 15 min. The medium should be boiled for a few minutes to drive off dissolved oxygen if it is not to be used the same day, unless the prereduced tubed media are used. Incubation in an anaerobic jar or under a petrolatum seal may be required for cultivation or maintenance of certain *Clostridium* species, except for prereduced tubed media.

CIN AGAR (*YERSINIA ENTEROCOLITICA* SELECTIVE AGAR)

(*Schiemann. 1982. Appl. Environ. Microbiol. 43:14.*)

1. Agar base (available commercially from Difco, Oxoid, and other suppliers) contains the following ingredients:

Yeast extract	2 g
Peptone	17 g
Proteose peptone (Difco)	3 g
Mannitol	20 g
Sodium deoxycholate	0.5 g
Sodium cholate	0.5 g
Sodium chloride	1 g
Sodium pyruvate	2 g
Magnesium sulfate, heptahydrate	10 mg
Agar (Bacto, Difco)	13.5 g
Neutral red	30 mg
Crystal violet	1 mg
Irgasan	4 mg

2. Add the ingredients to 1,000 ml distilled water. Heat to boiling to dissolve the powder.
3. Autoclave for 15 min at 121° C and cool to between 45°-50° C.

4. Aseptically add:

Cefsulodin	4 mg
Novobiocin	2.5 mg

5. Mix thoroughly and dispense into 90 mm diameter Petri plates, 20 ml per plate. Wrap plates tightly in plastic and store refrigerated for up to 1 month.

The antibiotics are available as premixed supplement solutions (CN, Difco, containing cefsulodin and novobiocin; SR109, Oxoid, containing irgasan, cefsulodin, and novobiocin). Colonies of *Yersinia* appear bright pink or red; most other bacteria are inhibited. One exception is certain strains of *Aeromonas hydrophila*; CIN agar has been found to aid in selective isolation of *Aeromonas* from stool.

CITRATE AGAR

(*Simmons. 1926. J. Infect. Dis. 39:209.*)

Agar	20 g
Sodium chloride	5 g
Magnesium sulfate	0.2 g
Ammonium dihydrogen phosphate	1 g
Dipotassium phosphate	1 g
Sodium citrate	2 g
Bromthymol blue	0.08 g
Distilled water	1,000 ml
(Final pH 6.9)	

Citrate agar is used to determine the utilization of citrate as the sole carbon source. Development of a blue color indicates a positive test.

COLUMBIA AGAR BASE

Polypeptone (BBL) or Pantone (Difco)	10 g
Biosate (BBL) or Bitone (Difco)	10 g
Myosate (BBL) or tryptic digest of beef heart	3 g
Cornstarch	1 g
Sodium chloride	5 g
Agar	13.5 g
Distilled or demineralized water	1,000 ml
(Final pH 7.3 ± 0.2)	

Heat with agitation until the medium boils. Dispense and autoclave at 121° C for 15 min.

COLUMBIA CNA AGAR

Polypeptone peptone (BBL)	10 g
Biosate peptone (BBL)	10 g
Myosate peptone (BBL)	3 g
Cornstarch	1 g
Sodium chloride	5 g
Agar, dried	13.5 g
Colistin	10 mg
Nalidixic acid	15 mg
Distilled water	1,000 ml

(Final pH 7.3±)

1. Suspend 42.5 g of dehydrated medium in water, heat with frequent agitation, and boil for 1 min.
2. Sterilize by autoclaving at 121° C for 15 min.
3. Cool to 50° C, add 5% defibrinated sheep blood, and pour plates.

This medium is excellent for the selective growth of gram-positive cocci, particularly streptococci, when gram-negative bacilli, especially *Proteus* species, tend to overgrow on conventional blood agar plates. This medium may be inhibitory for certain strains of staphylococci.

CORNMEAL AGAR

Yellow cornmeal	125 g
Distilled water	3,000 ml

Heat the cornmeal in water at 60° C for 1 h, filter through paper, make up to volume, and add 50 g of agar. Expose to flowing steam for 1 hr, filter through absorbent cotton, dispense in tubes, and autoclave at 121° C for 30 min. Cornmeal agar suppresses vegetative growth of many fungi while stimulating sporulation. With the addition of 1% Tween 80, it is useful in stimulating production of chlamydospores of *Candida albicans*. Some workers find that "homemade" media such as this give more consistent results.

CYCLOSERINE-CEFOXITIN FRUCTOSE AGAR (CCFA)

(George, et al. 1979. J. Clin. Microbiol. 9:214.)

Prepare 1 liter of egg yolk agar base, substituting 6 g of fructose for the glucose and adding 3 ml of 1% neutral red in ethanol. This base is dispensed in 100 ml quantities and sterilized at 121° C for 15 min. After cooling to 50° C, cycloserine base is added to a final concentration of 500 mg/ml, and cefoxitin base is added to a final concentration of 16 mg/ml. The egg yolk suspension is added as indicated for egg yolk agar. Alternatively, one may leave out the egg yolk suspension (the medium is effective without the egg yolk, but the lecithinase and lipase reactions cannot be determined directly, of course). This is a highly selective and differential medium for *Clostridium difficile*.

CYSTINE TELLURITE BLOOD AGAR

(Frobisher. 1937. J. Infect. Dis. 60:99.)

1. Melt 100 ml of sterile 2% infusion agar in a flask, and cool to 45°-50° C. Care should be taken to maintain this temperature throughout the following steps in the preparation of the medium.
2. Add aseptically 15 ml of sterile 0.3% solution of potassium tellurite in distilled water. The tellurite solution may be sterilized by autoclaving.
3. Add aseptically 5 ml of sterile blood, and mix well.
4. Add 3-5 mg of cystine. The dry powder is used and need not be sterilized. Since different lots of cystine vary, the optimal amount necessary to produce the best growth of *Corynebacterium diphtheriae* may vary from 3-5 mg/100 ml.
5. Thoroughly mix the medium, and pour into sterile Petri dishes. Since the cystine does not go entirely into solution, shake the flask frequently while pouring the plates.

This medium is used for the isolation of *C. diphtheriae.*

CYSTINE TRYPTICASE AGAR (CTA)

(Vera. 1948. J. Bacteriol. 55:531.)

Cystine	0.5 g
Trypticase	20 g
Agar	3.5 g
Sodium chloride	5 g
Sodium sulfite	0.5 g
Phenol red	0.017 g
Distilled water	1,000 ml

(Final pH. 7.3)

CTA is an excellent all-purpose medium for the growth of pathogenic organisms. It can be used for the maintenance of cultures (including fastidious organisms, held at 25° C), the determination of motility, and (with the addition of carbohydrates) the determination of fermentation reactions of fastidious organisms, including *Neisseria.* Sterilize at 115°-118° C (no more than 12 pounds pressure) for 15 min.

Fermentation Media for Neisseriae

1. Suspend 4.3 g of dehydrated CTA medium (available commercially or see above) in 150 ml of distilled water, and heat to boiling with frequent agitation.
2. Adjust to pH 7.4-7.6 with 1 N NaOH, dispense in 50 ml amounts in 250 ml Erlenmeyer flasks, and sterilize at no more than 118° C (12 pounds) for 15 min.
3. Prepare 20% solutions of glucose, lactose, maltose, and sucrose in distilled water; tube and sterilize by membrane filtration.
4. Add 2.5 ml of each carbohydrate to separate flasks of the 50 ml cooled CTA medium.
5. Mix and dispense in 2 ml amounts in sterile screw-capped tubes (13 × 100 mm) and refrigerate at 4° C.

DECARBOXYLASE TEST MEDIA

(Moeller. 1955. Acta Pathol. Microbiol. Scand. 36:161.)

Basal Medium (BBL, Difco, Gibco)

Peptone (Orthana special*)	5 g
Beef extract	5 mg
Bromcresol purple (1.6%)	0.625 ml
Cresol red (0.2%)	2.5 ml
Glucose	0.5 g
Pyridoxal	5 mg
Distilled water	1,000 ml

(Adjust to pH 6)

Divide the basal medium into four 250 ml amounts; one portion is tubed without addition of any of the amino acids (control). To another portion add 1% L-lysine dihydrochloride (Sigma or other chemical supplier), to a third add 1% L-arginine monohydrochloride, and to the fourth add 1% L-ornithine dihydrochloride. Adjust the ornithine portion to pH 6 with 1 N NaOH before sterilization. Tube the media in 3-4 ml amounts in small (13 × 100 mm) screw-capped tubes. Autoclave at 121° C for 10 min.

Inoculate all four tubes from an agar slant culture, and overlay each tube with 4-5 mm of sterile mineral oil.† If oil is not added, the reactions are not valid after 24 h. Some workers recommend the addition of 0.3% agar to the basal medium in place of an oil overlay.

Incubate all four tubes at 35° C, and read daily for not more than 4 days (most positive reactions with the enteric bacilli occur in 1-2 days). A **positive** reaction is indicated by alkalinization of the medium with a change in color from yellow (caused by the initial fermentation of glucose) to **violet** (caused by the decarboxylation of the amino acid). Therefore a **yellow** color after several days' incubation indicates a **negative** test, or the absence of the enzymes decarboxylase or dihydrolase. All positive tests

---

*Proteose peptone No. 3, 0.3%, has been found to be a suitable alternative.
†Sterilize in test tubes at 121° C for 45 min.

should be compared with the control tube, which remains grayish purple.

These media are used primarily for differentiating members of the Enterobacteriaceae.

DNA AGAR FOR TESTING *STAPHYLOCOCCUS AUREUS* FOR THERMOSTABLE NUCLEASE

(Zarzour and Belle. 1978. J. Clin. Microbiol. 7:133.)

Deoxyribonucleic acid (Difco)	0.3 g
Agar (Bacto agar, Difco)	10 g
NaCl	10 g

Add the above components to 1 liter of 0.05 M TRIS buffer pH 9.0 (hydroxymethylaminomethane, Sigma Chemical). Add 1 ml of 0.01 M anhydrous $CaCl_2$ (Mallinckrodt) and boil until dissolved.

Cool to 45° C and add 3 ml of 0.1 M toluidine blue O (Allied Chemical and Dye Corp.). Mix thoroughly.

Pour 15-20 ml into 100 mm diameter Petri dishes. After the agar has set, it may be stored at 4° C, tightly wrapped in plastic, for approximately 60 days.

Plates should be reincubated at 35°-37° C for 1 h before inoculating. Control organisms should be run on the same plate as test organisms.

DESOXYCHOLATE AGAR

(Leifson. 1935. J. Pathol. Bacteriol. 40:581.)

Peptone	10 g
Lactose	10 g
Sodium citrate	1 g
Ferric citrate	1 g
Sodium chloride	5 g
Dipotassium phosphate	2 g
Sodium desoxycholate	1 g
Agar	16 g
Neutral red	0.033 g
Distilled water	1,000 ml
(Final pH 7.2)	

Desoxycholate agar is used for the isolation of gram-negative enteric bacilli and the differentiation of lactose-fermenting and non-lactose-fermenting species.

DESOXYCHOLATE CITRATE AGAR

(Leifson. 1935. J. Pathol. Bacteriol. 40:581.)

Meat, infusion from	350 g
Peptone	10 g
Lactose	10 g
Sodium citrate	20 g
Ferric citrate	1 g
Sodium desoxycholate	5 g
Agar	17 g
Neutral red	0.02 g
Distilled water	1,000 ml
(Final pH 7.3)	

Desoxycholate citrate agar is used for the isolation of salmonellae and shigellae from stool and other specimens.

DEXTROSE ASCITIC FLUID SEMISOLID AGAR FOR SPINAL FLUID CULTURES

Phenol red broth base	4 g
Agar, powdered (weigh accurately)	0.5 g
Distilled water	250 ml

Suspend the ingredients in a 1-liter Erlenmeyer flask, plug with cotton, and autoclave at 121° C for 15 min. At the same time sterilize a rack of 18 × 125 mm screw-capped test tubes and a wrapped Cornwall automatic pipette.* Cool the medium, and add the following aseptically:

Ascitic fluid†	50 ml
Dextrose, sterile 20% solution	15 ml

Using the sterile pipette, tube in 5 ml amounts in screw-capped tubes, incubate overnight for sterility, and store at room temperature. This medium is poured over remaining spinal fluid sediment after smears and plate cultures have been made.

---

*Beckton-Dickinson's Cornwall Pipetting Unit with 5 ml syringe.
†Bacto-Ascitic Fluid, 10 ml ampules, Difco Laboratories.

EDWARD-HAYFLICK AGAR FOR ISOLATION OF MYCOPLASMA

(Clyde, Kenny, and Schachter. 1984. Cumitech 19; Laboratory diagnosis of chlamydial and mycoplasmal infections. Drew, Coordinating editor. American Society for Microbiology, Washington, D.C.)

1. Prepare base medium as follows:

Mycoplasma Broth Base (BBL)	21 g
Distilled water	700 ml
Noble agar (Difco)	8.5 g

   Stir the solids into boiling water until they dissolve. Dispense 350 ml into each of two 500 ml bottles and autoclave according to manufacturer's instructions. Store the agar at 4° C.
2. Before use, melt the agar base and cool to 56° C. Add the following supplements to each 500 ml bottle of base:

Aqueous yeast extract (prepared as described under *New York City medium*, below)	50 ml
Horse serum (gamma globulin–free, available commercially)	100 ml
Penicillin G sodium	500,000 U
or	
Ampicillin	1 mg/ml
Amphotericin B	0.25 g
Polymyxin B	250,000 U

   After addition of supplements, agar is poured into 90 mm diameter plastic Petri plates. Plates are poured thick (approximately 25 ml per plate) to prevent dehydration. They may be stored (tightly wrapped in plastic) up to 2 weeks at 4° C. Since lots of ingredients vary, be certain to test each new batch of agar with a quality control strain of *Mycoplasma* of known titer.

EGG YOLK AGAR

Add 10 ml of sterile yolk emulsion (Colab Laboratories) to 90 ml of melted and cooled blood agar base, and pour the plates.

Blood Agar Base

Proteose peptone No. 2	40 g
Sodium orthophosphate (Na_2HPO_4)	5 g
Potassium dihydrophosphate (KH_2PO_4)	1 g
Sodium chloride	2 g
Magnesium sulfate	0.1 g
Glucose	2 g
Hemin solution (see below; 5 mg/ml)	1 ml
Agar	25 g
Distilled water	1,000 ml
(Adjust to pH 7.6)	

Autoclave at 121° C for 15 min. This medium is used for the isolation and identification of members of the genus *Clostridium* and certain other anaerobes.

ELLINGHAUSEN, MCCULLOUGH, JOHNSON, AND HARRIS (EMJH) MEDIUM FOR CULTIVATION OF LEPTOSPIRES

(Johnson and Harris. 1967. J. Bacteriol. 94:27.)

1. Prepare stock solutions as follows:

a. NH_4Cl	25 g
Distilled water	100 ml
b. $ZnSO_4 \cdot 7H_2O$	0.4 g
Distilled water	100 ml
c. $CaCl_2 \cdot 2H_2O$	1 g
Distilled water	100 ml
d. $MgCl_2 \cdot 6H_2O$	1 g
Distilled water	100 ml
e. $FeSO_4 \cdot 7H_2O$	0.5 g
Distilled water	100 ml
f. $CuSO_4 \cdot 5H_2O$	0.3 g
Distilled water	100 ml
g. Glycerol	10 ml
Distilled water	90 ml
h. Tween 80	10 ml
Distilled water	90 ml
i. Thiamine (Sigma)	0.5 g
Distilled water	100 ml
j. Vitamin B_{12} (Sigma)	0.02 g
Distilled water	100 ml

2. Prepare basal medium as follows:

Na$_2$HPO$_4$	1 g
KH$_2$PO$_4$	0.3 g
NaCl	1 g
Stock NH$_4$Cl solution (solution a)	1 ml
Stock thiamine (solution i)	1 ml
Stock glycerol (solution g)	1 ml
Distilled water	997 ml

Adjust to pH 7.4 and autoclave for 20 min at 121°C.

3. Prepare albumin supplement as follows:

Bovine albumin, fraction V (Sigma)	20 g
Distilled water	100 ml

Add the albumin to the water in a 500 ml flask and place on a stirring platform. As the solution stirs, slowly add the following stock solutions.

Calcium chloride (solution c)	2 ml
Magnesium chloride (solution d)	2 ml
Zinc sulfate (solution b)	2 ml
Copper sulfate (solution f)	0.2 ml
Iron sulfate (solution e)	20 ml
Vitamin B$_{12}$ (solution j)	2 ml
Tween 80 (solution h)	25 ml

Adjust the pH to 7.4 and add enough distilled water to bring the volume to 200 ml. Sterilize by filtration through a 0.45 μm pore size membrane filter.

4. Add 1 part albumin supplement to 9 parts of basal medium.

Eosin-Methylene Blue Agar (EMB)

Peptone	10 g
Lactose	5 g
Sucrose	5 g
Dipotassium phosphate	2 g
Agar	13.5 g
Eosin Y	0.4 g
Methylene blue	0.065 g
Distilled water	1,000 ml

The agar concentration may be increased to 5% (use an additional 3.65 g of agar) to inhibit the spreading of *Proteus*. The Levine EMB agar, preferred by some workers, does not contain sucrose.

Lactose-fermenting, gram-negative bacteria may be distinguished from non-lactose-fermenting types by their appearance. Colonies of *Escherichia coli* usually have a characteristic metallic sheen. If the sucrose-containing medium is used, *Proteus* colonies also show this characteristic, provided they are inhibited from spreading by the higher agar concentration.

Esculin Agar, Modified

Esculin	1 g
Ferric citrate	0.5 g
Heart infusion agar (blood agar base)	40 g
Distilled water	1,000 ml

Heat to dissolve. Cool to 55° C, and adjust pH to 7.0. Dispense in 5 ml amounts in 16 × 125 mm screw-capped tubes. Autoclave at 121° C for 15 min. Cool in a slanted position.

Esculin hydrolysis is indicated when the medium turns black.

Fetal Bovine Serum Agar with Vancomycin for Isolation of *Haemophilus Ducreyi*

(Greenwood and Robertson. 1983. Haemophilus ducreyi. ASCP Check Sample MB 83-8 (MB-129). American Society for Clinical Pathology.)

Heart infusion agar base (Difco Laboratories)	80 g
Bacto agar (Difco)	10 g
Fetal bovine serum, not inactivated	200 ml
Vancomycin HCl (1,500 μg/ml; Sigma Chemical Co.)	4 ml
Distilled water	1,800 ml

Measure heart infusion agar into a 4 liter flask. Add 200 ml of cold distilled water and stir to a smooth paste. Add remaining water and heat the mixture on a hot plate with stirring until it boils. Autoclave for 15 min at 121° C. Cool to 50° C and add the fetal bovine serum and vancomycin aseptically. Mix solution thoroughly and pour agar plates of approximately 20 ml each.

FLETCHER'S SEMISOLID MEDIUM FOR *LEPTOSPIRA*

1. Sterilize 1.76 liters of distilled water by autoclaving at 121° C for 30 min.
2. Cool to room temperature, and add 240 ml of sterile normal rabbit serum.
3. Inactivate by incubation at 56° C for 40 min.
4. Add 120 ml of melted and cooled (no greater than 56° C) 2.5% meat extract agar at pH 7.4.
5. Dispense 5 ml amounts in sterile, 16 × 120 mm, screw-capped test tubes and 15 ml amounts in sterile, 25 ml, diaphragm-type, rubber-stoppered vaccine bottles.
6. Inactivate at 56° C for 60 min on 2 successive days.

GELATIN MEDIUM

To veal extract or infusion broth add 12% gelatin. Heat in an Arnold sterilizer or a double boiler until the gelatin is thoroughly dissolved. Adjust reaction to pH 7. Tube and autoclave at 121° C (15 pounds pressure) for 15 min. Sodium thioglycolate, 0.05%, may be added for cultivation of certain species of clostridia in an external aerobic environment.

GELATIN MEDIUM (DILUTE) FOR DIFFERENTIATION OF *NOCARDIA* AND *STREPTOMYCES*

(Centers for Disease Control.)

Gelatin	4 g
Distilled water	1,000 ml

(Adjust to pH 7)

Dispense in tubes, approximately 5 ml per tube. Autoclave at 121° C for 5 min. Inoculate with a small fragment of growth from a Sabouraud dextrose agar slant. Incubate at room temperature for 21-25 days. Examine for quantity and type of growth.

Nocardia asteroides exhibits no growth or very sparse, thin, flaky growth. *N. brasiliensis* shows good growth and round compact colonies. *Streptomyces* species show poor to good growth (stringy or flaky).

GN BROTH

(Hajna. 1955. Pub. Health Lab. 13:83.)

Peptone	20 g
Glucose	1 g
D-Mannitol	2 g
Sodium citrate	5 g
Sodium desoxycholate	0.5 g
Dipotassium phosphate	4 g
Monopotassium phosphate	1.5 g
Sodium chloride	5 g
Distilled water	1,000 ml

(Final pH 7)

Dissolve the dehydrated medium in distilled water and autoclave at 116° C (10 pounds steam pressure) for 15 min or steam for 30 min at 100° C.

This broth medium is used as an enrichment for isolating salmonellae and shigellae in fecal specimens.

HEKTOEN ENTERIC AGAR

Proteose peptone	12 g
Bile salts	9 g
Yeast extract	3 g
Lactose	12 g
Salicin	2 g
Sucrose	12 g
Sodium chloride	5 g
Sodium thiosulfate	5 g
Ferric ammonium citrate	1.5 g
Agar	14 g
Acid fuchsin	0.1 g
Bromthymol blue	0.065 g
Distilled water	1,000 ml

Suspend 76 g of dehydrated medium, if using the commercial product, in 1,000 ml of distilled water. Heat to boiling, and continue until the medium dissolves. **Do not autoclave.** Cool to 50° C, and pour into Petri dishes.

This medium is useful for the isolation and differentiation of gram-negative enteric pathogens. The coliforms are usually salmon to orange, whereas the salmonellae and shigellae are bluish-green.

HEMIN SOLUTION

Hemin solution is used as a medium supplement in a final concentration of 5 μg/ml. To prepare, dissolve 0.5 g of hemin (Sigma and others) in 10 ml of commercial ammonia water (or 1 N sodium hydroxide), bring volume to 100 ml with distilled water, and autoclave at 121° C for 15 min. A stock solution is 5 mg/ml.

As a supplement for anaerobic media, 1 ml of hemin solution is added per liter of agar or broth.

HORSE BLOOD–BACITRACIN AGAR (SELECTIVE) FOR RECOVERY OF HAEMOPHILUS SPECIES FROM RESPIRATORY CULTURES

(Klein and Blazevic. 1970. Am. J. Med. Technol. 36:97.)

Heart infusion agar (Difco)	40 g
Cornstarch (Argo)	1 g
Distilled water	1,000 ml

Add ingredients to water and heat to boiling to dissolve. Autoclave for 15 min at 121° C. Cool to 45° C in a water bath. Add the following ingredients aseptically:

Fildes enrichment (Difco)	20 ml
Defibrinated horse blood (GIBCO)	50 ml
Supplement B (Difco)	10 ml
Bacitracin standard laboratory powder (Upjohn)	375 μg/ml

Pour into Petri plates, approximately 20 ml per plate. Do not flame surfaces of plates to remove bubbles, since the heat may destroy the V factor. Store tightly wrapped in the refrigerator.

HUMAN BLOOD BILAYER MEDIUM (HBT) FOR SELECTIVE AND DIFFERENTIAL ISOLATION OF GARDNERELLA VAGINALIS

(Totten et al. 1982. J. Clin. Microbiol. 15:141.)

1. Prepare basal agar layer as follows:

Columbia agar base with colistin and nalidixic acid (CNA) (BBL)	44 g

Proteose peptone No. 3 (Difco)	10 g
Distilled water	1,000 ml

Suspend the agar in the water, mix thoroughly and heat to boiling to dissolve. Autoclave for 15 min at 121° C and cool to 55° C. Add amphotericin B to a final concentration of 2 μg/ml and 0.075 ml Tween 80 (BBL). Mix thoroughly and pour one-third of the CNA agar into 90 mm diameter Petri plates, 7 ml per plate.

2. Prepare overlayer as follows: Add freshly outdated human blood of any type (obtained from the hospital blood bank) to the remaining molten CNA agar base with Tween 80 and amphotericin to make a final concentration of 5% blood. Pour directly over the basal agar in the Petri plates, 14 ml per plate.

3. Plates should be stored in the refrigerator, wrapped tightly in plastic bags. They should last approximately 1 month, but should be discarded if they appear hemolyzed.

INDOLE-NITRITE MEDIUM

Trypticase	20 g
Disodium phosphate	2 g
Glucose	1 g
Agar	1 g
Potassium nitrate	1 g
Distilled water	1,000 ml
(pH 7.2)	

This medium is used to demonstrate indole production and nitrate reduction by aerobes and anaerobes.

KANAMYCIN-VANCOMYCIN BLOOD AGAR (KVBA)

1. Preparation of base:

Trypticase soy agar	40 g
Agar	2.5 g
Distilled water	1,000 ml
Kanamycin base (Bristol Laboratories)	100 mg

Sterilize by autoclaving at 121° C for 15 min, and cool to 50° C.

2. Add aseptically*:

Defibrinated sheep blood	50 ml
Vancomycin (Eli Lilly)	7.5 mg
Vitamin K_1 solution (see below, Vitamin K_1 solution)	1 ml

Mix well, pour plates (approximately 20 ml per plate), and store at room temperature.

This medium is extremely useful for primary inoculation of clinical specimens for selective isolation of anaerobes, particularly *Bacteroides*, but a nonselective medium (*Brucella* blood agar plate) should always be used as well.

KANAMYCIN-VANCOMYCIN LAKED BLOOD AGAR (KVLBA)

KVLBA is the same as KVBA, except that the final concentration of kanamycin is 75 μg/ml and the blood is laked (hemolyzed) by freezing whole blood overnight and then thawing. This medium is particularly useful for isolating the pigmented *Bacteroides*.

KELLY'S MEDIUM (NONSELECTIVE MODIFIED) FOR ISOLATION OF *BORRELIA BURGDORFERI* AND OTHER SPIROCHETES

(*Steere et al. 1983. N. Engl. J. Med. 308:733.*)

1. Prepare basal medium as follows:

CMRL-1066 with glutamine, 10 × tissue culture medium (GIBCO)	100 ml
Sterile distilled water	900 ml
Proteose peptone no. 2 (Difco)	5 g
Tryptone (Difco)	1 g
Bacto autolyzed yeast (Difco)	1 g
HEPES buffer, acid form (Sigma)	6 g
Glucose alpha-D(+) (Sigma)	3 g
Sodium citrate (Sigma)	0.7 g
Sodium pyruvate (Sigma)	0.8 g
Sodium bicarbonate (Sigma)	2.2 g
N-acetyl glucosamine (Sigma)	0.4 g
$MgCl_2 \cdot 6H_2O$ (Sigma)	0.3 g

---

*Hemin may also be added (1 ml of hemin solution).

Add all ingredients together, adjust pH to 7.6 with 5 N NaOH.

Filter sterilize through a 0.45 μm pore size membrane filter.

2. Prepare gelatin solution as follows:

Gelatin (Fisher Scientific)	14 g
Distilled water	200 ml

Add together and heat gently to cause gelatin to just go into solution. Autoclave for 15 min at 121° C. Allow to cool to 50°-55° C.

3. Add the gelatin to the basal medium. To this medium add 143 ml of a 35% solution of bovine serum albumin (Sigma) in sterile distilled water and 86 ml of membrane-filtered, heat-inactivated rabbit serum (GIBCO).

4. Dispense aseptically into 8 ml screw-cap test tubes, at least 7 ml per tube. The large volume of medium in the tube prevents excessive oxygenation of the medium.

KELLY'S MEDIUM (SELECTIVE MODIFIED) FOR ISOLATION OF *BORRELIA BURGDORFERI*

(*Johnson, S., et al. 1984. J. Clin. Microbiol. 19:81.*)

1. Prepare basal medium as follows:

1066 Connaught Medical Research Laboratories medium with glutamine, 10 × (GIBCO)	100 ml
Double distilled water	900 ml
Neopeptone (Difco)	5 g
Bovine serum albumin fraction V (Sigma)	50 g
N-2-hydroxyethylpiperazine-N'-2-ethane sulfonic acid buffer (Sigma)	6 g
Sodium citrate	0.7 g
Glucose	5 g
Sodium pyruvate (Sigma)	0.8 g
N-Acetylglucosamine (Sigma)	0.4 g
Sodium bicarbonate	2.2 g

Add all ingredients separately, dissolving each ingredient completely before the next is added. Adjust pH to 7.6 with 1 N NaOH.

2. Prepare gelatin solution as follows:

Gelatin (Difco)	14 g
Distilled water	200 ml

Warm the solution gently while stirring until gelatin just goes into solution.

3. Add the warm gelatin solution to the basal medium.
4. Sterilize the entire solution by filtration through a 0.45 μm membrane filter.
5. Add 70 ml of partially hemolyzed sterile rabbit serum (Hazleton) to produce a final serum concentration of 6%.
6. Add kanamycin laboratory standard powder (Bristol Laboratories) to a final concentration of 8 μg/ml and 5-fluorouracil laboratory standard powder (Roche Laboratories) to a final concentration of 230 μg/ml, using methods described in Chapter 13.
7. Final pH of the medium should be 7.7.

KLIGLER'S IRON AGAR

See Triple Sugar Iron Agar.

LÖFFLER COAGULATED SERUM SLANTS FOR CULTIVATION OF CORYNEBACTERIUM DIPHTHERIAE

(Löffler. 1887. Zentralbl. Bakt. 2:105.)

Add 3 volumes of beef, hog, or horse serum (collected as cleanly as possible) to 1 volume of glucose infusion broth (1% glucose). Dispense in tubes, slant, and inspissate for about 2 h at 75°-85° C on each of 3 successive days. The medium also may be sterilized in a slanted position in a horizontal autoclave. Close the autoclave tightly, and without allowing the air to escape, autoclave at 15 pounds pressure for 15 min to coagulate the medium. Then allow the air to escape slowly, and admit steam so that the pressure is maintained at 15 pounds. When an atmosphere of pure steam has been obtained, close the outlet valve tightly, and sterilize the medium with steam under 15 pounds pressure (121° C) for 15 or 20 min.

LOWENSTEIN-JENSEN (L-J) MEDIUM

Salt solution	
Monopotassium phosphate	2.4 g
Magnesium sulfate · 7H$_2$O	0.24 g
Magnesium citrate	0.6 g
Asparagine	3.6 g
Glycerol, reagent grade	12 ml
Distilled water	600 ml
Potato flour	30 g
Homogenized whole eggs	1,000 ml
Malachite green (2% aqueous)	20 ml

Add the potato flour to the flask of salt solution, and autoclave the mixture at 121° C for 30 min. Clean fresh eggs, no more than 1 week old, by vigorous scrubbing in 5% soap solution, and allow them to remain in it for 30 min. Place the eggs in running cold water until the water becomes clear. Immerse the washed eggs in 70% alcohol for 15 min, remove, and break into a sterile flask; homogenize completely by shaking with glass beads. Then filter the homogenate through four layers of sterile gauze.

Add 1 liter of the homogenized egg suspension to the flask of cooled potato flour–salt solution. Add the malachite green to this emulsion, and mix thoroughly. Dispense the medium aseptically with a sterile aspirator bottle in 6 ml amounts into sterile, screw-capped 150 mm glass tubes. Inspissate the tubes at 85° C for 50 min, and check for sterility by incubating at 35° C for 48 h. Store in a refrigerator, where the medium will keep for at least 1 month if the tubes are tightly sealed to prevent loss of moisture.

This medium is used for the cultivation of *Mycobacterium tuberculosis*.

LYSINE-IRON AGAR

(Edwards and Fife. 1961. Appl. Microbiol. 9:478.)

Peptone	5 g
Yeast extract	3 g
Glucose	1 g

L-Lysine	10 g
Ferric ammonium citrate	0.5 g
Sodium thiosulfate	40 mg
Bromcresol purple	20 mg
Agar	15 g
Distilled water	1,000 ml

(Adjust to pH 6.7)

Dispense 4 ml amounts into 13 × 100 mm tubes, and sterilize at 121° C for 12 min. Slant tubes to obtain a deep butt and a short slant. This medium is inoculated by using a straight wire to stab the butt twice and to streak the slant. Incubation is at 35° C for 18-24 h. If necessary, incubate for 48 h.

This medium is useful for determining whether members of the family Enterobacteriaceae can decarboxylate or deaminate lysine. However, this medium is not to be considered as a substitute for the Moeller method. A **positive** reaction is indicated by an alkaline or **purple** reaction in the butt of the tube. The absence of lysine decarboxylase is indicated by an acidic or **yellow (negative)** reaction in the butt of the tube caused by fermentation of glucose. Tryptophane deaminase is indicated by the formation of a **red** slant and is characteristic of the tribe Proteeae. It should be noted that H_2S-producing *Proteus* species do not blacken this medium. Furthermore, *Morganella morganii* does not consistently produce a red slant after 24 h incubation.

MacConkey Agar

Peptone	17 g
Proteose peptone	3 g
Lactose	10 g
Bile salts	1.5 g
Sodium chloride	5 g
Agar	13.5 g
Neutral red	0.03 g
Crystal violet	0.001 g
Distilled water	1,000 ml

The agar concentration may be increased to 5% (use an additional 3.65 g of agar) to inhibit the spreading of *Proteus*. The medium is inhibitory for gram-positive bacteria and differential rather than selective. Coliforms (lactose fermenting) produce red colonies on the medium, whereas nonlactose fermenters produce colorless colonies.

Malonate (Sodium) Broth

(Leifson. 1933. J. Bacteriol. 26:329. Ewing et al. 1957. Pub. Health Lab. 15:153.)

Yeast extract	1 g
Ammonium sulfate	2 g
Dipotassium sulfate	0.6 g
Monopotassium phosphate	0.4 g
Sodium chloride	2 g
Sodium malonate	3 g
Glucose	0.25 g
Bromthymol blue	0.025 g
Distilled water	1,000 ml

(Final pH 6.7)

Sterilize in small tubes in 3 ml amounts at 121° C for 15 min. Inoculate from TSI slants or broth cultures; incubate cultures at 35° C for 48 h.

The medium is used to test for utilization of sodium malonate by members of the Enterobacteriaceae. A **positive** test is shown by a change of the indicator from green to a **Prussian blue.**

Mannitol Salt Agar

Beef extract	1 g
Proteose peptone No. 3	10 g
Sodium chloride	75 g
Mannitol	10 g
Agar	15 g
Phenol red	0.025 g
Distilled water	1,000 ml

Sterilize the medium at 15 pounds pressure for 15 min, cool to 48° C, and pour into sterile Petri dishes. Use 15-20 ml per plate.

This medium is used for the selective isolation of pathogenic staphylococci, since many other bacteria are inhibited by the high salt concentration. Colonies of potentially pathogenic staphylococci are surrounded by a **yellow** halo, indicating mannitol fermentation.

MARTIN-LEWIS AGAR

(Same as Thayer-Martin agar except that anisomycin is substituted for nystatin and the concentration of vancomycin is increased from 3 to 4 μg/ml. Notice that some strains of *Neisseria gonorrhoeae* may be susceptible to vancomycin at either concentration. See Chapter 26.)

McBRIDE MEDIUM, MODIFIED, FOR THE CULTIVATION OF *LISTERIA*

(J. Lab. Clin. Med. 1960. 55:153.)

Phenylethanol agar*	35.5 g
Glycine, anhydride	10 g
Lithium chloride	0.5 g
Distilled water	1,000 ml

Dissolve with the aid of heat and sterilize at 121° C for 20 min.

METHYL RED–VOGES-PROSKAUER MEDIUM (MR-VP) (CLARK AND LUBS MEDIUM)

Buffered peptone	7 g
Glucose	5 g
Dipotassium phosphate	5 g
Distilled water	1,000 ml
(Final pH 6.9)	

This medium is used for the methyl red test and the Voges-Proskauer test (production of acetylmethylcarbinol). See Chapter 27 for a description of performance of the test.

MIDDLEBROOK 7H10 AGAR WITH OADC ENRICHMENT

The preparation of 7H10 oleic acid-albumin agar as originally described is extremely tedious and complicated. Its preparation may be simplified by the use of a combination of six stock solutions prepared in advance, as described in the handbook *Tuberculosis Labora-*

*Available from several commercial media suppliers. See *Phenylethanol agar*, below.

*tory Methods of the Veterans Administration.** However, for the average diagnostic microbiology laboratory, it is strongly recommended that **commercially prepared** 7H10-OADC complete medium be used whenever possible. For purposes of orientation, the ingredients of each medium are listed, but the directions are intended solely for preparation from dehydrated medium and prepared enrichment.

Middlebrook 7H10 Agar

Ammonium sulfate	0.5 g
D-Glutamic acid	0.5 g
Sodium citrate	0.4 g
Disodium phosphate	1.5 g
Monopotassium phosphate	1.5 g
Ferric ammonium phosphate	0.04 g
Magnesium sulfate	0.05 g
Pyridoxine	0.001 g
Biotin	0.0005 g
Malachite green	0.001 g
Agar	15 g

Middlebrook OADC Enrichment

Oleic acid	0.5 g
Bovine albumin, fraction V	50 g
Glucose	20 g
Beef catalase	0.04 g
Sodium chloride	8.5 g
Distilled water	1,000 ml

To rehydrate the 7H10 agar, suspend 20 g in 1 liter of cold distilled water containing 0.5% reagent grade glycerol and heat to boiling to dissolve completely. Distribute in 180 ml amounts in flasks; sterilize by autoclaving at 121° C for 10 min; cool to 50°-55° C; add 20 ml of OADC enrichment aseptically to each flask; and dispense in sterile plastic Petri dishes. Store at 4° C in the dark for no longer than 2 months in a plastic bag to prevent dehydration.

*Obtainable from the Superintendent of Documents, U.S. Government Printing Office, Washington, D.C.

MIDDLEBROOK 7H11 AGAR FOR SUSCEPTIBILITY TESTING OF MYCOBACTERIA

Middlebrook 7H10 agar base (Difco)	19 g
Casein hydrolysate (Sigma)	1 g
Glycerol (Difco)	5 ml
Distilled water	1,000 ml

Add ingredients together and heat gently to dissolve. Autoclave for 10 min at 121° C. Allow to cool to 55° C, and add 100 ml of OADC Enrichment (Difco). Mix gently and pour into Felson quadrant Petri plates (Falcon Laboratories) containing antimicrobial agent impregnated filter paper disks, as described in Chapter 13. Add 5 ml agar to each quadrant.

MILK MEDIA
Skimmed Milk

Fresh, clean, skimmed cow's milk may be used. This is dispensed in tubes and sterilized either by tyndallization (flowing steam for 30 min on 3 successive days) or in the autoclave at 10 pounds pressure for 10 min.

Commercial dehydrated skimmed milk is also completely satisfactory. The concentration used is 10% in distilled water. The method of sterilization is as before.

Litmus Milk

Skimmed milk powder	100 g
Litmus	5 g
Distilled water	1,000 ml

Autoclave at 10 pounds pressure for 10 min.

Reactions in litmus milk. Pink color of litmus indicates an acid reaction caused by fermentation of lactose. A purple or blue color (alkaline) indicates no fermentation of lactose. White color (reduction) results when litmus serves as an electron acceptor and is reduced to its leuco base. Coagulation (clot) is caused by precipitation of casein by the acid produced from lactose. Coagulation may also be caused by the conversion of casein to paracasein by the enzyme rennin.

Peptonization (dissolution of the clot) indi-cates digestion of the curd or milk proteins by proteolytic enzymes.

Litmus Milk with a Reducing Agent for Determination of Litmus Milk Reactions of Clostridium Species

Skimmed milk powder	100 g
Peptone	10 g
Sodium thioglycolate	0.5 g
Litmus	5 g
Distilled water	1,000 ml

Autoclave as above.

Methylene Blue Milk for Identification of Enterococci

Skimmed milk powder	10 g
Methylene blue (1% aqueous)	10 ml
Distilled water	90 ml

MOTILITY TEST MEDIUM*

Beef extract	3 g
Gelysate peptone	10 g
Sodium chloride	5 g
Agar	4 g
Distilled water	1,000 ml
(Final pH 7.3)	

1. Suspend 22 g of dehydrated medium in water, and add 0.05 g triphenyltetrazolium. Heat with frequent agitation; boil 1 min to dissolve ingredients.
2. Dispense in screw-capped tubes, and sterilize by autoclaving at 121° C for 15 min.
3. Tighten caps when cool; store at room temperature.

This medium is stabbed once to a depth of approximately 1 cm below the surface and read after 1-2 days' incubation at 35° C. Motile organisms spread out from the line of inoculation; nonmotile organisms grow only along the stab.

If the results are negative, follow with fur-

---

*Discussion adapted from Paik. 1980. In Lennette, Balows, Hausler, and Truant, editors. Manual of clinical microbiology, ed. 3. American Society for Microbiology, Washington, D.C.

ther incubation at 21°-25° C for 5 days. For special purposes, such as enhancement of the motility and flagellar development in poorly motile cultures, it is often advisable to pass cultures first through a semisolid medium containing 0.2% agar tubed in Craigie tubes or in U tubes. Subsequent passages may be made in 0.4% agar medium.

Motility media containing concentrations higher than 0.3% agar produce gels through which many motile organisms cannot spread. Spreading in a semisolid medium is judged by macroscopic examination of the medium for a diffuse zone of growth emanating from the line of inoculation. Many aerobic pseudomonads fail to grow deep in semisolid medium in a test tube. Organisms possessing "paralyzed" flagella are nonmotile and cannot spread in the medium. Some filamentous organisms spread in or on semisolid media but are nonmotile and nonflagellated. Although cultures may grow at 37° C or higher temperatures, the flagellar proteins of some organisms are not synthesized optimally at this temperature; hence, motility medium should be incubated at temperatures near 18°-20° C. These observations require judicious interpretation of motility and limit, to some extent, the reliability of using spreading in semisolid agar as the sole taxonomic criterion to delineate related species.

MOTILITY TEST SEMISOLID AGAR FOR *LISTERIA*

Bacto-tryptose (Difco)	10 g
Sodium chloride	5 g
Agar	5 g
Glucose	1 g
Distilled water	1,000 ml

Dissolve with the aid of heat, distribute in tubes, and sterilize at 121° C for 20 min.

Inoculate by stabbing with a 24 h broth culture. Incubate the tubes at 25° and 35° C, and observe for growth away from the stab line (motile).

MUELLER-HINTON AGAR

(Proc. Soc. Exp. Biol. Med. 1941. 48:330.)

Beef, infusion from	300 g
Peptone	17.5 g
Starch	1.5 g
Agar	17 g

(Final pH 7.4)*

Suspend the medium in distilled water, mix thoroughly, and heat with frequent agitation. Boil for about 1 min, dispense, sterilize by autoclaving at 116°-121° C (12-15 pounds steam pressure) for **no longer than 15 min,** and cool by placing immediately in a 50° C water bath before pouring.

The medium is used primarily for the disk-agar diffusion method of testing for antimicrobial susceptibility of microorganisms. Commercial dry powder is recommended for consistent results. It has also been used to detect starch hydrolysis by *Streptococcus bovis* (Lee. 1976. J. Clin. Microbiol. 4:312) and for culturing the Legionnaires' disease agent.

Five percent defibrinated animal blood may be added as enrichment.

MUELLER-HINTON BROTH (CATION SUPPLEMENTED)

(National Committee for Clinical Laboratory Standards. 1983. M7-T, Methods for dilution antimicrobial susceptibility tests for bacteria that grow aerobically. NCCLS, Villanova, Pa.)

1. Prepare Mueller-Hinton Broth as recommended by the manufacturer. After autoclaving, cool to 4° C in the refrigerator or in an ice bath.
2. Prepare stock magnesium solution as follows:

$MgCl_2 \cdot 6H_2O$	8.36 g
Deionized water	100 ml

*Check by using a surface electrode, if available, after gelling, or with other methods as discussed in Chapter 8.

Sterilize by membrane filtration and store at 4° C. The Mg^{++} concentration is 10 mg/ml.

3. Prepare stock calcium solution as follows:

$CaCl_2 \cdot 2H_2O$	3.68 g
Deionized water	100 ml

Sterilize by membrane filtration and store at 4° C. The Ca^{++} concentration is 10 mg/ml.

4. Add 2.5 ml of cold magnesium stock solution and 5 ml of cold calcium solution per liter of cold Mueller-Hinton broth for a final concentration of:

25 mg/liter Mg^{++} and 50 mg/liter Ca^{++}.

MYCOPLASMA MEDIA

Also see *Edward-Hayflick agar, SP-4 mycoplasma medium, Ureaplasma agar,* and *Ureaplasma broth.*

MYCOPLASMA HOMINIS AGAR AND BROTH

(Clyde, Kenny, and Schachter. 1984. Cumitech 19: Laboratory diagnosis of chlamydial and mycoplasmal infections. Drew, coordinating editor. American Society for Microbiology, Washington, D.C.)

1. Prepare 1% phenol red by dissolving 1 g of phenol red (sodium salt) in 100 ml of water. Autoclave for 15 min at 121° C.
2. Prepare stock penicillin solution by dissolving 1,000,000 U of penicillin G (sterile for injection) in 50 ml sterile water. Store in aliquots of 1.2 ml at −20° C.
3. Prepare basal medium as follows:

Soy peptone	20 g
NaCl	5 g
Phenol red (1%)	1 ml
Distilled water	1,000 ml

Adjust the pH to 7.3. A second broth base medium without phenol red indicator should also be prepared at the same time. For preparation of agar, add 10 g of agarose per liter after adjusting pH and mix to dissolve. Dispense the media in 100 ml bottles, 70 ml per bottle. Sterilize both broth and agar base solutions at 121° C for 15 min. Store at 4° C.

4. To broth base or to melted and cooled (to 50° C) agar base, add the following supplements:

Horse serum (unheated, sterile)	20 ml
Stock penicillin	1 ml
Fresh yeast extract (prepared as described for New York City medium, below)	10 ml

5. Dispense the broths aseptically into 16 × 125 mm screw-capped test tubes (5 ml per tube) and tighten caps. Store at 4° C for no longer than 1 week.
6. Pour agar into 35 mm diameter Petri dishes, 5 ml per dish. Store tightly wrapped in plastic at 4° C and use plates within 1 week of preparation.

NEW YORK CITY MEDIUM FOR ISOLATION OF MYCOPLASMA HOMINIS AND NEISSERIA GONORRHOEAE

(Adapted from Phillips and Nash. 1985. Culture media. In Lennette et al., editors. Manual of clinical microbiology, ed. 4. American Society for Microbiology, Washington, D.C.)

1. Prepare basal medium as follows:
   a. Agar base

Bacto-agar (Difco)	20 g
Distilled water	400 ml

Place the solution in an Arnold steam sterilizer (Chapter 8) or heat with continuous stirring on a hotplate until the agar has melted.

   b. Cornstarch

Cornstarch (Argo)	1 g
Distilled water	40 ml

Mix thoroughly on a magnetic stirrer-hotplate before heating. Heat on the hotplate with continuous stirring or in an Arnold steam sterilizer until the mixture is smooth and creamy.

c. Peptone and salt solution

Proteose peptone no. 3 (Difco)	15 g
Dipotassium phosphate (Sigma)	4 g
Monopotassium phosphate (Sigma)	1 g
Sodium chloride	5 g
Distilled water	200 ml

Bring peptone and salts to boiling on a magnetic stirrer-hotplate.

d. Add melted agar, cornstarch, and peptone and salts solutions together in a liter flask. Mix thoroughly on a magnetic stirrer-hotplate. Autoclave for 15 min at 121° C. The final pH should be 7.1 ± 0.1.

2. Prepare the following supplements:
   a. Yeast dialysate

Baker's yeast (available from grocery stores)	908 g
Distilled water	2,500 ml

Mix the yeast and the water to a smooth paste in a 4-liter flask. Autoclave the mixture for 10 min at 121° C and allow to cool to room temperature. Soak 2-inch (5 cm) diameter dialysis tubing in water to soften it and make at least 2 knots in one end of the tubing. Pour the yeast mixture into the other end of the dialysis tubing (a total length of about 1 yard of tubing is needed; several different lengths can be prepared), tie the tops of each length of tubing, and rinse the outside of the tubing and the knots to remove any yeast. Dialyze all of the lengths of tubing together against 2 liters of cold distilled water in a 4-liter flask for 48 h (in a cold room). Discard the dialysis tubing and the yeast mixture inside and dispense the dialysate (the solution remaining in the flask) in 25 ml amounts (in autoclavable 50 ml bottles or large screw-capped glass tubes). Autoclave the dialysate for 15 min at 121° C and store frozen at −20° C. The dialysate is stable at this temperature.

b. Glucose solution

Glucose (Difco)	50 g
Distilled water	100 ml

Mix thoroughly, filter sterilize by passing through a 0.45 μm pore size membrane filter, and dispense aseptically in 10 ml amounts into sterile 16 × 125 mm glass screw-capped tubes. Store refrigerated.

c. 3% hemoglobin solution

Add 6 ml of the sedimented red blood cells that remain in a collection bag after the plasma has been removed (packed human erythrocytes, available from the hospital blood bank) to 200 ml sterile distilled water at room temperature. The cells will lyse, creating the 3% hemoglobin solution.

d. Citrated horse plasma

Sodium citrate (Sigma)	1,200 g
NaCl	64 g
Distilled water	to 8 liters

Place 600 ml of the citrate solution in a blood collection bottle for horses and draw blood up to 6 liters, making a final concentration of 10% citrate in the blood.

e. Antibiotic mixture

Vancomycin	2 μg/ml
Colistin (Polymyxin)	5.5 μg/ml
Amphotericin B	1.2 μg/ml
Trimethoprim lactate	3 μg/ml

Prepare the antibiotic mixture in 5 ml total volume, using methods outlined in Chapter 13. If a larger quantity is prepared initially, it should be stored frozen at temperatures below −20° C in aliquots of 5 ml each.

3. To the 640 ml basal medium that has been melted from a previously prepared solution or freshly autoclaved and cooled to 55° C, the supplements are added in the following amounts:

Citrated horse plasma	120 ml
3% hemoglobin solution	200 ml
50% glucose solution	10 ml

| Yeast dialysate | 25 ml |
| Antibiotic mixture | 5 ml |

4. Mix all ingredients thoroughly (the final volume is 1 liter) and pour into Petri plates, approximately 20 ml per plate. Store plates tightly wrapped in plastic bags in the refrigerator. Medium is stable for approximately 10 weeks.

Modified New York City Medium (Henderson Formulation) for Isolation of Neisseria gonorrhoeae

See Chapter 19.

NITRATE BROTH FOR NITRATE REDUCTION TEST

Tryptone	5 g
Neopeptone	5 g
Distilled water	1,000 ml
Potassium nitrate (reagent grade)	1 g
Glucose	0.1 g

Before adding the potassium nitrate and glucose, boil the other ingredients in the water and adjust pH to 7.3-7.4. Dispense 5 ml per tube and sterilize at 15 pounds pressure for 15 min. The reagents and tests for nitrate reduction are listed in Chapter 44.

NUTRIENT AGAR

Beef extract	3 g
Peptone or Gelysate pancreatic digest of gelatin	5 g
Agar	15 g
Distilled water	1,000 ml

(Final pH 6.8)

Autoclave at 121° C for 15 min.

ONPG (BETA-GALACTOSIDASE) TEST

The ability of certain gram-negative bacilli to ferment lactose is a useful criterion for identifying certain members of the family Enterobacteriaceae. Since some coliform organisms, the so-called paracolon bacteria, ferment this carbohydrate slowly or not at all, they have been confused with the enteric pathogens.

Lactose fermentation is dependent on two enzymes: **permease,** which allows lactose to enter the bacterial cell, and **beta-galactosidase,** which splits lactose into glucose and galactose. The slow lactose fermenters are deficient in permease, and the demonstration of beta-galactosidase in such organisms permits more rapid identification of a lactose fermenter. This enzyme can be detected conveniently by the use of a tablet of *ortho*-nitrophenyl-beta-galactopyranoside (ONPG)* dissolved in distilled water and inoculated with a heavy suspension of the organism to be tested. The test is incubated at 35° C for 6 h; hydrolysis of ONPG is detected by the liberation of *ortho*-nitrophenol, with its characteristic **yellow** color, often within 30 min. Thus, a **positive** ONPG test indicates that the organism contains lactose-fermenting enzymes and may be classed as a lactose fermenter.

OXGALL (40%)

Dissolve 40 g oxgall in 100 ml of distilled water, autoclave at 121° C for 15 min, and refrigerate. Oxgall is available from media and chemical suppliers.

OXIDATIVE-FERMENTATIVE (O-F) BASAL MEDIUM

(Hugh and Leifson. 1953. J. Bacteriol. 66:24.)

See Chapter 28 for preparation and use of this medium.

PEPTIC DIGEST AGAR

Add 5% Fildes enrichment to trypticase soy agar base. This is a very good medium for demonstrating *Haemophilus influenzae.* Colonies are translucent blue.

*Key Scientific Products Co. or other products as mentioned in Chapter 27.

PHENOL RED BROTH BASE

Trypticase	10 g
Sodium chloride	5 g
Phenol red	0.018 g
(Final pH 7.4)	

Phenol red broth base can be used as a base for determining carbohydrate fermentation reactions. Carbohydrates can be added to the medium in 0.5%-1% concentrations before dispensing and sterilization. Durham tubes should be inserted into the tubed medium for detection of gas formation.

See *"Carbohydrate broth"* for further information.

PHENYLALANINE AGAR

(Ewing et al. 1957. Pub. Health Lab. 15:153.)

Yeast extract	3 g
DL-Phenylalanine	2 g
(or L-phenylalanine)	1 g
Disodium phosphate	1 g
Sodium chloride	5 g
Agar	12 g
Distilled water	1,000 ml

Dispense 3 ml amounts in small tubes, and sterilize at 121° C for 10 min. Allow to solidify in a slanted position.

This medium is used to test for deamination of phenylalanine to phenylpyruvic acid by members of the Enterobacteriaceae.

After incubation of the culture for 18-24 h at 35° C, allow 4-5 drops of fresh 10% ferric chloride solution to run down over the growth on the slant. If acid has been formed, a **green** color immediately develops on the slant and in the fluid at the base of the slant.

PHENYLETHANOL (PHENYLETHYL ALCOHOL, PEA) AGAR

(Lilley and Brewer. 1953. J. Am. Pharm. Assoc. [Scient. Ed.] 42:6.)

Trypticase	15 g
Phytone	5 g
Sodium chloride	5 g
Beta-phenylethyl alcohol	2.5 g
Agar	15 g
Distilled water	1,000 ml
(Final pH 7.3)	

Suspend the powder in the water, mix thoroughly, heat with agitation, and boil 1 min. Dispense in 16 × 150 mm screw-capped tubes. Sterilize at 118°-121° C (12-15 pounds pressure) for 15 min. If desired, 5% blood may be added to the cooled medium (45°-50° C) before pouring plates.

Phenylethyl alcohol agar is useful for the isolation of gram-positive cocci and the inhibition of gram-negative bacilli (particularly *Proteus*) when these are found in mixed culture.

PHOSPHATE-BUFFERED SALINE

See under Viral Media: Reagents and Solutions, p. 899.

POLYMYXIN *STAPHYLOCOCCUS* MEDIUM

(Finegold and Sweeney. 1961. J. Bacteriol. 81:636.)

Nutrient agar	23 g
Tween 80	10.2 ml
Lecithin	0.7 g
Polymyxin*	75 mg
Distilled water	1,000 ml

Autoclave at 15 pounds pressure for 15 min. Pour plates.

Coagulase-negative staphylococci, micrococci, and most gram-negative rods are inhibited. In addition to *S. aureus*, *Proteus* will grow; the latter can be recognized by translucent colonies. *Proteus* does not swarm on this medium.

POTATO-CARROT AGAR

Carrots, peeled	20 g
Potatoes, peeled	20 g
Distilled water	1,000 ml
Agar	15 g
Tween 80	5 ml

---

*75 mg = 75,000 μg, or 750,000 U of activity.

Wash potatoes and carrots, mash them, and place them in distilled water for 1 h. Boil for 5 min, filter through paper, make up to 1,000 ml of volume, and add 15 g of agar and 5 ml of Tween 80. Dispense in tubes, autoclave at 121° C for 20 min, slant, and cool. Potato-carrot agar is an excellent medium for demonstrating color characteristics of a fungal colony.

POTATO-DEXTROSE AGAR

Potatoes, infusion from	200 g
Glucose	20 g
Agar	20 g
Distilled water	1,000 ml

Boil potatoes in water for 15 min, filter through cotton, and make up to volume with water. Add dry ingredients, and dissolve agar with heat. No pH adjustment is required. Dispense as desired, and autoclave at 121° C for 10 min. The agar is used to stimulate spore production of fungi.

PURPLE BROTH BASE FOR TESTING CARBOHYDRATE FERMENTATION BY ENTEROBACTERIACEAE

Peptone: proteose or peptic digest of animal tissue USP	10 g
Beef extract	1 g
Sodium chloride	5 g
Bromcresol purple	0.015 g
Distilled water	1,000 ml
(Final pH 6.8)	

Autoclave at 121° C for not more than 15 min. Add sugars and alcohols to 1% (w/v).

See *Carbohydrate broth* for further information.

RESAZURIN

Use as an Eh indicator in PRAS media. Dissolve one tablet (Difco) in 44 ml of distilled water. Store the stock solution at room temperature.

RICE GRAIN MEDIUM

White rice	8 g
Distilled water	25 ml

Place in a 125 ml Erlenmeyer flask, and autoclave at 121° C for 15 min.

Rice grain medium is used for differentiation of *Microsporum* species. *M. canis* and *M. gypseum* grow and sporulate well in this medium; *M. audouinii* grows poorly. Conidial formation is stimulated in some of the *Trichophyton* species.

RINGER'S SOLUTION FOR DISSOLVING CALCIUM ALGINATE SWABS

Sodium chloride	8.5 g
Potassium chloride	0.2 g
Calcium chloride · 2H$_2$O	0.2 g
Sodium carbonate	0.01 g
Distilled water	1,000 ml
(pH 7.0)	

Sterilize by autoclaving at 121° C for 15 min. To use in dissolving calcium alginate swabs, prepare in one-quarter strength, and add 1% sodium hexametaphosphate. Approximately 10 min of shaking usually suffices for complete dissolution of the swab.

SABHI AGAR

(Gorman. 1967. Am. J. Med. Technol. 33:151.)

Calf brain, infusion from	100 g
Beef heart, infusion from	125 g
Proteose peptone	5 g
Neopeptone	5 g
Glucose	21 g
Sodium chloride	2.5 g
Disodium phosphate	1.25 g
Agar	15 g
Distilled water	1,000 ml
(Final pH 7.0)	

1. Suspend 59 g of commercial powder in 1,000 ml of distilled water and heat to boiling to completely dissolve medium.
2. Sterilize by autoclaving at 121° C for 15 min.
3. Cool to 50°-55° C, and add 1 ml of sterile chloramphenicol solution (100 mg/ml), prepared using methods discussed in Chapter 13.

4. Mix well, and dispense in sterile, cotton-plugged 25 × 150 mm Pyrex test tubes.
5. Slant, allow to harden, and refrigerate.

Sabhi is an equal mixture of Sabouraud dextrose agar and brain-heart infusion agar and has proved useful for isolation of clinically significant fungi, particularly from specimens containing bacteria, such as sputum.

Sabouraud Dextrose Agar (SAB)

Sabouraud dextrose agar	32.5 g
Agar, powdered	2.5 g
Distilled water	500 ml

Suspend ingredients in water, dissolve by heating to boiling, and dispense in approximately 20 ml amounts in cotton-plugged, 25 by 150 mm Pyrex test tubes (without lips). If antimicrobial agents are to be added, this may be done after heating the medium and before autoclaving. The following amounts are recommended (CDC):

Cycloheximide	250 mg dissolved in 5 ml acetone
Chloramphenicol	25 mg dissolved in 5 ml 95% ethanol

Mix well, and distribute into tubes or bottles as indicated. Autoclave at 118° C for **no longer than 10 min.** Slant, allow to harden, and refrigerate. This selective medium is used primarily for primary isolation of dermatophytes. It is available commercially as Mycobiotic agar (Difco) and Mycosel agar (BBL). Zygomycetes are unable to grow on this medium.

Sabouraud Dextrose Broth

Dextrose	40 g
Peptone	10 g
Distilled water	1,000 ml

Dissolve ingredients, dispense in 10 ml amounts in 18 × 150 mm tubes, and autoclave at 121° C for 10 min. Sabouraud dextrose broth is useful for differentiation of *Candida* species.

Salmonella-Shigella (SS) Agar

Beef extract	5 g
Peptone	5 g
Lactose	10 g
Bile salts mixture	8.5 g
Sodium citrate	8.5 g
Sodium thiosulfate	8.5 g
Ferric citrate	1 g
Agar	13.5 g
Brilliant green	0.33 g
Neutral red	0.025 g
Distilled water	1,000 ml

Dissolve by boiling. **Do not autoclave.**

Salmonella-Shigella agar is used primarily as a selective medium for isolation of salmonellae and shigellae, while inhibiting coliform bacilli. It can also differentiate lactose-fermenting from non-lactose-fermenting strains.

Schneider's *Drosophila* Medium

(Gibco)

(Supplemented with 30% v/v fetal calf serum)

Schneider's *Drosophila* medium is used for primary isolation as well as routine maintenance of a wide variety of leishmanial and trypanosomal species.

Scott's Modified Castañeda Media and Thioglycolate Broth for Blood Cultures

Agar Bottle—Slant

Trypticase soy agar*	40 g
Agar, granulated	15 g
Distilled water	1,000 ml

Heat in autoclave at 121° C for 5 min to melt agar or heat on a hot plate with a magnetic stirring bar.

Agar Bottle—Broth

Trypticase soy broth†	30 g
Sodium polyanethole sulfonate (SPS) ("Grobax," 5% sterile solution SPS)†	5 ml
Distilled water	1,000 ml

---

*Available in dehydrated form from Difco, BBL, and Gibco.
†Roche Diagnostics (No. 43000).

Thioglycolate Medium

Thioglycolate broth*	30 g
Sucrose	100 g
Sodium polyanethole sulfonate (SPS)	5 ml
Distilled water	1,000 ml

(pH of all media after autoclaving
should be 7.2 ± 0.2)

1. Dispense agar medium (slant) in the melted state in approximately 20 ml amounts into each of 50 clean, non-chipped, 4-ounce, square, clear-glass, screw-capped bottles (10 ml in 2-ounce bottles).†

2. Insert the disposable rubber diaphragms in the special screw caps, which are then applied loosely on the bottle tops.

3. Dispense the thioglycolate medium into 50 clean bottles, approximately 75 ml per bottle (30 ml in 2-ounce bottles), and apply screw caps as noted earlier.

4. Make up trypticase broth in a 2-liter flask and plug. Prepare a dispensing buret (a 300 ml Salvarsan tube‡ or satisfactory substitute) to the end of which are attached a 2-foot length of rubber tubing, a needle holder, and a 1½-inch, 21-gauge needle, in that order. Insert the attached needle, together with a portion of the rubber tubing, in the top of the buret, and make fast by plugging, thus assuring a closed unit during sterilization.

5. Autoclave all media and equipment at 118°-121° C for 12-15 min.

6. As soon as the pressure reaches zero, open the autoclave, remove all bottles rapidly, and tightly fasten the screw caps. The hands must be protected from the hot bottles by asbestos gloves.

7. Place the bottles containing the agar on their sides on a cool table top to permit hardening of the agar layer. After about 1 h, place bottles upright, and sterilize tops with alcohol sponges.* (The agar does not become detached from the sides of the bottles.)

8. Clamp the sterile dispensing buret to a ring stand. Using aseptic technique, fill the buret with sterile trypticase broth.

9. To each agar slant bottle add 60 ml of broth (25 ml in 2-ounce bottles) by puncturing the rubber diaphragm with the sterile needle. The partial vacuum in each bottle will readily permit addition of this amount.

10. Incubate agar slant bottles at 35° C for 48 h to ensure sterility. The thioglycolate bottles do not need incubation for a sterility check.

11. Inspect bottles, label, and store at room temperature (shelf-life is 6 months).

SELENITE-F ENRICHMENT MEDIUM

(Leifson. 1936. Am. J. Hyg. 24:423.)

Sodium hydrogen selenite (anhydrous)	0.4%
Sodium phosphate (anhydrous)	1%
Peptone	0.5%
Lactose	0.4%

(Final pH 7.0)

Dissolve ingredients in distilled water. Sterilize gently; 30 min in flowing steam in an autoclave is sufficient. It is important to note that the medium should not be autoclaved. This medium is used for the selective isolation of *Salmonella* and some strains of *Shigella*.

---

*BBL Microbiology Systems.

†Blood culture bottles (St. Louis Health Dept. type) with special screw caps and disposable rubber diaphragms, 4-ounce and 2-ounce sizes, can be obtained from several suppliers.

‡Arthur H. Thomas Co.

*At the Wilmington Medical Center the use of a loose application of a piece of steam autoclave tape (No.1222-3M) to the bottle top, which is then fastened down after sterilization, obviates the need for disinfection of the diaphragm when filling with broth (step 8) or when collecting the blood culture.

SELLERS DIFFERENTIAL AGAR

(Sellers. 1964. J. Bacteriol. 87:46.)

Yeast extract	1 g
Peptone	20 g
L-Arginine	1 g
D-Mannitol	2 g
Bromthymol blue	0.04 g
Phenol red	0.008 g
Sodium chloride	2 g
Sodium nitrate	1 g
Sodium nitrite	0.35 g
Magnesium sulfate	1.5 g
Dipotassium phosphate	1 g
Agar	15 g

To rehydrate the medium, suspend 45 g in 1,000 ml of cold distilled water, and heat to boiling to dissolve the medium completely. Dispense into test tubes, and stopper with cotton plugs or loosely fitting caps. Sterilize in the autoclave for 10 min at 15 pounds pressure (121° C). Allow the tubes to cool in the slanted position to give approximately 1½-inch butts and 3-inch slants. **Immediately before inoculating,** add 2 large drops or 0.15 ml of a sterile 50% glucose solution to each tube by letting it run down the **side of the tube opposite the slant.** Inoculate the tubes by stabbing deep into the butt and streaking the slant. Incubate for 24 h at 35° C. The final reaction of the medium will be pH 6.7 at 25° C.

Sellers differential agar is useful for differentiating and identifying nonfermentative gram-negative bacilli that produce an alkaline reaction on TSI agar (or KIA). The dehydrated medium is prepared according to the formula of Sellers and is recommended. This medium is particularly useful in differentiating *Pseudomonas aeruginosa, Acinetobacter calcoaceticus,* and *Alcaligenes faecalis* (Table 45.1).

SODIUM BICARBONATE

Sodium bicarbonate is used as a medium supplement for anaerobes in a final concentration of 1 mg/ml. To prepare, dissolve 2 g in 100 ml of distilled water, and filter sterilize. The stock solution is 20 mg/ml. For use, add 0.5 ml to 10 ml of medium.

SODIUM CHLORIDE BROTH (6.5%)

Brain-heart infusion broth	100 ml
Sodium chloride	6 g

Brain-heart infusion broth contains 0.5% sodium chloride. Thus, by adding an additional 6%, the desired concentration is obtained. The medium is selective for enterococci and other salt-tolerant organisms and is useful in identification as well.

SÖRENSEN pH BUFFER SOLUTIONS

Buffer solutions may be added to culture media to prevent a significant change in hydrogen ion concentration. Sörensen buffers, prepared from potassium and sodium phosphates, are readily prepared from the anhydrous salts or purchased from commercial sources.

TABLE 45.1
Reactions Produced on Sellers Medium by Nonfermentative Gram-Negative Bacilli

ORGANISM	SLANT COLOR	BUTT COLOR	BAND COLOR	FLUORESCENT SLANT	NITROGEN GAS
Pseudomonas aeruginosa	Green	Blue or no change	Sometimes blue	Yellow-green	Produced
Acinetobacter calcoaceticus var. anitratus	Blue	No change	Yellow	Absent	Absent
A. calcoaceticus var. lwoffi	Blue	No change	Absent	Absent	Absent
Alcaligenes faecalis	Blue	Blue or no change	Absent	Absent	Produced

Reagents

Solution A
  M/15 Na$_2$PO$_4$

Dissolve 9.464 g of the anhydrous salt, previously dried at 130° C, in distilled water, to make 1 liter of solution.

Solution B
  M/15 KH$_2$PO$_4$

Dissolve 9.073 g of the anhydrous salt, previously dried at 110° C, in distilled water to make 1 liter of solution. Mix solutions A and B as indicated.

pH	SOLUTION A	SOLUTION B
5.29	0.25 ml	9.75 ml
5.59	0.5 ml	9.5 ml
5.91	1 ml	9 ml
6.24	2 ml	8 ml
6.47	3 ml	7 ml
6.64	4 ml	6 ml
6.81	5 ml	5 ml
6.98	6 ml	4 ml
7.17	7 ml	3 ml
7.38	8 ml	2 ml
7.73	9 ml	1 ml
8.04	9.5 ml	0.5 ml

SP-4 *MYCOPLASMA* MEDIUM FOR PRIMARY ISOLATION OF *MYCOPLASMA*

1. Prepare base as follows:

Mycoplasma Broth Base (BBL)	3.5 g
Tryptone (Difco)	10 g
Bacto-Peptone (Difco)	5 g
Dextrose (50% aqueous solution, filter sterilized)	10 ml
Distilled water	615 ml

Stir the solids into boiling water to dissolve them and adjust the pH to 7.5. Autoclave according to the manufacturer's instructions. Cool to 56° C before adding supplements. To prepare the agar necessary for making biphasic media, add 8.5 g Noble agar (Difco) to the basal medium ingredients.

2. Add the following supplements for each 625 ml of base to make a final volume of 1 liter:

CMRL 1066 tissue culture medium with glutamine, 10 × (GIBCO)	50 ml
Aqueous yeast extract (prepared as described in New York City medium, above)	35 ml
Yeastolate (Difco; 2% solution)	100 ml
Fetal bovine serum (heat inactivated at 56° C for 30 min)	170 ml
Penicillin G sodium	1,000,000 U
or	
Ampicillin	1 mg/ml
Amphotericin B	0.5 g
Polymyxin B	500,000 U

Dispense 1 ml of SP-4 agar aseptically into the bottom of sterile 4 ml screw-capped vials. Allow the agar to set and dispense 2 ml of SP-4 broth above the agar layer in each vial. Seal caps tightly and store at −20° C indefinitely.

STARCH AGAR MEDIUM

Bacto-agar	20 g
Bacto-peptone	5 g
Beef extract	3 g
Sodium chloride	5 g
Soluble starch	20 g
Distilled water	1,000 ml

(Final pH 7.2)

1. Dissolve the agar in 300 ml of water with heat.
2. Dissolve the beef extract and peptone in 200 ml of water.
3. Mix the solutions in steps 1 and 2, and make up to 1,000 ml volume.
4. To this mixture add the starch, dissolve, and autoclave at 121° C for 15 min.

The medium may be dispensed in tubes (15-20 ml amounts) or flasks convenient for pouring plates and should be stored in a refrigerator. For pouring of plates, melt the medium in tubes or flasks as required. **If poured plates of starch agar are refrigerated, the medium becomes opaque.**

Starch agar is useful in developing smooth cultures by streaking borderline rough strains on the surface of the medium. It also may be used for testing cultures for starch hydrolytic activity.

STOCK CULTURE AND MOTILITY MEDIUM

(Hugh. 1974. In ASM Man. Clin. Microbiol., ed. 2, p. 263.)

Casitone	10 g
Yeast extract	3 g
Sodium chloride	5 g
Agar	3 g
Distilled water	1,000 ml

1. Suspend the ingredients in distilled water; heat to boiling to completely dissolve agar.
2. Dispense in 13 × 100 mm screw-capped tubes, 4 ml per tube.
3. Sterilize by autoclaving at 121° C for 15 min; store as butts.

This medium is used for motility testing by stabbing the inoculum once into the agar and incubating overnight at 35° C. Motility is indicated by growth spreading out from the line of stab.

The medium is also excellent for preserving stock cultures of nonfermenting and fermenting gram-negative rods (up to 6 months). After inoculation and overnight incubation, the caps are sealed with tape and the tubes refrigerated.

STUART'S TRANSPORT MEDIUM (MODIFIED FOR USE WITH DACRON OR RAYON SWABS)

Sodium glycerophosphate	10 g
Sodium thioglycolate	1 g
Calcium chloride dihydrate	0.1 g
Distilled water	1,000 ml

Mix thoroughly. Dispense into 16 × 125 mm screw-capped test tubes, 0.5 ml per tube. Autoclave for 10 min at 121° C. Tighten caps and store tubes at room temperature.

SUCROSE (5%) BROTH OR AGAR FOR TESTING VIRIDANS STREPTOCOCCI

See Chapter 25.

TELLURITE REDUCTION TEST MEDIUM FOR MYCOBACTERIA
Medium

1. Suspend 4.7 g of Middlebrook 7H9 dehydrated base in 900 ml of distilled water, and add 0.5 ml of Tween 80.
2. Autoclave at 121° C for 15 min, cool to 55° C, and add aseptically 100 ml ADC enrichment (Difco, BBL).
3. Dispense aseptically in 5 ml amounts in 20 × 150 mm screw-capped tubes, check for sterility, and refrigerate.

Tellurite Solution

1. Dissolve 0.2 g of potassium tellurite in 100 ml of distilled water.
2. Dispense in 2-5 ml amounts, and sterilize by autoclaving at 121° C for 10 min.

This medium is used to test the ability of certain nonphotochromogens to reduce tellurite rapidly to the **black,** metallic tellurium.

To perform the test, incubate the test organism for a minimum of 7 days (until the broth becomes turbid) in the broth medium. Add 2 drops of tellurite solution to each broth culture and incubate (37° C) for 4 more days. A **black precipitate** indicates a positive reaction.

TETRATHIONATE BROTH

Proteose peptone (Difco)	5 g
Bile salts	1 g
Calcium carbonate	10 g
Sodium thiosulfate	30 g
Distilled water	1,000 ml

Dispense the medium in 10 ml amounts, and heat to boiling. **Before use** add 0.2 ml of iodine solution (6 g of iodine crystals and 5 g of potassium iodide in 20 ml of water) to each tube.

This is a selective liquid enrichment medium for use in the isolation of *Salmonella*, except *S. typhi*. The sterile base **without iodine** may be stored in a refrigerator indefinitely.

THAYER-MARTIN AGAR

GC agar base (Difco) (double strength)	72 g
Agar	10 g
Distilled water	1,000 ml

1. Suspend the dehydrated medium in water, mix well, and heat with agitation. Boil for 1 min.
2. Sterilize by autoclaving at 121° C for 15 min.
3. At the same time, autoclave a suspension of 20 g of dehydrated hemoglobin in 1,000 ml water for 15 min (suspension must be **smooth** before sterilizing).
4. Cool both to 50° C, mix aseptically, and then add 20 ml of IsoVitaleX enrichment (BBL) and 20 ml of V-C-N inhibitor (BBL). Pour plates, using 20 ml per plate. Refrigerate.

This medium is recommended for the isolation of *Neisseria gonorrhoeae* from all sites that might contain a mixed flora, as well as for the recovery of *N. meningitidis* from nasopharyngeal and throat cultures.

Modified Thayer-Martin Medium for Isolation of Neisseria gonorrhoeae *and* N. meningitidis

(Modified from the Difco Manual, ed. 10. Difco Laboratories, Detroit.)

(Trimethoprim lactate and increased agar content inhibit swarming *Proteus* species.)
1. Prepare GC medium base as follows:

Bacto GC medium base (Difco)	36 g
Dextrose	1.5 g
Bacto agar (Difco)	10 g
Bacto supplement VX (Difco)	10 ml

Suspend the GC medium base, the agar, and the dextrose in 500 ml of distilled water. Heat to boiling to dissolve the ingredients

and autoclave for 15 min at 121° C. Cool the solution to 55° C in a waterbath and aseptically add the supplement VX. Allow the medium to remain in the waterbath until all components have been added together.
2. Prepare Bacto hemoglobin as follows:

Bacto hemoglobin (Difco)	10 g
Distilled water	500 ml

Place the hemoglobin in a dry liter beaker on a stirring platform with a stir bar. Add the distilled water in 100 ml amounts, stirring vigorously. Break up clumps with a spatula. Transfer to a liter flask and autoclave for 15 min at 121° C. Cool to 55° C in a water bath.
3. Aseptically add the warm GC medium base to the hemoglobin solution, swirling to mix thoroughly.
4. Rehydrate a vial of Bacto antimicrobic vial CNVT (containing 7,500 μg of colistin sulfate, 12,500 U of nystatin, 3,000 μg of vancomycin, and 5,000 μg of trimethoprim lactate) by aseptically adding 10 ml of sterile distilled or deionized water to the vial. Mix well.
5. Add the CNVT to the warm agar base mixture, mix thoroughly, and pour into Petri plates, approximately 20 ml per plate.

THIOGLYCOLATE MEDIUM WITHOUT INDICATOR* (THIO)

(Brewer. 1940 and 1943. J. Bacteriol. 39:10 and 46:395.)

Peptone	20 g
L-Cystine	0.25 g
Glucose	6 g
Sodium chloride	2.5 g
Sodium thioglycolate	0.5 g
Sodium sulfite	0.1 g
Agar	0.7 g
Distilled water	1,000 ml
(Final pH 7.2)	

*This may be enriched by the addition of 10% normal rabbit or horse serum when cool.

Dispense the medium in 15 ml amounts in 16 × 125 mm test tubes, making a column of medium 7 cm high. Autoclave for 15 min at 121° C. **Store at room temperature.**

Enriched THIO

Enriched THIO is prepared by adding to the freshly prepared and autoclaved medium (or to previously prepared medium that has been boiled for 10 min and then cooled) vitamin K_1 solution, 0.1 μg/ml; sodium bicarbonate, 1 mg/ml; and hemin, 5μg/ml. Rabbit or horse serum (10%) or Fildes enrichment (5%) may also be added. See Vitamin K_1 solution (below) and Hemin solution (above) for preparation of these supplements. Enriched thioglycolate medium is often used for susceptibility testing of anaerobes by the broth-disk method of Kurzynski (Chapter 13).

THIONINE OR BASIC FUCHSIN AGAR

(Huddleson et al. 1939. Brucellosis in man and animals, The Commonwealth Fund, New York.)

Trypticase soy agar may be used as a base for differential media containing thionine and basic fuchsin.

Prepare the dyes, thionine and basic fuchsin, in 0.1% stock solutions in sterile distilled water. These stock solutions may be stored indefinitely. Before adding to the media, heat the dye solutions in flowing steam in an autoclave for 20 min, shake well, and while still hot, add to melted agar. In trypticase soy agar the final concentration of the dye should be 1:100,000 (10 ml/liter of medium). Thoroughly mix the dyes (added individually) and the melted agar, and pour immediately into Petri dishes, one set containing thionine and one containing basic fuchsin. Place the plates in a 35° C incubator until the water of condensation disappears, at which time they are ready for use. Inoculate plates within 24 h of preparation.

Streak the surface of plates with a heavy suspension of *Brucella* prepared from a 48-72 h trypticase soy agar slant culture. It is advisable to streak plates in duplicate, incubating one set aerobically and the other in 10% CO_2. Incubate plates for 72 h, and observe for inhibition of growth by thionine or basic fuchsin or both. See Chapter 29 for further information.

TINSDALE AGAR, MOORE AND PARSONS, MODIFIED

Proteose No. 3 (Difco) or Thiotone peptic digest of animal tissue USP (BBL)	20 g
L-Cystine	0.24 g
Sodium chloride	5 g
Sodium thiosulfate	0.43 g
Agar, dried	14 g
or not dried	20 g
Distilled water	1,000 ml
(Final pH 7.4)	

1. Heat with agitation, and boil for 1 min. Dispense.
2. Autoclave at 121° C for 15 min. Cool to 56° C, and to each 100 ml of base add:

Sterile serum (e.g., bovine)	10 ml
Potassium tellurite, 1% aqueous	3 ml

3. Alternatively, the thiosulfate may be dissolved in 1.7 ml of water and added separately. It must be prepared fresh each time the medium is prepared. The cystine may be dissolved in 6 ml of 0.1 N HCl and added separately, in which case it may be necessary to add 6 ml of 0.1 N NaOH to make sure that the final pH is correct.

TODD-HEWITT BROTH, MODIFIED

(J. Pathol. Bacteriol. 1932. 35:973.)

Beef heart infusion	1,000 ml
Neopeptone	20 g

Adjust to pH 7 with normal sodium hydroxide and add:

Sodium chloride	2 g
Sodium bicarbonate	2 g
Disodium phosphate	0.4 g
Glucose	2 g

(Final pH 7.8)

Mix the chemicals in broth, and bring to a slow boil. Boil for 15 min, filter through paper, dispense in tubes, and autoclave at 115° C for 10 min.

Modified Todd-Hewitt broth is used for growing streptococci for serologic identification.

TRANSPORT MEDIA

See Amies transport medium, Cary and Blair transport medium, and Stuart's transport medium.

TRIPLE SUGAR IRON (TSI) AGAR

(Hajna, 1945. J. Bacteriol. 49:516.)

Peptone	20 g
Sodium chloride	5 g
Lactose	10 g
Sucrose	10 g
Glucose	1 g
Ferrous ammonium sulfate	0.2 g
Sodium thiosulfate	0.2 g
Phenol red	0.025 g
Agar	13 g
Distilled water	1,000 ml

(Final pH 7.3)

TSI agar is used for determining carbohydrate fermentation and hydrogen sulfide production as a first step in the identification of gram-negative bacilli.

This medium is considered to be a modification of KIA. The only difference between the two is that sucrose is not included in KIA. It should be stressed that pH changes in the butt and in the slant of the medium must be recorded only after 18-24 h of incubation. See Chapter 9 for further information on inoculation of these media and interpretation of the reactions.

TRYPTICASE SOY AGAR

Trypticase	15 g
Phytone	5 g
Sodium chloride	5 g
Agar	15 g
Distilled water	1,000 ml

(Final pH 7.3)

Trypticase soy agar is an excellent blood agar base and can be used for the isolation and maintenance of all organisms, except some with very special nutritional requirements.

TRYPTICASE SOY BROTH

Trypticase	17 g
Phytone	3 g
Sodium chloride	5 g
Dipotassium phosphate	2.5 g
Glucose	2.5 g
Distilled water	1,000 ml

(Final pH 7.3)

Trypticase soy broth is excellent for the rapid (6-8 h) growth of most organisms and supports growth of pneumococci and streptococci without the addition of blood or serum. It also supports growth of *Brucella*. However, fermentation of the glucose present will cause a drop in pH, and acid-sensitive organisms, particularly pneumococci, may die in 18-24 h.

TRYPTOPHAN BROTH

Tryptophan broth is a popular medium for the detection of indole production. Trypticase (BBL) or tryptone (Difco) is recommended, in 1% aqueous solution. Follow label directions for preparation.

TYROSINE OR XANTHINE AGAR

Nutrient agar	23 g
Tyrosine	5 g
or xanthine	4 g
Demineralized water	1,000 ml

1. Dissolve the nutrient agar in the water.
2. Add tryosine or xanthine, and mix to distribute the crystals evenly.

3. Adjust to pH 7.0, and autoclave at 121° C for 15 min.
4. Dispense in plates, 20 ml per plate, with the crystals evenly distributed.

Tyrosine or xanthine agar is recommended for differentiation of species of aerobic actinomycetes. Its use is similar to that of casein agar.

TWEEN 80–ALBUMIN BROTH FOR CULTIVATION OF SPIROCHETES

See Ellinghausen, McCullough, Johnson, and Harris medium.

UREA AGAR—UREASE TEST MEDIUM

(Christensen. 1946. J. Bacteriol. 52:461.)

Peptone	1 g
Glucose	1 g
Sodium chloride	5 g
Monopotassium phosphate	2 g
Phenol red	0.012 g
Agar	20 g
Distilled water	1,000 ml

(Final pH 6.8-6.9)

Prepare the agar base, and sterilize in the autoclave at 121° C for 15 min in flasks containing 100-200 ml amounts. Store until needed. Prepare a 29% solution of urea. Sterilize by filtering through a sterile bacteriologic filter. Add the sterile urea solution in a final concentration of 10% to a flask of the agar base that has been melted and cooled to a temperature of 50° C. Mix well, and distribute aseptically in sterile small tubes in amounts of 2-3 ml. Allow the medium to solidify in a slanting position in such a way as to obtain an agar butt of ½ inch and an agar slant of 1 inch.

Urea agar can be used to demonstrate urease production by species of *Proteus*. It also detects the small amounts of urease produced by other enteric bacilli, thus differentiating them from urease-negative *Salmonella* and *Shigella*. It also may be used to detect urease production by *Cryptococcus* species.

UREAPLASMA AGAR AND BROTH FOR CULTIVATION OF U. UREALYTICUM

Several components of both ureaplasma agar and broth must be made in advance, as described below.

1. Prepare MES buffer as follows:

2-(N-Morpholino) ethanesulfonic acid (acid form; Behring Diagnostics)	195 g
Distilled water	800 ml

Adjust pH to 6.0 at 37° C with concentrated NaOH (6 M), make volume up to 1 liter with water and sterilize through a membrane filter. Store at room temperature in the dark.

2. Prepare 1% phenol red by dissolving 1 g of phenol red (sodium salt) in 100 ml of water. Autoclave for 15 min at 121° C.
3. Prepare urea by dissolving 60 g of ultrapure urea (Schwartz/Mann) in 1 liter of distilled water to make a 1 M solution. Filter sterilize and store at room temperature.
4. Prepare stock penicillin solution by dissolving 1,000,000 U of penicillin G (sterile for injection) in 50 ml of sterile water. Store in aliquots of 1.2 ml at −20° C.
5. Prepare sodium sulfite solution as follows:

Sodium sulfite (use a fresh bottle of powder with no evidence of caking)	0.063 g
Phenol red solution (1%)	0.5 ml

Dispense 10 ml each into 16 × 125 mm screw-capped test tubes. Autoclave for 15 min at 121° C, and as soon as they are removed from the autoclave, tighten the caps. Store at room temperature. The tubes should be purple; if air has leaked into the medium the indicator will turn orange because of oxidation of sodium sulfite to the neutral sodium sulfate.

6. Prepare agar base as follows:

Soy peptone	20 g
NaCl	5 g

MES buffer	4.25 g
Phenol red (1%)	1 ml
Distilled water	1,000 ml
Agarose (Difco)	10 g

Heat the water to dissolve the agarose, and then add the other ingredients. Adjust to pH 6.0 at 37° with 1 N NaOH. Distribute the agar base into 100 ml bottles, 70 ml per bottle. Autoclave at 121° C for 15 min. Store bottles at room temperature.

7. Prepare agar medium by aseptically adding the components as follows:

Agar base (melted and cooled to 50° C)	70 ml
Yeast dialysate (prepared as in New York City agar, above)	10 ml
Sterile horse serum, unheated	20 ml
Urea (1 M)	0.2 ml
Stock penicillin solution	1 ml
Lincomycin solution (10,000 μg/ml, made fresh)	0.5 ml

Pour into 35 mm diameter plastic Petri plates, 5 ml per plate. Store tightly wrapped in plastic for no longer than 2 weeks at 4° C.

Ureaplasma Broth for Cultivation of U. urealyticum

1. Prepare urea broth base as follows:

Soy peptone	20 g
NaCl	5 g
Phenol red (1%)	1 ml
Distilled water	1,000 ml

Add ingredients together and adjust pH to 6.0 with 1 N HCl. Dispense into 100 ml bottles, 87.5 ml per bottle, and autoclave for 15 min at 121° C.

2. To each bottle, add the following supplements:

1 M MES buffer, pH 6.0	1 ml
1 M urea	0.5 ml
Sterile horse serum, unheated	10 ml
Stock penicillin solution	1 ml
Lincomycin (freshly made)	50 μg/ml

Store the bottle in the refrigerator for no longer than 2 weeks. Dispense in 4 ml vials, 3 ml per vial. Just before use, add 1 ml of sodium sulfite (100 mM) per 100 ml of broth (0.03 ml per vial).

UREASE TEST BROTH

(McKay, Edwards, and Leonard. 1947. Am J. Clin. Pathol. 17:479. Rustigian and Stuart. 1941. Proc. Soc. Exp. Biol. Med. 47:108. Stuart, Van Stratum, and Rustigian. 1945. J. Bacteriol. 49:437.)

Urea	20 g
Monopotassium phosphate	9.1 g
Disodium phosphate	9.5 g
Yeast extract	0.1 g
Phenol red	0.01 g
(Final pH 6.8)	

Use 3.87 g/100 ml of distilled water. **Do not heat.** When the powder has dissolved, filter the medium through a sterile bacteriologic filter. Distribute the broth in 0.5-2 ml amounts in small sterile tubes. Large amounts may be used if desired, but reactions are slower. If a filter is not available, it is possible to sterilize the medium in an autoclave, if the tubes are not tightly packed and the steam pressure is held at 5 pounds for 20 min or at 8 pounds for 7 min.

In addition, the medium generally gives reliable results without sterilization, if prepared and inoculated immediately. This strongly buffered medium is suitable for determining urease reactions of the strongly positive *Proteus, Morganella,* and *Providencia* species. There is a similar medium using the following concentrations of phosphates:

| Monopotassium phosphate | 0.091 g |
| Disodium phosphate | 0.095 g |

It may be used to detect the presence of urease in other bacteria.

Urease test broth may be inoculated from TSI agar (or KIA), trypticase soy agar, or other agar slants having heavy growth. It is recommended that large inocula be employed when it is desirable to obtain results rapidly. Incubate at 35° C. Normally the finished medium has a pale pink or pinkish-yellow color and a neutral pH of about 6.8-7.0. In cultures that attack urea, ammonia is formed during incubation and makes the reaction of the medium alkaline, with a **deep purple** or bluish-red color.

Urease test broth may be used in the same manner for the detection of urease activity of such organisms as members of the genera *Brucella*, *Bacillus*, *Sarcina*, and *Mycobacterium*. Incubation usually should be longer than for enteric bacilli.

NOTE: Both prepared broth and dehydrated base should be stored in the refrigerator. If the seal on the bottle has been broken, the bottle should preferably be stored with desiccant in a sealed container.

See Chapter 9 for a rapid urease test procedure.

VIRAL MEDIA: REAGENTS AND SOLUTIONS
Antibiotic Mixtures for Treatment of Viral Culture Specimens

1. *Antibiotic Mixture for Urine Specimens*

Gentamicin is used in preference to penicillin and streptomycin because of its broader antibacterial spectrum. Amphotericin B is used to control fungal contamination.

Gentamicin (50 mg/ml)	4 ml
Amphotericin B (250 μg/ml)	10 ml

Dispense 0.3 ml aliquots into test tubes (enough for 40 tubes) and store at −20° C until needed. To each tube of thawed mixture, add 5-10 ml of urine.

2. *Antibiotic Mixture for Other Viral Specimens*

MEM without bicarbonate in EBSS (see below) (1 × concentrate)	100 ml
Gentamicin (10 mg/ml)	1.5 ml
Amphotericin B (250 μg/ml)	3 ml
7.5% NaHCO$_3$	3 ml

Dispense 5 ml aliquots into sterile tubes containing eight glass beads. This mixture is used to suspend tissues and to treat stool and other specimens that require decontamination prior to inoculation.

Cell Culture Media

The following cell culture media, used to grow and maintain culture cells, are prepared with Eagle's minimum essential medium (MEM) without bicarbonate in Earle's balanced salt solution (EBSS). Both maintenance and growth media are prepared in 1,000 ml volumes, aliquoted into sterile, plastic 250 ml flasks, and stored at 4° C until needed. Routine quality control includes pH determination, assay for milliequivalents of Na$^+$, Cl$^-$, and culture for bacterial, mycoplasmal, and fungal contamination.

1. *Growth Medium*

MEM without bicarbonate in EBSS (10 × concentrate)	100 ml
Gentamicin (50 mg/ml)	0.2 ml
Amphotericin B (250 μg/ml)	10 ml
7.5% NaHCO$_3$	10 ml
Glutamine (200 mM)	10 ml
Fetal bovine serum (inactivated 30 min at 56° C)	100 ml
Distilled water (sterile) to bring final volume to 1,000 ml	

We have found it convenient to prepare this medium by adding the concentrate of MEM in EBSS to 1 liter of sterile distilled water from which 230 ml has been removed and then adding appropriate amounts of the remaining ingredients.

2. *Maintenance Medium for Primary Monkey Kidney (PMK) Cells*

MEM without bicarbonate in EBSS (10 × concentrate)	100 ml
Gentamicin (50 mg/ml)	1 ml
Amphotericin B (250 μg/ml)	10 ml
7.5% NaHCO$_3$	10 ml
Distilled water (sterile) to bring final volume to 1,000 ml	

Glutamine is omitted from this medium because it is toxic to monkey cells. Fetal bovine serum is omitted because it may contain substances inhibitory to myxoviruses.

3. *Maintenance Medium for HFD and Hep-2 Cells*

MEM without bicarbonate in EBSS (10 × concentrate)	100 ml
Gentamicin (50 mg/ml)	1 ml
Amphotericin B (250 µg/ml)	10 ml
Glutamine (200 mM)	10 ml
7.5% NaHCO₃	30 ml
Fetal bovine serum (inactivated 30 min at 56° C)	30 ml
Distilled water (sterile) to bring final volume to 1,000 ml	

Hanks' Balanced Salt Solution (BSS) with Antibiotics for Washing Cell Monolayers and Making Dilutions of Virus

Hanks' BSS without bicarbonate (1 × concentrate)	100 ml
Gentamicin (50 mg/ml)	0.1 ml
Amphotericin B (250 µg/ml)	0.5 ml
7.5% NaHCO₃	0.47 ml

Phosphate-Buffered Saline (PBS) Solutions

1. *PBS (pH 7.5) for Diluting Trypsin and Washing Monolayers*

NaCl	8 g
KCl	0.2 g
KH₂PO₄	0.12 g
NaH₂PO₄ (anhydrous)	91 g
Distilled water (sterile) to bring final volume to 1,000 ml	

2. *PBS (pH 7.2-7.5) for Fluorescent Antibody Wash*
   a. Stock solution (10 ×)
   Dissolve the following in 2,000 ml distilled water. Shake well after each addition of salt.

NaH₂HPO₄ · H₂O	6.65 g
Na₂HPO₄	35 g
NaCl	255 g

Distilled water (sterile) to bring final volume to 3,000 ml

Add 40% NaOH until pH is 7.2-7.5.
   b. Working solution (1 ×)

10 × stock solution	1.5 liter
Distilled water (sterile)	13.5 liter

70% Sorbitol (Holding Medium for CMV Specimens)

Sorbitol	70 g
Distilled water (sterile)	100 ml

Filter sterilize, and store at 4° C. To use, mix equal volumes of 70% sorbitol solution and urine specimen and freeze at −70° C. Solid specimens, such as tissue, can be immersed in the solution and then frozen to −70° C prior to shipping on dry ice.

0.25% Trypsin

Trypsin (2.5%)	5 ml
PBS (pH 7.5)	45 ml

Dispense in 2 ml aliquots and refrigerate (4° C).

VITAMIN K₁ SOLUTION

Vitamin K₁ solution is used as a medium supplement in a final concentration of 0.1 µg/ml for liquid media and 10 µg/ml for agar media. To prepare, weigh out 0.2 g of vitamin K₁ (Sigma Chemical Co. and other suppliers) on a small piece of sterile aluminum foil, and aseptically add it to 20 ml of absolute ethanol in a sterile tube or bottle. The stock solution is 10 mg/ml. The stock solution can be further diluted for use in sterile distilled water. Refrigerate in a tightly closed container protected from light.

Add 1 ml of stock solution per liter of agar and 0.01 ml/liter of broth (dilute stock solution in water).

XANTHINE AGAR

See Tyrosine Agar, above.

XYLOSE LYSINE DEOXYCHOLATE (XLD) AGAR

(Taylor. 1965. Am J. Clin. Pathol. 44:471.)

This medium may be prepared by use of the dehydrated xylose lysine agar base (BBL, Difco, Gibco, Inolex) and adding the sodium thiosulfate, ferric ammonium citrate, and sodium deoxycholate (procedure recommended by some workers) or by utilizing the complete (XLD) agar.

Xylose	3.5 g
L-Lysine	5 g
Lactose	7.5 g
Sucrose	7.5 g
Sodium chloride	5 g
Yeast extract	3 g
Phenol red	0.08 g
Agar, dried	13.5 g
Sodium deoxycholate	2.5 g
Sodium thiosulfate	6.8 g
Ferric ammonium citrate	0.8 g
Distilled water	1,000 ml

(Final pH 7.4)

Suspend the medium in distilled water, and heat with frequent agitation just to the boiling point. **Do not boil.** Transfer immediately to a 50° C water bath, and pour plates as soon as the medium has cooled. The medium should be red-orange and clear, or nearly so. Excessive heating or prolonged holding at 50° C may cause precipitation, which could lead to some differences in colony morphology.

This medium is useful for the isolation of enteric pathogens, especially shigellae.

YERSINIA SELECTIVE AGAR

See CIN Agar.

46 Formulas for Commonly Used Stains

Although a number of the more important staining formulas and procedures are presented in this chapter, space does not permit a comprehensive review of the subject. Many other staining procedures are presented throughout the text where appropriate. Further details are available in the *Manual of Clinical Microbiology** and other references. The solubilities of some of the more widely used stains and dyes, in water and in alcohol, are shown in Table 46-1. Most stains are also available commercially (readymade).

ACID FAST STAINS

See also Rhodamine-Auramine Flurochrome Stain for Acid Fast Cells.

Kinyoun Carbol-Fuchsin Method Reagents

See also Chapters 7 and 41.

(Kinyoun. 1915. Am. J. Pub. Health 5:867.)

Basic fuchsin	4 g
Phenol	8 ml
Alcohol (95%)	20 ml
Distilled water	100 ml

Dissolve the basic fuchsin in the alcohol, and add the water slowly while shaking. Melt

---

*Lennette, E.H., et al., editors. 1980 and 1985. Manual of clinical microbiology, eds. 3 and 4. American Society for Microbiology, Washington, D.C.

TABLE 46.1
Solubility of Stains

| STAIN | PERCENT SOLUBLE AT 26° C | |
	IN WATER	IN 95% ETHANOL
Bismarck brown	1.36	1.08
Congo red	0	0.19
Crystal violet (chloride)	1.68	13.87
Eosin Y	44.2	2.18
Fuchsin, basic (chloride)	0.26	5.93
Malachite green (oxalate)	7.60	7.52
Methylene blue (chloride)	3.55	1.48
Neutral red (chloride)	5.64	2.45
Safranin O	5.45	3.41
Thionin	0.25	0.25

Data from Conn, J.G. 1928. Biological stains, Commission on Standardization of Biological Stains. W.F. Humphrey Press, Geneva, N.Y.

the phenol in a 56° C water bath, and add 8 ml to the stain, using a pipet with a rubber bulb.

Stain the fixed smear for 3-5 min (no heat necessary), and continue as with Ziehl-Neelsen stain.

By the addition of a detergent or wetting agent the staining of acid fast organisms may be accelerated. Tergitol No. 7 (Sigma Chemical Co.) may be used. Add 1 drop of Tergitol No. 7 to every 30-40 ml of the Kinyoun carbol-fuchsin stain.

Acid fast bacteria stain red with carbol-fuchsin stains. The background color is dependent on the counterstain; methylene blue imparts a blue color to non–acid fast material, whereas brilliant green results in green background and picric acid results in yellow. More information about the appearance of acid fast organisms is found in Chapters 33 and 41.

Partial Acid Fast Stain

See Chapter 33. Other modifications include performing the standard Ziehl-Neelsen procedure (Chapter 7) with the substitution of 1% aqueous sulfuric acid or 0.5% acid alcohol for the standard 3% acid alcohol decolorizer. Par-

tially acid-fast organisms, such as *Nocardia* species, will stain red to reddish-purple.

Ziehl-Neelsen Reagents

Carbol-fuchsin Stain

Basic fuchsin	0.3 g
Ethanol (95%)	10 ml

Mix these with the following:

Phenol, melted crystals	5 ml
Distilled water	95 ml

Acid Alcohol

Hydrochloric acid, concentrated	3 ml
Ethanol (95%)	97 ml

Counterstain

Methylene blue	0.3 g
Distilled water	100 ml

Some workers may prefer 0.5% aqueous brilliant green or a saturated solution of picric acid as a counterstain; the latter is pale and does not selectively stain cellular material.

The technique for performance of the stain is given in Chaper 7.

ACRIDINE ORANGE STAIN

(McCarthy and Senne. 1980. J. Clin. Microbiol. 11:281.)

1. Prepare stock stain solution as follows:

Acridine orange (Fisher Scientific Co.)	1 g
Distilled water	100 ml

   Store in the dark at 4° C. Solution is stable for 6 months.
2. Prepare working stain solution daily by adding 0.05 ml of stock solution to 5 ml of 0.2 M acetate buffer (pH 4.0).
3. Prepare smears as usual and air dry. Fix with absolute methanol or heat fix.
4. Flood slides with working stain solution and allow to stand for 1 min.
5. Rinse with tap water and air dry.
6. Examine under oil immersion (1,000 ×) and ultraviolet light for bacteria.

Bacteria and yeast stain bright red-orange, and leukocytes stain pale apple green. Slides may be screened under low power for suspicious areas. Smears may be Gram stained directly without prior decolorization as long as all immersion oil is removed with xylene.

AURAMINE-RHODAMINE STAIN

See Rhodamine-Auramine Stain.

CALCOFLUOR WHITE

See Chapters 7 and 43.

CAPSULE STAINS
Anthony Method

1. Make a thin even smear of a culture in skimmed milk or litmus milk by spreading with a glass slide or an inoculating needle bent at a right angle. If it is not a milk culture, a loopful of the material may be mixed with a loopful of skimmed milk and then spread to give a uniform background.
2. Air dry. Do not fix with heat.
3. Stain with 1% aqueous crystal violet for 2 min.
4. Wash with a solution of 20% copper sulfate.
5. Air dry in a vertical position, and examine under the oil immersion lens. The capsule is unstained against a purple background; the cells are deeply stained.

Hiss Method

Mix a loopful of physiologic saline suspension of growth with a drop of normal serum on a glass slide. Allow the smear to air dry and heat fix. Flood the smear with crystal violet (1% aqueous solution). Steam the preparation gently for 1 min, and rinse with copper sulfate (20% aqueous solution). Capsules appear as faint blue halos around dark blue to purple cells.

India Ink Method*

In the India ink method, the capsule displaces the colloidal carbon particles of the ink and appears as a clear halo around the microorganism. The procedure is especially recommended for demonstrating the capsule of *Cryptococcus neoformans*.

1. To a small loopful of saline, water or broth on a clean slide, add a **minute amount of growth** from a young agar culture, using an inoculating needle. Spinal fluid may be used directly.
2. Mix well; then add a small loopful of India ink and immediately cover with a thin coverglass, allowing the fluid to spread as a thin film beneath the coverglass.
3. Examine immediately under the oil immersion objective, reducing the light considerably by lowering the condenser. Capsules, when present, stand out as **clear halos** against a dark background.

Muir Method
Muir Mordant

Tannic acid, 20% aqueous solution	2 parts
Saturated aqueous solution of mercuric chloride	2 parts
Saturated aqueous solution of potassium alum	5 parts

1. Prepare a thin even film of bacteria; allow to dry in air.
2. Cover the film with a piece of filter paper the size of the smear, and flood the slide with Ziehl-Neelsen carbolfuchsin.
3. Heat to steaming with a low Bunsen flame for 30 seconds.
4. Rinse gently with 95% ethanol and then with water.

---

*Not all India inks are suitable. Pelikan India ink made by Gunther Wagner of Hanover, Germany, is recommended; add about 0.3% thimerasol (Sigma Chemical Co.) as a preservative.

5. Add the mordant for 15-30 seconds; wash well with water.
6. Decolorize with ethanol to a faint pink; wash with water.
7. Counterstain with 0.3% methylene blue for 30 seconds.
8. Air dry and examine under the oil immersion lens. The cells are stained red and the capsules blue.

CARBOL-FUCHSIN COUNTERSTAIN FOR *LEGIONELLA PNEUMOPHILA*

See also Gram Stains.

Solution A

Basic fuchsin	0.3 gm
Ethyl alcohol	10 ml

Solution B

Phenol (melted crystals)	5 ml
Distilled water	95 ml

Prepare the counterstain by mixing solutions A and B together. Stain the smears according to the standard Gram stain. Counterstain with carbol-fuchsin solution for 1 min. Examine the smears microscopically using an oil immersion objective (100 ×).

FLAGELLA STAINS

See also Chapter 28.

(Gray. 1926. Bacteriol. 12:273.)

Mordant

Potassium alum, saturated aqueous solution	5 ml
Tannic acid, 20% aqueous solution	2 ml
Mercuric chloride, saturated aqueous solution	2 ml

Mix and add 0.4 ml of a saturated alcoholic solution of basic fuchsin. Make up fresh mordant for use each day.

Gray Method

1. Using a grease-free, well-cleaned slide that has been flamed and cooled, spread a drop of distilled water on the slide to cover an area of approximately 2 cm^2.

2. Select part of a colony from a younger agar culture or take a small amount of growth from a slant with an inoculating needle and **touch gently** into the drop of water at several places on the slide; then gently rotate the slide.
3. Allow to **air dry. Do not heat.**
4. Add the mordant, and allow it to act for 10 min.
5. Wash gently with distilled water or clean tap water.
6. Add Ziehl-Neelsen carbolfuchsin, and leave it on for 5-10 min.
7. Wash with tap water, air dry, and examine under oil.

Silver Stain for Flagella

Solution A (Mordant or Prestain)

Saturated aqueous solution of aluminum potassium sulfate (approximately 14 g/100 ml of water) (maintain as stock)	25 ml
Tannic acid, 10%	50 ml
Ferric chloride solution, 5% (maintain as stock)	5 ml

Combine and store in dark bottle at room temperature. The solution will remain stable for several months.

Solution B (Silver Stain)

1. Prepare 100 ml of 5% silver nitrate solution.
2. Add concentrated ammonium hydroxide (2-5 ml) dropwise to 90 ml of the 5% silver nitrate solution until the brown precipitate formed just redissolves.
3. Add some of the remaining 5% silver nitrate dropwise to the solution until a faint cloudiness persists.
4. Store the solution in a dark bottle at room temperature. The solution will remain stable for several months.

Staining Procedure

1. Label and flame commercially cleaned slides to burn off any residue. While the slides are hot, a heavy line may be

drawn with wax pencil to reduce the amount of stain needed (optional).

2. Using growth from 18-24 h cultures on heart infusion or trypticase soy agar slants incubated at 35° C, prepare a light suspension of organisms in 3 ml of sterile distilled water.* Suspension should be only slightly cloudy and less than 0.5 McFarland standard.

3. Place one large loopful of culture suspension on the flamed slide, and allow it to run to the end. Allow to air dry. Do not fix.

4. Place the slide on staining rack, and flood with solution A. Leave it for 4 min, and then rinse with distilled water.

5. Flood the slide with solution B, and heat just until steam is emitted by running a burner under the slide on a rack. Remove the burner, allow the slide to stain 4 min, rinse with distilled water, and slant to dry.

DIRECT FLUORESCENT ANTIBODY STAINS FOR *BORDETELLA PERTUSSIS* AND *LEGIONELLA*

See Chapters 16 and 39.

GIEMSA STAIN FOR CHLAMYDIAE

(Schachter. 1980. In Lennette et al., editors: Manual of clinical microbiology, ed. 3. American Society for Microbiology, Washington, D.C.)

Giemsa stain is prepared by dissolving 0.5 g of powder in 33 ml of glycerol at 55°-60° C for 1½-2 h. To this is added 33 ml of absolute methanol, acetone free. The solution is mixed thoroughly and allowed to sediment and then is stored at room temperature as stock. Dilutions of the stock stain are made with neutral distilled water or buffered water in a ratio of 1 part of stock Giemsa solution to 40 or 50 parts of diluent.

---

*Note: Do not use any fluid for suspension other than distilled water or nutrient broth.

The smear is air dried, fixed with absolute methanol for at least 5 min, and again dried. It is then covered with the diluted Giemsa stain (freshly prepared each day) for 1 h. The slide is then rinsed rapidly in 95% ethanol to remove excess dye, dried, and examined for the presence of the typical basophilic intracytoplasmic inclusion body.

GIEMSA STAIN FOR MALARIA

See Chapter 44.

GIMÉNEZ STAIN FOR CHLAMYDIAE AND RICKETTSIAE

(Hendrickson. 1985. Reagents and stains. In Lennette et al., editors: Manual of clinical microbiology, ed. 4. American Society for Microbiology, Washington, D.C.; and Giménez. 1984. ASM News 50:292.)

1. Prepare stock carbol-fuchsin as follows:

Basic fuchsin (total dye content >94%)	10 g
95% ethanol	100 ml
4% aqueous phenol	250 ml
Distilled water	650 ml

Hold this solution at 37° C for at least 48 h before using.

2. Prepare 0.2 M phosphate buffers as follows:

a. NaH_2PO_4	2.84 g
Distilled water	100 ml
b. Na_2HPO_4	2.76 g
Distilled water	100 ml

3. Prepare 0.1 M working phosphate buffer solution (pH 7.45) as follows:

0.2 M NaH_2PO_4	3.5 ml
0.2 M Na_2HPO_4	15.5 ml
Distilled water	19 ml

4. Prepare working buffered stain solution as follows:

Stock carbol-fuchsin stain	3 ml
Working phosphate buffer	10.5 ml

This working stain solution must be filtered immediately (Whatman No. 2 paper filters) and again before each use (see below). It is usable for approximately 3 days.

5. Prepare malachite green counterstain as follows:

Malachite green oxalate	0.8 g
Distilled water	100 ml

6. Air dry the smear and heat fix.
7. Drop working stain solution through a filter (Whatman no. 2) directly onto the slide. Allow to stand for 1-2 min.
8. Wash thoroughly with tap water.
9. Cover the smear with malachite green and allow to stand for 6-9 seconds, then wash with tap water.
10. Cover the smear a second time with malachite green for 6-9 seconds. Again wash thoroughly with tap water.
11. Examine slides under oil immersion (1,000 ×) for characteristic red-staining organisms and a green background.

GRAM STAINS

Although the reagents given below have yielded the most reproducible results, the dilution of the safranin counterstain and the makeup of the decolorizer vary among users. The classic (and longest) method is given in Chapter 7. A rapid modification is presented below. Other counterstains (usually containing carbol-fuchsin) are found under Carbol-fuchsin counterstain for *Legionella pneumophila*, above and below.

Gram Stain (Hucker Modification)

Reagents

Stock crystal violet	
Crystal violet (85% dye)	20 g
Ethanol (95%)	100 ml
Stock oxalate solution	
Ammonium oxalate	1 g
Distilled water	100 ml

Working solution. Dilute the stock crystal violet solution 1:10 with distilled water, and mix with 4 vol of stock oxalate solution. Store in a glass-stoppered bottle.

Gram iodine solution	
Iodine crystals	1 g
Potassium iodide	2 g

Dissolve these completely in 5 ml of distilled water; then add:

Distilled water	240 ml
Sodium bicarbonate, 5% aqueous solution	60 ml

Mix well; store in an amber-glass bottle.

Decolorizer	
Ethanol (95%)	250 ml
Acetone	250 ml

Mix; store in a glass-stoppered bottle.

Counterstain (stock safranin)	
Safranin O	2.5 g
Ethanol (95%)	100 ml

Working solution. Dilute stock safranin 1:5 or 1:10 with distilled water; store in a glass-stoppered bottle.

The principles of the Gram stain are discussed in Chapter 7. The following procedure is for the **rapid method:**

1. Prepare a thin film of the material to be examined; dry and fix as previously described.
2. Flood the slide with crystal violet stain, and allow it to remain on the slide for 10 seconds.
3. Pour off the stain, and wash off the remainder with the iodine solution.
4. Flood with iodine solution, and allow to mordant for 10 seconds.
5. Rinse off with running water. Shake off excess.
6. Decolorize with alcohol-acetone solution or 95% alcohol (an alcohol-acetone solution may prove to be too rapid) until no further color flows from the slide. This usually takes from 10-20 seconds, depending on the thickness of the smear.

Care should be taken not to overdecolor-ize the film, since this may result in an incorrect reading of the stain.

7. Counterstain with safranin for 10 sec-onds; then wash off with water.

8. Blot between clean sheets of bibulous paper and examine under oil immersion.

Carbol-Fuchsin Gram Stain Counterstain for Pale-Staining Bacteria

Prepare Kinyoun's carbol-fuchsin as de-scribed above under Acid fast stains. Dilute this stain 1:20 in distilled water (5 ml of carbol-fuchsin stain and 95 ml of distilled water) and use instead of safranin in the Gram stain. Or-ganisms known to stain poorly (*Legionella, Bor-detella,* etc.) may require as long as 3 min of the counterstain, whereas most gram-negative bacteria stain readily in 10 seconds.

GROCOTT'S GOMORI–METHENAMINE–SILVER NITRATE STAIN FOR ACTINOMYCETES AND FUNGI IN TISSUE SECTIONS

See also Chapter 16.

Solution A

Borax, 5%	8 ml
Distilled water	100 ml

Solution B

Silver nitrate, 10%	7 ml
Methenamine, 3%	100 ml

Add equal parts of solutions A and B to make a working methenamine–silver nitrate solution. These solutions should be made up fresh.

Stock Light Green Solution

Light green SF (yellow)	0.2 g
Distilled water	100 ml
Glacial acetic acid	0.2 ml

Deparaffinize and bring to distilled water. Oxidize in 5% chronic acid for 1 h. Wash in running tap water for a few seconds. Rinse in 1% sodium bisulfite for 1 min to remove resid-ual chromic acid. Wash in tap water for 5-10 min. Wash in three or four changes of distilled water. Place in working methenamine–silver nitrate solution in oven (58°-60° C) for 30-60 min. When the section turns yellowish-brown, use paraffin-coated forceps to remove the slide from the silver nitrate solution. Dip the slide in distilled water, and check with a microscope for adequate silver impregnation. Fungi should be dark brown at this stage. Rinse in six changes of distilled water. Tone in 0.1% gold chloride for 2-5 min. Rinse in distilled water. Remove the unreduced silver with 2% sodium thiosulfate for 2-5 min. Wash in tap water. Counterstain for 1 min with fresh 1:5 dilution in distilled water of stock light green solution. Dehydrate, clear, and mount.

IODINE SOLUTIONS FOR WET MOUNT PREPARATIONS

Iodine solutions are used to stain protozoan cysts in wet mounts. A weak rather than a strong iodine solution is best. The strong io-dine tends to coagulate the fecal particles and to destroy the refractile nature of the organism.

Several iodine solutions can be used satis-factorily. The two described below have been widely used and are simply prepared. The one recommended by Dobell and O'Connor is a weak iodine that should be prepared fresh about every 10 days for best results. Lugol io-dine must be diluted about five times with dis-tilled water, since the full-strength solution is too strong. Lugol iodine should be prepared fresh about every 3 weeks. Gram iodine used for bacteriologic work is not satisfactory for staining protozoan cysts.

Dobell and O'Connor Iodine Solution

(Dobell and O'Connor. 1921. Intestinal protozoa of man. William Wood, New York.)

Iodine (powdered crystals)	1 g
Potassium iodide	2 g
Distilled water	100 ml

The KI is dissolved in the distilled water, and the iodine crystals are added slowly and shaken thoroughly. Filter or decant.

Lugol Iodine Solution

Iodine (powdered crystals)	5 g
Potassium iodide	10 g
Distilled water	100 ml

The KI is dissolved in the distilled water, and the iodine crystals are added slowly and shaken until dissolved. Filter, and place in tightly stoppered bottle. Dilute to 1:5 with distilled water for use in staining protozoan cysts.

A small portion of feces is comminuted in a drop of the iodine solution, mounted with a coverslip, and sealed with a heated paraffin-petrolatum mixture.

In a correctly stained cyst the glycogen appears reddish-brown, the cytoplasm appears yellow, and the nuclei stand out as lighter refractile bodies. The location of karyosomes may be more easily determined, but the chromatoid bodies are less visible than in saline solution. Since glycogen is a reserve food, it does not usually appear in older cysts.

See Chapter 44 for further information.

IRON-HEMATOXYLIN STAIN

See Chapter 44.

KOH STAIN

See Potassium Hydroxide.

LACTOPHENOL COTTON BLUE FOR FUNGI

Phenol crystals	20 g
Lactic acid	20 g
Glycerin	40 g
Distilled water	20 ml

Dissolve these ingredients by heating gently over a steam bath. Add 0.05 g of cotton blue dye (Poirier's blue). This may be used for yeasts as well as molds and serves as both a mounting fluid and a stain.

1. Place a drop of fluid on a clean slide.
2. Place a small amount of culture in this drop. If the culture is on agar, remove a piece of the medium with the embedded growth.
3. Cover with a coverglass, and press down gently to flatten.
4. Warm gently to remove air bubbles if necessary.
5. Examine under the microscope with high-dry or oil immersion objectives.
6. Ring edges of coverglass with nail polish if a permanent mount is required.

METACHROMATIC GRANULE STAINS FOR CORYNEBACTERIUM SPECIES
Albert Stain (Christensen Modification)

(Clark, editor. 1981. Staining procedures, ed. 4. Williams & Wilkins, Baltimore.)

The Albert stain is a differential stain and is recommended for its simplicity in staining Corynebacterium diphtheriae.

1. Prepare stain as follows:

Toluidine blue O	0.15 g
95% ethanol	2 ml
Glacial acetic acid	5 ml
Distilled water	100 ml

Dissolve the toluidine blue O in the ethanol and then add the distilled water. Add the glacial acetic acid as the final step.
2. Prepare a thin smear of the organism in distilled water, air dry, and heat fix.
3. Flood the slide with acidic toluidine blue and allow to stand for 1 min. Rinse in tap water.
4. Flood the slide with Gram's iodine (above) and allow to stand for 1 min. Rinse in tap water.
5. Counterstain with Gram's safranin counterstain (above) and allow to stand for 1 min. Rinse in tap water and blot dry.
6. Examine under oil immersion ($1,000 \times$).

Granules appear blue-black; the bands appear blue to blue-green; and the cytoplasm appears green. The stain is excellent for demonstrating volutin granules in other bacteria as well.

METHYLENE BLUE STAIN (LOEFFLER'S)

Methylene blue	0.3 g
Ethyl alcohol (95%)	30 ml

When dissolved add:

Distilled water	100 ml

Cover the fixed smear with staining solution, and stain for 1 min. Wash with water, and blot dry with blotting paper.

Loeffler methylene blue stain, as formerly used, was prepared by adding alkali to the foregoing solution. Current commercial preparations of methylene blue do not require the addition of alkali. The older preparations contained acid impurities.

This is a simple stain. Prepare a smear of the organism, and fix with heat. Flood smear with Loeffler methylene blue, and allow to react for 1 min. Wash and blot dry. The granules readily absorb the dye and appear deep blue. Overstaining lessens the contrast.

PERIODIC ACID–SCHIFF STAIN FOR OBSERVATION OF FUNGI IN DIRECT SMEARS

(Hendrickson. 1985. Reagents and stains. In Lennette et al., editors: Manual of clinical microbiology, ed. 4. American Society for Microbiology, Washington, D.C. p. 1105.)

The periodic acid step in this stain method hydrolyzes cell wall aldehydes, which are then able to combine with the modified Schiff reagent (the carbol-fuchsin and the hydrosulfite solutions), coloring the cell wall carbohydrates red. Either zinc or sodium hydrosulfite may be used, and either picric acid or light green counterstain may be used in this method with good results. A control slide (a suspension of hyphal forms of yeast is adequate) should be run concurrently with each patient specimen.

1. Prepare basic fuchsin solution as follows:

Basic fuchsin	0.1 g
95% ethanol	5 ml
Distilled water	95 ml

Mix together and store at room temperature in tightly capped Coplin jars.

2. Prepare zinc (or sodium) hydrosulfite solution as follows:

Zinc (or sodium) hydrosulfite	1.0 g
Tartaric acid	0.5 g
Distilled water	100 ml

Mix together and store at room temperature in tightly capped Coplin jars.

3. Prepare saturated aqueous picric acid as follows:
Place 100 ml of distilled water into a flask and stir continuously on a slightly warm hotplate stirrer. Add crystals of picric acid slowly until the crystals no longer go into solution. Store tightly stoppered at room temperature.

4. Prepare light green counterstain as follows:

Light green	1 g
Glacial acetic acid	0.25 ml
80% ethanol	100 ml

Mix together and store at room temperature.

5. Prepare the slides by spreading material thinly (respiratory secretions, body fluids, and other viscous specimens), air dry, and heat gently to fix. For skin scrapings and dry material, fix the material to the slide with a small amount of 10% albumin.

6. Flood the slide with 95% alcohol (or immerse in the alcohol in a Coplin jar) for 1 min.

7. Immerse the slide in a Coplin jar containing 5% periodic acid.

8. Immerse the slide in basic fuchsin for 2 min and rinse gently in tap water.

9. Counterstain with either the aqueous picric acid for 2 min or light green for 5 seconds. Rinse thoroughly in tap water.

10. Dehydrate in 95% ethanol for 10 seconds followed by 100% ethanol for 1 min.

11. Clear through two quick changes in xylene and mount with Permount or other mount-

ing medium while the slide is still wet with xylene.

12. Examine for the presence of fungal elements, which stain bright red or purplish against an orange (picric acid) or green (light green) background.

POTASSIUM HYDROXIDE (10% KOH) WET PREPARATION FOR DIRECT OBSERVATION OF FUNGI IN CLINICAL MATERIAL

See also Chapters 7 and 43.

1. Prepare 10% KOH as follows:

Potassium hydroxide	10 g
Glycerin	10 ml
Distilled water	80 ml

Mix together and store at room temperature. Dispense into small dropper bottles for use.

2. Place the material to be stained on the slide and add a drop of 10% KOH. Equal amounts of 10% KOH and viscous material (sputum, etc.) should be mixed on the slide.

3. Cover the material with a coverslip, and allow to remain at room temperature for approximately 10 min. Gentle heating may hasten the breakdown of protein and allow better visualization of fungal elements.

4. Examine under all objectives for hyphal elements, budding cells, spherules, and other fungal morphologies. Reducing the light passing through the condensor or using phase microscopy may be helpful (Chapter 7).

PPLO (MYCOPLASMA) STAIN

(Dienes and Weinberger. 1951. Bacteriol. Rev. 15:245.)

Reagents

Methylene blue	2.5 g
Azure II	1.25 g
Maltose	10 g
Sodium carbonate	0.25 g
Distilled water	100 ml

Dissolve the ingredients in the water.

1. Spread a drop of stain on a grease-free coverglass, and allow it to dry.

2. With a sterile scalpel, cut out a small block of agar medium containing a few *Mycoplasma* colonies and place, with colonies up, on a clean glass slide.

3. Lay coverglass, stain side down, carefully on the agar block, without rubbing.

4. Seal the preparation with a mixture of 3 parts petrolatum and 1 part paraffin to prevent drying.

5. Examine under low-power objective.

Mycoplasma colonies are quite distinct with dense blue centers and light blue peripheries.

RHODAMINE-AURAMINE FLUOROCHROME STAIN FOR ACID FAST CELLS

See also Chapter 7.

Rhodamine-Auramine Fluorochrome Stain (Truant Method)

(Truant, Brett, and Thomas. 1962. Henry Ford Hosp. Med. Bull. 10:287.)

By staining a smear with fluorescent dyes, such as auramine and rhodamine, and examining by fluorescence microscopy using an ultraviolet light source, acid fast bacilli, when present, appear to glow with a **yellow-orange** color. They are visible under lower magnifications of the microscope; thus, a stained smear can be examined in much less time than is required by conventional methods. Numerous modifications of the procedure have been introduced; that reported by Truant and co-workers is recommended.

Auramine O*	1.5 g
Rhodamine B†	0.75 g

---

*Chroma 1B339, Chroma Gesellschaft, Schmid GmbH, available from Roboz Surgical Instrument Co., Washington, D.C.

†Matheson, Coleman, and Bell. CI 45170. Norwood, Ohio.

Glycerol	75 ml
Phenol	10 ml
Distilled water	50 ml

Combine the solutions, mix well (using a magnetic stirring device for 24 h or heating until warm and stirring vigorously for 5 min), filter through glass wool, and store in a glass-stoppered bottle at 4° C. The stain is stable for several months under refrigeration.

1. Heat fix on a slide warmer* at 65° C for 2 h or overnight.
2. Cover the smear with the auramine-rhodamine solution.
3. Stain for 15 min at room temperature or at 35° C.
4. Rinse off with distilled water.
5. Decolorize with 0.5% hydrochloric acid in 70% ethanol for 2-3 min, then rinse thoroughly with distilled water.
6. Flood the smear with counterstain, a 0.5% solution of potassium permanganate (filter and store in amber bottle), for 2-4 min (no longer—excessive exposure results in loss of brilliance).
7. Rinse with distilled water, dry, and examine.

Ultraviolet Light Source

The smears are examined under a binocular microscope using an ultraviolet light source. The Leitz, Zeiss, and Reichert fluorescent microscopy units are highly recommended and are equipped with Osram HBO 200 maximum pressure mercury vapor lamps as light sources, BG 12 (3 or 4 mm) or C 5113 (2 mm) violet exciter filters, and OG 1 deep yellow barrier filters in the eyepieces. This recommended filter combination results in **bright yellow-orange** staining bacilli against a dark background; nonspecific background debris fluoresces a pale yellow, quite distinct from the yellow-orange bacilli.

---

*Microslide staining and drying bath are available from Scientific Products, Division of American Hospital Supply Corp., McGaw Park, Ill.

It is suggested that a drop of immersion oil be placed on the darkfield condenser, the slide inserted, and the microscope first focused under bright light until a clear central area is seen on the slide. The microscope should then be switched over to the ultraviolet source. Smears may be rapidly examined under low- or high-power objective (25 or 40 ×) with a 10 × eyepiece; after a little practice, all smears may be examined at these magnifications or lower in a matter of seconds. Occasionally, it may be necessary to switch to the oil immersion objective to confirm typical morphologic characteristics, such as beading and cording. It is recommended that microscopic examination be carried out in a darkened room for maximum efficiency.

Quartz-Halogen Illuminator

(Runyon et al. 1980. In Lennette et al., editors: Manual of clinical microbiology, ed. 3. American Society for Microbiology, Washington, D.C.)

Excellent demonstration of fluorochrome-stained mycobacteria is obtained by use of a microscope equipped with a quartz-halogen illuminator and the proper combinations of primary (exciter) and secondary (barrier) filters. This system provides the same benefits as ultraviolet apparatus with the added advantages that the **blue light apparatus** does not require a special dark room (though subdued lighting is recommended), does not require oil on the condenser or slide, is simpler and more economical, and does not present radiation hazards. The following recommendations based on use of the Zeiss RA 38 microscope and attachments are applicable to other equipment having comparable features.

The equipment needed is a standard binocular microscope with an illuminator containing a collector lens and a 12 V, 100 W quartz-halogen lamp or high-intensity tungsten bulb, front-surface reflecting mirrors, brightfield condenser, low-power objectives (10 or 25 ×) for scanning, and high-dry (63 ×) planachromat (flat field; if the high-dry objective is corrected for coverslip, then a coverslip must be placed, not mounted, over the smear), a 100 × oil immersion objective for more critical examination of acid fast (fluorescent) bodies, and 10 × compensating eyepieces. A turret or intermediate tube with holders for secondary filters located in the tube body between the objectives and the eyepieces facilitates filter changing. The optics and light path must be precisely aligned to avoid loss of light intensity. The light source is adjusted for Köhler illumination by centering and focusing the lamp filament on the closed iris diaphragm of the condenser. Maximal intensity is obtained by making small adjustments of the condenser while viewing an auramine-stained mycobacterial smear.

Combinations of primary and secondary filters are selected to provide good contrast between a dark background and the fluorescing, yellow bacillus. However, the background must be sufficiently light that nonfluorescing debris can be seen for maintaining focus while scanning the slide. A BG 12 primary filter transmitting only wavelengths less than about 500 nm (peak 404 nm) in combination with secondary filters that transmit only wavelengths above 500 or 530 nm, as Zeiss No. 50 or 53, respectively, provides satisfactory demonstration of fluorescing mycobacteria. The particular combination of complementary exciter and barrier filters determines the color of the background. The greater the overlap of transmission curves, the lighter the background, and vice versa. Therefore, the user should have on hand BG 12 filters of various thicknesses (1, 1.5, 2, and 3 mm; Fish-Schurman Corp.) for neutral density purposes and secondary filters having transmission cutoffs at 500, 515, and 530 nm to determine which combinations provide optimal background-contrast qualities. The following exciter and barrier filter combinations have been found to be excellent for demonstrating fluorochrome-stained mycobacteria: 3 mm BG 12 and No. 50, light green background; 4 mm BG 12 and No. 50, dark green; 3 mm BG 12 and No. 53, light brown; 3.5 mm BG 12 and No. 53, dark brown. Another primary filter, the fluorescein isothiocyanate (FITC) interference filter, used in combination with a 3 mm BG 12 and a No. 50 or 53 barrier filter, results in excellent dark green and dark red-brown backgrounds, respectively. The FITC laminated to a BG 38 (to reduce red transmission) and in combination with a 1.5 mm BG 12 produces a reddish-tinged gray background with the No. 50 and a red field with the No. 53.

RICKETTSIAL STAINS
Castañeda Stain

Reagents

Solution A

Potassium phosphate (KH_2PO_4) (1% aqueous)	100 ml
Sodium phosphate (Na_2HPO_4 $12H_2O$) (25% aqueous)	100 ml

Mix and add 1 ml of formalin.

Solution B

Methyl alcohol	100 ml
Methylene blue	1 g

Mix 20 ml of solution A with 0.15 ml of solution B and add 1 ml of formalin.

Solution C (counterstain)

Safranin O (0.2% aqueous)	25 ml
Acetic acid (0.1%)	75 ml

1. Prepare a homogeneous film, and dry in air.
2. Cover film with stain (mixture of solutions A and B).
3. Drain off stain. Do not wash.
4. Counterstain with safranin O (solution C) for 1 to 4 seconds.
5. Wash with tap water. Blot dry.
6. Examine under oil immersion lens.

The rickettsiae stain blue, whereas the cellular elements stain red.

Giemsa Method*

1. Prepare a homogeneous film on a clean glass slide. Air dry.
2. Flood with methyl alcohol for 1 min.
3. Drain off alcohol, and allow to dry.
4. Cover film with Giemsa stain (15 drops), and allow to react for 1 min.
5. Add distilled water (30 drops), and continue staining for 5 min. Drain off.
6. Wash with distilled water.
7. Place slide on end, and allow to dry in air.
8. Examine under oil immersion lens. The rickettsiae stain a bluish-purple.

SILVER STAINS

See also Grocott-Gomori methenamine–silver nitrate stain (above) and Chapter 16 for the rapid 80° C modification of the Gomori methenamine–silver nitrate (GMS) stain for visualization of *Pneumocystis carinii* in respiratory specimens. These GMS stains also stain fungal elements very well. Fungal elements appear black or gray to black against a turquoise and gray background.

The Warthin-Starry silver stain for visualization of the agent of cat-scratch disease is described in Chapter 40.

SPORE STAINS
Dorner Method

1. Make a heavy suspension of organisms in distilled water in a test tube, and add an equal volume of freshly filtered carbol-fuchsin (Kinyoun, above).
2. Place tube in boiling water bath for 5-10 min.
3. Mix a loopful of the aforementioned combination with a loopful of boiled and filtered 10% aqueous solution of nigrosin on a clean slide.

---

*This stain may also be used for spirochetes, which stain blue.

4. Spread out and dry film quickly with gentle heat.
5. Examine under oil. The spores stain red, and the bacterial cells are almost colorless against a dark gray background.

A modification of the Dorner method may be employed whereby a smear of the culture is prepared and fixed. The smear is then covered with a strip of filter paper to which carbol-fuchsin is added. The dye is heated to steaming for 5-7 min with a Bunsen burner, and the filter paper is removed. Wash with water, blot dry, and cover with a thin film of nigrosin using a second slide or a needle. The appearance of the cells is as previously described.

Wirtz-Conklin Method

(Paik. 1980. In Lennette et al., editors: Manual of clinical microbiology, ed. 3. American Society for Microbiology, Washington, D.C.)

Flood the entire slide with 5% aqueous malachite green. Steam for 3-6 min, and rinse under running tap water. Counterstain with 0.5% aqueous safranin for 30 seconds. Spores are seen as green spherules in red-stained rods or with red-stained debris.

SUDAN BLACK B FAT STAIN FOR *BACILLUS* SP. AND OTHER BACTERIA

(Burdon. 1946. J. Bacteriol. 52:665.)

Sudan black B	0.3 g
Ethanol, 70%	100 ml

Shake the solution thoroughly at intervals during the day, and allow it to stand overnight before use. Dry and fix the smear with heat. Stain the slide with Sudan black for 10 min, drain, and blot dry. Wash and clear the smear with xylene. Counterstain with a 0.5% aqueous solution of safranin for 10-15 seconds. Wash in tap water; blot dry. The cells stain red; the highly refractile poly-beta-hydroxybutyrate granules are blue-black. For *Legionella pneumophila,* counterstain for 1 min.

TOLUIDINE BLUE O FOR *PNEUMOCYSTIS*

See Chapters 16 and 44.

TRICHROME STAIN FOR INTESTINAL PROTOZOA

See Chapter 44.

WARTHIN-STARRY STAIN

See Chapter 40.

WAYSON STAIN

Dissolve 0.2 g of basic fuchsin and 0.75 g of methylene blue in 20 ml of absolute ethanol. Add the dye solution to 200 ml of a 5% solution of phenol in distilled water. Filter. Stain smears for a few seconds. Wash, blot, and dry. This stain is useful in detecting polar staining morphology.

WRIGHT STAINS

These stains are used for demonstrating parasites in blood and occasionally in tissue. Because of its superior staining characteristics, the Giemsa stain (above) is used more frequently. The stain given below yields sharper results than the classic Wright formula does. Because of differences in lots of Wright stain, control slides should be stained with the reagents to ensure suitable results.

Wright Stain (Lille's Modification)

(Clark, editor. 1981. Staining procedures, ed. 4. Williams & Wilkins, Baltimore.)

1. Prepare stock Wright stain as follows:

Wright stain powder* (available commercially)	1 g
Glycerol	50 ml
Methanol (100%)	50 ml

Mix the alcohol and glycerol together before adding the stain powder. Store at room temperature.

---

*Biological Stain Commission certified.

2. Prepare working solution immediately before use as follows:

Stock stain solution	4 ml
Acetone	3 ml
Phosphate buffer (1/15 M, pH 6.5)	2 ml
Distilled water	31 ml

Mix together in a Coplin jar. The solution may be used for two staining procedures if they are performed one after the other.

3. Prepare blood or tissue films by spreading material thinly over slide using a second slide. Fix immediately in absolute methanol for 2 to 3 min.
4. Allow the fixed slides to air dry.
5. Immerse the slides in a Coplin jar containing the working solution for 5 min.
6. Wash gently in distilled water and air dry.
7. Examine for parasitic forms under several different magnifications. Structures appear blue, purplish, and red.

Wright-Giemsa Method for Staining Conjunctival Scrapings

The Wright-Giemsa stain, along with a Gram stain of the scrapings, gives immediate information to the ophthalmologist regarding conjunctivitis of bacterial origin, inclusion body conjunctivitis and trachoma, or eosinophilia of allergic conjunctivitis.

1. Two slide preparations of scrapings are made; one is stained by the Gram method and one by the Wright-Giemsa technique.
2. To carry out staining by the Wright-Giemsa technique, apply Wright stain to the slide for 1 min. Add an equal volume of neutral distilled water (pH 7.0), and stain for 4 min.
3. Shake off stain; then apply dilute Giemsa stain (1 drop to 1 ml of neutral distilled water), and allow to stain for 15 min.
4. Shake off, decolorize lightly with ethanol, and air dry (do not blot).

Appendix

Selected Product Suppliers for Clinical Microbiology

Although we have attempted to list many major sources of products, not all manufacturers or suppliers are listed here. Regional supply houses and other sources should be considered.

ANAEROBIC BACTERIAL PRODUCTS
General Supplies

Anaerobe Systems, Inc.
3074A Scott Blvd.
Santa Clara, CA 95054

Bartels Immunodiagnostics
12729 North East 20th St.
Bellevue, WA 98005

BBL Microbiology Systems
P.O. Box 243
Cockeysville, MD 21030

Bellco Glass, Inc.
340 Edrudo Rd.
Vineland, NJ 08360

Kontes (Kimble div. of Owens-Illinois)
1022 Spruce St.
Vineland, NJ 08360

Oxoid U.S.A., Inc.
9107 Red Branch Rd.
Columbia, MD 21045

Scott Laboratories, Inc.
771 Main St.
Fiskeville, RI 02823

Identification Systems

Analytab Products
200 Express St.
Plainview, NY 11803

BBL Microbiology Systems
P.O. Box 243
Cockeysville, MD 21030

Innovative Diagnostic Systems, Inc.
3404 Oakcliff Rd., Suite C-1
Atlanta, GA 30340

ANTIBIOTICS

See Chapter 13.

ANTIBODY DETECTION SYSTEMS

Abbott Laboratories
Abbott Park 6C4, Dept. 49B
Abbott Park, IL 60064

American Dade
P.O. Box 520672
Miami, FL 33152

Analytab Products
200 Express St.
Plainview, NY 11803

Behring Diagnostics
10933 N. Torrey Pines Rd.
La Jolla, CA 92037

Bio-Diagnostic Systems, Inc.
1 Wall St., Research Park
Princeton, NJ 08540

Calbiochem-Behring Corp.
10933 N. Torrey Pines Rd.
La Jolla, CA 92037

Cetus Corp.
1400 53rd St.
Emeryville, CA 94608

Clinical Sciences Inc.
30 Troy Rd.
Whippany, NJ 07981

Cooper Biomedical, Inc.
One Technology Court
Malvern, PA 19355

Cordis Laboratories, Inc.
2140 North Miami Ave.
Miami, FL 33127

DuPont Co.
Barley Mill Plaza
Wilmington, DE 19898

Electro-Nucleonics, Inc.
7101 Riverwood Dr.
Columbia, MD 21046

Flow Laboratories, Inc.
7655 Old Springhouse Rd.
McLean, VA 22102

Gull Laboratories
890 East 5400 South
Salt Lake City, UT 84107

Hynson, Westcott & Dunning
Charles and Chase Streets
Baltimore, MD 21201

ICL Scientific (Hybridoma Sciences, Inc.)
18249 Euclid St.
Fountain Valley, CA 92708

Immuno-Mycologics, Inc.
P.O. Box 1151
Norman, OK 73070

International Diagnostic Technology, Inc.
2050 Concourse Dr.
San Jose, CA 95131-1701

Kallestad Laboratories Inc.
2000 InterFirst Tower
Austin, TX 78701

Labsystems
P.O. Box 48723
Chicago, IL 60648

Litton Bionetics, Inc.
2020 Bridge View Dr.
Charleston, SC 29405

Meloy Laboratories Inc.
6715 Electronic Dr.
Springfield, VA 22151

Meridian Diagnostics
3471 River Hills Dr., P.O. Box 44216
Cincinnati, OH 45244

Ortho Diagnostic Systems
Route 202
Raritan, NJ 08869

Sclavo Inc.
5 Mansard Court
Wayne, NJ 07470

Syva Co.
900 Arastradero Rd.
Palo Alto, CA 94303

Travenol-Genentech Diagnostics
600 Memorial Dr.
Cambridge, MA 02139

Wampole Laboratories
Half Acre Rd.
Cranbury, NJ 08512

Whittaker M.A. Bioproducts
P.O. Box 127, Biggs Ford Rd.
Walkersville, MD 21793

Zeus Scientific, Inc.
St. John and Elizabeth Streets
Raritan, NJ 08869

ANTIBODY SEPARATION FILTERS

Isolab, Inc.
Drawer 4350
Akron, Ohio 44321

ANTIGEN DETECTION SYSTEMS

Abbott Laboratories
Abbott Park 6C4, Dept. 49B
Abbott Park, IL 60064

Ames (div. of Miles Laboratories)
P.O. Box 70
Elkhart, IN 46515

Antibodies Incorporated
P.O. Box 1560
Davis, CA 95617

BioDx
100 Ford Rd.
Denville, NJ 07834

Burroughs-Wellcome Co.
(see Wellcome Diagnostics Division)

Diagnostic Products Corp.
5700 West 96th St.
Los Angeles, CA 90045

Difco Laboratories, Inc.
P.O. Box 1058
Detroit, MI 48232

Electro-Nucleonics, Inc.
7101 Riverwood Dr.
Columbia, MD 21046

Enzo Biochem, Inc.
325 Hudson St.
New York, NY 10013

Flow Laboratories, Inc.
7655 Old Springhouse Rd.
McLean, VA 22102

Genetic Systems
3005 First Ave.
Seattle, WA 98121

Gen-Probe, Inc.
9620 Chesapeake Dr.
San Diego, CA 92123

Gibco Laboratories
231 Sutton St.
North Andover, MA 01845

Hynson, Westcott & Dunning
Charles and Chase Streets
Baltimore, MD 21201

Immuno-Mycologics, Inc.
P.O. Box 1151
Norman, OK 73070

International Diagnostic Technology, Inc.
2050 Concourse Dr.
San Jose, CA 95131-1701

Litton Bionetics, Inc.
2020 Bridge View Dr.
Charleston, SC 29405

Marion Scientific
9233 Ward Parkway, Suite 350
Kansas City, MO 64114

Meridian Diagnostics
3471 River Hills Dr., P.O. Box 44216
Cincinnati, OH 45244

Microbiological Associates
(see Whittaker M.A. Bioproducts)

Micro-Media Systems
6200 El Camino Real
Carlsbad, CA 92008

Northeast Biomedical, Inc.
R.R. no. 1, Inland Farm Dr.
South Windham, ME 04082

Orion Research, Inc.
(Medical Technology Corp.)
71 Veronica Ave.
Somerset, NJ 08873

Ortho Diagnostic Systems
Route 202
Raritan, NJ 08869

Ramco Laboratories, Inc.
3801 Kirby Dr., Suite 170
Houston, TX 77098

Syva Co.
900 Arastradero Rd.
Palo Alto, CA 94303

Ventrex Laboratories, Inc.
217 Read St.
Portland, ME 04103

Wampole Laboratories
Half Acre Rd.
Cranbury, NJ 08512

Wellcome Diagnostics Division
3030 Cornwallis Rd.
Research Triangle Park, NC 27709

Whittaker M.A. Bioproducts
P.O. Box 127, Biggs Ford Rd.
Walkersville, MD 21793

Zeus Scientific, Inc.
St. John and Elizabeth Streets
Raritan, NJ 08869

ANTISERA

BBL Microbiology Systems
P.O. Box 243
Cockeysville, MD 21030

Burroughs-Wellcome Co.
(see Wellcome Diagnostics Division)

Dan-Serum Inc. (div. of Statens Seruminstitut)
2920 Wolff St.
Racine, WI 53404

Difco Laboratories, Inc.
P.O. Box 1058
Detroit, MI 48232

Fisher Scientific Co.
711 Forbes Ave.
Pittsburgh, PA 15219

Flow Laboratories, Inc.
7655 Old Springhouse Road
McLean, VA 22102

Immuno-Mycologics, Inc.
P.O. Box 1151
Norman, OK 73070

Kallestad Laboratories Inc.
2000 InterFirst Tower
Austin, TX 78701

Meridian Diagnostics
3471 River Hills Dr., P.O. Box 44216
Cincinnati, OH 45244

Northeast Biomedical, Inc.
R.R. no. 1, Inland Farm Dr.
South Windham, ME 04082

Roach Laboratories Inc.
Route 5, Donald Dr.
Loganville, GA 30249

Scott-Nolan Laboratories
4958 Hammermill Rd.
Tucker, GA 30084

Statens Seruminstitut (see also Dan-Serum Inc.)
Amager Blvd. 80
DK 2300 Copenhagen S
Denmark

Wellcome Animal Health
P.O. Box 6036
Kansas City, KS 66106

Wellcome Diagnostics Division
3030 Cornwallis Rd.
Research Triangle Park, NC 27709

Whittaker M.A. Bioproducts
P.O. Box 127, Biggs Ford Rd.
Walkersville, MD 21793

Automated Microbiology Systems (Detection, Identification, Susceptibility, etc.)

Abbott Laboratories, Analytical Systems
P.O. Box 152020
Irving, TX 75015

American MicroScan
200 Corporate Dr.
Mahwah, NJ 07430

Analytab Products
200 Express St.
Plainview, NY 11803

Analytical Luminescence Laboratory
11760 Sorrento Valley Rd., #E
San Diego, CA 92121

BBL Microbiology Systems
P.O. Box 243
Cockeysville, MD 21030

Difco Laboratories, Inc.
P.O. Box 1058
Detroit, MI 48232

General Diagnostics
201 Tabor Rd.
Morris Plains, NJ 07950

Gibco Laboratories
231 Sutton St.
North Andover, MA 01845

Hewlett-Packard Co.
Route 41
Avondale, PA 19311

Johnston Laboratories
P.O. Box 20086
Towson, MD 21204

Marion Scientific
9233 Ward Parkway, Suite 350
Kansas City, MO 64114

MCT Diagnostics
1997 Sloan Pl., Suite 26
St. Paul, MN 55117

Micro-Media Systems
6200 El Camino Real
Carlsbad, CA 92008

Turner Designs
2247 Old Middlefield Way
Mountain View, CA 94043

Vitek Systems, Inc.
595 Anglum Dr.
Hazelwood, MO 63042

Bacterial and Fungal Identification Reagents
Single Test Reagents

Analytab Products
200 Express St.
Plainview, NY 11803

Austin Biological Laboratories, Inc.
6620 Manor Rd.
Austin, TX 78723

Carr-Scarborough Microbiologicals, Inc.
P.O. Box 1328
Stone Mountain, GA 30086

Difco Laboratories, Inc.
P.O. Box 1058
Detroit, MI 48232

DuPont Co.
Barley Mill Plaza
Wilmington, DE 19898

E-Y Laboratories, Inc.
127 N. Amphlett Blvd.
San Mateo, CA 94401

Key Scientific Co.
P.O. Box 66307
Los Angeles, CA 90066

Micro-Bio-Logics
217 Osseo Ave. North
St. Cloud, MN 56301

Remel
12076 Santa Fe Dr.
Lenexa, KS 66215

Scott Laboratories, Inc.
771 Main St.
Fiskeville, RI 02823

Wampole Laboratories
Half Acre Rd.
Cranbury, NJ 08512

Immunologic Reagents (Except Antisera)

American MicroScan
200 Corporate Dr.
Mahwah, NJ 07430

BBL Microbiology Systems
P.O. Box 243
Cockeysville, MD 21030

Burroughs-Wellcome Co.
(see Wellcome Diagnostics Division)

General Diagnostics
201 Tabor Rd.
Morris Plains, NJ 07950

Meridian Diagnostics
3471 River Hills Dr., P.O. Box 44216
Cincinnati, OH 45244

Organon Diagnostics
375 Mt. Pleasant Ave.
West Orange, NJ 07052

Pharmacia Inc.
800 Centennial Ave.
Piscataway, NJ 08854

Scott Laboratories, Inc.
771 Main St.
Fiskeville, RI 02823

Syva Co.
900 Arastradero Rd.
Palo Alto, CA 94303

Wellcome Diagnostics Division
3030 Cornwallis Rd.
Research Triangle Park, NC 27709

Multicomponent Systems

American MicroScan
200 Corporate Dr.
Mahwah, NJ 07430

Analytab Products
200 Express St.
Plainview, NY 11803

Austin Biological Laboratories, Inc.
6620 Manor Rd.
Austin, TX 78723

Bartels Immunodiagnostics
12729 North East 20th St.
Bellevue, WA 98005

BBL Microbiology Systems
P.O. Box 243
Cockeysville, MD 21030

DuPont Co.
Barley Mill Plaza
Wilmington, DE 19898

Flow Laboratories, Inc.
7655 Old Springhouse Rd.
McLean, VA 22102

General Diagnostics
201 Tabor Rd.
Morris Plains, NJ 07950

Innovative Diagnostic Systems, Inc.
3404 Oakcliff Rd., Suite C-1
Atlanta, GA 30340

Roche Diagnostic Systems
340 Kingsland St.
Nutley, NJ 07110

Winfield Laboratories, Inc.
670 International Parkway
Suite 150, P.O. Box 2616
Richardson, TX 75080

BLOOD CULTURE SYSTEMS

BBL Microbiology Systems
P.O. Box 243
Cockeysville, MD 21030

Difco Laboratories, Inc.
P.O. Box 1058
Detroit, MI 48232

DuPont Co.
Barley Mill Plaza
Wilmington, DE 19898

Johnston Laboratories
P.O. Box 20086
Towson, MD 21204

Roche Diagnostic Systems
340 Kingsland St.
Nutley, NJ 07110

CHEMICALS

Aldrich Chemical Co.
P.O. Box 355
Milwaukee, WI 53201

Allied Chemical and Dye Co.
1411 Broadway
New York, NY 10018

American Can Co. (Parafilm Products)
American Lane 2A3
Greenwich, CT 06830

Baker Chemical Co.
(see J.T. Baker)

Behring Diagnostics Division,
American Hoechst Corp.
10933 N. Torrey Pines Rd.
La Jolla, CA 92037

Bio Spec, Inc.
6499 Sierra Ln.
Dublin, CA 94566

Boehringer Mannheim
9115 Hague Rd.
Indianapolis, IN 46250

Colab Laboratories, Inc.
3 Science Rd.
Glenwood, IL 60425

E. Merck Darmstadt
480 Democrat Rd.
Gibbstown, NJ 08027

Eastman Chemical Co.
343 State St.
Rochester, NY 14650

Fisher Scientific Co.
711 Forbes Ave.
Pittsburgh, PA 15219

Hazleton Research Products, Inc.
Box 7200
Denver, PA 17517

ICN Pharmaceuticals, Inc.
222 N. Vincent Ave.
Covina, CA 91722

J.T. Baker Chemical Co.
600 N. Broad St.
Phillipsburg, NJ 08825

Mallinckrodt, Inc.
675 McDonnell Blvd.
St. Louis, MO 63134

Marion Scientific Corp.
9233 Ward Parkway, Suite 350
Kansas City, MO 64114

Medical Chemical Corp.
P.O. Box 445
Santa Monica, CA 90404

Merck Chemical Co.
P.O. Box 2000
Rahway, NJ 07065

Meridian Diagnostics
P.O. Box 44216
3471 River Hills Dr.
Cincinnati, OH 45244

Polysciences, Inc.
400 Valley Rd.
Warrington, PA 18976

Sargent-Welch Scientific Co.
7300 N. Linder Ave., P.O. Box 1026
Skokie, IL 60077

Sigma Chemical Co.
3050 Spruce St.
St. Louis, MO 63103

Trend Scientific, Inc.
13895 Industrial Park Blvd., Suite 175
Minneapolis, MN 55441

Winthrop Laboratories
90 Park Ave.
New York, NY 10018

DISINFECTANTS

Alcide Corporation
125 Main St.
Westport, CT 06880

National Laboratories
225 Summit Ave.
Montvale, NJ 07645

Sporicidin Co.
4000 Massachusetts Ave. N.W.
Washington, D.C. 20016

Stanbio Laboratory, Inc.
2930 E. Houston St.
San Antonio, TX 78202

FILTERS
See Membrane Filters.

INOCULATING LOOPS

Elkay Products, Inc.
800 Boston Turnpike
Box 5247, Turnpike Station
Shrewsbury, MA 01545

Microdiagnostics
601 Stones Levee
Cleveland, OH 44113

INSTRUMENTS (OTHER)

Bellco Glass, Inc.
340 Edrudo Rd.
Vineland, NJ 08360

Biotek Instruments
Highland Industrial Park
Winooski, VT 05404

Cetus Corp.
1400 53rd St.
Emeryville, CA 94608

Dynatech Laboratories, Inc.
900 Slaters Lane
Alexandria, VA 22314

New Brunswick Scientific Co., Inc.
44 Talmadge Rd., P.O. Box 986
Edison, NJ 08817

Spiral System Instruments, Inc.
4853 Cordell Ave., Suite A10
Bethesda, MD 20814

Tekmar Co.
P.O. Box 37202
Cincinnati, OH 45222

Ultra-Violet Products, Inc.
5100 Walnut Grove
San Gabriel, CA 91778

LIMULUS AMEBOCYTE LYSATE ASSAYS

Mallinckrodt, Inc.
675 McDonnell Blvd.
St. Louis, MO 63134

Polysciences, Inc.
400 Valley Rd.
Warrington, PA 18976

Sigma Chemical Co.
3050 Spruce St.
St. Louis, MO 63103

Whittaker M.A. Bioproducts, Inc.
Biggs Ford Rd., Building 100
Walkersville, MD 21793

MEDIA (PREPARED AND DRY)
Bacteriologic Media

Anaerobe Systems, Inc.
3074A Scott Rd.
Santa Clara, CA 95054

BBL Microbiology Systems
P.O. Box 243
Cockeysville, MD 21030

Carr-Scarborough Microbiologicals, Inc.
P.O. Box 1328
Stone Mountain, GA 30086

Difco Laboratories, Inc.
P.O. Box 1058
Detroit, MI 48232

Edge Diagnostics
P.O. Box 1198
Memphis, TN 38111

Flow Laboratories, Inc.
7655 Old Springhouse Rd.
McLean, VA 22102

Gibco Laboratories
(Life Technologies, Inc.)
421 Merrimack St.
Lawrence, MA 01843

Hana Biologicals, Inc.
626 Bancroft Way
Berkeley, CA 94710

Micro-Bio-Logics
217 Osseo Ave. North
St. Cloud, MN 56301

Oxoid U.S.A., Inc.
9107 Red Branch Rd.
Columbia, MD 21045

Remel
12076 Santa Fe Dr.
Lenexa, KS 66215

Scott Laboratories, Inc.
771 Main St.
Fiskeville, RI 02823

Viral Culture Media

Bartels Immunodiagnostics
12729 North East 20th St.
Bellevue, WA 98005

Difco Laboratories
P.O. Box 1058
Detroit, MI 48232

Earl-Clay Laboratories, Inc.
7075 Redwood Blvd.
Novato, CA 94947

Flow Laboratories, Inc.
7655 Old Springhouse Rd.
McLean, VA 22102

Genus Diagnostics
225 Wildwood
Woburn, MA 01801

Northeast Biomedical, Inc.
R.R. no. 1, Inland Farm Dr.
South Windham, ME 04082

Ortho Diagnostic Systems
Route 202
Raritan, NJ 08869

Viromed Laboratories, Inc.
5100 Gamble Dr., Suite 55
Minneapolis, MN 55416

Whittaker M.A. Bioproducts, Inc.
Biggs Ford Rd., Building 100
Walkersville, MD 21793

MEMBRANE FILTERS

Amicon Corporation
17 Cherry Hill Dr.
Danvers, MA 01923

Gelman Sciences, Inc.
600 South Wagner Rd.
Ann Arbor, MI 48106

Millipore Corporation
Ashby Road
Bedford, MA 01730

Nuclepore Corporation
7035 Commerce Circle
Pleasanton, CA 94566-3294

Sartorius Filters Inc.
30940 San Clemente, Bldg. D
Hayward, CA 94544

MICROORGANISMS (FOR QUALITY CONTROL)

American Type Culture Collection
12301 Parklawn Dr.
Rockville, MD 20852

Difco Laboratories, Inc.
P.O. Box 1058
Detroit, MI 48232

Micro-Bio-Logics
217 Osseo Ave. North
St. Cloud, MN 56301

Remel
12076 Santa Fe Dr.
Lenexa, KS 66215

Roche Diagnostic Systems
340 Kingsland St.
Nutley, NJ 07110

Scott Laboratories, Inc.
771 Main St.
Fiskeville, RI 02823

PARASITE CONCENTRATING DEVICES

Evergreen Scientific
2300 East 49th St.
Los Angeles, CA 90058

Trend Scientific Inc.
P.O. Box 41203
Minneapolis, MN 55441

PLASTICS

American Scientific Products
1430 Waukegan Rd.
McGaw Park, IL 60085

Becton Dickinson & Co.
299 Webro Rd.
Parsippany, NJ 07054

Corning Glass Works: Science Products
P.O. Box 1150
Elmira, NY 14902-9944

Costar
205 Broadway
Cambridge, MA 02139

Dynalab Corporation
P.O. Box 112
Rochester, NY 14692

Falcon Plastics (Becton-Dickinson)
1950 Williams Dr.
Oxnard, CA 93030

Miles Scientific
2000 N. Aurora Rd.
Naperville, IL 60566

Nunc InterMed
Postbox 280, Kamstrup-DK
4000 Roskilde, Denmark
Distributed by:
Vangard International, Inc.
1111-A Green Grove Rd.
Neptune, NJ 07753

SPECIMEN-TRANSPORT SYSTEMS
Culture Collection Devices and Environmentally Controlled Transport Systems

BBL Microbiology Systems
P.O. Box 243
Cockeysville, MD 21030

Becton-Dickinson Vacutainer Systems
301 Route 17 North
Rutherford, NJ 07070

Evergreen Scientific
2300 East 49th St.
Los Angeles, CA 90058

Marion Scientific
9233 Ward Parkway, Suite 350
Kansas City, MO 64114

Masterseal Corporation
711 W. 17th St.—G6
Costa Mesa, CA 92627

Micro-Bio-Logics
217 Osseo Ave. North
St. Cloud, MN 56301

Microdiagnostics
601 Stones Levee
Cleveland, OH 44113

Precision Dynamics Corp.
13880 Del Sur St.
San Fernando, CA 91340-3490

Remel
12076 Santa Fe Dr.
Lenexa, KS 66215

Sage Products, Inc.
680 Industrial Dr.
Carey, IL 60013

Scott Laboratories, Inc.
771 Main St.
Fiskeville, RI 02823

Spectrum Diagnostics, Inc.
3 Science Rd.
Glenwood, IL 60425

Trend Scientific, Inc.
P.O. Box 41203
1848 Berkshire Lane North
Minneapolis, MN 55441

Culture and Transport System for Gonococci

Flow Laboratories, Inc.
7655 Old Springhouse Rd.
McLean, VA 22102

Micro-Bio-Logics
217 Osseo Ave. North
St. Cloud, MN 56301

Viral Collection, Transport, and Isolation

Bartels Immunodiagnostics
12729 North East 20th St.
Bellevue, WA 98005

Difco Laboratories, Inc.
P.O. Box 1058
Detroit, MI 48232

Electro-Nucleonics, Inc.
368 Passaic Ave.
Fairfield, NJ 07006

Ortho Diagnostic Systems, Inc.
Route 202
Raritan, NJ 08869

Scott Laboratories, Inc.
771 Main Street
Fiskeville, RI 02823

Glossary

DRGs Diagnosis related groups; system introduced to control rising medical costs under which hospitals are reimbursed for costs of caring for patients based on the primary diagnoses of the patients and what is considered to be a fair dollar value for treatment of usual patients with those diagnoses.

Dx Diagnosis.

ELISA Enzyme-linked immunosorbent assay; similar to RIA but uses enzymes to produce a reaction with a visually discernible endpoint rather than a radioactive element.

EMB Eosin–methylene blue (agar plate).

FTA Fluorescent treponemal antibody.

FTA-ABS Fluorescent treponemal antibody absorption test.

FUO Fever of unknown origin.

GC Gonococcus.

GLC Gas-liquid chromatography.

GN Gram-negative (broth).

HAA Hepatitis-associated antigen.

HAI Hemagglutination inhibition.

HEPA High-efficiency particulate air filter; used in biological safety cabinets to trap pathogenic microorganisms.

HPLC High-pressure (or performance) liquid chromatography.

ID Infectious disease; identification.

IE Infectious endocarditis.

IFA Indirect fluorescent antibody; immunofluorescent antibody.

Ig, IgG, etc. Immunoglobulin, immunoglobulin G, etc.

K Alkaline.

KIA Kligler's iron agar (tube).

KOH Potassium hydroxide.

LPA Latex particle agglutination.

LPS Lipopolysaccharide; see endotoxin in Glossary Terms.

MAC MacConkey (agar plate).

MBC Minimum bactericidal concentration.

MIC Minimum inhibitory concentration.

NFB Glucose nonfermenting gram-negative bacteria.

NGU Nongonococcal urethritis.

O & P Ova and parasites.

O-F Oxidation-fermentation medium.

ONPG O-nitrophenol-β-galactopyranoside (β-galactosidase test).

PID Pelvic inflammatory disease.

PPD Purified protein derivative (skin test antigen for tuberculosis).

PPNG Penicillinase-producing (i.e., penicillin-resistant) *Neisseria gonorrhoeae*.

PRAS Prereduced, anaerobically sterilized.

QC Quality control.

QNS Quantity nonsufficient.

RIA Radiometric immunoassay (radioimmunoassay).

RNA Ribonucleic acid.

SBA Suprapubic bladder aspiration.

SBE Subacute bacterial endocarditis.

SPIA Solid-phase immunosorbent assay.

Stat Statim (Latin); immediately.

STD Sexually transmitted disease.

T cells Lymphocytes involved in cellular immunity.

TB Tuberculosis.

T-M Thayer-Martin (agar plate).

TORCH Toxoplasmosis, rubella, cytomegalovirus infection, and herpes infection; used for illnesses or tests.

TSI Triple sugar iron (agar tube).

TSS Toxic shock syndrome.

TTA Transtracheal aspiration.

URI Upper respiratory tract infection.

UTI Urinary tract infection.

VD Venereal disease.

V-P Voges-Proskauer.

TERMS

abscess Localized collection of pus.

accessioning Receipt and recording of specimens delivered to laboratory.

accolé Early ring form of *Plasmodium falciparum* found at margin of red cell.

acid-fast Characteristic of certain bacteria, such as mycobacteria, that involves resistance to decolorization by acids when stained by an aniline dye, such as carbol fuchsin.

acute serum Serum collected for antibody determination early in course of an illness when there would have been little or no antibody produced.

acute urethral syndrome Lower urinary tract infection that may be difficult to differentiate from cystitis; seen most commonly in younger, sexually active females and caused by *E. coli* (counts as low as 100/ml may be significant in this situation), *Chlamydia*, and other organisms.

aerobe, obligate Microorganism that lives and grows freely in air and cannot grow anaerobically.

aerogenic Producing gas (in contrast to anaerogenic—non-gas-producing).

aerosol Atomized particles suspended in air; in context of this book, microorganisms suspended in air.

aerotolerant Ability of an anaerobic microorganism to grow in air, usually poorly, especially after anaerobic isolation.

affinity Inherent attraction and relationship.

agglutination Aggregation or clumping of particles, such as bacteria when exposed to specific antibody.

alopecia Baldness.

aminoglycosides Group of related antibiotics including streptomycin, kanamycin, neomycin, tobramycin, gentamicin, and amikacin.

amniotic Pertaining to the innermost fetal membrane forming a fluid-filled sac.

anaerobe, obligate Microorganism that grows only in complete or nearly complete absence of air or molecular oxygen.

anaerogenic Non-gas-producing.

analytic reagent (AR) Grade of chemical.

anamnestic response More rapid production of antibodies in response to exposure to an antigen previously encountered.

anergy Absence of reaction to antigens or allergens.

antagonism Diminution of activity of one drug by a second one.

antibiogram Distinctive pattern of susceptibility of an organism to a battery of antimicrobial agents.

antibiotic Substance, produced by a microorganism, that inhibits or kills other microorganisms. A broad-spectrum antibiotic is therapeutically effective against a wide range of bacteria.

antibody Substance (immunoglobulin), formed in blood or tissues, that interacts only with antigen that induced its synthesis (e.g., agglutinin).

antigen Molecular structure that is capable of stimulating production of antibody.

antigenic determinant Antigen.

antimicrobial Chemical substance, either produced by a microorganism or by synthetic means, that is capable of killing or suppressing growth of microorganisms.

antiseptic Compound that stops or inhibits growth of bacteria without necessarily killing them.

arboviruses Arthropod-borne viruses.

arthritis, septic Infection of synovial tissue and joint fluid of one or more joints; characterized by joint pain, stiffness, swelling, and fever.

arthroconidium Spore formed by septation of a hypha and subsequent separation at septa.

ascitic fluid Serous fluid in peritoneal cavity.

assimilation Utilization of nutrients. Assimilation tests are used to determine whether yeasts are able to grow with only a single carbohydrate or nitrate; these tests are useful for classification of yeasts.

autotroph Organism that can utilize inorganic carbon sources (CO_2).

auxotroph Differing from the wild strain (prototroph) by an additional nutritional requirement.

avidity Firmness of union of two substances; used commonly to describe union of antibody to antigen.

bacteremia Presence of viable organisms in blood.

bacterial vaginosis Annoying, noninflammatory condition in vagina characterized by foul-smelling vaginal discharge.

bactericidal Term used to describe a drug that kills microorganisms.

bacteriocins Antibiotic-like substances, produced by bacteria, that exert a lethal effect on other bacteria.

bacteriophage Virus that infects a bacterial cell, sometimes bringing about its lysis.

bacteriostatic Term used to describe a drug that inhibits growth of an organism without killing it.

bacteriuria Presence of bacteria in urine.

benign tertian malaria Malaria caused by *Plasmodium vivax*.

beta-lactamases Enzymes that destroy penicillins and/or cephalosporins and are produced by a variety of bacteria.

bifurcated Divided into two branches.

biological safety cabinet Enclosure in which one can work with relatively dangerous organisms without risk of acquiring or spreading infection due to them. These cabinets, also called biosafety hoods, vary in design according to nature of agents to be worked with. The simpler ones maintain a negative pressure within the work area and a laminar air curtain, both of which operate to prevent escape of organisms from interior of hood. Air that is exhausted may be passed through a high-efficiency bacterial filter that will trap all microorganisms that are anticipated or may be passed through a furnace that will incinerate any organisms. (see Chapter 2 for more information.)

bioluminescence Light generation by living organisms.

biopsy Removal of tissue from a living body for diagnostic purposes (e.g., lymph node biopsy).

biotype Biological or biochemical type of an organism. Organisms of the same biotype will display identical biological or biochemical characteristics. Certain key markers are used to define and recognize biotypes in tracing the spread of organisms in the environment and in epidemics or outbreaks.

blackwater fever Condition in which the diagnostic symptom is passage of reddish or red-brown urine, which indicates massive intravascular hemolysis (*Plasmodium falciparum*).

blastoconidium A spore formed by budding, as in yeasts.

blepharitis Inflammation of eyelids.

blind loop A condition in which continuity of the bowel has been interrupted in such a way that a segment of bowel receives material from higher in the bowel in the usual way but cannot empty normally because it ends in a blind sac. This leads to proliferation of microorganisms, especially anaerobes, in the blind loop of bowel and may produce profound pathophysiologic effects. There are other situations in which there may be bacterial overgrowth in a segment of the bowel by other mechanisms.

B-lymphocytes (or B cells) Bursa-derived lymphocytes important in humoral immunity.

break point Level of an antibacterial drug achievable in serum; organisms inhibited by this level of drug are considered susceptible. In certain situations, clinicians strive to achieve serum or body fluid levels several times the MIC of an organism.

bronchial lavage Similar to bronchial washings but this term implies instillation of a larger volume of fluid before aspiration.

bronchial washings Fluid that may be aspirated from bronchial tree during bronchoscopy.

bronchitis Inflammation of mucous membranes of bronchi; often caused by infectious agents, viruses in particular.

bronchoscopy Examination of bronchi through a bronchoscope, a tubular illuminated instrument introduced through the trachea (windpipe).

bubo Inflammatory enlargement of lymph node, usually in the groin or axilla.

buffy coat Layer of white blood cells and platelets above red blood cell mass when blood is sedimented.

bullae Large blebs or blisters, filled with fluid, in or just beneath the epidermal layer of skin.

bursitis Inflammation of a bursa, which is a small sac lined with synovial membrane and filled with fluid interposed between parts that move on each other.

butt Lower portion of medium in a tube that has the medium dispensed in such a way that the lower portion fills the tube entirely while the upper portion is distributed in the form of a slanted surface leaving an air space between the slant and the opposite wall of the tube.

calibrated loop Bacteriological loop that is carefully calibrated to deliver a specified volume of fluid providing that directions are followed carefully and the loop has not been damaged; used as a simple means of quantitating the number of organisms present, especially for urine culture.

candle jar A jar with a lid providing a gas-tight seal in which a small white candle is placed and lit after the culture plates have been placed inside. Candle will burn only until the oxygen concentration has been lowered to the point where it will no longer support the flame. Atmosphere of such a jar has a lower oxygen content than room air and a carbon dioxide content of about 3%.

cannula An artificial tube for insertion into a tube or cavity of the body.

capneic incubation Incubation under increased CO_2 tension, as in a candle extinction jar (approximate 3% CO_2).

capnophilic Term used to describe microorganisms that prefer an incubation atmosphere with increased carbon dioxide concentration.

capsule Gelatinous material surrounding bacterial cell wall, usually of polysaccharide nature.

carrier One who harbors a pathogenic organism but is not affected by it.

caseation necrosis Tissue death with loss of cell outlines and a cheeselike, amorphous appearance.

catalase Bacterial enzyme that breaks down peroxides with liberation of free oxygen.

catheter Flexible tubular (rubber or plastic) instrument used for withdrawing fluids from (or introducing fluids into) a body cavity or vessel (e.g., urinary bladder catheter).

cation A positive ion.

cell line, continuous Line of tissue cells that is maintained by serial culture of an established cell line.

cell line, primary Line of tissue cells established by cutting up fresh tissue, often kidney, into tiny pieces, trypsinizing, and putting in a flask with appropriate medium.

cellulitis Inflammation of subcutaneous tissue.

cerebriform With brainlike folds.

cervical Pertaining either to the neck or to the cervix of the uterus.

Charcot-Leyden crystals Slender crystals shaped like a double pyramid with pointed ends, formed from the breakdown products of eosinophils and found in feces, sputum, and tissues; indicative of an immune response that may have parasitic or nonparasitic causes.

chemotherapeutic Chemical agent used in the treatment of infections (e.g., sulfonamides).

chlamydospore Thick-walled spore formed from a vegetative cell.

chromatography Method of chemical analysis by which a mixture of substances is separated by fractional extraction or adsorption or ion exchange on a porous solid.

chromogen Bacterial species whose colonial growth is pigmented (e.g., *Flavobacterium* species, yellow).

chromogenic Giving rise to color, as chromogenic substrates for colored products of biochemical reactions or chromogenic bacteria that produce pigmented colonies.

clavate Club shaped.

clone Group of microorganisms of identical genetic makeup derived from a single common ancestor.

coagglutination Agglutination of protein A–containing cells of *Staphylococcus aureus* coated with antibody molecules when exposed to corresponding antigen.

colitis Inflammation of mucosa of colon.

colony Macroscopically visible growth of a microorganism on a solid culture medium.

colorimetry Chemical analysis by color determination.

commensal Microorganism living on or in a host but causing the host no harm.

complement fixation test Antigen-antibody test based on fixation of complement in the presence of both elements and use of an indicator system to determine whether or not complement has been fixed.

congenital Existing before or at birth.

conjunctivitis Inflammation of the conjunctivae or membranes of the eye and eyelid.

convalescent serum Serum collected later in the course of an illness than the acute serum, usually at least 2 weeks after initial collection.

Creutzfeld-Jakob disease Debilitating prion-caused disease characterized by dementia, ataxia, delirium, stupor, coma, and death; has been transmitted by organ transplant.

croup Inflammation of upper airways (larynx, trachea) with respiratory obstruction, often due to virus infections in children.

culdocentesis Aspiration of fluid from the cul-de-sac by puncture of the vaginal vault.

cystitis Inflammation of urinary bladder, most often caused by bacterial infection.

cytotoxin Toxin that produces cytopathic effects in vivo or in a tissue culture system.

darkfield microscopy Technique used to visualize very small microorganisms or their characteristics by a system that permits light to be reflected or refracted from surface of objects being viewed.

debridement Surgical or other removal of nonviable tissue.

decontamination Process of rendering an object or area safe for unprotected people by removing or making harmless biological or chemical agents.

decubitus ulcer A craterlike defect in skin and subcutaneous tissue caused by prolonged pressure on the area. This occurs primarily over bony prominences of the lower back and hips in individuals who are unable to care for themselves well and unable to roll or move periodically; also known as pressure sores or bedsores.

definitive host Host in which the sexual reproduction of a parasite occurs.

dermatophyte A fungus parasitic on skin, hair, or nails.

desquamation Shedding or scaling of skin or mucous membrane.

dichotomous Branching in two directions.

diluent Fluid used to dilute a substance.

dimorphic fungi Fungi with both a mold phase and a yeast phase.

direct wet mount A preparation from clinical material suspended in sterile saline or other liquid medium on a glass slide and covered with a coverslip; used for microscopic examination to detect microorganisms in clinical material and, in particular, to detect motility directly.

disinfectant Agent that destroys or inhibits microorganisms that cause disease.

DNase Deoxyribonuclease, an enzyme that depolymerizes DNA, an essential component of all living matter, which contains the genetic code.

droplet nucleus A tiny aerosolized particle that, because of its lack of mass, may stay suspended in air for extended periods of time.

dysentery Inflammation of the intestinal tract, particularly the colon, with frequent bloody stools (e.g., bacillary dysentery).

dysgonic Growing poorly (bacterial cultures).

ectoparasite Organism that lives on or within skin.

ectothrix Outside of hair shafts.

edema Excessive accumulation of fluid in tissue spaces.

effusion Fluid escaping into a body space or tissue (e.g., pleural effusion).

Eh Oxidation-reduction potential.

elementary body The infectious stage of *Chlamydia*; a cellular inclusion body of a viral disease.

elephantiasis Condition caused by inflammation and obstruction of the lymphatic system, resulting in hypertrophy and thickening of the surrounding tissues, usually involving the extremities and external genitalia (filariasis).

elution Process of extraction by means of a solvent.

empyema Accumulation of pus in a body cavity, particularly empyema of the thorax or chest.

encephalitis Inflammation of the brain.

endocarditis A serious infection of the endothelium of the heart, usually involving leaflets of the heart valves where destruction of valves or distortion of them by formation of vegetations may lead to serious physiologic disturbances and death; also, an inflammation of the endocardial surface (much less common).

endocervix Mucous membrane of the cervical canal.

endogenous Developing from within the body.

endoparasite Parasite that lives within the body.

endophthalmitis Inflammation of internal tissues of eye; may rapidly destroy the eye.

endothelium Squamous epithelium lining blood vessels.

endothrix Within the hair shaft.

endotoxin Substance containing lipopolysaccharide complexes found in the cell wall of bacteria, principally gram-negative bacteria; felt to play an important role in many of the complications of sepsis such as shock, DIC, and thrombocytopenia.

enteric fever Typhoid fever; paratyphoid fever.

enteroinvasive Capable of invading the mucosal surface and sometimes the deeper tissues of the bowel.

enterotoxigenic Producing an enterotoxin (e.g., enterotoxigenic *E. coli*).

enterotoxin Toxin affecting the cells of the intestinal mucosa.

epidemiology The study of the occurrence and distribution of disease and factors that control presence or absence of disease.

epididymitis Inflammation of the epididymis characterized by fever and pain on one side of the scrotum; seen as a complication of prostatitis and cystitis.

epiglottitis Inflammation of the epiglottis, a structure that prevents aspirating swallowed food and fluids into the tracheobronchial tree; a serious infection because the swollen epiglottis may block the airway.

epithelium Tissue composed of contiguous cells that forms the epidermis and lines hollow organs and all passages of the respiratory, digestive, and genitourinary systems.

erysipelas An acute cellulitis caused by group A streptococci.

erythema Redness of the skin from various causes.

erythema chronicum migrans Characteristic radial skin lesion of Lyme disease.

erythrasma A minor, superficial skin infection.

erythrocytic cycle Developmental cycle of malarial parasites within red blood cells.

eschar A dry scar, particularly one related to a burn.

etiology Cause or causative agent.

eugonic Growing luxuriantly (bacterial cultures).

eukaryotic Organisms with a true nucleus, in contrast to bacteria and viruses.

exanthem Skin eruption as a symptom of an acute disease, usually viral.

exoerythrocytic cycle Portion of the malarial life cycle occurring in the vertebrate host in which sporozoites, introduced by infected mosquitoes, penetrate the parenchymal liver cells and undergo schizogony, producing merozoites, which then initiate the erythrocytic cycle.

exogenous From outside the body.

exotoxin A toxin produced by a microorganism that is released into the surrounding environment.

exudate Fluid that has passed out of blood vessels into adjacent tissues or spaces; high protein content.

facultative anaerobe Microorganism that grows under either anaerobic or aerobic conditions.

fascia Membranous covering of muscle.

favus Dermatophyte infection of the scalp produced by *Trichophyton schoenleinii.*

fermentation Anaerobic decomposition of carbohydrate.

filamentous Threadlike.

fimbriae Proteinaceous fingerlike surface structures of bacteria that provide for adherence to host surfaces.

fistula Abnormal communication between two surfaces or between a viscus or other hollow structure and the exterior.

Fitz-Hugh–Curtis syndrome Inflammation of the capsule of the liver that may be seen in course of gonococcal or chlamydial infection in the female.

floccose Cottony, in tufts.

flocculation test Antigen-antibody test in which a precipitin end product forms macroscopically or microscopically visible clumps.

fluorescent Emission of light by a substance (or a microscopic preparation) while acted on by radiant energy, such as ultraviolet rays, as in the immunofluorescent procedure.

fluorescent immunoassay Similar to RIA but employs fluorescent molecules as labels.

fluorochrome A dye that becomes fluorescent or self-luminous after exposure to ultraviolet light.

fomite Any inanimate object that may be contaminated with disease-causing microorganisms and thus serve to transmit disease.

fungemia Presence of viable fungi in blood

fusiform Spindle shaped, as in the anaerobe *Fusobacterium nucleatum.*

gangrene Death of a part or tissue resulting from disease, injury, or failure of blood supply.

gastric aspirate Fluid that may be aspirated from the stomach via a tube placed in the stomach by way of the nose or mouth.

gastroenteritis Inflammation of the mucosa of the stomach and intestines.

germicide An agent that destroys germs.

germ tube Tubelike process, produced by a germinating spore, that develops into mycelium.

glabrous Smooth.

glove box A device with flexible, semirigid, or rigid plastic walls used for cultivation of anaerobic bacteria. Bacteriologist must work by way of glove ports, and materials are brought into and out of the anaerobic work area by way of an interchange (airlock) that can be evacuated and refilled with an anaerobic atmosphere repeatedly until it itself is anaerobic. The interchange has one door leading into the glove box per se and another door to the outside. Some glove boxes have incubators within them. Also called anaerobic chamber or anaerobic cabinet.

granulocytopenia Reduced number of granulocytic white blood cells in the blood.

granuloma Aggregation and proliferation of macrophages to form small (usually microscopic) nodules.

halophilic Preferring high halide (salt) content.

headspace gas Gas generated during growth of an organism in a closed tube that accumulates between the upper surface of the broth in the tube and the top of the tube.

hemagglutination Agglutination of red blood cells caused by certain antibodies, virus particles, or high molecular weight polysaccharides.

hematogenous Disseminated by the bloodstream.

hemolysis, alpha Partial destruction of or enzymatic damage to red blood cells in a blood agar plate leading to greenish discoloration about the colony of the organism producing the alpha hemolysin.

hemolysis, beta Total lysis of red blood cells about a colony on a blood agar plate leading to a completely clear zone surrounding the colony.

hemolysis, gamma No hemolysis is seen with organisms classed as gamma hemolytic; nonhemolytic would be a better designation.

herpes Inflammation of the skin characterized by clusters of small vesicles (e.g., caused by herpes simplex).

heterotroph Organism that requires an organic carbon source.

hidradenitis suppurativa Inflammation of certain sweat glands leading to formation of abscesses and draining sinuses.

hilum of lung Central area where major vessels and bronchi begin to branch.

humidophilic Organisms preferring or requiring an increased moisture content; can be achieved by placing cultures in sealed jars or bags. For some organisms that do better in a candle jar than in the ambient atmosphere, it is the increased moisture content rather than the change in the gas content that is important.

humoral immunity Immunity effected by antibody.

hyaline Colorless, transparent.

hybridoma The product of fusion of an antibody-producing cell and an immortal malignant antibody-producing cell.

hydrolysis Breakdown of a substrate by an enzyme that adds the components of water to key bonds within the substrate molecule.

hyperalimentation Process by which nutrition (literally, extra nutrition) is provided; typically done by the intravenous route in subjects who are not able to absorb foods well from the gut because of disease of the bowel, in subjects in whom it is desirable to put the bowel "at rest" to promote healing, and in malnourished individuals to improve the nutritional status (e.g., before surgery); usually done over an extended period of time and requires use of a special access IV catheter such as a Hickman catheter.

hyperemia Increased blood in a part, resulting in distention of blood vessels.

hypertonic Hyperosmotic.

hypertrophy Increased size of an organ resulting from enlargement of individual cells.

hypha Tubular cell making up the vegetative portion or mycelium of fungi.

hypoxia Decreased oxygen content of tissues.

immunofluorescence Microscopic method of determining the presence or location of an antigen (or antibody) by demonstrating fluorescence when the preparation is exposed to a fluorescein-tagged antibody (or antigen) using ultraviolet radiation.

immunoglobulin Synonymous with antibody; five distinct classes have been isolated: IgG, IgM, IgA, IgE, and IgD.

immunoperoxidase stain Combination of an enzyme that catalyzes production of a colored product with an antibody to facilitate detection of certain antigens, particularly viral antigens.

immunosuppression Depression of the immune response caused by disease, irradiation, or administration of antimetabolites, antilymphocyte serum, or corticosteroids.

impedance Apparent resistance of a circuit to the flow of an alternating electric current.

impetigo Acute inflammatory skin disease, caused by streptococci or staphylococci, characterized by vesicles and bullae that rupture and form yellow crusts.

inclusion bodies Microscopic bodies, usually within body cells; thought to be virus particles in morphogenesis.

indigenous flora Normal or resident flora.

induced malaria Malaria infection acquired by parenteral inoculation (e.g., blood transfusion or sharing of needles by drug addicts).

induration Abnormal hardness of a tissue or part resulting from hyperemia or inflammation, as in a reactive tuberculin skin test.

infection Invasion by and multiplication of microorganisms in body tissue resulting in disease.

inhibitory quotient Ratio of the average peak achievable level of antibiotic in a body fluid from which an organism was isolated to the MIC of that organism.

inspissation Process of making a liquid or semisolid medium thick by evaporation or absorption of fluid.

intermediate host Required host in the life cycle in which essential larval development must occur before a parasite is infective to its definitive host or to additional intermediate hosts.

intertrigo Erythematous skin eruption of adjacent skin parts.

intramuscular (intraperitoneal, intravenous) Within the muscle (peritoneum, vein), as in intramuscular injection.

in vitro Literally, within glass (i.e., in a test tube, culture plate, or other nonliving material).

in vivo Within the living body.

involution forms Abnormally shaped bacterial cells occurring in an aging culture population.

ion exchange chromatography Chromatography based on the reversible exchange of ions in a solution with ions present in an ion exchanger.

isotonic Of the same osmolality of body tissues, red blood cells, bacteria, etc.

Kawasaki disease Mucocutaneous lymph node syndrome; disease of children that may involve more serious phenomena such as cardiac disease.

keratitis Inflammation of the cornea.

Köhler illumination Modification of brightfield microscopy in which a substage condenser is used to avoid glare from illuminating source.

lag phase Period of slow microbial growth that occurs following inoculation of the culture medium.

laked blood Hemolyzed blood; hemolysis may be effected in various ways, but alternate freezing and thawing is a simple method.

laminar flow Nonturbulent flow of air in layers (flowing in a vertical direction in the case of a biosafety hood).

latent Not manifest: potential.

latex agglutination Agglutination of latex particles coated with antibody molecules when exposed to the corresponding antigen.

Leishman-Donovan body Small, round intracellular form (called amastigote or leishmanial stage) of *Leishmania* species and *Trypanosoma cruzi.*

leukocytosis Elevated white blood cell count.

leukopenia Low white blood cell count.

L form Cell wall–deficient form of a bacterium.

Limulus **amebocyte lysate** Product of white blood cells of the horseshoe crab used in an assay for endotoxin.

liposome Small closed vesicle consisting of a single lipid bilayer.

logarithmic phase Period of maximal growth rate of a microorganism in a culture medium.

lysis Disintegration or dissolution of bacteria or cells.

lysogeny Process by which a viral genome is integrated into that of its host bacterium.

malignant tertian malaria Malaria caused by *Plasmodium falciparum.*

meconium Pasty greenish mass in intestine of fetus; made up of mucus, desquamated cells, bile, and such.

media, differential Media that permit ready recognition of a particular organism or group of organisms by virtue of facilitating recognition of a natural product of the organism being sought or by incorporating an appropriate substrate and indicator system so that organisms possessing certain enzymes will be readily recognized.

media, enrichment Media, usually liquid, that favor the growth of one or more organisms while suppressing most of the competing flora in a specimen with a mixture of organisms.

media, selective Culture media that contain inhibitory substances or unique growth factors such that one particular organism or group of organisms is conferred a real advantage over other organisms that may be found in a mixture. Efficient selective media will select out only the organism or organisms being sought, with little or no growth of other types of organisms.

media, supportive Culture media that provide adequate nutrition for most nonfastidious microorganisms and that permit each organism to grow normally without conferring any special advantage to one organism over another.

mediastinum Space in the middle of the chest between the medial surfaces of the two pleurae.

meningitis Inflammation of the meninges, the membranes that cover the brain and spinal cord (e.g., bacterial meningitis).

merozoite Product of schizogonic cycle in malaria that will invade red blood cells.

mesenteric adenitis Inflammation of mesenteric lymph nodes.

mesentery A fold of the peritoneum that connects the intestine with the posterior abdominal wall.

metastatic Spread of an infectious (or other) process from a primary focus to a distant one via the bloodstream or lymphatic system.

microaerophile, obligate Microorganism that grows only under reduced oxygen tension and cannot grow aerobically or anaerobically.

microcalorimetry Study of microcalories, a measure of heat production.

microconidia Small, single-celled fungal spores.

microfilaria Embryos produced by filarial worms and found in the blood or tissues of individuals with filariasis.

microscopy, brightfield Conventional microscopy in which the object to be viewed is illuminated from below.

miliary Of the size of a millet seed (0.5 to 1.0 mm); characterized by the formation of numerous lesions of the above size distributed rather uniformly throughout one or more organs.

mixed culture (pure culture) More than one organism growing in or on the same culture medium, as opposed to a single organism in pure culture.

monoclonal antibody Antibody that is derived from a single cell producing one antibody molecule type that reacts with a single epitope.

monolayer A confluent layer of tissue culture cells one cell thick.

mucopurulent Term used to describe material containing both mucus and pus (e.g., mucopurulent sputum).

mucosa A mucous membrane.

multiple myeloma Malignancy involving antibody-producing plasma cells.

mycelium Mass of hyphae making up a colony of a fungus.

mycetoma chronic infection, usually of feet, caused by various fungi or by *Nocardia* or *Streptomyces*, resulting in swelling and sinus tracts; pulmonary mycetoma is a mass of fungal hyphae ("fungus ball") growing in a cavity from previous tuberculosis or other pathologic condition.

mycoses Diseases caused by fungi (e.g., dermatomycosis, fungal infection of the superficial skin).

myocarditis Inflammation of the heart muscle.

myositis Inflammation of a muscle, sometimes caused by infection as in pyomyositis, an infection due to *S. aureus* that leads to small abscesses within the muscle substance.

nares External openings of nose (i.e., nostrils).

nasopharyngeal Pertaining to the part of the pharynx above the level of the soft palate.

necrosis Pathologic death of a cell or group of cells.

necrotizing fasciitis A very serious, painful infection involving the fascia (membranous covering) of one or more muscles; may spread widely in short periods of time since there is no anatomic barrier to spread in this type of infection.

neonatal First 4 weeks after birth.

nephelometry Determination of the degree of turbidity of a fluid by light scatter.

neuritis Inflammation of a nerve; most often not caused by an infectious agent.

neurotrophic Having a selective affinity for nerve tissue. Rabies is caused by a neurotrophic virus.

nonphotochromogens Slow-growing, nonpigmented mycobacteria.

nonsporulating Does not produce spores.

nosocomial Pertaining to or originating in a hospital, as nosocomial infection.

nucleic acid hybridization Process by which the single-stranded probe unites with complementary DNA in an unknown sample.

nucleic acid probe Piece of labeled single-stranded DNA used to detect complementary DNA in clinical material or a culture and thus to specifically identify the presence in these materials of an organism identical to that used to make the probe; also known as a DNA probe.

octal numbers Numbers employed in computer data bases to identify biochemical profiles of organisms and thus their identification.

oil immersion microscopy Use of immersion oil to fill the space between the slide being studied and the special objective of the microscope; this keeps the light rays from dispersing and provides good resolution at high magnification (total magnification of $1,000\times$).

operculated ova Ova possessing a cap or lid.

opsonize To facilitate destruction of pathogens by phagocytic ingestion or lysis by complement through the action of adherent antibodies.

osteomyelitis Inflammation of the bone and the marrow.

otitis Inflammation of the ear from a variety of causes, including bacterial infection; otitis media, inflammation of the middle ear.

oxidation A metabolic pathway of a microorganism that involves use of oxygen as a terminal electron acceptor. This type of reaction occurs in air.

oxidation-reduction potential Electromotive force exerted by a nonreacting electrode in a solution containing the oxidized and reduced forms of a chemical, relative to a standard hydrogen electrode; the more negative the value, the more anaerobic conditions are.

pandemic Epidemic over a wide geographic area, or even worldwide.

paracentesis fluid Fluid obtained by tapping the peritoneal cavity.

parasite Organism that lives on or within and at the expense of another organism.

parenteral Route of administration of a drug other than by mouth; includes intramuscular and intravenous administration.

paronychia Purulent inflammation about margin of a nail.

parotitis Inflammation of the parotid gland, the largest of the salivary glands; mumps is the most common cause of this.

paroxysm Rapid onset (or return) of symptoms; term usually applies to cyclic recurrence of malaria symptoms, which are chills, fever, and sweating.

pathogenic Producing disease.

pathologic Caused by or involving a morbid condition, as a pathologic state.

penicillinase (beta-lactamase I) Enzyme produced by some bacterial species that inactivates the antimicrobial activity of certain penicillins (e.g., penicillin G).

percutaneous Performed through the skin (e.g., percutaneous bladder aspiration).

pericarditis Inflammation of the covering of the heart (pericardium).

perineum The portion of the body bounded by the pubic bone anteriorly, the coccyx posteriorly, and the bony prominences (tuberosities) of the ileum on both sides.

peritoneal cavity Space between the visceral and parietal layers of the peritoneum; the serous membrane lining the abdominal cavity and surrounding the contained viscera.

peritonitis Inflammation of the peritoneal cavity, most often caused by bacterial infection.

petechiae Tiny hemorrhagic spots in the skin or mucous membranes.

phase-contrast microscopy Technique for direct observation of unstained material in which light beams pass through the object to be visualized and are partially deflected by the different densities of the object. These light beams are deflected again when they impinge on a special objective lens, increasing in brightness when aligned in phase.

photochromogens Mycobacteria that produce pigment after exposure to light but whose colonies remain buff colored in the dark.

pili Structures in bacteria similar to fimbriae that participate in bacterial conjugation and transfer of genetic material.

pilonidal cyst Hair-containing cyst in the skin or subcutaneous tissue, often with a sinus tract, commonly in the sacrococcygeal area.

plasma Fluid portion of blood; obtained by centrifuging anticoagulated blood.

plasmids Extrachromosomal DNA elements of bacteria carrying a variety of determinants that may permit survival in an adverse environment or successful competition with other microorganisms of the same or different species.

pleomorphic Having more than one form, usually widely different forms, as in pleomorphic bacteria.

pleura The serous membrane enveloping the lung and lining the internal surface of the thoracic cavity.

pleuropulmonary Pertaining to the lungs and pleura.

pneumonia Inflammation of the lungs, primarily caused by infectious agents.

pneumonia, aspiration Pneumonia caused by aspiration of oropharyngeal or gastric contents.

pneumothorax Introduction of air (usually inadvertently) into the pleural space leading to collapse of the lung on that side.

prion Proteinaceous infectious agent responsible for Creutzfeld-Jakob disease and perhaps other chronic, debilitating central nervous system diseases.

proctitis Inflammation of the rectum.

prodromal Early manifestations of a disease before specific symptoms become evident.

proglottid Segments of the tapeworm containing male and female reproductive systems; may be immature, mature, or gravid.

prognosis Forecast as to the possible outcome of a disease.

progressive bacterial synergistic gangrene Serious mixed infection of skin and soft tissue, often a postoperative complication, involving a mixture of microaerophilic streptococci and *Staphylococcus aureus* classically. At times the streptococci are anaerobic or gram-negative bacilli are seen in lieu of the staphylococci.

prokaryotic Organisms without a true nucleus.

prophylaxis Preventive treatment (e.g., the use of drugs to prevent infection).

prostatitis Inflammation of the prostate gland, usually due to infection; characterized by fever, low back or perineal pain, and at times urinary frequency and urgency; a common background factor for recurrent cystitis in males.

prosthesis An artificial part such as a hip joint or eye.

prototroph Naturally occurring or wild strain.

pseudomembrane Necrosis of mucosal surface simulating a membrane.

psychrophilic Cold loving (e.g., microorganisms that grow best at low [4° C] temperatures).

purulent Consisting of pus.

pus Product of inflammation, consisting of fluid and many white blood cells; often bacteria, cellular debris, and such are also present.

pyelonephritis Infection of the kidney and renal pelvis and the late effects of such infection.

pyoderma Any of the pus-producing lesions of the skin such as boils or impetigo.

pyogenic Pus producing.

quartan malaria Malaria caused by *Plasmodium malariae*.

radiometric analysis Determination of an element that is not itself radioactive by means of an interaction with a radioactive element.

reagin An antibody that reacts in various serologic tests for syphilis.

reservoir Source from which an infectious agent may be disseminated; for example, humans are the only reservoir for *M. tuberculosis*.

resin Plant product composed largely of esters and ethers of organic acids and acid anhydrides.

reticulate body The metabolically more active form of elementary bodies.

reticuloendothelial system Macrophage system, which includes all the phagocytic cells of the body except for the granulocytic leukocytes.

R factor A plasmid that carries gene coding for resistance to one or more antibacterial agents.

rheumatoid factor IgM antibodies produced by some patients against their own IgG.

rhizoid Rootlike absorbing organ.

saccharolytic Capable of breaking down sugars.

saprophytic Nonpathogenic.

schizogony Stage in the asexual cycle of the malaria parasite that takes place in the red blood cells of humans.

sclerotic Hard, indurated.

Scolex (pl., scolices) Head portion of a tapeworm; may attach to the intestinal wall by suckers or hooklets.

scotochromogens Mycobacteria that are pigmented even in the absence of exposure to light.

septate Having cross walls.

septic shock Acute circulatory failure caused by toxins of microorganisms; often leads to multiple organ failure and is associated with a relatively high mortality.

septicemia (sepsis) Systemic disease associated with presence of pathogenic microorganisms or their toxins in the blood.

sequestrum A detached or dead piece of bone within a cavity, abscess, wound, or area of osteomyelitis.

serosanguineous Like serous but with some blood present grossly.

serous Like serum.

serum Cell- and fibrinogen-free fluid after blood clots.

serum bactericidal level Lowest dilution of a patient's serum that kills a standard inoculum of an organism isolated from that patient; this, of course, is related to antibiotic level achieved in the patient's serum and the bactericidal activity of the drug being employed.

sinus Suppurating tract; paranasal sinus, hollows, or cavities near the nose (e.g., frontal and maxillary sinuses).

slant See definition of "butt." The slant is the upper surface of the medium in the tube described. It is exposed to air in the tube.

somatic Pertaining to the body (of a cell) (e.g., the somatic antigens of *Salmonella* species).

spore Reproductive cell of bacteria, fungi, or protozoa; in bacteria may be inactive, resistant forms within the cell.

sporogony Stage in the sexual cycle in the malarial parasite that takes place in the mosquito.

sporozoite Slender, spindle-shaped organism that is the infective stage of the malarial parasite; it is inoculated into humans by an infected mosquito and is the result of the sexual cycle of the malarial parasite in the mosquito.

sputum Material discharged from the surface of the lower respiratory tract air passages and expectorated (or swallowed).

stab culture Culture in which the inoculation of a tube of solid medium is made by stabbing with a needle to encourage anaerobic growth in the bottom.

stat (Do) immediately.

stationary phase Stage in the growth cycle of a bacterial culture in which the vegetative cell population equals the dying population.

sterile (sterility) Free of living microorganisms (the state of being sterile).

strobila Entire chain of tapeworm proglottids, excluding the scolex and neck.

substrate A substance on which an enzyme acts.

sulfur granule Small colony of organisms with surrounding clublike material; yellow-brown; resembles grain of sulfur.

superinfection Strictly speaking, this refers to a new infection superimposed on another being treated with an antimicrobial agent. The new infecting agent is resistant to the therapy initially employed and thus survives and causes persistence of the infection (now resistant to the treatment) or a new infection at a different site. Term is also used to indicate persistence or colonization with a new organism without any evidence of resulting infection.

suppuration Formation of pus.

suprapubic bladder aspiration Obtaining urine by direct needle puncture of the full bladder through the abdominal wall above the pubic bone.

syndrome Set of symptoms occurring together (e.g., nephrotic syndrome).

synergism Combined effect of two or more agents that is greater than the sum of their individual effects.

synovial fluid Viscid fluid secreted by the synovial membrane; found in joint cavities, bursae, and so forth.

tenesmus Painful, unsuccessful straining in an attempt to empty the bowels.

therapy, antimicrobial Treatment of a patient for the purpose of combating an infectious disease.

thermolabile Adversely affected by heat (as opposed to thermostable, not affected by heat).

thoracentesis Drainage of fluid from the pleural space.

thoracic Pertaining to the chest cavity.

thrush A form of *Candida* infection that typically produces white plaquelike lesions in the oral cavity.

tinea Dermatophyte infection (tinea capitis, tinea of scalp; tinea corporis, tinea of the smooth skin of the body; tinea cruris, tinea of the groin; tinea pedis, tinea of the foot).

titer Level of substance such as antibody or toxin present in material such as serum; reciprocal of the highest dilution at which the substance can still be detected.

T-lymphocytes (or T cells) Thymus-derived lymphocytes important in cell-mediated immunity.

tolerance A form of resistance to antimicrobial drugs; of uncertain clinical importance.

trachoma Serious eye infection caused by *Chlamydia trachomatis;* often leads to blindness.

transposon Genetic material from a plasmid that can move between plasmids or from a plasmid to a chromosome; so-called "jumping genes."

transtracheal aspiration Passage of needle and plastic catheter into the trachea for obtaining lower respiratory tract secretions.

transudate Similar to exudate but with low protein content.

trophozoite Feeding, motile stage of protozoa.

typing Methods of grouping organisms, primarily for epidemiologic purposes (e.g., biotyping, serotyping, bacteriophage typing, and the antibiogram).

urethritis Inflammation of the urethra, the canal through which urine is discharged (e.g., gonococcal urethritis).

vector An arthropod or other agent that carries microorganisms from a sick individual to another.

vegetation In endocarditis, the aggregates of fibrin and microorganisms on the heart valves or other endocardium.

vesicle A small bulla or blister containing clear fluid.

villi Minute, elongated projections from the surface of intestinal mucosa that are important in absorption.

Vincent's angina An old term, seldom used presently, referring to anaerobic tonsillitis.

viremia Presence of viruses in the bloodstream.

virulence Degree of pathogenicity or disease-producing ability of a microorganism.

viscus (pl., viscera) Any of the organs within one of the four great body cavities (cranium, thorax, abdomen, and pelvis).

Whipple's disease A disease thought to be caused by a bacterium and characterized by diarrhea, arthritis, and neurologic manifestations.

xenodiagnosis Procedure involving the feeding of laboratory-reared triatomid bugs on patients suspected of having Chagas' disease; after several weeks, the feces of the bugs are checked for intermediate stages of *Trypanosoma cruzi*.

zoogleal mass Jellylike matrix in which microorganisms may be embedded.

zoonoses Diseases of lower animals transmissible to humans (e.g., tularemia).

Index

Cocci
  aerobic gram-negative, 388-396; see also *Aerobic gram-negative cocci*
  anaerobic, 545-550
Coccidia, 78, 833
Coccidioides, 701, 702
  handling of cultures of, 16
  latex particle agglutination tests and, 163
  pleural fluid and, 316
Coccidioides immitis, 317, 718 (Plate), 730-731, 760
  antifungal agents and, 771
  direct examination of, 687
  exoantigen test for, 727
  identification of, 681, 703, 704, 705, 707
  incubation of, 726
  meningitis and, 228
  pathogenic mechanism and, 209
  pneumonia and, 248
  potassium hydroxide and, 692
  pulmonary infection and, 248
  rhinospiridiosis and, 589
  serology and, 767, 768
Coccidioidomycosis, 718 (Plate), 729-733
Coccobacilli
  urease test and, 411
  lactobacilli and, 497
Code of Federal Regulations, 62
Coelomycetes, 701
Coenurus, 811
Cold acid fast stain, 603
Cold agglutinins, 557
Cold enrichment, 484
Coliform
  clostridia and, 526, 526
  introitus and, 280-281
Colistin, 88
  Columbia base agar and, 271
  Enterobacteriaceae and, 420
  quality control and, 25
  manufacturer of, 178
  Neisseria and, 390
  special potency antibiotic disks and, 505, 507
Colistin nalidixic acid agar
  components and purpose and, 88
  quality control and, 25
Colitis, pseudomembranous, 262-263, 270 (Plate), 277, 530
  clostridia and, 277, 524
Collection kit
  sputum, 600
  fecal, 781-782
College of American Pathologists
  quality control and, 27
  workload recording unit, 31
Colon cancer, 372
Colonization, 238
Colonizers, abnormal, 54-55
Colony, 54-55, 238
  automated counter and, 147
  gram-negative bacilli and, 534
  identification of isolates and, 507
  morphology and, 613
Colony-forming units, 143
  determination of, 182
Colorado tick fever, 663
Colorimetry, 142, 143-144
  immunologic probe detection and, 170
  particle detection and, 146

Colostomy, 66
Columbia agar base, 271, 869-870
Columbia agar colistin-nalidixic acid
  blood and, 98
  components and purpose and, 88
  formula and preparation of, 870
  streptococci and, 372
Column chromatography, 520-521
Comma-shaped colony outgrowths, 477
Commercial supplier, 24
Complement, 157
Complement fixation, 157
  for antibody detection, 166-168
  Blastomyces and, 768
  genital tract infection and, 302
  Histoplasma and, 769
  parasites and, 808-811
  virus and, 671-672
Computer
  automated systems and, 152-154
  data base system and, 123-124
  diagnosis related groups and, 38-39
  on line capability and, 23
Concentration
  minimum bactericidal, 182-183
  minimum lethal, 183
Concentration procedures for fecal specimens, 788
Conception, products of, 301-302
Condenser, 71
Congenital disease
  fluorescent antibody test and, 663
  hepatitis and, 341
  immune deficiency and, 343
  infection and, 339
  isolation specimen and, 640
  rubella and, 674
  syphilis and, 340
Conidia, 696, 697, 698
  brown, 743
  sperm-shaped, 724
Conidiobolus, 744
Conidiophores, 696, 724, 725
Conjunctival membrane, 329
Conjunctival scraping, 914
Conjunctivitis, 330
  diphtheritic, 331, 336
  direct visual examination and, 336
  fluorescent antibody and, 663
  gonococcal, 331
  Haemophilus and, 444
  inclusion, 552, 555
  purulent, 335
  viral, 336
Conosporium, 703
Consulting microbiologist, 8
Contact transmission, 42-43
Containers, specimen collection, 55, 59
Contamination
  banked blood and, 219
  blood culture and, 215
  intravenous fluid and, 346
  Limulus amebocyte lysate assay and, 127
  mycobacteria and, 605-610
  specimen, 4, 54
  tissue culture and, 323
Continuous cell line, 102, 104
  hep-2, 644

Litmus milk broth, 492, 881
Liver abscess, 801-803
L-J medium, 26
Loa Loa, 208, 778, 856
Loboa loboi, 590
Lobomycosis, 590
Loculoascomycetes, 700
Loeffler agar, 91
  diphtheria and, 78, 245
Loeffler coagulated serum slant, 878
Loeffler's methylene blue, 73, 74
Loeffler's stain, 909
Lombard Dowell agar, 89
Lombard-Dowell Presumpto 1 plate, 512
Loop
  calibrated, 286
  inoculating, A8
Lorian, 37
Louse, 471, 472
Low peptone medium, 425, 426
Löwenstein-Jensen medium
  characteristics of, 99
  components and purpose and, 89
  formula and preparation of, 878
  mycobacteria and, 611, 613, 622 (Plate)
    culture and, 610-611
  sterilization and, 91
Lower respiratory tract infection, 249-258; *see also* Respiratory tract infection
  acute, 247-249
  Branhamella catarrhalis and, 388
  chronic, 249
  culture and, 252-258
  direct visual examination and, 251-252
  nonculture methods for diagnosing, 258
Luciferin, 145
Ludwig's angina, 334 (Plate)
Lugol iodine solution, 73
  Chlamydia trachomatis and, 556
  formula for, 908
Lukens trap, 250
Lumac Bacteriuria Screening System, 145, 146
Luminometer, 145
Lumpy jaw, 334 (Plate)
Lung abscess, 801-803
Lung biopsy
  Legionella and, 577
  open, 251
Lyme disease, 319, 472, 586
Lymph gland, 300
Lymph node syndrome, 591-592
Lymphadenitis, suppurative, 309
Lymphadenopathy, 208, 348
Lymphadenopathy-associated virus, 208
Lymphocyte
  B, 157, 159
  T, 156
Lymphocytic choriomeningitis virus
  encephalitis and, 228
  isolation specimen and, 640
  serology and, 671
Lymphogranuloma venereum, 552, 553-554
Lyophilized antimicrobial, 185
Lysine
  Acinetobacter and, 433
  Enterobacteriaceae and, 411
Lysine decarboxylase
  Plesiomonas and, 466-467

Lysine decarboxylase—cont'd
  quality control and, 26
Lysine iron agar, 412
  formula and preparation of, 878-879
Lysis-centrifugation
  bacteremia and, 221
  cost savings and, 35
  fungal infection and, 209
Lysogenic infection, 486
Lysostaphin, 357
Lysozyme resistance, 495

M

M protein, 369
  adherence and, 238
MacConkey agar, 405
  Aeromonas and, 465-466
  Alcaligenes and, 433
  characteristics of, 98
  components and purpose and, 89
  cost savings and, 33, 35
  flavobacteria and, 435
  formula and preparation of, 879
  gram-negative bacilli and, 462 (Plate)
  lactose-fermenting and non-lactose fermenting colonies on, 110 (Plate), 462 (Plate)
  lower respiratory tract infections and, 255
  Moraxella and, 434
  mycobacteria and, 624
  nonfermenters and, 425
  peritoneal dialysis and, 318
  Pseudomonas aeruginosa and, 428
MacConkey plate, 234
Macrobroth dilution test, 184-185
Macroconidia, 698
  Epidermophyton and, 710, 719
  Microsporum and, 73, 718-720
  Trichophyton and, 713
  tuberculate, 734
Macrophage, 241
Macular exanthem, 663
Maculopapular exanthem, 663
Madurella, 701
  direct examination of, 689
Madurella grisea, 689
Madurella mycetomatis, 689
Magnesium sulfate, 781
Mailing of biologicals, 17, 62-63
Malaria, 835-838
  laboratory diagnosis of, 811-813
  parasite and, 208
  serology and, 808
Malassezia furfur, 704, 718 (Plate)
  direct examination of, 687
  potassium hydroxide and, 690
Malassezia pachydermatis, 709
Malignancy
  identification of, 6
  infection and, 343-344
  pustule and, 477
Malonate broth, 879
Malthus Instruments, 147
Maltose, 569
Mannan antigen, 210
Mannitol salt agar
  components and purpose and, 89
  formula and preparation of, 879
  Staphylococcus, 356